MEDIAN HEIGHTS AND WEIGHTS AND RECOMMENDED ENERGY INTAKES (UNITED STATES)

AGE (YEARS)	WEIGHT (kg)	WEIGHT (lb)	HEIGHT (cm)	HEIGHT (inches)	REE[a] (cal/day)	Multiples of REE[b]	cal per kg	cal per day[c]
INFANTS								
0.0-0.5	6	13	60	24	320		108	650
0.5-1.0	9	20	71	28	500		98	850
CHILDREN								
1-3	13	29	90	35	740		102	1300
4-6	20	44	122	44	950		90	1800
7-10	28	62	132	52	1130		70	2000
MALES								
11-14	45	99	157	62	1440	1.70	55	2500
15-18	66	145	176	69	1760	1.67	45	3000
19-24	72	160	177	70	1780	1.67	40	2900
25-50	79	174	176	70	1800	1.60	37	2900
51 +	77	170	173	68	1530	1.50	30	2300
FEMALES								
11-14	46	101	157	62	1310	1.67	47	2200
15-18	55	120	163	64	1370	1.60	40	2200
19-24	58	128	164	65	1350	1.60	38	2200
25-50	63	138	163	64	1380	1.55	36	2200
51 +	65	143	160	63	1280	1.50	30	1900
PREGNANT (2ND AND 3RD TRIMESTERS)								+300
LACTATING								+500

[a]REE (resting energy expenditure) represents the energy expended by a person at rest under normal conditions.

[b]Recommended energy allowances assume light-to-moderate activity and were calculated by multiplying the REE by an activity factor.

[c]Average energy allowances have been rounded.

SOURCE: Reprinted with permission from *Recommended Dietary Allowances: 10th edition.* Copyright 1989 by the National Academy of Sciences. Courtesy of the National Academy Press. Washington, D.C.

DAILY VALUES (USED ON FOOD LABELS)

DAILY REFERENCE VALUES (DRVs)[a]

Food Component	DRV
fat	65g[d]
saturated fat	20 g
cholesterol	300 mg[a]
total carbohydrate	300 g
fiber	25 g
sodium	2,400 mg
potassium	3,500 mg
protein[b]	50 g

REFERENCE DAILY INTAKES (RDIs)[c]

Nutrient	Amount	Nutrient	Amount
vitamin A	5,000 International Units (IU), 1000 RE	vitamin B_6	2.0 mg
		folate	0.4 mg
vitamin C	60 mg	vitamin B_{12}	6 μg[f]
thiamin	1.5 mg	phosphorus	1.0 g
riboflavin	1.7 mg	iodine	150 μg
niacin	20 mg	magnesium	400 mg
calcium	1.0 g	zinc	15 mg
iron	18 mg	copper	2 mg
vitamin D	400 IU, 10 μg	biotin	0.3 mg
vitamin E	30 IU, 10 mg αTE	pantothenic acid	10 mg

[a]Based on 2,000 calories a day for adults and children over 4 only.

[b]DRV for protein does not apply to certain populations; Reference Daily Intake (RDI) for protein has been established for these groups: children 1 to 4 years: 16 g; infants under 1 year: 14 g; pregnant women: 60 g; nursing mothers: 65 g.

[c]Formerly the U.S. RDA, based on National Academy of Sciences 1968 Recommended Dietary Allowances.

[d](g) grams

[e](mg) milligrams

[f](μg) micrograms

SOURCE: R. Kunzwell. 'Daily Values' encourage healthy diet, *FDA Consumer,* May 1993, pp. 40-45.

ESTIMATED SAFE AND ADEQUATE DAILY DIETARY INTAKES OF ADDITIONAL SELECTED VITAMINS AND MINERALS (UNITED STATES)[a]

Age (years)	VITAMINS	
	Biotin (μg)	Pantothenic Acid (mg)
INFANTS		
0–0.5	10	2
0.5–1	15	3
CHILDREN		
1–3	20	3
4–6	25	3–4
7–10	30	4–5
11 +	30–100	4–7
ADULTS	30–100	4–7

Age (years)	TRACE ELEMENTS[b]				
	Chromium (μg)	Molybdenum (μg)	Copper (mg)	Manganese (mg)	Fluoride (mg)
INFANTS					
0–0.5	10–40	15–30	0.4–0.6	0.3–0.6	0.1–0.5
0.5–1	20–60	20–40	0.6–0.7	0.6–1.0	0.2–1.0
CHILDREN					
1–3	20–80	25–50	0.7–1.0	1.0–1.5	0.5–1.5
4–6	30–120	30–75	1.0–1.5	1.5–2.0	1.0–2.5
7–10	50–200	50–150	1.0–2.0	2.0–3.0	1.5–2.5
11 +	50–200	75–250	1.5–2.5	2.0–5.0	1.5–2.5
ADULTS	50–200	75–250	1.5–3.0	2.0–5.0	1.5–4.0

[a]Because there is less information on which to base allowances, these figures are not given in the main table of the RDA and are provided here in the form of ranges of recommended intakes.

[b]Because the toxic levels for many trace elements may be only several times usual intakes, the upper levels for the trace elements given in this table should not be habitually exceeded.

SOURCE: *Recommended Dietary Allowances,* © 1989 by the National Academy of Sciences, National Academy Press, Washington, D.C.

ESTIMATED MINIMUM REQUIREMENTS OF SODIUM, CHLORIDE, AND POTASSIUM

AGE (YEARS)	SODIUM[a] (MG)	CHLORIDE (MG)	POTASSIUM[b] (MG)
INFANTS			
0.0–0.5	120	180	500
0.5–1.0	200	300	700
CHILDREN			
1	225	350	1000
2–5	300	500	1400
6–9	400	600	1600
ADOLESCENTS	500	750	2000
ADULTS	500	750	2000

[a]Sodium requirements are based on estimates of needs for growth and for replacement of obligatory losses. They cover a wide variation of physical activity patterns and climatic exposure but do not provide for large, prolonged losses from the skin through sweat.

[b]Dietary potassium may benefit the prevention and treatment of hypertension and recommendations to include many servings of fruits and vegetables would raise potassium intakes to about 3500 mg/day.

SOURCE: *Recommended Dietary Allowances,* © 1989 by the National Academy of Sciences, National Academy Press, Washington, D.C.

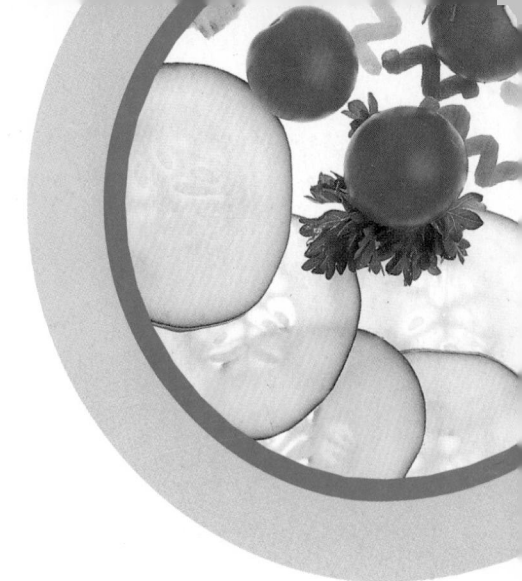

Personal Nutrition

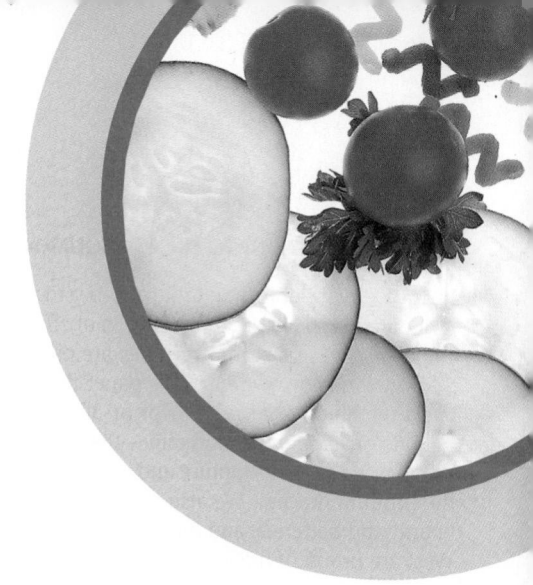

Personal Nutrition

Third Edition

Marie A. Boyle

Gail Zyla
Tufts University
Diet & Nutrition Letter

WEST PUBLISHING COMPANY   MINNEAPOLIS   ST. PAUL   NEW YORK   LOS ANGELES   SAN FRANCISCO

WEST'S COMMITMENT TO THE ENVIRONMENT

In 1906, West Publishing Company began recycling materials left over from the production of books. This began a tradition of efficient and responsible use of resources. Today, 100% of our legal bound volumes are printed on acid-free, recycled paper consisting of 50% new paper pulp and 50% paper that had undergone a de-inking process. We also use vegetable-based inks to print all of our books. West recycles nearly 27,700,000 pounds of scrap paper annually—the equivalent of 229,300 trees. Since the 1960s, West has devised ways to capture and recycle waste inks, solvents, oils, and vapors created in the printing process. We also recycle plastics of all kinds, wood, glass, corrugated cardboard, and batteries, and have eliminated the use of polystyrene book packaging. We at West are proud of the longevity and the scope of our commitment to the environment.

West pocket parts and advance sheets are printed on recyclable paper and can be collected and recycled with newspapers. Staples do not have to be removed. Bound volumes can be recycled after removing the cover.

Copyediting	Deborah Cady
Composition	Carlisle Communication
Artwork	Miyake Illustration, Sandra McMahon
Text Design	Janet Bollow
Indexing	Northwind Editorial Services
Cover Image	"Fruit Fireworks II" by Angela J. Graefenhain, 414 Sagebrush Road, Naperville, IL 60565

Production, Prepress, Printing and Binding by West Publishing Company.

British Library Cataloguing-in-Publication Data. A catalogue record for this book is available from the British Library.

COPYRIGHT ©1989, 1992   BY WEST PUBLISHING COMPANY
COPYRIGHT ©1996   BY WEST PUBLISHING COMPANY
610 Opperman Drive
P.O. Box 64526
St. Paul, MN 55164-0526

Library of Congress Cataloging-in-Publication Data

Boyle, Marie A. (Marie Ann)
    Personal nutrition / Marie A. Boyle, Gail Zyla. — 3rd ed.
        p.   cm.
    Includes bibliographical references and index.
    ISBN 0-314-06380-3 (soft : alk. paper)
    1. Nutrition.   I. Zyla, Gail.   II. Title.
RA784.B65   1996
613.2—dc20   95–45675
                                             CIP

To my brother,
Bob,
with hope and love
in words unspoken

Marie Boyle

For Pearl Woods

Gail Zyla

Marie A. Boyle, Ph.D., R.D., received her B.A. in Psychology from the University of Maine in 1975, her M.S. in nutrition from Florida State University in 1985, and her Ph.D. in nutrition from Florida State University in 1992. She has taught undergraduate and graduate nutrition and health-related courses at Edison Community College in Naples, Florida, the University of Florida in Gainesville, and Florida State University in Tallahassee. She is co-author of the senior-level textbook *Community Nutrition in Action: An Entrepreneurial Approach.* Her other professional activities include teaching a community-based "Culinary Hearts Cooking" class for the American Heart Association, developing a community workshop on "Nutrition and Health Fraud," and serving on the local Dietetic Association's Hunger Committee. She presently works as a consultant, writer, and nutrition/health educator in Atlanta, Georgia, where she teaches nutrition and health classes at Life College and Kennesaw State College. She maintains memberships with the American Dietetic Association, Georgia Dietetic Association, Florida Association of Professional Health Educators, and the American Public Health Association, and serves as a reviewer for the *American Journal of Health Promotion* and the *Florida Journal of Public Health.*

Gail Zyla, M.S., R.D., received her B.S. in Home Economics from Valparaiso University, Valparaiso, Indiana, in 1985 and completed her dietetic internship at Massachusetts General Hospital, Boston, in 1986. She received her M.S. in nutrition and communications from Boston University in 1988. Currently she serves as senior editor of the *Tufts University Diet & Nutrition Letter* in Boston, a position she has held since 1988. She is also a contributing editor for *Parenting* magazine, and she writes about nutrition for a variety of other consumer publications. In addition, she is an instructor at the Tufts University Schools of Medicine and Dental Medicine.

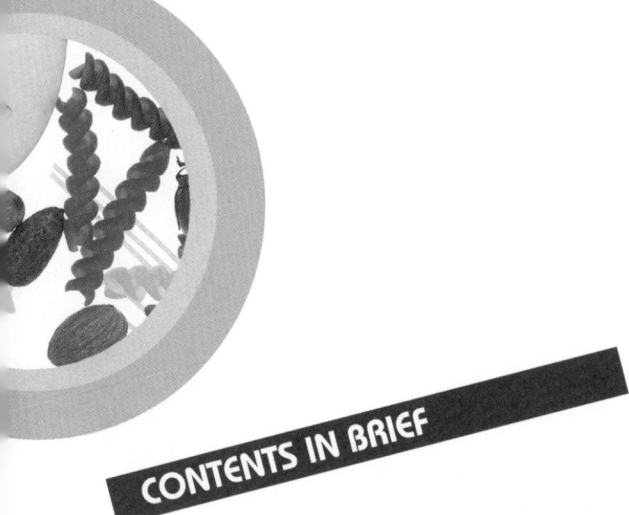

CONTENTS IN BRIEF

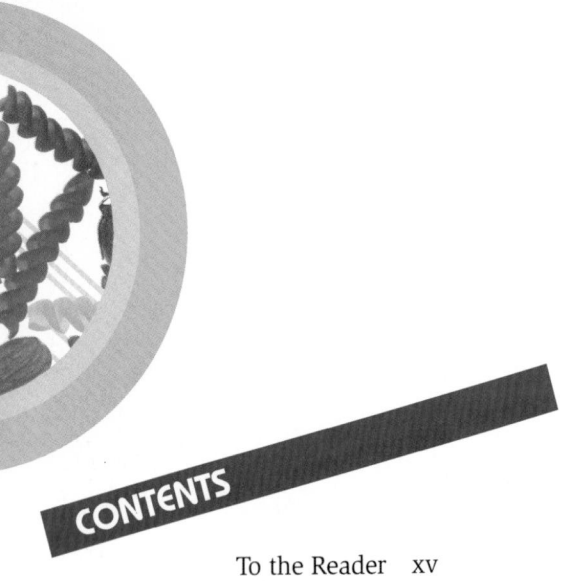

CONTENTS

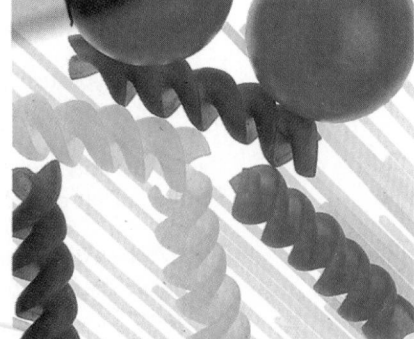

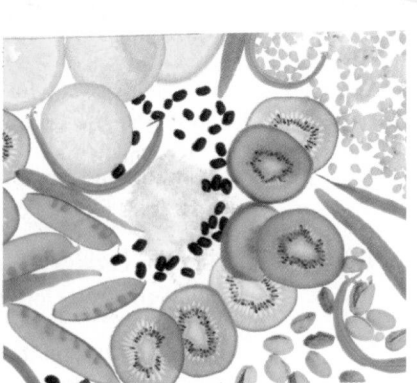

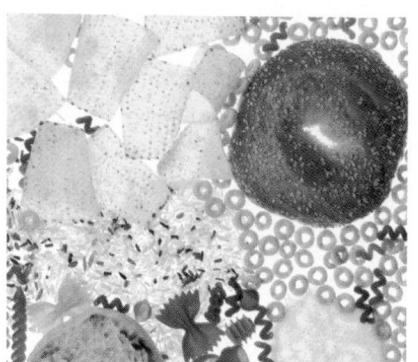

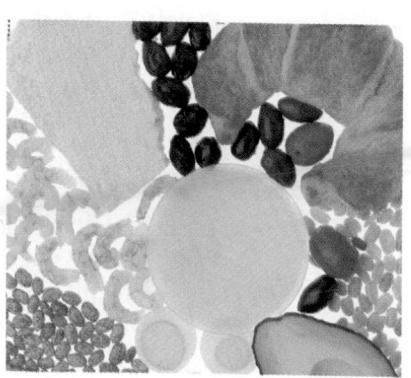

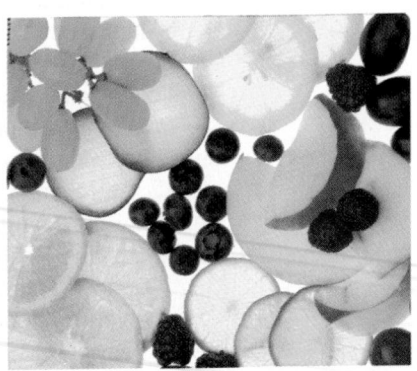

SEVEN   **THE MINERALS AND WATER   229**

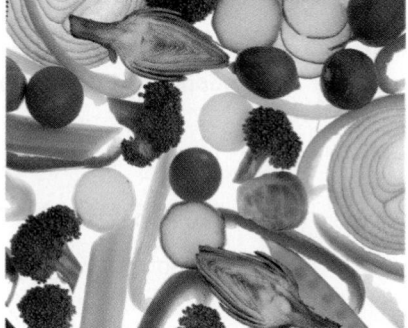

EIGHT   **WEIGHT CONTROL   269**

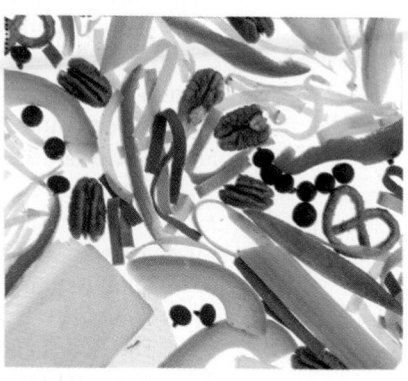

NINE   **NUTRITION AND FITNESS**   315

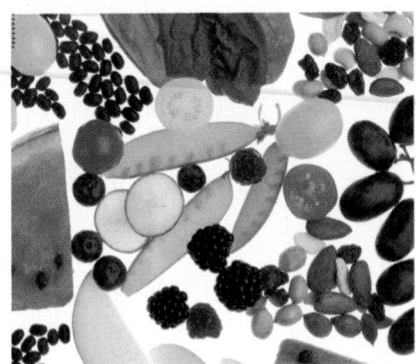

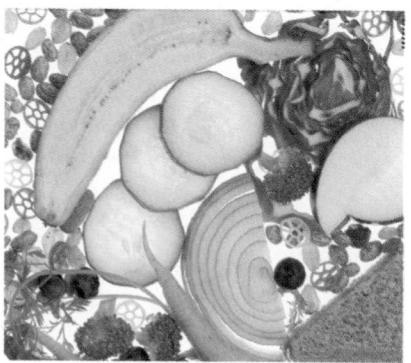

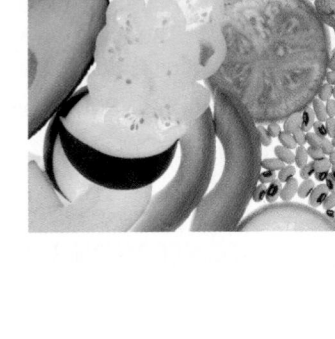

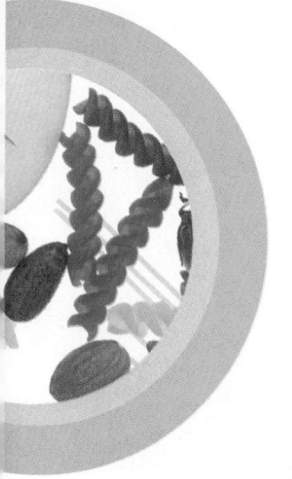

With this third edition of *Personal Nutrition,* we continue to develop the vision we had in writing the earlier editions of this book—that is, to apply basic nutrition concepts to personal everyday life. This edition reflects not only the many changes that have taken place in the field of nutrition in recent years, but also the increasing demands of our readers for practical nutrition information useful for making healthful decisions both now and in the future. Our challenge has been to teach the facts about nutrition as well as how to evaluate them and, most importantly, to motivate readers to apply what they learn in daily life. It is our hope that you will benefit from the new and fundamental information presented in this edition and enjoy its exciting and colorful new design.

Nutrition is a subject that is forever changing, and it is important that you, as a consumer of nutrition information, have the knowledge to evaluate the nutrition issues and controversies that confront you, both today and tomorrow. Newspapers are quick to print nutrition breakthroughs, new fad diets appear monthly on the magazine racks, and television advertising extols the wonders of products of questionable value. Nutrition claims bombard us frequently, and we must evaluate and assess them. This edition of *Personal Nutrition* continues to provide a sieve through which to separate the valid nutrition claims from the rest.

Chapter 1 provides a personal invitation to eat well for optimum health and assists the reader in becoming a sophisticated consumer of new information about nutrition. It also includes a new section that explores the factors that affect food choices, including the media, advertising, and cultural factors. Chapter 2 introduces the basic nutrients the body needs along with the nutrition tools and most recent guidelines needed to help make sound food choices. Beginning with Chapter 3, and continuing through each of five chapters, is a new and practical feature on "Checking Out the Food Label," which provides pointers for understanding the information found on food labels. Another new feature to these same chapters is the colorful "Pyramid Pointers" graphic which offers selection tips from the Food Guide Pyramid for building a healthful diet. Chapters 3 through 7 present the nutrients and show how they all work together to nourish the body. In addition, Chapter 3 includes a new section on various international and ethnic cuisines that highlights the multicultural heritage of our country. The chapters on vitamins and minerals spotlight the emerging importance of the antioxidant nutrients and phytochemicals and also feature colorful new food photos depicting food sources for individual vitamins and minerals. Chapter 8 discusses weight loss and weight gain and includes a new summary table that compares the major weight-loss diets and programs, and many of the popular diet books. Chapter 9 addresses the relationships between nutrition and personal fitness. Chapter 10 describes the special nutrition needs and concerns that arise during the various stages of the life cycle from conception through old age. Chapter 11 addresses consumer concerns about the safety of our food supply and provides a glimpse at some of the newer food technologies on the horizon.

The *Nutrition Action* features that appear in every chapter are magazine-style essays that keep you abreast of current topics important to the nutrition-conscious consumer. The *Nutrition Action* features address topics such as fast food, smart snacking, dental health, sweet alternatives to sugar, the trans fatty acid controversy, amino acid supplements, nutrition savvy in cooking to preserve vitamins in foods, calcium and osteoporosis, diet and blood pressure, the "never say diet" approach to weight loss, behavior modification, nutrition and stress, caffeine, the organic foods industry, and recycling and the environment.

Each chapter continues to provide a *Consumer Tips* feature that contains practical suggestions for healthful eating. They include stocking your cupboards with nutritious staple goods, supermarketing, choosing healthful ethnic foods, modifying recipes, packing healthful bag lunches, selecting a vitamin-mineral supplement, seasoning foods without excess salt, dining defensively, adding exercise to your day, making meals for one, and using the microwave oven safely.

Scorecards are hands-on features included in every chapter. *Scorecards* allow readers to evaluate their own nutrition behaviors and knowledge in many areas. Some of the *Scorecards* assist readers in assessing their longevity, diet, calcium intake, weight, exercise habits, and food safety knowhow.

The *Ask Yourself* sections at the beginning of each chapter contain a set of true-false questions designed to provide readers with a preview of the chapter's contents. New to this edition is the *Check Yourself* section at the end of each chapter, which includes review questions designed to test readers' comprehension of the chapter material.

The final special feature of each chapter is the *Spotlight*—many are brand new to this edition, and the others have been updated. Each addresses a common concern people have about nutrition. *Spotlight* topics include nutrition and the media, food labels, ethnic cuisines and multiculturalism, diet and heart disease, the vegetarian diet, antioxidant nutrients and phytochemicals, water safety, eating disorders, alcohol and nutrition, and nutrition and cancer prevention. The final *Spotlight* covers the many factors that influence nutrition and food insecurity among the people of the world and underscores that the practical suggestions offered throughout this book for attaining the ideals of personal nutrition are the very suggestions that best support the health of the whole earth as well. The *Spotlights* continue in their question and answer format to encourage the reader to ask further questions about nutrition issues. We encourage you to ask us questions, too, in care of the publisher.

The *Appendixes* have been updated. Appendix A contains an invaluable listing of general nutrition resources as well as current electronic sources of nutrition information; Appendix B provides a colorfully illustrated introduction to the workings of the human body; Appendix C includes the Canadian Dietary Guidelines and other recommendations; Appendix D presents aids to calculations, including how to calculate the percentage of calories from fat in one's diet; Appendix E provides both the U.S. and Canadian Food Exchange Systems; Appendix F includes the chapter reference notes; Appendix G supplies a guide to the West *Diet Analysis Plus* software; Appendix H provides answers to selected *Check Yourself* questions at the end of each chapter; and Appendix I includes our *Table of Food Composition*. The *Glossary* of terms that follows the Appendixes provides a quick reference to the nutrition terminology defined in the margins of the text and can be used as a review tool.

We welcome you to the fascinating subject of nutrition. We hope that the book speaks to you personally and that you find it practical for your everyday use. We hope, too, that by reading it you may enhance your own personal nutrition and health.

Marie Boyle
Gail Zyla

ACKNOWLEDGMENTS

We are grateful to the many individuals who have made contributions to the development of this third edition of *Personal Nutrition.* We thank our families and friends for their continued support and encouragement throughout this endeavor. We appreciate the insights and support provided by our colleagues—especially Diane Morris, Ph.D., R.D., Jean Kressy, Anne Fletcher M.S., R.D., and Mary Thang. Also, a word of special thanks goes to Larry Lindner of the *Tufts University Diet & Nutrition Letter* for his patience and generous support throughout this endeavor and countless others. Thanks also to Bob Geltz and Betty Hands and their staff at ESHA research for creating the food composition table (Appendix I), and the computerized diet analysis program that accompanies this book.

Special thanks to our editorial team of Pete Marshall, Becky Tollerson, and Brenda Owens for ensuring the quality of this production. We appreciate the work of our copyeditor, Deborah Cady, and the artwork of Randy Miyake. We also owe much to the following professionals who provided expert reviews of the manuscript, not only for their ideas and suggestions, many of which made their way into the text, but also for their continued support and interest in *Personal Nutrition:* Ellen Brennan, San Antonio College; Velma Butler, Northeast Louisiana University; Deborah Cohen, Creighton University; Dorothy Coltrin, De Anza Community College; Diane Fletcher, Pacific Union College; Diana Polley-Fugitt, University of Central Oklahoma; Caroline Knutson, Clackamas Community College; Lorrie Miller Kohler, Minneapolis Community College; Joan Magee, Henry Ford Community College; Rose Martin, Arizona State University; John Orta, California State University—Los Angeles; Carol Seaborn, University of Wisconsin-Stout; Kathy Talis, Aquinas College; Ann VanBeber, Texas Christian University; and Suzanne Vieira, Johnson and Wales University.

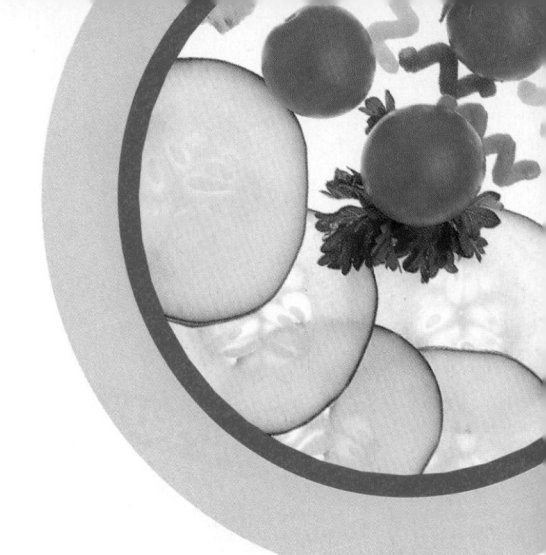

Tell me what you eat, and I will tell you what you are.

Anthelme Brillat-Savarin
(1755–1826, French politician and gourmet;
author of *Physiology of Taste*)

The Art of Understanding Nutrition

ONE

Contents

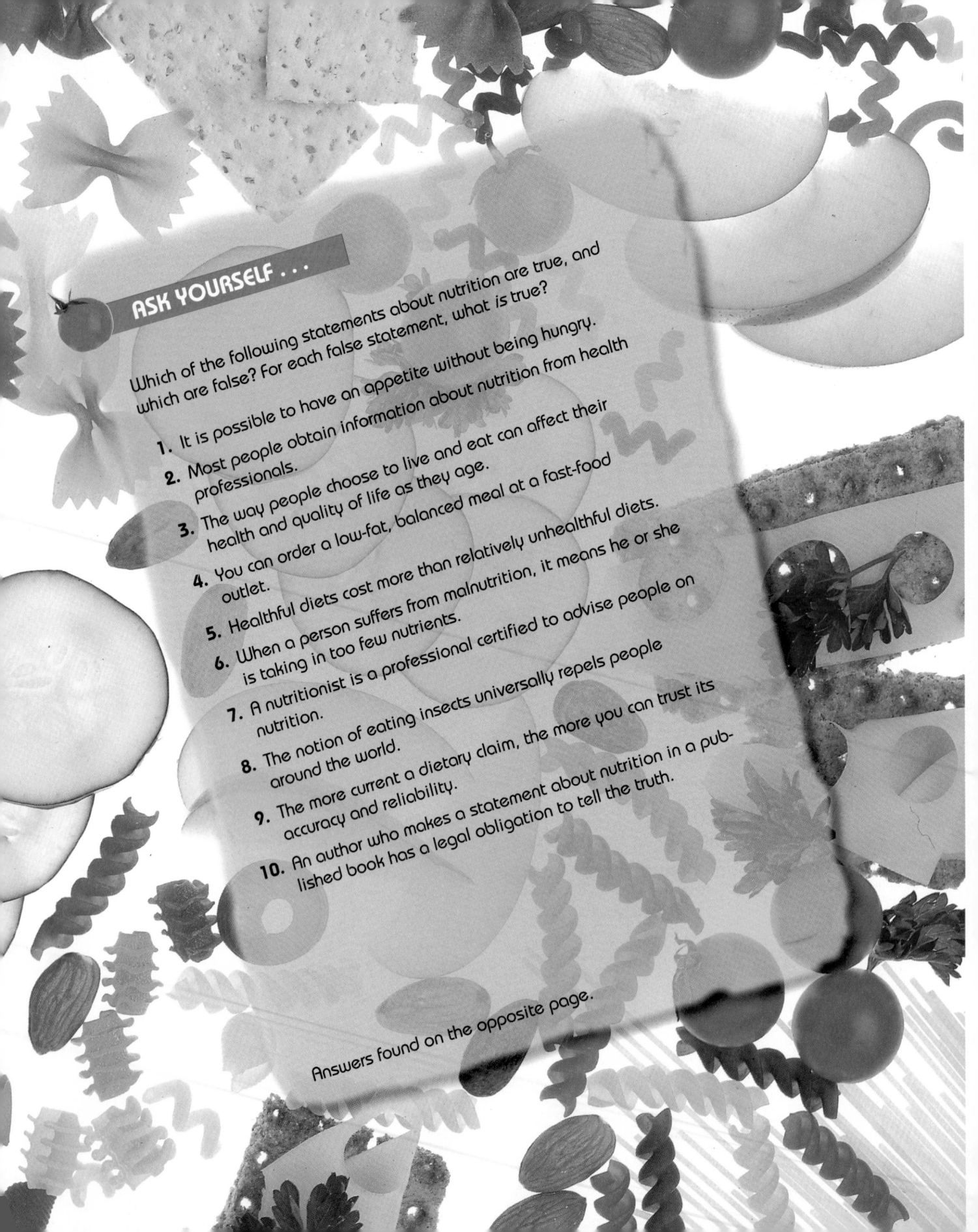

Which of the following statements about nutrition are true, and which are false? For each false statement, what *is* true?

1. It is possible to have an appetite without being hungry.

2. Most people obtain information about nutrition from health professionals.

3. The way people choose to live and eat can affect their health and quality of life as they age.

4. You can order a low-fat, balanced meal at a fast-food outlet.

5. Healthful diets cost more than relatively unhealthful diets.

6. When a person suffers from malnutrition, it means he or she is taking in too few nutrients.

7. A nutritionist is a professional certified to advise people on nutrition.

8. The notion of eating insects universally repels people around the world.

9. The more current a dietary claim, the more you can trust its accuracy and reliability.

10. An author who makes a statement about nutrition in a published book has a legal obligation to tell the truth.

Answers found on the opposite page.

Stroll down the aisle of any supermarket, and you'll see all manner of foods touting such claims as "reduced-fat," "low-calorie," and "fat-free." Flip through the pages of just about any magazine, and you're likely to find advice on how to lose weight. Walk into any gym, and you'll probably hear members discussing the merits of one performance-enhancing food or another. Pick up a newspaper, and you might notice headlines here and there regarding the federal government's ongoing debate with the supplement industry about the marketing of vitamin and mineral pills. What this all boils down to is that nutrition has become part and parcel of the American lifestyle.

It wasn't always that way, however. The field of nutrition is a relative newcomer on the scientific block. Although Hippocrates recognized diet as a component of health back in 400 B.C., only in the past one hundred years or so have researchers begun to understand that carbohydrates, fats, and proteins are needed for normal growth. The next nutrition breakthrough—the discovery of the first vitamin—occurred in the early 1900s. And it wasn't until 1934, when an organization called the American Institute of Nutrition was formed, that nutrition was officially looked upon as a distinct field of study.[1]* It took several more decades before nutrition achieved its current status as one of the most talked about scientific disciplines around.

Today we spend billions of dollars each year to investigate the many aspects of nutrition, a science that encompasses the study of not only vitamins, minerals, and the like but also such diverse subjects as alcohol, caffeine, and pesticides. In addition, nutrition scientists continually expand our understanding of the impact food has on our bodies by examining research in chemistry, physics, biology, biochemistry, immunology, and other nutrition-related fields.

A number of disciplines have made contributions to the study of nutrition. Related fields include psychology, anthropology, geography, agriculture, ethics, economics, sociology, and philosophy.

At the same time that science has shown that to some extent we really are what we eat, many consumers have become more confused than ever about how to translate the steady stream of new findings about nutrition into healthful eating. As Table 1–1 illustrates, people's priorities regarding diet have changed dramatically over the past decade. Each additional nugget of nutrition news that comes

---

ASK YOURSELF ANSWERS: 1. True. **2.** False. Most Americans look first to magazines for nutrition information, then to television, and finally to newspapers. **3.** True. **4.** True. **5.** False. People can save money when they switch from a typical high-fat diet to the grain-based, produce-rich diet recommended by health experts. **6.** False. Malnutrition can be caused either by taking in too few nutrients or by consuming an excess of nutrients. **7.** False. A nutritionist is a person who claims to specialize in the study of nutrition, but some are self-described experts whose training is questionable. **8.** False. It's true that most people in the United States and Canada find the idea of eating insects repulsive because the practice is not part of the American culture. But people in many other countries, because they have been brought up in cultures in which insects have long been a traditional food, consider dishes prepared with insects a delicacy. **9.** False. If a nutrition claim is too new, it may not have been adequately tested. Findings must be confirmed many times over by experiment and considered in light of other knowledge before they can be translated into recommendations for the public. **10.** False. Authors who write about nutrition are morally but not legally obligated to tell the truth.

---

*Reference notes for each chapter are in Appendix F.

along raises new concerns: Is caffeine bad for me? Should I take vitamin supplements? Do diet pills work? Can a sports drink improve my performance? Are pesticides posing a hazard?

Some manufacturers and media outlets feed into the confusion by offering health-conscious consumers unreliable products and misleading dietary advice. For example, in 1970 and 1989, General Nutrition, Inc. (GNC), the largest retailer of nutritional supplements in the United States, was charged with making unsubstantiated claims for a number of nutritional products, including supplements touted as fat melters, muscle builders, and energy boosters. In 1994, however, the U.S. Federal Trade Commission (FTC)—the arm of the government that monitors advertising—alleged that GNC had continued making spurious claims for more than 40 such products, despite FTC orders not to do so. As a result, GNC agreed to pay $2.4 million in penalties—the largest civil penalty for violating an advertising order in the FTC's history.[2]

Unfortunately, misinformation continues to run rampant in the marketplace. Americans spend some $30 billion annually on medical and nutritional **health fraud** and **quackery,** up from only $1 billion to $2 billion in the early 1960s.[3] Consider that college athletes alone may spend as much as $400 a month on nutritional supplements, even though most of the products pitched to serious exercisers are useless and, in some cases, potentially harmful.[4] The problem is so widespread that the U.S. Food and Drug Administration (FDA) has ranked false nutritional schemes and food products such as bee pollen and over-the-counter herbal remedies among the top ten health frauds. Also making the list were weight-loss gimmicks—skin patches, herbal capsules, grapefruit diet pills, and even magic weight-loss earrings.[5]

To be sure, the widespread interest in nutrition has generated some positive changes in the marketplace. Whereas the sale of low-fat items such as frozen yogurt was virtually unheard of ten years ago in fast-food chains, those eateries couldn't survive in the current nutrition-conscious environ-

Table 1–1
NATURE OF SHOPPERS' CONCERNS ABOUT DIET

While consumers have long placed importance on the nutritional profile of their diets, the nature of their concerns has changed over the years. The following figures show how respondents to a national survey answered this question in 1983 and in 1994. **What is it about the nutritional content of what you eat that most concerns you and your family?**

	1983 TOTAL PERCENTAGE	1994 TOTAL PERCENTAGE	PERCENTAGE POINT CHANGE
Fat content, low fat	9	59	+50
Cholesterol levels	5	21	+16
Salt content, less salt	18	18	0
Calories, low calories	6	7	+1
Sugar content, less sugar	21	14	−7
Vitamin/mineral content	24	6	−18
Preservatives	22	10	−12
Making sure we get a balanced diet	10	2	−8
Chemical additives	27	8	−19
Freshness, purity, no spoilage	14	5	−9
As natural as possible, not overly processed	12	4	−8
No harmful ingredients, nothing that causes illness/cancer	10	1	−9
Desire to be healthy, eat what's good for us	0	4	+4
Ingredients/content	0	2	+2
Excess food coloring, dyes	6	1	−5

SOURCE: The Food Marketing Institute, *Trends: Consumer Attitudes and the Supermarket*, 1990 and 1994 editions (Washington, D.C.: The Research Department, Food Marketing Institute).

HEALTH FRAUD conscious deceit practiced for profit, such as the promotion of a false or an unproven product or therapy.

QUACKERY fraud. A quack is a person who practices health fraud.
quack = to boast loudly

ment without offering such healthful fare. (See the Nutrition Action feature later in the chapter for tips on eating healthfully at fast-food outlets.) By the same token, food manufacturers have responded to consumer concern about diet by developing new technologies, such as the creation of fat substitutes, to provide shoppers with an unprecedented number of choices at the supermarket.

With the amount of nutrition information and the number of food alternatives ever on the rise, choosing a healthful diet can seem like a daunting task. Fortunately, you don't need a degree in nutrition to put the principles of the science to use in your own life. A basic understanding of nutrition can go a long way in

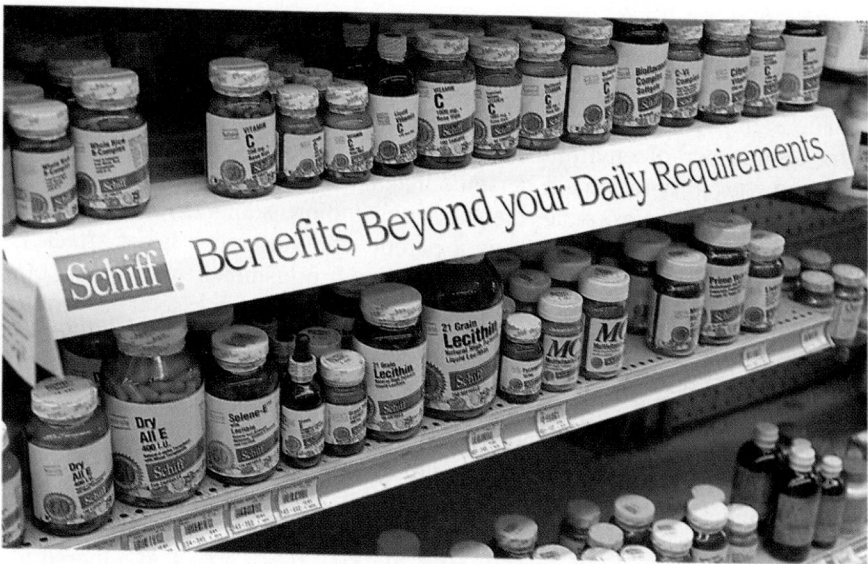

Some stores sell pills and potions touted as fat melters, energy boosters, and muscle builders.

helping you protect your health (and your wallet). This book will lay the foundation you need to take the science out of the laboratory and move it into your kitchen, both today and tomorrow. It will act as a sieve through which you can separate valid nutrition information from the rest as you confront the new issues and controversies that are sure to arise. The first step is exploring the current thrust of the field of nutrition.

Nutrition and Health Promotion

Time was when scientists investigating the role that diet plays in health zeroed in on the consequences of getting too little of one nutrient or another. Until the end of World War II, in fact, nutrition researchers concentrated on eliminating deficiency diseases such as **goiter,** a condition in which the thyroid gland swells from lack of the mineral iodine, and **pellagra,** inflammation of the skin caused by deficiency of the B vitamin niacin.

These days, the focus is just the opposite. Deficiency diseases have been virtually eliminated in America because of our country's abundant food supply and the practice of fortifying food with essential nutrients (adding iodine to salt, for example). Yet diseases related to **malnutrition** in the form of dietary excess and imbalance run rampant. Four of the ten leading causes of death—heart disease, cancer, stroke, and diabetes—have been linked to diet. Another three are associated with excessive alcohol consumption—accidents, suicide, and homicide.[6*] **Overnutrition** contributes to other ills as well, including high blood pressure and dental disease. Poor dietary habits and a

GOITER (GOY-ter) enlargement of the thyroid gland caused by iodine deficiency.

PELLAGRA (pell-AY-gra) niacin deficiency characterized by diarrhea, inflammation of the skin, and, in severe cases, mental disorders.

MALNUTRITION any condition caused by an excess, deficiency, or imbalance of calories or nutrients.

OVERNUTRITION calorie or nutrient overconsumption severe enough to cause disease or increased risk of disease; a form of malnutrition.

*The ten leading causes of death in the United States, in order of predominance, are heart disease, cancer, stroke, lung disease, accidents, pneumonia and flu, diabetes, HIV infection, suicide, and homicide.

sedentary lifestyle together account for an estimated 300,000 deaths each year, not to mention hospitalizations, lost time on the job, and poor quality of life among many Americans (see Table 1–2).[7]

This is not to say that diet is the sole culprit responsible for these conditions. A number of environmental, behavioral, social, and genetic factors work together to determine a person's likelihood of suffering from a **degenerative disease.** For example, diet notwithstanding, someone who smokes, doesn't exercise regularly, and has a parent who suffered a heart attack is more likely to end up with heart disease than a nonsmoker who works out regularly and does not have a close relative with heart disease. The way to alter disease risk is to concentrate on changing the day-to-day habits that can be controlled. The results can be significant.

Consider that researchers who monitored the habits and health of a group of some 7,000 Californians for nearly two decades were able to pinpoint seven common lifestyle elements associated with optimal quality of life and longevity: avoiding excess alcohol, not smoking, maintaining desirable weight, exercising regularly, sleeping seven to eight hours a night, not snacking between meals, and eating breakfast. In fact, after 20 years, those who had adhered to the healthful habits were only half as likely to have died as those who hadn't. They were also half as likely to have suffered disabilities that interfere with day-to-day living. Granted, the researchers speculated that the last three habits—sleeping seven to eight hours a night, not eating between meals, and eating breakfast—are not necessarily as beneficial as, say, the habit of exercising regularly. Rather, regular eating and sleeping habits are most likely signs that people take the time and have enough control of their lives to take care of their health.[8]

These findings illustrate that you can change the probable length and quality of your life. Since nutrition is involved in at least half of the preceding lifestyle recommendations, it no doubt plays a key role in maintaining good health. The Longevity Game Scorecard further demonstrates the point.

In 1988, recognizing diet's vital influence on health, the Surgeon General released a landmark statement called *The Surgeon General's Report on Nutrition and Health,* which outlines ways to improve health with sound nutrition practices.[9] A year later, a committee of scientists brought together by the National Research Council pub-

DEGENERATIVE DISEASE chronic disease characterized by deterioration of body organs as a result of misuse and neglect; poor eating habits, smoking, lack of exercise, and other lifestyle habits often contribute to degenerative diseases, including heart disease, cancer, osteoporosis, and diabetes.

TABLE 1–2
CONTRIBUTORS TO AND CAUSES OF DEATH IN THE UNITED STATES

Many of the major killers, such as heart disease, are influenced by a number of factors, including a person's genetic make-up, eating and exercise habits, and exposure to tobacco. The following chart provides a rough estimate of the number of U.S. deaths influenced primarily by certain contributing factors.

CONTRIBUTOR/CAUSE	ESTIMATED NUMBER OF DEATHS	PERCENTAGE OF TOTAL DEATHS[a]
Tobacco	400,000	19
Diet/activity patterns	300,000	14
Alcohol misuse	100,000	5
Infections[b]	90,000	4
Toxic agents[c]	60,000	3
Firearms	35,000	2
Unprotected sex	30,000	1
Motor vehicle injuries	25,000	1
Illicit drug use	20,000	<1

[a]Note that the percentages do not add up to 100 because this chart shows only the major contributors. Other variables that are more difficult to pinpoint, such as income and lack of access to health care, are not included here.

[b]Does not include infection with human immunodeficiency virus (HIV), which causes AIDS. Deaths related to HIV infection are accounted for under unprotected sex.

[c]Refers to environmental pollutants and contaminants of food and water.

SOURCE: Adapted from J. M. McGinnis and W. H. Foege, Actual causes of death in the United States, *Journal of the American Medical Association* 270 (1993): 2208.

 You can't look into a crystal ball to find out how long you will live. But you can get a rough idea of the number of years you're likely to survive based largely on your lifestyle today as well as certain givens, such as your family history. To do so, play the Longevity Game.

Start at the top line—age 74, the average life expectancy for adults in the United States today. For each of the 11 lifestyle areas add or subtract years as instructed. If an area doesn't apply, go on to the next one. If you are not sure of the exact number to add or subtract, make a guess. Don't take the score too seriously, but do pay attention to those areas where you lose years; they could point to habits you might want to change.

START WITH _____74_____

1. Exercise _____
2. Relaxation _____
3. Driving _____
4. Blood Pressure _____
5. 65 and working _____
6. Family history _____
7. Smoking _____
8. Drinking _____
9. Gender _____
10. Weight _____
11. Age _____

Your final score _____

1. **Exercise.** If your job requires regular, vigorous activity or if you work out each day, add three years. If you don't get much exercise at home, on the job, or at play, subtract three years.

2. **Relaxation.** If you have a laid-back approach to life (you roll with the punches), add three years. If you're aggressive, hard-driving, or anxious (you suffer from sleepless nights or bite your nails), subtract three years. If you consider yourself unhappy, subtract another year.

3. **Driving.** Drivers under age 30 who have received traffic tickets in the past year or who have been involved in an accident should subtract four years. Other violations, minus one. If you always wear seatbelts, add a year.

4. **Blood pressure.** While high blood pressure is a major contributor to common killers—heart attacks and strokes—it can be lowered effectively through drugs and changes in lifestyle. The problem is that rises in blood pressure can't be felt, so many victims don't know they have it and therefore never receive lifesaving treatment. If you *know* your blood pressure, add one year.

5. **65 and working.** If you are at the traditional retirement age or older and still working, add three.

6. **Family history.** If any grandparent has reached age 85, add two; if all grandparents have reached age 80, add six. If a parent died of a stroke or heart attack before age 50, minus four. If a parent or brother or sister has (or had) diabetes since childhood, minus three.

7. **Smoking.** Cigarette smokers who finish more than two packs a day, minus eight; one or two packs a day, minus six; one-half to one pack, minus three.

8. **Drinking.** If you drink two cocktails (or beers or glasses of wine) a day, subtract one year. For each additional daily libation, subtract two.

9. **Gender.** Women live longer than men. Females add three years; males subtract three years.

10. **Weight.** If you avoid eating fatty foods and don't add salt to your meals, your heart will probably remain healthy longer, entitling you to add two years.

    Now, weigh in: overweight by 50 pounds or more, minus eight; 30 to 40 pounds, minus four; 10 to 29 pounds, minus two.

11. **Age.** How long you have already lived can help predict how much longer you'll survive. If you're under 30, the jury is still out. But if your age is 30 to 39, plus two; 40 to 49, plus three; 50 to 69, plus four; 70 or over, plus five.

SOURCE: From "The Longevity Game," by Northwestern Mutual Life Insurance Company, with permission.

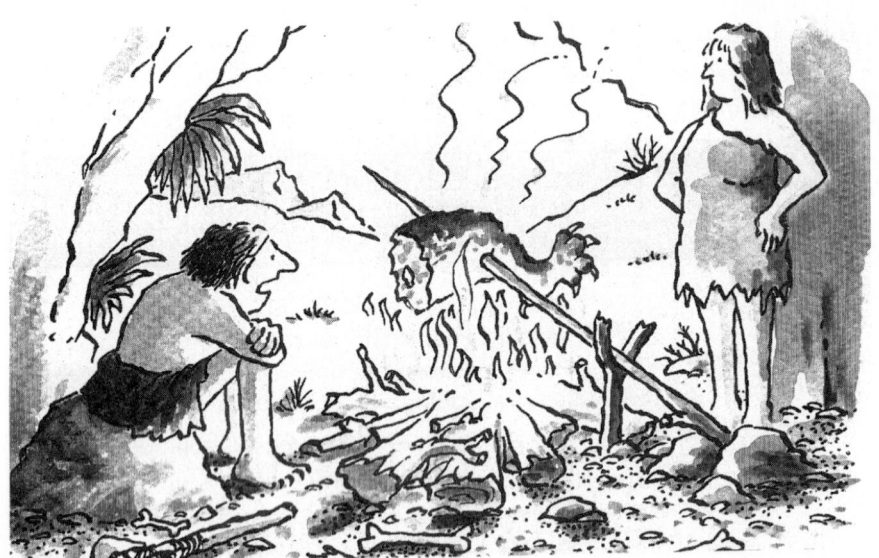

John Jonik

"You figure it. Everything we eat is 100 percent natural, yet our life expectancy is only 31 years."

lished an equally important document titled *Diet and Health,* which provides similar guidelines for reducing disease risk through diet.[10]

Table 1–3 summarizes the dietary recommendations of these two sources. As you read Table 1–3, keep in mind that while everyone can benefit from eating a healthful diet that complies with the guidelines, some people stand to gain more than others. Those who have high blood cholesterol levels, for instance, are already at risk for heart disease, thereby making it especially important for them to eat a low-fat diet and maintain a healthful weight. By the same token, those who have close relatives with, say, diabetes, would do well to keep their weight down and pay particular attention to the other nutrition guidelines that help stave off the condition. (The chapters that follow explain the link between diet and chronic diseases in more detail and offer advice on how to follow each dietary recommendation.)

The exact proportion that dietary factors contribute to each health problem can only be estimated, but some experts speculate that they account for a third or more of all cases of both cancer and heart disease.[11] Moreover, some elements appear to play a more integral role than others in determining disease risk. A high-fat diet, for instance, raises the risk of some types of cancer, heart disease, and obesity, which in turn contributes to a number of other problems, including diabetes and high blood pressure.

The relative importance of certain dietary recommendations is underscored by their appearance in the U.S. Department of Health and Human Services' official strategy for improving the nation's health during the 1990s. Dubbed *Healthy People 2000: National Health Promotion and Disease Prevention Objectives,* the plan of action includes a number of nutritional goals geared toward increasing the span of healthy life for Americans:[12]

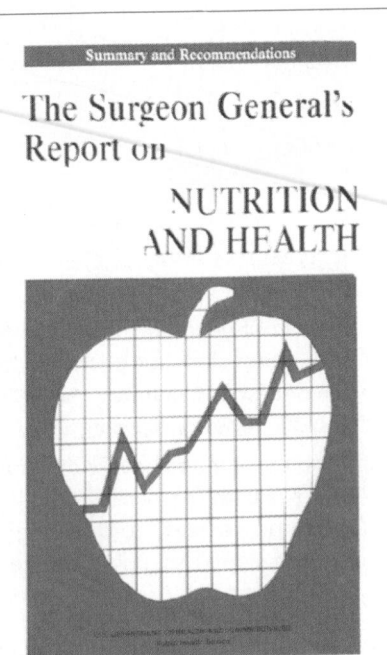

TABLE 1–3
EATING TO BEAT THE ODDS

DIETARY RECOMMENDATION	TO HELP REDUCE THE RISK OF
Fat: Reduce total fat intake to 30% or less of calories. Reduce saturated fat intake to less than 10% of calories and the intake of cholesterol to less than 300 milligrams daily.[a]	Some types of cancer, obesity, heart disease, and possibly gallbladder disease.
Weight: Achieve and maintain a desirable weight.[a]	Diabetes, high blood pressure, stroke, cancers (especially breast and uterine), and gallbladder disease.
Carbohydrates and fiber: Increase consumption of fruits, vegetables, legumes, and whole grains.[a]	Diabetes, heart disease, and some types of cancer.
Sodium: Limit daily intake of salt (sodium chloride).[b]	High blood pressure and stroke.
Alcohol: Avoid completely or drink only in moderation.[a]	Heart disease, high blood pressure, liver disease, stroke, some forms of cancer, and malformations in babies born to mothers who drink alcohol during pregnancy.
Sugar: Limit consumption and frequency of use.	Cavities.
Calcium: Maintain adequate intake.	Osteoporosis and bone fractures.
Fluoride: Maintain optimal intake.	Cavities.

[a]Pay particular attention to this guideline if you have glucose intolerance, high blood cholesterol or high triglyceride levels, or high blood pressure.

[b]Pay particular attention to this guideline if you have high blood pressure.

SOURCE: Adapted from *Surgeon General's Report on Nutrition and Health: Summary and Recommendations* (Washington, D.C.: U.S. Government Printing Office, 1988), pp. 8–17; and *Diet and Health: Implications for Reducing Chronic Disease Risk—Executive Summary* (Washington, D.C.: National Academy Press, 1989), pp. 10–15.

- Reduce dietary fat consumption among people aged two and older from 36 percent of total calories to an average of not more than 30 percent of calories.*

- Increase the number of servings of fruits and vegetables from two and a half a day to five or more, and increase the daily servings of grain products (bread and cereals) from three to at least six.

- Decrease salt consumption by increasing the proportion of people who avoid using salt at the table from 68 percent to 80 percent and by increasing the number of cooks who season dishes without salt.

- Reduce the prevalence of overweight among adults from 26 percent to 20 percent.

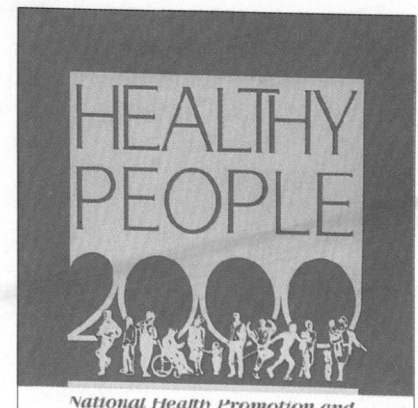

National Health Promotion and Disease Prevention Objectives

Although these are just a few of the goals for nutrition spelled out in *Healthy People 2000*, they represent some of the priorities for maintaining good health. Much of the practical information presented later in this chapter and in those that follow is aimed at guiding you toward developing eating and lifestyle habits that will help you achieve the goals.

*The comparison figures are based on survey results gathered in the 1970s and 1980s and serve as rough estimates of the way Americans presently eat and the current prevalence of overweight.

Fast Guide to Eating on the Run

Chances are you've stood in line for a burger and fries, a slice of pizza, a taco, or a muffin and coffee at least once this week. You're not alone. Every day one out of two Americans orders food served or prepared outside the home, and much of this food is takeout fare. In fact, fast food is the fastest-growing segment of the restaurant industry.[13]

McDonald's golden arches, Domino's Pizza deliveries, and Burger King's "Have It Your Way" slogan are as much a part of American culture as baseball and apple pie. But while a meal eaten on the run fits easily into a busy schedule, it's not necessarily so simple to work it into the dietary guidelines recommended by major health organizations. Two all-beef patties with special sauce and other requisite trimmings, an order of fries, and a milkshake, for example, can chalk up anywhere from 1,000 to 1,500 calories, more than 1,000 milligrams of sodium, and 65-plus grams of fat—more than the amount in half a stick of butter.

The good news is that in the past several years, McDonald's and other fast-food giants have begun offering such items as low-fat dairy products and salads that can fit more easily into the high-carbohydrate, low-fat diet that experts are recommending for good health. With just a little bit of nutrition know-how, you can combine new alternatives with old favorites to place orders more in keeping with today's dietary guidelines. A regular burger, tossed salad, and cup of low-fat milk, for instance, supply only a third of the calories and a quarter of the fat of a standard double-burger-with-fries-and-a-shake order. (Table 1–4 gives the nutritional breakdown of other fast-food meals.) The following tips can guide you in trimming fat and calories from fast-food meals:

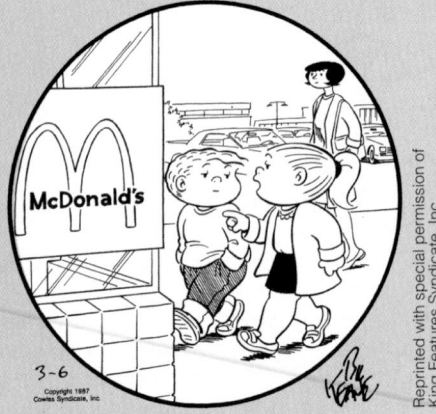

"Before he opened this he had a farm."

- Select an English muffin, bagel, or toast with margarine for breakfast rather than a Danish, doughnut, or muffin. You'll save upwards of 150 calories and take in about three times less fat. A three-inch bagel topped with two teaspoons of jelly contains only about a gram of fat, while many takeout muffins contain in the neighborhood of 13 grams of fat.

- Buy breakfast sandwiches or entrees with Canadian bacon or ham instead of sausage. Whereas a three-inch sausage patty provides 200 calories and 17 grams of fat, two slices of Canadian bacon contribute only 85 calories and 4 grams of fat. Three slices of cured bacon supply about 110 calories and 9 grams of fat.

- Sweeten your pancakes with syrup or spread your toast with jelly or marmalade, but hold the butter. Each tablespoon of butter you spread on your pancakes contributes 100 calories, virtually all of which come from fat. A tablespoon of syrup or jelly, on the other hand, adds only 50 calories and not a trace of fat.

- Hold the mayo. Each dollop of that condiment adds about 100 calories, nearly all of which are fat. Most fast-food sandwiches contain more than just one spoonful of mayo in their toppings and special sauces. The same goes for tartar sauce. Order a fish sandwich without it, and you'll trim at least 70 fat-laden calories (the amount in just one tablespoon) from your meal.

- Opt for a side salad moistened with reduced-calorie dressing with your burger instead of French fries and ketchup. You'll trim at least 150 calories and a good deal of fat from your meal.

- Wash your meal down with low-fat milk instead of a milkshake, thereby cutting the fat and calorie count at least in half.

- Satisfy your sweet tooth with a cup of hot chocolate. Whereas the hot chocolate contains about 100 to 200 calories per cup, sundaes, pies, milkshakes, and other sweets contribute 300 or more calories per serving (and little else in the way of nutrients).

- Don't let the word *chicken* or *fish* fool you. Granted, many health-conscious consumers have heard the advice to choose skinless poultry and fish instead of relatively high-fat red meat. But when it comes to chicken nuggets and fish patties coated with batter and deep fried, it is a different story. Six chicken nuggets, for example, typically contain as many calories (about 300) as an entire burger. What's more, many chicken- and fish-patty sandwiches chalk up as much fat as a pint and a half of ice cream. Even rotisserie-style chicken contains a large amount of fat and calories if you don't remove the skin before eating it.

- When ordering a pizza, hold the sausage and pepperoni and ask for mushrooms, green peppers, and onions instead. Pizza is an excellent

TABLE 1–4
WHAT'S IN AN ORDER?[a]

	CALORIES	GRAMS OF FAT	MILLIGRAMS OF SODIUM
FAT AND CALORIES TO GO			
Double burger with sauce	625	40	880
Milkshake	410	10	190
French fries (regular size)	240	15	120
Total	1,275	65	1,190
Fish sandwich with cheese and tartar sauce	495	25	676
Soda (12 ounces)	150	0	15
French fries (regular size)	240	15	120
Total	885	40	811
Chicken nuggets (6)	310	20	700
Apple pie	280	15	400
Coffee with cream	65	5	15
Total	655	40	1,115
SLIM PICKIN'S			
Single burger	290	13	435
Tossed salad with low-calorie dressing	50	1	445
Low-fat milk (8 ounces)	105	2	125
Total	445	16	1,005
Baked potato (plain)	150	trace	5
Margarine (1 pat)	35	4	45
Tossed salad with low-calorie dressing	50	1	445
Low-fat milk (8 ounces)	105	2	125
Total	340	7	620
Cheese pizza (1 slice)	155	5	455
Tossed salad with low-calorie dressing	50	1	445
Orange juice (8 ounces)	110	0	0
Total	315	6	900

[a]Figures represent the average nutrient values for similar items from three or more fast-food chains.

SOURCE: Adapted from C. Roberts, Fast-food fare: Consumer guidelines, *New England Journal of Medicine* 321 (1989): 754.

source of calcium—that bone-building mineral many Americans don't get enough of—as well as protein, carbohydrate, and a number of vitamins and minerals. Two slices of *pepperoni* pizza, however, can easily contain 100 more calories and twice as much fat as the same amount topped with onions, green peppers, and mushrooms.

- Cover your plate with fresh greens, fruits, and vegetables at the salad bar, but go easy on some of the toppings. A tablespoon here and a tablespoon there of "fixings," such as bacon bits or rich dressing, can turn a low-fat, low-calorie meal into a high-fat, high-calorie extravaganza (see Table 1–5).

- Ask for lots of lettuce and tomatoes and less sour cream and guacamole on your nachos and tacos. A tablespoon of either sour cream or guacamole adds about 25 calories to Mexican fare. A few extra chunks of tomato, on the other hand, supply a negligible number of calories, no fat, and a good deal of vitamin C.

- Order a plain baked potato with a pat of margarine. While a potato with margarine has fewer than 200 calories, spuds covered with bacon and cheese, sour cream, or chili and cheese can contain as many calories and as much fat as a double burger.

- Choose frozen yogurt instead of ice cream, but remember that many "mix-ins" rack up additional fat and calories. Two tablespoons of sprinkles, or "Jimmies," contain about 250 calories and 6 grams of fat (see Table 1–6).

TABLE 1–5
TOPPING IT OFF

	CALORIES PER TABLESPOON	GRAMS OF FAT PER TABLESPOON
Creamy Italian dressing	70	8
Reduced-calorie Italian dressing	15	2
Imitation bacon bits	30	2
Sunflower seeds	50	4
Chopped egg	15	1
Grated process cheese	25	2
Seasoned croutons	5	trace
Raisins	28	trace

SOURCE: U.S. Department of Agriculture, Human Nutrition Information Service, Home and Garden Bulletin No. 232–11, *Eating Better When Eating Out Using the Dietary Guidelines*, p. 9.

TABLE 1–6
FROZEN YOGURT "MIX-INS"

	CALORIES PER TABLESPOON	GRAMS OF FAT PER TABLESPOON
Sprinkles (Jimmies)	122	3
Yogurt-covered raisins	67	2
Chocolate syrup	46	<1
Fudge topping	62	2
Crumbled chocolate chip cookie	66	3
Crumbled Heath Bar	71	4
Reese's Pieces	69	3
m&m's	68	3
Mixed nuts	85	7
Granola	35	2
Fresh strawberries	3	<1

Understanding Our Food Choices

The choices you make about what to eat can have a profound impact on your health, both now and in your later years. The healthful eater resists disease and other stresses better than a person with poor dietary habits and is more likely to enjoy an active, vigorous lifestyle for a greater number of years. Even so, the nutritional profile of various foods ranks as only one of many factors that influence your eating habits. Whether you realize it or not, each time you sit down to a meal you bring to the table such factors as your own personal preferences, cultural traditions, and economic considerations. These influences exert as great an impact on your eating habits as does **hunger**—the physiological need for food—and **appetite**—the psychological desire for food, which may arise in response to the sight, smell, or thought of food even when you're not hungry. The following sections examine some of the most influential factors in making food choices.

HUNGER the physiological need for food.

APPETITE the psychological desire to eat, which is often but not always accompanied by hunger.

Availability

Our diets are limited by the types and amounts of food available through the food supply, which in turn is influenced by many forces. Because we have the geographical area, climate, soil conditions, labor, and capital necessary to maintain a large agricultural industry, Americans enjoy what is arguably the most abundant food supply in the world. In addition, unlike many other less wealthy countries, the United States and Canada have the resources needed to import and distribute a wide variety of foods from other countries—everything from kiwi from New Zealand to mangoes from the tropics.

History has shown, however, that when it comes to health, an abundant food supply can be a double-edged sword. Access to many types of foods allows people to choose high-fat diets rich in meats, eggs, and other fatty foods, which can contribute to increased rates of heart disease and other problems. That's one of the reasons why degenerative diseases are sometimes referred to as diseases of affluence.

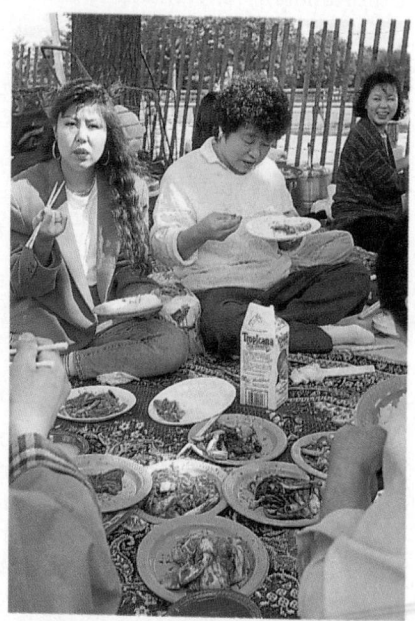

Many factors influence our food choices, including advertising, early experiences, economics, and cultural traditions.

UNDERNUTRITION severe underconsumption of calories or nutrients leading to disease or increased susceptibility to disease; a form of malnutrition.

Income and Food Prices

As most college students know firsthand, the amount of money available to spend on food can mean the difference between ordering pizza every night and resigning yourself to a steady diet of peanut butter and jelly sandwiches. Extremely low incomes can make it difficult for people to buy enough food to meet their minimum nutritional needs, thereby putting them at risk for **undernutrition.**

A consumer's *perception* of the cost of various foods can also play a role in his or her choices. For example, one barrier that prevents people from adopting healthful eating habits is the belief that it would be too expensive. In fact, 40 percent of consumers who answered one survey said that fruits, vegetables, seafood, and other elements of a low-fat, nutrient-rich diet would strain their budgets.[14] But some research has shown that switching from a high-fat diet to one that is lower in fat can reduce food costs.[15] Just cutting back on the amount of meat and poultry—from which much of the fat in the American diet comes and on which many of our food dollars are spent—goes a long way in trimming food budgets.

Advertising and the Media

Television and radio commercials as well as magazines and newspapers play an extremely powerful role in influencing our food choices and our knowledge of nutrition.[16] Given today's health-conscious environment, food manufacturers are promoting the nutritional merits of their products more than ever before. In fact, in some of the most popular women's magazines, the number of food and beverage ads containing nutrition claims increased by nearly 100 percent between 1975 and 1990.[17] Unfortunately, advertising is not always created with the consumer's best interest in mind. Much of the food advertising that we're exposed to from the earliest ages is aimed at selling products that aren't the optimal choices for regular inclusion in a healthful diet. For example, the great majority of television commercials geared to children and aired on Saturday mornings promote high-fat, sugary foods such as candy and sugar-coated cereals.[18] Yet commercials promoting good nutrition are relatively few and far between.

Along with advertising, the media rank among the most influential sources of diet and nutrition information, which in turn affects our food choices. Consider that most Americans look first to magazines as a source of nutrition information, then to television, and finally to newspapers.[19] The downside is that the reliability of information delivered by the media varies considerably. For instance, Table 1–7 shows how the nutrition information in some of the most popular magazines in the United States was judged by the American Council on Science and Health.[20] The council's assessment emphasizes the importance of learning how to evaluate the nutrition information you receive via the media. The Spotlight at the end of the chapter will help you to learn techniques for critiquing articles.

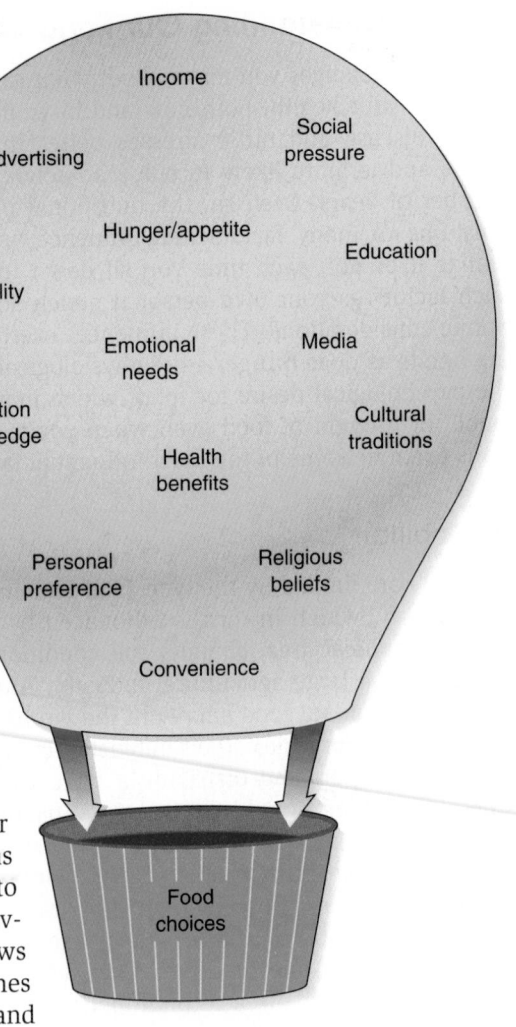

Income
Social pressure
Advertising
Hunger/appetite
Education
Availability
Emotional needs
Media
Nutrition knowledge
Cultural traditions
Health benefits
Personal preference
Religious beliefs
Convenience
Food choices

See Appendix A for a complete list of publications that contain reliable nutrition information.

Social and Cultural Factors

The social and cultural groups to which a person belongs make a strong impact on food choices. **Social groups** such as families, friends, and co-workers tend to exert the most influence. The family, particularly the wife/mother, plays one of the most powerful roles in determining our food choices.[21] That makes sense, as the family is both the first social group a person encounters and the one to which he or she typically belongs for the longest period of time. The values, attitudes, and traditions of our family can have a lasting effect on our food choices. Think of the holiday food traditions

SOCIAL GROUP a group of people, such as a family, who depend on one another and share a set of norms, beliefs, values, and behaviors.

in your own family and your friends' families. Treasured recipes or rituals surrounding holiday meals are often passed from one generation to the next.

Friends, co-workers, and members of other social networks also influence our food choices and eating behavior. For instance, many weight-loss programs feature group sessions made up of people who are in the same boat so that they can support one another in their efforts to lose weight. Social pressure can also push us to eat meals we might not choose on our own. For example, as a guest in another country or in a friend's home, your choosing not to partake of the food and drink that's offered might be considered rude. By the same token, it's natural to join your friends on a spontaneous trip for ice cream or pizza even when you're not hungry.

Culture also determines our food choices to a large extent. Many of our eating habits arise from the traditions, belief systems, technologies, values, and norms of the culture in which we live. For example, in the United States and Canada, the idea of eating insects is generally considered repulsive. But many people throughout the rest of the world relish dishes prepared with various bugs, including locust dumplings (northern Africa), red-ant chutney

CULTURE knowledge, beliefs, customs, laws, morals, art, and literature acquired by members of a society and passed along to succeeding generations.

TABLE 1–7

HOW DOES YOUR FAVORITE MAGAZINE RATE?

Here's how a panel of experts judged the reliability of the nutrition information and recommendations found in some of the most popular American magazines. Keep in mind that the content of magazines sometimes varies a great deal from year to year, as editors come and go. Still, some of the best magazines, such as *Cooking Light,* consistently provide accurate nutrition information.

	SCORE (OUT OF 100)		SCORE (OUT OF 100)
EXCELLENT		**FAIR**	
Cooking Light	91	*Family Circle*	77
GOOD		*Harper's Bazaar*	77
American Health	88	*Runner's World*	77
Consumer Reports	88	*Self*	76
Good Housekeeping	88	*Health*	75
Better Homes & Gardens	87	*Mademoiselle*	75
Glamour	86	*Vogue*	75
Parents	85	*Ladies' Home Journal*	74
Reader's Digest	85	*New Woman*	74
McCall's	80	**POOR**	
Prevention	80	*Cosmopolitan*	62
Redbook	80		
Woman's Day	80		

SOURCE: Adapted from D. Woznicki and A. G. Case, *Nutrition Accuracy in Popular Magazines* (New York: American Council on Science and Health, Inc., 1994).

(India), water beetles in shrimp sauce (Laos), and fried caterpillars (South Africa).[22]

One of the ways people of different cultures often come together to share their heritage is by sampling each other's traditional foods. American consumers are particularly fortunate in that they don't have to travel far to get a taste of the food of different cultures. **Ethnic cuisine** ranging from Chinese to Mexican to Italian to Indian food has become embedded in American culture. (The Spotlight in Chapter 3 discusses in detail the foodways of different cultures.)

One aspect of culture that affects the food choices of millions of people worldwide is religion. The practice of giving and abstaining from food has long been used by many cultures as a way to show devotion, respect, and love to a supreme being or power. While the food choices of Christians in the West tend not to be dictated by church doctrine, dietary customs play a major role in the practice of many other of the world's major religions. As Table 1–8 shows, many religions specify which foods their followers may eat and how the foods must be prepared.

Other Factors That Affect Our Food Choices

One of the main reasons you choose to eat certain foods is your preferences for certain tastes. Just about everyone enjoys sweet foods, for example, because humans are born with an affinity for sugar.[23] In addition, we usually prefer foods with which we have happy associations—special foods prepared for birthdays or holiday gatherings, those given to us by a loved one when we were children, or those eaten by an admired role model. By the same token, intense aversion to certain foods—say, foods you were given when you were sick or foods you were forced to eat—can be strong enough to last a lifetime. Your parents may have taught you to prefer certain foods and pass up others for reasons of their own, without even being aware they were doing so.

Food habits are also intimately tied to deep psychological needs, such as an infant's association of food with a parent's love. Yearnings, cravings, and addictions with profound meaning and significance sometimes surface as food behavior. Some people respond to stress—positive or negative—by eating; others use food to fill a void, such as lack of satisfying personal relationships or fulfilling work.

Some people adopt a certain way of eating or make specific choices based on a larger worldview. For instance, many environmentally conscious people, believing that raising animals for human consumption strains the world's

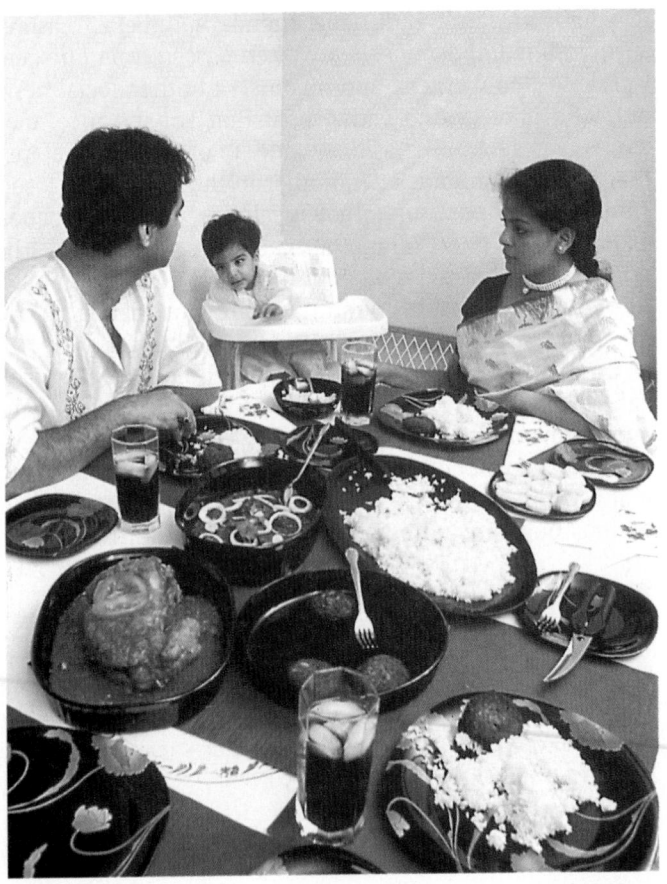

Many of our eating habits stem from the culture in which we live.

ETHNIC CUISINE the traditional foods eaten by the people of a particular culture.

TABLE 1–8
DIETARY PRACTICES OF SEVERAL MAJOR RELIGIONS

RELIGION	DIETARY PRACTICES
BUDDHISM	The central tenet of Buddhism is vegetarianism. In the eyes of Buddhists, to eat meat is to destroy the seeds of compassion. All plant foods are considered appropriate to eat except for the "five pungent foods": garlic, leek, scallion, chives, and onion. These foods are considered unclean and are believed to generate lust when eaten cooked and to induce rage when eaten raw.
HINDUISM	Hindus believe that food was created by the Supreme Being for the benefit of humans. Beef is prohibited, and many Hindu followers are vegetarians.
ISLAM	Islamic food laws prohibit the consumption of "unclean" foods such as swine, animals killed in a manner that prevents their blood from being fully drained from their bodies, carnivorous animals with fangs (such as lions and wolves), birds with sharp claws (including falcons and eagles), and land animals without ears (frogs and snakes, for example).
JUDAISM	The traditional dietary laws of Judaism prohibit the consumption of swine, carrion eaters, and shellfish and specify other practices, such as the ritual slaughtering of animals. The term *kosher* indicates that the food was prepared according to certain methods. For example, the meat was salted to help remove the blood, or milk and meat were prepared using separate utensils.
SEVENTH-DAY ADVENTISM	Vegetarianism is the foundation of Seventh-Day Adventist dietary practices. In addition, dietary standards call for abstaining from alcohol and avoiding caffeine. Followers typically eat a wholesome diet consisting of whole grains, fruits, nuts, vegetables, a little milk, and occasional eggs.

SOURCE: Adapted from M. A. Boyle and D. H. Morris, *Community Nutrition in Action* (St. Paul: West Publishing Company, 1994), p. 245.

supply of land and water, choose to abstain from meat as much as possible in an effort to preserve the earth's resources. Others may choose to boycott certain manufacturers' items for political reasons, perhaps because they disagree with a company's advertising practices.

It all boils down to the fact that the influences on people's eating habits are as many and varied as the individuals themselves. Our food choices reflect our own unique cultural legacies, philosophies, and beliefs. To think about food as nothing more than a source of nutrients would be to deny food's rich symbolism and meaning and would take away from much of the pleasure of breaking bread with friends and family. As you read this book and consider ways to improve your own eating habits, take time to reflect on your own unique background and think about how you can integrate your knowledge of nutrition into your cultural heritage and philosophies.

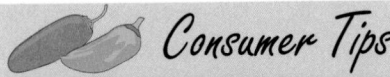 *Consumer Tips*

Stocking Up for Healthful Eating

To prepare healthful meals, you need to have the proper ingredients. It helps to keep staples on hand to save time and last-minute trips to the grocery store. Keeping a well-stocked pantry or refrigerator containing the following items will make it easier to put to practice the dietary advice and guidelines that appear later in the book.

Flour, Cereal, and Other Grains

- bran flakes (and other cold cereals)
- bread
- brown and white rice
- cornmeal
- graham crackers
- regular or quick-cooking oats
- spaghetti and macaroni
- whole all-purpose flour
- whole-wheat flour

Leavening and Thickening Agents

- baking powder
- baking soda
- cornstarch

Sweeteners

- brown sugar
- honey
- molasses
- white sugar

Seasonings and Condiments

- basil
- bay leaves
- black pepper
- chili powder
- cinnamon
- dillweed
- lemon juice
- mustard
- nutmeg
- onion powder
- oregano
- paprika
- garlic cloves and powder
- ginger
- ketchup
- salt
- vanilla extract
- vinegar

Other Basics

- beans and peas (dry and/or canned)
- carrots
- cheese
- evaporated skim milk
- nonfat milk powder
- nuts
- onions
- peanut butter
- plain low-fat or nonfat yogurt
- popcorn
- potatoes
- raisins
- tomato paste
- tomato sauce
- vegetable oil

When it comes to storing your staple goods, keep a few tips in mind:[24]

- Rotate foods already in your cupboard or refrigerator with new items to ensure that the older foods are used first.
- Keep staples, including flour, sugar, and cereal, in airtight containers to prevent bug infestation; store whole-wheat flour in the refrigerator or freezer.
- Store frozen foods in airtight containers, freezer bags, or heavy duty freezer wrap or foil in a freezer kept at zero degrees Fahrenheit or colder.
- Maintain the refrigerator temperature below 40 degrees Fahrenheit and keep foods in airtight containers to prevent the spread of odors or flavors. Keep items far enough from one another to allow air to circulate.
- Place dry foods in clean, cool, dark, and dry shelves above the floor and away from water pipes and air ducts.

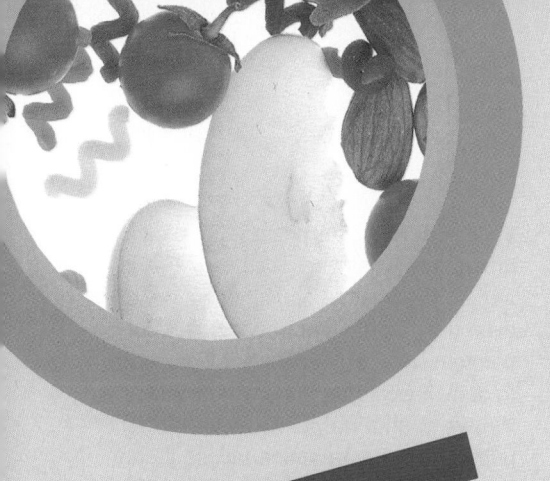

Separating Nutrition Fact from Fiction

You've just watched a television commercial for a vitamin supplement guaranteed to produce a laundry list of benefits, including fewer colds, a better complexion, and a decreased risk of cancer. Should you buy it? You've just read a magazine article with a plan for quick weight loss. Should you believe it? Someone who plays the same sport as you says that improving your diet will help your game. Where do you go for help?

We all find ourselves faced with such dilemmas at one time or another. It's essential to know how to handle them to protect ourselves from nutrition misinformation. As we pointed out earlier, health fraud costs consumers some $30 billion each year. At the same time, the sale of weight-loss programs and products—not all of them sound—has become a 32-billion-dollar industry.[25] Media attention to "hot" foods and nutritional supplements generally causes spending on those items to soar.

Money down the drain is just one of the problems stemming from misleading dietary information. While some fraudulent claims about nutrition are harmless and might make for a good laugh, others can lead to tragic consequences. Swallowing false claims about nutritional products has been known to bring about malnutrition, birth defects, mental retardation, and even death in extreme cases. Negative effects from following false claims can come about in two ways. One is that the product in question causes direct harm. Even a seemingly innocuous substance such as vitamin A can cause severe liver damage over time if taken in large enough doses. The other way that using spurious nutritional remedies can cause problems is that such remedies build false hope and may keep a consumer from obtaining sound, scientifically tested medical treatment. A person who relies on a so-called anti-cancer diet as a cure for the disease, for example, might forego possible life-saving interventions such as surgery or chemotherapy.

The following questions and answers should help you learn to evaluate the nutrition information you see in the newspapers or on labels. It should enable you to develop the skills with which to view nutrition claims with a skeptic's eye or, at the very least, find a qualified professional who can.

Judging by what I've read in newspapers, it seems as if nutritionists are always changing their minds. One week the headlines say take vitamins to prevent cancer, and the next week they say vitamins may cause cancer. Why is there so much controversy? Part of the confusion stems from the way the media interpret the findings of scientific research. A good case in point is the controversy over whether people should take supplement pills containing large doses of beta-carotene, vitamin C, and vitamin E—collectively known as antioxidants. (The way antioxidants work in the body as well as their role in your diet is discussed in detail in the Chapter 6 Spotlight.) Since the early 1990s, the media have delivered a steady stream of news stories hailing the benefits of antioxidants in, among other things, preventing cancer. Supplement manufacturers were quick to get on the bandwagon, offering consumers an ever-growing assortment of antioxidant pills.

In 1994, a flurry of headlines, such as "To swallow or not to swallow: that is the new vitamin question," threatened to pull the pedestal out from under antioxidants.[26] A study published in the *New England Journal of Medicine,* one of the most prestigious medical journals, suggested that antioxidant supplements did nothing to prevent cancer. Even worse, people who took supplements ended up with higher cancer rates than those who didn't.[27] In other words, the new study and some of the news reports that discussed it were implying that scientists had deceived the public by overstating the value of antioxidants.[28]

The antioxidant story illustrates how news reports based on just one study can leave the public with the impression that scientists can't make up their minds. It seems as if one week scientists are saying that antioxidants are good, and the next week the word is that antioxidants are harmful. The truth is that few experts and no major health organizations have recommended that the general public take antioxidant supplements because, as the one study that created such a stir underscored, the answers on antioxidants are not all in. Most scientists have been emphasizing all along that eating fruits and vegetables is the key to reaping any potential benefits from antioxidants.

Contrary to what some headlines imply, reputable scientists do not base their dietary recommendations for the public on the findings of just one or two studies. Scientists are still conducting research to determine whether antioxidant supplements do in fact help to prevent disease and, if so, in what dosages. Scientists design their research to test theories, such as the notion that taking a vitamin tablet is associated with a lower risk of cancer. Other factors, however, often confound the matter at hand. The alarming study previously mentioned involved only smokers. Had the same research been carried out among a group of nonsmokers, the outcome may have been different.[29]

Even if an experiment is carefully designed and carried out perfectly, its findings cannot be considered definitive until they have been confirmed by other research. Testing and retesting reduce the possibility that the outcome was simply the result of chance or an error or oversight on the part of the experimenter. Every study should be viewed as preliminary until it becomes just one addition to a significant body of evidence pointing in the same direction.

When making dietary recommendations for the public, experts pool the results of different types of studies, such as analyses of food patterns of groups of people and carefully controlled studies on people in hospitals or clinics. Before drawing any conclusions, they then consider the evidence from all of the research. In fact, the dietary guidelines spelled out in the 1,300-page *Diet and Health* report are based on the results of hundreds of studies. The bottom line is that if you read a report in the newspaper or watch one on television that advises

making a dramatic change in your diet or lifestyle based on the results of one study, don't take it to heart. The findings may make for a good story, but they're not worth taking too seriously.

What about animal studies? If I hear on the news that a substance in food makes rats sick, should I stop eating it? Not necessarily. It's wise to be leery of media stories based solely on animal experiments. Admittedly, conducting animal research is a logical first step in gathering information about how chemicals, drugs, or devices may affect living things. It's not practical or ethical to gather this knowledge by allowing humans to use untested products. Translating the findings of animal studies to humans, however, can be just as dangerous and unethical. While different species may respond in some way for better or for worse to a treatment, the same response will not necessarily occur in humans.

For example, suppose rats became sick when injected with the amount of substance X that a person would normally consume in a year's time. A researcher might correctly conclude that substance X could cause illness. But in a case like this, remember that a rat is a tiny animal with a different physical make-up than a human being. Moreover, the rodent received a huge dose of substance X all at once. Thus, the experiment does not indicate whether small amounts of substance X taken by a person over the course of a year would produce the same harmful effect. A news story that implies otherwise misses the mark.

Why doesn't the government do something to prevent the media from delivering misleading nutrition information? The government lacks the power to do so because the **First Amendment** guarantees freedom of

the press. Thus, it is possible for people to express whatever views they like in the media, whether sound, unsound, or even dangerous. This freedom is a cornerstone of the U.S. Constitution, and to deny it would be to deny democracy. Writers cannot be punished by law for publishing misinformation unless it can be proved in court that the information has caused a reader bodily harm.

Fortunately, most professional health groups maintain committees to combat the spread of health and nutrition misinformation. A list of organizations that provide reliable scientific information appears in Appendix A, and any of these organizations can serve as sources for your own inquiries about the authenticity of scientific information in their areas.*

Does the First Amendment also make it legal for companies to say whatever they want about the products they sell? No. Unlike journalists, purveyors of products are bound by law to make only true statements about their wares. The Food and Drug Administration (FDA) holds the authority to prosecute companies that display false nutrition information on product labels or enclosures, and the Federal Trade Commission (FTC) can take to task manufacturers who make fraudulent or misleading statements in their advertise-

---

*If you have questions about a medical book, product, or service, contact the American Medical Association; about an anticancer book, product, or service, the American Cancer Society; about a heart disease treatment, the American Heart Association; about a diet or nutritional supplement, the American Dietetic Association; and so forth. Many professional organizations have banded together to form the National Council Against Health Fraud (NCAHF), which has branches in many states. The NCAHF monitors radio, television, and other advertising and investigates complaints. You can write to the NCAHF at P.O. Box 1276, Loma Linda, CA 92354.

ments. Nevertheless, combating health fraud is an overwhelming job requiring enormous amounts of time and money. As one FDA official has put it, "Quack promoters have learned to stay one step ahead of the laws either by moving from state to state or by changing their corporate names."[30]

How can I tell whether a product is bogus? It's not always easy. Given that many misleading claims are supposedly backed by scientific-sounding statements, it is difficult for even informed consumers to separate fact from fiction. The following red flags can help you spot a quack:

• *The promoter claims that the medical establishment is against him or her and the government won't accept this new "alternative" treatment.*

If the government or medical community doesn't accept a treatment, it's because the treatment hasn't been proven to work. Reputable professionals don't suppress knowledge about fighting disease. On the contrary, they welcome new remedies for illness, provided the treatments have been carefully tested.

• *The promoter uses testimonials and anecdotes from satisfied customers to support claims.*

Valid nutrition information comes from careful experimental research, not from random tales. A few people's reports that the product in question "works every time" are never acceptable as sound scientific evidence.

• *The promoter uses a computer-scored questionnaire for diagnosing "nutrient deficiencies."*

Those computers are programmed to suggest that just about everyone has a deficiency that can be reversed with the supplements the promoter just happens to be selling, regardless of the consumer's symptoms or health.

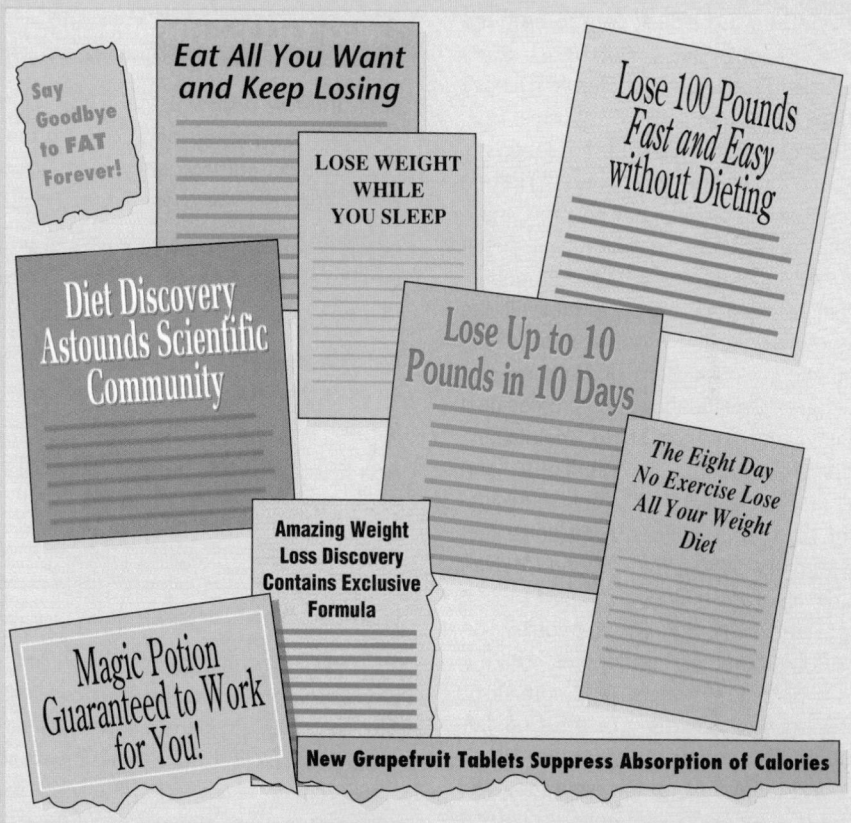

If it sounds too good to be true, it probably is.

• *The promoter claims the product will make weight loss easy.*

Unfortunately, there is no simple way to lose weight. In other words, if a claim sounds too good to be true, it probably is.

• *The promoter promises that the product is made with a "secret formula" available only from this one company.*

Legitimate health professionals share their knowledge of proven treatments so that others can benefit from it.

• *The treatment is available only through the back pages of magazines, over the phone, or by mail-order ads in the form of news stories or 30-minute commercials (known as infomercials) in talk-show format.*

Results of studies on credible treatments are reported first in medical journals and administered through a doctor or other health professional. If information about a treatment appears only elsewhere, it probably can't withstand scrutiny.*

---

*If you think you've been duped by a quack, write the FDA, Office of Consumer Affairs and Information, HFC-110, 5600 Fishers Lane, Rockville, MD 29857; your state Attorney General's office; the Federal Trade Commission, Correspondence Branch, Sixth and Pennsylvania Avenues, N.W., Washington, DC 20580; and/or the newspaper, magazine, or TV or radio station running the ad. If you ordered the product by mail, call the U.S. Postal Service at 202-636-2300 and ask for a fraud packet. If you've been seriously harmed and you want to take legal action, write or call the National Council Against Health Fraud's Task Force on Victim Redress at P.O. Box 1747, Allentown, PA 18105, 215-437-1795.

If I do buy a product, say, to help me lose weight, but I still need some advice about dieting, should I check with a nutritionist? To answer that question, first consider the following. About ten years ago, Charlie Herbert became a professional of the International Academy of Nutrition Consultants. Another member of the household, Sassafras Herbert, met all the requirements for membership in the American Association of Nutrition and Dietary Consultants, a "professional association dedicated to maintaining ethical standards in nutritional and dietary consulting." The only qualification for membership is a 50-dollar fee, regardless of your background (or even your species). Charlie Herbert is a cat, and Sassafras is a poodle. The two obtained their "credentials" with the help of Victor Herbert, M.D., professor of medicine, chairman of the Committee to Strengthen Nutrition at Mount Sinai School of Medicine, New York City, and a leader in combating nutrition

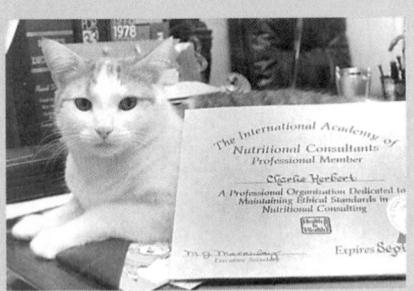

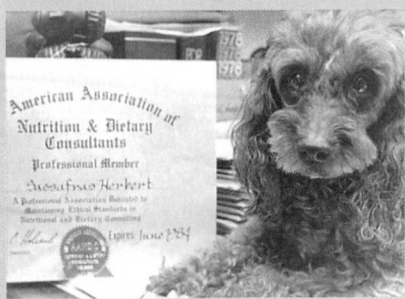

Charlie and Sassafras display their professional credentials.

MINIGLOSSARY

ACCREDITATION approval; in the case of hospitals or university departments, approval by a professional organization of the educational program offered. There are phony accrediting agencies; the genuine ones are listed in a directory called *Accredited Institutions of Postsecondary Education.*

CORRESPONDENCE SCHOOL a school from which courses can be taken and degrees granted by mail. Schools that are accredited offer respectable courses and degrees.

DIPLOMA MILL a correspondence school that grinds out degrees—sometimes worth no more than the cost of the paper they are printed on—the way a grain mill grinds out flour.

FIRST AMENDMENT the amendment to the U.S. Constitution that guarantees freedom of the press.

NUTRITIONIST a person who claims to be capable of advising people about their diets. Some nutritionists are registered dietitians, whereas others are self-described experts whose training is questionable.

REGISTERED DIETITIAN (R.D.) a professional who has graduated from a program of dietetics approved by the American Dietetic Association (ADA), has passed a registration examination, has served an internship program or the equivalent to gain practical skills, and maintains competencies through continuing education. Some states require licensing for dietitians; that is, they have legislation in place obligating anyone who wants to use the title "dietitian" to receive permission by passing a state examination. Other states do not require dietitians to be licensed. R.D. (the abbreviation for registered dietitian) is often used to refer to such a professional in the same way M.D. designates a medical doctor.

fraud. Dr. Herbert had his pets added to the membership rosters of those organizations to demonstrate how easy it is for anyone to get fake nutrition credentials. This is because in most states, the term **nutritionist** is not at present legally defined.

During the past decade, the situation doesn't seem to have improved much. In 1994, a 32-state survey sponsored by the National Council Against Health Fraud found that consumers who turn to the Yellow Pages to find a nutrition counselor have about a 50-50 chance of finding someone with legitimate training. Many so-called practitioners calling themselves nutritionists or nutrition-oriented physicians hold

bogus degrees and dispense bad advice and pricey supplements.[31]

Before you pay a fee or follow a nutritionist's advice, inquire about the person's credentials. Some "nutritionists" obtain their diplomas and titles without undergoing the rigorous training required to obtain a legitimate degree in nutrition. Lax state laws make it possible for irresponsible **correspondence schools**—also called **diploma mills**—to grant degrees to unqualified individuals for nothing more than a fee.

How can I check a nutritionist's credentials? You can call the institution that the person claims has awarded the degree. To find out about the existence or reputation of an institution of higher learning, you can go to any library and ask for a directory of colleges and universities called *Accredited Institutions of Postsecondary Education,* published by the American Council on Education. Be suspicious of diplomas or degrees issued by institutions that cannot prove that they have **accreditation** from the Council on Education.

Another option is to find out whether the person is a special type of nutritionist, known as a **registered dietitian (R.D.).** The R.D., an especially meaningful credential, has a standard definition—a professional who has fulfilled coursework required by the American Dietetic Association (ADA), including courses in chemistry, anatomy, physiology, advanced nutrition, diet therapy, food science, and food service administration. In addition, the R.D. has completed an internship that includes on-the-job training counseling people about diet and has passed a national registration exam. All registered dietitians must keep their credentials current by completing regular continuing education requirements.

You can check on any R.D. by asking for that person's registration number and calling the ADA's Commission on Dietetic Registration (312-899-0040). If you'd like to contact an R.D. but don't know where to find one, call the ADA's Consumer Nutrition Hot Line at 1-800-366-1655 for a referral.

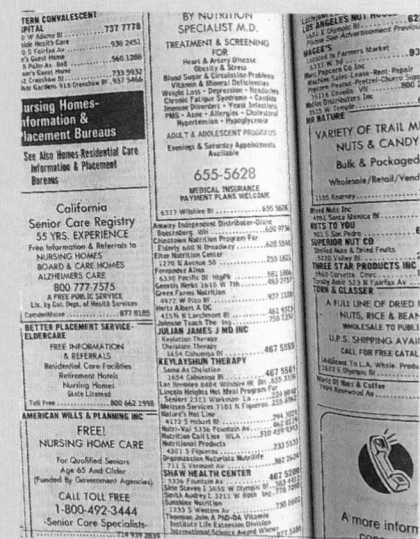

If you're looking for a credible nutritionist, be careful when you "let your fingers do the walking" through the Yellow Pages.

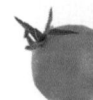

CHECK YOURSELF...

1. Name three diseases associated with overnutrition.

2. Describe the difference between a nutritionist and a registered dietitian.

3. Name four factors that affect your eating habits.

4. Define health fraud.

5. Identify three ways you can cut fat and calories from fast food.

6. Describe three red flags that can help you spot a nutrition quack.

7. Explain how culture influences eating habits.

8. Name three factors besides diet that affect longevity.

9. Describe the role of the Food and Drug Administration and of the Federal Trade Commission in monitoring sellers of nutrition-related products.

10. Name two government reports that recognize the role of nutrition in health.

Answers to selected Check Yourself questions are found in Appendix H.

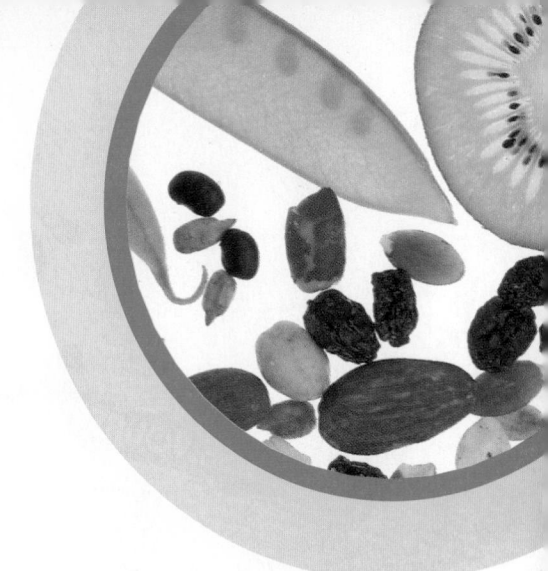

> If the doctors of today will not become the nutritionists of tomorrow, the nutritionists of today will become the doctors of tomorrow.
>
> Thomas Edison
> (1847–1931, American inventor)

The Pursuit of an Ideal Diet

TWO

Contents

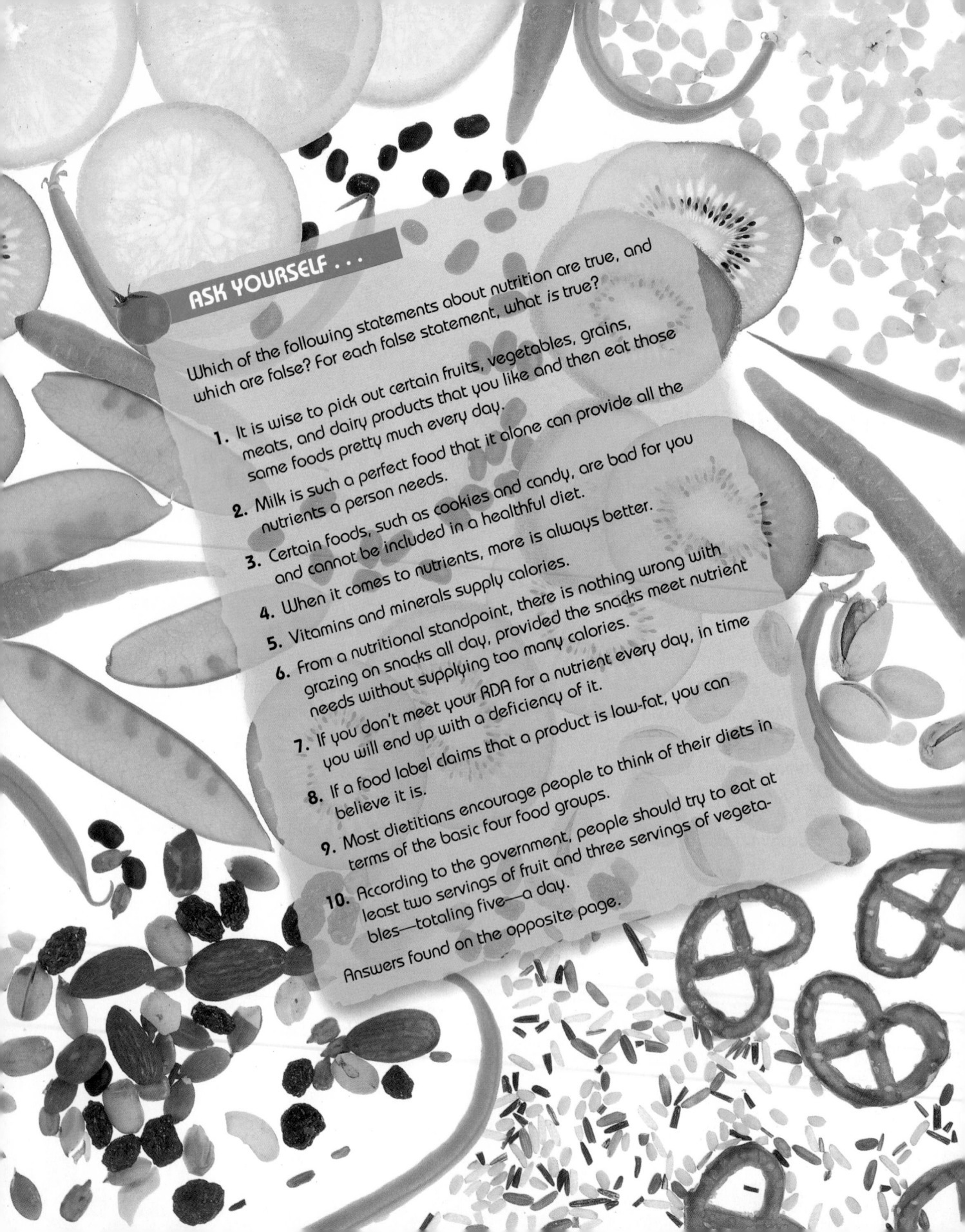

ASK YOURSELF . . .

Which of the following statements about nutrition are true, and which are false? For each false statement, what *is* true?

1. It is wise to pick out certain fruits, vegetables, grains, meats, and dairy products that you like and then eat those same foods pretty much every day.

2. Milk is such a perfect food that it alone can provide all the nutrients a person needs.

3. Certain foods, such as cookies and candy, are bad for you and cannot be included in a healthful diet.

4. When it comes to nutrients, more is always better.

5. Vitamins and minerals supply calories.

6. From a nutritional standpoint, there is nothing wrong with grazing on snacks all day, provided the snacks meet nutrient needs without supplying too many calories.

7. If you don't meet your RDA for a nutrient every day, in time you will end up with a deficiency of it.

8. If a food label claims that a product is low-fat, you can believe it is.

9. Most dietitians encourage people to think of their diets in terms of the basic four food groups.

10. According to the government, people should try to eat at least two servings of fruit and three servings of vegetables—totaling five—a day.

Answers found on the opposite page.

For most people, eating is so habitual that they give hardly any thought to the foods they choose to eat. Yet, as Chapter 1 emphasized, the foods you select can have a profound effect on the quality and possibly even the length of your life. Given all the statistics and government mandates presented so far, however, designing a healthful diet may seem like a complicated matter involving a rigid regimen that excludes certain foods from the diet. Fortunately, that's not the case. The government, as well as many major health organizations, has devised dietary guidelines and tools such as food labels to help you choose the most healthful diet for you. This chapter provides an overview of some of the best guides and tools and shows you how to use them.

As you read the following pages, keep in mind that one of the biggest misconceptions about planning a healthful diet is that some foods, say, carrots and celery sticks, are "good," while others, like cookies and candy, are "bad." People who class foods this way often feel guilty every time they "splurge" on a so-called bad food. The overall diet is what counts, however. A diet consisting of nothing but carrot sticks is just as unhealthful as one made up of only candy bars. The trick is choosing a healthful balance of foods. The ideal diet contains primarily foods that supply adequate nutrients, fiber, and calories without an excess of fat, sugar, sodium, or alcohol.

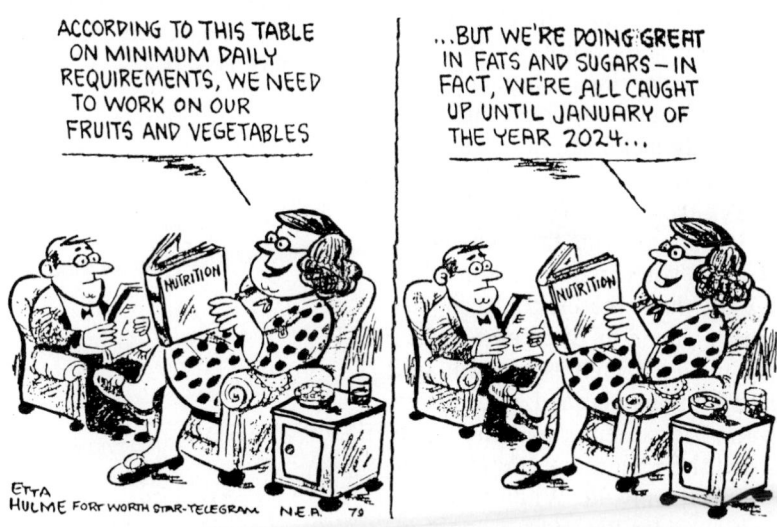

ETTA HULME. Reprinted by permission of Newspaper Enterprise Association, Inc.

ASK YOURSELF ANSWERS: **1.** False. It is unwise to eat the same foods day in and day out; your diet will lack variety and probably will not supply all the nutrients your body needs. **2.** False. Milk rates as an excellent source of nutrients such as calcium and protein, but it contains only very small amounts of iron and several other nutrients. **3.** False. Any food can fit into a healthful eating plan. It's the total diet, not individual foods, that can be either good or bad for health. **4.** False. Too much or too little of a nutrient is often equally harmful. **5.** False. Only protein, carbohydrate, and fat supply calories. **6.** True. **7.** False. Even if you don't meet your RDA for a nutrient, you still may be consuming a sufficient amount of the nutrient. **8.** True. **9.** False. Dietitians today encourage people to think about eating from the five food groups in the Food Guide Pyramid. **10.** True.

The ABCs of Eating for Health

When you plan a diet for yourself, try to make sure it has certain characteristics: **adequacy** (it will provide enough of the essential nutrients, fiber, and energy—in the form of calories); **balance** (it will not overemphasize any food type or nutrient at the expense of another); **calorie control** (it will supply the amount of energy you need to maintain desirable weight—not more, not less); **moderation** (it will not contain excess amounts of unwanted constituents, such as fat, salt, or sugar); and **variety** (it will be made up of different foods rather than the same meals day after day). Equally important, it will suit you; that is, it will consist of foods that fit your personality, family and cultural traditions, lifestyle, and budget. At best, it will be a source of both pleasure and good health.

Any nutrient could be used to demonstrate the importance of dietary *adequacy*. Consider iron, an essential nutrient that your body loses daily and must be replaced continually via iron-rich foods. If your diet does not provide adequate iron—that is, it lacks food sources of the mineral—you can develop a condition known as iron-deficiency anemia. If you add iron-rich foods such as meat, fish, poultry, and legumes to your diet, the condition will most likely soon disappear. (More information about iron appears in Chapter 7.)

To appreciate the importance of *balance*, consider a second essential nutrient. Calcium plays a vital role in building a strong frame that can withstand the gradual loss of bone that occurs with age. Thus, adults are advised to consume daily at least two, and preferably more, servings of milk or milk products—the best sources of the bone-building mineral—to meet their calcium needs. Foods that are rich in calcium typically lack iron, however, and vice versa, so you have to balance the two in your diet.

Balancing the whole diet is a juggling act that, if successful, provides enough, but not too much, of every one of the 40-odd nutrients the body needs for good health. As you will see later in the chapter, you can design a diet that is both adequate and balanced by using food group plans that help you choose from various groups specific amounts of foods that should be eaten each day.

Because not all foods that supply essential nutrients such as calcium and iron contain the same number of calories, diets must be planned with *calorie control* in mind. A cup and a half of ice cream, for example, has about the same amount of calcium as a cup of milk, but the ice cream may contain more than 500 calories, while the milk may supply only 90. When it comes to iron, a three-ounce serving of beef pot roast provides the same amount of the mineral as a three-ounce serving of canned water-packed tuna. But whereas the beef contains 325 calories, the tuna adds only 175 to the diet. The choice of which one to eat depends on personal preferences as well as the calorie content of the other foods in the diet.

Those who are trying to limit the number of calories they take in each day should be sure to include foods that are rich in nutrients (protein, vitamins, and minerals) but relatively low in calories and fat. Such foods are referred to as **nutrient dense.** Nonfat milk, for example, contains more calcium, protein, vitamin D, and vitamin A for its calories than ice cream. Hence, it is more nutrient dense. Figure 2–1 compares the nutrient density of ice cream and plain low-fat yogurt.

ADEQUACY characterizes a diet that provides all of the essential nutrients, fiber, and energy (calories) in amounts sufficient to maintain health.

BALANCE a feature of a diet that provides a number of types of foods in balance with one another, such that foods rich in one nutrient do not crowd out of the diet foods that are rich in another nutrient.

CALORIE CONTROL control of consumption of energy (calories); a feature of a sound diet plan.

MODERATION the attribute of a diet that provides no unwanted constituent in excess.

VARIETY a feature of a diet in which different foods are used for the same purposes on different occasions—the opposite of *monotony*.

NUTRIENT DENSE refers to a food that supplies large amounts of nutrients relative to the number of calories it contains. The higher the level of nutrients and the fewer the number of calories, the more nutrient dense the food is.

FIGURE 2-1
NUTRIENT DENSITY OF ICE CREAM AND YOGURT

The figures show the contribution that ½ cup of ice cream and 1 cup of plain, low-fat yogurt make to the Reference Daily Intakes for protein, vitamin A, vitamin C, thiamin, riboflavin, niacin, calcium, and iron. While both contain about the same number of calories, the yogurt provides nearly seven times as much protein, three times the riboflavin and almost five times as much calcium as the ice cream. Thus, the yogurt has a higher nutrient density.

SOURCE: Courtesy National Dairy Council™ *Comparison Cards,* 1990.

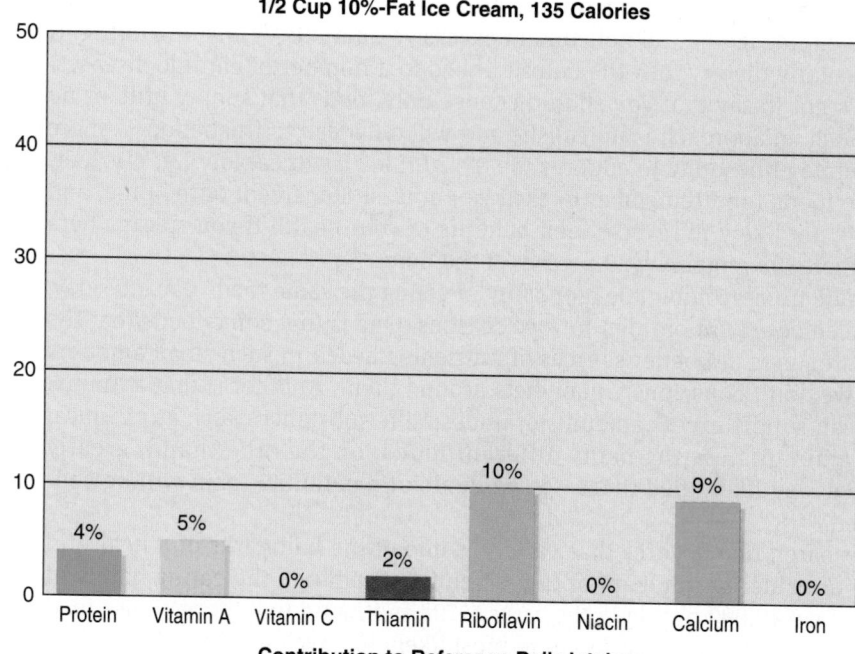

1/2 Cup 10%-Fat Ice Cream, 135 Calories
Contribution to Reference Daily Intakes

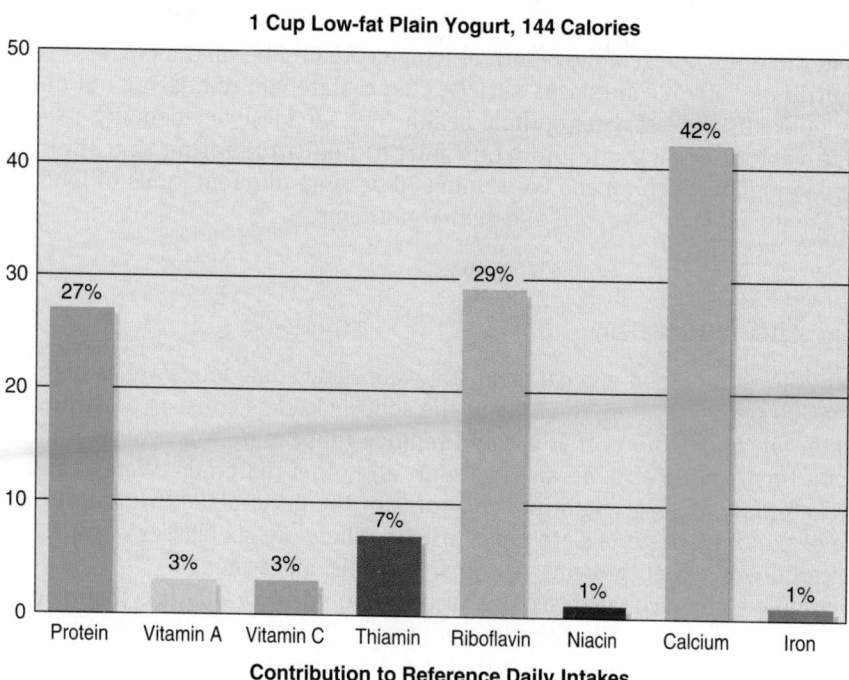

1 Cup Low-fat Plain Yogurt, 144 Calories
Contribution to Reference Daily Intakes

Another characteristic of a healthful diet is *moderation.* In other words, try to eat meals that do not contain excessive amounts of any one nutrient, particularly dietary fat—the culprit linked to a number of chronic diseases. That's not to say that you should choose only foods that supply little or no fat. Such an approach is unrealistic and will only lead to frustration. A more moderate philosophy to adopt is the 80/20 rule: Try to eat low-fat, nutrient-dense foods (and remember to exercise) at least 80 percent of the time, and you're not likely to reverse their benefits to your health if you splurge here and there the remaining 20 percent of the time.

Aside from avoiding the monotony of eating the same foods day after day, we need *variety* in our diet for two reasons. One is that some foods that the body requires are better sources of nutrients needed in such small amounts that we don't consciously plan diets around them. Another is that a limited diet can supply excess amounts of undesirable substances such as chemical contaminants. Eating many different foods, on the other hand, greatly reduces the likelihood that large amounts of a potential toxin will be consumed.

Research underscores that variety is one of the hallmarks of a healthful diet. Consider that a team of U.S. scientists examined the eating habits of more than 10,000 people in the early 1970s and found that those whose food choices were the least varied were most likely to have died 20 years later. In addition, they found that many of the people surveyed failed to regularly include items from major food groups in their meals. About 25 percent left out calcium-rich dairy products, and 17 percent went without fruit while 46 percent did not eat vegetables—both of which contain fiber and many essential nutrients.[1] If your diet lacks variety, chances are you're missing out on many nutrients necessary for optimal health. The Japanese, incidentally, recognize variety as such an important part of healthful eating that their dietary guidelines recommend consuming 30 or more different kinds of food every day to achieve a balance of essential nutrients.[2]

The Nutrients

Almost any food you eat is mostly water, and some foods are as high as 99 percent water. The bulk of the solid materials consists of carbohydrate, fat, and protein. If you could remove these materials, you would detect a tiny residue of minerals, vitamins, and other materials. Water, carbohydrate, fat, protein, vitamins, and some of the minerals are **nutrients.** Some of the other materials are not nutrients. There are six classes of nutrients: carbohydrate, fat, protein, vitamins, minerals, and water.

A complete chemical analysis of your body would show that it is made of similar materials in roughly the same proportions as most foods. For example, if you weigh 150 pounds (and that is a desirable weight for you), your body contains about 90 pounds of water and some 30 pounds of fat. The other 30 pounds consist of mostly protein, carbohydrate, and the major minerals of your bones—calcium and phosphorus. Vitamins, other minerals, and incidental extras constitute a fraction of a pound.

Diet planning principles:

- Adequacy—enough of each type of food.
- Balance—not too much of any type of food.
- Calorie control—not too many or too few calories.
- Moderation—not too much fat, salt, or sugar.
- Variety—as many different foods as possible.

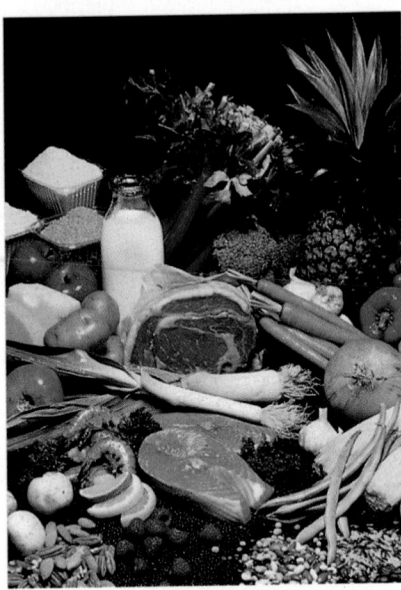

Variety fosters good nutrition.

NUTRIENTS substances obtained from food and used in the body to promote growth, maintenance, and repair.

The six classes of nutrients:

- carbohydrate
- fat
- protein
- vitamins
- minerals
- water

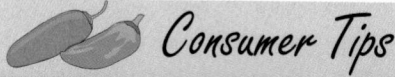

Consumer Tips

Ten Tips for Supermarketing

The first step in preparing a nutritious meal often begins at the supermarket. It takes both preparation and some label-reading skills to leave the grocery store with the necessary items for a well-balanced diet. Next time you're shopping for groceries, keep in mind these smart-shopping tips.

1. Use the weekly food section of your local newspaper to give you ideas for the best seasonal buys and special sale items.

2. Make eating healthfully a fun experience. For example, buy at least one new nutritious item and try one new recipe each week.

3. Check to see what foods you already have on hand. Plan to use items that are close to their expiration date or peak freshness.

4. Shop from a list to limit extra trips to the store and to help avoid buying unnecessary items. Keep a running list in your kitchen for noting items you need to replace.

5. Read the nutrition panel and ingredients list to compare different brands and types of foods. Ingredients are listed in order of quantity.

6. When available, use unit pricing to determine the best buy per serving.

7. Redeem coupons for items you normally buy to save money.

8. Avoid shopping when you are hungry, since everything looks good on an empty stomach.

9. Use product dating information to assure quality and freshness.

10. Learn to shop using the perimeter of the grocery store. Many of the low-fat, high-carbohydrate foods on your list will be located around the edges of the store—fresh produce, dairy products, whole-grain breads, and meat, poultry, or fish.

When referring to nutrients, scientists use the words *nonessential* and *essential* to distinguish between those that the body must obtain from food and those that the body can produce using its own resources. For instance, some of the oils and fats in the body are nonessential because they can be made from any of several different raw materials. Likewise, carbohydrate is nonessential because the body can convert some of the materials in protein into carbohydrate when needed. In contrast, about 40 nutrients are known to be **essential;** that is, they are compounds that the body cannot make for

ESSENTIAL NUTRIENTS nutrients that must be obtained from food because the body cannot make them for itself.

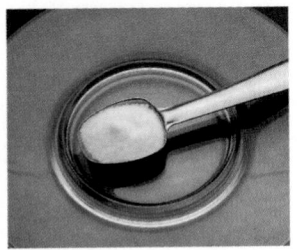

Remember that 1 gram is a very small amount. For instance, one teaspoon of sugar weighs roughly 5 grams.

itself but are indispensable to life processes. Essential nutrients belong to a different class than "necessary" nutrients. Many compounds the body makes for itself are necessary for good health. What distinguishes an essential nutrient is that it must be obtained through foods. How can you be sure you're getting all the nutrients you need? The rest of this chapter will help you design a diet that covers all your body's needs.

The Energy-Yielding Nutrients

On being broken down in the body, or digested, three of the nutrients—carbohydrate, protein, and fat—yield the **energy** that the body uses to fuel its various activities. In contrast, vitamins, minerals, and water, once broken down in the body, do not yield energy but perform other tasks, such as maintenance and repair.

The body uses energy from carbohydrate, fat, and protein to do work or generate heat. This energy is measured in **calories**—familiar to most everyone as markers of how "fattening" foods are. If your body doesn't "burn" the energy you obtained from a food soon after you've eaten it, it stores it, usually as body fat, for use later. If excess amounts of protein, fat, or carbohydrate are eaten fairly regularly, the stored fat builds up over time and leads to obesity. Too much of any food, whether lean meat (a protein-rich food), potatoes (a high-carbohydrate food), or peanuts (a fatty food), can contribute excess calories that result in overweight.

Only one other compound that people consume provides calories, and that is alcohol. Alcohol is not considered a nutrient, however, because it does not help maintain or repair body tissues the way nutrients do.

ENERGY the capacity to do work, such as moving or heating something.

The energy-yielding nutrients:
- carbohydrate
- fat
- protein

CALORIE the unit used to measure energy. Technically, when we see the term *calorie* on food labels or talk about the amount of calories our bodies need, we are referring to *kilocalories* (*kcal*)—the amount of heat required to raise the temperature of one kilogram of water one degree Celsius. Use of the term *kilocalorie*, however, tends to be reserved for laboratories and technical journals. Throughout this book, we will use the term *calorie* rather than kilocalorie.

color = heat

Keep in mind that 1 gram of carbohydrate yields 4 calories, 1 gram of fat yields 9 calories, and 1 gram of protein yields 4 calories. Alcohol is a nonnutrient that provides energy (see Chapter 9 for a detailed discussion about alcohol). One gram of alcohol provides 7 calories.

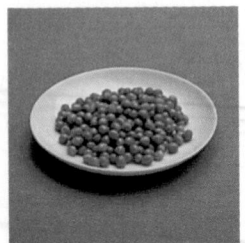

Calorie Values of Carbohydrate, Fat, and Protein

If you know the number of grams of carbohydrate, fat, and protein in a food, you can calculate the number of calories in it. Simply multiply the carbohydrate grams by 4, the fat grams by 9, and the protein grams by 4. Add the totals together to obtain the number of calories. For example, a half cup of cooked peas contains about 11 grams of carbohydrate, 4 grams of protein, and barely a trace of fat:

11 grams carbohydrate × 4 calories	= 44 calories
4 grams protein × 4 calories	= 16 calories
Trace of fat	= 0 calories
Total	60 calories

Amounts of Nutrients Eaten Daily

If you could extract and purify the carbohydrate, fat, and protein from your daily diet, they would fill two or three measuring cups, even though the foods they come in weigh much more and occupy much more space. For instance, a half cup of vegetables contains only 10 or so grams of energy-yielding nutrients, the rest being water, fiber, and other noncaloric materials.

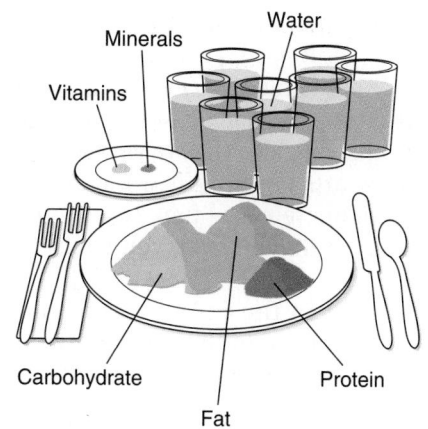

Vitamins, Minerals, and Water

Unlike carbohydrate, fat, and protein, **vitamins** and **minerals** do not supply energy, or calories. Instead, they regulate the release of energy and other aspects of metabolism. As Table 2–1 shows, there are 13 vitamins, each with its special roles to play. Vitamins are divided into two classes: water-soluble (the B vitamins and vitamin C) and fat-soluble (vitamins A, D, E, and K). This distinction has many implications for the kinds of foods the different vitamins are found in and the way the body uses them, as you will see in Chapter 6.

The minerals also perform important functions. Some, such as calcium, make up the structure of bones and teeth. Others, including sodium, float

VITAMINS organic, or carbon containing, essential nutrients vital to life and needed in minute amounts.
  vita=life
  amine =containing nitrogen

MINERALS inorganic compounds, some of which are essential nutrients.

Vitamins and minerals—play regulatory roles.

Water—provides the medium for life processes.

TABLE 2–1
THE VITAMINS AND MINERALS

THE VITAMINS		THE MINERALS	
The water-soluble vitamins:	The fat-soluble vitamins:	The major minerals:	The trace minerals:
B vitamins	Vitamin A	†Calcium Potassium	**Chromium **Manganese
Thiamin Vitamin B$_{12}$	Vitamin D	Chloride Sodium	**Copper **Molybdenum
Riboflavin Folate	Vitamin E	†Magnesium Sulfur	**Fluoride †Selenium
Niacin *Biotin	Vitamin K	†Phosphorus	†Iodine †Zinc
Vitamin B$_6$ *Pantothenic acid			†Iron
Vitamin C			

*Vitamins for which Estimated Safe and Adequate Daily Dietary Intakes have been set.

†Minerals for which RDA have been set.

**Minerals for which Estimated Safe and Adequate Daily Dietary Intakes have been set.

Note: A number of trace minerals are currently under study to determine possible dietary requirements for humans. These include arsenic, boron, cadmium, cobalt, lead, lithium, nickel, silicon, tin, and vanadium.

about in the body's fluids, where they help regulate crucial bodily functions, such as heartbeat and muscle contractions.

Often neglected but equally vital, water is the medium in which all the body's processes take place. Some 60 percent of your body's weight is water, which carries materials to and from cells and provides the warm, nutrient-rich bath in which cells thrive. It also transports hormonal messages from place to place. When energy-yielding nutrients release "fuel," they break down to water and other simple compounds. Without water, you could live only a few days.

Because each day your body loses water in the form of sweat and urine, you must replace large amounts of it daily—on the order of two to three quarts a day. To be sure, you don't need to drink that much water daily, because the foods and other beverages you consume supply it in abundance.

RECOMMENDED DIETARY ALLOWANCES (RDA) a set of daily nutrient and calorie consumption levels intended to meet the nutritional needs of virtually all healthy people living in the United States.

RECOMMENDED NUTRIENT INTAKES (RNI) nutrition guidelines set forth by the Canadian government for the Canadian people; similar to the RDA used in the United States. (See Appendix C for a full listing of the RNI.)

Nutrient Recommendations

At this point, knowing that foods are made of so many different combinations of nutrients, you may be wondering how to determine whether you are eating the right amount to supply the right balance of nutrients. Obviously, if your diet lacks any of the essential nutrients, you may develop deficiencies. Even if you don't develop a full-blown deficiency disease, if you are less than optimally nourished, you may get sick more easily and suffer other health problems.

To help prevent such problems and provide a benchmark for people's nutrient needs, the U.S. government devised the **Recommended Dietary Allowances (RDA).** In Canada, a similar set of standards, known as the **Recommended Nutrient Intakes (RNI),** is used (see Appendix C).

The Recommended Dietary Allowances (RDA)

A committee of nutrition experts gathered by the National Academy of Sciences/National Research Council meets periodically to set forth the RDA—a set of daily nutrient standards based on the latest scientific evidence regarding diet and health. The first set was published in 1943 and has been revised ten times since then, most recently in 1989 (see the inside front cover of this book).

While the RDA are widely used, many people have misconceptions about their meaning and intent. To get a proper perspective about the RDA, consider the following facts:

- The RDA are designed to evaluate the diets of *populations,* such as urban dwellers or elementary school children. They are not intended to be nutrient requirements *individuals* must meet day in and day out.

- The RDA are recommendations, not requirements, and they include a substantial margin of safety. That is, they take into account differences among individuals and establish a range within which most people's nutritional needs will be covered. (See Figure 2–2.)

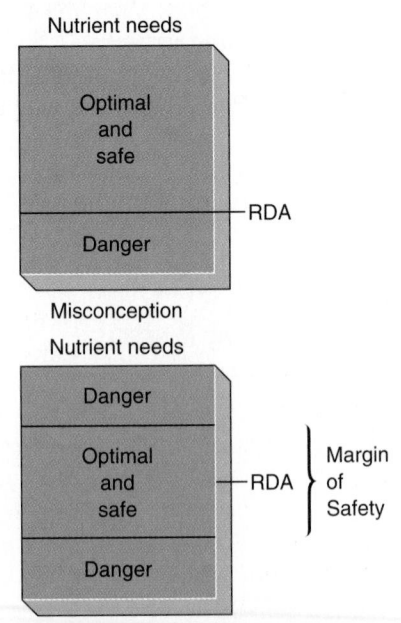

FIGURE 2–2
THE CORRECT VIEW OF THE RDA

People often think that more is better when it comes to nutrients. Too much of a good thing can be dangerous, however, so the RDA fall within an optimal margin of safety.

- The RDA estimate the needs of *healthy* people. People with certain medical problems often have different nutritional needs.
- The government-funded committee that determines the RDA consists of scientists representing a variety of nutrition-related specialties. This committee revises the RDA periodically using the most current scientific research available.
- Separate recommendations are made for different groups of people. For instance, the committee puts forth one set of recommendations for children ages 4 to 6, another set for adult men, another for pregnant women, and so on.

The RDA for Nutrients

While the RDA are best suited to evaluating the nutrient consumption of populations, they are often used as a way of assessing an individual's diet. Using the RDA as such, however, has certain limitations. Consider an example of how scientists determine the RDA for a nutrient.

Suppose we were the committee members, and we were called upon to set the RDA for nutrient X. First, we would try to find out how much of that nutrient the average healthy person needs. To do so, we could review scientific research exploring how the body stores the nutrient, what the consequence of a deficiency might be, what causes depletion of the nutrient, and other factors that affect a person's need for it. We could conduct a type of research known as a **balance study,** in which scientists feed people a controlled diet containing a specific amount of nutrient X and then measure the amount they excrete. Provided nutrient X isn't changed in the body prior to excretion, a balance study can give a good idea of a person's **requirement** for nutrient X. If the amount of the nutrient in the diet falls below the requirement, the person would slip into *negative balance.* Over time, his or her body's stores of nutrient X would begin to dwindle and deficiency symptoms would eventually set in. It would become clear that different people have different requirements. Mr. A might need an average of 40 units of nutrient X daily; Ms. B might need 35; Mr. C, 65. If we looked at enough people, we might find that their nutrient requirements were distributed as shown in Figure 2–3, with most clustered together in the middle, and a few extremes on either side.

After conducting balance studies, our next step would be to decide what amount of nutrient X to recommend for everybody. One option would be to set it at the average requirement for nutrient X (shown in Figure 2–3 at 45 units). But if we did so and people took us literally, half the population— Mr. C and everyone else whose requirement is greater than 45—would

BALANCE STUDY a laboratory study in which a person is fed a controlled diet to measure the intake and excretion of a nutrient. If the nutrient is not changed in the body and a person excretes more of it than is consumed over time, the person slips into *negative balance.*

REQUIREMENT the minimum amount of a nutrient in the diet that will prevent the development of deficiency symptoms. Requirements differ from the RDA, which include a substantial margin of safety to cover the requirements of different individuals.

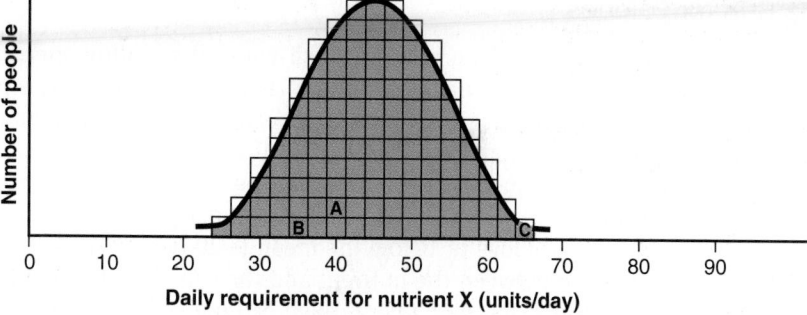

FIGURE 2–3

NUTRIENT REQUIREMENTS VARY FROM PERSON TO PERSON

Each square represents a person: A, B, and C are Mr. A, Ms. B, and Mr. C.

eventually develop deficiencies. Another alternative would be to set the RDA at or above the extreme—say, at 70 units a day—so that everyone would be covered. That might work in theory, but if nutrient X is expensive or scarce, setting the RDA so high might put an unnecessary strain on the majority of people, such as Ms. B, whose needs fall well below 70. Or it might mislead people into eating an excess of foods that contain nutrient X while excluding foods that contain other important nutrients.

To benefit the most people, we would probably set the RDA at a point high enough to cover the bulk of the population without recommending an excess. In this case, a reasonable choice might be 63 units. In choosing that amount, we would have added a generous safety margin to ensure that just about all healthy people are covered.

Going through the steps scientists take in setting the RDA underscores the limitations of using them as nutritional "goals" to be met daily. You can't know your exact nutrient requirements. And the RDA not only include a large margin of safety but also are based on certain assumptions. For instance, when scientists set the requirement for a nutrient, they assume that your diet already contains sufficient calories, protein, and other nutrients.

As you read the RDA tables, note that for some vitamins and minerals the committee has set forth recommendations called Estimated Safe and Adequate Daily Dietary Intakes. Because scientists have less knowledge about these nutrients than the others, they have devised a range of intakes rather than one number. The range is considered sufficient to cover most people's needs without posing a hazard. The committee also established Estimated Minimum Requirements for sodium and chloride—two nutrients that people's bodies appear to respond to differently when consumed in excess—and potassium. The role of these minerals in the body is discussed in detail in Chapter 7.

The bottom line is that the RDA are best suited for use with populations. The dietary guidelines introduced in Chapter 1 and discussed later in this chapter were developed with the RDA in mind, and you can use the RDA to get a feel for the adequacy of your own diet. Just remember that the RDA are group recommendations and not individual nutrient prescriptions.

RDA are set for

- Energy (calories)
- Protein
- Vitamins: A, C, D, E, K, thiamin, riboflavin, niacin, B_6, B_{12}, and folate
- Minerals: calcium, phosphorus, magnesium, iron, zinc, iodine, and selenium

Ranges of estimated safe and adequate daily dietary intakes are set for

- Vitamins: biotin and pantothenic acid
- Minerals: copper, manganese, fluoride, chromium, and molybdenum

Estimated minimum requirements are given for

- Minerals: sodium, potassium, and chloride

The RDA for Calories

The RDA committee took a different approach when it set allowances for energy, or calories, than it did for the nutrients. That's because while small excesses of protein, vitamins, and most minerals are harmless for the majority of people, excess calories can lead to obesity. Too few calories can cause undesirable weight loss. Thus, the committee set the RDA for calories at the mean for each group, with the stipulation that for most people, an acceptable amount of variation above or below the mean is 20 percent. Figure 2–4 illustrates the difference between the nutrient and the calorie RDA. The RDA for calories, in particular, offer only a very rough estimate of individual calorie needs, which vary tremendously as a result of factors that cannot be accounted for in the RDA, such as a person's ratio of muscle to fat and activity level. If you want to know the number of calories needed to, say, lose or gain weight, you're better off getting a thorough assessment from a health professional than checking the RDA for calories.

Protein is the only calorie-yielding nutrient for which RDA are set. No RDA are given for carbohydrate or fat because the committee assumes that you will need to obtain a certain number of calories from protein and derive the rest from a balance of carbohydrate, fat, and, in some cases, alcohol. The best way to do so is discussed later in the chapter.

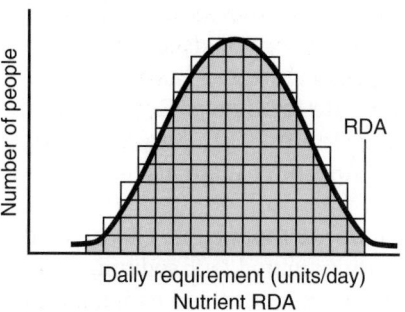 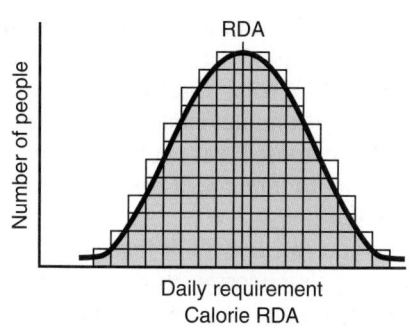

FIGURE 2–4

THE DIFFERENCES BETWEEN THE RDA FOR NUTRIENTS AND THE RDA FOR CALORIES

The nutrient RDA are intended to meet nearly all people's requirements. The calorie RDA, on the other hand, are set at a point at which half the population's requirements will fall below and half will fall above.

Other Recommendations

Different nations and international groups have set forth different sets of standards similar to the RDA. The Canadian recommendations—the Recommended Nutrient Intakes (RNI)—differ from the RDA in some respects, partly because of the way the data on which they are based are interpreted and partly because they are set with the particular diets and lifestyles of the Canadian population in mind.

Another widely used set of recommendations comes from two international organizations: the Food and Agriculture Organization (FAO) and the World Health Organization (WHO). The FAO/WHO recommendations are considered sufficient to address the needs of nearly all people around the world. They differ from the RDA in that they are devised with slightly different priorities and purposes in mind. They assume, for example, that most people's diets contain protein of a lower quality than the protein in the diets of people in the United States. As a result, they recommend higher amounts of that nutrient (Chapter 5 discusses protein quality). The FAO/WHO recommendations also take into consideration the fact that worldwide, people are generally smaller and more physically active than people in the United States.

The Challenge of Dietary Guidelines

While the RDA make specific recommendations for protein, vitamin, and mineral consumption, they provide only general guidelines for calorie intake. What's more, they do not address the hazards of nutrient excesses, such as too much fat in the diet. Yet, as Chapter 1 pointed out, health authorities are as concerned today about widespread nutrient excesses among Americans as they used to be about nutrient deficiencies. This is where dietary guidelines come into play. Unlike the RDA, these guidelines consist of suitable recommendations for individuals to follow with ease. Among the most widely used are the *Surgeon General's Report* and the

National Research Council's *Diet and Health* report (discussed in Chapter 1—see Table 1–3 on page 9). Others include the *Dietary Goals for the United States*, the *Dietary Guidelines for Americans* (see Figure 2–5) as well as recommendations devised by the American Institute for Cancer Research and the American Heart Association (listed in Table 2–2). The *Nutrition Recommendations for Canadians* presented in Appendix C are also commonly used.

As you can see, all of these guidelines recommend that people choose diets with low to moderate amounts of fat (particularly saturated fat), sodium, sugar, cholesterol, and alcohol while maintaining a healthy weight and eating plenty of fruits, vegetables, and grains. The goal of the recommendations is to help people decrease their risk of some forms of cancer, heart disease, obesity, diabetes, high blood pressure, stroke, and liver disease—the so-called **lifestyle diseases.** Following such recommendations certainly makes sense, given the considerable potential health benefits they confer. Eating healthfully may also benefit the earth, as will be explored in later chapters.

LIFESTYLE DISEASES conditions that may be aggravated by modern lifestyles that include too little exercise, poor diets, and excessive drinking and smoking. Lifestyle diseases are also referred to as diseases of affluence.

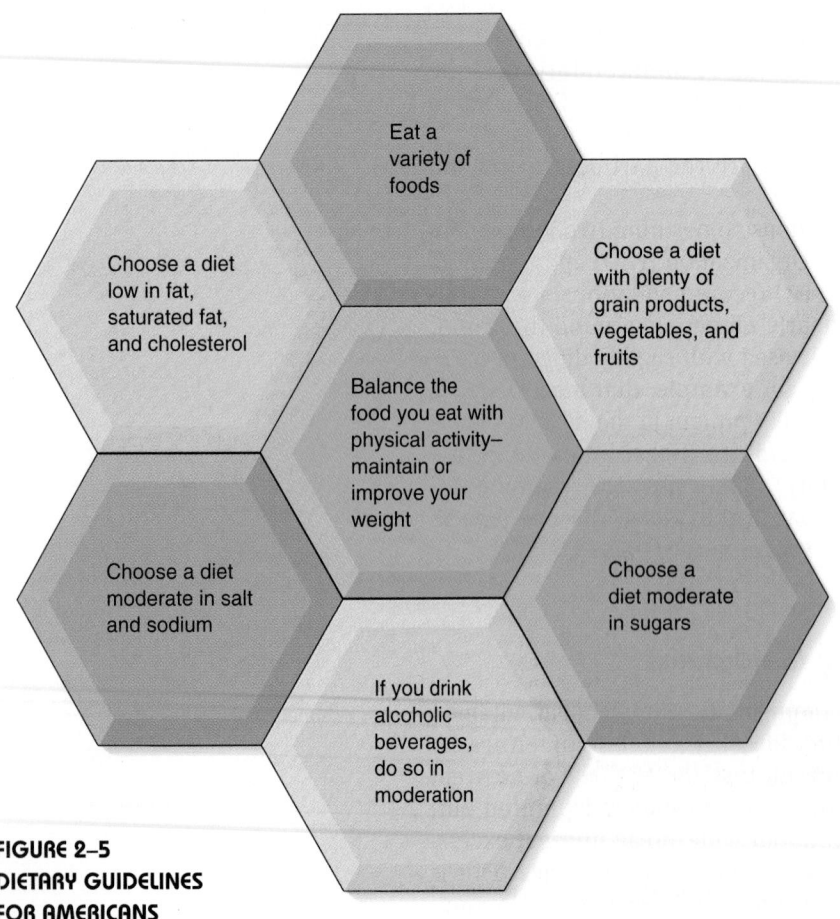

FIGURE 2–5
DIETARY GUIDELINES
FOR AMERICANS

Use the seven guidelines together to choose a healthful and enjoyable diet.

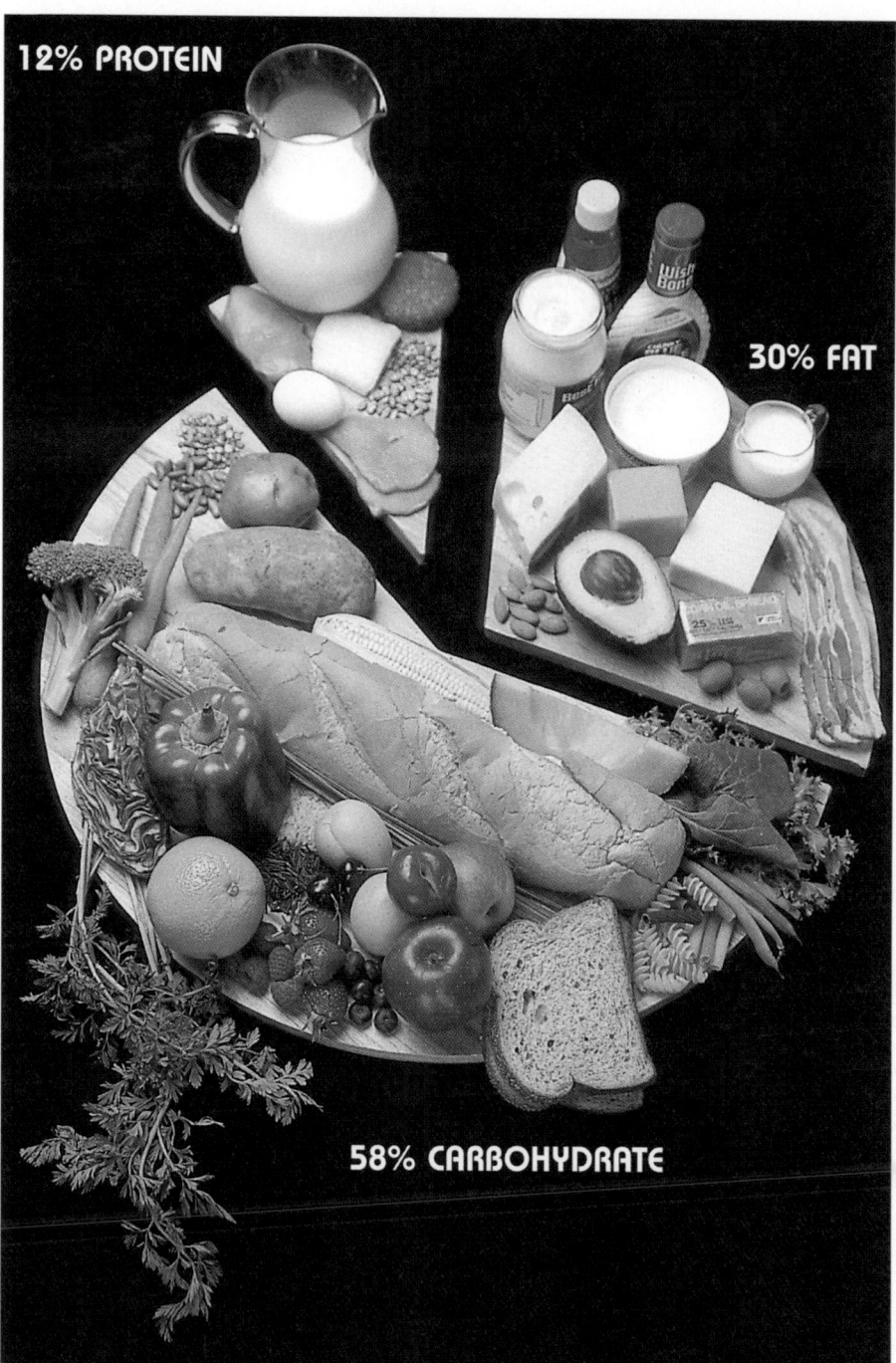

Dietary Goals for the United States

A balanced diet is composed of 12% protein from animal and vegetable sources, about 58% carbohydrate, and no more than 30% fat calories, including the fat from meats, whole milk, eggs, cheese, vegetable oils, and nuts.

TABLE 2–2
CURRENT DIETARY RECOMMENDATIONS

DIETARY GUIDELINES FOR AMERICANS	AMERICAN HEART ASSOCIATION	AMERICAN INSTITUTE FOR CANCER RESEARCH	SUGGESTIONS FOR FOOD CHOICES
Balance the food you eat with physical activity— maintain or improve your weight.	Consume sufficient calories to maintain recommended body weight.	Avoid obesity.	Control overeating. Eat fewer fatty foods and sweets. Eat more foods low in calories and high in nutrients.
Eat a variety of foods.	Consume a wide variety of foods.		Include these foods every day: fruits and vegetables; whole-grain and enriched breads and cereals and other products made from grains; milk and milk products; meats, fish, poultry, and eggs; and dried peas and beans.
Choose a diet low in fat, saturated fat, and cholesterol.	Limit total fat intake to less than 30% of calories. Limit saturated fat intake to less than 10% of calories. Limit cholesterol intake to 300 milligrams per day.	Reduce the intake of total dietary fat from the current average of about 37% to a level of no more than 30% of total calories and, in particular, reduce the intake of saturated fat to less than 10% of total calories.	Choose low-fat protein sources such as lean meats, fish, poultry, and dried peas and beans. Use eggs and organ meats in moderation. Limit intake of fats on and in foods. Trim fats from meats. Broil, bake, or boil— don't fry. Limit breaded and deep-fried foods. Read food labels for fat content.
Choose a diet with plenty of grain products, vegetables, and fruits.	Consume at least 50% to 55% of calories from carbo-hydrate sources, especially complex-carbohydrate sources.	Increase the consumption of fruits, vegetables, and whole grains.	Substitute starchy foods for foods high in fats and sugars. Select whole-grain breads and cereals, fruits and vegetables, and dried peas and beans to increase fiber and starch intake.
Choose a diet moderate in sugars.			Use less sugar, syrup, and honey. Eat fewer concentrated sweets such as candy, soft drinks, and cookies. Read food labels for sugar content.
Choose a diet moderate in salt and sodium.	Sodium intake should be no more than 3,000 milligrams (3 grams) per day.		Learn to enjoy the flavors of unsalted foods. Flavor foods with herbs, spices, and lemon juice. Reduce salt in cooking. Add little or no salt at the table. Limit salty foods. Read food labels for salt or sodium content.

continued

TABLE 2–2
continued

DIETARY GUIDELINES FOR AMERICANS	AMERICAN HEART ASSOCIATION	AMERICAN INSTITUTE FOR CANCER RESEARCH	SUGGESTIONS FOR FOOD CHOICES
If you drink alcoholic beverages, do so in moderation.	If alcoholic beverages are consumed, limit intake to 1 to 2 oz of ethanol per day.	Drink alcoholic beverages only in moderation, if at all.	For individuals who drink, limit alcoholic beverages to one or two drinks per day. "One drink" means 12 oz of beer, 5 oz of wine, or 1½ oz of distilled spirits. (Pregnant women should not use alcohol. If you drink, do not drive.)
	Consume approximately 15% of calories from protein sources.		
		Eat foods rich in vitamins A and C.	*For Vitamin A:* Eat dark green and deep yellow vegetables, cabbage, spinach, carrots, broccoli, tomatoes, and Brussels sprouts.
			For Vitamin C: Eat citrus fruits, berries, peaches, melons, green and leafy vegetables, tomatoes, cauliflower, red and green peppers, and sweet potatoes.
		Consume salt-cured, salt-pickled, and smoked foods only in moderation.	

SOURCE: U.S. Department of Agriculture, U.S. Department of Health and Human Services, *Nutrition and Your Health: Dietary Guidelines for Americans,* 3rd ed. (Washington, D.C.: U.S. Government Printing Office, 1990); Nutrition Committee, *Dietary Guidelines for Healthy American Adults: A Statement for Physicians and Health Professionals* (Dallas: American Heart Association, 1991); American Institute for Cancer Research, *Dietary Guidelines to Lower Cancer Risk* (Washington, D.C.: AICR, 1990).

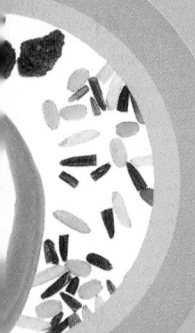

Grazer's Guide to Smart Snacking

Government surveys show that just about everyone reaches for a little something between meals. In fact, Americans spend some $14.7 billion annually on snack foods such as popcorn and potato chips.[3] But while **grazing** is in, many people feel a twinge of guilt now and then about between-meal munching. Perhaps the parental warnings of childhood that snacks can spoil a meal linger in the back of many minds. Nevertheless, nutritious nibbling can make it easier for many people to eat healthfully.

Snacks can supply essential vitamins, minerals, and calories to the diets of little children, whose small stomachs and appetites often cannot handle larger meals. As for teenagers, who typically don't seem to have the time (or the inclination) to eat regularly as they go to school, baseball practice, or music lessons or engage in other activities, snacks account for upwards of a third of the calories they eat and as much as 20 percent of their vitamin and mineral consumption.[4] Snacks also contribute to the nutritional needs of adults, who may find fitting meals into a busy schedule difficult. Even senior citizens, whose lifestyles tend to be less hectic, can benefit from grazing. That's because lack of activity, certain medications, and isolation can blunt a formerly hearty appetite, making frequent, small meals more desirable than large breakfasts, lunches, and dinners.

At any age, the key to healthful snacking is to choose low-fat, high-fiber, nutrient-rich foods such as fruits, low-fat cheese and yogurt, whole-grain crackers, and plain popcorn. Cakes, cookies, candy, and potato chips are harder to fit into a healthful eating plan because they add fat and calories to the diet and little else in the way of nutrients.

Some snacks that appear nutritious may be deceiving. For example, fruit drinks, mixes, and punches are loaded with sugar and are more similar to soft drinks than to fruit juice. Fruit rolls and bars are nutritionally similar to jams and jelly, not to fresh fruit. Sugar is added, and most of the nutrients in the

GRAZING eating small amounts of food at intervals throughout the day rather than—or in addition to—eating regular meals.

TABLE 2–3
SMART SNACKING

INSTEAD OF	TRY
Fruit drinks	Fruit juice
Soft drinks	Fruit juice concentrate and sparkling water
Milk shakes	Shakes made with nonfat milk and fresh fruit
Potato chips	Pretzels (try low salt)
Chips and sour cream dip	Vegetables and buttermilk dip
Granola bars	Homemade oatmeal cookies (reduce the fat and sugar)
Frosted cake	Angel food cake and fruit
Pie	Fruit cobblers
Cookies	Vanilla wafers, gingersnaps, graham crackers

fruit are lost when it is processed with heat. Granola bars can also be deceiving because, like candy bars, many are loaded with sugar and fat. Even some varieties of microwave popcorn don't rate well as snacks because they contain lots of oil and salt. (You can easily make your own popcorn in the microwave oven without adding an excess of extras.) When you feel like snacking, try some of the alternatives offered in Table 2–3. Use Table 2–4 as a guide to see how some of your favorite snacks rate in terms of calories and fat. In addition, consider the following tips next time you're in the mood to grab a snack.

- Stock your refrigerator and kitchen cupboards with nutritious foods such as fruit juices, low-fat yogurt, fresh fruits and vegetables, plain popcorn, pretzels, whole-grain crackers, and low-fat cheeses so that they are close at hand. Nibblers often reach for a snack just to have something to munch on rather than because of a desire for the food itself. If nutritious choices are easy to get to, chances are that's what you'll eat.

- Carry fresh fruit and crackers and cheese, or even half a sandwich, in your backpack or briefcase so you won't have to resort to buying candy from a vending machine when you get the urge to munch.

- Create your own snacks. Mix together one cup each pretzels, peanuts, raisins, and sunflower seeds to take with you on your next bicycle trip or hike. As a substitute for cream cheese, blend ½ cup drained low-fat yogurt with ½ cup low-fat cottage cheese. Add a bit of chopped pineapple, strawberries, or other fruit and spread this mixture on crackers, bagels, English muffins, or rice cakes.

TABLE 2–4
WHAT'S IN A MUNCHER'S MENU?

FOOD	GRAMS OF FAT	CALORIES
½ cup corn chips	4	70
1 cup plain popcorn	trace	30
1 cup buttered and salted popcorn	2	50
2 graham cracker squares	1	60
4 saltine crackers	1	50
2 bread sticks	1	75
1 3½"-round bagel	2	200
1 2½"-round bran muffin	6	125
10 thin pretzel sticks	trace	10
2 carrot and 2 celery sticks	trace	5
6 fluid ounces tomato juice	trace	30
10 potato chips	7	105
10 French fries	8	160
Small apple	trace	60
Banana	1	105
1 small box raisins (about 1½ tbsp)	trace	40
1 ounce process American cheese	9	105
1 cup nonfat milk	1	90
8-ounce carton low-fat yogurt with fruit	2	230
¼ cup roasted peanuts	18	210
2 tablespoons peanut butter	16	190
½ cup frozen yogurt	2	105
½ cup ice cream	7	135
2 2⅓"-round chocolate chip cookies	6	90
2 chocolate or vanilla sandwich-type cookies	4	100
2 fig bars	2	105
Frosted cream-filled cupcake	4	160
Cake-type doughnut	12	210
1½-ounce chocolate candy bar	14	220
12 fluid ounces regular cola soft drink	0	160

SOURCE: Adapted from Muncher's Guide in *Making Bag Lunches, Snacks, & Desserts Using the Dietary Guidelines* (U.S. Department of Agriculture Human Nutrition Information Service, Home and Garden Bulletin No. 232–9): pp. 7–8.

● Make new versions of old favorites, such as **Frozen Bananas,**[5] **Chili Popcorn,** and **Mexican Snack Pizzas.**[6]

FROZEN BANANAS

Mix 1 tablespoon peanut butter with 1/4 cup evaporated skim milk. Roll a banana, cut in half, in the peanut butter mixture. Then roll the coated banana halves in bran cereal. Place in the freezer until frozen. Makes two banana halves, each of which supplies about 165 calories, 4 grams of fat, and 149 milligrams of sodium.

CHILI POPCORN

Mix 1 quart popped popcorn with 1 tablespoon melted margarine. In a separate bowl, mix 1 1/4 teaspoons chili powder, 1/4 teaspoon cumin, and a dash of garlic powder. Sprinkle seasonings over popcorn and mix well. Makes about four 1-cup servings, each of which contains approximately 50 calories, 3 grams of fat, and 42 milligrams of sodium.

MEXICAN SNACK PIZZAS

Split two English muffins and toast lightly. Mix 1/4 cup tomato paste, 1/4 cup canned, drained, chopped kidney beans, 1 tablespoon each chopped onion and chopped green pepper, and 1/2 teaspoon oregano. Spread mixture on muffin halves. Top with 1/4 cup shredded part-skim mozzarella cheese and broil until cheese is bubbly (about two minutes). Garnish with 1/4 cup shredded lettuce. Makes 4 servings, each of which contains 95 calories, 2 grams of fat, and 300 milligrams of sodium.

● Snack with a friend. If you're craving a candy bar or chips and nothing else will do, try splitting a bar or a bag with a friend. That way you'll satisfy your craving without going too far overboard on calories, fat, or salt.

● Try to brush your teeth—or at least rinse your mouth thoroughly—after snacking to prevent tooth decay. (See the Nutrition Action feature in Chapter 3 for a detailed explanation of the role of diet in dental health.)

Tools Used in Diet Planning

While the RDA and the various dietary guidelines provide good frameworks for healthful eating, planning daily menus requires use of other, more specific tools. Dietitians and other nutrition experts often rely on a number of tools that you, too, can use to assess and plan your own diet.

Food Group Plans

One of the most helpful, easy-to-use diet planning tools is the **food group plan,** which separates foods into specific groups and then spells out the number of **servings** from each group to eat each day. The most well-known example of such a plan is the Four Food Group Plan, devised in the 1950s and taught to consumers for nearly four decades. Several years ago, however, scientists updated this plan, taking into consideration new nutrition knowledge gained over the years. The revised version, shown in Figure 2–6, is called the Food Guide Pyramid. It contains five food groups rather than four; the tip is not considered to be a major food group because the foods found there provide extra calories and little else in the way of nutrients.

FOOD GROUP PLAN a diet-planning tool, such as the Food Guide Pyramid, that groups foods according to similar origin and nutrient content and then specifies the number of foods from each group that a person should eat.

SERVING the amount of food a person might eat, similar to a helping.

The pyramid was designed to help consumers choose foods that supply a good balance of nutrients, but not too much total fat, saturated fat, sugar, sodium, or alcohol, in keeping with the U.S. government's *Dietary Guidelines for Americans.* The placement of the five food groups on the pyramid emphasizes their role in the diet. The grains that form the base should serve as the foundation of a healthful diet because breads, cereals, rice, and pasta are generally high in carbohydrate and low in fat. The grains are followed by fruits and vegetables, which supply the vitamins, minerals, and fiber many people's diets lack. The next level suggests eating smaller amounts of dairy products as well as meat, poultry, fish, beans, eggs, and nuts. While foods from these groups provide protein, calcium, iron, zinc, and other nutrients, they often contain large amounts of fat as well as saturated fat.

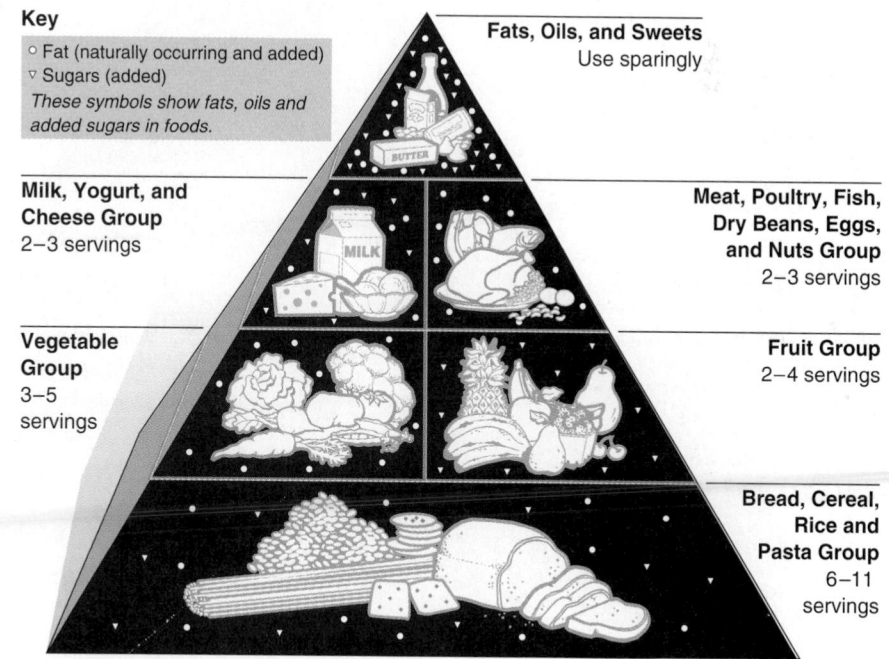

Key

○ Fat (naturally occurring and added)
▽ Sugars (added)
These symbols show fats, oils and added sugars in foods.

Fats, Oils, and Sweets
Use sparingly

Milk, Yogurt, and Cheese Group
2–3 servings

Meat, Poultry, Fish, Dry Beans, Eggs, and Nuts Group
2–3 servings

Vegetable Group
3–5 servings

Fruit Group
2–4 servings

Bread, Cereal, Rice and Pasta Group
6–11 servings

FIGURE 2–6
EATING FROM THE BOTTOM UP: THE FOOD GUIDE PYRAMID

The pyramid shows the proportions of foods that should make up a healthful diet. Those found in the bottom half—grains, fruits, and vegetables—should make up the bulk of the diet. Those in the top half, including fats and sweets, should be eaten in moderate amounts.

Thus, choosing wisely from these groups goes a long way in limiting the fat content of your diet.

Not considered one of the food groups, the tip of the pyramid consists of fats, oils, and sweets—foods such as butter, margarine, salad dressing, oils, candy, soda pop, and other similar items—which typically supply lots of fat and calories and few nutrients. As their placement in the tip suggests, these items should be added to the diet sparingly.

Note that alcohol is not included in any portion of the pyramid, but like the foods in the tip, it provides calories and no nutrients to speak of. The *Dietary Guidelines* recommend that consumers have no more than one or two alcoholic drinks a day. A standard drink is a 12-ounce can or bottle of beer, a 5-ounce glass of wine, or a 1½-ounce shot of liquor.

Using the pyramid to assess and plan your own diet requires an understanding of what amount of food counts as one serving from the various food groups. For instance, one slice of bread, one half a bagel, and a half cup of pasta each counts as a serving from the bread, cereal, rice, and pasta group. When it comes to vegetables, a half cup of raw or cooked vegetables or one cup of leafy raw vegetables chalks up one serving. Figure 2–7 shows

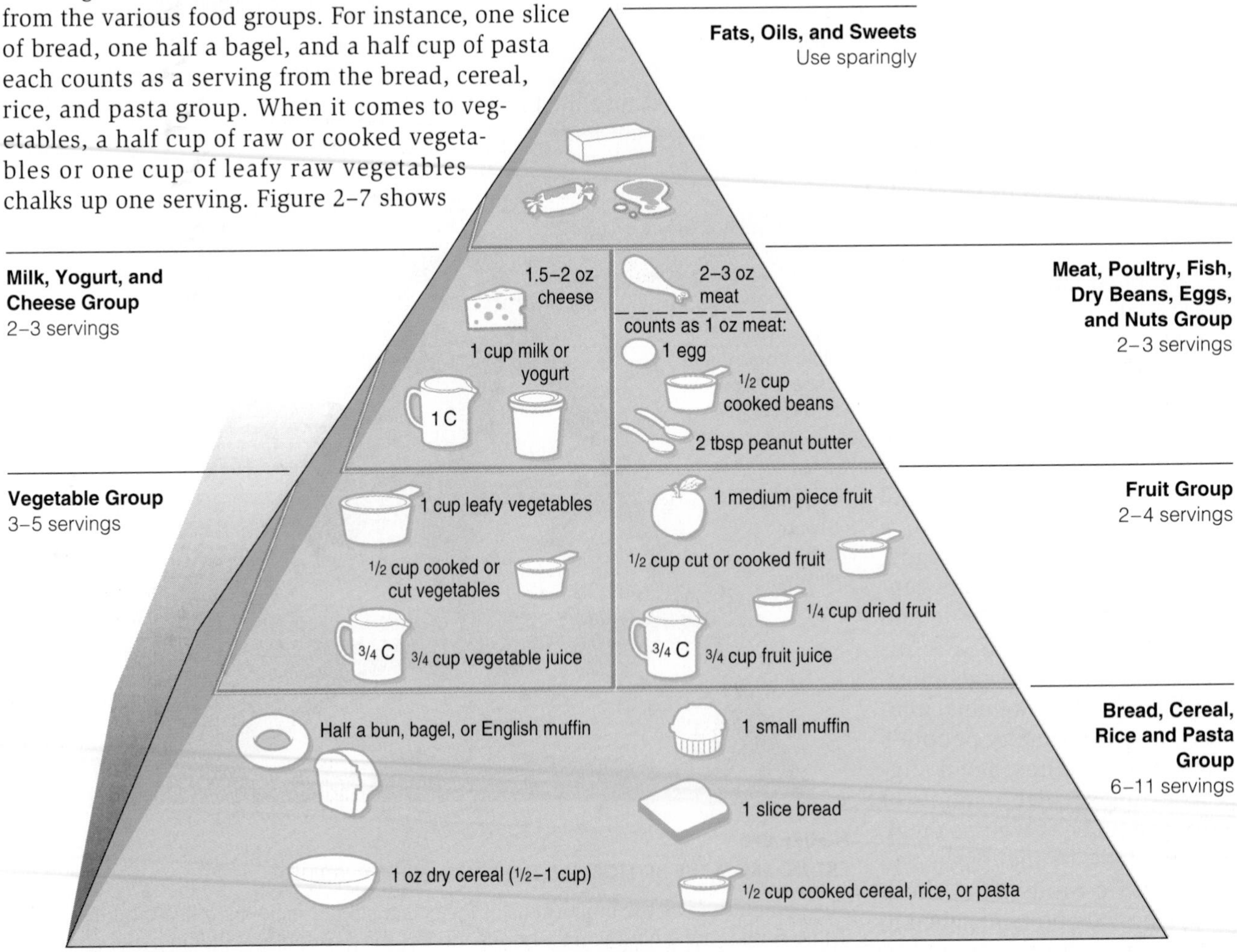

The pyramid isn't the only food group plan. Canada has one of its own—Canada's Food Guide (shown in Appendix C).

Fats, Oils, and Sweets
Use sparingly

Milk, Yogurt, and Cheese Group
2–3 servings

1.5–2 oz cheese

1 cup milk or yogurt

1 C

Meat, Poultry, Fish, Dry Beans, Eggs, and Nuts Group
2–3 servings

2–3 oz meat
counts as 1 oz meat:
1 egg
½ cup cooked beans
2 tbsp peanut butter

Vegetable Group
3–5 servings

1 cup leafy vegetables

½ cup cooked or cut vegetables

3/4 C 3/4 cup vegetable juice

1 medium piece fruit

½ cup cut or cooked fruit

¼ cup dried fruit

3/4 C 3/4 cup fruit juice

Fruit Group
2–4 servings

Bread, Cereal, Rice and Pasta Group
6–11 servings

Half a bun, bagel, or English muffin

1 small muffin

1 slice bread

1 oz dry cereal (½–1 cup)

½ cup cooked cereal, rice, or pasta

FIGURE 2–7   WHAT COUNTS AS A SERVING?

SOURCE: Adapted from the *Pyramid Packet* © 1993, Penn State Nutrition Center, 417 East Calder Way, University Park, PA 16801; (814)865-6323.

the portions that count as a serving from each of the various food groups, and Figure 2–8 shows where some hard-to-place foods fit on the pyramid. When considering your own diet, you may want to look at some measuring cups to get a good idea of just how much a cup really is. You may be surprised to learn how much you're really eating. In fact, most people tend to over- or underestimate serving sizes.

Note that certain foods within each group are relatively low in fat and added sugars. Since these foods are generally the most nutrient dense choices within the group, it makes sense to select them the majority of the time. For example, consider the meat, poultry, fish, dry beans, eggs, and nuts group. Since lean cuts of meat, skinless poultry, and fish rank lower in fat than ground beef and chicken with skin, the leaner items should be chosen more often than the high-fat selections. Dry beans, which contain only a trace of fat, are good choices to add to the diet even more often. When it comes to the milk group, low-fat and nonfat dairy products make the best choices.

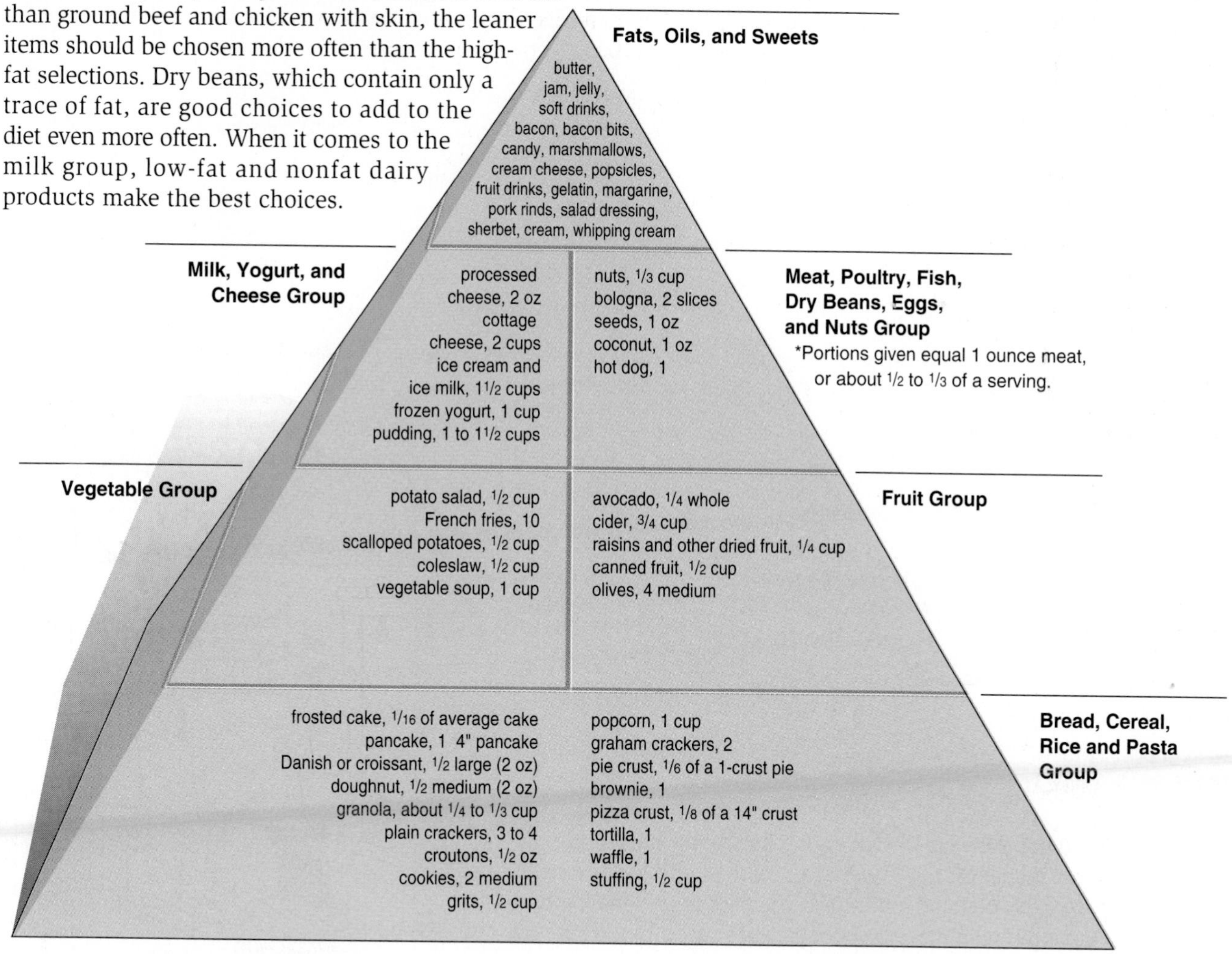

To get an idea of how your current diet compares with the Food Guide Pyramid, try the Rate Your Plate Scorecard on the following page.

Fats, Oils, and Sweets

butter, jam, jelly, soft drinks, bacon, bacon bits, candy, marshmallows, cream cheese, popsicles, fruit drinks, gelatin, margarine, pork rinds, salad dressing, sherbet, cream, whipping cream

Milk, Yogurt, and Cheese Group

processed cheese, 2 oz
cottage cheese, 2 cups
ice cream and ice milk, 1 1/2 cups
frozen yogurt, 1 cup
pudding, 1 to 1 1/2 cups

nuts, 1/3 cup
bologna, 2 slices
seeds, 1 oz
coconut, 1 oz
hot dog, 1

Meat, Poultry, Fish, Dry Beans, Eggs, and Nuts Group

*Portions given equal 1 ounce meat, or about 1/2 to 1/3 of a serving.

Vegetable Group

potato salad, 1/2 cup
French fries, 10
scalloped potatoes, 1/2 cup
coleslaw, 1/2 cup
vegetable soup, 1 cup

avocado, 1/4 whole
cider, 3/4 cup
raisins and other dried fruit, 1/4 cup
canned fruit, 1/2 cup
olives, 4 medium

Fruit Group

frosted cake, 1/16 of average cake
pancake, 1 4" pancake
Danish or croissant, 1/2 large (2 oz)
doughnut, 1/2 medium (2 oz)
granola, about 1/4 to 1/3 cup
plain crackers, 3 to 4
croutons, 1/2 oz
cookies, 2 medium
grits, 1/2 cup

popcorn, 1 cup
graham crackers, 2
pie crust, 1/6 of a 1-crust pie
brownie, 1
pizza crust, 1/8 of a 14" crust
tortilla, 1
waffle, 1
stuffing, 1/2 cup

Bread, Cereal, Rice and Pasta Group

FIGURE 2–8 HARD-TO-PLACE FOODS

The serving sizes that follow the various foods are the equivalent of one serving from the group in which the food has been placed. Note that the placement of the foods on this pyramid was reviewed by the U.S. Department of Agriculture's Human Nutrition Information Service. Certain items in each group, particularly the high-fat choices, may be difficult to fit into a healthful eating plan on a regular basis. In the chapters that follow, we will explore the food groups in more detail to see how the items within them rate.

SOURCE: Adapted from the *Pyramid Packet* © 1993, Penn State Nutrition Center, 417 East Calder Way, University Park PA 16801; (814)865-6323.

 To see how your diet measures up to the recommendations in the Food Guide Pyramid, follow these steps.

Step 1: Write down everything you ate yesterday, including both meals and snacks. Make note of portion sizes as well.

Step 2: Identify the food group to which each item you ate belongs (refer to Figures 2–6, 2–7, and 2–8 for help).

Step 3: Determine the number of servings from the five food groups that are right for you. The Food Guide Pyramid shows a range of recommended number of servings for each food group. The optimal amount for you depends on the number of calories you need, which in turn is influenced by a number of factors such as your age and activity level. The following chart gives sample daily diets for three different calorie levels to help you get a rough estimate of the type of diet that might work for you. Note that 1,600 calories is a good estimate for sedentary women and some older adults; 2,000 to 2,200 is about right for most children, teenage women, and many sedentary men; and 2,800 is a generous estimate for many teenage boys, active men, and very active women.

SAMPLE DIETS FOR A DAY

	1,600 calories	2,000 to 2,200 calories	2,800 calories
Bread group servings	6	8–9	11
Vegetable group servings	3	4	5
Fruit group servings	2	3	4
Milk group servings	2–3[a]	2–3[a]	2–3[a]
Meat group[b] (ounces)	5	5–6	7

[a]Pregnant or breastfeeding women, teenagers, and young adults up to 24 years of age need three servings from the milk group.
[b]Meat group servings are given in total ounces. That is, five servings from this group means 5 ounces.

Step 4: Circle the estimated number of servings that are right for you in the left column. In the right column, write down the number of servings you ate yesterday (refer to Figures 2–7 and 2–8 to help determine what counts as a serving). Compare the two columns to see how your diet rates.

	NUMBER OF SERVINGS YOU SHOULD EAT	NUMBER OF SERVINGS YOU ATE
Bread group servings	6 7 8 9 10 11	_____
Vegetable group servings	3 4 5	_____
Fruit group servings	2 3 4	_____
Milk group servings	2 3	_____
Meat group (ounces)	5 6 7	_____

Step 5: Decide what changes in your eating habits will make your diet more healthful. If your diet is "top heavy," with lots of foods coming from the top of the pyramid rather than the middle and the bottom, you may want to make gradual changes, such as eating more fruits and vegetables. The chapters that follow offer tips on how to do so.

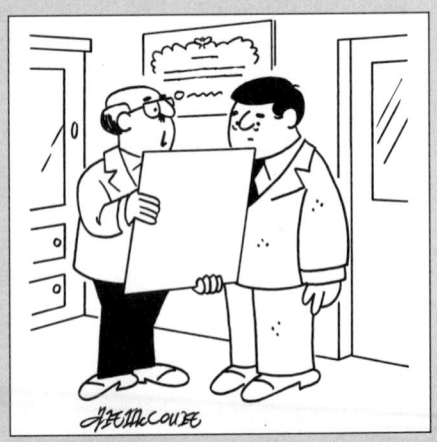

"Here's your problem . . .You've been reading the Food Pyramid upside down!"

SOURCE: Adapted from *USDA's Food Guide Pyramid* (U.S. Department of Agriculture Human Nutrition Information Service, Home and Garden Bulletin Number 249): pp. 9, 28–29.

Exchange Lists

While food group plans provide sufficient detail to help most healthy people plan a good diet, **exchange lists** take meal planning a step further. As their name implies, exchange lists are simply lists of categories of foods, such as fruit, with portions specified in a way that allows the foods to be mixed and matched or exchanged with one another in the diet. For instance, you might strive to eat two servings of fruit each day, and the exchange list shows you that a half cup of orange juice, half a banana, or a small apple each counts as a fruit.

Portion sizes within groups are determined by considering the calorie, protein, carbohydrate, and fat content of the food. For example, one fruit contains about 60 calories and 15 grams of carbohydrate. One starch, on the other hand, provides about 80 calories, 15 grams of carbohydrate, 3 grams of protein, and a trace of fat. This breakdown makes exchange lists particularly useful tools for people who need to follow carefully planned diets as a result of a health problem, such as Type I diabetes.

Exchange lists are also useful for people who are following calorie-controlled diets to lose weight. Dietitians sometimes give clients tailor-made diets centered on the exchange lists—say, a 1,500-calorie daily diet that might include 8 starches, 3 vegetables, 2 fruits, and so forth. A person can take such a framework and use the exchange lists to choose a wide variety of foods that fit into the basic eating plan. Table 2–5 shows the seven common exchange lists. Typical portions used in the list are as follows:

Starch: 1 small potato/1 slice bread—80 calories

Fruit: 1 small orange—60 calories

Milk: 1 cup nonfat milk—90 calories

Other Carbohydrates: 3 gingersnaps—80 calories (but calories in this list vary)

Vegetable: ½ cup green beans—25 calories

Meat and meat substitutes: 1 ounce lean meat or low-fat cheese—55 calories

Fat: 1 teaspoon butter—45 calories

The complete exchange lists shown in Appendix E can give you a better understanding of the nutritional profile of various foods.

EXCHANGE LISTS lists of foods with portion sizes specified; the foods on a single list are similar with respect to nutrient and calorie content and so can be mixed and matched in the diet.

TABLE 2–5
THE EXCHANGE LISTS

Carbohydrate Group
  Starch
  Fruit
  Milk
    Skim (nonfat)
    Low-fat
    Whole
  Other carbohydrates
  Vegetable
Meat and Meat Substitute Group
  Very lean
  Lean
  Medium-fat
  High-fat
Fat Group

Food Composition Tables

You now have an understanding of the tools you need to set up a healthful eating plan for yourself. You may find useful yet another tool: **food composition tables,** which list the exact number of calories, grams of fat, milligrams of sodium, and other nutrients found in commonly eaten foods. In fact, you may already be familiar with one of the many books of food composition sold in supermarkets and bookstores and geared to consumers.

Appendix I provides a food composition table that profiles the nutrient content of more than 1,900 different foods. Such tables offer the health-conscious eater a wealth of useful information—everything from the amount of vitamin C in an orange to the number of calories in an order of French fries to the amount of calcium in various cheeses. To be sure, the nutritional content of foods listed in food composition tables varies depending on cooking

FOOD COMPOSITION TABLES tables that list the nutrient profile of commonly eaten foods.

methods and other factors, and not every table lists every single nutrient. Still, food composition tables give fairly precise estimates of the nutrients in the foods you eat.

See Appendix I for a listing of the nutrient content of more than 1,900 foods.

Computer buffs can take advantage of one of the many software packages containing a database that is, in essence, a food composition table. Simply plug in the foods you eat, and the computer will generate a profile of your daily diet. Dietitians often use such software to analyze both people's diets and recipes. More and more reasonably priced, reliable nutrition-analysis software is becoming widely available.

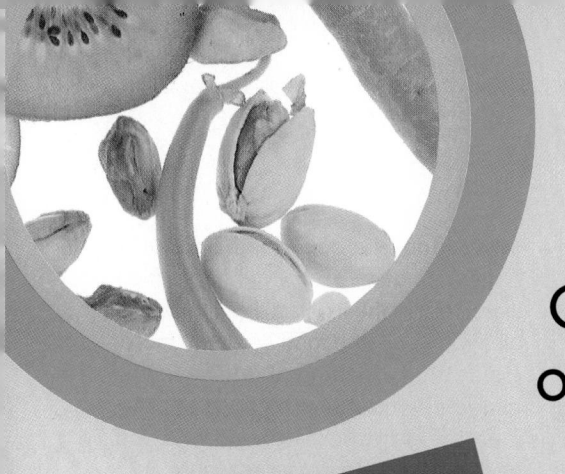

Close-Up on Food Labels

In 1990, Congress passed one of the most important pieces of legislation of the twentieth century. Known as the Nutrition Labeling and Education Act, the law called for sweeping changes in the way foods are labeled in the United States. Officials at the Food and Drug Administration, the nation's food industry watchdog, spent several years devising regulations aimed at revamping the food label. Finally, in January 1993, the organization issued its guidelines. By May 1994, food manufacturers had to relabel some 300,000 packaged foods sold in American supermarkets.[7]

For consumers, the law ensures that food companies provide the kind of nutrition information that best allows people to select foods that fit into a healthful eating plan. Considering the great variety of packaged foods available, using the food label to understand the nutrients a food supplies or lacks is essential (see Figure 2–9). The label is one of the most important tools you can use to eat healthfully, and the following questions and answers will help you understand it.

What will the label tell me? By law, all labels must contain the following:

The package must always state the product name, the name and address of the manufacturer, and the weight or measure.

The label may state information about sodium, calories, fat, or other constituents.

Approved health claims may be made but only in terms of total diet.

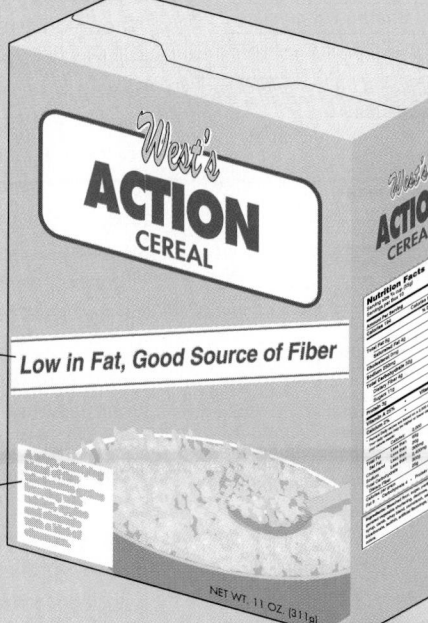

**FIGURE 2–9
ANATOMY OF A FOOD LABEL**

Calorie/gram reminder

Ingredients in descending order of predominance

Nutrition Facts

Serving size ³/₄ cup (55g)
Servings per Box 5

Amount Per Serving

Calories 167	Calories from Fat 27

	% Daily Value*
Total Fat 3g	5%
Saturated Fat 1g	5%
Cholesterol 0mg	0%
Sodium 250mg	10%
Total Carbohydrate 32g	11%
Dietary Fiber 4g	16%
Sugars 11g	
Protein 3g	

Vitamin A 25%	•	**Vitamin C** 25%
Calcium 2%	•	**Iron** 25%

*Percent Daily values are based on a 2,000 calorie diet. Your daily values may be higher or lower depending on your calorie needs:

	Calories:	2,000	2,500
Total Fat	Less than	65g	80g
Sat Fat	Less than	20g	25g
Cholesterol	Less than	300mg	300mg
Sodium	Less than	2,400mg	2,400mg
Total Carbohydrate		300g	375g
Dietary Fiber		25g	30g

Calories per gram
Fat 9 • Carbohydrate 4 • Protein 4

Ingredients: Whole oats, milled corn, enriched wheat flour (contains niacin, reduced iron, thiamin mononitrate, riboflavin), dextrose, maltose, high fructose corn syrup, brown sugar, partially hydrogenated cottonseed oil, coconut oil, walnuts, vitamin C (sodium ascorbate), vitamin A (palmitate), iron.

Serving size and calorie information

Percentage of Daily Value for nutrients

Reference values

This allows comparison of some values for nutrients in a serving of the food with the needs of a person requiring 2,000 or 2,500 calories per day to show how the product fits into the daily diet.

- The name of the food, also known as the statement of identity.
- The name of the manufacturer, packer, or distributor, as well as the firm's city, state, and zip code.
- The net quantity, which tells you how much food is in the container so that you can compare prices. Net quantity has to be stated in both inch or pound units and metric units.

- The **ingredients list,** with items listed in descending order by weight. The first ingredient listed makes up the largest proportion of all the ingredients in the food, the second, the second largest amount, and so on. If the first ingredient in the list is sugar, for example, you know the food contains more sugar than anything else. The list is especially useful in helping people identify ingredients they avoid for health, religious, or other reasons.

- The **Nutrition Facts panel,** unless the package is small—no larger than 12 square inches of surface area, or about the size of a small candy bar or a roll of breath mints; small packages must carry a telephone number or address consumers can contact to obtain nutrition information (see Figure 2–10).

Which nutrients must be included on the Nutrition Facts panel? The Nutrition Facts panel must indicate the amount of certain mandatory nutrients that one serving of the food contains. When you consider the nutrition information, keep serving sizes in mind. Based on the amount of food most people eat at one time, the FDA has set forth a list of serving sizes for more than 100 food categories. Manufacturers must use these recommended serving sizes on food labels. For instance, the serving size for product X must always be 8 ounces. This ensures that consumers can easily compare one brand of the product to another without going through the calculations that would be necessary if serving sizes varied—say, if another brand's label had a 6-ounce serving size. The nutrient information that must appear on the Nutrition Facts panel is calories, calories from fat, total fat, saturated fat, cholesterol, sodium, total carbohydrate, dietary fiber, sugars, protein, vitamin A, vitamin C, calcium, and iron (in that order).

These nutrients were chosen to appear on the Nutrition Facts panel because they address today's health

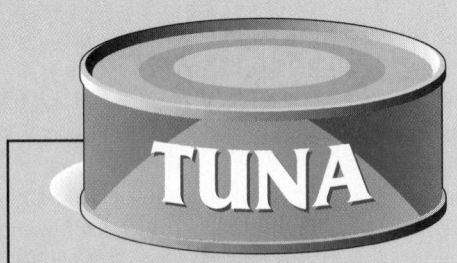

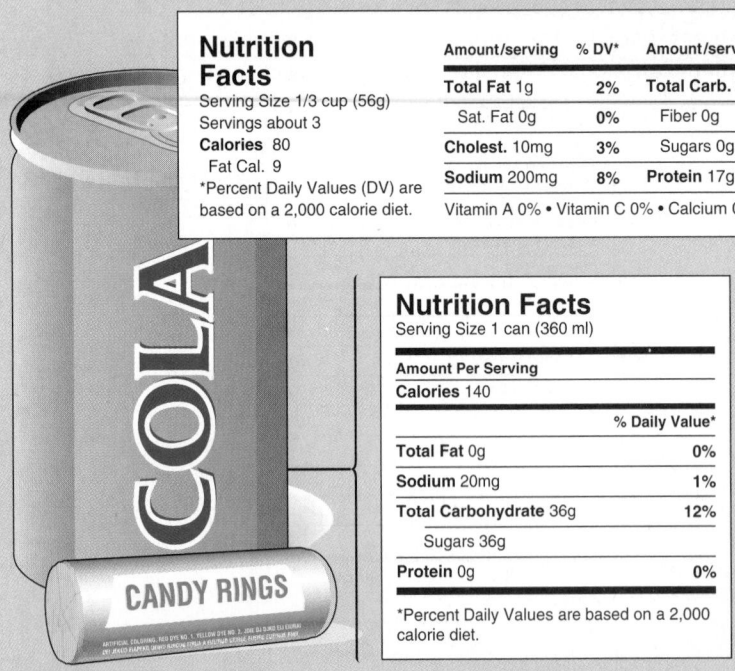

FIGURE 2–10
TYPES OF FOOD LABELS

A container with less than 40 square inches of surface area for nutrition labeling can present fewer facts in the format shown on the can of tuna. A simplified format, shown on the can of cola, is allowed on foods that do not contain significant amounts of nutrients. Packages with less than 12 square inches of surface area, such as small candy bars, need not carry nutrition information, though they must provide a telephone number or address for contacting the company to obtain nutrition information.

concerns. In fact, many of the vitamins and minerals that were included in the old food labels no longer appear because most people obtain plenty of them. Today, many people need to be concerned about getting an excess of certain nutrients, such as fat, rather than too few vitamins and minerals.

The ranking of the required nutrients as listed previously was spelled out by the Food and Drug Administra-tion to ensure that the label reflects the government's dietary priorities for the public. For example, fat falls near the top of the list because most consumers need to pay closer attention to the amount of fat in their diet. Most people eat too much fat, which raises the risk of developing heart disease, obesity, and cancer—chronic problems suffered by millions of Americans. Protein, on the other hand, appears near the bottom of the label, because the amount of protein most people eat does not rate as a major health concern.

Note that only vitamins A and C, iron, and calcium appear on the nutrition panel. Those are the only vitamins and minerals (except for sodium) required to be on food labels, unless a manufacturer makes a nutrition claim about another one. For instance, if a manufacturer says that a cereal is **forti-fied** with niacin, the amount of niacin in the product must appear on the label.[8]

What are the % Daily Values listed in the righthand column? The % **Daily Values** are based on the idea that a healthful diet should consist of certain amounts of fat, saturated fat, sodium, and so on. For instance, since no more than 30 percent of total calories should come from fat, the % Daily Value tells you the percentage of fat that a serving of the food contributes to a 2,000-calorie eater's fat "allowance." A 2,000-calorie diet was chosen as a

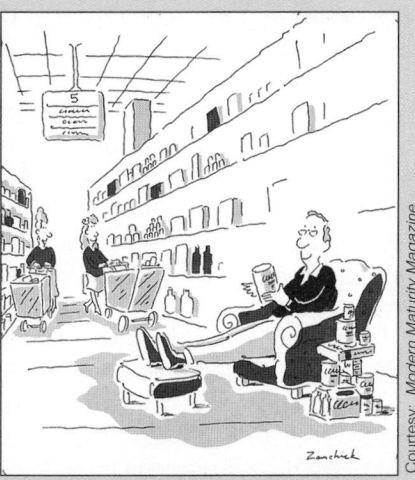

Courtesy: Modern Maturity Magazine.

"Henry likes nothing more than to curl up with a good label."

good point of reference because that's about the amount eaten by most moderately active women, teenage girls, and sedentary men. Of course, more calories may be appropriate for many men, teenage boys, and active women. This is why the nutrition panel also shows **Daily Values** for a 2,500-calorie diet (refer to the bottom of the Nutrition Facts panel in Figure 2–9).

To understand how the Daily Values for fats, sodium, carbohydrates, and fiber are calculated, let's go through an example. First, look for the grams of total fat and the % Daily Value for the cereal shown in Figure 2–9. The label shows that a serving supplies 3 grams of fat, with a Daily Value of 5 percent. This means that a serving of the cereal contributes 5 percent of the total fat that a person eating 2,000 calories a day should consume.

Now look at the bottom of the Nutrition Facts panel, which indicates that someone eating 2,000 calories a day should take in no more than 65 grams of fat. Divide 3—the number of fat grams in a serving of the cereal—

by 65. Multiply that number by 100 to obtain a percentage. The answer is 5, that is, 5 percent of the total fat.

The Daily Values for fats, sodium, carbohydrates, and fiber are calculated according to what experts deem a healthful diet:

- no more than 30 percent of calories as fat
- no more than 10 percent of calories as saturated fat
- fewer than 300 milligrams of cholesterol
- fewer than 2,400 milligrams of sodium
- at least 60 percent of calories as carbohydrate
- 11.5 grams of fiber per 1,000 calories

But if I don't eat 2,000 calories a day, how can I use the % Daily Values to choose foods? You can use the % Daily Values to get a good idea of how various foods fit into a healthful diet, regardless of the number of calories you eat. Consider a student who eats only 1,800 calories a day. If she snacks on two servings of potato chips with a Daily Value of 15 percent fat per serving, she's already taken in 30 percent of the fat someone eating *2,000* calories should have in an entire day. Because she eats less than 2,000 calories, the potato chips contribute slightly more than 30 percent. Thus, the 30 percent Daily Value shows that potato chips chalk up a lot of fat for a snack. If she checks the % Daily Value for fat on a label of pretzels, on the other hand, she might see that a serving supplies only about 3 percent. If she eats two servings, she's only up to less than 10 percent of the fat she can have, leaving her much less likely to go overboard on fat throughout the rest of the day. In other words, the % Daily Value column can give you a good idea of how different foods fit into the overall diet.

You can also use the Daily Values to comparison shop. For example, if you're looking for a high-fiber cereal to increase the amount of fiber in your diet, you can check the % Daily Value for fiber on the labels of several brands of cereal. If a serving of Brand X's cereal has a Daily Value of 16 percent for fiber and Brand Y supplies only 5 percent, Brand X is higher in fiber and the best bet for any fiber seeker, regardless of the number of calories he or she usually consumes.

I'm trying to cut back on the fat in my diet. Is there another way I can use the food label to help me do that? Some people find it easiest to bypass the % Daily Values and simply check the grams of total fat a serving of food supplies to see how much it adds to a daily fat tally. Let's say a man eats 2,000 calories a day and therefore should consume no more than 65 grams of fat a day. If he eats a muffin (15 grams of fat) and coffee with cream (10 grams) in the morning, he's up to 25 grams of fat. That means he can have about 40 more grams during the rest of the day to stay within his fat "budget."

Once you determine the maximum number of fat grams you should have in a day, you can use the food label to get a good idea of how many grams of total fat the items you buy add to your daily tally. To figure out your fat allowance, check Table 4–10 on page 143.

What about the % Daily Values for vitamins and minerals—are they based on the RDA? Not exactly. The % Daily Values for those nutrients are calculated using what is known as the **Reference Daily Intakes (RDI)**, designed specifically for use on food labels. Shown on the inside cover of this book, the RDI table is a listing of essential nutrients and one recommended amount for each nutrient. The RDI were created to help manufacturers avoid a stumbling block they face as they label foods. Since manufacturers don't know whether you're an 18-year-old woman or a 30-year-old man, they don't know exactly what your nutritional needs are. You may recall that the RDA include a different set of vitamin and mineral recommendations for each gender and age group.

To help get around the problem, the nutrient recommendations used in the RDI represent the highest of all the RDA to ensure that virtually everyone in the population is covered. For most nutrients, the highest RDA is for an adult man. When it comes to iron, however, the RDA for women is the highest (women require more iron than men), so the women's RDA is used for the RDI.

The protein Daily Values used on the food label are also based partly on the RDI, which include two values for protein. If the protein in the food is of high quality, say, from meat, the RDI is 50 grams. If it's of lower quality, say, from beans, the RDI is 65 grams. (See Chapter 5 for more about protein quality.)

One limitation of the RDI is that they were compiled back in 1968 (at that time they were called the U.S. Recommended Daily Allowances, or U.S. RDA). Since that time, as scientists have gathered more knowledge about people's nutritional needs, the RDA have been updated several times. Yet the RDI haven't changed to keep pace with current knowledge. The FDA is reconsidering use of the RDI in the future.

Lots of foods in the grocery store are marked low-fat. Do I have to check the Daily Values to see whether the foods really are low-fat? No, you don't need to scrutinize all the numbers on the food labels as you shop. You can believe the claims you see on food packages. By law, foods carrying terms called **nutrient content claims—**low-fat, low-calorie, light, and so forth—must adhere to specific definitions spelled out by the Food and Drug Administration. For instance, a serving of a food dubbed low-fat must contain no more than 3 grams of fat. An item touted as low-calorie may provide no more than 40 calories per serving. Table 2–6 lists the claims commonly used on food labels and their legal definitions.

I noticed that the label of some macaroni and cheese I bought says something about osteoporosis and calcium. Does that mean it protects against osteoporosis? The statement you see on the label is known as a **health claim,** or a statement linking the nutritional profile of a food to a reduced risk of a particular disease. The FDA has set forth very strict rules governing the use of such health claims. For example, if a food's label bears health claims regarding calcium, a serving of the product must contain at least 20 percent of the Daily Value for calcium, among other restrictions. What's more, the manufacturers are allowed to imply only that the food "may" or "might" reduce risk of disease. They must also note the other factors, such as exercise, that play a role in prevention of the disease. Finally, they must phrase the claim so that the consumer can understand the relationship between the nutrient and the disease.

For example, a health claim on a food low in fat, saturated fat, and cholesterol might read: "While many factors affect heart disease, diets low in saturated fat and cholesterol may reduce the risk of this disease." See Figure 2–11 for an example of the type of health claim you might see on a package of macaroni and cheese. Note that the manufacturer is not allowed to state that the food protects against osteoporosis.[9]

TABLE 2–6
DEFINITIONS OF NUTRIENT CONTENT CLAIMS

Free means a product contains none or only negligible amounts of fat, saturated fat, cholesterol, sodium, sugar, and/or calories. For instance, "calorie-free" means fewer than 5 calories per serving.

Low indicates the food can be eaten frequently without exceeding dietary guidelines for fat, saturated fat, cholesterol, sodium, and/or calories. More specifically:

low-fat: 3 grams or fewer per serving*

low saturated fat: no more than 1 gram per serving

low sodium: no more than 140 milligrams per serving*

very low sodium: no more than 35 milligrams per serving

low cholesterol: no more than 20 milligrams and no more than 2 grams of saturated fat per serving*

low-calorie: no more than 40 calories per serving*

Lean and **extra lean** describe the fat content of meat, poultry, seafood, and game meats:

lean: fewer than 10 grams of fat, no more than 4.5 grams of saturated fat, and fewer than 95 milligrams of cholesterol per serving (or 100 grams)

extra lean: fewer than 5 grams of fat, fewer than 2 grams of saturated fat, and fewer than 95 milligrams of cholesterol per serving (or 100 grams)

High used when a serving of a food contains 20 percent or more of the Daily Value for a particular nutrient.

Good source indicates that a serving of the food supplies 10 percent to 19 percent of the Daily Value for a particular nutrient.

Reduced denotes a product that has been nutritionally altered and contains 25 percent less of a nutrient such as fat or calories than the regular, unaltered product. A product cannot be dubbed "reduced," however, if the regular version of the food already meets the requirements for a "low" claim. That is, if a food is "low-fat" to begin with, it cannot be called "reduced" if manufacturers take even more fat out of it.

Less means that a food contains 25 percent less of a nutrient or calories than a comparable food. For example, pretzels containing 25 percent less fat than potato chips carry a "less fat" claim. "Fewer" can be used in the same way.

Light carries several meanings:

First, that a nutritionally altered food contains one-third fewer calories or half the fat as the regular product. If fat supplies 50 percent or more of the calories to begin with, it must be reduced by half to be called "light."

Second, that the sodium content of a low-fat, low-calorie food has been reduced by 50 percent. If the food is not low in fat and calories but the sodium has been decreased by half, it must be labeled "light in sodium."

Third, "light" can be used to describe a food's color and/or texture, as long as the label explains the intent. For example, "light brown sugar."

More means that a serving of the food contains at least 10 percent more of the Daily Value of a particular nutrient than the regular food. The label on calcium-fortified bread can state that the product contains "more calcium" than regular bread.

Percent fat free is an indication of the amount of a food's weight that is fat-free, which can be used only on foods that are low-fat or fat-free to begin with. For instance, a food that weighs 100 grams with 3 grams from fat can be labeled "97 percent fat-free." Note that this term refers to the amount that is fat-free by weight, not calories. If that same food supplies 100 calories, the 3 grams of fat contribute 27 of them (1 gram of fat contains 9 calories). This means that 27 of the 100 calories, or 27 percent of the total calories, come from fat.

Made with oat bran, no tropical oils claims, known as implied claims, are prohibited if they mislead consumers into believing a product supplies (or lacks) significant levels of nutrients. For example, a manufacturer can say a product is "made with oat bran" only if it contains enough oat bran to meet the definition for "good source" of fiber.

Healthy indicates that a food is low in fat and saturated fat; contains no more than 60 milligrams of cholesterol per serving; and provides at least 10 percent of the Daily Value for vitamin A, vitamin C, protein, calcium, iron, or fiber (main dishes must supply at least two of the six nutrients). In addition, by 1998, the food must meet sodium requirements: no more than 360 milligrams of sodium per serving of individual foods and no more than 480 milligrams per main dish meal.[12]

Fresh indicates that a food is raw or unprocessed. That is, it has never been frozen or reheated and contains no preservatives (irradiation at low levels is allowed, however). "Fresh frozen," "frozen fresh," and "freshly frozen" can be used on foods that are quickly frozen while still fresh.

---

*On meals and main dish products such as frozen dinners, "low-calorie" can be used if the dish contains no more than 120 calories in 100 grams, or about 3.5 ounces; "low sodium" means the dish supplies no more than 140 milligrams per 100 grams; and "low cholesterol" indicates a maximum of 20 milligrams and 2 grams saturated fat per 100 grams. "Light" means the dish or meal is low-fat or low-calorie.

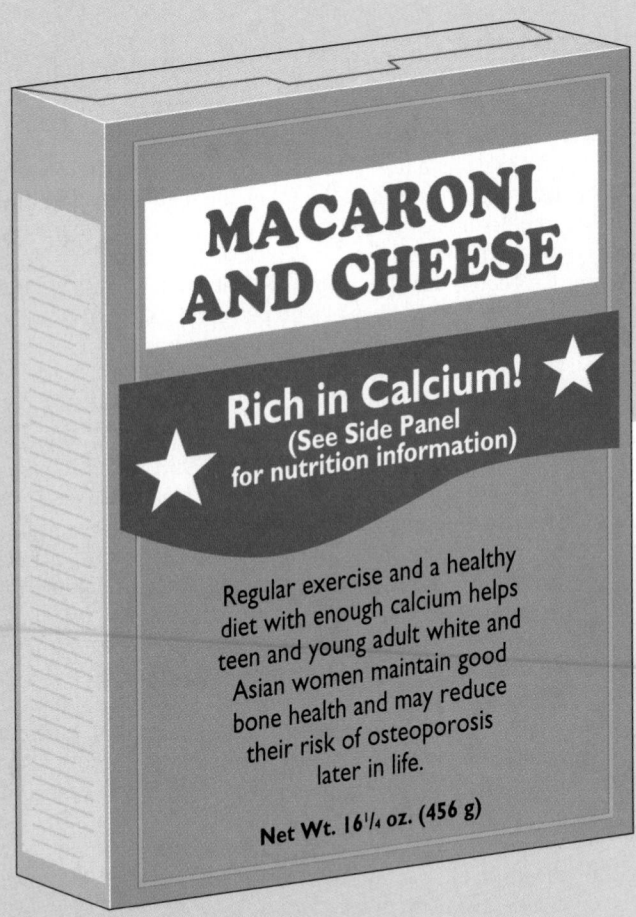

FIGURE 2–11
HEALTH CLAIMS: LINKING FOOD AND HEALTH

The following are the seven nutrient/disease relationships about which health claims can be made:

- calcium and osteoporosis
- fat and cancer
- saturated fat and cholesterol and heart disease
- fiber-containing grain products, fruits, and vegetables and cancer
- fruits, vegetables, and grain products that contain fiber and heart disease
- sodium and high blood pressure
- fruits and vegetables and cancer

The FDA has also authorized the use of a health claim about the relationship between folic acid, a form of the vitamin folate (see page 205 in Chapter 6) and the risk of birth defects called neural tube defects. The claim is allowed for use on folic-acid containing supplements and foods naturally high in folic acid. However, the FDA is still con-sidering whether to allow a similar health claim on foods fortified with folic acid.

Why don't foods such as meat and chicken carry Nutrition Facts panels?
Unlike almost all processed foods, packages of raw meat and poultry such as beef roasts and chicken breasts are not required by law to carry nutrition labels. The same goes for fresh fruits and vegetables. However, as more and more shoppers have become interested in nutrition, a growing number of supermarkets have begun providing nutrition information about such products on posters and brochures.[10]

I've noticed that some fast-food chains post nutrition information. Are the others supposed to as well?
By law, fast-food outlets, delicatessens, and other restaurants needn't provide nutrition information via, say, posters or brochures. The only exception under consideration is foods for which a nutritional claim has been made. For instance, the government is proposing that if a restaurant puts a symbol such as a little red heart next to a menu item to claim that the selection is heart healthy, the restaurant must have on hand reasonable proof that the item meets the government's requirements for that particular claim.[11]

Most fast-food chains now provide nutrition information brochures to patrons who ask for such information. If you frequent one or another of the chains, obtaining a copy of their brochure is certainly not a bad idea. (Refer also to the Nutrition Action feature, "Fast Guide to Eating on the Run," in Chapter 1.)

MINIGLOSSARY

DAILY VALUES the amount of fat, sodium, fiber, and other nutrients health experts say should make up a healthful diet. The % **Daily Values** that appear on food labels tell you the percentage of a nutrient that a serving of the food contributes to a healthful diet.

FORTIFIED FOOD a food to which manufacturers have added 10 percent or more of the Daily Value for a particular nutrient.

HEALTH CLAIM a statement on the food label linking the nutritional profile of a food to a reduced risk of a particular disease, such as osteoporosis or cancer. Manufacturers must adhere to strict government guidelines when making such claims.

INGREDIENTS LIST a listing of the ingredients in a food, with items listed in descending order of predominance by weight. All food labels are required to bear an ingredients list.

NUTRIENT CONTENT CLAIMS claims such as "low-fat" and "low-calorie" used on food labels to help consumers who don't want to scrutinize the Nutrition Facts panel get an idea of a food's nutritional profile. These claims must adhere to specific definitions set forth by the Food and Drug Administration.

NUTRITION FACTS PANEL a detailed breakdown of the nutritional content of a serving of a food that must appear on virtually all packaged foods sold in the United States.

REFERENCE DAILY INTAKES (RDI) a table devised in 1968 listing one suggested daily intake for vitamins, minerals, and protein. The RDI are not intended as nutritional goals that everyone should meet. Rather, they are for use on food labels to help people get an idea of the amount of nutrients a serving of the product contributes to the diet. The RDI were known as the U.S. RDA (the U.S. Recommended Daily Allowances) until the food labels were revamped in 1993.

CHECK YOURSELF...

1. Name two characteristics of a healthful diet.

2. Describe the concept of nutrient density.

3. Identify the five food groups shown in the Food Guide Pyramid and the approximate number of servings you need from each group.

4. Name six of the nutrients that must appear on virtually all food labels (excluding small labels and other exceptions).

5. Explain how the % Daily Value column on food labels can be used.

6. Name the seven dietary guidelines for Americans.

7. Explain the limitations of using the RDA to evaluate individual diets.

8. List three examples of relatively low-fat snacks.

9. Describe the order in which ingredients are listed on food labels.

10. List the three calorie-yielding nutrients.

Answers to selected Check Yourself questions are found in Appendix H.

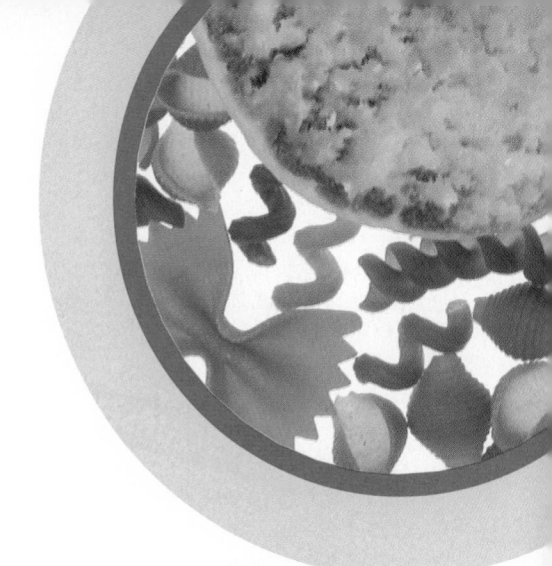

Rabbit said, "Honey or condensed milk with your bread?" [Pooh] was so excited that he said, "Both," and then, so as not to seem greedy, he added, "But don't bother about the bread, please."

from *Winnie the Pooh*, A. A. Milne
(1882–1956, children's book author)

The Carbohydrates: Sugar, Starch, and Fiber

THREE

Contents

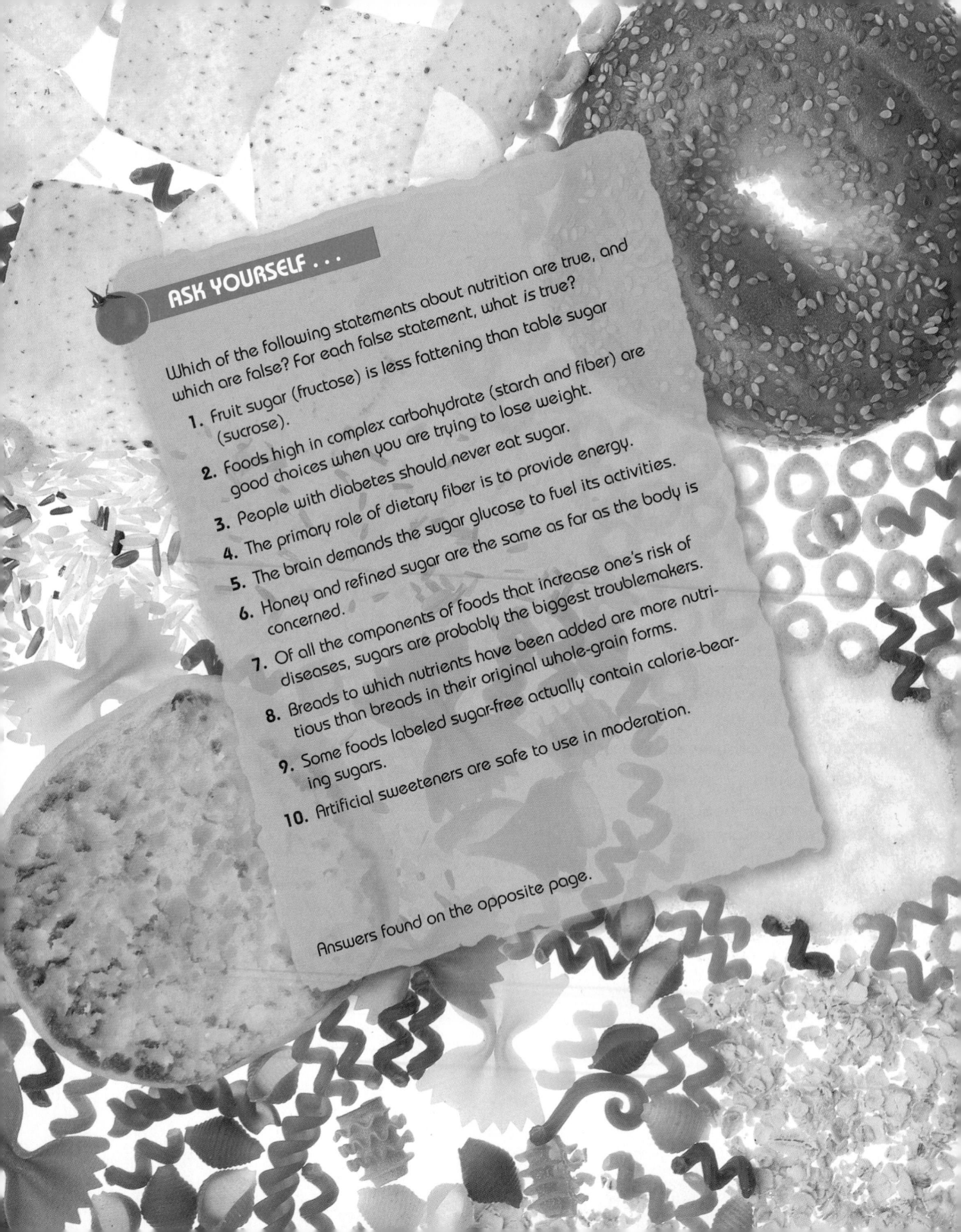

ASK YOURSELF . . .

Which of the following statements about nutrition are true, and which are false? For each false statement, what *is* true?

1. Fruit sugar (fructose) is less fattening than table sugar (sucrose).

2. Foods high in complex carbohydrate (starch and fiber) are good choices when you are trying to lose weight.

3. People with diabetes should never eat sugar.

4. The primary role of dietary fiber is to provide energy.

5. The brain demands the sugar glucose to fuel its activities.

6. Honey and refined sugar are the same as far as the body is concerned.

7. Of all the components of foods that increase one's risk of diseases, sugars are probably the biggest troublemakers.

8. Breads to which nutrients have been added are more nutritious than breads in their original whole-grain forms.

9. Some foods labeled sugar-free actually contain calorie-bearing sugars.

10. Artificial sweeteners are safe to use in moderation.

Answers found on the opposite page.

Once upon a time, bread, potatoes, pasta, and other starchy foods were placed on the dieter's list of most-fattening or "illegal" foods. This unattractive image doubtless comes from the practice of serving many carbohydrate-rich foods laden with fat—potatoes with sour cream and butter, vegetables or pasta with rich cream sauces, toast with butter, and salads with fat-rich dressings. People who need to lose weight must limit high-calorie foods, but they are ill-advised to try to avoid all **carbohydrate.** It is the fat, not the carbohydrate, that raises the calorie count the most.

CARBOHYDRATES compounds made of single sugars or multiples of them and composed of carbon, hydrogen, and oxygen atoms.

$carbo$ = carbon (C)
$hydrate$ = water (H_2O)

This chapter invites you to learn to distinguish between certain carbohydrates, such as starch and fiber, and others, such as concentrated sugars. You will learn to choose your calories by the company they keep (see Table 3–1).

Carbohydrate Basics

The primary role of carbohydrates is to provide the body with energy (calories), and for certain body systems (for example, the brain and the nervous system), carbohydrates are the preferred energy source. Carbohydrates are the ideal fuel for the body. There are only two alternative calorie sources: protein and fat. Protein-rich foods are usually expensive and provide no advantage over carbohydrates when used to provide fuel for the body. Fat-rich foods might be less expensive, but fat cannot be used efficiently as fuel by the brain and nerves, and diets high in fat are associated with many chronic diseases. Thus, of all alternative food-energy sources, carbohydrates are preferred; they provide most of the day's energy for most of the world's people.

Of the three energy nutrients, carbohydrates are the one we are told to increase in our diet. A balanced diet would ideally contain about 58 percent carbohydrate, 12 percent protein, and not more than 30 percent fat.

TABLE 3–1

CHOOSING CARBOHYDRATES BY THE COMPANY THEY KEEP

FOOD	CALORIES	GRAMS OF FAT
TOAST (2 SLICES)		
with margarine (2 tsp)	188	9
with low-sugar jelly/fruit spread (2 tsp)	139	2
POTATO (MEDIUM)		
with margarine (1 tsp) and sour cream (1 tbsp)	287	10
with yogurt cheese* (2 tbsp)	223	0
BAGEL (MEDIUM)		
with regular cream cheese (2 tbsp)	263	11
with fat-free cream cheese (2 tbsp)	188	1
PASTA (1 CUP)		
with Alfredo sauce (⅓ c)	390	20
with tomato and mushroom sauce (⅓ c)	232	4

*To make yogurt cheese: Drain nonfat plain yogurt through cheesecloth to thicken to consistency of cream cheese. Add herbs for flavor. Or, try the *fat-free* sour cream now on the market.

SOURCE: Adapted from *Environmental Nutrition* Vol. 17, February 1994, p. 2.

Alcohol can provide calories but has the same disadvantages as fat as well as others; it is not a nutrient in any sense (see Chapter 9's Spotlight).

ASK YOURSELF ANSWERS 1. False. Fructose and sucrose are equally fattening because they have the same number of calories per gram. **2.** True. **3.** False. People with diabetes need to watch the total carbohydrate in their diets, but they can choose foods with sugar as a small portion of that total. **4.** False. Although certain fibers may provide negligible calories to the diet, fiber's primary role is in providing bulk for the digestive tract. **5.** True. **6.** True. **7.** False. Of all the things in foods associated with risk of diseases, fat is by far the biggest troublemaker. **8.** False. Breads to which nutrients have been added are *less* nutritious than breads in their original forms because more nutrients have been lost than are added. **9.** True. **10.** True.

It's not the potatoes that are fattening; it's the butter, sour cream, or gravy that they put on us!

Carbohydrates are divided into two categories: complex carbohydrates and simple carbohydrates. **Complex carbohydrates** include starch and fiber. Starches make up a large part of the world's food supply—mostly as grains (breads and pastas). Consider such staples as wheat, rice, and corn, which are rich sources of starch. Fiber is found abundantly in plants, especially in the outer portions of cereal grains, and in fruits, legumes, and most vegetables. **Simple carbohydrates** include naturally occurring sugars in fresh fruits and some vegetables and in milk and milk products and added sugars in concentrated form, as in honey, corn syrup, or sugar in the sugar bowl. All of these carbohydrates have characteristics in common, but they are of different merit nutritionally. The only carbohydrates we are told to limit are the concentrated forms in sweeteners, not the dilute sugars in fruits, other plant foods, or milk. Table 3–2 introduces the different types of carbohydrates.

COMPLEX CARBOHYDRATES long chains of sugars (glucose) arranged as starch or fiber. Also called polysaccharides.
poly = many
saccharides = sugar unit

SIMPLE CARBOHYDRATES (sugars) the single sugars (monosaccharides) and the pairs of sugars (disaccharides) linked together.

Glycogen is another type of complex carbohydrate composed of glucose but one that is not a major source of energy; glycogen is made and stored by liver and muscle tissues of human beings and animals as a storage form of glucose.

All carbohydrates, with the exception of fiber, provide the same number of calories as protein—4 per gram—as compared with the 9 calories per gram of fats or the 7 per gram of alcohol.

TABLE 3–2
CATEGORIES AND SOURCES OF CARBOHYDRATE

CARBOHYDRATE TYPE	COMMON NAMES	FOOD SOURCES
MONOSACCHARIDES		
Glucose	Dextrose, blood sugar	Fruits, sweeteners
Fructose	Fruit sugar, levulose	Fruits, honey, high-fructose corn syrup
Galactose	—	Part of lactose, found in milk
DISACCHARIDES		
Sucrose (glucose + fructose)	Table sugar	Beet and cane sugar, fruit
Lactose (glucose + galactose)	Milk sugar	Milk and milk products
Maltose (glucose + glucose)	Malt sugar	Germinating grains
POLYSACCHARIDES		
Starches	Dextrins	Potatoes, legumes, corn, wheat, rye, and other grains
Dietary fiber	Roughage, bulk: Hemicellulose Pectins Cellulose Gums Mucilages Psyllium	Whole grains, legumes, fruits, vegetables

The Simple Carbohydrates

Carbohydrate-rich foods are obtained almost exclusively from plants. Milk is the only animal-derived food that contains significant amounts of carbohydrate. All carbohydrates are composed of single sugars, alone or in various combinations. All contain the simple sugar **glucose** and other sugars much like it in composition and structure.

The Single Sugars: Monosaccharides

All of the carbohydrates are made of simple sugars, and all carbohydrates but fiber can quickly be converted to glucose in the body. Green plants make glucose from carbon dioxide and water through a process known as **photosynthesis** in the presence of **chlorophyll** and sunlight, as illustrated in the margin.

Glucose is not a very sweet sugar, but plants can rearrange its atoms to form another sugar, **fructose,** which is sweet to the taste. Fructose is found mostly in fruits, in honey, and as part of another sugar—table sugar. Glucose and fructose are the most common single sugars in nature.

The Double Sugars: Disaccharides

Some sugars are double sugars, made by bonding two single sugars together. When glucose and fructose are bonded together, they form **sucrose,** or table sugar, the product most people refer to when they use the term *sugar.* The sweet taste of sucrose comes primarily from the fructose in its structure. It occurs naturally in many fruits and vegetables. Sugar cane and sugar beets are two sources from which sucrose is purified and granulated to various extents to provide the brown, white, and powdered sugars available in the supermarket. Sucrose is one of the two most caloric ingredients of candy, cakes, pastries, frostings, cookies, pre-sweetened ready-to-eat cereals, and other concentrated sweets. (The other major calorie contributor is fat, discussed in Chapter 4.)

Another double sugar, **maltose,** appears wherever starch is being broken down. It occurs in sprouting seeds and arises during the digestion of starch in the human body. Maltose consists of two glucose units. The malt found in

In the presence of chlorophyll and the energy of the sun, plants make glucose. Water, absorbed here by the plant's roots, and carbon dioxide, absorbed through the plant's leaves, combine to form a molecule of glucose.

GLUCOSE (GLOO-koce) the building block of carbohydrate; a single sugar used in both plant and animal tissues as quick-energy currency. A single sugar is known as a **monosaccharide.**
mono = one

The chemical structure of glucose.

PHOTOSYNTHESIS a process in which plants use the green pigment chlorophyll to trap the energy of the sun and produce glucose from carbon dioxide and water.

CHLOROPHYLL green pigment of plants necessary for photosynthesis.

FRUCTOSE (FROOK-toce) fruit sugar—the sweetest of the single sugars. Another single sugar, **galactose** (ga-LACK-toce), occurs bonded to glucose in the sugar of milk. A double sugar is known as a **disaccharide.**
di = two

SUCROSE (SOO-crose) a double sugar composed of glucose and fructose.

MALTOSE a double sugar composed of two glucose units.

beer contains maltose. Enzymes used in the brewing process break down the long chains of starch in barley and wheat into maltose units. Dry heat can also be used to break down long glucose chains to form maltose. Bread tastes sweeter after toasting for this reason.

Finally, there is **lactose,** the major sugar in milk, a double sugar made by mammals from galactose and glucose units. A human baby is born with the digestive enzymes necessary to split lactose into its two simple sugars—glucose and galactose—so that they can be absorbed. Lactose facilitates the absorption of calcium and promotes the growth of beneficial bacteria in the intestines. Breastmilk and infant formula, which contain lactose, are ideal foods for babies because they provide a simple, easily digested carbohydrate to meet an infant's energy needs.

When you eat a food containing lactose, an **enzyme** in your small intestine first splits the double sugar into single sugars so that they can enter your bloodstream. Your liver then quickly converts galactose to glucose or to smaller pieces that can serve as building blocks of either glucose or fat.

Many people can lose the ability to digest lactose during or after childhood. Thereafter, the person may experience nausea, bloating, abdominal pain or cramping, diarrhea, or excessive gas after drinking milk or eating lactose-containing products because the intestinal bacteria will use the lactose for energy, producing gas and other products that irritate the intestine. This condition—**lactose intolerance**—is inherited by about 80 percent of the world's people. It is most common in African-Americans, Greeks, Native Americans, and Asians, and less common in people of northern European origin.[1] It also can develop temporarily in anyone who is malnourished or sick, making the avoidance of milk and milk products temporarily necessary. Because milk is an almost indispensable source of calcium for growth, a milk substitute must be found for children who are lactose intolerant. Chapter 7 describes ways to find substitutes for milk when necessary.

How the Sugars Rate

The single sugar fructose is sold in purified, crystalline form and advertised as a "natural" sugar that—unlike the "unnatural" sugar sucrose—won't cause weight gain. This is just a sales pitch. What's natural about *any* purified, concentrated sugar? The calories in fructose are used for energy, just as those in ordinary table sugar are, and too much of either can cause weight gain if calories are excessive.

Some people believe that honey is more nutritious than white table sugar

> **LACTOSE** a double sugar composed of glucose and galactose; commonly known as milk sugar.
>
> **ENZYMES** protein catalysts. A catalyst facilitates a chemical reaction without itself being altered in the process. (Proteins are discussed in Chapter 5; digestive enzymes in Appendix B).
>
> **LACTOSE INTOLERANCE** inability to digest milk sugar as a result of a lack of the necessary enzyme lactase; a genetic flaw that can occur at any age. Symptoms include nausea, abdominal pain, diarrhea, or excessive gas that occurs anywhere from 30 minutes to a couple of hours after consuming milk or milk products.

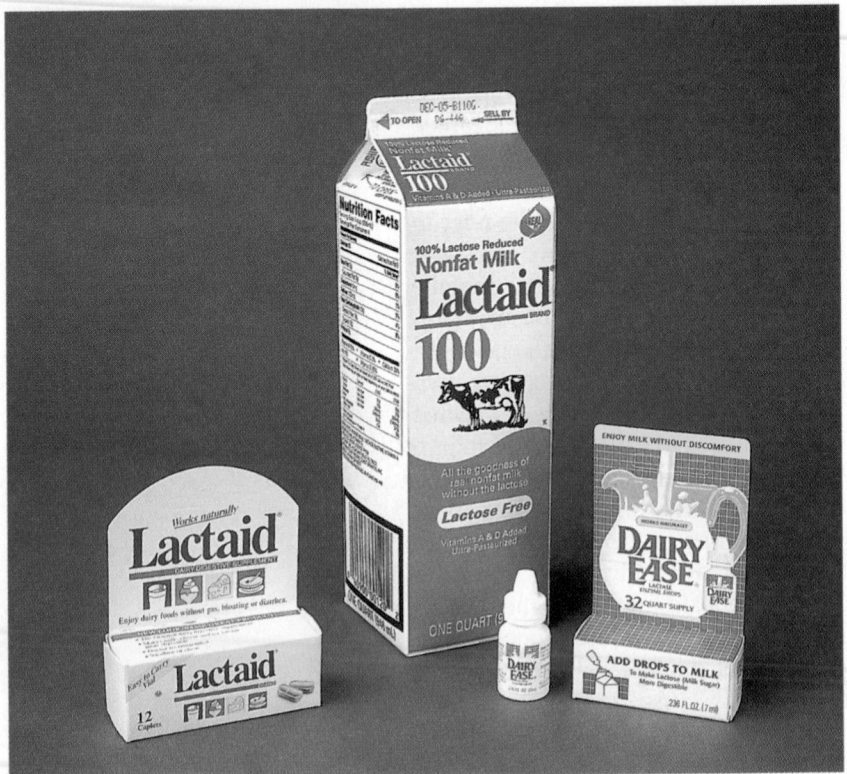

Lactose-reduced milk, enzyme solutions containing lactose for treating dairy products, and lactose tablets are available to help reduce the symptoms of lactose intolerance.

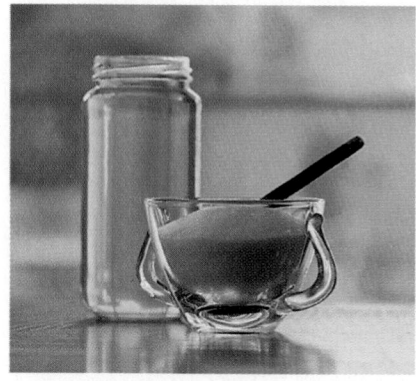 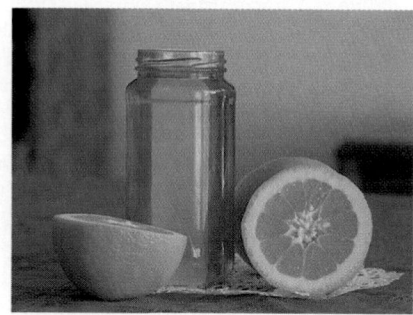

Honey and sucrose contain the same monosaccharides, but in sucrose they are linked together. Compared with honey or sugar, fruit is more nutrient dense.

because it is "natural." As a matter of fact, chemically, honey and table sugar are almost indistinguishable. Honey contains the two monosaccharides glucose and fructose in approximately equal amounts. Table sugar contains the same monosaccharides, but joined together to form the double sugar sucrose. In the body, after digestion, table sugar and honey are identical. Spoon for spoon, however, table sugar contains *fewer* calories than honey because sugar's dry crystals take up more space than the crystals of honey dissolved as a liquid.

When people learn that fruit's energy comes from sugars, they may think that eating fruit is the same as consuming concentrated sweets such as candy or soft drinks. However, fruits differ from candy and soft drinks in important ways. Their sugars are diluted in large volumes of water, packaged in fiber, and mixed with many vitamins and minerals needed by the body. In contrast, concentrated sweets such as honey and table sugar are merely—as the popular phrase calls them—**empty-calorie foods.**

The preceding examples illustrate that the most significant difference between sugar sources is not between "natural" and "purified" sugar but between concentrated sweets and the dilute sugars of fruits and vegetables. When you are advised to decrease sugar consumption, it is primarily concentrated sugars such as sucrose and corn syrup that you are supposed to limit. How much sugar *do* you eat? Try the Carbohydrate Consumption Scorecard on the next page, which checks your diet for sugar, starch, and fiber, to find out.

EMPTY-CALORIE FOODS a phrase used to indicate that a food supplies calories but negligible nutrients. When many empty-calorie foods are eaten regularly, they displace nutrient-dense foods from the diet and contribute to both poor nutritional health and obesity.

Sugar and Health

Sugar is often in the headlines and has been accused of contributing to a host of human ills such as tooth decay, obesity, diabetes, heart disease, hyperactive behavior in children, and even criminal behavior. Nevertheless, research studies have not shown a direct link between sugar and any of these conditions, except tooth decay (see the Nutrition Action feature starting on page 72).[2] However, eating a lot of sugar could mean that you are eating an inadequate amount of foods containing essential nutrients. Conversely, if you eat a lot of sugar without eating less of other foods, you might be getting too many calories.

Rating Your Diet: How Sweet Is It?

Now that you are aware of some of the sources of added sugars, let's take a look at *your* diet. Check the box that most closely describes your eating habits to see how the foods you choose affect the amount of added sugars in your diet.

How often do you	SELDOM OR NEVER	1 OR 2 TIMES A WEEK	3 TO 5 TIMES A WEEK	ALMOST DAILY
1. Drink soft drinks, sweetened fruit drinks, or punches?	☐	☐	☐	☐
2. Choose sweet desserts and snacks, such as cakes, pies, cookies, and ice cream?	☐	☐	☐	☐
3. Use canned or frozen fruits packed in heavy syrup or add sugar to fresh fruit?	☐	☐	☐	☐
4. Eat candy?	☐	☐	☐	☐
5. Add sugar to coffee or tea?	☐	☐	☐	☐
6. Use jam, jelly, or honey on bread or rolls?	☐	☐	☐	☐

How Did You Do? The more often you choose the items listed above, the higher your diet is likely to be in sugars. You may need to cut back on sugar-containing foods, especially those you checked as "3 to 5 times a week" or more. This does not mean eliminating these foods from your diet. You can moderate your intake of sugars by choosing foods that are high in sugar less often and by eating smaller portions.

Check Your Diet for Starch and Fiber

How often do you eat	SELDOM OR NEVER	1 OR 2 TIMES A WEEK	3 TO 4 TIMES A WEEK	ALMOST DAILY
1. Several servings of breads, cereals, pasta, or rice?	☐	☐	☐	☐
2. Starchy vegetables such as potatoes, corn, or peas or dishes made with dried beans or peas?	☐	☐	☐	☐
3. Whole-grain breads or cereals?	☐	☐	☐	☐
4. Several servings of vegetables?	☐	☐	☐	☐
5. Whole fruit with skins and/or seeds (berries, apples, pears, etc.)?	☐	☐	☐	☐

How Did You Do? The best answer for all of the above is ALMOST DAILY. Breads, cereals, and other grain products and starchy vegetables provide starch. Whole-grain products, legumes, fruits, and vegetables, especially those with edible skins and seeds, are good sources of fiber.

SOURCE: USDA Home & Garden Bulletin.

Excess calories from any energy nutrient, even protein, are stored as body fat. Evidence from population studies in many countries shows that obesity rates rise as sugar consumption increases. One reason may be that many sugary foods, such as candy bars, are also high in fat.

There is no reason to believe that moderate consumption of sugar (5 percent to 10 percent of calories) is dangerous to a healthy human being. The guideline to limit sugar to less than 10 percent of total calories does not apply to *all* sugars in the diet. The diluted *naturally occurring* sugars found in milk and fruits should not be confused with concentrated refined sugars, such as table sugar, honey, and corn syrup. These concentrated sweets should be avoided if they displace needed nutrients.

After digestion, purified, refined white sugar—sucrose—yields a 50-50 mixture of glucose and fructose. In the body, the mixture becomes equivalent to pure glucose (because fructose is converted to glucose). As such, it differs in no way from the glucose that comes from starch. However, starch usually comes in foods with other nutrients, whereas sugar itself contains no other nutrients—no protein, vitamins, or minerals—and so can be termed an empty-calorie food. If you have 200 calories to "spend" on something and you spend them on sugar, you get very little value in terms of nutrients for your outlay. If 200 calories equal 10 percent of your total energy allowance, they ought to bring 10 percent of your total needed nutrients with them. If you spend your 200 calories on three slices of whole-wheat bread instead, you get 18 percent of the protein, 18 percent of the thiamin, and 12 percent of the niacin recommended for a day, as well as comparable amounts of many other nutrients (see Table 3–3). Whether you can afford to eat sugar, then,

TABLE 3–3

SAMPLE NUTRIENTS IN SUGARS AND OTHER CARBOHYDRATE-RICH FOODS

The indicated portion of any of these foods would provide approximately 100 calories. Notice what nutrients the eater receives along with the energy.

FOOD	SIZE OF 100-CALORIE PORTION	GRAMS OF CARBOHYDRATE	Protein	Fiber	PERCENTAGE OF DAILY VALUE* Calcium	Iron	Vitamin A	Vitamin C
Shredded wheat (spoon-size)	⅔ c	27	6	12	1	5	0	0
Kidney beans	½ c	22	13	32	4	13	<1	3
Watermelon	4″×8″ wedge	23	4	8	3	12	50	60
Whole-wheat bread	1½ slices	20	9	16	4	7	0	0
Sugar, white	2 tbsp	24	0	0	0	0	0	0
Blackstrap molasses	2 tbsp	22	0	0	27	35	0	0
Cola beverage	1 c	26	0	0	0	0	0	0
Honey	1½ tbsp	26	0	0	0	0	0	0
Jelly	2 tbsp	26	0	0	0	0	0	0
Recommended Daily Values		300 g	50 g	25 g	1,000 mg	18 mg	1,000 RE	60 mg

*Percentages are rounded to the nearest whole number. The Daily Values shown are recommended adult intakes based on a 2,000-calorie diet.

depends on the overall nutrient density of your diet and the number of calories you have to spend altogether.

It is theoretically possible, with careful food selection, to obtain all the needed nutrients within an allowance of about 1,500 calories—but this is not easy for most people. For example, a teenage boy needs as many as 4,000 calories to get all the energy he needs. If he eats some very nutritious foods, perhaps the empty calories of soft drinks are an acceptable part of his diet. On the other hand, since many teenage girls eat 1,200 calories or even less, they can afford to take in only the most nutrient-dense foods and should avoid empty-calorie foods. Overconsumption of sugar can clearly cause malnutrition, not by any positive action of its own but by displacing nutrients that prevent malnutrition. Nutritious foods must come first.

Keeping Sweetness in the Diet

The taste of sweetness is a pleasure; the liking for it is innate. However, the *Dietary Guidelines for Americans* recommends that people use concentrated sweets only in moderation. To help with this task while still catering to the sweet tooth, consider the following pointers:

- Use less of all sugars, including white sugar, brown sugar, raw sugar, honey, and syrups.
- Eat less of foods containing large amounts of sugars, such as soft drinks, candy, ice cream, cakes, and cookies.
- Select fresh fruits or fruits canned without sugar or in light syrup rather than heavy syrup to satisfy your urge for sweets.
- Read ingredient lists on food labels for clues on sugar content—if the word *sucrose, glucose, maltose, dextrose, fructose,* or *syrup* appears first, the food contains a large amount of sugar (see Figure 3–1 on page 70). Use sparingly foods in which these sweeteners are among the first three ingredients listed. Table 3–4 shows the amounts of sugar in some common products.
- Remember, for dental health, how frequently you eat sugar is as important as—and perhaps more important than—how much sugar you eat at one time (see the Nutrition Action feature on page 72).

Alternatives to sweet desserts might be whole-grain crackers, low-fat cheese, and yogurt. Snacks for children could include fruits, raw vegetables, popcorn, unsalted nuts, homemade fruit juice popsicles, and other wholesome foods. Here are some other suggestions:

- Substitute fruit *juices* or plain water for fruit drinks, regular soft drinks, and punches that contain considerable amounts of sugar.
- Buy *unsweetened* cereals so that you can control the amount of sugar added. Many cereals are presweetened. Check the Nutrition Facts panel for the grams of sugar present (see Figure 3–1). Many list sugar first—or second and third—among their ingredients.
- Experiment with reducing the sugar in your favorite recipes. Some recipes taste just the same even after a 25 percent to 50 percent reduction in sugar content. Others taste different, but just as—if not more—delicious.

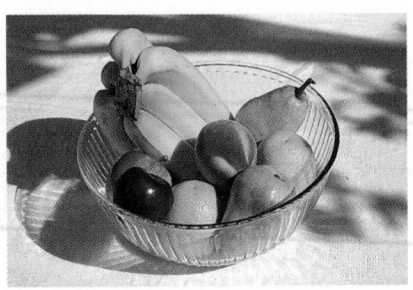

Naturally sweet foods like fruit can satisfy your sweet tooth.

● The sweet spices—allspice, anise, cardamom, cinnamon, cloves, fennel, ginger, and nutmeg—can replace substantial sugar in recipes. Use half as much sugar and increase one and a half times the amount of spice the recipe calls for. Increasing the amount of extracts like vanilla can enhance sweetness, too. Experiment with other extracts like maple, coconut, banana, and chocolate; add chopped dried fruit to baked goods for extra sweetness and nutrients as you decrease sugar.

For a fun dessert, put a whole ripe banana on a cookie sheet (leave the peel on) and bake at 350 degrees for 20 minutes. Split baked fruit with knife; sprinkle with cinnamon or nutmeg.

Still another alternative is to use sugary foods that convey nutrients as well as calories. Examples: rather than sugar cookies, serve oatmeal cookies; rather than brownies, eat apricot bars; and rather than table sugar as a topping, add raisins and banana slices, which are really very sweet.

Keep in mind that sugar is delicious and that you can use it with discretion, but use it in moderation. The person with nutrition sense and a taste for sweets can artfully combine the two by using sugar with creative imagination to enhance the flavors of nutritious foods.

You may wonder whether using artificial sweeteners to reduce some of the total sugar in your diet is a safe and recommended strategy. The Nutrition Action feature "Sweet Talk," starting on page 74, will help you decide.

TABLE 3–4 SUGAR IN SELECTED FOODS	
FOOD	**TEASPOONS OF SUGAR PER SERVING**
Angel food cake, (¹⁄₁₂ of cake)	5
Apple pie (⅙ of pie)	6
Applesauce, sweetened (½ c)	5
Cake, frosted (¹⁄₁₆ of cake)	6
Catsup (1 tbsp)	1
Cereal, sweetened (Sugar Pops, ¾ c)	4
Chewing gum (2 sticks)	1
Chocolate milk, 2 percent (1 c)	3
Chocolate shake (10 oz)	9
Cola (12 oz)	9
Cookie, Oreo type (1)	1
Dairy creamer (1 tbsp)	2
Doughnuts, glazed (1)	4
Doughnuts, plain (1)	2
Fig bars (2)	10
Fruit, canned in heavy syrup (½ c)	4
Fruit drink, ade (12 oz)	12
Fudge (1 oz)	5
Gelatin dessert (½ c)	4
Ice cream, ice milk, or frozen yogurt (½ c)	3
Jellybeans (10)	7
Sherbet (½ c)	5
Sugar, jam, or jelly (1 tsp)	1
Syrup or honey (1 tbsp)	3
Yogurt, fruit flavored (1 c)	7

FIGURE 3–1
USING THE INGREDIENTS LIST ON FOOD LABELS

The cereal shown contains sugars. To find out how much, start by checking the carbohydrate section of the Nutrition Facts panel for sugars. This number refers to both the sugars added by the manufacturer and the simple sugars naturally present in the food. Many cereals contain considerably more sugar than this cereal contains. Check labels and make your own comparisons. The more processed the food is, the more likely it is to contain sugar. Learn to read the ingredients list (see label at right). Labels list ingredients in order of amount by weight with the greatest amount of an ingredient present in the food listed first. Check labels for sugar terms, in addition to sucrose, listed in the accompanying Miniglossary. If one or more of these sweeteners are listed first, second, or third on the label, the food contains a large proportion of sugar. Use sparingly foods in which these sweeteners are among the first three ingredients listed.

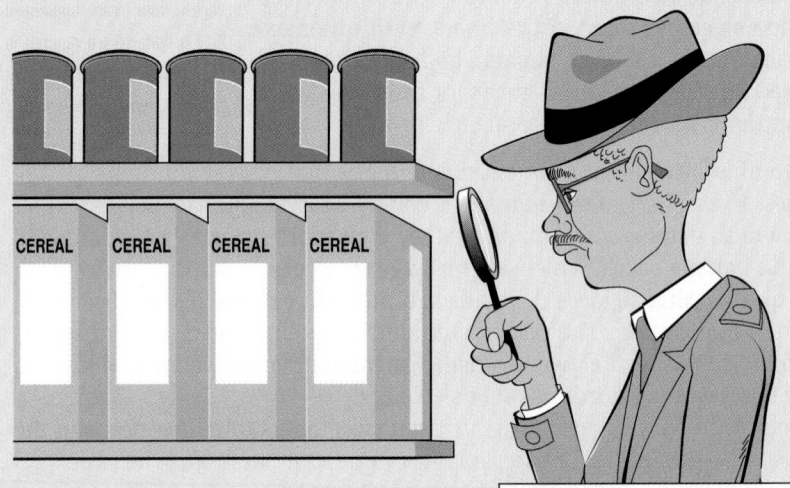

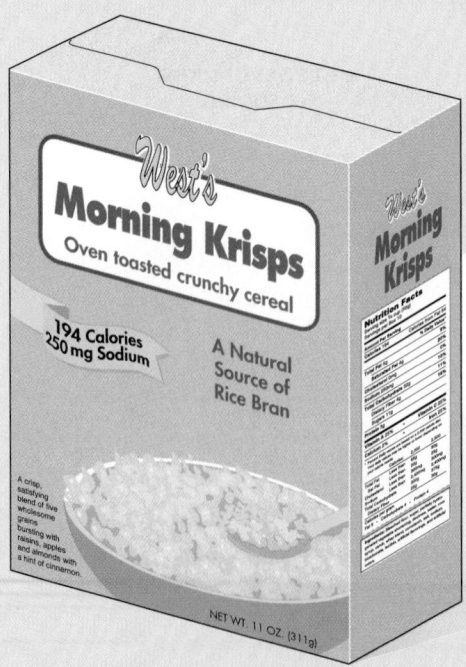

West's **Morning Krisps**
Oven toasted crunchy cereal

194 Calories
250 mg Sodium

A Natural Source of Rice Bran

NET WT. 11 OZ. (311g)

Nutrition Facts

Serving size ¾ cup (55g)
Servings per Box 5

Amount Per Serving

Calories 194	Calories from Fat 54

	% Daily Value*
Total Fat 6g	**9%**
Saturated Fat 4g	**20%**
Cholesterol 0mg	**0%**
Sodium 250mg	**10%**
Total Carbohydrate 32g	**11%**
Dietary Fiber 4g	**16%**
Sugars 11g	
Protein 3g	

Vitamin A 25%	•	**Vitamin C** 25%
Calcium 2%	•	**Iron** 25%

*Percent Daily Values are based on a 2,000 calorie diet. Your Daily Values may be higher or lower depending on your calorie needs.

	Calories:	2,000	2,500
Total Fat	Less than	65g	80g
Sat Fat	Less than	20g	25g
Cholesterol	Less than	300mg	300mg
Sodium	Less than	2,400mg	2,400mg
Total Carbohydrate		300g	375g
Dietary Fiber		25g	30g

Calories per gram
Fat 9 • Carbohydrate 4 • Protein 4

Ingredients: Brown rice, wheat gluten, sugar, partially hydrogenated vegetable shortening, dextrose, water, corn syrup, whey blend, cornstarch, salt, sodium bicarbonate, raisins, dehydrated apple, almond, and cinnamon.

MINIGLOSSARY OF SWEETENERS

BROWN RICE SYRUP similar to honey in taste and consistency; also available as a powder.

BROWN SUGAR white sugar with molasses added; about 95% pure sucrose.

CONCENTRATED FRUIT JUICE SWEETENER a concentrated sugar syrup made from dehydrated, deflavored fruit juice, commonly grape juice, used to sweeten products such as jams and cookies that can then claim to be "all fruit."

CONFECTIONERS SUGAR finely powdered sucrose; 99.9% pure sucrose.

CORN SWEETENERS corn syrup and sugars derived from corn.

CORN SYRUP a syrup produced by the action of enzymes on cornstarch; contains mostly glucose.

DEXTROSE another name for glucose.

FRUCTOSE, GALACTOSE, GLUCOSE the monosaccharides.

GRANULATED SUGAR common table sugar; crystalline sucrose—99.9% pure sucrose.

HIGH-FRUCTOSE CORN SYRUP (HFCS) the predominant sweetener used in processed foods and beverages; contains mostly fructose, with some glucose and maltose.

HONEY primarily a mixture of glucose and fructose made by bees from the sucrose in nectar.

INVERT SUGAR a mixture of glucose and fructose formed by splitting sucrose in processing; sold in liquid form and used as an additive to prevent crystallization of sucrose in candies and other confections.

LACTOSE, MALTOSE, SUCROSE the disaccharides.

LEVULOSE another name for fructose.

MALTITOL, MANNITOL, SORBITOL, XYLITOL sugar alcohols that can be derived from fruits or commercially produced from dextrose; absorbed more slowly and metabolized differently than other sugars in the human body. The sugar alcohols are not readily used by ordinary mouth bacteria and therefore are associated with less cavity formation. Although the sugar alcohols are used as sugar substitutes, they add the same amount of calories as sugar does to a food product. They are found in a wide variety of chewing gums, candies, and dietetic foods.

MAPLE SYRUP a concentrated form of sucrose purified from the sap of the sugar maple tree; maple sugar is made from the syrup.

MOLASSES a thick brown syrup; a leftover from the process of refining sucrose from sugar cane; blackstrap molasses contains certain minerals—notably iron—picked up from the machinery used to process it.

NATURAL SWEETENERS a term without a legal definition; refers to any sugar or sweetener other than refined table sugar.

RAW SUGAR the first crystals produced during the sugar refining process; not sold in the United States because of the presence of "filth" (dirt, insect fragments).

TURBINADO SUGAR raw sugar that has been washed to remove the filth.

WHITE SUGAR pure sugar; made by dissolving, concentrating, and recrystallizing raw sugar.

Keeping Out from Under the Dental Drill

For years, conventional wisdom has held that staying away from candy, cookies, sugary soda pop, and the like is the most important line of dietary defense against cavities. Even Aristotle asked in about 350 B.C., "Why do figs when they are sweet, produce damage to the teeth?"[3]

These days, dentists advise that cutting down on the amount of sugar eaten is not the only way to prevent **dental caries.** Every bit as—if not more—important to consider is whether a food clings to the teeth and lingers in the mouth as well as when and how often it's eaten. It has to do with the mouth's level of acid. Each time you bite into a food, the bacteria that live in your mouth feed on the sugar in it and release an acid that eats away at tooth enamel. When a large number of bacteria living in a film referred to as **dental plaque** produce enough acid to dissolve a "hole" in the enamel over a period of time, the result is a cavity.

While consuming sugary items such as soft drinks boosts acid production in the mouth, so does munching on starchy foods such as crackers or pretzels. This is because enzymes in the saliva can break the carbohydrate in the cracker or pretzel into the simple sugars that bacteria feast on. If a crumb or two from a starchy food gets caught between the teeth, it might provide enough carbohydrate for bacteria to feed on for hours, thereby prolonging the teeth's exposure to acid. In fact, some research indicates that even high-sugar foods such as chocolate bars and hot fudge sundaes are less likely to contribute to cavity formation than stickier, starchier items that are likely to linger in the mouth, such as potato chips and crackers.[4]

To be sure, the carbohydrate content and stickiness of a food are only two of the many factors that influence the food's effect on teeth. Another is how often you eat the food. Each time you eat a carbohydrate-containing food, your teeth are bathed in acids for about 20 minutes. Thus, the more often you eat, the longer your teeth are exposed to harmful acids.[5]

Yet another factor is what you eat along with the food. Starchy, sugary foods tend to be less harmful to the teeth when eaten with a meal than when consumed alone. One reason may be that the mouth makes more saliva during a full meal. That's crucial, because even though saliva helps make sugar for bacteria, it also clears food particles from the mouth and neutralizes destructive acids before they can dissolve the teeth. Consider that one study at the University of Iowa's College of Dentistry found that after people nibbled on foods with a strong tendency to produce acid, such as raisins and chocolate bars, and then chewed sugarless gum, within ten minutes the gum helped stimulate the release of enough saliva to neutralize the acid flow that the sweets had caused.[6] In addition, some research suggests that, like sugarless chewing gum,

DENTAL CARIES decay of the teeth, or cavities.

caries = rottenness

DENTAL PLAQUE a colorless film, consisting of bacteria and their by-products, that is constantly forming on the teeth.

such foods as cheese and peanuts help fight acid attacks stimulated by eating carbohydrate-rich foods.[7]

Of course, while saliva helps fight cavities, the best way to ensure good dental health is to brush your teeth as soon as possible after eating, or at least swish the mouth with water or milk after a meal to help rinse the teeth and dislodge stuck particles. Flossing daily is also important because flossing rids the mouth not only of food but also of plaque before it becomes so widespread that it produces tooth-threatening levels of acid. Regular visits to the dentist play a role in keeping dental health up to snuff. In addition, drinking water containing fluoride, a mineral that helps strengthen tooth enamel, can prevent cavities. People whose drinking water does not supply fluoride should check with a dentist about the need for fluoride supplements.

Along with practicing good dental hygiene, eating a balanced diet helps keep the mouth healthy. One reason is that if the diet lacks essential nutrients, mouth tissues can become compromised, leaving them particularly vulnerable to infection. In fact, some experts believe that **periodontal disease** is especially severe among people who have poor diets.[9] Another reason to eat an adequate diet, particularly for children, is that it helps to ensure proper development of the teeth.[10] Similarly, eating well should rank as a high priority for a pregnant woman, whose unborn baby's teeth, among other things, start forming after just six weeks and begin to harden between the first and second trimester of pregnancy.[11]

Incidentally, parents should never allow an infant to sleep with a bottle filled with sweetened liquids, fruit juices, milk, or formula. Little ones allowed to do so often develop what is known as **nursing bottle syndrome.** As a baby sucks on a bottle, the tongue pushes outward slightly and covers the lower teeth. If the infant falls asleep with the bottle in the mouth, the liquid bathes the teeth, particularly the upper teeth not protected by the tongue, thereby literally soaking them in cavity-causing carbohydrates for hours at a time.

PERIODONTAL DISEASE inflammation or degeneration of the tissues that surround and support the teeth.

NURSING BOTTLE SYNDROME (also called baby bottle tooth decay) decay of all the upper and sometimes the back lower teeth that occurs in infants given carbohydrate-containing liquids when they sleep. The syndrome can also develop in babies given bottles of liquid to carry around and sip all day.

For optimal dental health, the American Dental Association (ADA) recommends:[8]

- Eat a balanced diet.

- Keep snacking to a minimum, if possible. The ADA recognizes that some people, such as people with diabetes, may require snacks. For others, however, the ADA suggests limiting the number of snacks if brushing the teeth is not possible shortly after eating them.

- Eat sweets with meals rather than between them.

- Brush and floss thoroughly each day to remove dental plaque.

- Use an ADA-accepted fluoride toothpaste and mouth rinse and talk to your dentist about the need for supplemental fluoride.

- Visit a dentist regularly.

- Do not allow infants to sleep with bottles in their mouth that contain sweetened liquids, fruit juices, milk, or formula.

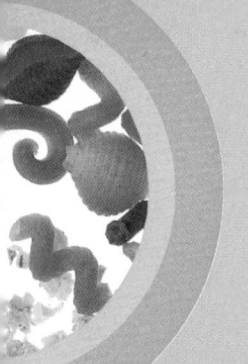

Sweet Talk: Alternatives to Sugar

It all started back in 1879—the year that a substance called saccharin was first discovered and found to be able to sweeten foods without adding calories. Since that time, the sale of **artificial sweeteners** for use in tabletop sweeteners, such as Sweet 'N Low and Equal, and in artificially sweetened soft drinks, yogurt, and numerous other products has become a $1.4-billion-a-year business.[12] But despite the ever-growing popularity of such sweeteners, doubts about their safety have stirred a good deal of controversy over the years. In addition, confusion about the characteristics of the various alternatives to sugar (see Table 3–5) and their role in fighting problems such as obesity and tooth decay prevail among the millions of Americans who use them. The following assumptions about sugar substitutes and the facts behind them should help put matters into perspective.

ARTIFICIAL SWEETENERS nonnutritive sugar replacements such as acesulfame K, aspartame, and saccharin.

TABLE 3–5
HOW SWEET IT IS

NAME (TRADE NAME)	SWEETENERS COMPARED WITH SUCROSE	CHARACTERISTICS[a]
SWEETENERS APPROVED FOR USE IN THE UNITED STATES		
Acesulfame K (Sunette/Sweet One)	200 times sweeter	Stable in high temperatures; soluble in water
Aspartame[b] (NutraSweet/Equal)	180 times sweeter	Loses sweetness at high temperatures and may lose sweetness over time; cannot be used in baking or cooking but can be added to cooked products after heating
Saccharin (Sweet'N Low)	300 times sweeter	Stable at high temperatures
SWEETENERS FOR WHICH U.S. APPROVAL IS PENDING		
Alitame (Novasweet)	2,000 times sweeter	Stable at high temperatures and in both acidic and nonacidic foods; highly soluble in water
Cyclamate[c]	30 times sweeter	Stable at high temperatures; long shelf life
Sucralose[d] (Splenda)	600 times sweeter	Stable at various temperatures

[a]In addition to the characteristics listed, all of the sweeteners have a synergistic effect when combined with other sweeteners. In other words, together they enhance each other's sweetness, yielding a combined sweetness greater than the sum of all the substances' sweetness.

[b]The NutraSweet Company held the patent on aspartame from 1981 to 1992. NutraSweet is still the most common trade name for aspartame, but others may become common in the future.

[c]Cyclamate was banned in the United States in 1970 because studies suggested that it may cause cancer in rats. The validity of the studies has been questioned, however. Currently, a petition is before the FDA to reapprove cyclamate for use in the United States. In Canada, cyclamate has been approved for use in tabletop sweeteners and as a sweetening agent in drugs.

[d]In 1991, Canada became the first country to approve sucralose for use in foods.

SOURCE: Calorie Council Sweetener Fact Sheets: acesulfame K, alitame, aspartame, cyclamate, saccharin, and sucralose; American Council on Science and Health, *Low-Calorie Sweeteners* (New York: American Council on Science and Health, 1993), pp. 3–28.

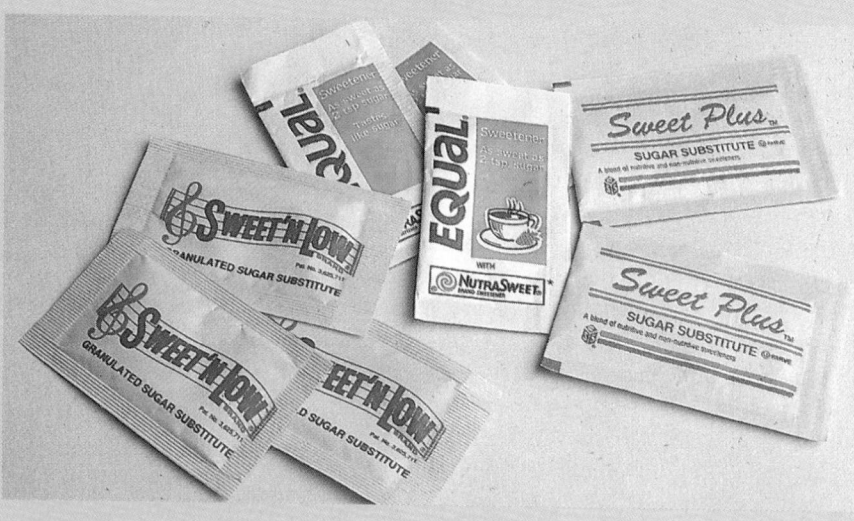

Small Amounts of Saccharin Cause Cancer

This assumption has never been proven. It's true that some studies of **saccharin,** the sweetener in Sweet 'N Low, have found that it can cause bladder cancer in laboratory rats. A human, however, would have to drink 850 cans of soft drinks a day to take in a dose equivalent to what the rats in those studies were given. Moreover, some research suggests that while very high doses of saccharin may promote bladder cancer in rats, the sweetener does not have the same impact on mice, hamsters, monkeys, or humans.[13] In addition, investigations of large groups of people have yet to establish any clear-cut link between saccharin consumption and the risk of cancer. One study conducted by the National Cancer Institute and involving more than 9,000 men and women showed no association between saccharin use and bladder cancer.[14] Thus, it appears that the health risks, if any, posed by saccharin are minuscule at most. Those fearful of getting cancer would be better off quitting smoking or reducing the amount of fat in their diet than worrying about putting Sweet 'N Low in their coffee now and then. As the American Medical Association's Council on Scientific Affairs has stated, "In humans, available evidence indicates that the use of artificial sweeteners, including saccharin, is not associated with an increased risk of bladder cancer."[15]

Aspartame Can Be Used to Sweeten Baked Goods

Not so. **Aspartame,** the artificial sweetening agent most often marketed under the trade name NutraSweet, cannot be used in products that require cooking or baking because it breaks down upon heating and releases tiny amounts of methyl alcohol, which imparts a sour flavor. It can be used only to sweeten warm and cold foods and liquids or can be added to foods once they have already been cooked.

Saccharin, on the other hand, can withstand the high temperatures needed for cooking or baking. The same goes for **acesulfame potassium** (or acesulfame K, the chemical symbol for potassium), marketed as Sunette.

SACCHARIN a zero-calorie sweetener discovered in 1879 and used in the United States since the turn of the century. A possible link to bladder cancer has led to saccharin's being banned as a food additive in Canada, although it is available there as a tabletop sweetener; it is used with a warning label in the United States and is the sweetening agent in Sweet 'N Low.

ASPARTAME a dipeptide (see Chapter 5) containing the amino acids aspartic acid and phenylalanine and used in the United States and Canada since 1981. While it is digested as protein and supplies calories, it is so sweet that only small amounts, which contribute negligible calories, are needed to sweeten foods. Thus, it is classified as a nonnutritive sweetener. Often sold under the trade name NutraSweet, aspartame is blended with lactose and an anticaking agent and sold commercially as Equal.

ACESULFAME K (AY-see-sul-fame) a derivative of acetoacetic acid approved for use in the United States in 1988 (approval in Canada is still under consideration). Since it is not metabolized by the body, acesulfame K does not contribute calories and is excreted from the body unchanged. It is currently approved for use in more than 70 countries and found in more than 100 international products, including chewing gum, gelatins, nondairy creamers, powdered drink mixes, and puddings.

Aspartame Causes Headaches

Not in most people. While the Food and Drug Administration has received numerous complaints from consumers who claim to suffer from headaches, nausea, anxiety, and other symptoms after consuming aspartame-containing foods or beverages, scientific studies have never confirmed that the sweetener is truly the culprit. Consider that scientists at Duke University who conducted carefully controlled research into the matter concluded that tablets containing the amount of aspartame in about four liters of diet soft drinks were no more likely to prompt headaches in people than **placebo** pills administered for the sake of comparison.[16] Furthermore, numerous careful scientific investigations carried out both before and after aspartame first appeared on the market have indicated that the product brings about adverse health effects only in a small group of people with a rare metabolic disorder known as **phenylketonuria,** or PKU. People born with PKU must carefully control their consumption of phenylalanine—one of the two amino acids that make up aspartame—to prevent health problems as severe as mental retardation. The American Medical Association's Council on Scientific Affairs, the Centers for Disease Control and Prevention, the Food and Drug Administration, The American Dietetic Association, and numerous other health organizations all consider the sweetener safe for use except by people with PKU.[17] Table 3–6 shows how to determine the amount of aspartame in your diet.

PLACEBO (plah-SEE-bo) a sham treatment given to a control group; an inert, harmless "treatment" that the group's members cannot recognize as different from the real thing. This will minimize the chance that an effect of the treatment will appear to have occurred due to the **placebo effect**—the healing effect that the belief in the treatment, rather than the treatment itself, often has.

PHENYLKETONURIA an inborn error of metabolism, detectable at birth, in which the body lacks the enzyme needed to convert the amino acid phenylalanine to the amino acid tyrosine. As a result, derivatives of phenylalanine accumulate in the blood and tissues, where they can cause severe damage, including mental retardation.

TABLE 3–6
CHECKING THE ASPARTAME IN YOUR DIET

The Food and Drug Administration has set forth an "acceptable daily intake" of 50 milligrams of aspartame per kilogram (2.2 pounds) of body weight. Most people, however, take in much less—on the order of fewer than 5 milligrams per kilogram daily. To reach the FDA's limit, consider that a 150-pound adult would have to consume about 19 12-ounce cans of diet soda pop or 97 packets of Equal, and a 50-pound child would have to consume six 12-ounce cans of diet soft drinks or 32 packets of Equal. To see how much aspartame you're getting in your diet, check the following numbers for the average amount of aspartame found in typical artificially sweetened foods.

ASPARTAME-SWEETENED FOOD	MILLIGRAMS OF ASPARTAME
1 packet Equal tabletop sweetener	35
12 ounces diet soda pop	180
4 ounces gelatin dessert	95
6 ounces hot chocolate	50
4 ounces pudding	25
1 cup cereal	55
8 ounces iced tea made with instant, sweetened mix	80
12 ounces wine cooler	89
8 ounces yogurt	124

SOURCES: Position of the American Dietetic Association: Use of nutritive and nonnutritive sweeteners, *Journal of The American Dietetic Association* 93 (1993): 818; Approximate aspartame content in Food and Drug Administration–approved categories, The NutraSweet Company.

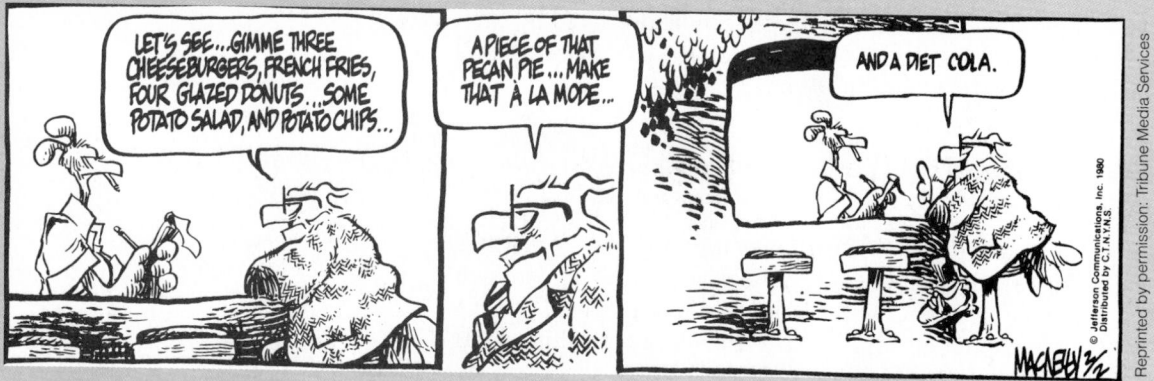

Use of Artificial Sweeteners Will Bring About Weight Loss

If only it were that simple. Obviously, because artificially sweetened foods typically contain fewer calories than their sugar-sweetened counterparts, substituting a low-calorie alternative for a sugar-laden one can help a person who is trying to lose weight enjoy sweet-tasting foods and save calories. But simply *adding* foods sweetened with sugar substitutes to the diet will not do the trick. Moreover, eating artificially sweetened foods to have an excuse to splurge on a high-calorie food defeats the purpose. A person who drinks diet soda pop to justify eating an ice cream sundae later is reaping little, if any, benefit. In other words, it's the way in which you fit artificial sweeteners into the rest of your diet that counts.

On the flip side, some consumers may be under the impression that artificial sweeteners bolster the appetite. Back in 1986, a report that aspartame sends mixed signals to the brain and thereby increases appetite as well as food consumption spawned the notion that artificial sweeteners can interfere with weight loss.[18] That report was based on comparisons of the effects of drinking plain water and drinking aspartame- and sugar-sweetened water, however, rather than consuming actual foods or beverages that are typically sweetened with aspartame. Moreover, the researchers did not measure how much food people ate after drinking the liquids. Thus, the study did not show how consuming aspartame-sweetened foods influences appetite and eating behavior in the "real world."

Since that time, about a dozen investigations into the relationship between appetite and foods and beverages sweetened with the substances have indicated that aspartame either lessens, or doesn't affect, feelings of hunger or the amount of food ultimately eaten.[19] So for now, at least, it appears that aspartame's impact on appetite need not be of concern to those trying to lose weight.

Foods Sweetened with Sugar Substitutes do not Contribute to Tooth Decay

Not necessarily. As pointed out earlier, any carbohydrate-containing food, be it sugar sweetened or otherwise, can promote tooth decay. When you eat a sugary food, the millions of bacteria lurking on the surfaces of and between your teeth feast on the sugar and, in the process, release an acid that eats away at tooth enamel. Once inside the mouth, carbohydrates can be devoured by cavity-causing bacteria because enzymes in the saliva break the complex carbohydrates into simple sugars, which bacteria thrive on.

People with Diabetes Should Eat Foods Sweetened Only with Sugar Substitutes

That depends. It is often assumed that because one of the hallmarks of diabetes is high blood sugar (glucose), sugar from foods is the major culprit behind high blood sugar and should therefore be off limits for people with diabetes. But it's not that simple. The total amount of carbohydrate, including both simple and complex, exerts the most influence on blood glucose levels. What's more, many other factors, including the amount of fat and fiber in a food, affect the body's blood glucose response to it. That's why people with diabetes do not have to limit themselves to only artificially sweetened foods. Sugar-containing items can be incorporated into a carefully designed eating plan.

Another reason that blanket statements about the use of sugar substitutes are not made for people with diabetes is that the various types of sweeteners behave differently in the body. A group of sugar substitutes known as **alternative sweeteners** (fructose, sorbitol, mannitol, and xylitol), for instance, contain calories but used to be frequently recommended for people with diabetes because the body generally absorbs them more slowly than it does table sugar. Most, however, have side effects that detract from their desirability. Some research suggests, for example, that large amounts of fructose may contribute to rises in blood cholesterol levels, making fructose a poor choice for the many people whose diabetes goes hand in hand with heart disease. By the same token, some people experience diarrhea after consuming large amounts of sorbitol, mannitol, and xylitol, and those sweeteners' overall effect on blood glucose control is insignificant, according to the American Diabetes Association. Thus, the role sugar substitutes play in the overall diet is a decision that should be made individually with the help of a dietitian and a physician.[20]

ALTERNATIVE SWEETENERS nutritive (calorie-containing) sweeteners such as fructose, sorbitol, mannitol, and xylitol.

Sugar-free Chewing Gum Doesn't Contain Any Calories

Not so. Sugar-free chewing gum is sweetened with certain alternative sweeteners, such as xylitol and sorbitol, also known as sugar alcohols. While sugar alcohols impart a sweet taste and supply calories (about eight per stick), unlike sucrose, they do not promote tooth decay.

The Complex Carbohydrates and Health

Complex carbohydrates are thought to be our most valuable energy nutrient. The *Dietary Guidelines for Americans* includes the following suggestions:

- Choose a diet with plenty of grain products, vegetables, and fruits.
- Choose a diet moderate in sugars.

If you have been exposed to as much anticarbohydrate propaganda as most people have been, the statement that we need to consume more carbohydrates rather than less may be startling. Yet much evidence supports it. Figure 3–2 compares the number of servings of carbohydrates Americans actually consume with the recommended number of servings from the Food Guide Pyramid.[21] As you can see, the shape of the pyramid actually consumed is somewhat top-heavy, with liberal amounts of servings from the *Fats, Oils, and Sweets Group,* and is rather lean with servings from the groups offering complex carbohydrates—notably the *Bread, Cereal, Rice, and Pasta Group, Vegetable Group,* and *Fruit Group.* Table 3–7 presents pointers on how to build a more stable pyramid.

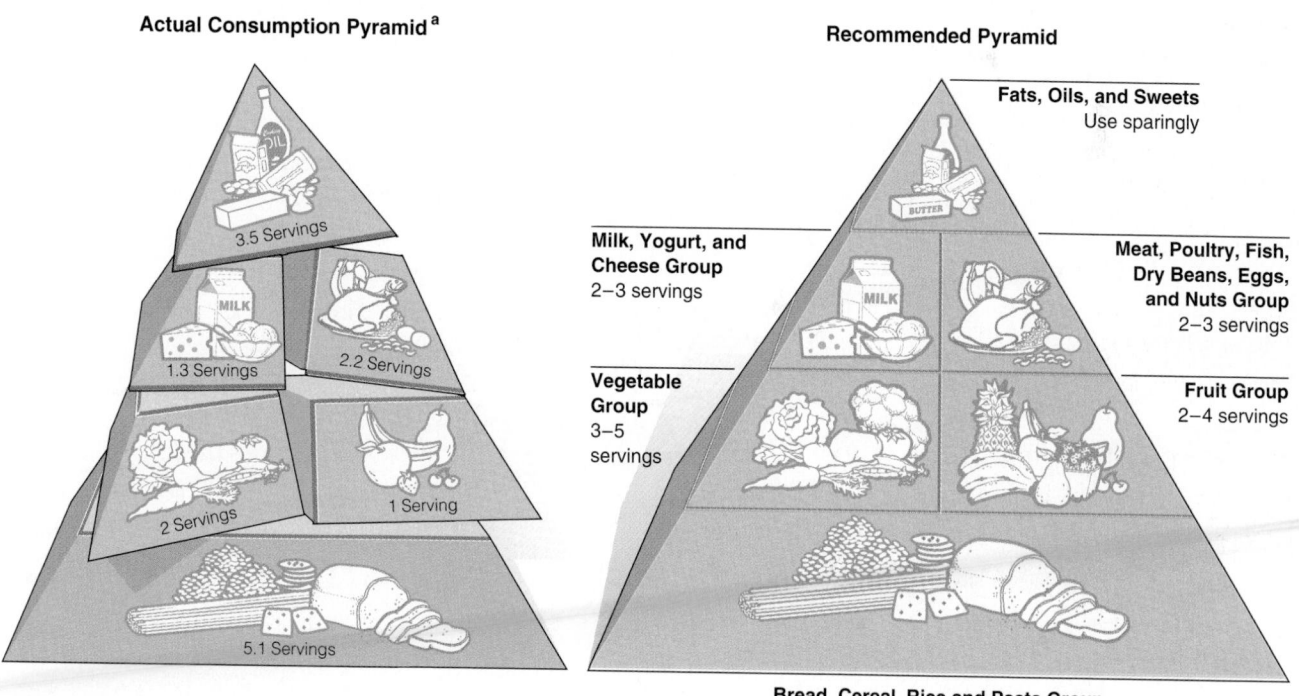

FIGURE 3–2 COMPARING PYRAMIDS: ACTUAL CONSUMPTION VERSUS RECOMMENDED SERVINGS OF CARBOHYDRATE IN THE DIET

While total carbohydrate in the diet is supposed to increase, sugar as a percentage of the total carbohydrate is supposed to decrease. The figure shows the actual servings being consumed from the Food Guide Pyramid compared to the recommended number of servings.

[a]The Actual Consumption Pyramid is from: *Eating in America,* Edition II (EAT II) (Chicago: National Livestock and Meat Board, 1994), p. 4.

TABLE 3–7
PYRAMID POINTERS: SELECTION TIPS FOR CARBOHYDRATES IN THE DIET[a]

BREAD, CEREAL, RICE, AND PASTA GROUP

Good source of complex carbohydrate, riboflavin, thiamin, niacin, iron, protein, magnesium, and fiber

- To get the fiber you need, choose several servings a day of foods made from whole grains.
- Go easy on the fats and sugars you add as spreads, seasonings, or toppings.
- Choose most often from the Best Choices column; those foods contain little fat.

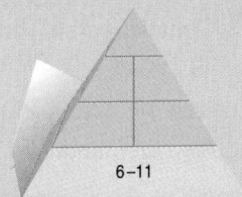

6–11

Best Choices (<3 g fat per serving)	Fair Choices (3 to 5 g fat per serving)	Use-Sparingly Choices (> 5 g fat per serving)
angel food cake	biscuit	cake
bagel	cookies: brownie, chocolate chip	cheese curls
breadsticks	flour tortilla (not fried)	chow mein noodles
crackers: animal crackers, matzoh crackers, melba toast, oyster crackers, rye crackers, saltines	croutons	cornbread
	muffin	corn chips
cookies: fig bars, gingersnaps, graham crackers, vanilla wafers	pizza crust	croissant
	popcorn (commercially popped, plain)	cupcake
corn tortilla (not fried)	presweetened cereals	doughnut
couscous		fried rice
English muffin		granola
enriched breads		pastry
farina		popcorn (commercially popped, buttered)
grits		stuffing
pancakes		toaster pastry
pasta		tortilla (fried)
pita bread		waffle
popcorn (air popped)		
pretzels		
ready-to-eat cereals		
rice		
rice cake		
taco shell		
whole-grains (wheat, oats, barley, bulgur, millet, rye)		

[a]This table includes four of the five pyramid groups that contain carbohydrate. The milk group also provides carbohydrate as lactose, a naturally occurring sugar. Refer to page 46 in Chapter 2 for serving sizes.

continued

TABLE 3–7
continued

VEGETABLE GROUP

Good source of vitamin A, vitamin C, folate, potassium, magnesium, and fiber

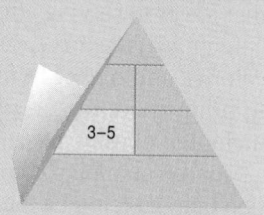

- Different types of vegetables provide different nutrients. Eat a variety.
- Go easy on the fat you add to vegetables at the table or during cooking.
- Include dark green leafy vegetables and legumes several times a week—they are especially good sources of dietary fiber, vitamins, and minerals.
- Choose most often from the Best Choices column; those foods contain little fat.

Best Choices (<2 g fat per serving)	Fair Choices (2 to 3 g fat per serving)	Use-Sparingly Choices (> 3 g fat per serving)
most vegetables (served raw, steamed, or microwaved and without butter, oil, or salt) vegetable juices vegetable soup (with fat removed)	vegetables served with a reduced-fat sauce	coleslaw French fries fried vegetables hash browns mashed potatoes potato chips potato salad scalloped potatoes

FRUIT GROUP

Good source of vitamin A, vitamin C, potassium, and fiber

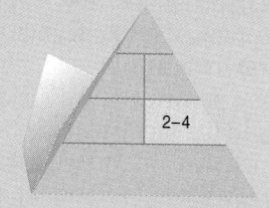

- Eat whole fruits often—they are higher in fiber than fruit juices.
- Go easy on fruits canned or frozen in heavy syrups and sweetened fruit juices.
- Count only 100 percent fruit juice as fruit. Punches, ades, and most fruit "drinks" contain only a little juice and lots of added sugars.
- Choose most often from the Best Choices column; those foods contain little fat.

Best Choices (< 2 g fat per serving)	Fair Choices (2 to 3 g fat per serving)	Use-Sparingly Choices (> 3 g fat per serving)
fresh fruits fruit juice frozen fruits without added sugar or syrup canned fruits packed in juice or water	olives	avocado

FATS, OILS, AND SWEETS GROUP

Use sparingly

- Go easy on sugars and fats added to foods in cooking or at the table—butter, margarine, gravy, salad dressing, sugar, and jelly.
- Choose fewer foods that are high in sugars—candy, sweet desserts, and soft drinks.

SOURCE: The foods listed in the table are adapted from Pyramid Packet, © 1993, Penn State Nutrition Center, 417 East Calder Way, University Park, PA 16801.

The health benefits to be expected from such a change would be many. A diet lower in servings from the *Fats, Oils, and Sweets Group* and higher in foods containing complex carbohydrates would almost necessarily be lower in fat and calories and higher in fiber. Working together, these factors might be expected to bring about or contribute to lower rates of the so-called lifestyle diseases—including obesity, heart disease, diabetes, cancer, and malnutrition.

Foods containing complex carbohydrates are usually lower in calories per portion than protein-rich foods because the latter often include considerable fat. A diet high in complex carbohydrates might be more beneficial for weight loss than a diet of comparable calories that is high in fat. Researchers report that altering the composition of the diet to achieve a higher carbohydrate-to-fat ratio may actually decrease the incidence of obesity.[22] One reason is that switching to a high complex carbohydrate (high-fiber) diet tends to make you feel full faster, which may reduce caloric intake.

Most health recommendations tell us to make reductions in four areas: fats and cholesterol, sodium, alcohol, and body weight. In contrast, complex carbohydrates are the nutrient most promoted by these health recommendations.

Complex Carbohydrates: Starch

All starchy foods are plant foods. **Starch** is made up of many glucose units bonded together—3,000 or so in each molecule of starch. Seeds such as grains, peas, and beans are the richest starch source. Most societies have a primary or **staple grain** that provides most of the people's food energy. In many Asian nations, the staple grain is rice. In Canada, the United States, and Europe, the staple grain is wheat. If you consider all the food products made from wheat—bread (and other baked goods made from wheat flour), cereals, and pasta—you will realize how all-pervasive this grain is in the food supply. The staple grains of other peoples include corn, millet, rye, barley, and oats.

STARCH a plant polysaccharide composed of glucose, digestible by human beings.

STAPLE GRAIN a grain used frequently or daily in the diet—for example, corn (in Mexico) or rice (in Asia).

A second important source of starch is the legume family, including such dried beans and peas as butter beans, kidney beans, pinto beans, navy beans, black-eyed peas, chick-peas (garbanzo beans), lentils, and soybeans. These vegetables are about 40 percent starch by weight and contain abundant protein. Root vegetables (such as yams) and tubers (such as potatoes) are other sources of starch that are important in many societies.

Starch can be broken down during food processing to shorter chains of glucose units known as dextrins. The word *dextrins* sometimes appears on food labels, because dextrins can be used as thickening agents in foods.

Adding Whole Foods to the Diet

As it happens, most of the nutrition goals and guidelines offered to date have had one point in common. They tend to favor a return toward a more whole-food, plant-based diet. The Worldwatch Institute (a private organization) has taken the position that the only known risk of such a trend would be to the food industry, whereas important benefits to the economy would counterbalance this effect. An increase in the consumption of fruits, vegetables, and whole grains and a decrease in the consumption of empty-calorie fats, oils, alcohol, and sugar would increase the nutrient density of our diet, thereby reducing malnutrition, including overnutrition.

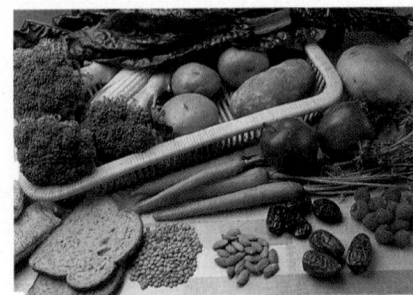

We are advised to increase our intakes of complex carbohydrates. The best way to get enough complex carbohydrates in your diet is to eat plenty of fruits, vegetables, legumes, and whole grains.

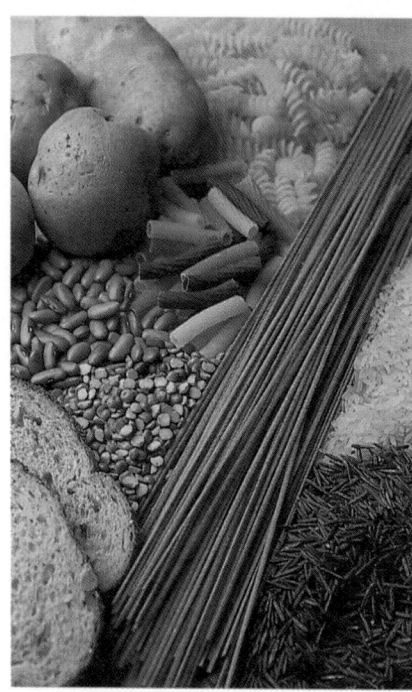

Foods such as potatoes, dried beans and peas, rice and whole-grain breads, cereals, and pastas are especially nutritious because of their starch, fiber, vitamin, and mineral content—and because they are virtually fat and cholesterol free.

Generally speaking, the more a food resembles the original, farm-grown product, the more nutritious it is likely to be. During processing, some nutrients may be lost, and often nutrient-poor additions such as sugar, salt, and fat are made. For example, a potato contains 20 milligrams of vitamin C, the same number of calories in French fries contain only about 7 milligrams, and the same number of calories in potato chips contain only 2 milligrams of vitamin C.

When you want to choose nutritious foods, a useful guideline is to choose **whole, natural foods.** But you don't have to do this all the time. Not every potato product you use must be recognizably potato. A principle that helps with making food choices is to ask, "What am I using this food for?" or "How big a part of my diet is this food?" The more you depend on a food as a **staple food,** the more important is its wholesomeness. If, for example, bread is one of your staple foods, whole-grain bread is certainly a better choice than refined, white bread (as the next section of this chapter demonstrates).

WHOLE FOOD a food that is altered as little as possible from the plant or animal tissue from which it was taken—such as beets, milk, or oats.

NATURAL FOOD one that has been altered as little as possible from the original farm-grown state. As used on labels, this term may misleadingly imply unusual power to promote health; it has no legal definition.

STAPLE FOOD a food used frequently or daily in the diet—for example, potatoes (in Ireland) or rice (in the Far East).

Conversely, the less often or heavily you use a food, the less its quality matters. An example is candy bars. If you eat them only on picnics and you picnic only once a year, they'll hardly detract from your nutrition on a year-round basis. But if you are eating nothing but candy bars for breakfast and lunch every day, they are a staple item in your diet and a very poor choice indeed.

Whether you choose to adopt these recommendations as your own goals is, of course, up to you. If you do, you will find the new food label a useful tool for locating foods that measure up to the current recommendations. Figure 3–3 examines the food label and the Nutrition Facts panel as they relate to carbohydrates in the diet.

The high-fiber, nutrient-dense foods from plants are most often lower in fat than animal-derived foods. People who eat mostly the former can therefore enjoy a nutritious diet that is low in fat, but only if other high-fat foods like nuts, olives, and butter are limited, too. Both the Consumer Tips feature on pages 100 and 101 and the Spotlight at the end of this chapter show how to include nutritious foods from various international cuisines.

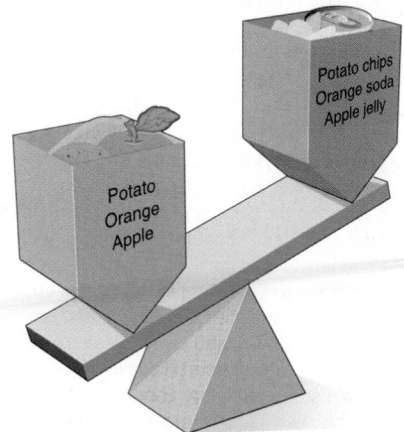

The whole food has the nutritional advantage. The nutrients supplied by the potato, orange, and apple far outweigh those from their empty-calorie processed forms.

FIGURE 3–3 CHECKING OUT THE FOOD LABEL: CARBOHYDRATE POINTERS

■ **Check the Nutrition Facts panel**, usually on the side or back of the package. The panel will give more complete nutrition information about the food.

■ **Serving Size and Calories per Serving**
First, look at the *serving size.* Since it is about the same for similar items, it is easy to compare the nutritional qualities of your favorite foods. Next, look at the *calories per serving.* The typical adult shopper for whom the Nutrition Facts panels are designed needs about 2,000 calories per day. A serving of this vegetable would therefore provide less than 2 percent of the consumer's daily calorie need.

■ **Nutrient Content Claims and Health Claims**
Look for claims (such as those shown at right), usually on the front of the package, describing a food's nutritional content or stating a health benefit. Food labels may carry health claims for fiber and disease risk. For example, foods that contain at least 0.6 g of soluble fiber per serving *and* are low-fat, low-saturated fat, and low-cholesterol may claim to reduce the risk of heart disease. Foods that are a *good* source of dietary fiber (contain at least 2.5 g of fiber per serving) *and* are low in fat may claim to reduce cancer risk. Such claims must state that the risk of heart disease or cancer depends on many factors.

■ **Total Carbohydrate**
Listing of *Total Carbohydrate, Dietary Fiber,* and *Sugars* is mandatory for most labels. The *Total Carbohydrate* value refers to the amounts of starch, dietary fiber, and sugar in a serving of the food. Some manufacturers voluntarily list soluble and

Nutrition Facts

Serving Size 3 oz
(84g/about 1/2 stalk)
Servings Per Container about 2.5

Amount Per Serving

Calories 30	Calories from Fat 0

	% Daily Value
Total Fat 0g	**0%**
Saturated Fat 0g	**0%**
Cholesterol 0mg	**0%**
Sodium 20mg	**1%**
Total Carbohydrate 5g	**2%**
Dietary Fiber 3g	**12%**
Soluble Fiber 1g	
Sugars 0g	
Protein 3g	

Vitamin A 25%	•	**Vitamin C** 110%
Calcium 4%	•	**Iron** 4%

*Percent Daily Values are based on a 2,000 calorie diet. Your Daily Values may be higher or lower depending on your calorie needs.

	Calories:	2,000	2,500
Total Fat	Less than	65g	80g
Sat Fat	Less than	20g	25g
Cholesterol	Less than	300mg	300mg
Sodium	Less than	2,400mg	2,400mg
Total Carbohydrate		300g	375g
Dietary Fiber		25g	30g

Ingredients: Broccoli cuts.

insoluble dietary fiber along with total dietary fiber in this section of the panel. *Sugars* include both *naturally occurring sugars* in fruits, vegetables, milk products, and other wholesome foods and added sugars — the sugar and other caloric sweeteners added by manufacturers during processing. Some manufacturers voluntarily list sugar alcohols here as well. Check the ingredients list on the package to identify added sugars. (Recall that the ingredients are listed in order of predominance by weight.) When the term *Other Carbohydrates* appears on the label, it refers to the complex carbohydrate content — total carbohydrate minus any sugar (monosaccharides and disaccharides) or dietary fiber in a serving of the food.

■ **% Daily Value**
Look at the column labeled *% Daily Value.* This column compares the total carbohydrate, dietary fiber, and other nutrients in a serving of the food with a person's daily need. The % Daily Value tells you whether the food has large or small amounts of total carbohydrate, dietary fiber, sugars, and other nutrients. Note at the bottom of the Nutrition Facts panel that for a person requiring 2,000 calories a day, the Daily Value for carbohydrate is 300 g and the Daily Value for dietary fiber is 25 g. The reference value of 300 g of carbohydrate for a 2,000-calorie-per-day diet is derived from the recommendation for health that states that 60% of our calories should come from carbohydrate. A serving of the vegetable shown here would provide 2 percent of the Daily Value for total carbohydrate and 12 percent of the Daily Value for dietary fiber. For total carbohydrate and dietary fiber, a higher % Daily Value is better. Your goal is to select foods that will meet or exceed 100% of the Daily Value over the course of your day for these nutrients. (Your goal for fat, cholesterol, and sodium would be *not* to exceed 100% of the Daily Value.) If, for individual foods, the % Daily Value is 5 or less, the food is generally considered low in that nutrient. Foods with 10 percent or more of the Daily Value for fiber are considered *good* sources of dietary fiber. One serving of the broccoli shown here would be a good source of dietary fiber.

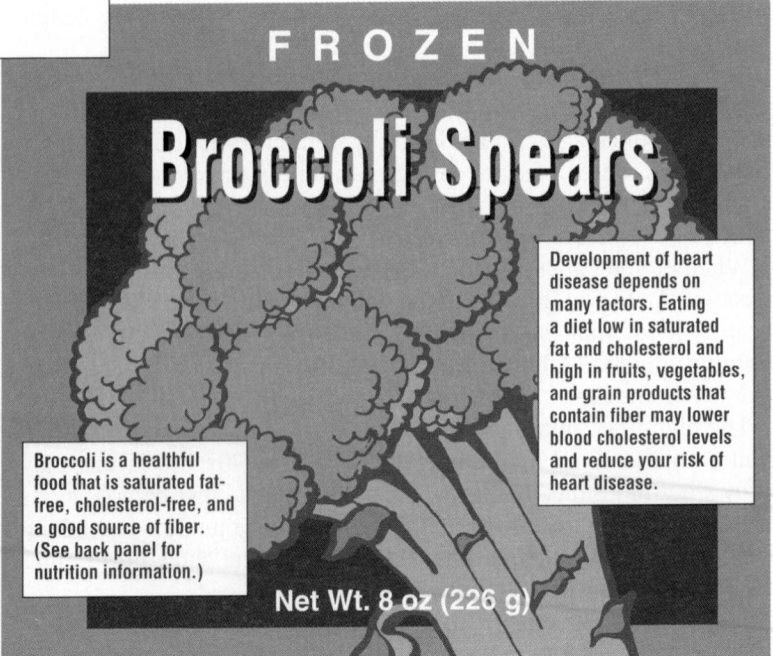

FROZEN

Broccoli Spears

Development of heart disease depends on many factors. Eating a diet low in saturated fat and cholesterol and high in fruits, vegetables, and grain products that contain fiber may lower blood cholesterol levels and reduce your risk of heart disease.

Broccoli is a healthful food that is saturated fat-free, cholesterol-free, and a good source of fiber. (See back panel for nutrition information.)

Net Wt. 8 oz (226 g)

The Bread Box: Refined, Enriched, and Whole-Grain Breads

For many people, grains supply much of the carbohydrate, or at least most of the starch, in a day's meals. Because grains have such a primary place in the diet, be sure that the grains you choose—wheat, rice, oats, or corn—contribute the nutrients you need. Learn the meanings of the words associated with the flours that make up the grain products you use—**refined, enriched, fortified,** and **whole grain.** This discussion of the nutritional differences between different

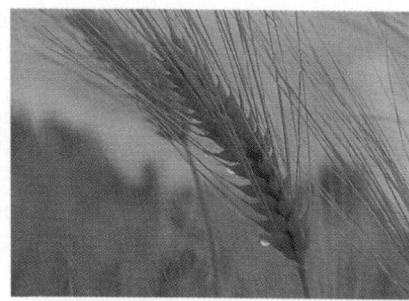

The nutrients present in the wheat plant at harvest are not always present in the wheat products you eat.

breads provides an example of an important principle of nutrition: foods far removed from the original state of wholeness may be lacking in significant nutrients.

The part of the wheat plant that is made into flour and then into bread and other baked goods is the kernel. About 50 kernels cluster in the grain head, where they stick tightly until fully ripe. These kernels are first separated from the stem and then further broken apart by the milling process.

The wheat kernel (a whole grain) has four main parts (see Figure 3–4). The **germ** is the part that grows into a wheat plant, and it contains concentrated food to support the new life. It is especially rich in protein, vitamins, and minerals. The **endosperm** is the soft, white inside portion of the kernel containing starch and protein. The **bran,** a protective coating around the kernel similar in function to the shell of a nut, is also rich in nutrients and fiber. The **husk,** commonly called chaff, is unusable for most purposes except for animal feed.

In earlier times, people milled wheat by grinding it between two stones, then sifting out the inedible chaff but retaining the nutrient-rich bran and germ as well as the endosperm. Improved milling machinery made it possible to remove the dark, heavy germ and bran as well, leaving a whiter, smoother-textured flour. People came to look on this flour as more desirable than the crunchy, dark-brown, "old-fashioned" flour but at first were unaware of the nutrition implications. Bread eaters suffered a tragic loss of needed nutrients in turning to white bread. A U.S. survey done in 1936 revealed that many people were suffering from deficiencies of the nutrients iron, thiamin, riboflavin, and niacin, which they had formerly received from bread. The Enrichment Act of 1942 standardized the return of these four lost nutrients to commercial flour. This doesn't make a single slice of bread "rich" in these four nutrients, but people who eat several or many slices of bread a day obtain significantly more of them than they would from unenriched white bread.

To a great extent, the enrichment of white flour eliminated the four then-known deficiency problems in the eaters of refined white bread. Today, you can assume that almost all breads, grains such as rice, wheat products such as macaroni and spaghetti, and cereals, both cooked and ready-to-eat, have been

REFINED refers to the process by which the coarse parts of food products are removed. For example, the refining of wheat into flour involves removing three of the four parts of the kernel—the chaff, the bran, and the germ—leaving only the endosperm (starch, with only a little protein).

ENRICHED refers to a process by which the B vitamins thiamin, riboflavin, and niacin and the mineral iron are added to refined grains and grain products at levels specified by law. After enrichment, a grain product has approximately the same amount of thiamin, niacin, and iron and about twice as much riboflavin as the original whole-grain product had.

ENRICHED FOODS wheat flour, cornmeal, grits, and polished rice.

FORTIFIED FOODS foods to which nutrients have been added. Examples: margarine with added vitamin A, milk with added vitamin D, certain brands of orange juice and bread with added calcium.

WHOLE GRAIN refers to a grain that is milled in its entirety (all but the husk), not refined. Whole grains include wheat, corn, rice, rye, oats, amaranth, barley, buckwheat, sorghum, and millet; two others—bulgur and couscous—are processed from wheat grains.

GERM the nutrient-rich and fat-dense inner part of a whole grain (removed during refining).

ENDOSPERM the bulk of the edible part of a grain; contains starch grains embedded in a protein matrix.

BRAN the fibrous protective covering of a whole grain and the chief source of fiber in grain (removed during refining). The bran covering actually includes four outer layers of the whole grain—primarily the *aleurone* and *pericarp* layers.

HUSK the outer, inedible covering of a grain.

enriched. Figure 3–5 on page 87 shows that although enrichment makes refined bread comparable to whole-grain bread with respect to the four mentioned nutrients, it does not do so with respect to other important nutrients. Therefore, although the enrichment of flour and other cereal products does improve them, it doesn't improve them enough: whole-grain products are still preferred over enriched products. If bread is a staple food in your diet—that is, if you eat it every day—you would be well advised to learn to like the hearty flavor of whole-grain bread.

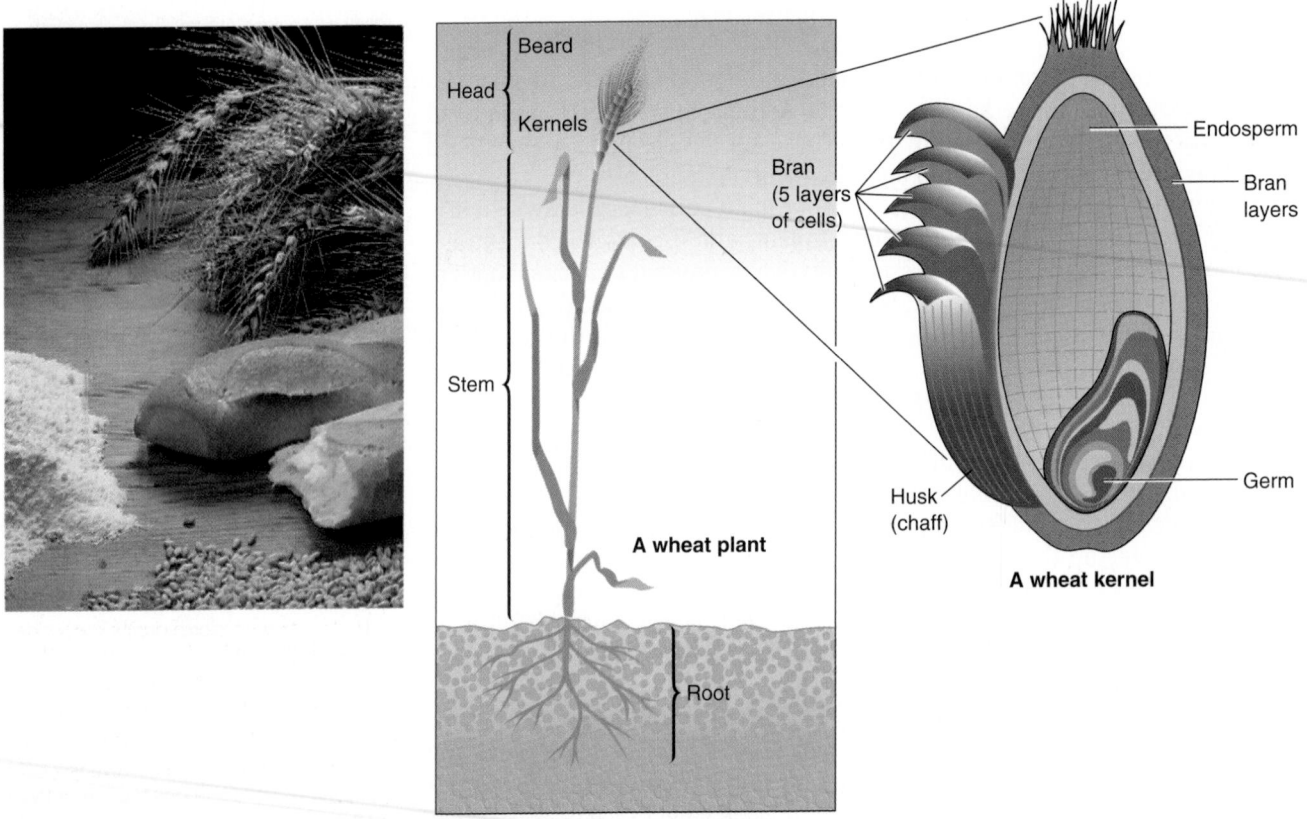

FIGURE 3–4   A WHOLE-GRAIN (WHEAT) PLANT AND A KERNEL OF WHEAT

To make flour and then bread, wheat kernels are first separated from the stem of the wheat plant and then further broken apart by the milling process. A wheat kernel (a whole grain) has four main parts: the germ or plant embryo (containing protein, unsaturated fats, thiamin, riboflavin, niacin, iron, and other nutrients), the endosperm (containing primarily starch, the storage form of glucose in plants), the bran (a rich source of fiber), and the husk (inedible).

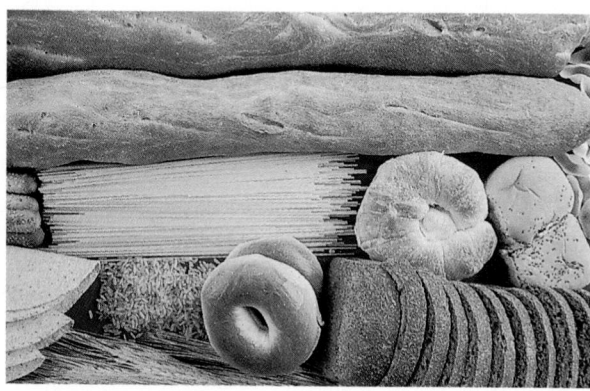

Enjoy the hearty flavor of whole grains.

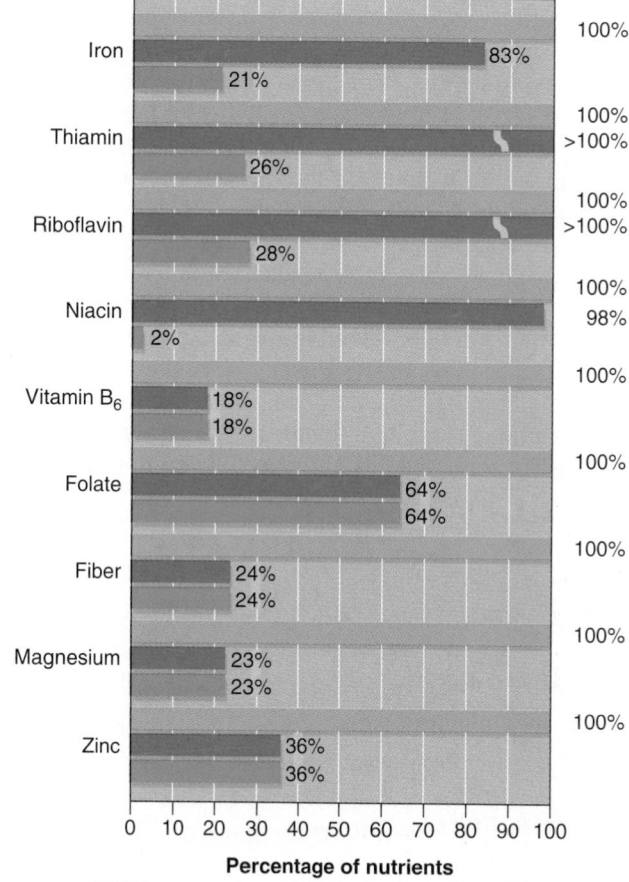

Nutrients in bread

Key:
□ = Whole-grain bread
■ = Enriched white bread
■ = Unenriched white bread

Iron 83% / 21% — 100%
Thiamin >100% / 26% — 100%
Riboflavin >100% / 28% — 100%
Niacin 98% / 2% — 100%
Vitamin B$_6$ 18% / 18% — 100%
Folate 64% / 64% — 100%
Fiber 24% / 24% — 100%
Magnesium 23% / 23% — 100%
Zinc 36% / 36% — 100%

0 10 20 30 40 50 60 70 80 90 100
Percentage of nutrients
(100% represents nutrient levels of whole-grain bread.)

FIGURE 3–5
NUTRIENTS IN WHOLE-GRAIN, ENRICHED WHITE, AND UNENRICHED WHITE BREADS

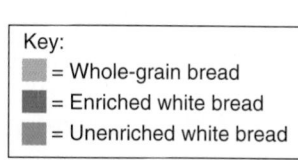

The Complex Carbohydrate Fiber

The **fibers** of a plant form the supporting structures of the plant's leaves, stems, and seeds. Most fibers are polysaccharides, just as starch is, but with different bonds between the glucose units— bonds that cannot be broken by human digestive enzymes. The term *fiber* is used by almost everyone as if it represented a single entity. It was known generations ago as **roughage.** However, there are many compounds, mostly carbohydrates, that make up fiber.* Such compounds are familiar as the strings of celery, the skins of corn kernels, and the membranes separating the segments in citrus fruits. Isolated from plants, they may be used to thicken jelly (citrus pectin), to keep salad dressing from separating (guar gum), to provide roughage (wheat and other brans), and to exert other effects on texture and consistency.

The bonds that hold the units of fiber together cannot be broken by human digestive enzymes, but some can be broken by the bacteria that reside in the human digestive tract. Therefore, we may obtain a trace amount of glucose and some related products from fiber molecules. Fibers exert important effects on people's health, as described in the following section.

FIBERS the indigestible residues of food, composed mostly of polysaccharides. Thus fibers are the nonstarch polysaccharides in foods. The term *dietary fiber* refers to nutritionally significant fiber in food—that is, the fiber that resists human digestive enzymes.

ROUGHAGE (RUFF-edge) the rough parts of food; an imprecise term that has been largely replaced by the term *fiber.*

The best known of the fibrous polysaccharides are **cellulose, hemicellulose, pectin,** and **gums.**

* The woody material of heavy stems and bark is the noncarbohydrate lignin, classed by some as a fiber.

The Health Effects of Fiber

Many health experts are encouraging consumers to eat more fiber. According to recent evidence, inadequate levels of fiber in the diet are associated with several diseases (see the Miniglossary on page 89), while consumption of recommended levels of fiber offers many health benefits. Recall that dietary fiber is found only in plant foods, such as fruits, vegetables, legumes, and grains, and it is the part of plant foods that human enzymes cannot digest. Fiber has two forms: **insoluble** and **soluble.** Table 3–8 shows the health benefits from these two types of fiber. As you can see from Table 3–8, not all fibers are created equal. Since insoluble and soluble fibers have different effects in the body, it is important to eat a variety of high-fiber foods to get both types.

Both types of fiber—soluble and insoluble—can help with weight control. In the stomach, they convey a feeling of fullness because they absorb water, and some of them delay the emptying of the stomach so that you feel fuller longer. If you eat many high-fiber foods, you are likely to eat fewer empty-calorie foods such as concentrated fats and sweets. Indeed, producers of some diet aids base

INSOLUBLE FIBER includes the fiber types called cellulose, hemicellulose, and lignin; insoluble fibers do not dissolve in water.

SOLUBLE FIBER includes the fiber types called pectin, gums, and mucilages; soluble fibers either dissolve or swell when placed in water. Psyllium seed husk is an ingredient in certain bulk-forming laxatives and contains soluble fiber.

TABLE 3–8
HEALTH BENEFITS AND SOURCES OF DIETARY FIBER

FOODS RICH IN INSOLUBLE FIBER		HEALTH PROBLEM	FIBER TYPE	POSSIBLE HEALTH BENEFITS
apples	rice bran	Obesity	Soluble Insoluble	Replaces calories from fat, provides satiety, and prolongs eating time because of chewiness of food
bananas	root vegetables			
brown rice	pears			
cabbage family	peaches			
cauliflower	plums			
corn bran	seeds	Digestive tract disorders: Constipation Diverticulosis Hemorrhoids	Insoluble	Provides bulk and promotes regularity
green beans	strawberries			
green peas	tomatoes			
legumes	wheat bran			
mature vegetables	whole-grain breads	Colon cancer	Insoluble	Speeds transit time through intestines and may protect against colon cancer[a]
nuts	and cereals			
FOODS RICH IN SOLUBLE FIBER				
apples	green peas	Diabetes	Soluble	May improve blood sugar tolerance by delaying glucose absorption
apricots	legumes			
bananas	oat bran			
barley	oatmeal			
black-eyed peas	pears	Heart disease	Soluble	May lower blood cholesterol
broccoli	potatoes			
cabbage	prunes			
carrots	rye			
cherries	seeds			
citrus fruits	sweet potatoes			
corn	zucchini			
grapes				

[a]This effect is based on epidemiologic studies and is usually observed along with a reduced-fat intake.

the success of their products on the ability of certain fibers in the products to provide bulk and make you feel full.

Insoluble fibers—the type in wheat bran—hold water in the colon, thus increasing bulk, which stimulates the muscles of the digestive tract so that they retain their health and tone. The toned muscles can more easily move waste products through the colon for excretion. This prevents **constipation, hemorrhoids** (in which veins in the rectum swell, bulge out, become weak, and bleed), and **diverticulosis** (in which the intestinal walls become weak and bulge out in places in response to pressure needed to excrete waste when bulk is inadequate). These fibers may also speed up the passage of food through the digestive tract, thus shortening the time of exposure of the tissue to agents in food that might cause certain cancers, such as **colon cancer.**[23]

Soluble fibers, the type in beans and oats, are credited with reducing the risks of heart and artery disease—**atherosclerosis**—by lowering the level of cholesterol in the blood. It appears that the products of bacterial digestion of soluble fiber in the colon are absorbed into the body and may inhibit the body's production of cholesterol, as well as enhance the clearance of cholesterol from the blood.[24] Cholesterol levels may also decrease if food sources of soluble fiber (for example, barley, lentils, peas, beans, oat bran, or psyllium-enriched cereal) are used as part of a low-fat, low-cholesterol diet.[25] Certain insoluble fibers also bind cholesterol compounds and carry them out of the body with the feces so that the whole body content of cholesterol is lowered.

Soluble fibers also improve the body's handling of glucose, even in people with diabetes, perhaps by slowing the digestion or absorption rate of carbohydrates. Blood glucose levels therefore stay moderate, helping to prevent symptoms of diabetes or hypoglycemia. The list of fiber's contributions to human health, therefore, is impressive.

When people choose high-fiber foods in hopes of receiving some of these benefits, they must choose with care. Wheat bran, which is composed mostly of cellulose, has no cholesterol-lowering effect, whereas oat bran and the fibers of legumes, carrots, apples, and grapefruits do lower blood cholesterol. On the other hand, the fiber of wheat bran in whole-wheat bread is one of the most effective stool-softening fibers that help prevent constipation and hemorrhoids. If a single practical conclusion were to be drawn from what is known about fiber, it would have to be that all whole plant foods seem to contain many kinds of fibers and so can be expected to have the whole range of

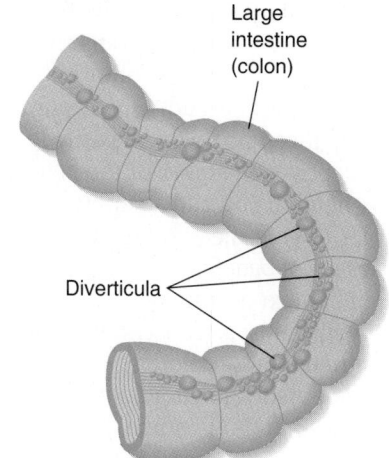

Diverticulosis.

The outpocketings of intestinal linings that balloon through the weakened intestinal wall muscles are known as **diverticula.**

MINIGLOSSARY OF DISEASES AND CONDITIONS ASSOCIATED WITH LACK OF FIBER IN THE DIET

APPENDICITIS inflammation and/or infection of the appendix, a sac protruding from the large intestine.

ATHEROSCLEROSIS (ATH-er-oh-scler-OH-sis) a type of cardiovascular disease; the most common kind of hardening of the arteries characterized by the formation of fatty deposits, or plaques, in their inner walls.

COLON CANCER cancer of the large intestine (colon), the terminal portion of the digestive tract (see Appendix B).

CONSTIPATION hardness and dryness of bowel movements associated with discomfort in passing them.

DIABETES a disorder characterized by insufficiency or relative ineffectiveness of insulin that renders a person unable to regulate the blood glucose level normally.

DIVERTICULOSIS (dye-ver-tic-you-LOCE-iss) outpocketings of weakened areas of the intestinal wall, like blowouts in a tire, that can rupture, causing dangerous infections.

HEMORRHOIDS (HEM-or-oids) swollen, hardened (varicose) veins in the rectum, usually caused by the pressure resulting from constipation.

OBESITY body weight high enough above normal weight to constitute a health hazard (see also Chapter 8).

effects previously mentioned. To obtain the greatest benefits from fiber, therefore, you have to eat a variety of foods that contain it rather than take doses of purified fiber such as bran from a single source.

The wholesale addition of purified fiber to foods is probably ill-advised because it can be taken so easily to extremes. Taking only one isolated type of fiber deprives the taker of the benefits the other types of fiber provide. On the other hand, if you add a variety of whole grains, legumes, nuts, fruits, and vegetables to your diet, you get the various types of fiber you need, together with a package of benefits—water, minerals, vitamins, and the energy nutrients. Fiber out of context is similar to sugar out of context: It can be viewed as nutrient-empty fiber, just as concentrated sugar is sometimes seen as nutrient-empty calories.

Adding one or two servings of oats, beans, or other form of soluble fiber helps lower fasting blood sugar levels in persons with diabetes.

Undoubtedly, including fiber in a daily meal plan has benefits—but how much is enough? Even fiber has potential to cause harm if taken in excess. Since fiber carries water out of the body, taking too much can cause dehydration and intestinal discomfort. Iron is mainly absorbed early during digestion, and because fiber speeds the movement of foods through the digestive system, it may limit the opportunity for the absorption of iron and other nutrients. Binders in some fibers link chemically with minerals such as calcium and zinc, making them unavailable for absorption by carrying them out of the body (more about this in Chapter 7). Too much bulk from the diet could reduce the total amount of food consumed and cause deficiencies of both nutrients and energy. The malnourished, the elderly, and children, because they eat small amounts of food anyway, are especially vulnerable to these concerns.

There is no RDA for fiber, and not everyone agrees on just how to measure a food's fiber content. Still, with all the uncertainties, the National Cancer Institute recommends that about 20 to 35 grams of dietary fiber daily is a desirable intake. The diet can supply that amount, given ample choices of whole foods (see Table 3–9). The diet does have to be high in fruits, vegetables, legumes, and grains, and moderate in meats, fats, and concentrated sugars—the same recommendations made in the *Surgeon General's Report* and in the *Dietary Guidelines*. Figure 3–6 contains two sample menus to show meals that provide the recommended fiber level at different calorie levels.

Adding Fiber to the Diet

As previously mentioned, current recommendations advise people to eat 20 to 35 grams of dietary fiber a day.[26] Most Americans, however, now eat only 11 to 13 grams of fiber a day, largely because refined foods, fats, and sweets have displaced the higher fiber foods our great grandparents used to enjoy—the basic, whole foods such as fruits, vegetables, legumes, and whole-grain breads and cereals. Adding fiber to your diet can be easier and tastier than you might think. The following easy tips will help you to include more fiber-rich foods in your diet:

- Increase consumption of a variety of fiber-rich foods, including fruits, vegetables, legumes, and whole-grain breads, cereals, and pastas (refer to Table 3–9 for the fiber content of various foods).

TABLE 3–9
LOOKING FOR FIBER IN THE FOOD GUIDE PYRAMID[a]

| FOOD GROUP | **FIBER CONTENT** | | |
	High (5–10 g per serving)	**Medium** (2–4 g per serving)	**Low** (# 1 g per serving)
BREAD, CEREAL, RICE, AND PASTA	bran cereals, ½ c Shredded Wheat, 1 c	oatmeal, 1 c whole-grain flakes, 1 c (e.g., Wheaties, Total) puffed wheat, 1½ c whole-wheat bread, 1 slice rye bread, 1 slice whole-grain crackers, 5 popped popcorn, 2 c brown rice, ½ c barley, ½ c	corn flakes, 1 c Special K, 1 c Rice Krispies, 1 c Cheerios, 1 c white rice, ½ c pasta, ½ c
VEGETABLE[b]	legumes	broccoli Brussels sprouts cabbage carrots corn eggplant green beans potato, with skin, 1 medium spinach tomatoes, 1 large	asparagus califlower celery lettuce onions peppers pickle, 1 large potato, without skin, 1 medium
FRUIT[c]		apple, 1 small apricot banana, 1 small berries, 1 c cantaloupe, ½ melon cherries, 16 large orange peach pear prunes, 2 raisins, ¼ c	canned fruit, 1 c juices, 1 c
MILK, YOGURT, AND CHEESE	0	0	0
MEAT, POULTRY, FISH, DRY BEANS, EGGS, AND NUTS	legumes, cooked or canned, ½ c	nuts and seeds, 1 oz peanut butter, 2 tbsp	

[a]Appendix I lists the grams of dietary fiber in more than 1,900 foods.
[b]The serving size for vegetables is ½ cup, unless otherwise noted.
[c]The serving size for fruits is one medium piece, unless otherwise noted.

1,300-Calorie Menu Plan

Breakfast	Grams of Dietary Fiber
1 scrambled egg	0.0
1 slice 100% whole-wheat bread	2.8
2 teaspoons margarine	0.0
1/2 grapefruit	1.6
1 cup coffee	0.0
Snack	
1/2 cup low-fat cottage cheese	0.0
1 peach	2.0
1/2 cup strawberries	1.6
Lunch	
2 slices 100% whole-wheat bread	5.7
2 tablespoons tuna salad (with celery)	0.1
4 carrot sticks	2.0
1/2 green pepper	0.5
1/2 stalk of celery	0.5
8 ounces club soda	0.0
Afternoon Snack	
1/2 cup raisin bran	3.5
1/2 cup 1% milk	0.0
Dinner	
1 cup "Black Beans on Rice" (recipe follows)	3.3
3 slices lean roast beef (5.5 oz)	0.0
1/2 cup applesauce	2.0
1 cup 1% milk	0.0

1323 calories   Carbohydrates: 47%
Protein: 20%   Fat: 33%
Dietary Fiber: 25.6 grams

1,800-Calorie Menu Plan

Breakfast	Grams of Dietary Fiber
1/2 cup Bran Chex cereal	3.9
1/2 cup 1% milk	0.0
1 slice 100% whole-wheat bread	2.8
1 teaspoon margarine	0.0
1 teaspoon jelly	0.0
1/2 cup orange juice	0.4
Snack	
1 apple, unpeeled (medium)	3.2
Lunch	
1 cup "Two Bean and Peas Salad" (recipe follows)	6.4
1 slice 100% whole-wheat bread	2.8
2 teaspoons margarine	0.0
8 ounces club soda	0.0
Afternoon Snack	
5 graham crackers	1.0
2 tablespoons peanut butter	2.8
1 packet raisins (1.2 oz)	1.2
Dinner	
1 baked potato, peeled	3.7
1 teaspoon sour cream	0.0
1 chicken breast	0.0
1 cup cooked broccoli	6.4
1/2 cup frozen yogurt	0.0
1 cup 1% milk	0.0

1842 calories   Carbohydrates: 48%
Protein: 22%   Fat: 30%
Dietary Fiber: 34.6 grams

Black Beans on Rice

1 pound dry black beans
6 cups boiling water
2 green peppers, chopped
6–8 green onions (scallions) with tops, chopped
1 clove garlic, minced
1/3 cup oil
2 teaspoons seasonings
1 pound brown rice, cooked

Cover the beans with the boiling water and cook for 1 hour. Saute the green peppers, green onion (reserve 1 to 2 teaspoons), and garlic in oil. Combine the vegetables with the beans, add the other seasonings (as desired), and cook until the beans are tender and the liquid is thick. Serve over brown rice. Garnish with the reserved chopped green onions. Yield: 16 servings, 3/4 cup each.

Calories: 160   Protein: 5 grams
Carbohydrates: 21 grams   Fat: 6.5 grams
Dietary Fiber: 3.3 grams

Source: Jane Brody: *Jane Brody's Nutrition Book.* Bantam Books, New York, 1987.

Two Beans and Peas Salad

2 cups cooked chickpeas
2 cups cooked kidney beans
2 cups cooked blackeyed peas
2 cups cooked green beans
1 chopped green bell pepper
1/4 cup diced onions
3 tablespoons olive oil
2 tablespoons vinegar
1/2 teaspoon salt
1/4 teaspoon pepper
1/4 teaspoon basil
1/4 teaspoon oregano

Cook the chickpeas, kidney beans, blackeyed peas, and green beans separately (you can also use one 16-ounce can of each). Mix olive oil, vinegar, salt, and the spices. Combine all ingredients and stir well. Serve over chopped lettuce. Makes 10 servings, 1 cup each.

Calories: 162   Protein: 8.8 grams
Carbohydrates: 22.3 grams   Fat: 4.8 grams
Dietary Fiber: 6.39 grams

SOURCE: Adapted from *Fiber Display Kit,* Penn State Nutrition Center, 417 East Calder Way, University Park, PA 16801.

- Select high-fiber foods when shopping for groceries—whole-grain cereals, breads, and snack foods, for example. Buy products that list a whole grain or whole-wheat or other whole-grain flour as the first ingredient. Check the food label for dietary fiber content.

- Choose whole fruits instead of juice. Look for nonwaxed varieties of fruits and vegetables so that you can leave the skin on the fruits and vegetables that you purchase.

- Add berries to muffin and pancake batters.

- Whenever possible, substitute whole-grain flour for all-purpose flour when baking.

- Use oats in place of flour in crumb toppings for fruit crisps; using a blender, grind whole-grain oats into flour, which you can then use to replace one-third or more of the all-purpose flour called for in recipes; try toasted whole-grain oats as a replacement for bread crumbs on top of casseroles, cooked vegetables, or fish fillets; add cinnamon to the toasted oats and sprinkle over fresh fruit and yogurt.

- Eat whole, baked, or boiled potatoes, including skins, instead of mashed.

- Use unpeeled vegetables in salads, soups, and stews.

- Experiment with legumes: add beans to salads, soups, stews, tacos, or burritos; one-half cup of cooked kidney beans in a bowl of chili adds about 8 grams of dietary fiber.

- Use brown rice instead of white rice for added fiber and nutrients.

- Eat high-fiber snacks—popcorn, fresh fruits, raw vegetables, dried fruits, and nuts (go easy on the nuts, however, since 1 cup of most nuts has 800 calories).

- Start your day with a high-fiber selection: a warm bowl of oatmeal with fresh fruit; bran cereals or shredded wheat with sliced fruit; banana bread; oat- or wheat-bran muffins; compote of prunes with citrus fruits; whole-grain English muffin.

- Remember to add high-fiber foods to the diet gradually (being sure to consume adequate fluids to allow your body to adjust).

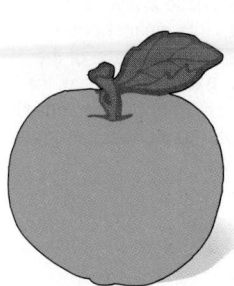 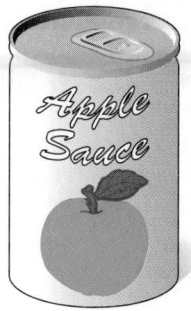 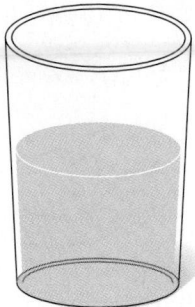

Large whole apple
with peel: 5.0 g fiber

Applesauce,
½ cup: 2.0 g fiber

Apple juice,
¾ cup: 0.2 g fiber

How the Body Handles Carbohydrates

Just as glucose is the original unit from which the variety of carbohydrate foods are made, so is glucose the basic carbohydrate unit that each cell of the body uses. Cells cannot use lactose, sucrose, or starch—they require glucose. The task of the digestive system, then, is to disassemble the double sugars and starch to single sugars and to absorb these monosaccharides into the blood. The liver converts to glucose those carbohydrates that are not already in the form of glucose so that they can be transported to the cells. The cells can then store this glucose, use it for energy, or convert it to fat.

The first digestive enzymes to work on starch are those in the saliva; they begin taking the starch apart, and enzymes in the intestines continue digestive action (see Figure 3–7). The enzymes release the individual glucose units, which are absorbed across the intestinal wall into the

> Cooking facilitates the digestive process by spreading out the tightly packaged chains of glucose so that during digestion the digestive enzymes can break the chains down into glucose units for absorption.

FIGURE 3–7
A SUMMARY OF CARBOHYDRATE DIGESTION AND ABSORPTION

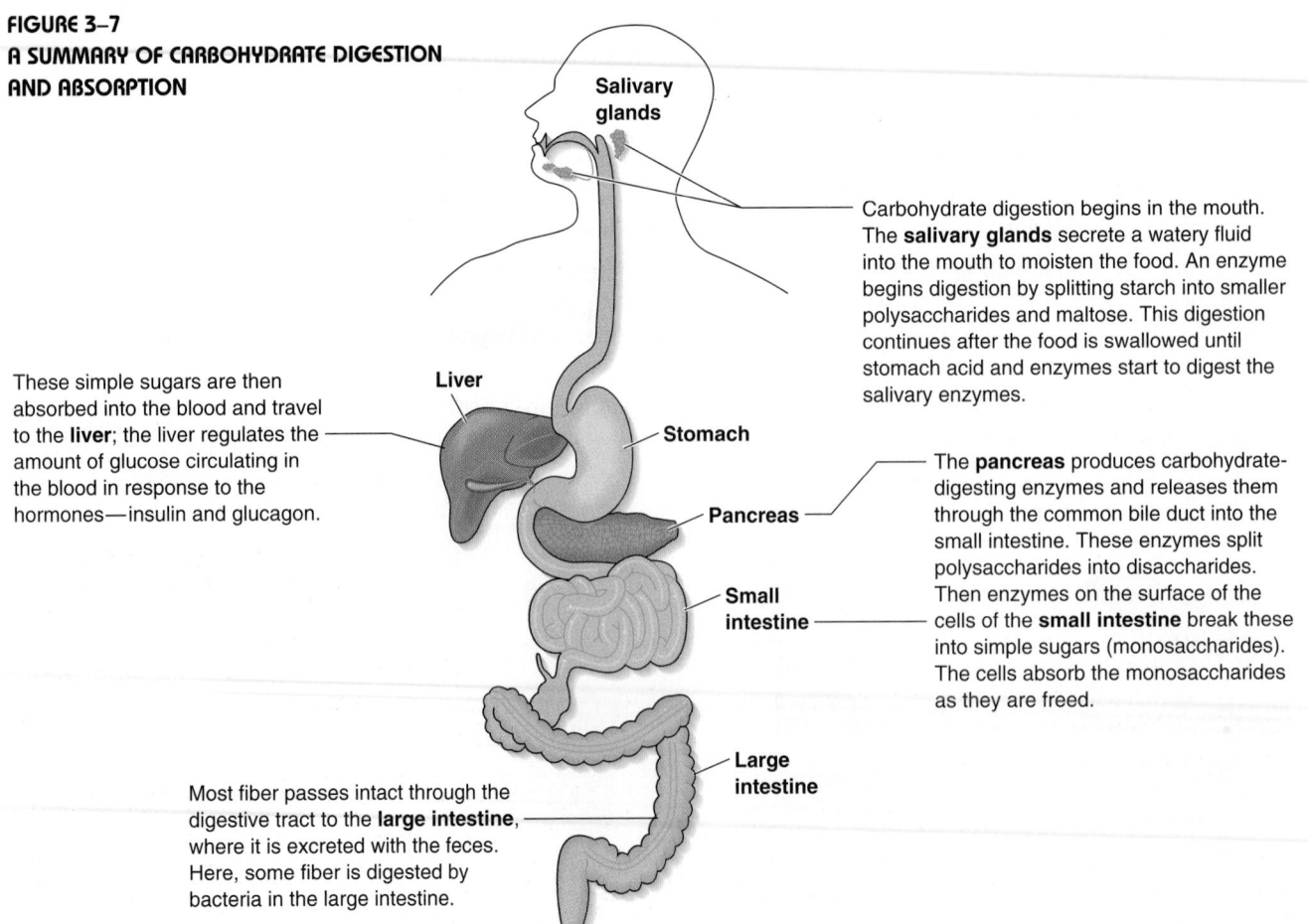

Salivary glands

Carbohydrate digestion begins in the mouth. The **salivary glands** secrete a watery fluid into the mouth to moisten the food. An enzyme begins digestion by splitting starch into smaller polysaccharides and maltose. This digestion continues after the food is swallowed until stomach acid and enzymes start to digest the salivary enzymes.

Liver

Stomach

These simple sugars are then absorbed into the blood and travel to the **liver**; the liver regulates the amount of glucose circulating in the blood in response to the hormones—insulin and glucagon.

Pancreas

The **pancreas** produces carbohydrate-digesting enzymes and releases them through the common bile duct into the small intestine. These enzymes split polysaccharides into disaccharides. Then enzymes on the surface of the cells of the **small intestine** break these into simple sugars (monosaccharides). The cells absorb the monosaccharides as they are freed.

Small intestine

Large intestine

Most fiber passes intact through the digestive tract to the **large intestine**, where it is excreted with the feces. Here, some fiber is digested by bacteria in the large intestine.

If you limit your carbohydrate intake drastically, the body will take glycogen from the liver + muscles — which deplete the muscles? p.97 can't protein change into a carbohydrate

why then 50 - 60% carbs?

blood (see Appendix B). One to four hours after a meal, all the starch has been digested and absorbed and is circulating to the cells as glucose.

If the blood delivers more glucose than the cells need, the liver and muscles take up the surplus to build the polysaccharide **glycogen.** The muscles hold two-thirds of the body's total store of this carbohydrate and use it during exercise. (Chapter 9 explores the relationship between glycogen and exercise and offers tips on how to make the most of glycogen stores.) The liver stores the other one-third, making it available to maintain the blood glucose level.

After the glycogen stores are full and the cells' immediate energy needs are met, the body takes a third path for using carbohydrates. Say you have eaten dinner that includes enough carbohydrates to fill your glycogen stores. Now, you watch a movie, eat popcorn, and drink a cola. Your digestive tract is delivering glucose from the popcorn and soda to your liver; your liver breaks these extra energy compounds into small fragments and puts them together into the more permanent energy-storage compound—fat. The fat is then released from the liver, carried to the fatty tissues of the body, and deposited there. (Fat cells, too, can utilize excess glucose to make fat for storage.) Unlike the liver cells, though, which can store only about half a day's worth of glucose as glycogen, the fat cells can store unlimited quantities of fat.

GLYCOGEN (GLY-co-gen) a polysaccharide composed of chains of glucose, manufactured in the body and stored in liver and muscle. As a storage form of glucose, glycogen can be broken down by the liver to maintain a constant blood glucose level when carbohydrate intake is inadequate.

This section refers to many body organs. To review them, turn to Appendix B.

Maintaining the Blood Glucose Level

The brain and nervous system are sensitive to the concentration of glucose in the blood. Normal blood glucose levels are important for a feeling of well-being. When your blood glucose level becomes too concentrated, you get sleepy; when the concentration falls too low, you get weak and shaky. Only when blood glucose is within the normal range can you feel energetic and alert. The person who wants to feel energetic and alert all day should make the effort to eat so as to maintain blood glucose levels in the normal range to fuel the critical work of the brain and nervous system.

The maintenance of a normal blood glucose level depends on two safeguards, as shown in Figure 3–8. When the level gets too high—for example, immediately after a meal—it can be corrected by siphoning off the excess into liver and muscle glycogen and into body fat. When it gets too low—for example, following an overnight fast—it can be replenished by drawing on liver glycogen stores.

When the blood glucose level rises, the body adjusts by storing the excess. The first organ to detect the excess glucose is the pancreas, which releases the hormone **insulin** in response. Most of the body's cells respond to insulin by taking up glucose from the blood to make glycogen or fat. Thus, the blood glucose level is quickly brought back down to normal as the body stores the excess. Insulin's opposing hormone, released by the pancreas when blood glucose is too low, is **glucagon,** which draws forth glucose from storage, making it available to supply energy. Insulin and glucagon both work to maintain

INSULIN a hormone secreted by the pancreas in response to high blood glucose levels; it assists cells in drawing glucose from the blood.

GLUCAGON (GLUE-cuh-gon) insulin's opposing hormone, released by the pancreas when blood glucose is too low; it draws forth glucose and other fuels from storage, making them available to supply energy to cells.

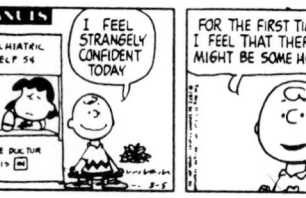
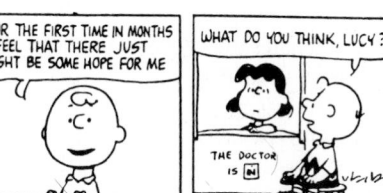
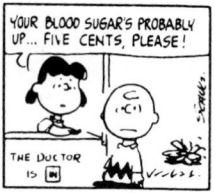

FIGURE 3–8
BLOOD GLUCOSE REGULATION

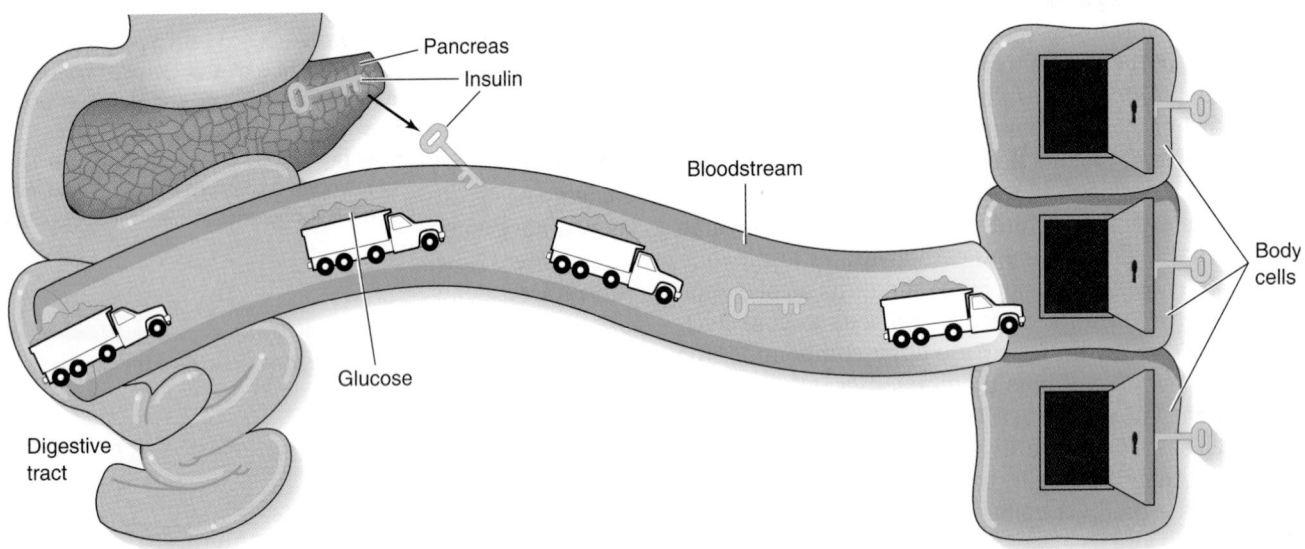

A. High blood glucose (sugar) stimulates the pancreas to release insulin. Insulin serves as a key for entrance of blood glucose into cells. Liver and muscle cells store the glucose as glycogen. Excess glucose can also be stored as fat.

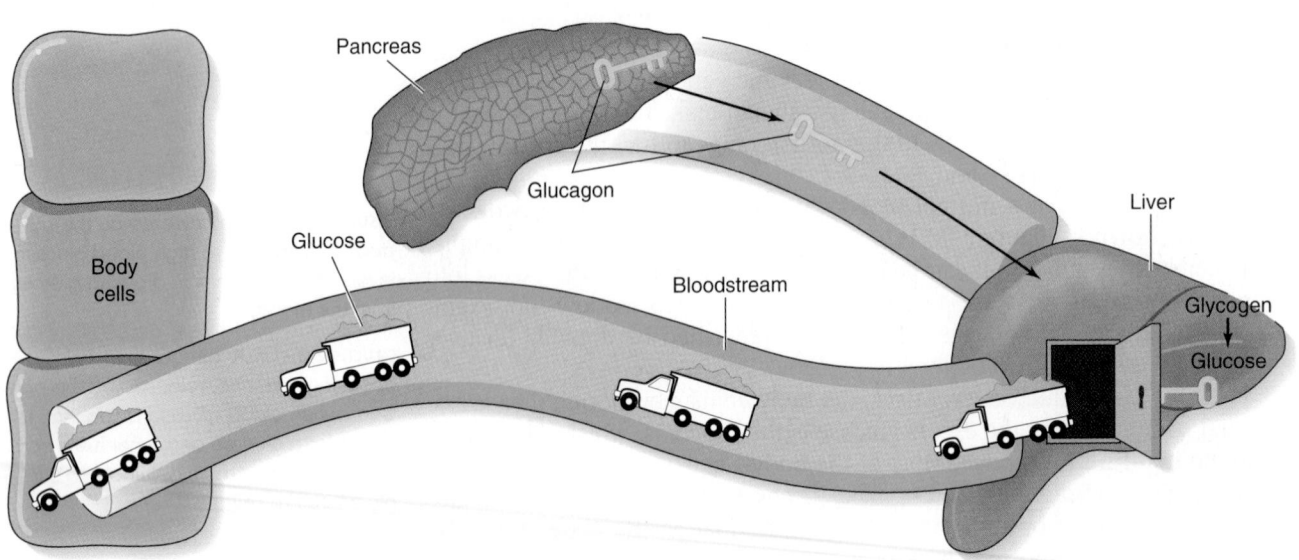

B. Later, low blood glucose stimulates the pancreas to release glucagon, which serves as the key for the liver to break down stored glycogen to glucose and release it into the blood.

the concentration of glucose in the blood within the normal range—neither too high nor too low.

Obviously, when the blood glucose level falls and stores are depleted, a meal or a snack can replenish the supply. An appropriate choice is to eat a **balanced meal** containing several different kinds of food that offer carbohydrate, protein, and fat:

- The carbohydrates in the meal provide a quick source of glucose. (Glucose, remember, is quickly put away by insulin.)

- The protein in the meal stimulates glucagon secretion, which opposes insulin and keeps it from putting away glucose too fast.

- The fat in the meal slows down digestion so that you receive a steady stream of nutrients rather than a sudden flood.

By these standards, a bowl of whole-grain cereal with fresh fruit and low-fat milk for breakfast (offering carbohydrate, protein, and fat) is a good choice. Eating well-spaced, carefully chosen meals that provide the balance of protein, carbohydrates, and fat recommended in the *Dietary Guidelines* can prevent rapid rises and falls in the blood glucose level.

Researchers rank foods according to their effects on blood glucose.[27] The effect of a food on the blood glucose level is important to people with abnormalities of blood glucose regulation, notably **diabetes** and **hypoglycemia**.* Rapid swings in blood glucose can affect the performance of both an athlete during an endurance event and an office employee following lunch. People are wise to eat well-balanced meals high in carbohydrate, adequate in protein, and low in fat.

Hypoglycemia

Suppose the blood glucose falls, the glycogen reserves are exhausted, and you do *not* eat. Gradually, your body will shift into a fasting state, breaking down its muscle to provide amino acids to the liver. The liver converts some of these into glucose to fuel the brain. The fat released from the muscle cells is used to fuel other cells. (Chapter 8 describes this state—ketosis—in more detail on page 286.) Most times, the transition is smooth and is not noticeable. But there may be times when your blood glucose level falls rapidly or below what is normal for you, and you may experience symptoms of glucose deprivation to the brain: anxiety, hunger, and dizziness. Your muscles become weak, shaky, and trembling, and your heart races in an attempt to speed more fuel to your brain. These symptoms of low blood glucose signify that your system is out of balance, but this is usually no cause for concern. All of us, at times, experience the ordinary type of hypoglycemia—low blood glucose levels occurring within six hours of a meal. The treatment consists of learning to eat promptly and properly.

BALANCED MEAL a meal containing sufficient but not excessive amounts of foods from each of the food groups and therefore sufficient but not excessive amounts of carbohydrates, fat, protein, vitamins, and minerals.

DIABETES (dye-uh-BEET-eez) a disorder (technically termed *diabetes mellitus*) characterized by insufficiency or relative ineffectiveness of insulin, which renders a person unable to regulate the blood glucose level normally.

HYPOGLYCEMIA (HIGH-po-gligh-SEEM-ee-uh) an abnormally low blood glucose concentration—below about 60 to 70 mg/100 ml.

*The effect of food on a person's blood glucose and insulin response is called the *glycemic effect*—how fast and how high the blood glucose rises and how quickly the body responds by bringing it back to normal. A *glycemic index* ranks foods on the basis of the extent to which the foods raise the blood glucose level as compared with pure glucose.

There is another type of hypoglycemia, however, that requires treatment. It is a rare and often serious condition in which abnormal amounts of hormones are secreted, perhaps because of a pancreatic tumor or other abnormalities. As a result, the person's blood glucose is constantly too low—independent of dietary intake. This kind of hypoglycemia causes symptoms (headache, confusion, fatigue, amnesia, seizures, or unconsciousness), even after only 8 to 14 hours without food (for example, overnight). A person with this kind of hypoglycemia urgently needs diagnosis and medical treatment.

Hypoglycemia has been a popular buzzword for many decades. It is not a single entity; it is a symptom, not a disease. It may be simple and easy to avoid, or it may be a serious matter. Diagnosis and treatment are properly left to a qualified professional. But for anyone who has a hard time making it from one meal to the next, there can be no harm in eating balanced, sustaining meals of a kind most likely to blunt the glycemic effect—meals containing adequate protein, a bit of fat, ample fluid, and abundant carbohydrate, including fiber, from vegetables, grains, fruits, and especially legumes.

Diabetes

Knowing how the blood glucose level is maintained, you can appreciate the problem of the person with diabetes whose insulin response is slow or ineffective. Most adults with diabetes fall into this category (see Table 3–10).* Even if the blood glucose level rises too high (**hyperglycemia**), glucose still fails to get into cells and so stays too high for an abnormally long time. The kidneys may respond by shifting some glucose out of the body into the urine so that it can be excreted. People with diabetes must be careful to eat regularly scheduled, balanced meals—providing a constant, steady, moderate flow of glucose to the bloodstream—so the insulin response can keep up. Recent research indicates that many people with diabetes actually do best on a diet that is high in complex carbohydrate-rich foods—as high as is recommended for any healthy person.[28] The starch and protein in these foods help to regulate the blood glucose level, as already described.

A common myth about diabetes is that too much sugar in the diet causes it—as if the person with diabetes had "overstrained the pancreas" in an effort to handle large amounts of sugar in the diet. However, sugar is not to blame. Research has suggested that the most common type of diabetes (Type II)—usually diagnosed in people over 40—is caused by genetic factors, too little insulin, or resistance to insulin.[29] The less common type of diabetes (Type I) is seen usually in children and has been linked to a possible immune system disorder. Neither type is caused by consuming excess sugar.

HYPERGLYCEMIA an abnormally high blood glucose concentration, often a symptom of both types of diabetes.

---

*Most diabetes is of the type known as Type II, or non-insulin-dependent diabetes mellitus (NIDDM). People with this form of diabetes secrete insulin, but the insulin is ineffective or the body's response is delayed. Often the diet can be adjusted to enable the body's own insulin to do its work so that no shots or drugs are needed. The rarer type of diabetes is called Type I, or insulin-dependent diabetes mellitus (IDDM), in which the person produces no insulin at all.

TABLE 3–10
DISTINCTIONS BETWEEN THE TWO MAJOR TYPES OF DIABETES

	TYPE I: INSULIN-DEPENDENT DIABETES	TYPE II: NON-INSULIN-DEPENDENT DIABETES
Incidence	10% of cases	90% of cases
Insulin deficiency	Yes, pancreas unable to make insulin to meet needs	In some cases there may be insufficient insulin, or cells may be unresponsive to insulin
Risk factors	Genetic predisposition plus environmental factor (for example, viral infection)	Genetic predisposition plus obesity (especially central-type obesity), family history
Treatment	Insulin injections, diet, and exercise	Weight loss, diet, and exercise

Recently, the American Diabetes Association eased its restriction on sugar use in the diets of people with diabetes because sucrose-containing foods do not seem to exert any higher of a glycemic response than do starchy foods.[30] Any foods containing sucrose must be used in place of other carbohydrate-containing foods and should not exceed 5 percent to 10 percent of the total carbohydrate calories. The key to controlling blood sugar, then, is not so much the type of carbohydrates but rather the total amount of carbohydrates in the diet.

People with Type II diabetes—those who make insulin but whose cells resist responding to it—tend to become obese, storing more fat than normal and being constantly hungry. This is because the liver takes up from the blood the glucose that the cells cannot take up, converts the glucose to fat, and then ships it out to the fat cells for storage. The fat cells respond—slowly, to be sure—but ultimately they store all the fat that is sent to them. Due to the insulin resistance of body cells, insulin does not move glucose into cells effectively, and the message that energy fuels are coming in from food is delayed, causing the person with diabetes to be constantly hungry. Unfortunately, the larger the fat cells become, the more resistant they may be to insulin, thus making the diabetes worse. People with diabetes in their family are urged not to gain excess weight, for it is likely to precipitate the onset of the disease.

The rarer type of diabetes (Type I) occurs in about 10 percent of all cases. It involves a total lack of insulin and requires insulin injections. The person who does not produce any insulin is likely to experience a sudden onset of the disease. Such a person may lose weight rapidly because without insulin, the cells cannot store glucose or fat. Thus, the two types of diabetes have opposite effects on body weight—one making the person fat; the other, thin.

Choosing Healthful International Cuisines

Every culture has its own typical foods and ways of combining foods into meals. The challenge for healthful ethnic dining is in learning to choose foods for good health without sacrificing good taste. The following tips guide you through a variety of international cuisines with this challenge in mind.

Chinese

Many Chinese dishes are based on an abundance of rice and vegetables, small portions of meat, and low-fat preparation methods, making them quite healthful. Here are a few things to look for when you buy or prepare Chinese food.

Limit

1. Foods prepared with whole eggs, such as lobster sauce, egg drop soup, and egg foo yung.
2. Fried foods, such as egg rolls, fried noodles, fried rice, "crispy" meat, poultry, or fish, and fried dumplings.
3. Fatty foods, such as duck, goose, poultry with skin, and spareribs.
4. Regular soy sauce, duck sauce, plum sauce, and MSG—they are high in sodium.

Try Instead

1. Dishes made with low-fat, cholesterol-free egg whites.
2. Foods cooked using the stir-fry method with a small amount of unsaturated oil, such as chicken with broccoli and shrimp with Chinese vegetables, or by steaming, such as dim-sum selections and steamed dumplings.
3. Lean cuts of meat, skinless poultry, all types of fish, and shellfish—also try bean curd (tofu) to replace or enhance meat.
4. Reduced-sodium soy sauce. Also, most Chinese restaurants will prepare food without MSG, if requested.

Japanese

Most Japanese cuisine fits easily into a healthful lifestyle with its emphasis on fresh fish and vegetables prepared with little fat. The basis for much of its flavor, however, is soy sauce (shoyu). This salty condiment may be a problem if you are watching your sodium intake.

Limit

1. Deep-fried foods, such as fish, meat, or vegetable tempura.
2. Bottled prepared sauces, such as soy sauce, teriyaki, or tempura. They can be high in sodium.
3. Commercial miso soups.

Try Instead

1. Steamed or grilled (kushiyaki) vegetable, fish, shellfish, or skinless poultry dishes with a little tempura dipping sauce on the side.
2. Reducing the amount you use, switching to a reduced-sodium soy sauce, or preparing daikon sauce. To make this sauce, grate fresh daikon radish and add lemon juice, chopped green onions, and a little reduced-sodium soy sauce (optional).
3. Preparing miso soup at home with a lower-salt miso paste.

Consumer Tips

African-American

The traditional African-American diet has copious amounts of healthful vegetables and whole-grain foods. Many dishes, though, also call for fatty meats and a fair amount of fat added during preparation. Try some of these alternatives.

Limit

1. Fried foods, such as fried chicken, fried fish, or beef livers with onions.

2. High-fat cuts of meat, such as pig feet, chitterlings (chitlins) and hogmaws, pig tails, spareribs, sausage, regular bacon, oxtails, goat, and ham hocks.

3. Vegetables and beans prepared with fat back, neck bones, salt pork, ham hocks, or coconut oil.

4. Hominy grits with butter, baked macaroni and cheese, and home fries.

5. Ice cream, frosted cake, and fruit cobbler made with lard or shortening.

Try Instead

1. Baked, broiled, or stewed chicken (no skin); baked, broiled, or steamed fish. Eat liver (chicken or beef) only occasionally and bake or broil instead of frying.

2. Lower-fat meats, such as skinless chicken or turkey, fish, lean stew beef, beef tenderloin, center-cut ham, Canadian bacon, pork tenderloin, and pork loin chops.

3. Vegetables and beans prepared with turkey parts (no skin) and selected herbs for seasoning.

4. Hominy grits with a little margarine, baked macaroni and low-fat cheese (5 or fewer grams of fat per ounce), or baked or boiled potatoes.

5. Low-fat frozen yogurt, ice milk, fruit ice, angel food cake with fruit instead of icing, or fruit cobbler made with a small amount of liquid vegetable oil or margarine.

Hispanic

Traditionally, Hispanic foods are hearty fare, relying heavily on rice, meat, tortillas, beans, salted fish, and fats. By making some simple ingredient and preparation changes, traditional Hispanic cuisine can be more healthful as well.

Limit

1. Corn chips (fried), pork skins (*chicharron*), and guacamole.

2. Butter, lard, shortening, coconut oil, palm oil, and salt pork.

3. Prepared sauces, such as *sofrito* and *mojo criollo*.

4. Fried foods, such as fried tortillas, fried vegetable fritters (*alcapurrias*), banana slices (*tostones*), fried pork or chicken with skin, and refried beans.

5. High-fat meats and salad dishes, such as roast pork (*lechon asado*), shrimp, tuna, and lobster salads made with mayonnaise, *picadillo* with ground beef, and chicken stew (*pollo asopao*).

6. Higher-fat ground beef-filled tacos, burritos, and enchiladas.

7. Malt beer and egg yolk (*malta*), coffee with cream or evaporated whole milk, and blender drinks with whole milk (*batidas*).

Try Instead

1. Baked tortillas, popcorn, regular salsa, or sauce made from low-fat or plain yogurt with tabasco and coriander.

2. Small amounts of corn, olive, safflower, canola, sunflower, soybean, cottonseed oils, or margarines/spreads made from these oils.

3. Homemade *sofrito* with a little liquid oil instead of lard. For *mojo criollo*, use garlic powder and seasonings, but no meat drippings.

4. Baked tortillas, boiled dumplings (*pasteles*), boiled bananas (*tuineo, platano*), baked or broiled meat or chicken without skin, and boiled beans.

5. Well-trimmed roast pork, salads with reduced-calorie mayonnaise or low-fat or nonfat plain yogurt, *picadillo* with lean ground turkey, or chicken stew with skinless chicken.

6. Lean beef-, chicken-, or bean-filled soft burritos, enchiladas, or tacos.

7. Plain malt beer, juice, coffee with nonfat or low-fat milk, and blender drinks with nonfat yogurt or nonfat milk.

SOURCE: Adapted from Ethnic and Healthful, *Nutrition Counselor,* Volume VII, 1990.

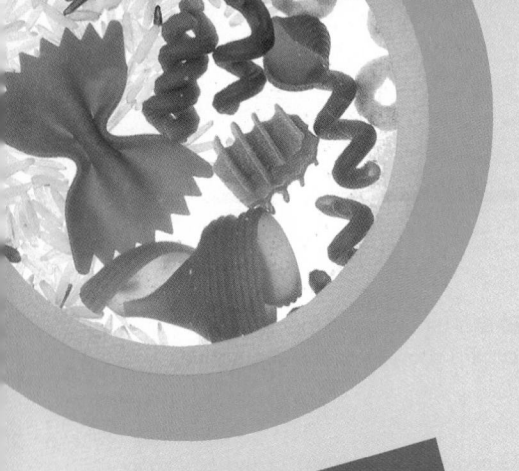

Dipping Into the Melting Pot

American cuisine is often described as nothing more than meat-and-potato meals or burgers, fries, hot dogs, and apple pie. But to define American food in this limited way does the United States an injustice. American eating habits are as diverse as the various ethnic and cultural groups that make up America's people. Throughout American history, immigrant groups—from Poles to Jews to Italians to Irish to Germans to Hispanics to African-Americans to Asians—have had and continue to have a profound effect on the collective American palate.

Certainly, it's not only the Americans who are members of various ethnic groups who enjoy their own traditional fare. Consider that in the past decade, more and more consumers from many different cultural backgrounds have begun to enjoy an ever increasing variety of ethnic foods. In fact, according to the National Restaurant Association, some 90 percent of restaurant menus now include ethnic dishes, and 80 percent use recipes from more than one national cuisine, a 35 percent increase from 1988.[31] What's more, **fusion cuisine**—the merging of elements from different ethnic cuisines to create a new dish—has been gaining in popularity in the past decade. For example, many restaurants are now offering items such as Mexican pizza, which borrows from both Hispanic and Italian food traditions.

As food writer and critic John Mariani has pointed out:

. . . the United States—a stewpot of cultures—has developed a gastronomy more varied. . . than that of any other country in the world. . . . In any major American city one will find restaurants representing a dozen national cuisines, including northern Italian trattorias, bourgeois French bistros, Portuguese seafood houses, Vietnamese and Thai eateries, Chinese dim sum parlors, Japanese sushi bars, and German rathskellers.[32]

This Spotlight examines some of the more prevalent ethnic and regional food practices to see how they originated and how they fit into a healthful eating plan.

I love to eat Mexican food, but I've heard that it is loaded with fat. Is that true? Do the Mexican people eat a lot of high-fat food? It's true that many menu selections in Mexican restaurants are loaded with high-fat ingredients such as cheese, ground beef, sour cream, guacamole, and fried tortillas. But most dishes eaten regularly in Chicano, or Mexican-American, homes are much simpler. Breakfast, for example, might be tortillas (flat, thin corn or wheat pancakes) served with fried beans, eggs, or cereal, and a beverage. Lunches and dinners often consist of beans and rice, bread or tortillas, meat/sausage (often as part of a stew), a vegetable or lettuce and tomato, and a beverage. The traditional Mexican diet, which draws largely from Spanish and Indian influences, was even simpler, containing mostly vegetables, including beans, squash, and maize (corn). In addition, it often included cactus parts, agave (a plant with spiny-margined leaves and flowers), chili peppers, **amaranth** (a grain), avocado, and **guava** (a sweet, juicy fruit with green or yellow skin and red or yellow flesh).

This emphasis on a diet high in complex carbohydrates, such as rice, and vitamin A- and C-rich fruits and vegetables is a particularly healthful aspect of the traditional Mexican way of eating. Consider that no Mexican meal is complete without salsa, a low-fat condiment consisting of vitamin-rich tomatoes, chilis, and onions. Another plus of the Mexican diet is the frequent use of beans, mostly the pinto variety, which rank as a particularly good source of fiber.

Among the downsides of the Mexican diet, however, is the heavy-handed use of oil and lard. Most foods, even beans and rice, are fried rather than baked or broiled. For example, frijoles refritos (refried beans) are usually fried in lard and contain about 270 calories and 3 grams of fat per cup. Most flour tortillas are also made with lard, sometimes 1 or 2 teaspoons' worth per tortilla. (Corn tortillas, on the other hand, typically contain very little fat.) Another drawback of the Mexican diet is the frequent consumption of high-fat meats, such as **chorizo** (spicy pork or beef sausage) and eggs, which are used in dishes such as **chiles rellenos** (roasted mild green chili pepper stuffed with cheese, dipped in egg batter, and fried), **burritos** (warm flour tortillas stuffed with a mixture of egg, meat, beans, and/or avocado), and **chilaquiles** (tortilla casserole often made with eggs or meat).

Fortunately, Mexican-food lovers can take advantage of the popular cuisine with a little knowhow. Instead of the usual American versions of Mexican fare, such as fried tortillas packed with ground beef and smothered in cheese and sour cream, opt for corn tortillas filled with, say, regular, unfried pinto beans mixed with chopped onion and topped with a sprinkle of shredded cheese and a generous portion of lettuce, salsa, a dollop of nonfat plain yogurt (a low-fat alternative to sour cream), and a garnish of sliced avo-

cado. Or, instead of serving high-fat commercial tortilla chips with salsa, try making "no-fry" chips: immerse several tortillas in warm water, drain quickly, cut into six to eight wedges, and place on a nonstick pan; bake in a 500-degree Fahrenheit oven for three to four minutes, flip, and continue to bake for another minute or two until golden brown.

Adventurous eaters who have access to a wide variety of exotic produce might want to try some of the different fruits and vegetables the Mexican people have enjoyed for decades, such as **jicama** (HE-cah-mah) (yam bean root—a vegetable that is tan outside and white inside, has a mild chestnut flavor, and is always eaten raw).[33] Figure 3–9 shows produce and other foods commonly eaten by Chicanos.

I always thought chop suey, egg rolls, and fortune cookies were traditional Chinese foods, but a Chinese-American friend of mine says they aren't. Is she right? Yes, it's true that chop suey and the like are American inventions. The tradi-

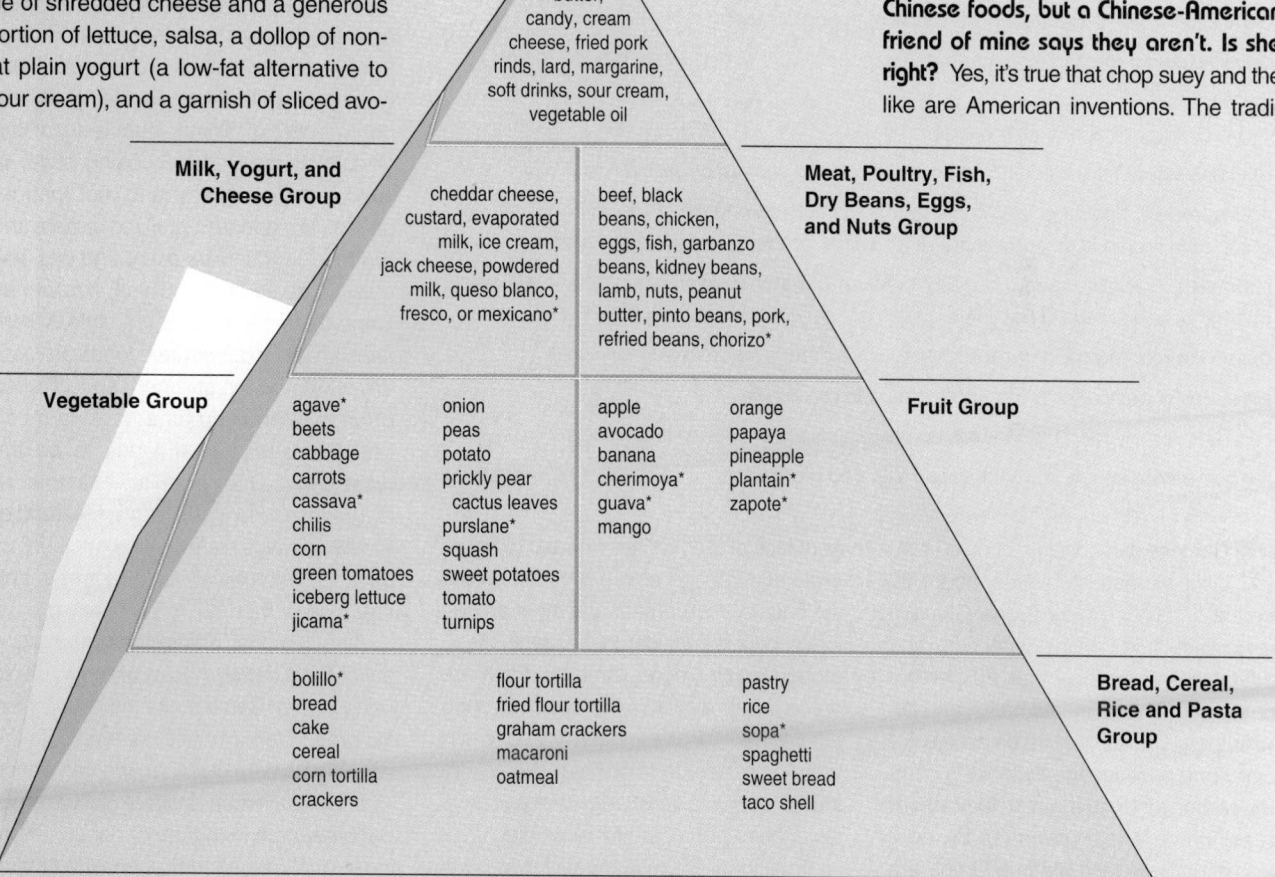

FIGURE 3–9
CHICANO FOODS AND THE FOOD GUIDE PYRAMID

*These foods are described in the Miniglossary.

SOURCE: Adapted from *Pyramid Packet,* © 1993, Penn State Nutrition Center, 417 East Calder Way, University Park, PA 16801.

MINIGLOSSARY

FUSION CUISINE a term used to describe food that combines the elements of two or more cuisines—say, European and Oriental—to create a new one.

CHICANO FOODS

AGAVE a plant with spiny-margined leaves and flower

BOLILLO a roll-like bread often used instead of tortillas or to make sandwiches

BURRITOS warm flour tortillas stuffed with a mixture of egg, meat, beans, and/or avocado

CASSAVA a starchy root that is never eaten raw because it must be cooked to eliminate its bitter smell

CHERIMOYA a fruit with a rough green outer skin and sherbetlike flesh

CHILAQUILES tortilla casserole often made with eggs or meat

CHILES RELLENOS roasted mild green chili pepper stuffed with cheese, dipped in egg batter, and fried

CHORIZO spicy beef or pork sausage

GUAVA a sweet juicy fruit with green or yellow skin and red or yellow flesh

JICAMA a crisp, bean root vegetable that is tan outside and white inside and is always eaten raw; jicama is as popular in Mexico as the potato is in the United States

PLANTAIN a greenish, starchy banana; because it is starchy even when ripe, it is never eaten raw and is usually pan-fried

QUESO BLANCO, FRESCO, or **MEXICANO** soft white cheese made of part-skim milk

SOPA rice or pasta that is fried and cooked in consomme

PURSLANE leafy vegetable that can be used in salads or cooked like spinach

ZAPOTE an apple-size fruit with green skin and black flesh

tional Chinese diet consists of much simpler, lower-fat dishes. Overall, about 80 percent of calories in traditional Chinese fare comes from grains, legumes, and vegetables, while the other 20 percent comes from animal meats, fruits, and fat. In southern China, rice can be easily produced and provides the bulk of the complex carbohydrate in the diet. In northern areas, where wheat grows readily, noodles, dumplings, and steamed buns are staples. In all regions of the country, fruits and vegetables are eaten in abundance. Typically, they are not eaten raw but rather are steamed, added to soups, or stir-fried in peanut or corn oil or, less frequently, lard. In addition, vegetables are often salted, pickled, and dried, a practice resulting from lack of the facilities needed to refrigerate and transport fresh produce across the country. As for meat and other protein foods, pork is considered the staple meat, though poultry, eggs, lamb, and fish are eaten when available. Tofu, or soybean curd, is another staple often added to stir-fries or fermented into sauces. Dairy foods, such as milk and cheese, have never been part of the Chinese diet.

Traditional Chinese meals follow basically the same pattern. Breakfast might be rice congee (rice gruel containing bits of meat), a salty side dish such as pickles, and tea. Lunch typically consists of soup, rice, and mixed dishes made with vegetables and fish, meat, or poultry, and dinner is usually a larger version of lunch, occasionally followed by fresh fruit.

Four schools of cooking have developed within China as a result of differences in climate, food production, religion, and custom: Peking, Shanghai, Szechwan or Hunan, and Cantonese. Peking cooking, which comes from the north and northeast part of China, is distinguished by use of garlic, leeks, and scallions and has given rise to familiar dishes such as Peking duck and spring rolls. Shanghai cuisine, from the east and coastal areas, is characterized by "red-cooking"—braising foods with large amounts of soy sauce and sugar. Pickled and salted vegetables are also frequently served with meat. In the west and central part of China, people favor the Szechwan or Hunan cooking style, in which chili peppers and hot pepper sauces are added liberally to dishes, and the food tends to be spicy and oily. The cuisine of southern China, known as Cantonese cooking, is the style Americans know best. Because foods are usually steamed or stir-fried and chicken broth is often used as a cooking medium, Cantonese food tends to be the least fatty. One popular example of Cantonese food is **dim sum,** steamed or fried dumplings stuffed with pork, shrimp, beef, sweet paste, or preserves and steamed or fried.[34]

The regional differences in cooking styles and eating habits among people living in rural China make the country fertile ground for scientific research into the effects of diet on disease. Another reason rural China is such an ideal place to conduct research is that most people residing in rural China today spend their entire lives within the vicinity of the community in which they were born. In addition, eating habits are dictated by climate and environment because the country has little or no means of transporting foods from one region to another. Thus, scientists have been able to carefully study eating patterns and disease rates in an attempt to see how the two are related. One of the largest such studies was led by T. Colin Campbell, Ph.D., of Cornell University. Begun in 1983, the research was carried out in 130 villages located in 65 counties of rural China and included 6,500 adults. While the data accumulated in this study are enormous and analyses are still underway, the findings suggest that the traditional, plant-based Chinese diet is associated with low rates of many of the chronic diseases that plague Americans, such as heart disease and some types of cancer.[35]

To be sure, Chinese food served in American Chinese restaurants is a far cry from the type eaten day in and day out by the rural Chinese people. Many

Chinese restaurant meals are swimming in oil and contain much more meat and poultry and fewer vegetables than "real" Chinese food. Consider that a typical American Chinese meal might include won ton soup, barbecued spareribs, chicken lo mein, and fried rice—chalking up some 1,400 calories and more than 80 grams of fat. A typical meal eaten in rural China, on the other hand, would likely contain a heaping portion of rice, along with fiber- and

nutrient-rich vegetables and less than an ounce of meat and fish and would thereby contain only a fraction of the fat.[36] Americans who want to enjoy both the flavor and the health benefits of traditional Chinese cuisine can "stretch" one of the many, delicious vegetable-based dishes with relatively large portions of rice and go easy on deep-fried appetizers such as egg rolls. People who enjoy cooking can also follow the Chinese people's lead and make low-fat, high-carbohydrate stir-fries with lots of vegetables, little oil, and small amounts of meat, poultry, or seafood. People who are sodium-conscious may also want to go easy on soy sauce, which con-

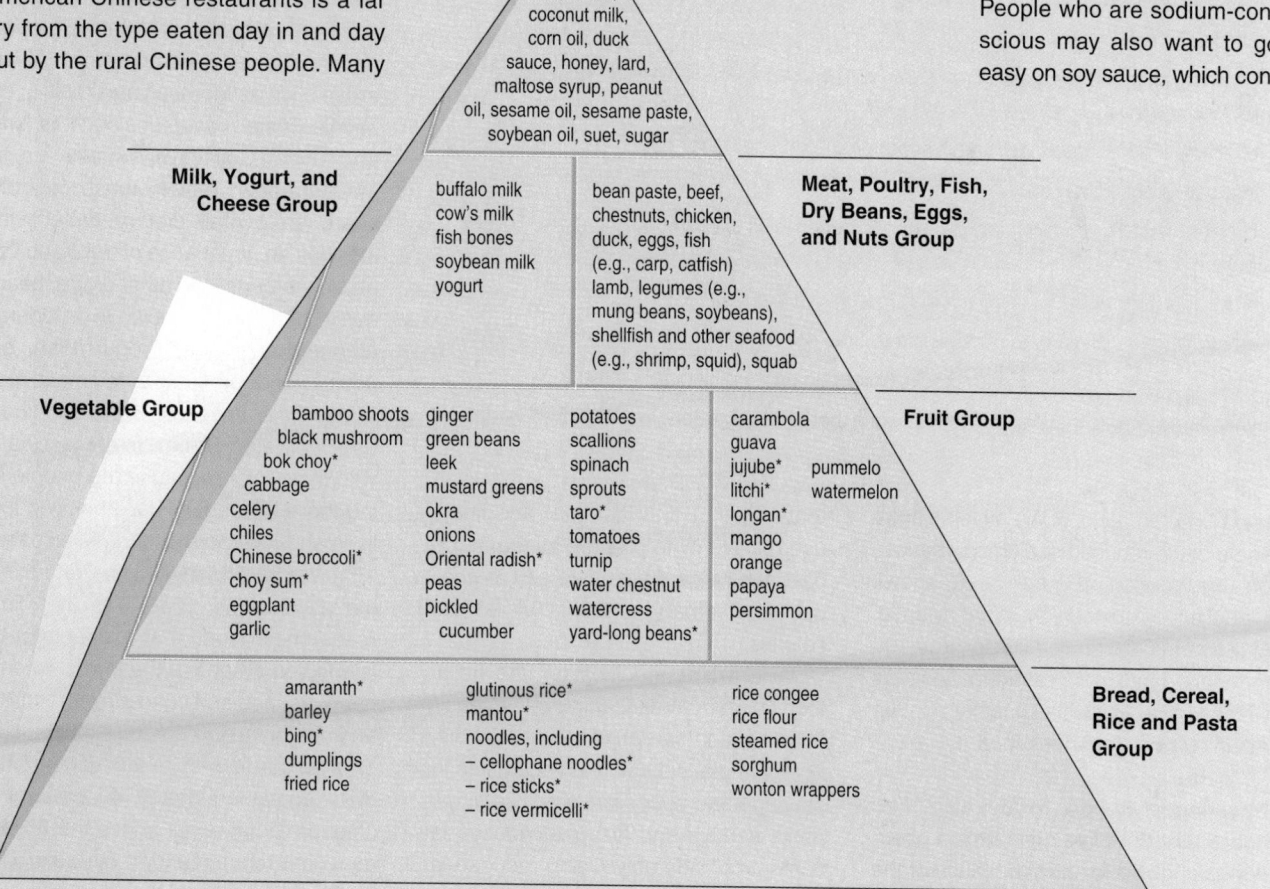

FIGURE 3–10
A CHINESE-AMERICAN FOOD GUIDE PYRAMID

SOURCE: Adapted from *Pyramid Packet,* © 1993, Penn State Nutrition Center, 417 East Calder Way, University Park, PA 16801.

MINIGLOSSARY

CHINESE-AMERICAN FOODS

AMARANTH a golden-colored grain

BING thin pancakes

BOK CHOY a vegetable with broad, white or greenish-white stalks and dark green leaves; also called Chinese chard

CELLOPHANE NOODLES thin, translucent noodles made from mung beans

CHINESE BROCCOLI a green leafy vegetable often stir-fried; also called Chinese kale

CHOY SUM a bright-green vegetable commonly stir-fried; also called field mustard or Chinese flowering cabbage

DIM SUM steamed or fried dumplings stuffed with pork, shrimp, beef, sweet paste, or preserves and steamed or fried

GLUTINOUS RICE short-grained, opaque, white rice that turns sticky when cooked

JUJUBE Chinese date

LITCHI small, round fruits with orange-red skin and opaque, white flesh; also called litchee or lychee

LONGAN a small, round fruit with smooth brown skin and clear pulp

MANTOU steamed bread

ORIENTAL RADISH large, cylindrically shaped vegetables with smooth skin; also called daikon

RICE STICKS flat, opaque, wide noodles made from rice flour

RICE VERMICELLI thin, white noodles made from rice flour

TARO a starchy vegetable with brown, hairy skin and a pink-purple interior

YARD-LONG BEANS thin, tender string beans that grow to as long as 18 inches

tains large amounts of the mineral, or try some of the reduced-sodium soy sauces on the market. Figure 3–10 shows Chinese foods placed on a food pyramid.

See the Consumer Tips on page 100 for more hints on preparing healthful Chinese food as well as another popular Asian cuisine, Japanese food.

How does Italian food rate? I've heard that the olive oil in Italian pasta dishes is good for health. Much of the Italian food served in the United States runs very high in fat and calories. Rich cream sauces in dishes such as fettucine alfredo, an abundance of cheese and sausage in entrees, including meat-topped pizza and lasagna, and liberal use of olive oil to prepare all manner of pasta and other Italian fare can all chalk up extraordinary amounts of fat and calories.

With a little modification, the Italian food so many Americans love can easily fit into a high-carbohydrate, low-fat diet. For example, substituting vegetables for sausage and pepperoni on pizza and in pasta sauces and lasagna reduces fat content considerably. Using reduced-fat cheeses, such as part-skim mozzarella and ricotta and low-fat cottage cheese, as substitutes for high-fat versions called for in many Italian recipes also helps skim some of the fat.

When it comes to olive oil, a staple in traditional Italian cuisine, it's true that using it instead of butter is preferable from a health standpoint. For reasons that we will explain in detail in Chapter 4, olive oil and other vegetable oils are less likely than certain other types of fat, such as butter and lard, to boost blood cholesterol levels. Some scientists even believe that people can eat large amounts of fat—in the neighborhood of 35 to 40 percent of total calories—without raising their risk of heart disease, as long as the predominant fat is olive oil. This line of thinking stems from research conducted in southern Italy and the Greek island of Crete, as well as southern regions of other European nations, including France; North African areas such as Morocco and Tunisia; and Middle Eastern countries such as Israel and Syria. Collectively known as the Mediterranean region, these countries share an overall dietary pattern that includes an abundance of fruits and vegetables, breads, and other grains, beans, nuts, and seeds; low to moderate amounts of cheese, yogurt, fish, and poultry; small amounts of red meat; moderate consumption of wine; and liberal use of olive oil. Scientists are fascinated with this region because the people living there historically have enjoyed long lives and low rates of chronic diseases. That was particularly true in Crete during the 1950s and 1960s. At that time, researchers found that residents of the island shared one of the lowest rates of heart disease and cancer ever recorded and one of the longest life expectancies. That held true despite the fact that their diets contained nearly 40 percent of calories as fat—well above the 30 percent limit recommended by major U.S. health organizations.[37]

With this historical perspective in mind, some scientists recommend that Americans adopt a "Mediterranean diet" that includes lots of fruits, vegetables, and grains; little meat and other flesh food; moderate amounts of wine; and generous amounts of olive oil. This advice has sparked a good deal of controversy within the scientific community, however. Many nutrition experts question the wisdom of recommending such a diet in America, where excess fat from olive oil and other sources might contribute to the epidemic of obesity in this country. In addition, many experts point out that diet is not the only lifestyle factor that may have promoted the long, healthy lives of the people of Crete and Italy several decades ago. For example, the residents of this region farmed the land and thereby engaged in far more physical activity than the average American, a factor that probably played a role in their health and longevity. In addition, unlike many modern-day Americans,

they enjoyed the social support of extended networks of family and friends, another part of their lifestyle that probably contributed to their well-being. Given these caveats, major U.S. health organizations, including The American Dietetic Association, the American Heart Association, and the U.S. Department of Health and Human Services, maintain that Americans should keep the amount of total fat—whether in the form of olive oil or anything else—to no more than 30 percent of total calories.

Our advice is that you consider adopting the aspects of the Mediterranean diet virtually all nutrition experts advocate: eat an abundance of produce, grains, and legumes combined with moderate amounts of dairy products, and relatively smaller amounts of meats, poultry, and fish.

What about "soul food"? Do most African-Americans eat lots of it? Soul food is a term that was coined in the mid-1960s to promote ethnic pride and solidarity among African-Americans.[38] But the origins of soul food date back to a much earlier time in history. Black-eyed peas, grits (coarsely ground cornmeal), collard greens, okra, and other soul foods evolved from the traditional diet of West African slaves living in the South. When West Africans were brought to the

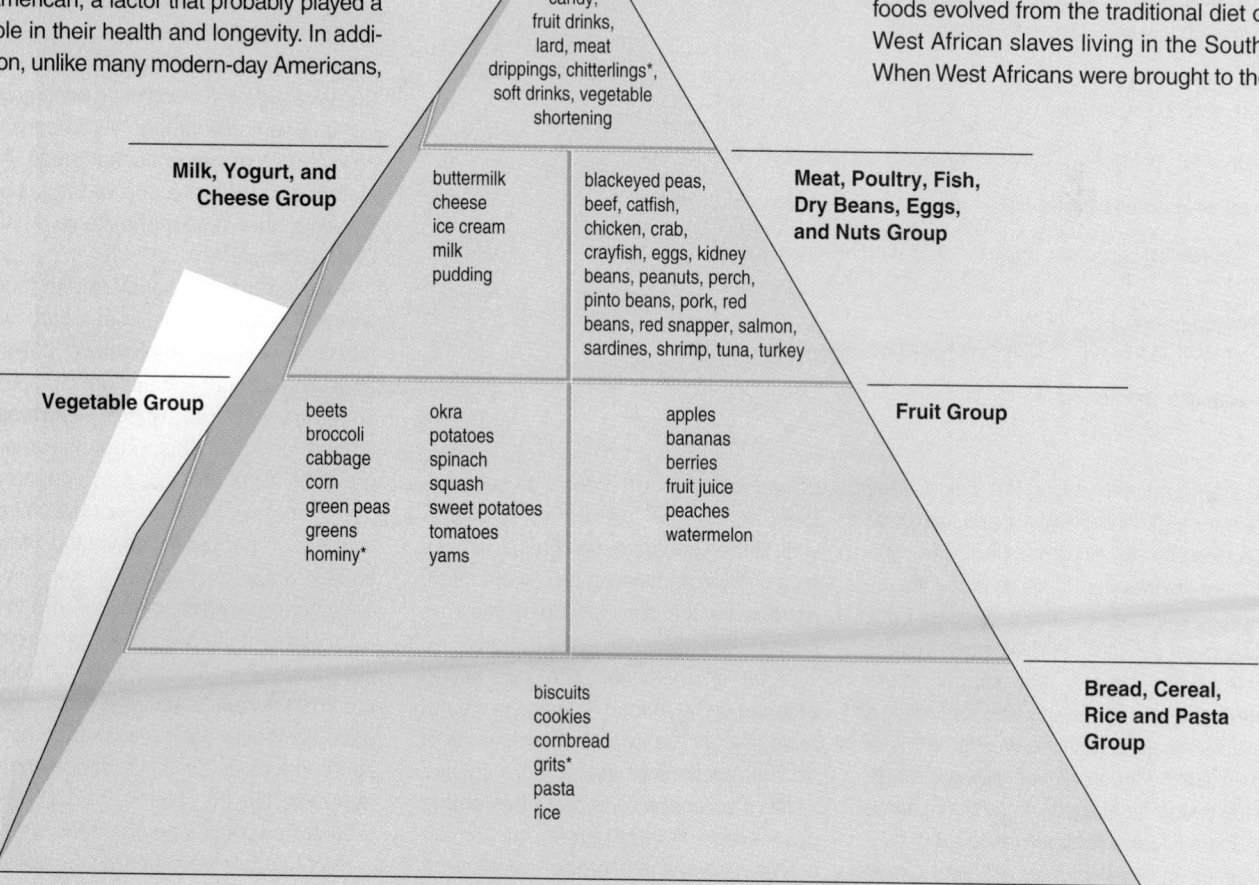

FIGURE 3–11
TRADITIONAL AFRICAN-AMERICAN FOODS AND THE FOOD GUIDE PYRAMID

SOURCE: Adapted from *Pyramid Packet*, © 1993, Penn State Nutrition Center, 417 East Calder Way, University Park, PA 16801.

MINIGLOSSARY

AFRICAN-AMERICAN FOODS AND TERMS

SOUL FOOD a term coined in the mid-1960s to promote ethnic pride and solidarity among African-Americans

GRITS coarsely ground cornmeal

HOMINY hulled, dried corn kernels with certain parts removed

CHITTERLINGS (chitlins) pig intestine

JEWISH-AMERICAN FOODS AND TERMS

BIALY a flat breakfast roll that is softer than a bagel

CHALLAH an egg-containing yeast bread, often braided, and served on the Sabbath and holidays

GELFILTE FISH a chopped fish mixture often made with pike and whitefish as well as matzoh crumbs, eggs, and seasonings

KASHA cracked buckwheat, barley, millet, or wheat that is served as a cooked cereal or potato substitute

KASHRUT biblical ordinances regarding which foods are fit to eat

KNISH a potato pastry filled with ground meat, potato, or kasha

KOSHER fit, proper, or in accordance with religious law

LOX smoked salmon

MATZOH a crackerlike bread eaten most often at Passover

SCHMALTZ chicken fat

United States to work the fields, their dietary habits revolved around the foods provided by slave owners. Corn was commonly given as a staple, and the slaves prepared it in many forms, such as grits, cornmeal pudding, and **hominy** (hulled, dried corn kernels with certain parts removed). Salt pork was also frequently a staple supplied to the slaves, so pork fat was used to fry and flavor greens, breads, stews, and other foods. In addition, some owners allowed their slaves to grow vegetables in small plots. Okra and black-eyed peas, two West African favorites, were introduced in the United States by the slaves who farmed such plots, and American vegetables, including cabbage,

collard and mustard greens, sweet potatoes, and turnips, were often grown as well. Other southern favorites, such as fried chicken and fried catfish, were made popular by the slaves who worked as cooks in the homes of slave owners.

After emancipation, the food-eating patterns of the African-Americans did not change significantly and represent much of what we think of as southern cuisine today. The underpinnings of this eating style, which is very high in fat, remain corn-based dishes, greens, pork, and pork products such as **chitterlings** (chitlins--pig intestines) and ham hocks. The food habits of African-Americans around the country tend to be influenced more

by economic status and geographic location than by heritage, although soul food remains a symbol of identity and heritage for many African-Americans.[39] Figure 3–11 shows traditional African-American foods in pyramid form.

I see lots of foods marked kosher in the supermarket, especially during Jewish holidays such as Passover. Are kosher foods better for health than regular items? Do other religious groups eat special foods? As pointed out in Chapter 1 (refer to Table 1–8 on page 17), food is part of the symbolism and traditions of many major religions. In the predominantly Christian United States, however, most people's eating habits are not dictated by religion to a large extent.

Nevertheless, during the past few decades "Jewish" foods have been growing in popularity among Americans of all different religious backgrounds. For instance, bagels are one of the fastest growing breakfast menu items in the United States.[40]

Most of the traditional Jewish foods eaten in America come from a particular group known as Ashkenazic Jews—Jews from central and eastern European countries such as Russia, Germany, Poland, and Romania. (The other major group is Sephardic Jews, who come mainly from Spain and Portugal.) While few Jewish people in the United States strictly abide by all the dietary laws Judaism prescribes, many adhere to at least some of the rules of **kashrut,** biblical ordinances specifying which foods are **kosher,** or fit to eat. The most widely used symbol to denote kosher certification on foods is the U, which designates approval by the Union of Orthodox Jewish Congregations of America.

Most people assume that the laws of kashrut were set forth to protect the health of the Jewish people. For example, a popular misconception is that kashrut forbids the consumption of pork products because eating undercooked pork can cause serious illness. In truth, however, Jewish dietary laws are considered divine commandments set forth to maintain spiritual, not physical, health. Foods labeled as kosher are not necessarily more healthful than their unmarked counterparts. Instead, the designation kosher indicates that a food has been prepared in accordance with the basic tenets of kashrut. For instance, one principle of kashrut is separation of milk and meat products, meaning that an item containing, say, both ground beef and cheese would not be kosher. Another tenet is selection of appropriate meat, poultry, and seafood items: Only animals with cloven hooves who chew their cud are allowed—cattle, sheep, goats, and

deer; chicken, turkey, goose, pheasant, and duck can be kosher, but birds of prey are not; and seafood with both fins and scales can be kosher, while shellfish is forbidden. Finally, keeping kosher requires eating only animal flesh that has undergone a ritual slaughtering process that usually includes covering the meat with large amounts of salt.

As a result of the salting process used to prepare kosher animal foods,

many traditional Jewish foods are high in sodium. Herring, smoked fish, canned beef, tongue, corned beef, and other deli-style meats are examples. Other traditional Jewish foods, many of which are high in fat, include **schmaltz** (chicken fat), **knishes** (potato pastry filled with ground meat or potato), cream cheese, and chopped liver.[41] Figure 3–12 shows how some traditional Jewish foods fit into the Food Guide Pyramid.

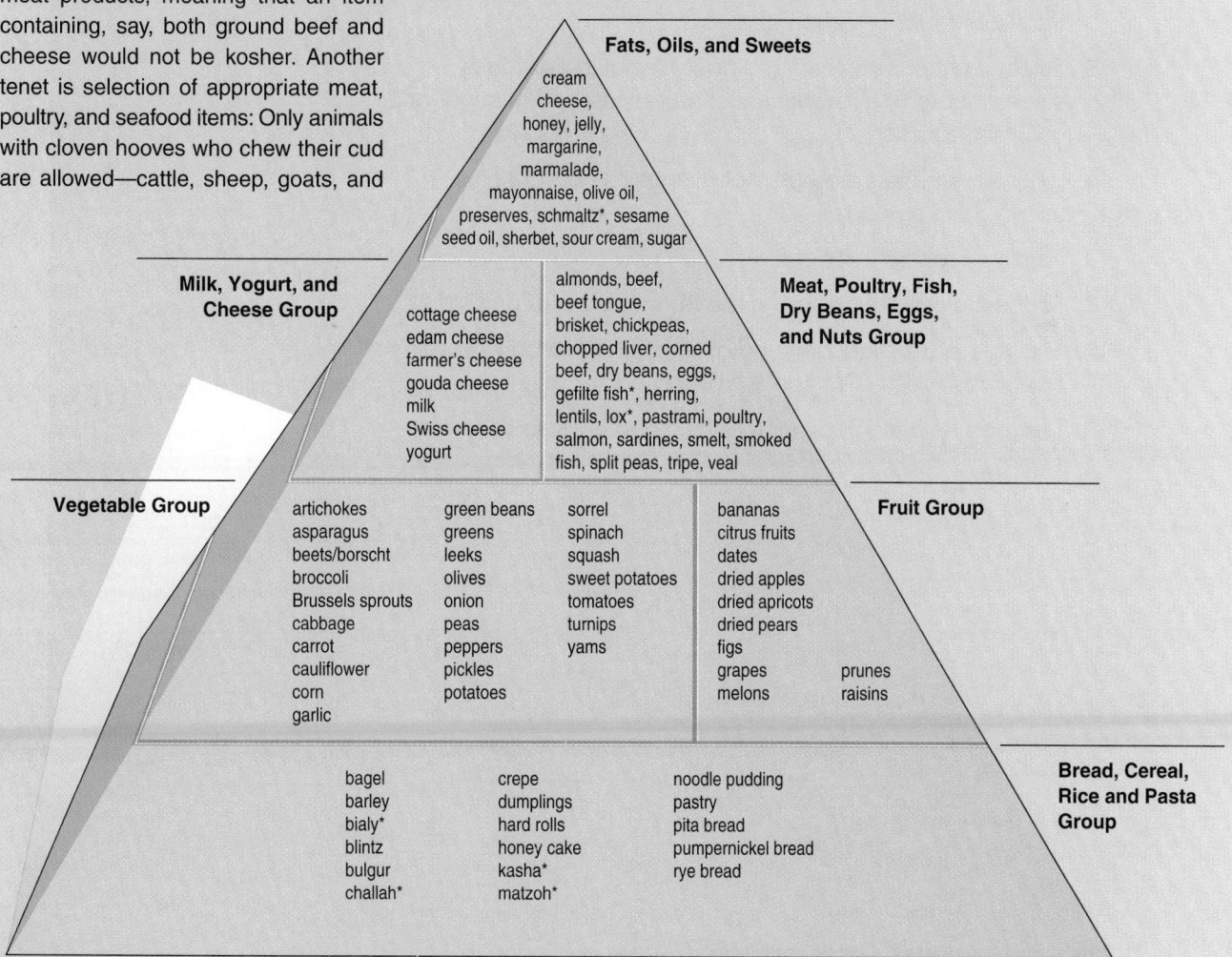

FIGURE 3–12

FITTING JEWISH-AMERICAN FOODS INTO THE FOOD GUIDE PYRAMID

SOURCE: Adapted from Pyramid Packet, © 1993, Penn State Nutrition Center, 417 East Calder Way, University Park PA 16801.

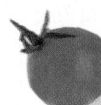

CHECK YOURSELF...

1. Which carbohydrates are described as simple and in which foods are they found?

2. Which carbohydrates are described as complex and in which foods are they found?

3. Why are carbohydrates the ideal fuel for the body?

4. What are the current dietary recommendations regarding the intake of complex carbohydrates and sugar?

5. State whether people with diabetes should eat foods sweetened only with sugar substitutes instead of sugar and give a rationale.

6. Why are enriched products not always as nutritious as whole-grain products?

7. List the health effects of fiber.

8. Suggest ways for increasing the fiber content of one's diet.

9. Summarize the digestion and absorption of carbohydrates in the body.

10. Describe how the body maintains blood glucose concentrations.

Answers to selected Check Yourself questions are found in Appendix H.

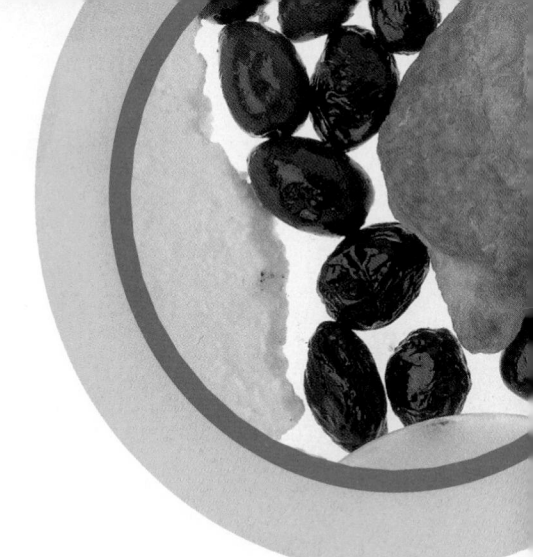

> The ultimate reality of nutrition rests with the chemistry of the food we eat and its effects on the processes of life.
>
> R. M. Deutsch
> (1928–1988, nutrition author and educator)

The Lipids: Fats and Oils

FOUR

Contents

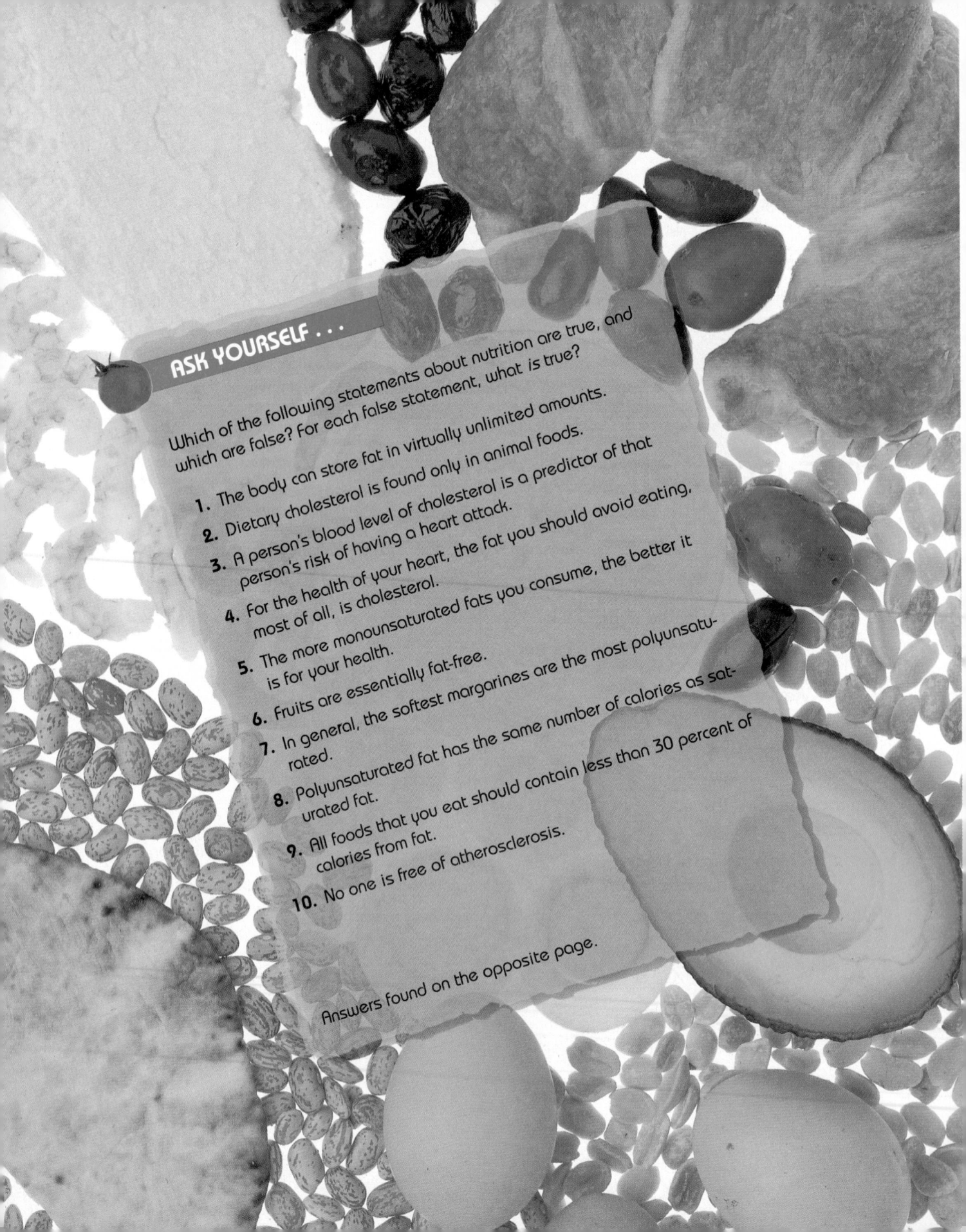

ASK YOURSELF . . .

Which of the following statements about nutrition are true, and which are false? For each false statement, what *is* true?

1. The body can store fat in virtually unlimited amounts.

2. Dietary cholesterol is found only in animal foods.

3. A person's blood level of cholesterol is a predictor of that person's risk of having a heart attack.

4. For the health of your heart, the fat you should avoid eating, most of all, is cholesterol.

5. The more monounsaturated fats you consume, the better it is for your health.

6. Fruits are essentially fat-free.

7. In general, the softest margarines are the most polyunsaturated.

8. Polyunsaturated fat has the same number of calories as saturated fat.

9. All foods that you eat should contain less than 30 percent of calories from fat.

10. No one is free of atherosclerosis.

Answers found on the opposite page.

While you and your friend are visiting a health fair at a local shopping mall, you learn that your blood cholesterol level is high. Your friend, a registered dietitian, urges you to see your health-care provider to request a blood test to determine the level of triglycerides and the ratio of "good" to "bad" cholesterol in your blood. As you are leaving the mall, you notice a bookstore display for a new diet book that urges you to cut fat intake to reduce cancer risk. Then you stop at the window of a health-food store. Your friend points to the freshly ground peanut butter, mentioning to you that it is not hydrogenated, while you stare at the bottles of antioxidant and fish oil supplements that line the wall. Later, during the evening news, your attention is drawn to a television commercial featuring a loving couple promising to use heart-healthy spreads on their morning muffins. "What does all of this mean?" you ask.

Actually you may know more than you think you do about the **lipids,** more commonly called **fats** and **oils.** The most obvious dietary sources of fat are oil, butter, margarine, and shortening. Other food sources that provide fat to the diet are meats, nuts, mayonnaise, salad dressings, eggs, bacon, gravy, cheese, ice cream, and whole milk. You may know that egg yolk and liver are high in cholesterol, and you probably know that the cholesterol in the body is in some way related to heart disease. However, you may be confused by the many terms related to the fat in your diet. This chapter explores the terminology of fat and describes how fats can both contribute to health and detract from it.

LIPIDS a family of compounds that includes triglycerides (fats and oils), phospholipids (lecithin), and sterols (cholesterol).

FATS lipids that are solid at room temperature.

OILS lipids that are liquid at normal room temperature.

A Primer on Fats

Most people have the impression that fat is bad for them, and it might come as a surprise that fats are valuable. More than valuable, some are absolutely essential, and some fats must be present in the diet for you to maintain good health. Even if you wanted to, it would be impossible to remove all the fat from your diet, because at least a trace of fat is found in almost all foods.

The Functions of Fat in the Body

Fat is the body's chief storage form for the energy (or calories) from food eaten in excess of immediate need. Fats provide most of the energy needed to perform much of the body's work, and especially muscular work.

Fat serves as an energy reserve. Whenever you eat, you store some fat, and within a few hours after a meal, you take the fat out of storage and use it for energy until the next meal. Thus, both glucose and fat are stored after meals, and both are released later when needed as fuel for the cells' work. However, whereas excess carbohydrate and protein can be converted to fat, they cannot be made from fat. Fat can serve only as an energy fuel for cells equipped to use it.

The body has scanty reserves of carbohydrate and virtually no protein to spare, but it can store fat in practically unlimited amounts. A pound of body fat

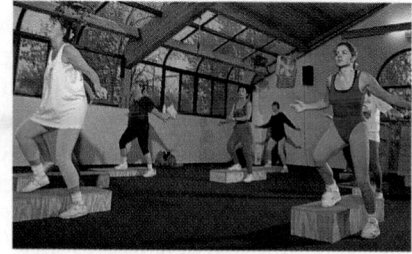

Muscles derive most of the fuel they need for work from body fat.

is worth 3,500 calories, and a person's body can easily carry 30 to 50 pounds of fat without appearing fat at all.

Both fats and oils are found in your body, and both help to keep your body healthy. Fat is important to all your body's cells as part of their cell membranes. Natural oils in the skin provide a radiant complexion; in the scalp they help to nourish the hair and make it glossy. Fat insulates the body and cushions the body's vital organs. It serves as a shock absorber. The fat blanket under the skin also provides insulation from extremes of temperature, thus achieving internal climate control. Table 4–1 summarizes the major functions of fats in the body.

The Functions of Fat in Foods

Fat is a nutrient found in many foods. As the most concentrated source of calories, fat contains more than twice as many calories, ounce for ounce, as protein or carbohydrate. High-fat foods may therefore deliver many *unneeded* calories in only a few bites to the person who is not expending much physical energy. Fats in foods also provide **satiety** by slowing the rate at which the stomach empties. This is the reason you feel fuller longer after eating meals that include fat.

Fat is important for another reason. Some essential nutrients are soluble in fat and therefore are found mainly in foods that contain it. These nutrients are the essential fatty acids (to be described shortly) and the fat-soluble vitamins—A, D, E, and K (described in Chapter 6). Fat also carries many dissolved compounds that give foods their aroma and flavor. This accounts for the aromatic smells associated with foods that are being fried, such as onions or French fries. It also helps explain why a plain doughnut is more flavorful than a plain roll—it is higher in fat. Table 4–2 summarizes the functions of fats in foods.

The Terminology of Fat

About 95 percent of the lipids in foods and in the human body are **triglycerides.** Other members of the lipid family are the **phospholipids** (of which **lecithin** is one) and the **sterols** (**cholesterol** is the best known of these). The **blood lipid profile** refers to a test analyzed by a medical laboratory that reveals the amounts of various lipids (especially triglycerides and cholesterol) found in the blood and the carriers (such as LDL and HDL, described later) in which they are found. The results of this test tell much about a person's risk of heart disease, or **cardiovascular disease** (**CVD**). The blood cholesterol level is especially telling, and it bears on the question of whether people should avoid foods containing fat, those containing cholesterol, or both.*

---

*Blood, plasma, and serum cholesterol all refer to about the same thing; this book uses the term blood cholesterol. Plasma is simply blood with the cells removed; serum has the clotting factors also removed. The concentration of cholesterol is not much altered by these treatments.

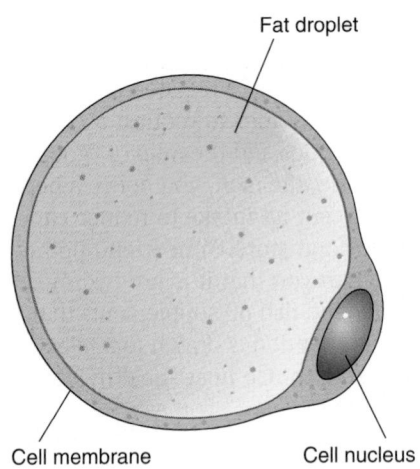

Fat droplet

Cell membrane   Cell nucleus

A Fat Cell

Within the fat cell, lipid is stored in a droplet. This droplet can greatly enlarge, and the fat cell membrane will grow to accommodate its swollen contents. (More about fat cells and obesity in Chapter 8.)

SATIETY the feeling of fullness or satisfaction that people feel after meals.

TABLE 4–1 THE ROLE OF FATS IN THE BODY
FATS IN THE BODY:
• Provide a concentrated source of energy
• Serve as an energy reserve
• Form the major components of cell membranes
• Nourish skin and hair
• Insulate the body from extremes of temperature
• Cushion the vital organs to protect them from shock

TABLE 4–2 THE ROLE OF FATS IN FOODS
FATS IN FOODS:
• Provide calories (9 calories per gram)
• Provide satiety
• Carry fat-soluble vitamins and essential fatty acids
• Contribute aroma and flavor

Two kinds of lipids in foods are:

- triglycerides (commonly called fat)
- cholesterol

Similarly, two kinds of lipids in the blood are:

- triglycerides
- cholesterol

A person's *blood* level of cholesterol is considered to be a predictor of that person's likelihood of suffering a heart attack or stroke. The fat in *food* that contributes most to a high blood cholesterol level is triglycerides (especially those that contain *saturated* fat), *not cholesterol*. People often fail to understand this point, and the question arises again and again: "Should I eat cholesterol?" When told, "It doesn't matter much," the questioner often jumps to the wrong conclusion—the conclusion that cholesterol doesn't matter. It does matter. High *blood* cholesterol is an indicator of risk for CVD, but the main *food* factor associated with it is a high *fat intake.***** One more distinction must be made clear about fats on the plate: they come in two varieties, saturated and unsaturated, and the saturated type is strongly implicated in raising blood cholesterol. The differences between saturated and unsaturated fats are described later.

A Closer View of Fats

Most of the fat, especially saturated fat, in our diet comes from animal flesh or animal products (see Figure 4–1). Animal fat, in turn, may have come from the fats and oils in plants; from the carbohydrate in plants, as you learned in the previous chapter; or from protein, discussed in Chapter 5. When the energy from any of the energy-yielding nutrients is to be stored as fat, it is first broken into fragments—small molecules made of carbon, hydrogen, and oxygen. These fragments are then linked together into chains known as **fatty acids**—the major building blocks of triglycerides, the chief form of fat.

Saturated Versus Unsaturated Fats

Fatty acids differ from one another in two ways: in chain length and in degree of saturation. Chain length refers to the number of carbons that are hooked together in the fatty acid.† Chain length is significant because it affects solubility of

TRIGLYCERIDES (try-GLISS-er-ides) the major class of dietary lipids, including fats and oils. A triglyceride is made up of three units known as fatty acids and one unit called glycerol.

PHOSPHOLIPIDS (FOSS-foh-LIP-ids) one of the three main classes of lipids; a lipid similar to a triglyceride but containing phosphorus.

LECITHIN (LESS-ih-thin) a phospholipid, a major constituent of cell membranes, manufactured by the liver and also found in many foods.

STEROLS (STEER-alls) one of the three main classes of lipids; a lipid with a structure similar to that of cholesterol.

CHOLESTEROL (koh-LESS-ter-all) one of the sterols, manufactured in the body for a variety of purposes and also found in animal-derived foods.

BLOOD LIPID PROFILE a test that determines the amounts and kinds of lipids in the blood, normally as part of a diagnosis for cardiovascular disease risk.

CARDIOVASCULAR DISEASE (CVD) disease of the heart and blood vessels. The two most common forms of CVD are *atherosclerosis* and *hypertension* (see this chapter's Spotlight).

FATTY ACIDS basic units of fat composed of chains of carbon atoms with an acid group at one end and hydrogen atoms attached all along their length.

---

*A few individuals have a hereditary inability to clear from their blood the cholesterol they have eaten and absorbed. This condition is rare but well-known in medical circles, because the study of it led to the discovery of how cholesterol is transported in the body. People with hereditary high blood cholesterol levels must refrain from eating cholesterol in foods. The vast majority of people can eat eggs and other cholesterol-containing foods in moderation without fear of incurring high blood cholesterol levels.

†Short-chain fatty acids contain 4 to 6 carbons; medium-chain fatty acids contain 8 to 10 carbons; long-chain fatty acids contain 12 or more carbons.

the fat in water—the short-chain fatty acids are somewhat soluble in water. Milk, butter, and cheese are rich in the short-chain fatty acids; vegetable oils and red meat contain triglycerides with long-chain fatty acids.

Of more significance than chain length is the degree of *saturation*, mentioned earlier in relation to heart disease. Saturation refers to the chemical structure—specifically to the number of hydrogens the fatty acid chain is holding. If every available bond from the carbons is holding a hydrogen, we say the chain is a **saturated fatty acid**—filled to capacity, or saturated, with hydrogen (see Figure 4–2).

Sometimes, especially in the fatty acids in plants and fish, there is a place in the chain where hydrogens are missing—an "empty spot," or **point of unsaturation** (see Figure 4–2). A chain that possesses a point of unsaturation is an **unsaturated fatty acid.** If there is one point of unsaturation, it is a **monounsaturated fatty acid.** If there are two or more points of unsaturation, it is a **polyunsaturated fatty acid.**

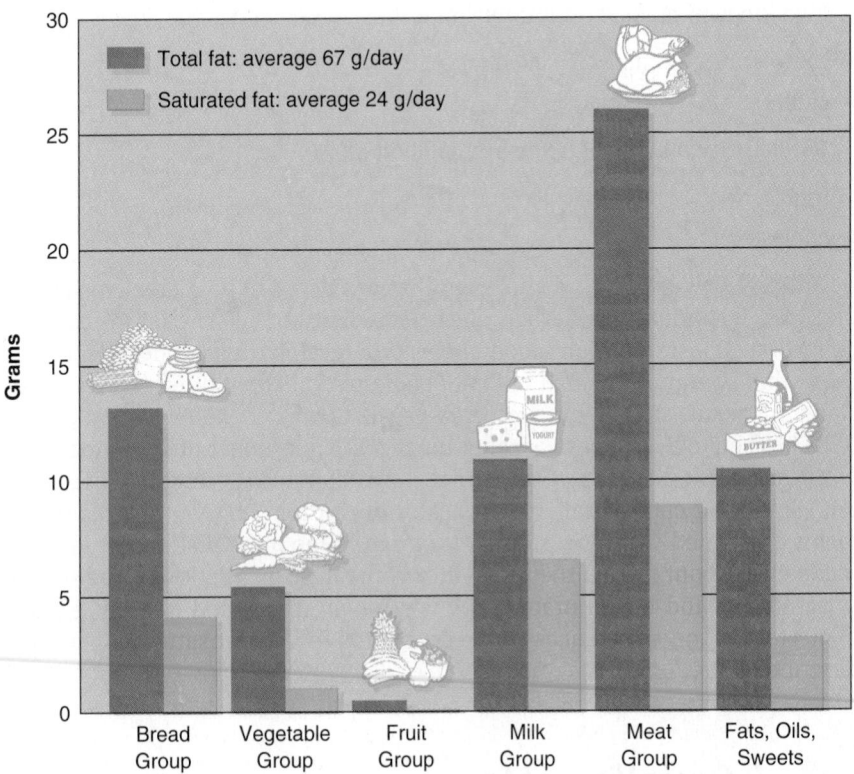

FIGURE 4–1

FAT AND SATURATED FAT CONTRIBUTED BY THE FOOD PYRAMID GROUPS IN THE U.S. DIET

SOURCE: *Eating in America Today: A Dietary Pattern and Intake Report/Edition II (Eat II)*, 1994, p. 13.

The Essential Fatty Acids

The human body can synthesize all the fatty acids it needs from carbohydrate, fat, or protein, except two—**linoleic acid** and **linolenic acid.** These two cannot be made from other substances in the body or from each other, and they must be supplied by the diet; they are, therefore, **essential fatty acids.** These fatty acids are polyunsaturated fatty acids, widely distributed in the diet, especially in plant and fish oils. To be sure, they are readily stored in the adult body, making deficiencies unlikely. Still, deficiency symptoms can appear in the person deprived of these acids—a characteristic skin rash and, in children, poor growth.

One further classification system for unsaturated fatty acids classifies the fatty acid as either an **omega-6** or an **omega-3** fatty acid (see Figure 4–2). Of the two essential fatty acids, linoleic acid is an omega-6 fatty acid, related to a whole series of others. Linolenic acid is an omega-3 fatty acid, with a similar family of its own.

Of interest in relation to dietary fat are findings on the omega-3 fatty acids found in fish oils, which offer a protective effect on health. Interest in fish oils was first kindled when someone thought to ask why the Eskimos of Greenland, who eat a

SATURATED FATTY ACID a fatty acid carrying the maximum possible number of hydrogen atoms (having no points of unsaturation). A saturated fat is one that is made up primarily of saturated fatty acids.

POINT OF UNSATURATION a site in a molecule where the bonding is such that additional hydrogen atoms can easily be added.

UNSATURATED FATTY ACID a fatty acid in which one or more points of unsaturation occur. An unsaturated fat is a triglyceride in which one or more of the fatty acids is unsaturated.

MONOUNSATURATED FATTY ACID (sometimes abbreviated MUFA) a fatty acid containing one point of unsaturation.

POLYUNSATURATED FATTY ACID (sometimes abbreviated PUFA) a fatty acid in which two or more points of unsaturation occur.

diet very high in fat, have such a low rate of heart disease. The trail led to the abundance of fish they eat, then to the oils in those fish, and finally to the omega-3 fatty acids—EPA and DHA—in the oils. Now scientists are unraveling the mystery of what those fatty acids do.[1]

The omega-3 fatty acids—found in highest amounts in fish that live in cold waters—have a profound effect on the synthesis of certain hormonelike compounds that play many regulatory roles in the body. They affect a number of body functions, including the formation of blood clots, the raising and lowering of blood pressure and blood lipid levels, the immune response, and the inflammatory response to injury and infection.* The types of these compounds made in the body determine the degree of vulnerability to certain diseases, including cardiovascular disease and cancer.[2] For example, an earlier study from the Netherlands reported that one or two fish meals a week in place of meat are all it takes to exert a significant positive effect.[3] The fatty acids in the fish appear to favorably alter the body's blood-clotting balance by reducing the ability of the blood to clot. These omega-3 fatty

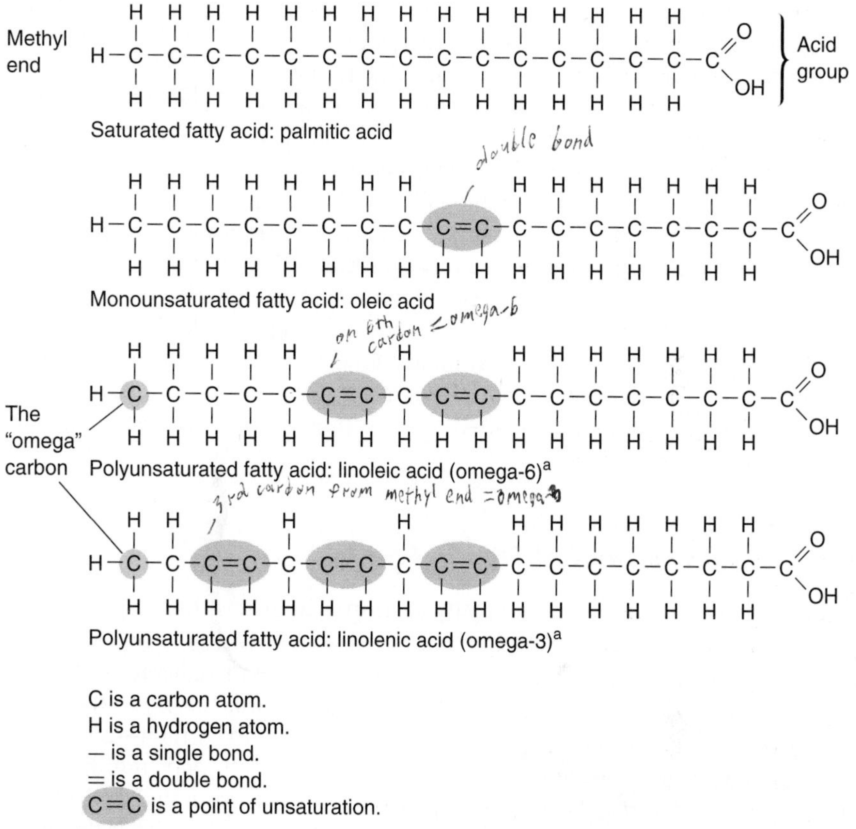

FIGURE 4–2
THE TYPES OF FATTY ACIDS

[a]The omega number (omega-6 or omega-3) designates the location of the first double bond, counting from the far end (the methyl [CH_3] end) of the fatty acid. Linoleic acid and linolenic acid are *essential* fatty acids.

acids provide protection against heart disease, possibly by producing substances that dilate the arteries, lower the blood pressure, and help to dissolve blood clots.[4] Researchers are currently trying to determine the appropriate amount of omega-3 fatty acids for a day's intake that might protect against heart disease.[5]

People who eat large amounts of fish tend to have lower blood cholesterol and triglyceride levels and slower clot-forming rates.[6] More than 70 studies have now documented other connections as well. Diets high in omega-3 fatty acids seem to bring about enhanced defenses against cancer (via the immune response) and reduced inflammation in arthritis and asthma sufferers. The Eskimos apparently did well using fish for food. Perhaps we, too, could benefit from eating fish in abundance.

LINOLEIC (lin-oh-LAY-ic) **ACID, LINOLENIC** (lin-oh-LEN-ic) **ACID** polyunsaturated fatty acids, essential for human beings.

ESSENTIAL FATTY ACID a fatty acid that cannot be synthesized in the body in amounts sufficient to meet physiological need.

OMEGA the last letter—the far end—of the Greek alphabet (ω), used by chemists to refer to the position of the end-most double bond in a fatty acid. The **omega-6** fatty acids have their end-most double bonds after the sixth carbon in the chain; the **omega-3** acids, after the third.

---

*The hormonelike compounds referred to here are the **eicosanoids** (eye-COSS-uh-noyds)—compounds that regulate blood pressure, clotting, and other body functions. Names of classes of eicosanoids are prostaglandins, thromboxanes, prostacyclins, and leukotrienes.

If our diets need modification, it is not by self-prescribing supplements of fish oils. Many hazards may be associated with the taking of such supplements. One reason is that they could unbalance the diet too far; you do need omega-6, too, remember. Too much fish oil might make a person susceptible to stroke or hemorrhage because of its effect of prolonging bleeding and clotting time. Fish oils—made from fish livers—may contain toxic amounts of fat-soluble vitamins and pesticide residues. These and other risks do not normally accompany the eating of a variety of fish. Furthermore, fish is both a good source of high-quality protein and relatively low in calories. The purified oils contain just oil, and oil is high in calories. If you tried to take enough fish oil to match the Eskimos' intake, you would need 300 to 500 calories a day—enough to gain about 25 pounds a year. Instead, substitute two or three fish meals a week for meals based on other protein-rich foods, and you may improve your health more safely.

Characteristics of Fats in Foods

The amount of unsaturated fatty acids in a fat affects the temperature at which the fat melts. The more unsaturated a fat, the more liquid it is at room temperature. In contrast, the more saturated a fat (the more hydrogen it has), the firmer it is. Thus, of three fats—beef fat, chicken fat, and corn oil—beef fat is the most saturated and the hardest; chicken fat is less saturated and somewhat soft; and corn oil, which is the most unsaturated, is a liquid at room temperature (and the only one of the three that comes from a plant). If your health-care provider tells you to use **monounsaturated fats** or **polyunsaturated fats,** you can usually judge which ones to choose by their hardness at room temperature. Fats and oils contain mixtures of saturated, monounsaturated, and polyunsaturated fatty acids; the fatty acids that predominate determine whether the fat is solid or liquid at room temperature. Figure 4–3 compares the most common fats and oils with regard to their percentages of the various types of fat.

Because fats differ chemically, they behave differently in foods. To control their characteristics, food manufacturers sometimes alter them—and sometimes the alterations have health consequences, as described in the Nutrition Action feature on page 120.

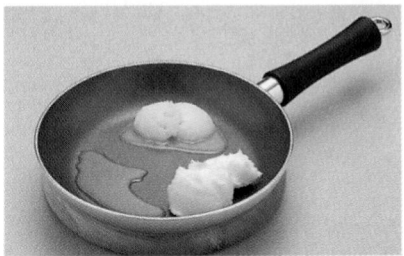

The more unsaturated a fat, the more liquid it is at room temperature. The more polyunsaturated the fat is, the sooner it melts.

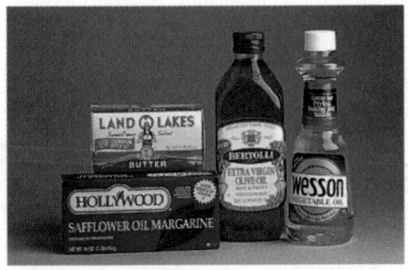

Fats in common use. The vegetable oil is polyunsaturated, the olive oil is monounsaturated, the butter is largely saturated, and the margarine, no doubt, is partially hydrogenated.

The fatty acids in fish oils include eicosapentaenoic (EYE-kossa-PENTA-ee-NOH-ic) acid (EPA) and docosahexaenoic (DOE-cosa-HEXA-ee-NOH-ic) acid (DHA), both of which are omega-3 fatty acids. In the future, we may see EPA and DHA classified as essential fatty acids.

SEAFOOD ESPECIALLY HIGH IN OMEGA-3 FATTY ACIDS (AT LEAST 1 GRAM OF OMEGA-3 FATTY ACIDS IN 3.5 OUNCES OF FISH): anchovies, Atlantic bluefish, herring, mackerel, sablefish, salmon (all varieties), sardines, sturgeon, tuna (white albacore—canned in water—or bluefin), and whitefish.

SEAFOOD MODERATELY HIGH IN OMEGA-3 FATTY ACIDS (0.5–0.9 GRAM IN 3.5 OUNCES OF FISH): pompano, rainbow trout, shark, smelt, striped bass, and swordfish.

OTHER SEAFOOD SOURCES OF OMEGA-3 FATTY ACIDS (0.5 GRAM OR LESS IN 3.5 OUNCES OF FISH): catfish, clams, cod, crab, crayfish, flounder, grouper, haddock, hake, halibut, lobster, mahi mahi, mullet, ocean perch, orange roughy, oysters, pike, pollock, rockfish, scallops, sea bass, sea trout, shrimp, snapper, and whiting.

OTHER MINOR SOURCES OF OMEGA-3 FATTY ACIDS (LINOLENIC ACID) BESIDES FISH AND SEAFOOD: canola oil, leafy vegetables, soybean oil, and walnuts.

MONOUNSATURATED FAT a triglyceride in which one or more of the fatty acids is monounsaturated.

POLYUNSATURATED FAT a triglyceride in which one or more of the fatty acids is polyunsaturated.

Points of unsaturation in fatty acids are like weak spots in that they are vulnerable to attack by oxygen. When the unsaturated points react with oxygen, the oils become rancid (see Figure 4–4). This is why unprocessed oils should be stored in tightly covered containers. If stored for long periods, they need refrigeration to prevent spoilage.

One way to prevent spoilage of oils containing unsaturated fatty acids is to change them chemically by **hydrogenation,** but this causes them to lose their unsaturated character and the health benefits that go with it. When food producers want to use a polyunsaturated oil such as corn oil to make a spreadable margarine, they hydrogenate the oil. Hydrogen is forced into the oil, some of the unsaturated fatty acids accept the hydrogen, and the oil becomes harder. The spreadable margarine that results is more saturated than the original oil but not as saturated as butter.

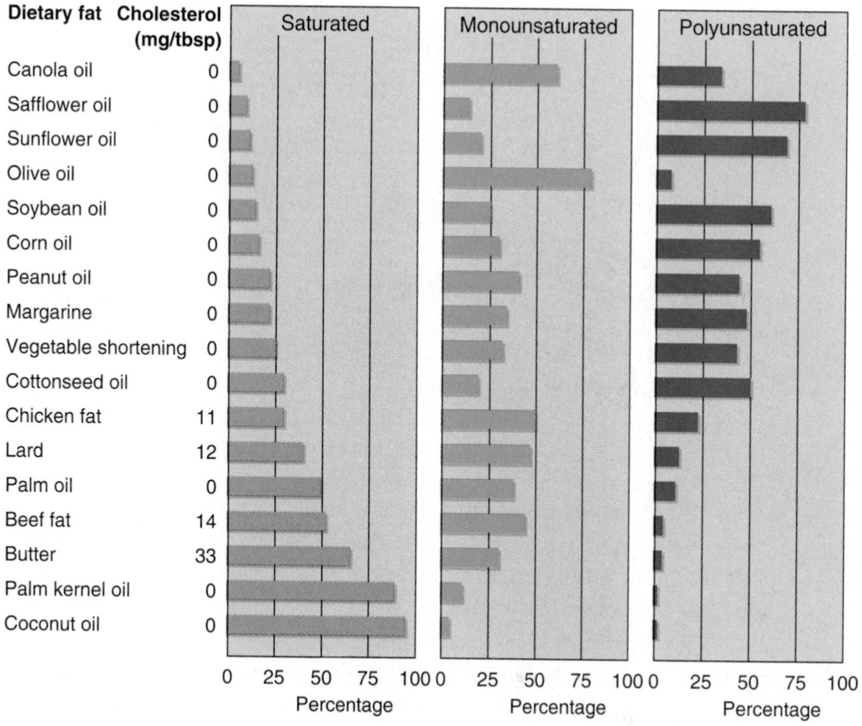
Dietary fat
Cholesterol (mg/tbsp)
Saturated
Monounsaturated
Polyunsaturated
Canola oil 0
Safflower oil 0
Sunflower oil 0
Olive oil 0
Soybean oil 0
Corn oil 0
Peanut oil 0
Margarine 0
Vegetable shortening 0
Cottonseed oil 0
Chicken fat 11
Lard 12
Palm oil 0
Beef fat 14
Butter 33
Palm kernel oil 0
Coconut oil 0
0 25 50 75 100
Percentage

FIGURE 4–3 COMPARISON OF DIETARY FATS

A second way to prevent spoilage of oils is to add a chemical that will compete for the oxygen and thus protect the oil. Such an additive is called an **antioxidant.** Examples are the well-known additives BHA and BHT listed on the labels of many processed foods, such as breakfast cereals and snack foods, and the natural antioxidants vitamin C and vitamin E. A third alternative, already mentioned, is to keep the product refrigerated.

For more information about the beneficial qualities of the antioxidant nutrients, see the Spotlight feature in Chapter 6.

Another way that the food industry alters natural fats and oils is by adding an **emulsifier** to a food product to allow fats and water to mix and remain mixed in a food product. Mayonnaise, margarines, salad dressings, and cake mixes often list an emulsifier on their labels. Mono- and diglycerides are good emulsifiers, as is the emulsifier found in egg yolk—lecithin.

HYDROGENATION (high-droh-gen-AY-shun) the process of adding hydrogen to unsaturated fat to make it more solid and more resistant to chemical change.

ANTIOXIDANT (anti-OX-ih-dant) a compound that protects other compounds from oxygen by itself reacting with oxygen.

EMULSIFIER a substance that mixes with both fat and water and can break fat globules into small droplets, thereby suspending fat in water.

FIGURE 4–4 OXIDATION

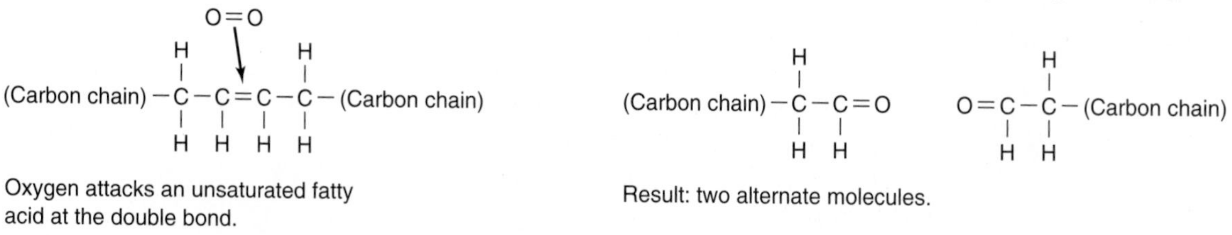
(Carbon chain)
(Carbon chain)
Oxygen attacks an unsaturated fatty acid at the double bond.
Result: two alternate molecules.

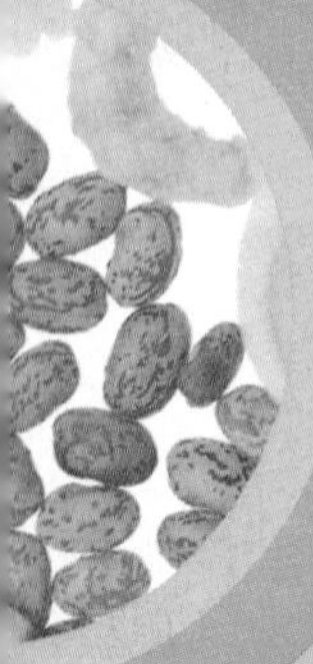

The Trans Fatty Acid Controversy: Is Butter Better?

NUTRITION ACTION

Conventional nutrition wisdom has long held that margarine is better than butter to use on food, including bagels and other breads. But in recent years, rumors have been spreading that margarine may not be the most healthful choice after all. The heart of the controversy is a growing body of research suggesting that a certain type of fat found in margarine may be as likely to boost blood cholesterol levels as the saturated fat found in butter.[7]

The alleged culprit, called **trans fatty acid,** is formed when margarine is processed. Consider that to make margarine, manufacturers take a highly unsaturated vegetable oil and partially hydrogenate (add hydrogen to) it; hydrogenation is what gives the spread its relatively solid consistency and helps protect against rancidity. During the hydrogenation process, however, a chemical "fluke" occurs. Hydrogenating the oil creates a new chemical configuration, known as a trans fatty acid, in which hydrogen atoms of the fat lie on opposite sides of the point of unsaturation in the carbon chain (see Figure 4–5). (You may recall that the body of a fatty acid molecule consists of a chain of carbon atoms to which hydrogen is attached, as shown in Figure 4–2 on page 117.)

Because trans fatty acids are formed whenever oils are hydrogenated, margarine isn't the only food on the market that contains trans fatty acids. Shortenings, baked goods, commercial frying fats used in fast-food outlets to cook French fries and other fried items, and any other foods that list "partially hydrogenated vegetable oil" among the ingredients contain trans fatty acids.

While nutrition experts have long advised that using margarine as a spread is preferable to using butter and that partially hydrogenated oils are the more healthful alternative to, say, lard, studies conducted during the past several years caught the attention of the media and sparked numerous news stories challenging that advice. The research suggests that high levels of trans fatty acids may raise blood levels of "bad" LDL-cholesterol nearly as much as saturated fats. What's more, the research suggests that in large amounts, trans fatty

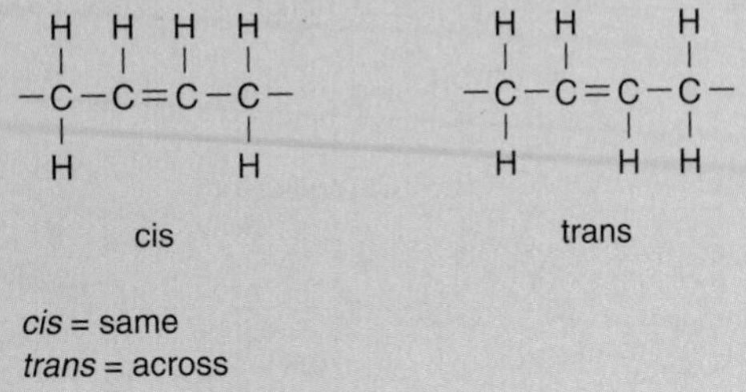

TRANS FATTY ACID a type of fatty acid created when an unsaturated fat is hydrogenated. Found primarily in margarines, shortenings, commercial frying fats, and baked goods, trans fatty acids have been implicated in preliminary research as culprits in heart disease.

cis = same
trans = across

FIGURE 4–5
TYPES OF UNSATURATED FATTY ACIDS: CIS VERSUS TRANS

Unsaturated fatty acids are either in *cis* form or in *trans* form, depending upon the way in which the hydrogen atoms are attached to the points of unsaturation in the carbon chain. If the hydrogen atoms are attached to the same side of the points of unsaturation, the arrangement is called cis. If the hydrogen atoms are attached to different sides, the arrangement is called trans.

acids lower "good" HDL-cholesterol in the blood.[8] One large-scale study even indicated that women who ate a diet high in trans fatty acid-containing foods, particularly margarine, were more likely to suffer heart disease than their counterparts who ate relatively little margarine and other trans fatty acid-containing foods. The study prompted a flurry of headlines and news reports questioning whether margarine was a healthful alternative after all.[9]

Fueling the controversy even further was an analysis by researchers at Harvard University suggesting that more than 30,000 American deaths each year are attributable to trans fatty acids. The authors of the report went so far as to call for government legislation mandating that manufacturers include trans fatty acid amounts on food labels and phase out the use of partially hydrogenated oils in the United States.[10]

Many major health organizations, including the American Heart Association, The American Dietetic Association, and the American Institute of Nutrition, have stated that the trans fatty acid brouhaha has been overblown. The organizations say that because only a handful of studies have been conducted on trans fatty acids, the research gathered to date doesn't warrant any changes in the way foods are labeled or recommendations for healthful eating.[11] What's more, the organizations point out that the trans fatty acid research does not indicate that consumers should switch back from eating margarine to eating butter, which contains an excess of saturated fat. That's because trans fatty acids account for only about two to eight percent of the total calories in a typical American diet, whereas saturated fat comprises some 12 percent to 14 percent of calories. Thus, the long-standing recommendation to keep to a minimum consumption of saturated fat, which a comprehensive body of research has clearly shown raises blood cholesterol levels, far outweighs concerns about trans fatty acids.

To be sure, continuing research may shed more light on the health effects of trans fatty acids. And while the evidence that has come to light doesn't warrant going back to butter, it does underscore the value of keeping the amount of

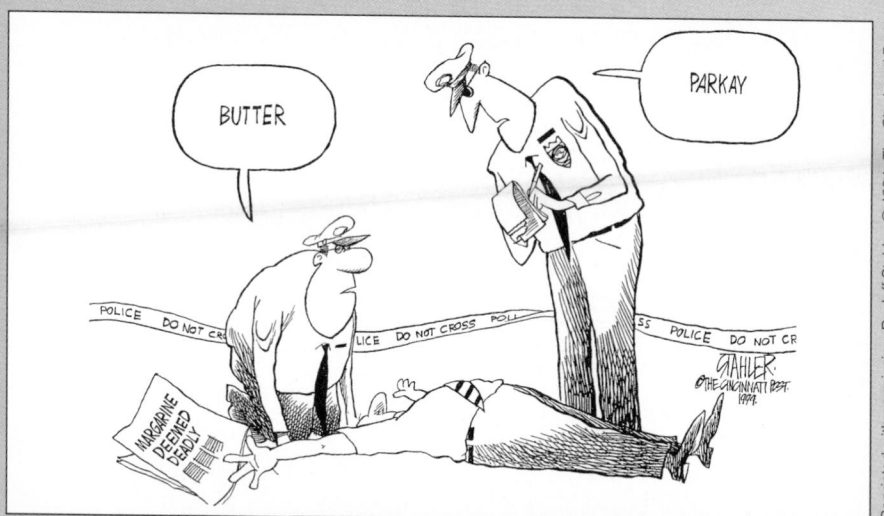

Reprinted with permission. By Jeff Stahler, © 1994, *The Cincinnati Post*.

total dietary fat to a minimum. The foods that contain large amounts of trans fatty acids—French fries, corn chips, deep-fat fried doughnuts—are also high in total fat (see Table 4–3). Thus, health-conscious eaters who want to hedge their bets against the possibility that trans fatty acids contribute to high blood cholesterol levels should stick with the same principles of low-fat eating that have been outlined throughout the book. They should also pay particular attention to the following:

- Shop for margarine containing no more than two grams of saturated fat per tablespoon, and choose soft tub or liquid forms over stick; "hard" stick margarines typically contain the most trans fatty acids.

- Limit total daily consumption of fats and oils to no more than five to eight teaspoons to keep both total fat and trans fatty acid consumption to a minimum.[12]

- Cook and bake with a vegetable oil, such as canola, olive, or corn oil, instead of butter, shortening, or margarine whenever possible.

- Check ingredients lists for "partially hydrogenated vegetable oil." The higher on the list it appears, the more of both total fat and trans fatty acids the product probably contains, and the more difficult it is to fit into a healthful diet. As an alternative, look for similar products made with unhydrogenated oils and smaller amounts of total fat.

- Remember that deep-fat fried foods such as French fries, doughnuts, chicken nuggets, and fried seafood contain excessive amounts of total fat as well as trans fatty acids and should be eaten in moderation.

TABLE 4–3
TUNING INTO TRANS FATTY ACIDS

Trans fatty acids occur naturally in meat, poultry, and dairy products. They show up in packaged and fast foods to which hydrogenated vegetable oils have been added. Note that high levels of trans fatty acids go hand in hand with high-fat foods. Thus, if you eat a low-fat diet, you will consume minimal amounts of trans fatty acids.

FOOD	GRAMS OF TRANS FATTY ACIDS*	GRAMS OF TOTAL FAT
ANIMAL FOODS		
5 oz beef	0.9	27.7
1 tsp butter	0.1	4.1
5 oz chicken	0.1	10.4
5 oz pork	0.1	21.7
VEGETABLE FATS		
1 tsp soft margarine	0.27	4
1 tsp stick margarine	0.62	4
1 tsp vegetable oil	0.02	4.5
1 tsp vegetable shortening	0.63	4.3
PACKAGED FOODS AND FAST FOODS		
1 piece yellow cake with chocolate frosting	1.04	11.2
1 oatmeal raisin cookie	0.86	3.3
1 oz corn chips	1.42	9.5
1 cake doughnut	3.19	10.8
4 oz deep-fat fried french fries	5.5	18.5
1 blueberry muffin	0.09	3.7
1 slice apple pie	1	13.8
1 slice cheese pizza	0.13	6.1
1 oz potato chips	0.11	9.8

*Figures represent the average values derived from several brands or varieties of the foods.

SOURCE: Adapted from L. Litin and F. Sacks, Trans-fatty-acid content of common foods, *New England Journal of Medicine* 329 (1994): 1969–1970.

The Other Members of the Lipid Family: Phospholipids and Sterols

Lecithin and other phospholipids are important components of cell membranes. Because of the way the phospholipids are constructed (see Figure 4–6), they can serve as emulsifiers in the body—joining with both water and fat so that they can help fats travel back and forth across the lipid-containing membranes of cells into the watery fluids on both sides. Due to its role as an emulsifier, lecithin is often listed in the ingredients list on food labels as a food additive. Food manufacturers add lecithin to foods such as margarine, chocolate, salad dressings, and frozen desserts to keep the fats dispersed with the other ingredients.

Magical properties are sometimes attributed to lecithin, and health-food advertisers try to persuade people to supplement their diets with it. But lecithin is widespread in food and is also made by the body in abundant quantities and therefore most people's diets contain adequate amounts.

Cholesterol is found only in animal foods and is also made and destroyed in the body, where it is an important compound with many functions (see Figure 4–7). It is a part of **bile,** which is necessary in the digestion of fats. It is the starting material from which the sex hormones and many other hormones are made. In the skin, one of its derivatives is made into vitamin D with the help of sunlight. It is an important lipid in the structure of brain and nerve cells. In fact, cholesterol is a part of every cell. But while it is widespread in the body and necessary to the body's function, it also is the major component of the plaque that narrows the arteries in the killer disease atherosclerosis (see the Spotlight at the end of the chapter for more on heart disease).

A molecule of lecithin is like a triglyceride but contains only two (polyunsaturated) fatty acids. The third position is occupied by choline (a compound related to the B vitamins). Two natural sources of lecithin include soybeans (soy lecithin) and eggs (egg yolk lecithin).

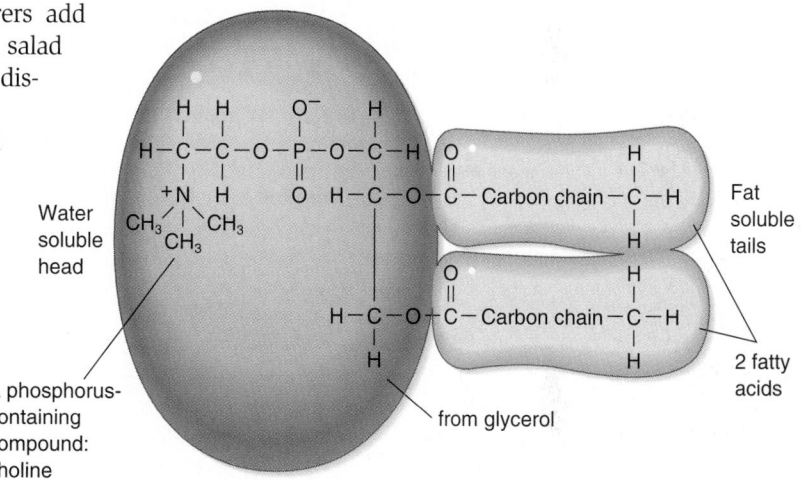

FIGURE 4–6
A PHOSPHOLIPID: LECITHIN

This phospholipid (lecithin) consists of a water-soluble head (with a phosphorus-containing compound) and a fat-soluble tail (made up of 2 fatty acids); thus, a phospholipid is a phosphorus-containing fat.

BILE a mixture of compounds, including cholesterol, made by the liver, stored in the gallbladder, and secreted into the small intestine. Bile emulsifies lipids to ready them for enzymatic digestion and helps transport them into the intestinal wall cells.

How the Body Handles Fat

When you eat carbohydrate or protein, some of it can be made into fat in the body (as already discussed for carbohydrate in Chapter 3). The carbohydrate is first digested to glucose. Some may be stored as glycogen, but some is broken down to fragments. Some of these fragments are used for energy; some are joined together to make fatty acids. The fatty acids are attached to **glycerol** to make triglycerides (see Figure 4–8). Finally, these are transported to the fat depots—muscles, breasts, the insulating fat layer under the skin, the abdominal region, and other areas.

GLYCEROL (GLISS-er-all) an organic compound, three carbons long, of interest here because it serves as the backbone for triglycerides.

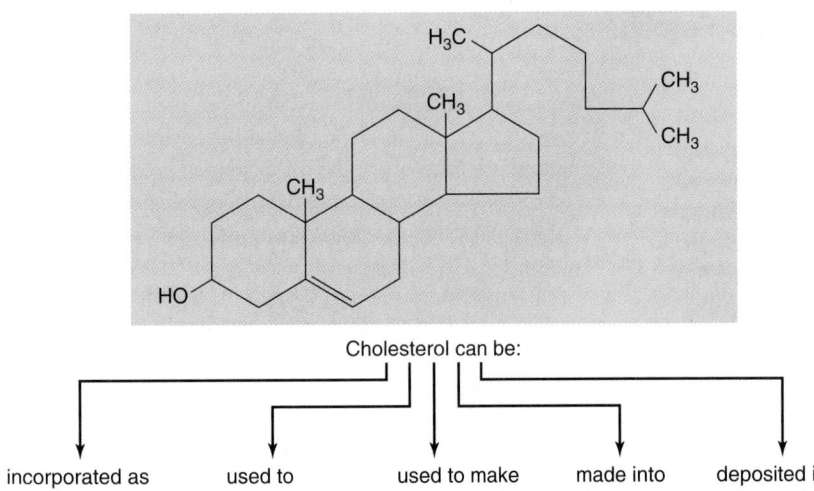

FIGURE 4–7 CHOLESTEROL

Notice how different the structure of cholesterol is from the structures of triglycerides and phospholipids.

Cholesterol can be:

| incorporated as an integral part of the structure of cell membranes | used to make bile for digestion | used to make sex hormones (estrogen and testosterone) | made into vitamin D | deposited in the artery walls leading to plaque buildup and heart disease |

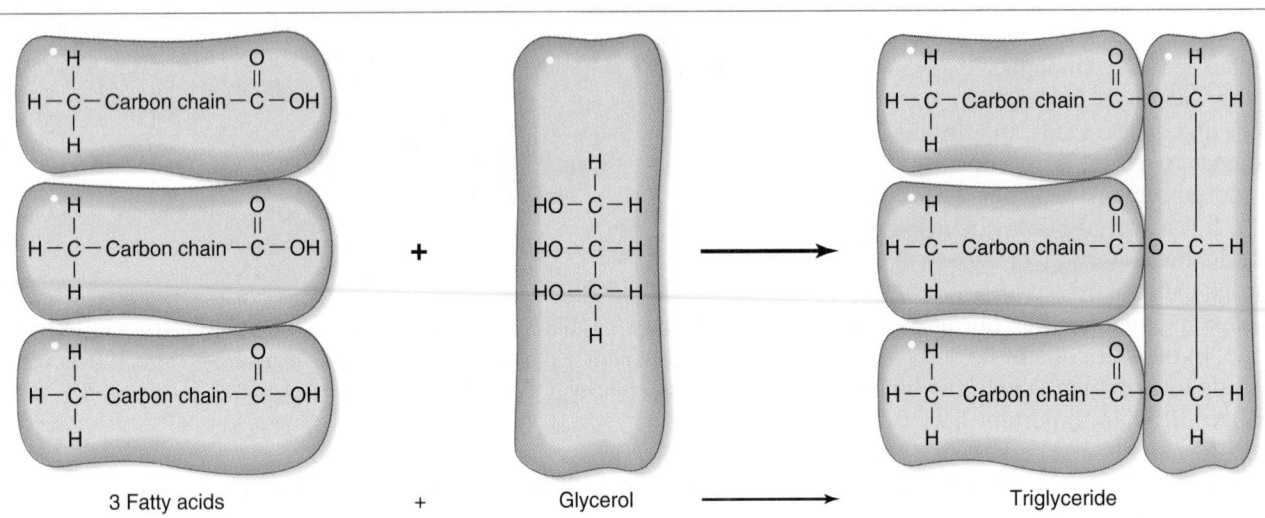

A triglyceride is made up of three fatty acids attached to a molecule of glycerol.

FIGURE 4–8 A TRIGLYCERIDE

When you eat animal flesh (meat, fish, or poultry) or animal products (milk, cheese, or eggs), you are eating a combination of fat and protein. Of the fat, 95 percent is triglyceride that has been made in the animal body, mostly from carbohydrate, the same way your body makes it. Animal fat can end up in fat stores in your own body, as can excess glucose or protein (see Figure 4–9), but first it has to be digested, absorbed, and transported to its cell destinations.

After digestion in the upper small intestine, the products of fat digestion—fatty acids, glycerol, and **monoglycerides**—must enter the bloodstream if they

MONOGLYCERIDE (mon-oh-GLISS-er-ide) one of the products of digestion of lipids; a glycerol molecule with one fatty acid attached to it.

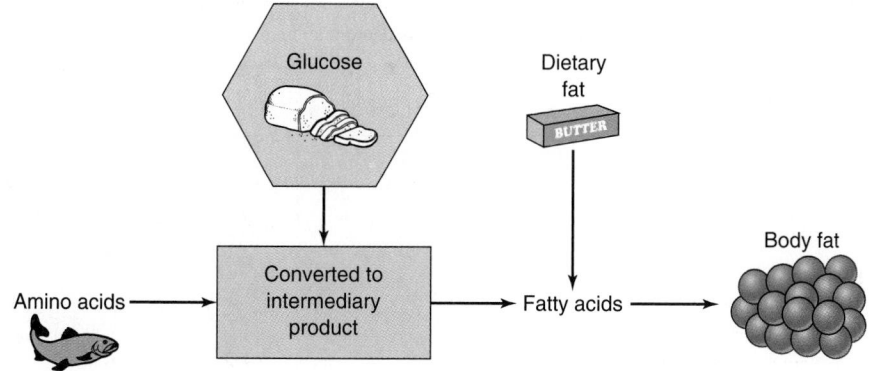

FIGURE 4–9
STORAGE OF EXCESS CALORIES FROM THE ENERGY NUTRIENTS (CARBOHYDRATE, PROTEIN, FAT) AS BODY FAT

are to be of use to the body's cells. The shortest free fatty acids pass by simple diffusion into the cells that line the intestine. Because these short-chain fatty acids are somewhat water soluble, they can, without any further processing, enter the body's capillaries. Like the products of carbohydrate digestion, the short-chain fatty acids are transported from these capillaries through collecting veins to the capillaries of the liver. The liver cells pick them up and convert them to other substances the body needs. The glycerol follows the same path as the short-chain fatty acids because it, too, is water soluble.

The larger products of fat digestion (long-chain fatty acids, cholesterol, and phospholipids) are insoluble in water, a difficulty that must be overcome. The body's fluids—**lymph** and blood—are watery and will not accept these larger molecules as they are. The longer-chain fatty acids do pass into the intestinal cells, but there they reconnect with glycerol or with monoglycerides, forming new triglycerides. Then the cells package them for transport before releasing them into the lymph system. Figure 4–10 summarizes this process.

The cells allow triglycerides and other lipids to form and combine with special proteins to make **chylomicrons,** one of the four types of **lipoproteins** found in the blood. Within the body, the larger fats always travel in lipoproteins. In this ingenious configuration, the water-soluble proteins enable the fats to travel in the watery body fluids. That way, when the tissues of the body need energy from fat, they can extract what they need from lipoproteins. The remnants that remain are picked up by the liver, which dismantles them and reuses their parts. The characteristics of the four types of lipoproteins circulating in the blood are shown in Figure 4–11 on page 128.

Lipoproteins are very much in the news these days. In fact, the health-care provider who measures your blood lipid profile is interested not only in the types of fats in your blood (triglycerides and cholesterol) but also in the lipoproteins that carry them. One distinction among types of lipoproteins is of great importance because it has implications for the health of the heart and blood vessels—the distinction between low-density lipoproteins (**LDL**) and high-density lipoproteins (**HDL**). The more protein in the lipoprotein molecule, the higher the density; a large percentage of lipids characterizes the lower-density molecules. Both LDL and HDL carry similar lipids around in the blood, but there is a functional difference between them (discussed shortly).

LYMPH (LIMF) the body fluid that moves from the bloodstream into tissue spaces and then travels in its own lymphatic vessels, which transport the products of fat digestion toward the heart and eventually drain back into the bloodstream; lymph consists of the same components as blood except red blood cells.

CHYLOMICRON (KIGH-loh-MY-cron) a type of lipoprotein (very low in density) made by the cells of the intestinal wall; serves as a means of transporting newly digested fat from the intestine through lymph and blood. Chylomicrons donate lipids to all body cells, and the remnants are ultimately cleared from the blood by liver cells.

LIPOPROTEINS (LIP-oh-PRO-teens) clusters of lipids associated with protein that serve as transport vehicles for lipids in blood and lymph. The four main types of lipoproteins are **chylomicrons, VLDL, LDL** and **HDL**.

VLDL (very-low-density lipoprotein) carries fats packaged or made by the liver to various tissues in the body.

LDL (low-density lipoprotein) carries cholesterol (much of it synthesized in the liver) to body cells. A high blood cholesterol level usually reflects high LDL.

HDL (high-density lipoprotein) carries cholesterol in the blood back to the liver for recycling or disposal.

FIGURE 4–10
A SUMMARY OF LIPID DIGESTION AND ABSORPTION

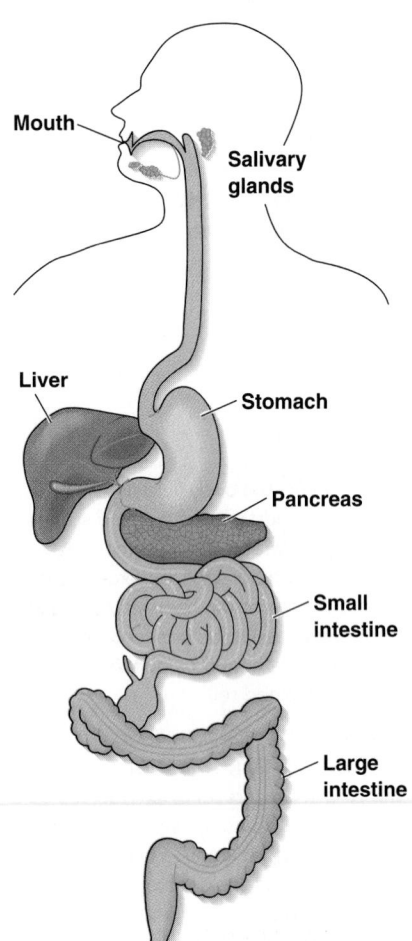

Mouth

Salivary glands

Liver

Stomach

Pancreas

Small intestine

Large intestine

A. Digestion of Fat.

Mouth
Some hard fats begin to melt as they reach body temperature.

Stomach
The stomach's churning action mixes fat with water and acid. A stomach enzyme accesses and breaks apart a small amount of fat. Fat is last to leave the stomach.

Small Intestine
Once in the small intestine, fat encounters **bile** (see B.), an emulsifier made in the liver. The gallbladder, a storage organ, squirts bile into the contents of the small intestine to blend the fat with the watery digestive secretions.

Pancreas
Fat-digesting enzymes from the pancreas (pancreatic lipase) enter the small intestine. The enzymes can attack fat only after emulsification by bile. They break down the triglycerides to fatty acids, glycerol, and monoglycerides.

Large intestine
Some fat and cholesterol, trapped in fiber, are carried out of the body with other wastes.

B. Emulsification of Fat.

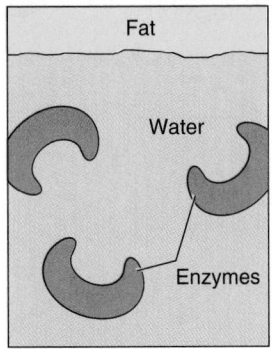

Fat

Water

Enzymes

A. Fats and water separate; enzymes are in water and can't get at the fat.

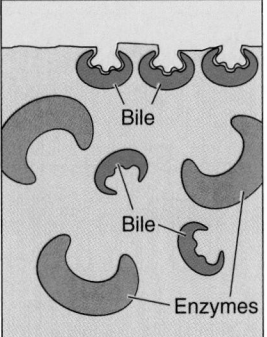

Bile

Bile

Enzymes

B. Bile (emulsifier) has affinity for fats and for water so it can bring them together.

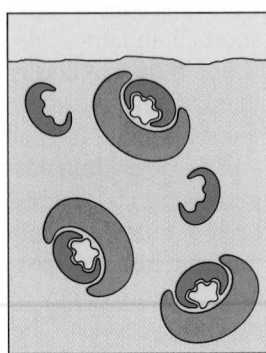

C. Small droplets of emulsified fat. The enzymes now have access to the fat, which is mixed in the water solution.

continued

FIGURE 4-10, *continued*

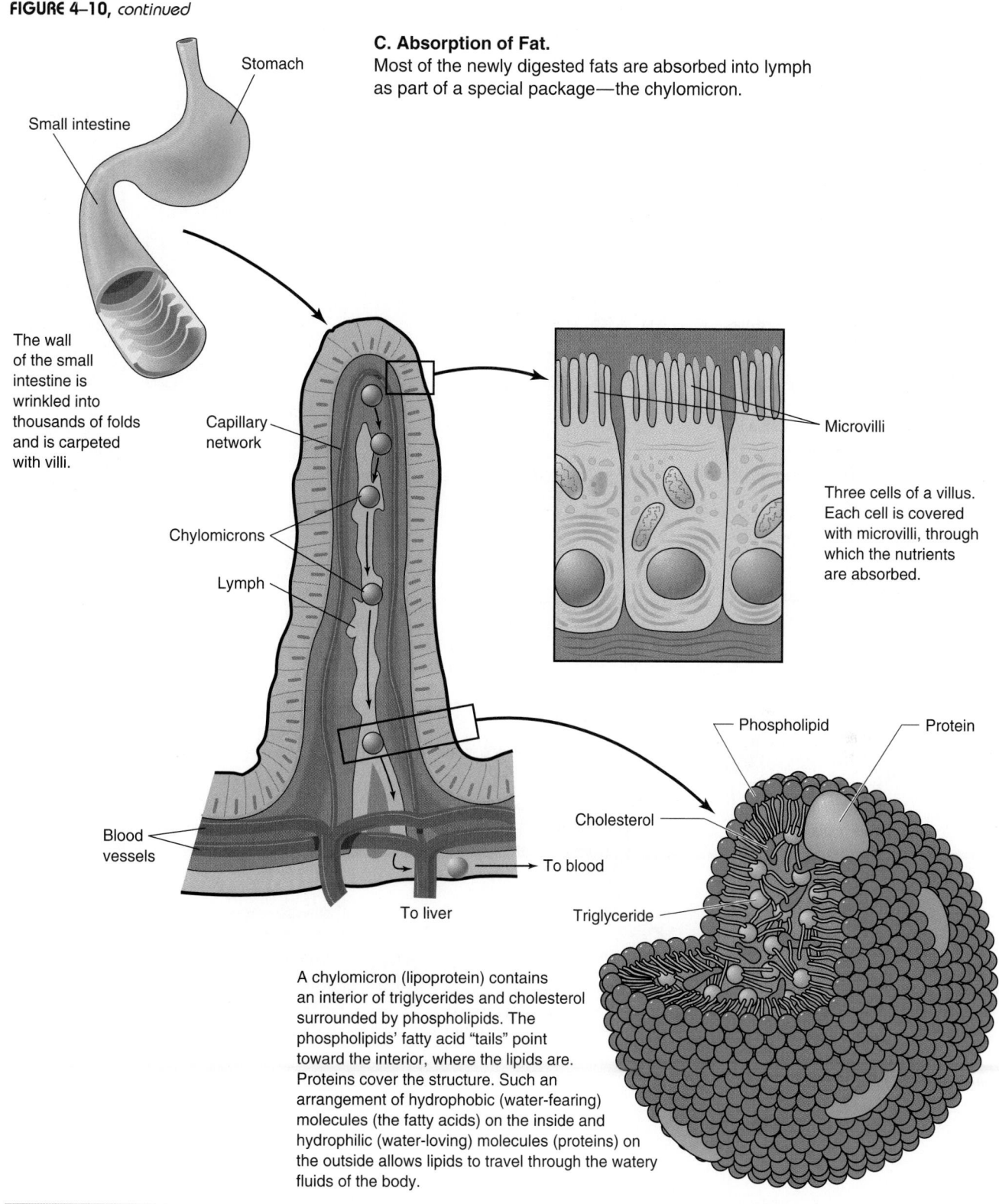

C. Absorption of Fat.
Most of the newly digested fats are absorbed into lymph as part of a special package—the chylomicron.

Stomach

Small intestine

The wall of the small intestine is wrinkled into thousands of folds and is carpeted with villi.

Capillary network

Chylomicrons

Lymph

Blood vessels

To liver

To blood

Microvilli

Three cells of a villus. Each cell is covered with microvilli, through which the nutrients are absorbed.

Phospholipid   Protein

Cholesterol

Triglyceride

A chylomicron (lipoprotein) contains an interior of triglycerides and cholesterol surrounded by phospholipids. The phospholipids' fatty acid "tails" point toward the interior, where the lipids are. Proteins cover the structure. Such an arrangement of hydrophobic (water-fearing) molecules (the fatty acids) on the inside and hydrophilic (water-loving) molecules (proteins) on the outside allows lipids to travel through the watery fluids of the body.

FIGURE 4–11 LIPOPROTEINS

A. Characteristics of Lipoproteins

Chylomicron (KIGH-loh-MY-cron), a type of lipoprotein (very low in density) made by the cells of the intestinal wall; serves as a means of transporting newly digested fat from the intestine through lymph and blood. Chylomicrons donate lipids to all body cells, and the remnants are ultimately cleared from the blood by liver cells.

VLDL (very-low-density lipoprotein)—carries fats made by the liver to various tissues in the body.

LDL (low-density lipoprotein)—carries cholesterol (much of it synthesized in the liver) to body cells. A high blood cholesterol level usually reflects high LDL.

HDL (high-density lipoprotein)—carries cholesterol in the blood back to the liver for recycling or disposal.

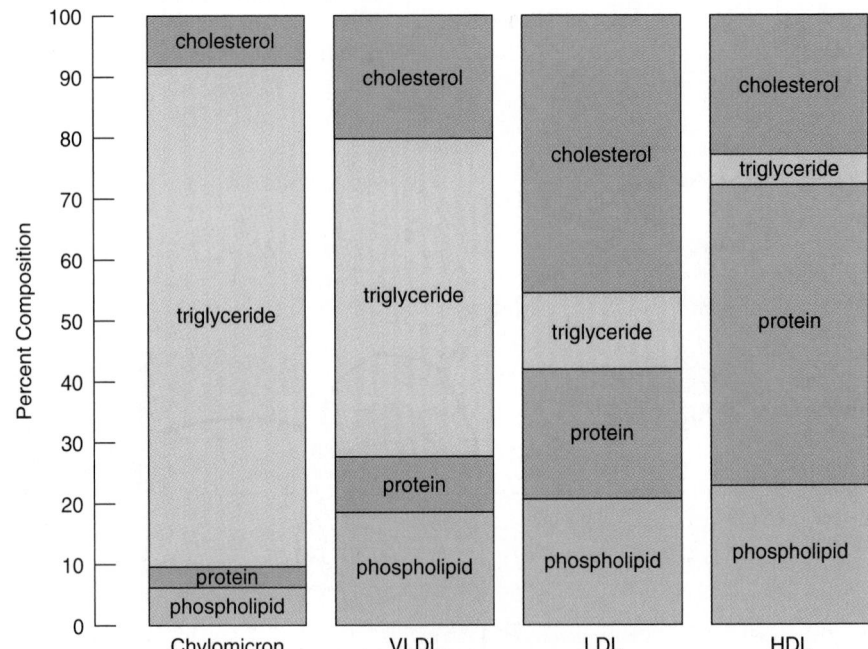

B. Functions and Interactions of Lipoproteins

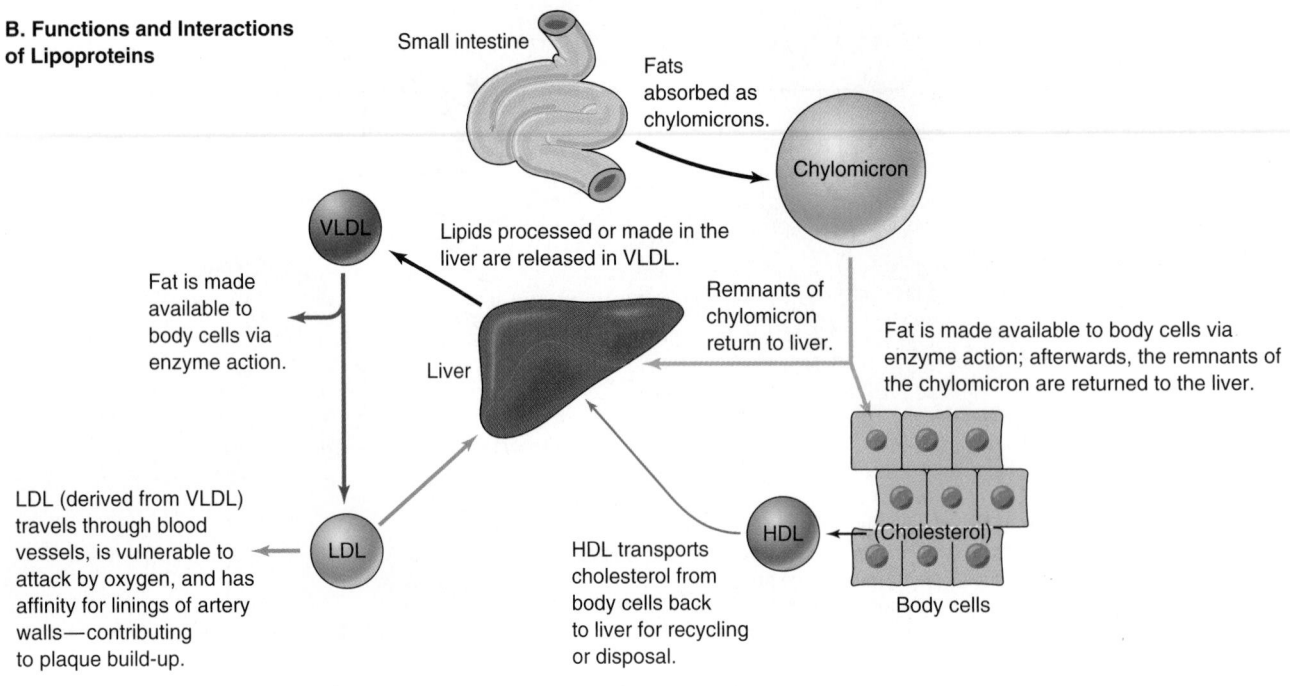

Small intestine

Fats absorbed as chylomicrons.

Chylomicron

Lipids processed or made in the liver are released in VLDL.

Fat is made available to body cells via enzyme action.

Remnants of chylomicron return to liver.

Liver

Fat is made available to body cells via enzyme action; afterwards, the remnants of the chylomicron are returned to the liver.

LDL (derived from VLDL) travels through blood vessels, is vulnerable to attack by oxygen, and has affinity for linings of artery walls—contributing to plaque build-up.

HDL transports cholesterol from body cells back to liver for recycling or disposal.

(Cholesterol)

Body cells

This description of the intestine's processing of fat has omitted the few other dietary fats, such as phospholipids and cholesterol, that may have entered the body in food. These fats enter the circulation the same way the triglycerides do and travel packaged in chylomicrons. After transport, they end up in the liver as part of the chylomicron remnants.

The Lipids and Health

The question of what kind of fat to include in the diet can be puzzling. Research has potentially linked the fat in the diet to several diseases, including breast and colon cancer, heart disease, arthritis, and gallbladder disease. For both cancer and heart disease, the most important strategy is to lower the total fat content of the diet.

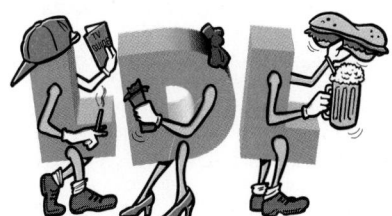

LDL, the "bad" cholesterol

"Good" Versus "Bad" Cholesterol

A silent, symptomless risk factor for heart disease is much talked about but little understood: elevated blood cholesterol levels. Blood cholesterol levels may be high for any of a number of reasons. Some people inherit tendencies to make too much cholesterol or to fail to destroy it on schedule. Others have high blood cholesterol

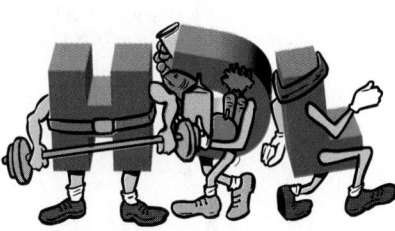

HDL, the "good" cholesterol

for any or all of the following lifestyle reasons: eating too much fat or too much saturated fat, exercising too little, or carrying too much weight. The blood lipid profile mentioned earlier can give you an idea of your standing as to this risk factor. Figure 4–12 shows how to interpret your blood cholesterol level.[13]

The underlying cause of heart disease is atherosclerosis—the narrowing of the arteries caused by a buildup of cholesterol-containing plaque in the arterial walls (this chapter's Spotlight further discusses atherosclerosis and heart disease). The initiating step in the process of atherosclerosis is some form of injury or inflammation in the artery wall. High blood pressure, high blood cholesterol levels, and cigarette smoke are potential sources of injury, as are other causes (see Table 4–4). Raised LDL concentrations in the blood are a sign of high heart attack risk because LDLs in the blood tend to deposit cholesterol in the arteries.[14]

TABLE 4–4
RISK FACTORS FOR HEART DISEASE

RISK FACTORS

- Age: Men ≥ 45
  Women ≥ 55 or premature menopause without estrogen replacement therapy
- High blood cholesterol (greater than 200 mg/dL)
- High LDL-cholesterol (greater than 130 mg/dL)
- Low HDL-cholesterol (less than 35 mg/dL)
- Cigarette smoking
- Hypertension (high blood pressure)
- Physical inactivity
- Obesity
- Diabetes
- Diet high in total fat and saturated fat
- Gender (males are at higher risk)
- Family history of heart disease before the age of 55
- Circulation disorders of blood vessels to the legs, arms, and brain

PROTECTIVE FACTORS

- High HDL-cholesterol level (≥ 60 mg/dL)
- Regular physical activity
- Low-fat, heart-healthy diet

SOURCE: Adapted from Expert Panel on Detection, Evaluation, and Treatment of High Blood Cholesterol in Adults, *Journal of the American Medical Association* 269 (1993): 3015–3023, and American Heart Association, *Position Statement on Exercise*, February 19, 1992.

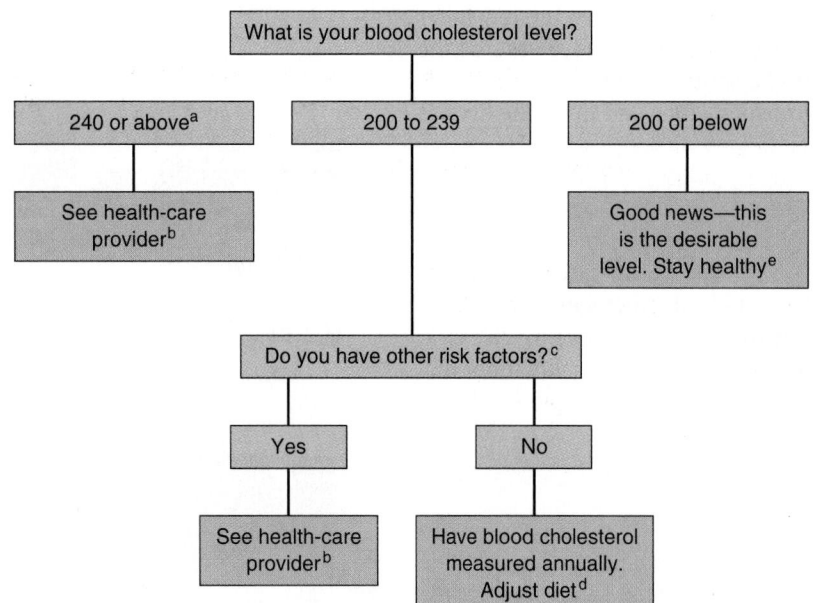

What is your blood cholesterol level?

240 or above[a]	200 to 239	200 or below

See health-care provider[b]

Good news—this is the desirable level. Stay healthy[e]

Do you have other risk factors?[c]

Yes — No

See health-care provider[b]

Have blood cholesterol measured annually. Adjust diet[d]

[a]Blood cholesterol is measured in milligrams per deciliter (mg/dL) of blood. 100 ml is sometimes called a dL. Values for blood cholesterol given in mg/100 ml are the same as those given in mg/dL.

[b]Ask to have your low-density-lipoprotein (LDL) level determined. If LDL is high, your health-care provider may suggest diet and/or drug therapy.

[c]Risk factors: being male, family history of premature death from heart disease, hypertension, smoking, obesity, sedentary lifestyle, diabetes, age (≥ 45 for males; ≥ 55 for females), history of stroke, low HDL levels.

[d]Reduce total fat, saturated fat, and cholesterol in the diet.

[e]A reading of 200 mg/dL or below is recommended. Stay heart-healthy with a nutritious diet and exercise. Re-check cholesterol every five years or with physical exams.

FIGURE 4–12
WHAT IS YOUR CHOLESTEROL LEVEL AND RISK FOR HEART DISEASE?

A diet high in fiber and complex carbohydrates and low in fats and cholesterol plus regular exercise can help you achieve heart-healthy cholesterol levels.

Researchers now theorize that LDL-cholesterol is damaging to the artery walls once it has been oxidized. Circulating LDL-cholesterol is more likely to settle along the linings of the artery walls after it first reacts with an unstable form of oxygen to become **oxidized LDL-cholesterol** (o-LDL) (see Figure 4–13).[15]

Researchers believe that scavenger cells from the immune system known as macrophages ingest more and more of the o-LDL particles and eventually become **foam cells**—so called because of their resemblance to seafoam. These foam cells eventually burst and deposit their accumulated cholesterol as debris in the arterial wall, leading to the development of fatty streaks—the precursors of plaque. Thus, scientists speculate that the oxidized form of LDL catalyzes the process of atherosclerosis in the artery walls by attracting these macrophages to the arterial area.

One of the key steps in the development of atherosclerosis is the accumulation of o-LDL in the walls of the artery. The more LDLs in the circulating blood, the greater the chance for oxidation to occur. This leaves more o-LDL available

OXIDIZED LDL-CHOLESTEROL (o-LDL) the cholesterol in LDLs that is attacked (oxidized) by reactive oxygen molecules inside the walls of the arteries; o-LDL is taken up by scavenger cells which are deposited in arterial plaque.

FOAM CELLS macrophage cells from the immune system containing scavenged oxidized LDL-cholesterol that are thought to initiate plaque formation and the development of atherosclerosis.

for ingestion by the scavenger cells and more debris left behind in the arterial wall. In theory then, steps to reduce the total amount of LDL circulating in the blood (reducing saturated fat in the diet) or steps to prevent the oxidation of LDL-cholesterol (ample antioxidants in the body) would reduce the formation of foam cells and cause less injury to arterial walls. Thus, the process of atherosclerosis could be slowed or possibly prevented.

A low HDL level is less than 35 mg/dL and is considered a risk factor for heart disease. An HDL level greater than or equal to 60 mg/dL is associated with a decreased risk of heart disease. LDL-to-HDL ratios greater than 5.0 for men and greater than 4.5 for women indicate risk for heart disease.

Most blood cholesterol is carried in LDL and correlates *directly* with heart disease risk, but some is carried in HDL and correlates *inversely* with risk. In fact, the most potent single predictor of heart attack risk may be the HDL level. Recent research indicates that an acceptable total blood cholesterol reading of 200 mg/dL or below may not be protective against heart disease if the HDL level is low.[16] Raised HDL concentrations relative to LDL represent cholesterol on its way out of the arteries back to the liver—and a reduced risk of heart attack. The Spotlight feature at the end of the chapter gives further tips on how to raise your HDL level and lower your LDL level.

Some cases of elevated blood cholesterol do not respond to changes in lifestyle. In such cases, cholesterol-lowering drugs might be prescribed. However, for many, a few simple changes in diet can improve cholesterol readings, as discussed next.

Lowering Blood Cholesterol Levels

Among the most influential diet-related factors that raise blood cholesterol levels are total fat intake, saturated fat intake, and obesity.[17] As it turns out, the changes in diet that reduce blood cholesterol concentrations mostly do so by reducing LDL-cholesterol. Dietary modifications that help lower LDL include substituting highly monounsaturated fats (canola, olive, and peanut oils) and highly polyunsaturated fats (vegetable oils and fish oils—see Table 4–5) for saturated fats.[18] As for dietary cholesterol itself, it raises LDL levels slightly for

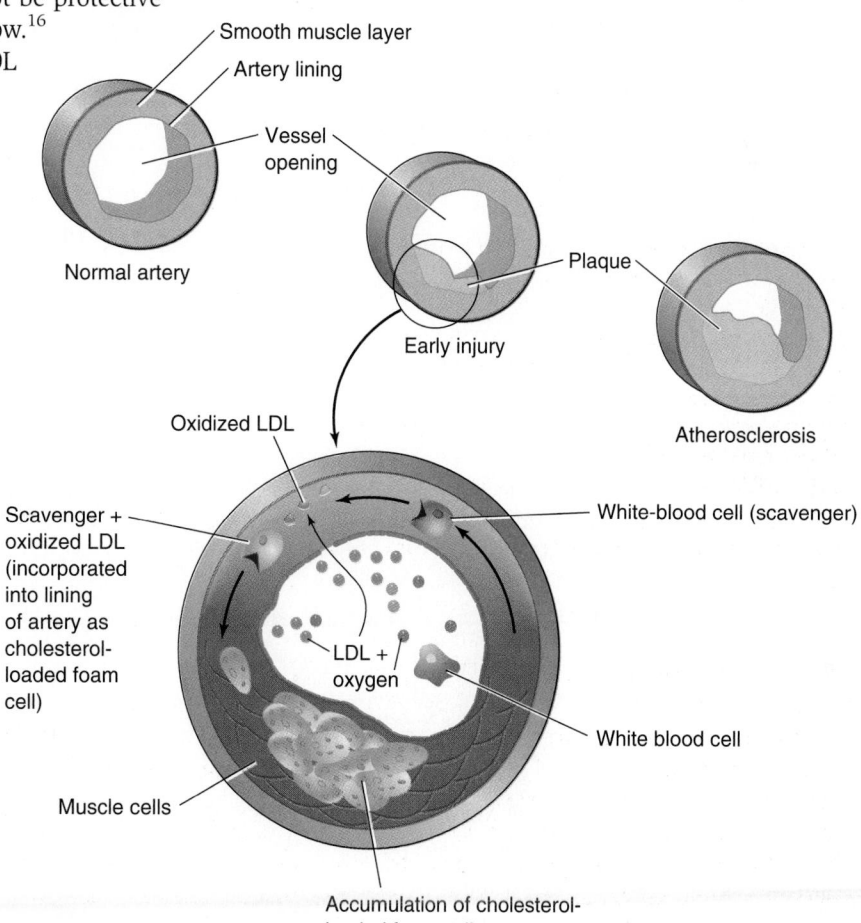

FIGURE 4–13 ATHEROSCLEROSIS

As LDL particles penetrate the walls of the arteries, they become oxidized-LDL and next are scavenged by the body's white blood cells. These foam cells are then deposited into the lining of the artery wall. This process, known as atherosclerosis, causes plaque deposits to enlarge, artery walls to lose elasticity, and the passage through the artery to narrow.

TABLE 4–5
THE EFFECTS OF VARIOUS KINDS OF FAT ON BLOOD LIPIDS

TYPE OF FAT*	DIETARY SOURCES	EFFECTS ON BLOOD LIPIDS
SATURATED FAT	All animal meats Beef tallow Butter Cheese Chocolate Cocoa butter Coconut oil Cream Hydrogenated oils Lard Palm oil Stick margarine Shortening Whole milk	Increases total cholesterol Increases LDL-cholesterol

MONOUNSATURATED FAT	Avocados
	Canola oil
	Cashews
	Olive oil
	Olives
	Peanut butter
	Peanut oil
	Peanuts
	Poultry
		If used to *replace* saturated fat in
		the diet, monounsaturated fats may:
		    Decrease total cholesterol
		    Decrease LDL-cholesterol without
		       decreasing HDL-cholesterol

POLYUNSATURATED FAT	Almonds
	Corn oil
	Cottonseed oil
	Filberts
	Fish
	Liquid/soft margarine
	Mayonnaise
	Pecans
	Safflower oil
	Sesame oil
	Soybean oil
	Sunflower oil
	Walnuts
		If used to *replace* saturated fat in
		the diet, polyunsaturated fat may:
		    Decrease total cholesterol
		    Decrease LDL-cholesterol
		    Decrease HDL-cholesterol

OMEGA-3 FAT	Canola oil
	Ocean fish
	Shellfish
	Some vegetables (spinach, broccoli, lettuce)
	Soybeans/tofu
	Walnuts
	Wheat germ
		If used to *replace* saturated fat in
		the diet, omega-3 fat may:
		    Decrease total cholesterol
		    Decrease LDL-cholesterol
		    Increase HDL-cholesterol

*All fats, whether classified as mainly saturated fat, monounsaturated fat, or polyunsaturated fat, contain mixtures of saturated and unsaturated fats and provide the same number of calories: 9 calories per gram.

some people, depending on the amount consumed and on the body's ability to compensate by making less.

The current recommendations for diet, based on these findings, include the following:

- Eat no more than 30 percent of calories as fat.
- Eat no more than 10 percent of calories as saturated fat.
- Eat no more than 10 percent of calories as polyunsaturated fats.
- Eat 10 percent to 15 percent of calories as monounsaturated fats (see Table 4–6).
- Limit daily cholesterol intake to no more than 300 milligrams.

Table 4–7 presents additional tips from the American Heart Association diet.

Researchers continue to debate which type of fat makes the best replacement for saturated fat in the diet.[19] For years, polyunsaturated fats were recommended as substitutes for saturated fats in the diet until evidence suggested that PUFAs play a role in the oxidation of LDL-cholesterol. A diet high in polyunsaturated fats (corn or vegetable oil) may increase the oxidation of LDL-cholesterol and therefore increase the risk of heart disease. Since the polyunsaturated fat (being transported on the LDL carrier) has several points of unsaturation, it is vulnerable to attack by oxygen or other oxidizing agents.[20] Monounsaturated fats (olive and canola oil) are more stable than the polyunsaturated fats because they have only one point of unsaturation.

Researchers have shown that the substitution of monounsaturated for saturated fatty acids in the diet brings about a significant decrease in blood levels of LDL-cholesterol, without the decrease in HDL-cholesterol seen when polyunsaturated fats (at intakes greater than 10 percent of calories) are substituted for saturated fats.[21] Some researchers warn, however, that diets rich in monounsaturated fat can be calorically dense and could worsen the problem of obesity in the United States and Canada.

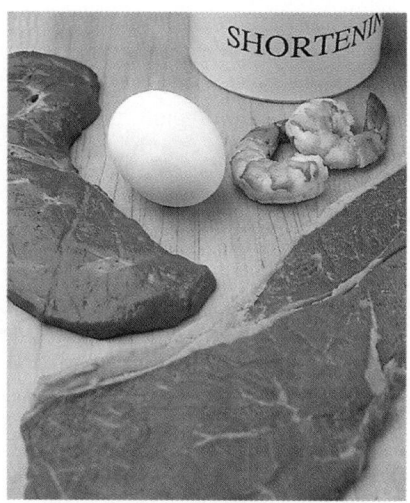

Saturated fats and cholesterol contribute to high blood cholesterol levels.

TABLE 4–6

TIPS FOR A HEART-HEALTHY DIET

Consider some of the following changes for your own diet:

- Use legumes as occasional alternatives to meat, poultry, and fish.
- Use small amounts of olive oil in cooking and in oil-and-vinegar dressings for salads.
- Try brushing a small amount of olive oil instead of butter or margarine on breads warm from the toaster or oven.
- Use canola oil in place of other fats in your favorite cookie, muffin, or cake recipes.
- Use *very small* quantities of nuts to add flavor to quick breads and other baked goods.
- Keep in mind that the goal is to *replace* saturated fats with monounsaturated fats, but not to exceed a healthful intake of total fat.
- Choose foods naturally rich in the antioxidant nutrients and other protective compounds by eating five or more servings of fruits and vegetables *every* day.

Still, researchers continue to investigate whether the high consumption of olive oil, typical in the Mediterranean region, may be partly responsible for the lower risk of heart disease seen among the people of Greece, France, Italy, and other Mediterranean countries. Other factors undoubtedly contribute to the lower incidence of heart disease in the Mediterranean region as implied in the following anecdote:[22]

> He's a shepherd or small farmer, a beekeeper or fisherman, or a tender of olives or vines. He walks to work daily and labors in the soft light of his Greek Isle. His midday, main meal is of eggplant, with large mushrooms, crisp vegetables, and country bread dipped in golden olive oil. Once a week there is a bit of lamb. Once a week there is chicken. Twice a week there is fish fresh from the sea. Other meals are hot dishes of legumes seasoned with meats and condiments. The main dish is followed by a tangy salad, then by dates, Turkish sweets, nuts, or fresh fruits. A sharp local wine completes the meal.

In understanding the paradox of how a high-fat diet (more than 30 percent of calories from mostly monounsaturated fats) can coexist with a low incidence of heart disease, it is important to note that people from the Mediterranean region in general are more physically active, have the social and emotional support found in extended networks of family and friends, eat more fruits, vegetables, legumes, and nuts and less meat and animal fat, use monounsaturated fat (found in vegetable oils such as olive or canola) more than saturated fat, and consume more of each day's calories earlier in the day than people in the United States and Canada. Any one of these factors may be significant for the lower incidence of heart disease in the region. A healthful eating pattern (with a Mediterranean twist) for most people in the United States and Canada is one that is lower in total fat and higher in complex carbohydrates and fiber (fruits, vegetables, whole grain breads and other grains, and legumes).

In the past few years, attention has focused on reducing heart disease risk by both reducing contributory factors in the diet—notably, saturated fat—and increasing

TABLE 4–7
THE AMERICAN HEART ASSOCIATION DIET

Control the amount and kind of fat you eat:

- Limit your intake of lean meat, seafood, and skinless poultry to no more than 6 oz/day.
- Try main dishes featuring pasta, rice, beans, and/or vegetables. Or create "low-meat" dishes by mixing these foods with small amounts of lean meat, poultry, or fish.
- Choose lean cuts of meat, trim all the fat you can see, and throw away the fat that cooks out of the meat.
- Use no more than a total of 5 to 8 tsp of fats and oils per day for cooking, baking, and salads.
- Use low-fat or nonfat dairy products.

Control your intake of cholesterol-rich foods to take in no more than 300 mg/day:

- Use no more than three to four egg yolks a week, including those used in cooking.
- Limit your use of organ meats such as liver, chitterlings, and gizzards.

Also control:

- Alcohol: Have no more than two drinks per day of wine, beer, or liquor, and only when caloric limits allow.
- Protein: consume no more than 15% of calories as protein.
- Sodium: use no more than 3,000 mg/day.
- Calories: eat just enough to maintain recommended weight.

To round out the rest of your eating plan:

- Eat five or more servings of fruits or vegetables per day.
- Eat six or more servings of breads, cereals, or grains per day.

SOURCE: Adapted from *The American Heart Association Diet, An Eating Plan for Healthy Americans,* a booklet (1991) available from the American Heart Association National Center, 7320 Greenville Ave., Dallas, TX 75231.

For more about the dietary customs and health status of the people living in the Mediterranean region, refer to the Spotlight feature in Chapter 3.

the intake of protective factors, such as the antioxidant vitamins. Antioxidants—beta-carotene, vitamins C and E, and the mineral selenium—act to strengthen the body's natural defenses against cell damage by blocking the potentially damaging **free radicals** that arise as a part of numerous normal cell activities. Free radicals—the chemical compounds that oxidize LDL-cholesterol—become a problem when there are too many of them.

Antioxidants in the body may reduce the amount of LDL-cholesterol that becomes oxidized because the antioxidants (particularly vitamin E) can neutralize the highly reactive oxygen before it gets a chance to oxidize the LDL particle, thereby lessening the buildup of plaque in the artery walls.[23] Scientists are now exploring the potential abilities of all the antioxidant nutrients to protect against heart disease.[24] Indeed, the role of the antioxidants in protecting against heart disease is a rapidly growing area of research.[25] Important questions remain unanswered: What is the optimal level of vitamin E (or beta-carotene or vitamin C) intake that confers the greatest benefit in reducing risk of heart disease? Also, can this amount be obtained from the diet, or will an antioxidant supplement be recommended?

> **FREE RADICALS** highly toxic compounds created in the body as a result of chemical reactions that involve oxygen. Environmental pollutants such as cigarette smoke and ozone also prompt the formation of free radicals.

> The Spotlight feature in Chapter 6 discusses the risks and benefits of supplement use and presents more on the role of antioxidants in reducing risks for chronic diseases such as heart disease and cancer.

While waiting for the results of this ongoing research, two suggestions can be made for the time being:

1. Keep blood cholesterol at or below the recommended levels. For every one percent reduction in a high blood cholesterol level, there is a two percent to three percent reduction in the risk of heart attack. Substitute monounsaturated fats and polyunsaturated fats for saturated fats in the diet because both lower LDL-cholesterol levels in the blood.

2. Eat generous amounts of fruits and vegetables—at least five servings a day—as a source of antioxidants and other protective compounds in the diet.

Fat in the Diet

The remainder of this chapter will help you to apply what you have learned about fats—that is, how to choose foods that supply enough but not too much of the right kinds of fat to support optimal health and provide pleasure in eating. To start, you must know where the fats are located in the Food Guide Pyramid (see Table 4–8). Three groups—the *Fats, Oils, and Sweets Group;* the *Meat, Poultry, Fish, Dry Beans, Eggs, and Nuts Group;* and the *Milk, Yogurt, and Cheese Group*—have traditionally accounted for about nine-tenths of the fat in the U.S. diet. Currently, the average American diet includes about 37 percent of its calories from fat with about 14 percent of calories from saturated fat.[26] Dietary guidelines recommend that *total* fat not exceed 30 percent of the day's total calories, and saturated fat contribute less than 10 percent.

"Fat on the plate" includes visible fats and oils, such as butter, the oil in salad dressing, and the fat you trim from a steak. It also refers to some you cannot see, such as the fat that marbles a steak or that is hidden in such foods as nuts, cheese, biscuits, crackers, doughnuts, cookies, muffins, avocados, olives, fried foods, and chocolate.

Typical intake

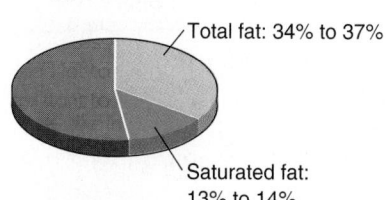

Total fat: 34% to 37%

Saturated fat: 13% to 14%

Recommended intake

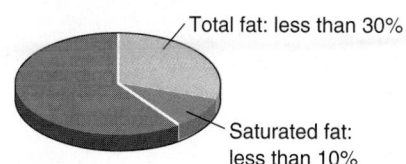

Total fat: less than 30%

Saturated fat: less than 10%

Typical versus recommended intake of fat, expressed as a percentage of total calories.

TABLE 4–8
PYRAMID POINTERS: SELECTION TIPS FOR FAT IN THE DIET

FATS, OILS, AND SWEETS GROUP

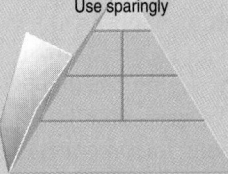

Use sparingly

- Go easy on fats added to foods in cooking or at the table—butter, margarine, gravy, salad dressing, shortening, cream, and cream cheese.
- Experiment with reduced-fat and fat-free products like fat-free mayonnaise and salad dressings, low-fat or nonfat margarine, sour cream, and cream cheese.
- Use part-skim ricotta cheese, low-fat Neufchatel cheese, or low-fat farmer's cheese in place of higher-fat mayonnaise and cream cheese in your favorite dip recipes.
- Choose low-fat sweets like frozen yogurt, sorbet, frozen fruit and juice bars, sherbet, fat-free or reduced-fat baked goods, and low-fat cookies like graham crackers, gingersnaps, or fig bars. Try reducing the amount of fat called for in your recipes by one-third or one-half (see Consumer Tips on page 151 for ideas on how to trim fat from recipes).

MEAT, POULTRY, FISH, DRY BEANS, EGGS, AND NUTS GROUP

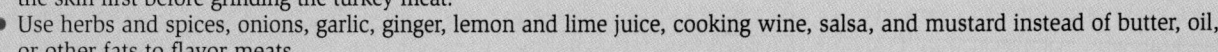

2–3

- Choose lean meat, poultry without skin, fish, and legumes often; they are the choices lowest in fat.
- Prepare meals in low-fat ways: trim away all the fat that you can see; remove skin from poultry; and broil, roast, bake, grill, or poach these foods rather than frying them.
- Nuts and seeds are high in fat, so eat them in moderation.
- Use low-fat luncheon meats containing no more than 1 gram of fat per ounce.
- Try substituting chicken, turkey, or fish in a recipe that normally calls for red meat. For example, try chili, meatloaf, or meatballs made with ground turkey; be sure to ask the butcher to remove the skin first before grinding the turkey meat.
- Use herbs and spices, onions, garlic, ginger, lemon and lime juice, cooking wine, salsa, and mustard instead of butter, oil, or other fats to flavor meats.
- After making a soup or stew containing meat or poultry, refrigerate it until the fat congeals. Remove the fat before heating or serving the soup or stew.
- Choose most often from the **Best Choice** column—these are the choices lowest in fat.

Best Choices (trace or < 3 g fat per ounce)	Fair Choices (3 to 5 g fat per ounce)	Use Sparingly Choices (> 5 g fat per ounce)
beef: flank, round, sirloin, or tenderloin steak Canadian bacon chicken cornish hen egg white fish: fresh, canned (in water), or frozen (unbreaded) some luncheon meat (check labels) pork: ham or tenderloin shellfish: clams, oysters, scallops turkey	beef: cubed, t-bone, extra-lean ground, lean ground, Lebanon bologna, rump, or porterhouse egg substitute fish (canned in oil) lamb: chop, leg, or roast pork: chop, cutlet, loin, or roast	beef: chuck, corned beef brisket, prime rib, regular ground, ribeye, or rib roast bacon egg yolk fried meat or fish lamb: ground luncheon meats organ meats sausage: breakfast type, hot dogs, Italian, pepperoni, Polish, or Vienna shellfish: crab, lobster, shrimp shortribs or spareribs

continued

TABLE 4–8
continued

MILK, YOGURT, AND CHEESE GROUP

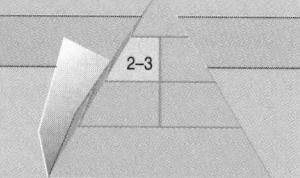

- Choose nonfat milk and nonfat yogurt instead of their whole milk counterparts.
- Choose part-skim or low-fat cheeses.
- Use lower-fat milk desserts like ice milk and frozen yogurt.
- Choose most often from the **Best Choice** column—these are the choices lowest in fat.

Best Choices (< 3 g fat per ounce)	Fair Choices (3 to 5 g fat per ounce)	Use Sparingly Choices (> 5 g fat per ounce)
cheese: diet (less than 56 calories per ounce), farmer's, imitation mozzarella, low-fat cottage, Parmesan, or part-skim ricotta milk : 1% fat or nonfat milk, nonfat buttermilk, evaporated nonfat milk or nonfat dry milk yogurt : 1% fat	cheese: cottage, light cream cheese, part-skim mozzarella, or processed cheese product milk: 2% fat or low-fat buttermilk yogurt: 2% fat or low-fat	cheese: American, blue, brick, Brie, cheddar, Colby, cream, Gouda, Gruyere, Monterey Jack, Muenster, Neufchatel, provolone, processed, or Swiss cream: half & half, heavy, light, sour, or whipped cream substitutes made with palm or coconut oil imitation sour cream milk: chocolate, condensed, evaporated, or whole

BREAD, CEREAL, RICE, AND PASTA GROUP

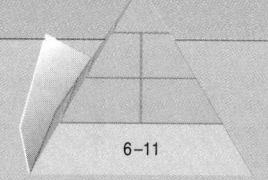

- Go easy on the fats you add as spreads, seasonings, or toppings.
- Choose most often from the **Best Choice** column—these are made with little fat.

Best Choices (< 3 g fat per serving)	Fair Choices (3 to 5 g fat per serving)	Use Sparingly Choices (> 5 g fat per serving)
angel food cake bagel breadsticks brown rice crackers: matzoh, melba toast, oyster, rye, saltines cookies: fig bars, gingersnaps, graham crackers, vanilla wafers corn tortilla (not fried) couscous English muffin enriched/whole grain breads grits pancakes pasta popcorn (air-popped) pretzels ready-to-eat cereals rice cakes taco shell	biscuit cookies: brownie, chocolate chip cookies flour tortilla (not fried) croutons muffin pizza crust popcorn (commercially popped, plain)	cake cheese curls chow mein noodles cornbread corn chips croissant cupcake doughnut fried rice granola pastry popcorn (commercially popped, buttered) stuffing toaster pastry tortilla (fried) waffle

continued

TABLE 4–8
continued

VEGETABLE GROUP

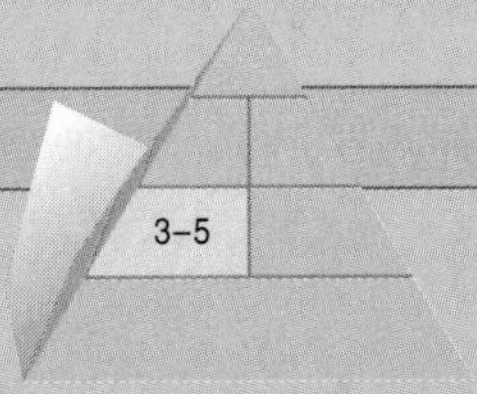

- Go easy on the fat you add to vegetables at the table or during cooking.
- Choose most often from the **Best Choice** column—these are made with little fat.

3–5

Best Choices (< 2 g fat per serving)	Fair Choices (2 to 3 g fat per serving)	Use Sparingly Choices (> 3 g fat per serving)
most vegetables (served raw, steamed, or microwaved and without butter or oil) vegetable juices vegetable soup (with fat removed)	vegetables served with a reduced-fat sauce	coleslaw French fries fried vegetables hash browns mashed potatoes potato chips potato salad scalloped potatoes

FRUIT GROUP

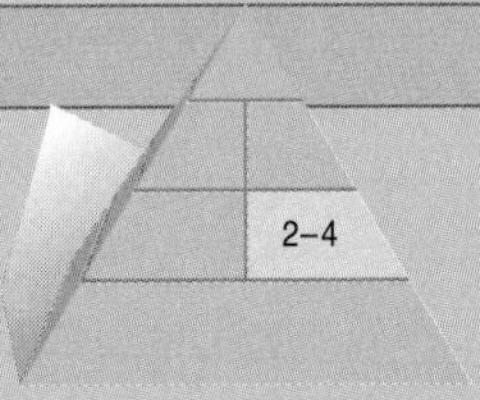

- Enjoy fruit for dessert; unprocessed fruits are virtually fat-free.
- Snack on raw fruits in place of high-fat snacks like potato chips.

2–4

SOURCE: The foods listed in the table are adapted from *Pyramid Packet*, © 1993, Penn State Nutrition Center, 417 East Calder Way, University Park, PA 16801.

The listings of foods in Table 4–8 show exactly where the fats are. Two groups always contain fat (the fats and the meats), and two sometimes contain fat (the milks and the breads). The unprocessed vegetables and fruits are, for the most part, fat-free.

Meats probably conceal most of the fat that people unwittingly consume. Many people, when choosing a serving of meat (or certain meat alternates), don't realize that they are electing to eat a large amount of fat (see Figure 4–14). Recently, some animal breeders have begun producing beef and pork that is lower in fat. This is a help to those people who choose lean cuts—they get less fat in the same quantity of meat. When selecting beef or pork, look for the words loin or round on the label—these words represent lean cuts from which the fat can be trimmed.

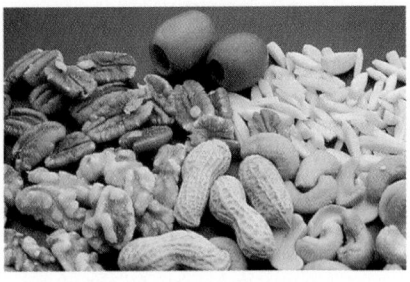

Nuts are rich in many nutrients but are also high in fat. Two whole walnuts or ten large peanuts contain the same amount of fat as is found in a teaspoon of butter or margarine (5 grams of fat and 45 calories).

Shopping for Fats

Generally speaking, vegetable and fish oils are rich in polyunsaturates; olive, peanut, and canola oils are rich in monounsaturates; and the harder fats—animal fats—are more saturated. However, not all vegetable oils are polyunsaturated. When you read food labels, be sure to note the amounts of total fat and saturated fat listed on the Nutrition Facts panel. You have to know your fats; it

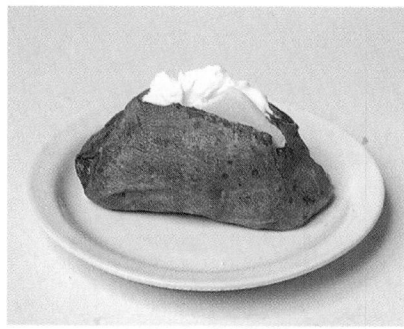

Large potato with 1 tablespoon butter and 1 tablespoon sour cream (14 grams fat, 350 calories).

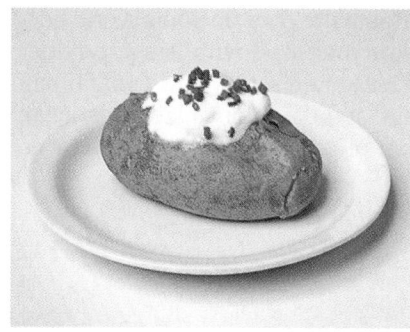

Plain large potato with 2 tablespoons nonfat plain yogurt seasoned with chives (less than 1 gram fat, 235 calories).

is not enough simply to use plant oils over animal fats. Remember, too, that some vegetable oils are hydrogenated to make them solid and are not much better than the saturated fats themselves. When buying margarines, choose the ones with the *lowest* amount of saturated fats and hydrogenated oils.

One strategy for using fats is to use a variety but to keep the amounts as low as possible. Try reducing the fat in recipes by a tablespoon at a time, and notice that you can do so and still get a good-tasting product. If you reduce fat by 1 tablespoon of butter or oil, you lower the total fat in the product by about 12 grams and at least 100 calories. Or, to reduce the fat even further, try substituting unsweetened applesauce for the oil called for in your favorite cake and cookie recipes.

Moderation is a good word to keep in mind when you find yourself wanting to butter foods. Be conscious of where you are adding the fat—often, it isn't necessary. For example, you don't really need to add butter (or mayonnaise) to the bread

FIGURE 4–14

COMPARE THE SATURATED FAT CONTENT OF FISH, POULTRY, AND BEEF*

	GRAMS PER 3 OZ SERVING[†]	
	Total fat	Saturated fat
Turkey breast, roasted (without skin)	1	<1
Halibut, baked	2.5	<1
Chicken breast, roasted (without skin)	3	1
Chicken breast, roasted (with skin)	7	2
Beef, top round, broiled	4	1.5
Beef, sirloin, broiled	6	2
Beef, ground lean	15	6
Turkey, ground	11	3
Beef, T-bone steak, broiled	10	4

*To compare the saturated fat and total fat content of other foods, see Table 4-14 in this chapter's Spotlight feature.

[†]How much is three ounces? A three-ounce portion of lean beef, chicken, or fish has roughly the dimensions of a deck of playing cards. Three ounces is also the approximate size of the palm of the average woman's hand.

when making a tuna salad or egg salad sandwich, nor do you need to add that oil to the pasta's cooking water. If you eat your toast with jam and butter, try using the jam without the butter. Most fruit butters and jams contain half the calories per teaspoon that butters contain, and the calories are from sugar, not from fat. More tips on cutting the fat out of your diet are offered later in the chapter.

Understanding Fat Substitutes

Fat-free ice cream, cookies, cakes, and salad dressings have long been the stuff that dieters' dreams are made of. The food industry has now made such fatless fare a reality. With more and more low-fat and fat-free items introduced daily into supermarkets across the country, sales of nonfat products are soaring.

The boom in both low-fat and fat-free products has to do with the country's expanding health consciousness. While most Americans have heard the warnings that fat can contribute to heart disease, cancer, and obesity, many people find low-fat diets particularly unpalatable since fat adds a desirable flavor and texture—known as "mouth feel"—to foods. With innovations in food chemistry, however, the food industry can concoct new recipes or ingredients that yield low-fat or nonfat products that retain the characteristic flavor and mouth feel of fat. Entenmann's, the manufacturer of a line of fat-free cakes and cookies, for example, makes those products by substituting egg whites for whole eggs and nonfat milk for whole milk as well as by removing the butter from its recipes. The end product: sweets that contain fewer calories and four to five fewer grams of fat per serving than the company's traditional desserts.[27] Table 4–9 compares regular foods with low-fat and nonfat foods.

Similarly, McDonald's cooked reduced-fat burger patties by adding an ingredient called **carrageenan** to beef. Derived from seaweed, carrageenan helps retain moisture, which in turn makes up for the loss of juiciness that accompanies a reduction in fat. Dubbed McLean Deluxe, the low-fat quarter-pound burger contained 11 fewer grams of fat and 99 fewer calories than the company's Quarter Pounder.[28] In February, 1996, however, McDonald's pulled McLean Deluxe from its menu due to poor sales.

Another technique manufacturers use to replace fat is to add starches, gums, and gels to their products. For example, Kraft uses cellulose gel, a complex carbohydrate, as a filler to make fat-free salad dressings and Sealtest nonfat dairy dessert.[29] Other companies add starches and gums—also complex carbohydrates—to items such as sauces and yogurts to skim fat from those foods. That's because starches and gums hold water and impart a smooth creamy texture similar to that of fat and add form and structure to foods. These substitutes cannot, however, replace the fat used for cooking and frying.[30]

Yet another more innovative approach the food industry has taken to provide fat-free fare is the development of fat substitutes. In 1990, a substance called **Simplesse**® became the first such product to gain the approval of the Food and Drug Administration. Six years in the making, Simplesse® is a mixture of food proteins such as egg white, whey, and milk protein that are cooked and blended to form tiny round particles that trap water. Inside the mouth, the particles roll over

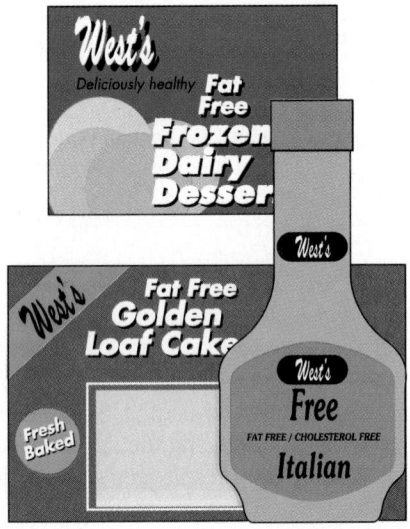

CARRAGEENAN a seaweed derivative used by food manufacturers to add "body" to numerous products, including ice cream, frozen yogurt, and salad dressings.

SIMPLESSE® the trade name for a protein-based, low-calorie artificial fat, approved by the FDA for use in foods such as frozen desserts; cannot be used for frying or baking.

OLESTRA an artificial fat derived from vegetable oils and sugar combined in such a way that the body cannot break them down. Sold under the brand name Olean®, olestra does not contribute calories to food. It can, however, prevent absorption of some nutrients. Thus, the FDA requires all products made with it to bear this warning: "This Product Contains Olestra. Olestra may cause abdominal cramping and loose stools. Olestra inhibits the absorption of some vitamins and nutrients. Vitamins A, D, E, and K have been added."

one another, and the tongue perceives them as a creamy, smooth liquid similar to fat.

The FDA allows use of Simplesse® in foods including cheese, baked goods, ice creams, frozen desserts, mayonnaise, salad dressings, yogurts, sour cream, and butter. Foods made with the fat substitute contain considerably less fat and fewer calories than their traditional fat-containing counterparts.[31] The reason is that while fat contains 9 calories per gram, Simplesse supplies only 1 to 2. Simplesse® cannot be used for frying or baking, since heat causes it to gel and lose its creaminess. Figure 4–15 illustrates the role of Simplesse in the reduction of fat and calories in the diet.

Another artificial fat recently approved for use in salty snacks and crackers is **olestra** (sold under the brand name Olean®). Created by Procter & Gamble, the olestra molecule resembles a triglyceride but is structured in a way that prevents its breakdown by digestive enzymes in the body, thereby allowing it to pass through the digestive tract completely unabsorbed. Many scientists have a number of concerns about olestra, however. One is that it interferes with the absorption of fat-soluble vitamins as well as beta-carotene and other nutrients. Another is that large amounts of the product can cause abdominal cramping and loose stools. Because of these issues, the FDA requires any product containing olestra to bear a warning label.[32]

Certainly, the growing number of fat-free foods and fat substitutes provides consumers with viable

TABLE 4–9
FAT-FREE FARE: BEFORE AND AFTER

CRACKERS/COOKIES/CAKES	GRAMS OF FAT	CALORIES
Better Cheddars Snack Crackers (22 crackers)	8	150
Reduced Fat Better Cheddars Snack Crackers (24)	6	140
Wheatsworth Stoned Ground Wheat Crackers (5)	3.5	80
SnackWell's Fat Free Wheat Crackers (5)	0	60
Fig Newtons (2)	2.5	110
Fat Free Fig Newtons (2)	0	100
Marshmallow Puffs Fudge Cookies (1)	4	90
SnackWell's Devil's Food Cookie Cakes (1)	0	50
Oreo cookies (3)	7	160
Reduced Fat Oreo cookies (3)	5	140
Hostess Chocolate Cup Cakes (1)	5	170
Hostess Chocolate Cup Cakes Light (1)	1.5	120
Entenmann's All Butter Pound Loaf (⅙ loaf)	10	220
Entenmann's Golden Loaf Cake (fat-free) (⅛ loaf)	0	130

DAIRY PRODUCTS		
Regular Swiss cheese, average (1 slice)	8	107
Kraft Singles Swiss Flavor (1.3 slice)	3	67
Weight Watchers Fat Free Swiss (1.3 slice)	0	40
Regular vanilla ice cream (½ cup)	7	133
Weight Watchers Oh! So Very Vanilla (½ cup)	2.5	120
Healthy Choice Premium Low Fat Ice Cream vanilla (½ cup)	2	100
Breakstone Sour Cream (2 tbsp)	5	60
Breakstone Fat-Free Sour Cream (2 tbsp)	0	35

CONDIMENTS		
Hidden Valley Ranch salad dressing (2 tbsp)	14	140
Hidden Valley Ranch Light salad dressing (2 tbsp)	7	80
Hidden Valley Fat Free Ranch salad dressing (2 tbsp)	0	45
Kraft Mayonnaise (1 tbsp)	11	100
Kraft Light Mayonnaise (1 tbsp)	5	50
Kraft Free Mayonnaise (1 tbsp)	0	10

MEATS		
Ground beef, regular (4 oz)	22	331
Ground beef, extra lean (4 oz)	18	300
Swift 95 Supreme Extra Lean ground beef (4 oz)	5	140
Oscar Mayer Wiener (1 link)	13	150
Oscar Mayer Light Wiener (1 link)	9	110
Oscar Mayer Free Hot Dog (1 link)	0	40

SOURCE: Manufacturer's information, product labels, and Reduced-fat foods: Dieter's dream or marketer's ploy? *Consumer Reports on Health,* July 1995, p. 79.

alternatives to fattier fare.* Nevertheless, many experts view the fat-free boom with skepticism. While reduced-fat foods can help lower the overall fat content of the diet, they *do* contain calories, and they are not a replacement for a healthful diet rich in whole grains and fresh fruits and vegetables. Nor are they likely to become the panacea that will prevent problems such as heart disease and obesity. Fit into a low-fat diet, however, they can help consumers reach and adhere to the goal of taking in no more than 30 percent of total calories as fat.

Using the Food Label

As a consumer, you need to remember two important points when reading food labels: the type of fat and the amount of fat in the food, since both can affect your blood cholesterol level. Health professionals recommend that total fat account for no more than 30 percent of total calories. Table 4–10 can help you to determine the amount of fat (in calories and in grams) you should be eating daily based on your total calorie intake. You can also determine what percentage of a food's calories comes from fat by following the steps in Figure 4–16. The Fit or Fat Scorecard on page 146 will help you rate your own dietary selections for fat.

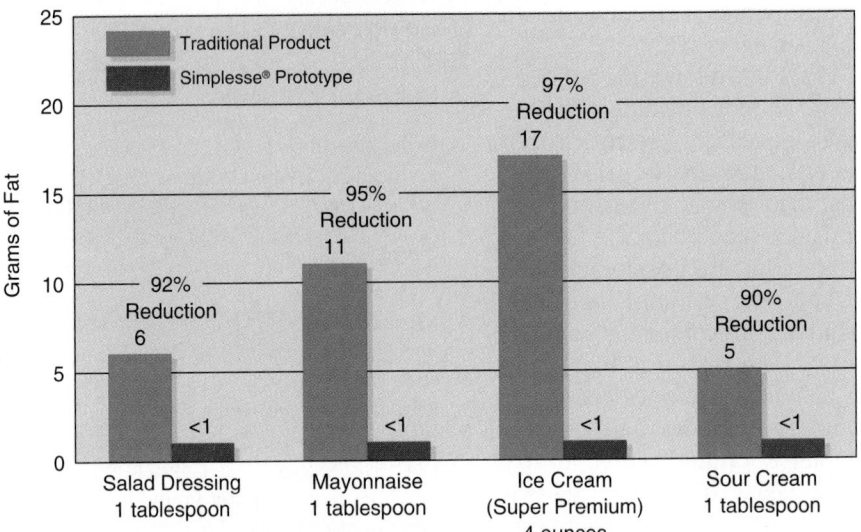

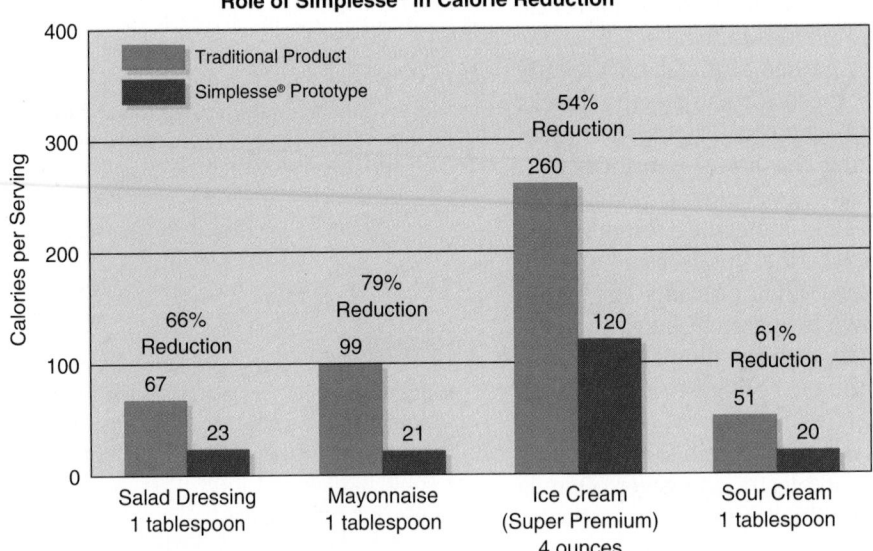

FIGURE 4–15
THE ROLE OF SIMPLESSE® IN FAT AND CALORIE REDUCTION

SOURCE: USDA Handbook No. 8; Hazleton Labs.

---

*The U.S. Food and Drug Administration also allows food manufacturers to market products made with other artificial fats. These include: *Stellar®* made from corn starch; *Oatrim®* made from oat flour; *Caprenin,®* designed to imitate the taste and feel of cocoa; and *Appetize,®* a blend of vegetable oil and animal fats (beef, pork, or milk) from which the cholesterol has been removed. In addition to these altered fats, many other artificial fats are currently under development.

TABLE 4–10
HOW TO DETERMINE TOTAL DAILY FAT ALLOWANCE

We are advised to limit our total daily fat intake to 30% *or less* of our total daily calories and to limit our saturated fat intake to no more than 10% of our total daily calories. Use this table to find your total daily fat and your daily saturated fat allowances. For instance, a 2,000-calorie diet could contain up to 67 grams of total fat (30% of total calories) and 22 grams of saturated fat (10% of total calories).

DAILY CALORIC INTAKE	CALORIES FROM FAT PER DAY	MAXIMUM GRAMS FAT PER DAY	MAXIMUM GRAMS SATURATED FAT PER DAY
1,200	360	40	13
1,400	420	47	16
1,500	450	50	17
1,600	480	53	18
1,800	540	60	20
2,000	600	67	22
2,200	660	73	24
2,400	720	80	27
2,600	780	87	29
2,800	840	93	31
3,000	900	100	33

Example: If you are eating 1,500 calories per day, multiply 1,500 by 30% to determine the maximum number of calories that should come from fat in one day (1,500 × .30 = 450 calories from fat). Since 1 gram of fat provides 9 calories, divide the calories from fat by 9 to see how many grams of fat you should have per day (450 ÷ 9 = 50 grams fat per day):

Total daily calories × .30 = total fat calories
Total fat calories ÷ 9 = total fat grams

To quickly estimate the number of fat grams allowed in a day, follow these three steps:
1. Estimate your daily calorie intake.
2. Drop the last digit.
3. Divide by 3 = Fat grams/day.

Example:

$$\frac{2,000}{3} = 67 \text{ g fat/day}$$

To determine your saturated fat goal: Multiply your total daily calories by 10% (1,500 × .10 = 150). Next divide the saturated fat calories by 9 (150 ÷ 9 = 17) to find out how many grams of saturated fat this equals:

Total daily calories × .10 = saturated fat calories
Saturated fat calories ÷ 9 = saturated fat grams

FIGURE 4–16
CHECKING OUT THE FOOD LABEL FOR FAT INFORMATION

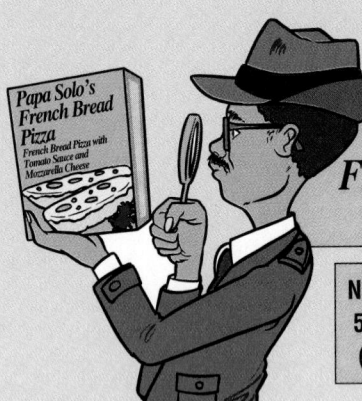

Papa Solo's French Bread Pizza
French Bread Pizza with Tomato Sauce and Mozzarella Cheese

NET WT. 5.6 OZ. (158g)

MAMA MIA's
Pepperoni Pizza-for-One

NET WT. 6¾ OZ. (191g)

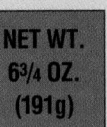

Calories from fat are now shown on the label to help consumers meet dietary guidelines that recommend people get no more than 30 percent of their calories from fat. See next page to figure "percent of calories from fat."

% Daily Value shows how a food fits into the overall daily diet.

The list of nutrients covers those most important to the health of today's consumers, most of whom need to worry about getting *too much* of certain items (fat, for example).

Daily Values are also something new. Some are maximums, as with fat (65 grams *or less*); others are minimums, as with carbohydrates (300 grams *or more*). The Daily Values on the label are shown for a daily diet of 2,000 and 2,500 calories. Individuals should adjust the values to fit their own calorie intake.

Nutrition Facts
Serving Size 1 pizza (158 g)
Servings per Container 1

Amount Per Serving

Calories 310	Calories from Fat 36
	% Daily Value*

	% Daily Value*
Total Fat 4g	**6%**
Saturated Fat 2g	**10%**
Polyunsaturated Fat 0.5g	
Monounsaturated Fat 1g	
Cholesterol 10mg	**3%**
Sodium 470mg	**20%**
Total Carbohydrate 49g	**16%**
Dietary Fiber 6g	**24%**
Sugars 3g	
Protein 20g	

Vitamin A 4% •	**Vitamin C** 0%
Calcium 30% •	**Iron** 15%

* Percent Daily Values are based on a 2,000 calorie diet. Your Daily Values may be higher or lower depending on your calorie needs:

	Calories:	2,000	2,500
Total Fat	Less than	65g	80g
Sat Fat	Less than	20g	25g
Cholesterol	Less than	300mg	300mg
Sodium	Less than	2,400mg	2,400mg
Total Carbohydrate		300g	375g
Dietary Fiber		25g	30g

Calories per gram
Fat 9 • Carbohydrate 4 • Protein 4

Ingredients: French bread (enriched unbleached wheat flour), water, wheat gluten, oat fiber, sugar, soybean oil, nonfat dry milk, mozzarella cheese, tomatoes. Contains 2% or less of each of the following: pizza spice mix (spices, salt, onion and garlic), sugar, coloring (dextrose, cabbage extract, annatto).

Nutrition Facts
Serving Size 1 pizza (191g)
Servings per Container 1

Amount Per Serving

Calories 520	Calories from Fat 243
	% Daily Value*

	% Daily Value*
Total Fat 27g	**42%**
Saturated Fat 10g	**50%**
Cholesterol 25mg	**8%**
Sodium 1,280mg	**53%**
Total Carbohydrate 53g	**18%**
Dietary Fiber 4g	**16%**
Sugars 6g	
Protein 19g	

Vitamin A 45% •	**Vitamin C** 0%
Calcium 30% •	**Iron** 10%

* Percent Daily Values are based on a 2,000 calorie diet. Your Daily Values may be higher or lower depending on your calorie needs:

	Calories:	2,000	2,500
Total Fat	Less than	65g	80g
Sat Fat	Less than	20g	25g
Cholesterol	Less than	300mg	300mg
Sodium	Less than	2,400mg	2,400mg
Total Carbohydrate		300g	375g
Dietary Fiber		25g	30g

Calories per gram
Fat 9 • Carbohydrate 4 • Protein 4

Ingredients: CRUST: Wheat flour with malted barley flour, water, partially hydrogenated vegetable oil (soybean and/or cottonseed oil) with soy lecithin, soybean oil, yeast, high fructose corn syrup, salt; TOPPING: Part-skim mozzarella cheese substitute, pepperoni (pork and beef, salt, water, dextrose, spices, sodium nitrite), part-skim mozzarella cheese; SAUCE: Tomato puree, water, green peppers, salt, lactose and flavoring, spices, corn oil, xanthum gum.

FIGURE 4–16

continued

- **Serving Size and Calories per Serving**

  First, look at the *serving size.* It is about the same for similar items, so it is easy to compare the nutritional qualities of your favorite pizzas or other similar foods. Next, look at the *calories per serving.* The typical adult shopper for whom the Nutrition Facts panels are designed needs about 2,000 calories per day. A serving of the French bread pizza would therefore provide 16 percent of the consumer's daily calorie need; the pepperoni pizza provides 26 percent of the calories needed for the day.

- **Percentage of Calories from Fat**

  The Nutrition Facts panel can be used to find out how many calories in a serving of the food come from fat. As you can see from the information found on these products' labels, the French bread pizza contains 36 (or 12%) of the calories from fat; the pepperoni pizza has 243 (or 47%) of the calories from fat.

  To determine percentage of calories from fat:

  $$\frac{\text{calories from fat}}{\text{total calories}} \times 100$$

  The recommendation itself to limit fat to no more than 30% of our total calories applies to the *total* daily intake of fat, and not to individual foods. For example, you may occasionally choose to eat a food with more than 30% of calories from fat, but you will need to balance it with other foods with a low percentage of calories from fat if you want your diet's average fat content to meet current recommendations to limit fat to 30% of total calories. Check Table 4-10 on page 143 to see the amount of fat (in grams) you should be eating daily based on your total calorie intake.

- **Total Fat**

  Total fat refers to all the fat in the food: saturated, monounsaturated, and polyunsaturated. Only total fat and saturated fat information is required on the label because high intakes of both are linked to high blood cholesterol levels, which in turn are linked to increased risk of heart disease. Listing the amount of monounsaturated and polyunsaturated fats in the food is voluntary.

- **% Daily Value**

  Look at the column called *"% Daily Value."* It compares the total fat, saturated fat, and cholesterol in a serving of the food with a person's daily need. The % Daily Value tells you if the food has large or small amounts of total fat, saturated fat, and cholesterol. Note at the bottom of the Nutrition Facts panel that the Daily Value for total fat is *less than* 65 grams for a person requiring 2,000 calories a day. The reference value of 65 grams for total fat is derived from the recommendation for health that states that 30% *or less* of our calories should come from fat. (For a 2,000 calorie diet, this amount would equal 65 grams—the Daily Value for total fat.) A serving of the French bread pizza shown here provides 6% of the Daily Value for total fat, 10% of the Daily Value for saturated fat, and 3% of the Daily Value for cholesterol; the pepperoni pizza provides 42% of the Daily Value for total fat, 50% of the Daily Value for saturated fat, and 8% of the Daily Value for cholesterol. The overall goal should be to select foods that together do *not* exceed 100% of the Daily Values for fat, saturated fat, and cholesterol over the course of your day for these nutrients.

FIT OR FAT SCORECARD

Do the foods you eat provide more fat than is good for you? Answer the questions below to see how your diet rates.

HOW OFTEN DO YOU EAT:	Seldom or Never	1-2 Times per Week	3-5 Times per Week	Almost Daily
1. Butter or margarine on vegetables, dinner rolls, and toast?	☐	☐	☐	☐
2. Salad dressings, mayonnaise, and guacamole?	☐	☐	☐	☐
3. Rich sauces and gravies?	☐	☐	☐	☐
4. Whole milk, cheese, and ice cream?	☐	☐	☐	☐
5. Whipped cream, sour cream, and cream cheese?	☐	☐	☐	☐
6. Croissants, biscuits, muffins, or other breakfast pastries?	☐	☐	☐	☐
7. Snacks such as potato chips, corn chips, cheese puffs, tortilla chips, buttered popcorn, and candy bars?	☐	☐	☐	☐
8. Desserts such as pies, pastries, cookies, and cakes.	☐	☐	☐	☐
9. Fried, deep-fat-fried, breaded, or battered foods such as refried beans, French fries, egg rolls, or taco shells?	☐	☐	☐	☐
10. Fatty meats such as bacon, sausage, hot dogs, ribs, and luncheon meats?	☐	☐	☐	☐
11. Heavily marbled steaks or chicken with the skin?	☐	☐	☐	☐
12. Nuts or seeds?	☐	☐	☐	☐

Scoring: Take a look at your answers. Several responses in the last two columns means you may have too much fat in your diet. Is it time to cut back on foods high in fat? If so, try following the strategies offered in the following section to help you reduce the amount of fat in your diet.

SOURCE: Adapted from USDA Home and Garden Publication 232-3.

Be Fat Wise

Ample evidence exists that people in developed countries continue to consume a high-fat diet and that this diet is causing an increase in chronic diseases such as heart disease, cancer of the breast and colon, obesity, gallbladder disease, and arthritis. With that in mind, the *Dietary Guidelines* advise us to choose a diet low in fat, saturated fat, and cholesterol. This broad guideline can be translated into food-specific behaviors with the following examples:[33]

- Eat more fresh fruits and vegetables, whole-grain breads and cereals, potatoes, rice, noodles, dried beans, peas, and lentils.
- Choose low-fat dairy products, including nonfat and 1%-fat milk, low-fat cheeses, and low-fat or nonfat yogurt.
- Choose lean meats and fish, and skinless chicken and turkey.

It is not the food itself but how you prepare it that often determines the total fat (and calories) in a food. Compare the fat in three ounces of broiled chicken (3 grams fat, 141 calories) versus three ounces of fried chicken (18 grams fat, 364 calories). What makes the difference in calories? Fat. The single most effective step you can take to reduce the calorie value of a food is to eat the food without the fat. This step is also an effective dietary weapon against high blood cholesterol levels.

Foods you purchase in the grocery store can tell you much about their fat content—if you take the time to read the Nutrition Facts panel on their labels. Figure 4–17 lists the definitions related to fat allowed on food labels that can alert you to the fat that foods contain. For example, if you see a food labeled "low-fat," you can be sure that it contains 3 grams or less of fat in one serving. Remember, too, that the ingredients on a food label are listed in order of predominance in the product; if fat is one of the first ingredients listed, you know you are holding in your hands a high-fat product. Whether or not to choose the food depends on how you intend to use it in your diet: as a staple item, as an occasional treat, or as a garnish for other foods.

The following list suggests a variety of ways to significantly reduce the fat content of your diet:

- Read manufacturers' labels to determine both the amounts and the types of fat contained in foods.
- Check the Nutrition Facts panel on the packages you buy—it lists the amount of fat in grams per serving. Each gram of fat you eliminate saves you 9 calories.
- Serve 4-ounce or smaller portions of lean meats and poultry, adding them to stews, soups, stir-fry recipes, or pasta.
- Choose the low-fat and lean varieties of processed meats (sausages, luncheon meats, bacon, and frankfurters).
- Choose water-packed canned fish rather than oil-packed varieties.
- Choose lean cuts of meat; remove "visible" fat from meat; remove skin from poultry.
- Include vegetable protein sources in your diet, such as dried peas, beans, and lentils.

FIGURE 4–17
TERMINOLOGY OF FAT ON FOOD LABELS

DESCRIPTOR	DEFINITION
Fat free	Contains less than 0.5 gram of fat per serving.
Low-fat	Contains 3 grams or less of fat per serving.
Reduced fat	A nutritionally altered product that contains 25% less fat than the regular or reference product. This cannot be used if the reference food already meets the criteria for a low-fat food.
Low in saturated fat	This may be used to describe a food that contains 1 gram or less of saturated fat per serving.
Reduced saturated fat	A nutritionally altered product that contains 25% less saturated fat than the regular or reference product. This cannot be used if the reference food already meets the criteria for a food low in saturated fat.
Cholesterol free	Contains less than 2 mg of cholesterol per serving.
Low cholesterol	Contains less than 20 mg of cholesterol per serving and no more than 2 grams saturated fat.
Reduced cholesterol	A nutritionally altered product that contains 25% less cholesterol than the regular or reference product. This cannot be used if the reference food already meets the criteria for a low-cholesterol food.
Lean	Contains less than 10 grams of fat, less than 4.5 grams of saturated fat, and less than 95 mg of cholesterol per serving and per 100 grams.
Extra lean	Contains less than 5 grams of fat, less than 2 grams of saturated fat, and less than 95 mg of cholesterol per serving and per 100 grams.

Percent fat free is an indication of the amount of a food's weight that is fat free, which can be used only on foods that are low-fat or fat free to begin with. For instance, if a food weighs 100 grams and 3 grams are from fat, it can be labeled "97 percent fat free." Note that this term refers to the amount that is fat free by weight, not calories. If that same food supplies 100 calories, the 3 grams of fat contribute 27 of them (1 gram of fat contains 9 calories). That means 27 of the 100 calories, or 27 percent, of the total calories come from fat.

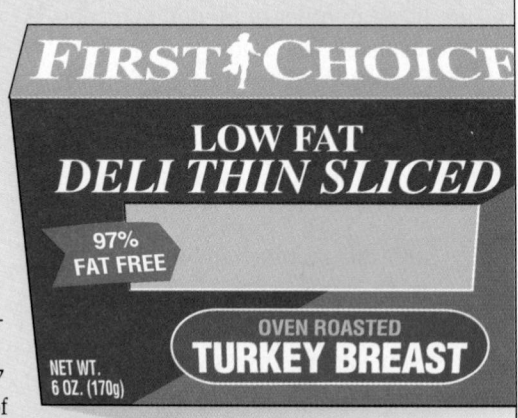

Nutrition Facts	
Serving Size 6 slices (54g)	
Servings per Container about 3	
Amount Per Serving	
Calories 60	60
Calories from Fat	14
	% Daily Value*
Total Fat 1.5g	2%
Saturated Fat 0.5g	3%
Cholesterol 20mg	7%
Sodium 480mg	20%
Total Carbohydrate 2g	1%
Dietary Fiber 0g	0%
Sugars 1g	
Protein 10g	20%
Vitamin A 0% • **Vitamin C** 0%	
Calcium 0% • **Iron** 0%	
*Percent Daily Values are based on 2,000 calorie diet.	

Ingredients: Turkey breast, water, modified food starch, dextrose, salt, sodium lactate, sodium phosphate, flavorings, celery juice.

Compare labels on packaged deli meats. This package of turkey breast slices states that it is "97% fat free." What this means is that 3% of the product's weight is contributed by fat. If you determine percentage of calories from fat, you will see that this does not mean that only 3% of the calories in a serving come from fat.

Applying the formula for percentage of calories from fat: $\dfrac{14 \text{ calories from fat}}{60 \text{ total calories}} \times 100 = 23\%$ calories from fat

- Eat fried foods sparingly; rather, **bake, braise, broil, steam, poach,** and **saute** (see Miniglossary of Cooking Terms). Cook meats on a rack so that the "invisible" fat can drain off.

- Experiment with some new low-fat, low-cholesterol recipes. (See Appendix A for a listing of recommended resources.)

- Use low-fat or nonfat dairy products. Learn to substitute: low-fat or nonfat milk for whole milk, low-fat or nonfat yogurt for sour cream, low-fat Neufchatel cheese for cream cheese, and part-skim ricotta and mozzarella cheese for whole-milk varieties.

MINIGLOSSARY OF COOKING TERMS

BAKE to cook in an oven surrounded by heat.

BRAISE to cook by browning in fat and then simmering in a covered container with a little liquid.

BROIL to cook quickly over or under a direct source of intense heat, allowing fats to drip away.

POACH to cook foods (fish, an egg without its shell, etc.) in water near the boiling point.

SAUTÉ (saw-TAY, the French word for stir-fry) to cook in a pan using little fat; foods are stirred frequently to prevent sticking.

STEAM to cook foods suspended over boiling water.

- Limit your intake of butter, cream, margarine, vegetable shortenings, coconut and palm oils, half-and-half, sour cream, and mayonnaise.

- Use polyunsaturated or monounsaturated vegetable oils and soft margarine containing these oils; use the low-fat or fat-free varieties of margarine, mayonnaise, and salad dressings now available on the market.

- When you use margarine, butter, or cream cheese, try the whipped varieties, which contain half the calories of the regular types.

- Use oil-and-vinegar salad dressings instead of creamy ones, which usually have a higher fat content.

- For flavor in sauces and dressings, experiment using herbs and spices, onions or garlic, salsa, ginger, lemon juice, plain nonfat yogurt with lemon juice, mustard, or butter-flavored granules instead of butter, margarine, or oil.

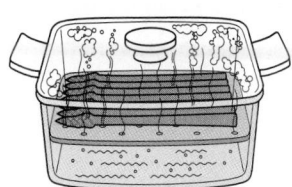
Bake, broil, poach, or steam.

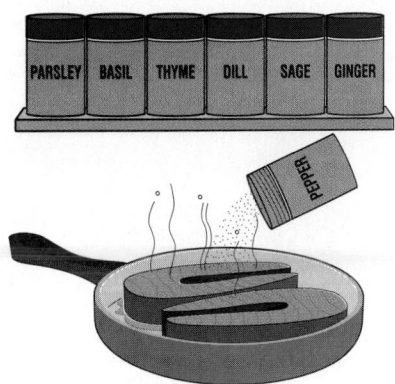
Season with herbs and spices.

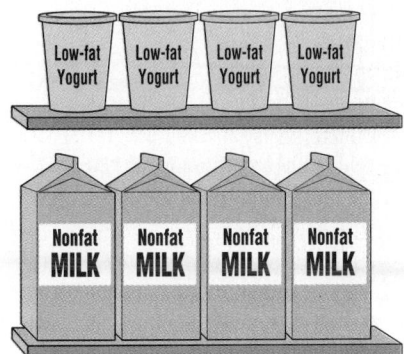
Buy low-fat foods.

- Use nonstick sprays rather than fat to coat cooking pans.
- If you are sauteing a vegetable such as onion in butter, margarine, or oil, try reducing the amount used and substitute water or cooking wine in its place.
- Eat fewer high-fat desserts (such as cheesecake, ice cream, brownies, pies, pastries, and butter- and cream-frosted cakes).
- Prepare broths, soups, and stews ahead of time, refrigerate them, and then skim off hardened fat from the surface. This also gives the flavors time to blend and develop.
- Use low-fat or nonfat milk when making cream soups.
- Learn to substitute. Table 4–11 offers some ways to reduce both fat and calories. The Consumer Tips feature offers more suggestions to help you lighten your favorite recipes.

TABLE 4–11
HOW TO CUT BACK ON FAT IN YOUR DIET

SUBSTITUTE THIS . . . Food	Fat (g)	WITH THIS . . . Food	Fat (g)	AND SAVE FAT/CALORIES Fat (g)	Calories*
Whole milk, 8 oz	8	Nonfat milk, 8 oz	Trace	8	72
Sour cream, 4 oz	22	Low-fat yogurt, 4 oz	2	20	180
Ice cream, 1 c	14	Sorbet, 1 c	0	14	126
Chicken breast, with skin, 3 oz	7	Chicken breast, skinless, 3 oz	3	4	36
Hamburger, 3 oz	17	Lean hamburger, 3 oz	10	7	63
Fish sticks, 5	10	Broiled fish, 3 oz	5	5	45
Biscuits, 2 dinner	6	Bread, 2 slices	2	4	36
Butter/margarine, 1 tbsp	12	Parmesan cheese, 1 tbsp	2	10	90
Mayonnaise, 1 tbsp	11	Fat-free mayonnaise, 1 tbsp	0	11	99
Asparagus, 1 c, with hollandaise sauce	18	Asparagus, 1 c, with lemon	0	18	162
French fries, 15	12	Baked potato with 1 pat butter	4	8	72
Fried egg, 1	9	Broiled or poached egg, 1	6	3	27
Bacon, 1 oz	14	Canadian bacon, 1 oz	2	12	108
Round steak, 8 oz	30	Round steak, 4 oz	15	15	135
Apple pie, 1 slice	18	Apple crisp, 1 portion	8	10	90
Potato chips, 2 oz (1 small bag)	24	Unbuttered popcorn, 3 c	2	22	198
Danish pastry, 1	15	English muffin with 1 tbsp jam	1	14	126
Yellow cake with icing, 1/12 cake	13	Angel food cake, 1/12 cake	Trace	13	117

*Grams of fat × 9.
SOURCE: Adapted from The Potato Board.

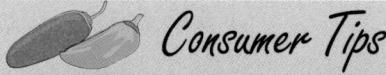

Consumer Tips

Recipe Modification

Use this substitution information to modify your own favorite recipes. They'll be more healthful but still look and taste as good as your originals!

INTEAD OF	SUBSTITUTE	RESULT
1 whole egg	2 whipped egg whites	less fat, less cholesterol, fewer calories
whole milk	nonfat milk	less fat, less cholesterol, fewer calories
evaporated milk	evaporated nonfat or low-fat milk	less fat, less cholesterol, fewer calories
sugar (baking)	use ⅓ less than called for in baking, add a small amount of vanilla, cinnamon or nutmeg	fewer calories
oil	use a vegetable oil spray for preventing foods from sticking	less fat, fewer calories
cake frosting	sprinkled powdered sugar	less sugar, less fat, fewer calories
heavy cream (which does not need to be whipped)	evaporated nonfat or low-fat milk	less fat, less cholesterol, fewer calories
sour cream	reduced-fat or nonfat sour cream or plain yogurt	less fat, less cholesterol, fewer calories
solid shortening (baking)	vegetable oil, margarine	less saturated fat
solid shortening (stir-frying)	peanut oil	less saturated fat
mayonnaise	reduced-fat or nonfat mayonnaise or plain yogurt (mixed with 1 tbsp mayo per cup yogurt)	less fat, less cholesterol, fewer calories
salt	use ½ the salt called for in recipes (try seasoning with herbs & other spices) except yeast breads	less sodium
cream cheese	reduced-fat or nonfat cream cheese	less fat, fewer calories
regular cheese	cheese made from part-skim milk (mozzarella, Swiss lace, farmer) or reduced-fat cheeses	less fat, less cholesterol, fewer calories
salad dressing	nonfat or oil-free salad dressings or reduced-calorie dressing	less fat, less cholesterol, fewer calories
white sauce (made with cream & butter)	use low-fat milk and cornstarch or flour by blending the starch into cold liquid to eliminate the need for fat	less fat, less cholesterol, fewer calories

Try a lower-fat guacamole: Blend 1 medium avocado with 1 cup low-fat (1%) cottage cheese; add 1 tbsp lime juice, 1 tsp chives, and ¼ tsp red pepper flakes. Per ¼ cup serving: 60 calories and 4 grams of fat—about half the fat of traditional guacamole.

Try oven-baked fries: (3 grams fat per serving) instead of traditional French fries (12 grams fat per serving): Place 4 medium russet potatoes (cut into wedges) into bowl and sprinkle with 1 tbsp vegetable oil, ¼ tsp black pepper, and a pinch of salt (optional); toss gently to combine; arrange potatoes in single layer on nonstick baking sheet sprayed with vegetable cooking spray. Bake in oven (425° F) for 35 minutes or until lightly browned. Serve with salsa or nonfat yogurt mixed with fresh herbs (serves 4).

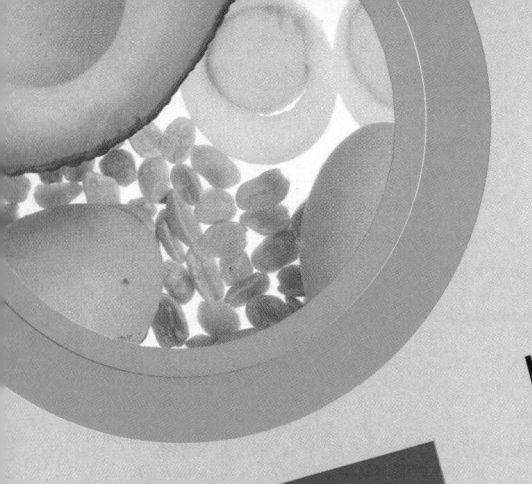

Diet and Heart Disease

SPOTLIGHT More than half the people who die in the United States each year die of heart and blood vessel disease. The underlying condition that contributes to most of these deaths is atherosclerosis, which leads to closure of the arteries that feed the heart and brain and thus to heart attacks and strokes. In terms of direct health care costs, lost wages, and lost productivity, heart disease costs the United States more than $60 billion a year.[34] There is little wonder, then, that much effort has been focused on preventing it.

The twin demons that lead to most forms of heart disease are atherosclerosis and hypertension. Atherosclerosis, the subject of this Spotlight, is the common form of hardening of the arteries; hypertension (discussed in the Nutrition Action feature of Chapter 7) is high blood pressure; and each aggravates the other.

How can I know whether I have atherosclerosis? No one is free of atherosclerosis. The question is not whether you have it but how far advanced it is and what you can do to retard or reverse it. As mentioned in the chapter, atherosclerosis usually begins with the accumulation of soft mounds of lipid, known as plaques, along the inner walls of the arteries, especially at the branch points (see Figure 4–18). These plaques gradually enlarge, making the artery walls lose their elasticity and narrowing the passage through them. Most people have well-developed plaques by the time they are 30.

Normally, the arteries expand with each heartbeat to accommodate the pulses of blood that flow through them. Because arteries hardened and narrowed by plaques cannot expand, the blood pressure rises. The increased pressure puts a strain on the heart and further damages the artery wall. At damaged points, plaques are especially likely to form; thus, the development of atherosclerosis is a self-accelerating process.

Hypertension makes atherosclerosis worse. A stiffened artery, already strained by each pulse of blood surging through it, is stressed even more if the internal pressure is high. Injured places develop more frequently, and plaques grow faster.

Also, atherosclerosis makes hypertension worse. By hardening the arteries, it makes the arteries unable to expand with each beat of the heart, so the pressure rises instead. This leads to further hardening of the arteries, as already explained. Hardened arteries also fail to let blood flow freely through the body's blood pressure-sensing organs—the kidneys—which respond as if the blood pressure were too low and raise it further.

How can I slow the process down? Learn your risk factors, and control the ones you can control. Among the many factors linked to heart disease are smoking, gender (being male), age (men older than 45 and women older than 55), postmenopausal status in women, heredity, diabetes, high blood pressure, lack of exercise, obesity, high blood cholesterol level, and low HDL-cholesterol level (see Table 4–12). Some

of the risk factors are powerful predictors of heart disease. If you have none of them, the statistical likelihood of your developing heart disease may be only one in 100. If you have three major ones, the chance may rise to over one in 20. The three factors that have emerged as the most powerful predictors of risk are high blood cholesterol, high blood pressure, and smoking.

The accompanying Heart Health Scorecard shows one way of calculating your risk score based on present knowledge. Such a quiz not only helps you look at what your risks may be but also points out areas that you can change to reduce your risk.

What can I do to improve my risk score? Obviously, some risk factors cannot be altered. Being born male or

TABLE 4–12
LEADING RISK FACTORS FOR HEART DISEASE

- High blood cholesterol (especially LDL-cholesterol)
- Cigarette smoking
- High blood pressure
- High-fat/high-saturated-fat diet
- Family history of early heart attack
- Diabetes
- Obesity
- Physical inactivity
- Gender (males are at higher risk)
- Low HDL-cholesterol

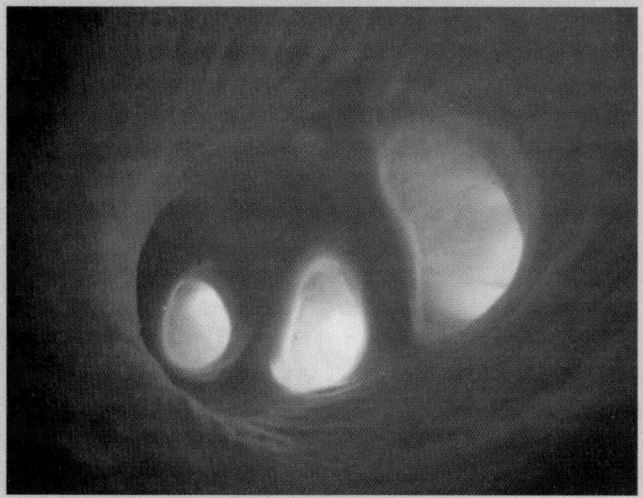

A normal artery provides open passage for blood to circulate.

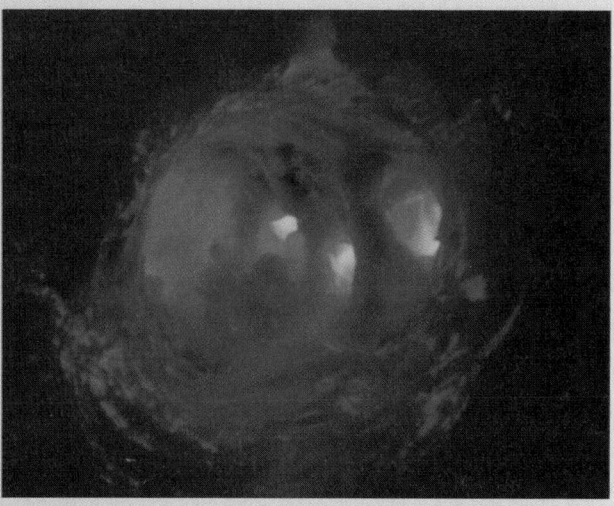

Plaques along an artery narrow the passage and obstruct blood flow.

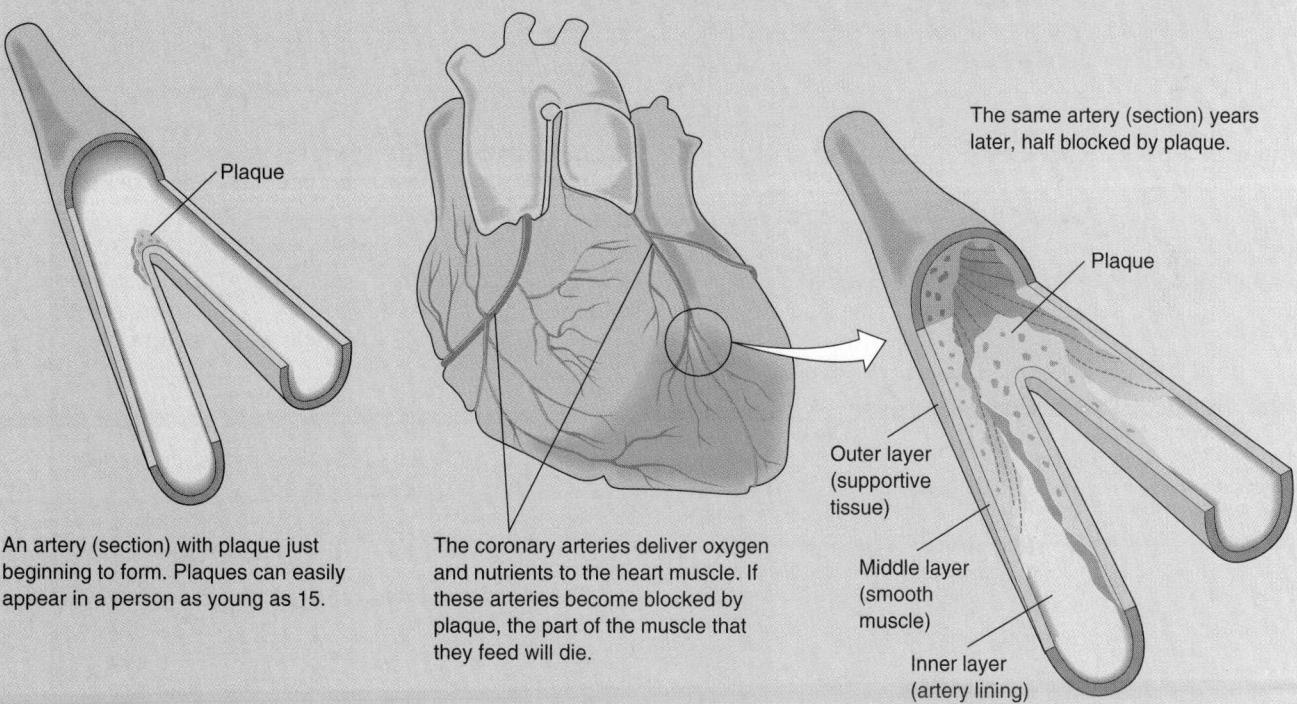

Plaque

An artery (section) with plaque just beginning to form. Plaques can easily appear in a person as young as 15.

The coronary arteries deliver oxygen and nutrients to the heart muscle. If these arteries become blocked by plaque, the part of the muscle that they feed will die.

The same artery (section) years later, half blocked by plaque.

Plaque

Outer layer (supportive tissue)

Middle layer (smooth muscle)

Inner layer (artery lining)

FIGURE 4–18
THE DEVELOPMENT OF ATHEROSCLEROSIS

Every disease has risk factors; those for heart disease are among the best known. The better you know the nature of the risks you face, the better you can decide what prevention measures may be appropriate. To determine your risk of heart disease, add up the numbers in each category that most nearly describe you:

	1	2	3	4	6
Heredity[a]	No known history of heart disease	One relative over 60 years old with heart disease	Two relatives over 60 years old with heart disease	One relative under 60 years old with heart disease	Two relatives under 60 years old with heart disease
	1	2	3	5	6
Exercise	Intensive exercise, work, and recreation	Moderate exercise, work, and recreation	Sedentary work and intensive recreational exercise	Sedentary work and moderate recreational exercise	Sedentary work and light recreational exercise
	1	2	3	4	6
Age	10 to 20	21 to 30	31 to 40	41 to 50	51 to 65
	0	1	2	4	6
Lb	More than 5 lb below standard weight	± 5 lb of standard weight	6 to 20 lb overweight	21 to 35 lb overweight	36 to 50 lb overweight
	0	1	2	4	6
Tobacco	Nonuser	Cigar or pipe	10 cigarettes or fewer per day	20 cigarettes or more per day	30 cigarettes or more per day
	1	2	3	4	6
Habits of eating fat[b]	No animal or solid fat	Very little animal or solid fat	Little animal or solid fat	Much animal or solid fat	Equal to the typical meat eater's diet

Your risk of heart attack:

4 to 9: Very remote	16 to 20: Average	26 to 30: Dangerous
10 to 15: Below average	21 to 25: Moderate	31 to 35: Urgent danger—reduce score!

Other conditions—such as stress, high blood pressure, and increased blood cholesterol level—detract from heart health and should be evaluated by your physician.

---

[a]Diabetes and hypertension in the family are also predictors.

[b]If you know your blood cholesterol level, use it instead. Below 180 = 0 points; 181 to 200 = 1; 201 to 235 = 2; 236 to 260 = 4; 261 to 300 = 5; over 300 = 6.

SOURCE: Courtesy of Loma Linda University.

inheriting a predisposition to develop high blood cholesterol or high blood pressure are factors beyond your control. Even so, you can make conscious choices that may reduce your risk of developing heart disease. Let's examine one of the two major risk factors related to diet—high blood cholesterol—with an eye toward learning which dietary and lifestyle changes will help reduce your heart disease risk.

To what extent does a high blood cholesterol level raise the risk of developing heart disease? The likelihood of a person's developing or dying from heart disease increases as blood cholesterol level rises. Figure 4–19 presents this relationship graphically: The number of deaths from heart disease increases steadily among those with elevated blood cholesterol levels, particularly when the level rises above 200 milligrams per deciliter. Individuals with a blood cholesterol level in the neighborhood of 300 milligrams per deciliter run four times the risk of dying from heart disease as those whose cholesterol level is lower than 200 milligrams per deciliter. Having a low HDL-cholesterol value is now also recognized as being a risk factor for heart disease. A low HDL value is defined as one below 35 milligrams per deciliter. A combined effort to lower LDL-cholesterol and raise HDL-cholesterol delivers a double punch in the fight against heart disease.

Reducing high blood cholesterol levels, particularly the "bad" LDL-cholesterol level, is thus an important strategy toward lowering the risk of heart disease. This is especially true for persons having one or more of the other major heart disease risk factors, such as smoking. Figure 4–12 on page 130 and Table 4–13 on page 157 provide information for determining what to do if your blood cholesterol level is high and whether you might need to seek treatment.

What sorts of dietary changes should I make to reduce my total cholesterol and LDL-cholesterol? Probably the most significant dietary change you can make is to reduce the amount of fat that you eat, particularly saturated fat, since high intakes of these dietary constituents are related to high blood levels of LDL-cholesterol. The goals to work toward are to reduce your intake of total fat to 30 percent of total calories or less and reduce your intake of saturated fat to 10 percent of total calories or less. Many Americans are on the right track toward reducing their intakes of fat and saturated fat and lowering their blood LDL-cholesterol levels.

In addition to reducing fat intakes, people can make other dietary changes that might also help lower LDL-cholesterol. Dietary fiber, for example, may confer benefits. People on high-fiber diets have been shown to excrete more cholesterol and fat than those on low-fiber diets. A 5 percent decrease in total cholesterol can be achieved with a 5- to 10-gram increase in soluble fiber intake.[35] One reason is that the high-fiber diet decreases food's transit time through the digestive tract, allowing less time for cholesterol to be absorbed. When cholesterol from the diet is thus reduced, the body must turn to its own supply for making necessary body compounds. Diets high in fiber are typically low in fat and cholesterol—another advantage to emphasizing fiber.

The various dietary fibers have varying effects on blood cholesterol. Rolled oats, oat bran, and psyllium-fortified cereals have favorable effects on blood cholesterol, whereas wheat bran does not appear effective.[36] Apples, pears, peaches, oranges, and grapes are good sources of pectin, another type of cholesterol-lowering fiber.

Should I also reduce my cholesterol intake? The *Dietary Guidelines* recommend that we limit the cholesterol in our daily diets to 300 milligrams. On the average, men consume 400 to 500 milligrams of cholesterol and women consume about 300 milligrams daily. The average for American men is above that consumed in countries with little heart disease.

Some experts say that all adults should cut their cholesterol intake; others say only those medically identified as at risk for heart disease should do so. The question remains open, but most people who develop heart-healthy eating habits, such as decreasing saturated fat, tend to lower their cholesterol intake along with their fat intake.

What factors determine my HDL-cholesterol level? One is gender. Women have higher HDL-cholesterol levels than men. However, heart disease is the major cause of death among women after menopause, when low levels of estrogen lead to a decrease in HDL levels along with an increase in LDL levels.[37] Another factor, interestingly, seems to be smoking habits. Nonsmokers have uniformly higher HDL levels than do smokers. Still another factor is weight reduction for those who are overweight.[38]

If there are dietary factors of any significance, one may be the use of some fish in the diet.[39] Another may be the use of foods containing soluble fibers that lower LDL levels selectively and leave HDL levels unchanged. By far the most powerful influence on HDL levels is not a dietary factor at all—it is regular exercise. The discovery that exercise raises HDL levels has given great impetus to the physical fitness movement—and especially to the popularity of running and walking. The earliest reports were of raised HDL levels in long-distance runners, and the continuing study of this elite group has repeatedly demonstrated that running does indeed elevate HDL. People do not, however, have to become competitive athletes to raise their HDL—moderate exercise such as walking may both lower LDL levels and raise HDL levels if the activity is consistently pursued for long enough periods. Evidently, then, almost all people are capable of exercising enough to reap this and many other benefits (see Chapter 9).

What about alcohol? I've heard that moderate alcohol intake can be beneficial to heart disease. The evidence with regards to alcohol and blood lipids points to a possible protective mechanism between moderate alcohol consumption and heart disease risk factors.[40] Investigators have reported that the consumption of moderate amounts of alcohol appears to raise HDL levels.[41] Moderate drinking is defined as no more than one drink a day for most women, and no more than two drinks a day for most men (see the Spotlight feature in Chapter 9). A strong association between moderate alcohol consumption and low rates of heart disease was first observed in France and then in other wine-drinking areas of the Mediterranean. Researchers have since identified antioxidants and other compounds that decrease blood clotting in red wine, which may help explain part of the "French paradox"—or how a region with high fat intakes could have such low rates of heart disease. Researchers are quick to point out, however, that other factors certainly may contribute to the paradox. For example, the French consume about 57 percent of their day's calories before 2 p.m., whereas most Americans have only consumed about 38 percent of their calories by that time.[42] Also, the French

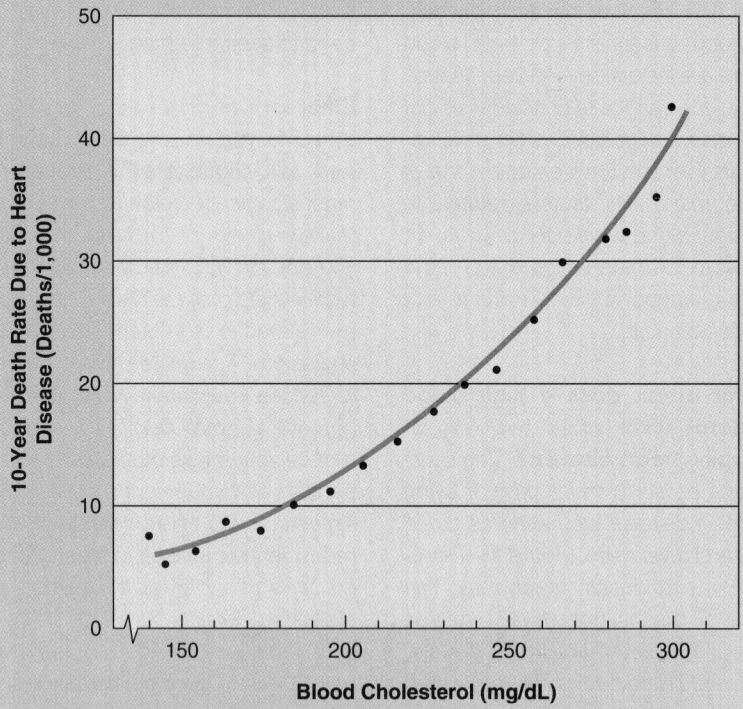

FIGURE 4–19
RELATIONSHIP BETWEEN BLOOD CHOLESTEROL LEVEL AND DEATH RATE FROM HEART DISEASE

Persons with blood cholesterol levels of 300 mg/dL are four times as likely to die from heart disease as those with blood cholesterol levels below 200 mg/dL.

SOURCE: Data from 361,662 men screened for the Multiple Risk Factor Intervention Trial (MRFIT). Adapted from National Cholesterol Education Program, *Report of the Expert Panel on Population Strategies for Blood Cholesterol Reduction*, Bethesda, Md.: U.S. Department of Health and Human Services, Public Health Service, National Institutes of Health, National Heart, Lung, and Blood Institute, NIH Publication No. 90-3046, November 1990, p. 7.

mostly consume their wine with meals and eat more fruits and vegetables and leaner cuts of meat.

Scientists warn that caution is needed in recommending moderate alcohol consumption to the public. Many people need to refrain from alcohol consumption altogether (pregnant women, recovering alcoholics, people under age 21, persons on certain medications, and those intending to drive a vehicle).[43] Keep in mind that alcohol can have profoundly negative effects on the body and is associated with many disease states (see the Chapter 9 Spotlight feature).

How do I translate these recommendations into a healthful eating pattern? Most people have a difficult time translating the dietary recommendations into actual meal patterns. What foods should you eat, for example, to achieve the goal of reducing your fat intake to 30 percent or less of total calories? It's virtually impossible to know exactly what your fat intake is without having your daily food intake analyzed using a computerized nutrient program. Even so, some general guidelines will help you make the heart-healthy food choices needed to achieve your goals. If you were to take all of the steps suggested, you would:

• Choose healthful portions of skinless poultry, lean meat, and fish, especially omega-3-fatty-acid-rich fish such as mackerel, salmon, and canned albacore tuna.

• Choose nonfat or low-fat dairy products, such as nonfat milk or low-fat or nonfat yogurt.

• Consume abundant legumes of many varieties, including soybeans, kidney beans, and lentils.

• Eat generous quantities of fiber-rich fruits and vegetables, including many raw ones.

• Eat whole grains (oats, wheat, corn, rice, pasta) often.

• Limit your use of foods particularly rich in saturated fat, such as fatty red meats (see Table 4–14). Trim away all visible fat from meats before cooking.

• Adopt low-fat cooking methods, such as broiling, roasting, steaming, braising, and stir-frying.

• Become a savvy supermarket shopper—learn to read food labels to help you choose low-fat and fat-free food products.

• Consume alcohol only in moderation, if at all.

It seems that the factors affecting the health of the heart are all tangled together. The exact relationships among them have not yet been worked out; we don't know which causes what, but all evidence points to the same general recommendations. For good health and to avoid heart disease, stop smoking; reduce blood pressure and weight, if necessary; eat a balanced, adequate, and varied diet; reduce total fat intake, especially saturated fat; and exercise regularly.

Attention to emotional health is also important in reducing the risk of heart

TABLE 4–13

STANDARDS FOR BLOOD CHOLESTEROL LEVELS AND RISK OF HEART DISEASE

EVALUATING BLOOD LIPID LEVELS

Total Cholesterol Levels	Classification
Less than 200 mg/dL	Desirable
200 to 239 mg/dL	Borderline high
240 mg/dL or higher	High

HDL-Cholesterol Levels

Less than 35 mg/dL	Increased risk for CHD (Coronary Heart Disease)
60 mg/dL or higher	Decreased risk for CHD

LDL-to-HDL Ratio

Men: greater than 5.0 indicates risk
Women: greater than 4.5 indicates risk

Triglyceride Levels

Less than 200 mg/dL	Desirable
200 to 400 mg/dL	Borderline high
400 to 1,000 mg/dL	High
1,000 mg/dL or higher	Very High

TREATING LDL-CHOLESTEROL LEVELS

Risk Status	Target/Recommendations for LDL-Cholesterol
Low-risk individuals[a]	Less than 160 mg/dL Begin dietary therapy at 160 mg/dL; consider drug therapy at 190 mg/dL in men over 45 and postmenopausal women. Begin drug therapy at 220 mg/dL in younger men and women.
High-risk individuals[b]	Less than 130 mg/dL Begin dietary therapy at 130 mg/dL; consider drug therapy at 160 mg/dL.
Very high risk individuals[c]	Less than 100 mg/dL Begin dietary therapy at 100 mg/dL; consider drug therapy if dietary therapy fails to reduce LDL-cholesterol levels below 100 mg/dL.

[a]Low-risk individuals are those with one or no risk factors for heart disease.

[b]High-risk individuals are those who have at least two risk factors for CHD. (Men over age 45 and postmenopausal women are considered to have one risk factor.)

[c]Very-high-risk individuals are those with known heart disease (history of heart attack or previous bypass surgery or angioplasty).

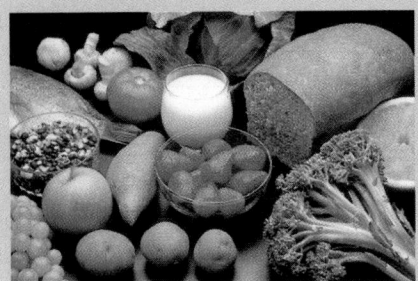

Enjoy a variety of low-fat foods for the health of your heart.

disease. Both love and affection seem to affect the heart. People with many social ties appear to develop less heart disease than people with few or none. Married men have less heart disease than single men, and pet owners (even owners of pet fish) have lower blood pressure than do people without pets. Clearly, the mystery of heart disease, like all the great human mysteries, involves the mind and spirit as well as the body. So nourish yourself in all ways—not just physically.

The verdict is not yet in as to whether following these suggestions will reverse the process of atherosclerosis. However, the evidence collected to date tends to show that following these suggestions will help to prevent the condition from getting any worse and may also begin to clear the arteries.

What about garlic? I've heard that garlic pills and whole cloves help lower blood cholesterol. A sizeable body of evidence from around the world suggests that garlic may help lower blood cholesterol. However, much of the research has been short-term, lasting no longer than several months. In addition, many studies linking garlic to reduced blood cholesterol levels have failed to account for other factors that can influence cholesterol levels, such as the amount of fat in the garlic consumers' diets or changes in weight.[44] While the research is promising, further studies are needed before scientists can come to any conclusions about the usefulness of fresh garlic or garlic pills, which vary a great deal in composition, in lowering blood cholesterol levels.

Should children, like their parents, eat low-fat diets for heart health? In 1991, a panel of experts representing 42 major U.S. health and professional organizations recommended that children aged two and older eat diets containing no more than 30 percent of total calories from saturated fat and no more than 300 milligrams of cholesterol daily. The reason is that hardening of the arteries often begins in childhood. However, from birth to two years of age, a child's fat consumption should not be restricted, because fat is a concentrated source of the calories needed to ensure proper physical development.

The panel also advised that youngsters or teens should get their blood cholesterol measured if they have one parent with a high blood cholesterol level. For children and adolescents, a total of 200 milligrams per deciliter or more is considered high, 170 to 199 is borderline high, and less than 170 is acceptable. In addition, youngsters born to families with a history of premature heart disease should have both total blood cholesterol and HDL-cholesterol checked.[45]

TABLE 4–14

COMPARISON OF SATURATED FAT, TOTAL FAT, AND CHOLESTEROL IN SELECTED FOODS[a]

The following foods within each grouping are ranked from low to high saturated fat.[b] The foods chosen for this chart are meant to be representative of their type. You will want to select most often the low saturated fat and cholesterol foods from the upper portion of each group.

	GRAMS OF SATURATED FAT	GRAMS OF TOTAL FAT	MILLIGRAMS OF CHOLESTEROL	TOTAL CALORIES
BEEF (3 1/2 OZ)				
Top round	1.7	5.0	90	199
Sirloin	2.6	6.8	89	191
Chuck, arm pot roast	2.8	7.6	101	210
Ground lean	7.2	18.5	87	272
Salami, about 4 slices	8.4	20.1	60	254
PORK (3 1/2 OZ)				
Ham steak, extra lean	1.4	4.2	45	122
Fresh tenderloin	1.7	4.8	93	166
Fresh, leg, rump half	3.7	10.7	96	221
LAMB (3 1/2 OZ)				
Leg	2.8	7.7	89	191
Loin chop	3.5	9.7	95	216
Arm chop	5.0	14.1	121	279
POULTRY (3 1/2 OZ)				
Turkey, fryer-roasters:				
Light meat without skin	0.4	1.2	86	140
Light meat with skin	1.3	4.6	95	164
Chicken, broilers:				
Light meat without skin	1.3	4.5	85	173
Dark meat without skin	2.7	9.7	93	205
Light meat with skin	3.0	10.9	84	222
Dark meat with skin	4.4	15.8	91	253
Ground turkey	3.8	13.8	69	229
FISH (3 1/2 OZ)				
Haddock	0.2	0.9	74	112
Halibut	0.4	2.9	41	140
Tuna	1.6	6.3	49	184
Salmon	1.9	11.0	87	216

[a]If you want to check whether you are eating 30 percent of your total calories from fat (or 10 percent of your total daily calories from saturated fat), use this table to add up the grams of fat (or saturated fat) you eat each day and refer to Table 4-10 to see the amount of fat and saturated fat you should be eating based on your total caloric intake.

[b]All values for meat, poultry, and fish are for products prepared by broiling, braising, roasting, or moist heat cooking methods rather than frying, unless otherwise indicated.

continued

TABLE 4–14

continued

	GRAMS OF SATURATED FAT	GRAMS OF TOTAL FAT	MILLIGRAMS OF CHOLESTEROL	TOTAL CALORIES
SHELLFISH (3 1/2 OZ)				
Lobster	0.1	0.6	72	98
Clam	0.2	2.0	67	148
Shrimp	0.3	1.1	195	99
Oyster	1.3	5.0	109	137
Clam, breaded and fried	2.7	11.2	61	202
MILK (8 OZ)				
Nonfat	0.3	0.4	4	86
Buttermilk	1.3	2.2	9	99
Low-fat, 1%	1.6	2.6	10	102
Low-fat, 2%	2.9	4.7	18	121
Whole	5.1	8.2	33	150
YOGURT (4 OZ)				
Plain nonfat yogurt	0.1	0.2	2	63
Plain yogurt	2.4	3.7	14	70
SOFT CHEESES (4 OZ)				
Cottage cheese, low-fat	0.7	1.2	5	82
Cottage cheese, creamed	3.2	5.1	17	117
Ricotta, part-skim	5.5	8.9	34	171
Ricotta, whole milk	9.3	14.5	57	216
HARD CHEESES (1 OZ)				
Mozzarella, part-skim	2.9	4.5	16	72
Mozzarella	3.7	6.1	22	80
Swiss	5.0	7.8	26	107
American processed	5.6	8.9	27	106
Cheddar	6.0	9.4	30	114
FROZEN DESSERTS (1 CUP)				
Orange sherbet	2.4	3.8	14	270
Vanilla ice milk	3.5	5.6	18	184
Vanilla ice cream	8.9	14.3	59	269
EGGS (1 LARGE)				
Egg white	0	trace	0	16
Egg yolk	1.6	5.1	213	59

continued

TABLE 4–14

continued

	GRAMS OF SATURATED FAT	GRAMS OF TOTAL FAT	MILLIGRAMS OF CHOLESTEROL	TOTAL CALORIES
FATS AND OILS (1 TBSP)				
Canola oil	1.0	14.0	0	124
Safflower oil	1.2	13.6	0	120
Peanut butter	1.5	7.9	0	94
Corn oil	1.7	13.6	0	120
Olive oil	1.8	13.5	0	119
Margarine, soft tub	2.1	11.4	0	101
Margarine, stick	2.1	11.4	0	101
Butter	7.1	10.8	31	101
NUTS AND SEEDS (1 OZ)				
Almonds	1.4	14.8	0	167
Pecans	1.5	19.2	0	190
Sunflower seeds	1.5	14.1	0	162
English walnuts	1.6	17.6	0	182
Pistachio	1.7	13.7	0	164
Peanuts	1.9	13.8	0	159
BREADS (1 WHOLE ITEM)				
Corn tortilla	0.1	1.0	0	65
English muffin	0.3	1.0	0	140
Bagel	0.3	2.0	0	200
Whole-wheat bread	0.4	1.0	0	70
Hamburger bun	0.5	2.0	trace	115
Croissant	3.5	12.0	13	235
SWEETS AND SNACKS				
Air-popped popcorn, 1 cup	trace	0	trace	30
Angel food cake, 1/12 cake	trace	trace	0	125
Vanilla wafers, 5	0.9	3.3	12	94
Fig bars, 4	1.0	4.0	27	210
Potato chips, 1 oz	2.6	10.1	0	147
Pound cake, 1/17 cake	3.0	5.0	64	110
Chocolate chip cookies, 4	3.9	11.0	18	185

SOURCE: Adapted from *Facts About Blood Cholesterol*, Bethesda, Md.: National Heart, Lung, and Blood Institute, U.S. Department of Health and Human Services, Public Health Service, National Institutes of Health, NIH Publication No. 90-2696, October 1990, pp. 12–16.

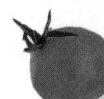

CHECK YOURSELF...

1. What are the functions of fat in the diet?

2. What are the functions of fat in the body?

3. Give an example of a food source of (a) a saturated fat, (b) a monounsaturated fat, (c) a polyunsaturated fat, and (d) cholesterol.

4. What does hydrogenation do to fats?

5. How do the four lipoproteins differ in function from one another in the body?

6. How do levels of HDLs and LDLs in the blood relate to risk of heart disease?

7. Describe the process of fat digestion in the body.

8. What are the current dietary recommendations regarding fat and cholesterol intake?

9. List four risk factors for heart disease.

10. What steps are recommended for raising one's HDL-cholesterol level in the blood?

Answers to selected Check Yourself questions are found in Appendix H.

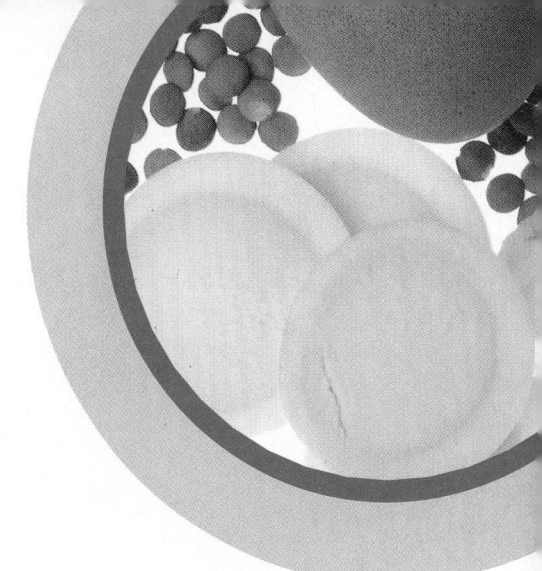

The amino acids of proteins are the raw materials of heredity, the keys to life chemistry, handed from generation to generation.

R. M. Deutsch
(1928–1988, nutrition author and educator)

The Proteins and Amino Acids

FIVE

Contents

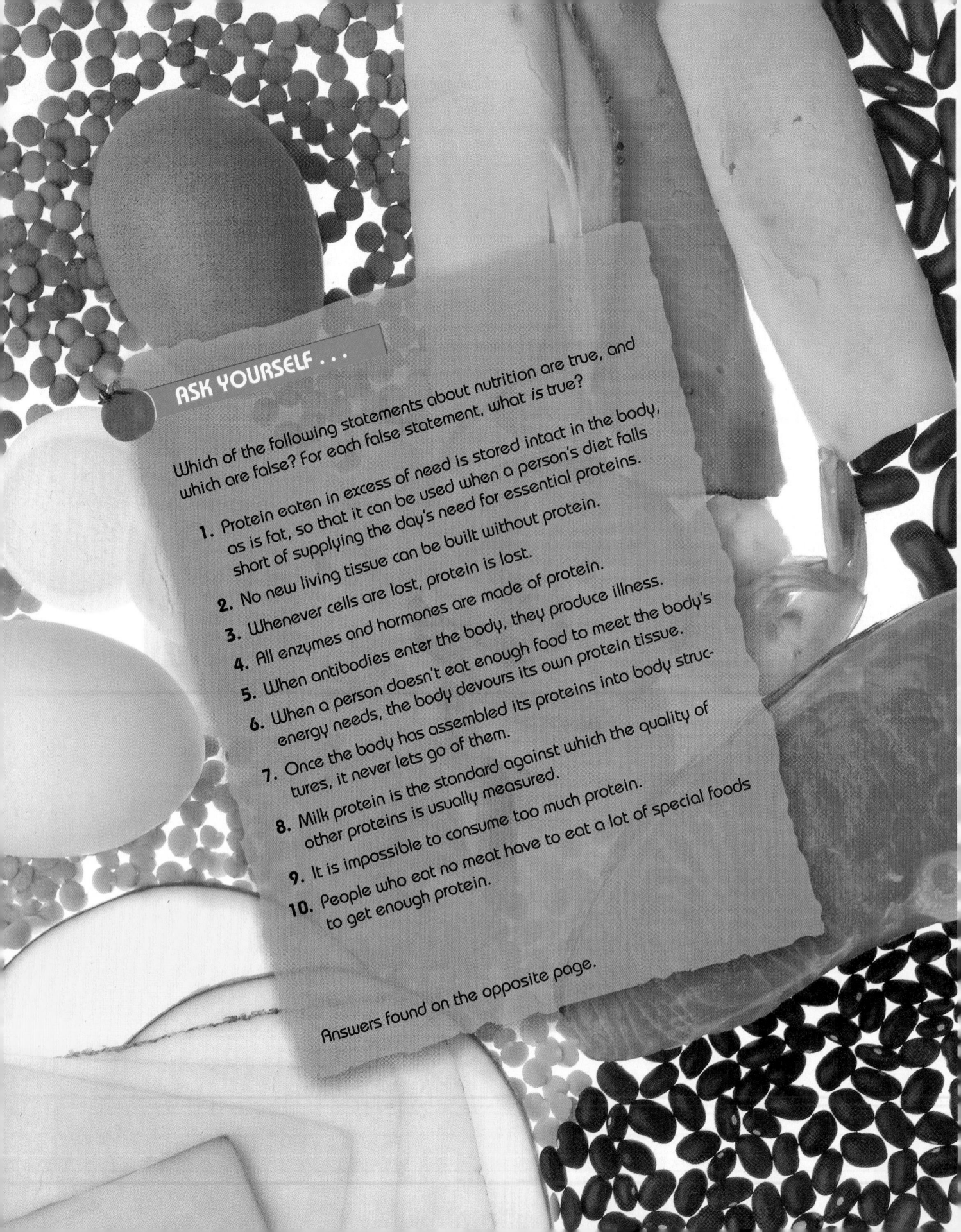

ASK YOURSELF . . .

Which of the following statements about nutrition are true, and which are false? For each false statement, what *is* true?

1. Protein eaten in excess of need is stored intact in the body, as is fat, so that it can be used when a person's diet falls short of supplying the day's need for essential proteins.

2. No new living tissue can be built without protein.

3. Whenever cells are lost, protein is lost.

4. All enzymes and hormones are made of protein.

5. When antibodies enter the body, they produce illness.

6. When a person doesn't eat enough food to meet the body's energy needs, the body devours its own protein tissue.

7. Once the body has assembled its proteins into body structures, it never lets go of them.

8. Milk protein is the standard against which the quality of other proteins is usually measured.

9. It is impossible to consume too much protein.

10. People who eat no meat have to eat a lot of special foods to get enough protein.

Answers found on the opposite page.

The **proteins** are perhaps the most highly respected of the three energy nutrients, and the roles they play in the body are far more varied than those of carbohydrate or fat. Without them, life would not exist. First named 150 years ago after the Greek word *proteios* ("of prime importance"), proteins have revealed countless secrets about the ways living processes take place, and they account for many nutrition concerns. How do we grow? How do our bodies replace the materials they lose? How does blood clot? What makes us able to become immune to diseases we have been exposed to? The answers to these and many other such questions arise to a great extent from an understanding of the nature of the proteins.

PROTEINS compounds—composed of atoms of carbon, hydrogen, oxygen, and nitrogen—arranged as strands of amino acids. Some amino acids also contain atoms of sulfur.

AMINO (a-MEEN-o) **ACIDS** building blocks of protein; each is a compound with an amine group at one end, an acid group at the other, and a distinctive side chain.

AMINE (a-MEEN) **GROUP** the nitrogen-containing portion of an amino acid.

What Proteins Are Made Of

To appreciate the many vital functions of proteins, we must understand their structure. One key difference from carbohydrate and fat, which contain only carbon, hydrogen, and oxygen atoms, is that proteins contain nitrogen atoms. These nitrogen atoms give the name *amino* ("nitrogen containing") to the **amino acids** of which protein is made. Another key difference is that in contrast to the carbohydrates—whose repeating units, glucose molecules, are identical—the amino acids in a strand of protein are different from one another.

All amino acids have the same, simple chemical backbone with an **amine group** (the nitrogen-containing part) at one end and an acid group at the other end. The differences between the amino acids depend on a distinctive structure—the chemical side chain—that is attached to the backbone (see Figure 5–1). It is the nature of the side chain that gives identity and chemical nature to each amino acid. Twenty amino acids with 20 different side chains make up most of the proteins of living tissue.

The side chains vary in complexity from a single hydrogen atom like that on glycine to a complex ring structure like that on phenylalanine (see Figure 5–2). Not only do these structures differ in composition, size, and shape, they also differ in electrical charge. Some are negative, some are positive, and some have no charge. These side chains help to determine the shapes and behaviors of the larger protein molecules that the amino acids make up.

Essential and Nonessential Amino Acids

The body can make about half of the amino acids (known as nonessential amino acids) for itself, given the needed parts: nitrogen to form the amine group, along with backbone fragments derived from carbohydrate or fat. But there are some amino acids that the healthy body cannot make. These are known as **essential**

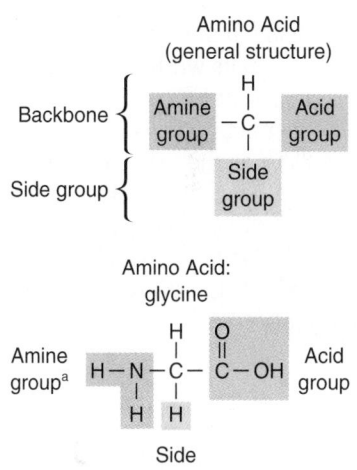

FIGURE 5–1
THE STRUCTURE OF AN AMINO ACID

The "backbone" of an amino acid is the same as that of carbohydrates or fats—two carbon atoms joined together. The structure includes an amine group, an acid group, and a side group of one or more atoms that is different for each amino acid.

[a]Note that the distinctive element of all amino acids—nitrogen—is in the amine group.

ASK YOURSELF ANSWERS: **1.** False. Protein eaten in excess of need is not stored in the body, as is fat, so it has to be eaten every day if it is not to become depleted. **2.** True. **3.** True. **4.** False. All enzymes, but not all hormones, are made of protein. **5.** False. Antibodies protect the body from illness caused by antigens. **6.** True. **7.** False. Your body loses protein every day. **8.** False. Egg white protein, not milk protein, is the standard against which the quality of other proteins is usually measured. **9.** False. It is possible to consume too much protein. **10.** False. People who eat no meat can easily get enough protein without eating a lot of special foods.

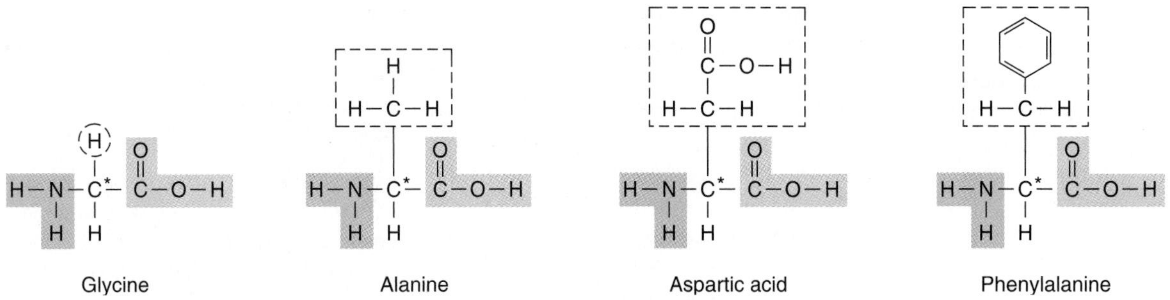

FIGURE 5–2 EXAMPLES OF AMINO ACIDS WITH DIFFERENT SIDE CHAINS
Note that the side chains are different in each amino acid. The asterisk denotes the central carbon.

amino acids. If the diet does not supply them, the body cannot make the proteins it needs to do its work. The indispensability of the essential amino acids makes it necessary for people to eat protein food sources every day.

The distinction between essential and nonessential amino acids is not quite as clear-cut as the list in the margin makes it appear.* Histidine often appears not to be essential, perhaps because the diet supplies it in abundance.[1] Arginine, under some conditions, may be synthesized too slowly to fully meet the human need for it.[2] States of illness can interfere with amino acid transformations in the body and so make other amino acids essential for certain individuals.[3]

Proteins as the Source of Life's Variety

In the first step of **protein synthesis,** each amino acid is hooked to the next. A bond, called a **peptide bond,** is formed between the amino end of one and the acid end of the next. Proteins are made of many amino acid units, from several dozen to many hundred.

A strand of protein is not a straight, but a tangled, chain. The amino acids at different places along the strand are attracted to one another, and this attraction causes the strand to coil into a shape similar to that of a metal spring. Not only does the strand of amino acids form a long coil, but the coil tangles, forming a globular structure (as shown in Figure 5–3).

The charged amino acids are attracted to water, and in the body fluids they orient themselves on the outside of the globular structure. The neutral amino acids are repelled by water and are attracted to one another; they tuck themselves into the center, away from the body fluid. All these interactions among the amino acids and the surrounding fluid result in the unique architecture of each type of protein. Additional steps may be needed for the protein to become functional. A mineral or a vitamin may be needed to complete the

ESSENTIAL AMINO ACIDS amino acids that cannot be synthesized by the body or that cannot be synthesized in amounts sufficient to meet physiological need.

The nine essential amino acids for human adults that must be obtained from the diet:

tryptophan	lysine
valine	phenylalanine
threonine	methionine
isoleucine	histidine
leucine	

The nonessential amino acids—also important in nutrition:

alanine	glutamine
arginine	glycine
aspartic acid	proline
cysteine	serine
cystine	tyrosine
glutamic acid	

PROTEIN SYNTHESIS the process by which cells assemble amino acids into proteins. Each individual is unique because of minute differences in the ways his or her body proteins are made. The instructions for making every protein in a person's body are transmitted in the genetic information the person receives at conception.

PEPTIDE BOND a bond that connects one amino acid with another.

---

*Cysteine and tyrosine normally are not essential because the body makes them from methionine and phenylalanine. However, if there are not enough of these precursors from which to make them, they have to be supplied in the diet. Likewise, glutamine is considered a conditionally essential amino acid during critical illness associated with inflammation and injury.

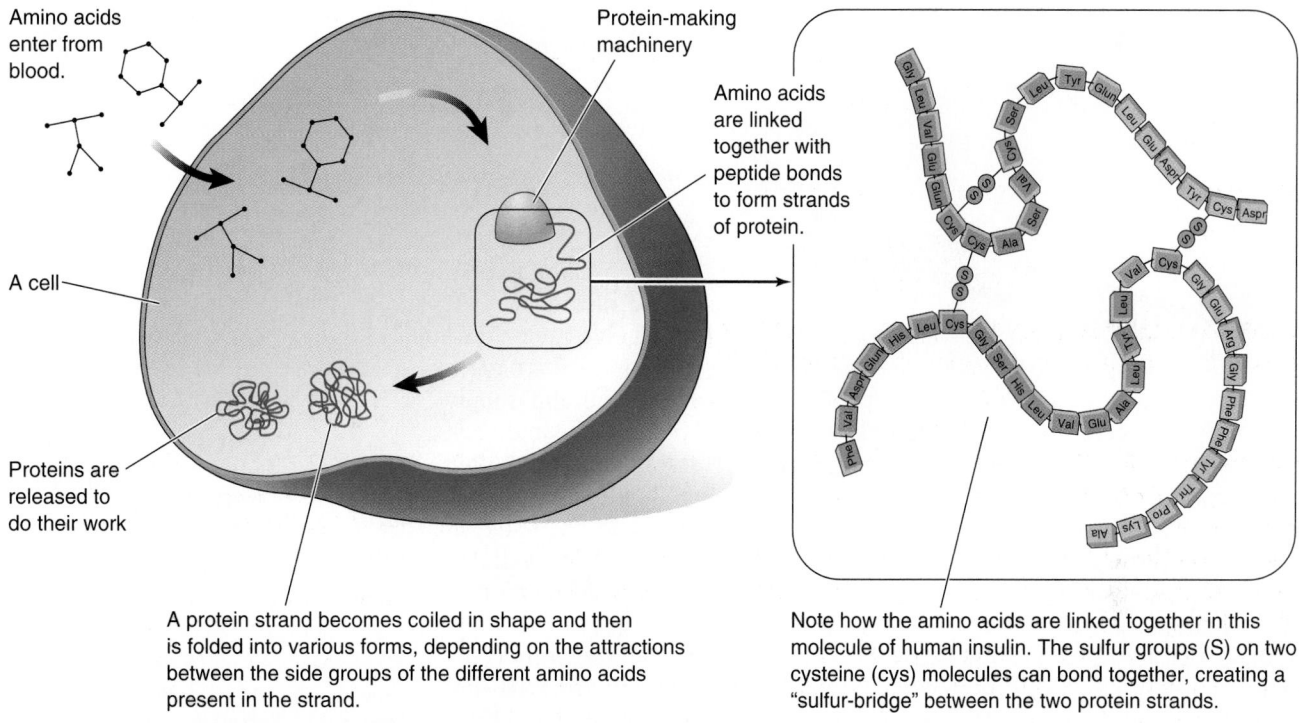

Amino acids enter from blood.

A cell

Proteins are released to do their work

A protein strand becomes coiled in shape and then is folded into various forms, depending on the attractions between the side groups of the different amino acids present in the strand.

Protein-making machinery

Amino acids are linked together with peptide bonds to form strands of protein.

Note how the amino acids are linked together in this molecule of human insulin. The sulfur groups (S) on two cysteine (cys) molecules can bond together, creating a "sulfur-bridge" between the two protein strands.

FIGURE 5–3 HOW THE BODY USES AMINO ACIDS TO MAKE PROTEIN

unit and activate it, or several proteins may gather to form a functioning group.

The differing shapes of proteins enable them to perform different tasks in the body. In proteins that give strength and elasticity to body parts, several springs of amino acids coil together and form ropelike fibers. Other proteins, like those in the blood, do not have such structural strength but are water soluble, with a globular shape like a ball of steel wool. Some are hollow balls that can carry and store minerals in their interiors. Still others provide support to tissues. Some—the enzymes—act on other substances to change them chemically.

Denaturation of Proteins

Proteins can undergo **denaturation,** resulting in distortion of shape by heat, alcohol, acids, bases, or the salts of heavy metals. The denaturation of a protein is the first step in the protein's breakdown. Denaturation is useful to the body in digestion. During the digestion of a food protein, an early step is denaturation by the stomach acid, which opens up the protein's structure, permitting digestive enzymes to cleave the peptide bonds. Denaturation can also occur during food preparation. For example, cooking an egg denatures the proteins of the egg and makes the egg firmer. Perhaps more important, cooking denatures two raw-egg proteins that bind the B vitamin biotin and the mineral iron, and another that slows the digestion of other proteins. Cooking eggs liberates biotin and iron and aids in protein digestion.

DENATURATION the change in shape of a protein brought about by heat, alcohol, acids, bases, or other agents. Many well-known poisons are salts of heavy metals such as mercury and silver; these salts alter the structure of proteins wherever they touch them.

Amino Acid Essentials

Dr. Gerald Gleich had a hunch. Back in 1989, the blood disorder expert from Minnesota's Mayo Clinic received telephone calls from several doctors baffled over the cause of a bizarre set of symptoms, including muscle pain, mouth sores, and abnormally high levels of a certain type of white blood cell in the blood of a handful of patients. But Dr. Gleich identified a suspect: a dietary supplement called **L-tryptophan,** which all of the victims had been taking before their symptoms appeared. One of the essential amino acids, L-tryptophan had been sold in supermarkets, drug stores, health food stores, and other retail outlets and had been self-prescribed for everything from sleeping problems to depression to stress to premenstrual syndrome to drug addiction.

Dr. Gleich contacted the Centers for Disease Control and Prevention, the Atlanta-based public-health watchdog, sparking a national investigation that confirmed his suspicions within two weeks and prompted the Food and Drug Administration to ban the supplement shortly thereafter.[4] Nevertheless, by 1992, more than 1,500 consumers had reported similar symptoms as a result of popping L-tryptophan supplements, and 38 deaths had been linked to the product.[5] The cause of the illness, dubbed **eosinophilia-myalgia syndrome (EMS),** was later suspected to be an impurity that contaminated a particular manufacturer's L-tryptophan supplements, though some experts theorize that the amino acid itself caused EMS in some people.[6]

The case of the contaminated tryptophan brought to the forefront concerns about the safety of amino acid supplements. Granted, the Food and Drug Administration had long cautioned that excesses of one or more of those building blocks of protein can be toxic and create imbalances of other amino acids in the body. That's why, in 1974, the FDA removed amino acids from its list of substances that are generally recognized as safe. (The only uses of amino acids approved by the FDA are (1) their addition to foods to improve the value of an item's protein and (2) their use in the making of special "medical foods" designed to be taken under a physician's supervision by people who require special protein formulations because of health problems such as kidney or liver disease.[7])

Still, as a result of the eosinophilia-myalgia syndrome scare, the FDA asked a panel of experts to review the safety of amino acids currently sold in the marketplace. The panel's conclusions underscore the need for better regulation of these supplements. For instance, the panel found that the labels of most amino acid supplements failed to carry vital information including suggested doses, shelf life, and contraindications for use of the product. In addition, the panel identified certain groups of people who may be at particularly high risk of suf-

L-TRYPTOPHAN an essential amino acid that has been sold in tablets, capsules, and powders as a dietary supplement.

EOSINOPHILIA-MYALGIA (ee-o-sin-o-FIL-ia my-AL-jia) **SYNDROME (EMS)** a disease characterized primarily by a high level of eosinophils, a type of white blood cell, as well as myalgia—that is, muscle pain and weakness.

If you would like more information about eosinophilia-myalgia syndrome, call the EMS Hotline at 1-800-367-2829.

fering health problems as a result of swallowing amino acid supplements. Children and teenagers, for example, may not grow properly if they take amino acid pills or powders. That's because young, underdeveloped bodies may metabolize amino acids differently than adult bodies, possibly leaving young people more vulnerable to harmful effects of excess amino acids. Other high-risk groups include pregnant or breastfeeding women, women of childbearing age, elderly people, people with medical conditions that alter the body's ability to metabolize amino acids, people who regularly consume low amounts of protein, smokers, and people with medical problems, particularly those that require medication.[8]

Safety hazards aren't the only problems that the panel identified. The panel also found that much of the advertising and product label information regarding the effectiveness of the amino acid supplements is questionable and based on anecdotes rather than grounded in careful, scientific research. In fact, the lack of data to support the usefulness of many amino acid supplements has been a source of concern for years. Consider that L-tryptophan has never been shown to relieve depression, insomnia, stress, premenstrual syndrome, or any other ills its manufacturers claim it treats.

The same goes for arginine, an amino acid that has been touted as "causing weight loss overnight" by stimulating secretion of a substance called human growth hormone, which in turn supposedly promotes weight loss. While it's true that arginine can prompt the release of the hormone, it will do so only when people take in whopping doses of it that are unlikely to be found in supplements. And even if a person were to take enough arginine to prompt a surge of the hormone into the body, he or she wouldn't automatically shed pounds; human growth hormone has not been found to cause weight loss. Thus, claims that arginine "burns fat" are spurious, at best. In 1978, an FDA advisory panel on over-the-counter weight-loss products investigated arginine along with 11 other amino acids touted as diet aids—namely, cystine, histidine, isoleucine, leucine, L-lysine, methionine, phenylalanine, threonine, tryptophan, tyrosine, and valine—and found no basis for the claims about the effectiveness of any of them in controlling weight.

Another popular amino acid supplement about which overblown claims are often made is lysine. Some research indicated that lysine could help treat herpes infections, a suggestion that has been used to hawk the substance. That evidence was based on poorly controlled studies, however, which carefully controlled research failed to confirm. Thus, lysine is not recommended by reputable professionals as a treatment for herpes.[9]

In addition to people suffering from health problems, athletes rank as prime targets of amino acid supplement manufacturers. Pick up any copy of one of the bodybuilding magazines, and you're likely to see ads for supplements packed with "free-form," "predigested," and "peptide-bond" amino acids touted as optimum sources of protein for athletes. Scientific-sounding names notwithstanding, such products have never been shown to increase muscle size or enhance athletic prowess. Consider that one comparison of Marine officer candidates given protein supplements with another set of trainees who received a placebo indicated that the groups performed equally well before, during, and after the program, regardless of supplement use or lack thereof.[10]

A panel of experts from the Federation of American Societies for Experimental Biology (FASEB) advises that the following groups are at a particularly high risk of harm as a result of long-term use of amino acid supplements:

- Infants, children, and teenagers
- Women of childbearing age
- Pregnant and breastfeeding women
- Elderly men and women
- People with medical conditions that alter the body's ability to metabolize amino acids
- People who consume low amounts of protein
- Smokers
- People with medical problems, especially if they take medications

Refer to the Spotlight feature in Chapter 1 for some tips on how to spot fraudulent nutritional products.

The latest group to begin swallowing fraudulent claims about amino acids is young professionals who down "smart drinks," made with amino acids such as phenylalanine, choline, taurine, and L-cysteine and touted as intelligence, energy, and memory boosters. Smart drinks started to become popular in the early 1980s, when the baby boom generation began coming of age and looking for ways to make career strides. But while the efficacy of these so-called intellect enhancers has never been proven, the side effects of taking smart drinks are well-known: Phenylalanine can make an otherwise healthy person irritable or lead to insomnia, choline can cause gastrointestinal illness, and L-cysteine can cause health problems for people who take antidepressants, to name a few such side effects.[11]

Health risks aside, consumers should note that special protein supplements command a high price. Foods, on the other hand, supply ample amounts of protein at a fraction of the cost. One glass of milk, a serving of rice and beans, or a three-ounce portion of chicken, for example, provides a generous helping of all nine essential amino acids for less than half the price of a dose of most amino acid tablets, liquids, or powders. That's why it's easy for most Americans to eat a diet that supplies the body with more than enough protein and amino acids. Table 5–1 compares costs of protein supplements with costs of high-protein foods.

Finally, consumers should be wary of companies that sell tests that measure the amino acid content of the blood and urine. Costing in the neighborhood of $150, these tests are then used to help sell concoctions designed to replace the "missing" amino acids. That practice, however, is completely fraudulent; amino acid levels in the blood and urine vary greatly from day to day and have no bearing on the body's supply or requirement for amino acids.[12]

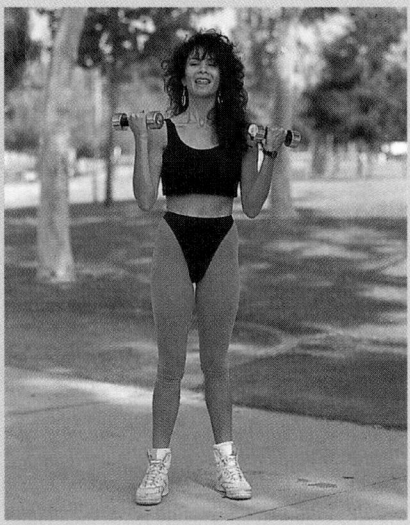

We cannot force extra protein into our muscles just by eating more of it—the way to make muscles grow is to make them work (see Chapter 9).

TABLE 5–1
THE HIGH COST OF PROTEIN SUPPLEMENTS

FOOD OR SUPPLEMENT	AMOUNT NEEDED TO OBTAIN ABOUT 15 GRAMS OF PROTEIN	COST[a]
Nonfat milk	2 cups	$ .44
Tuna (canned in water)	2 ounces	.40
Twinlab Amino Fuel Anabolic Liquid Amino Acid Concentrate	3 tablespoons	1.17
Twinlab Amino Fuel Tablets	15 tablets	2.50
Hot Stuff Fitness Enhancing Nutritional Powder	About 2 tablespoons	1.73

[a]Based on 1995 prices at Boston area stores.

SOURCE: Manufacturers' information; J. A. T. Pennington, *Bowes and Church's Food Values of Portions Commonly Used*, 16th ed., (Philadelphia: J. B. Lippincott Company, 1994).

The Functions of Body Proteins

No new living tissue can be built without protein, for protein is part of every cell. About 20 percent of our total body weight is protein. Proteins come in many forms: enzymes, antibodies, hormones, transport vehicles, oxygen carriers, tendons and ligaments, scars, the cores of bones and teeth, the filaments of hair, the materials of nails, and more (see Table 5–2). A few of the many vital functions of proteins are described here to show why they have rightfully earned their position of importance in nutrition.

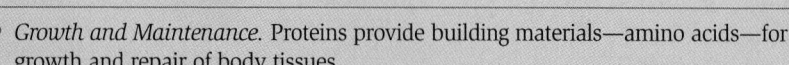

TABLE 5–2
THE FUNCTIONS OF PROTEINS IN THE BODY

- *Growth and Maintenance.* Proteins provide building materials—amino acids—for growth and repair of body tissues.
- *Enzymes.* Proteins facilitate numerous chemical reactions in the body; all enzymes are proteins.
- *Hormones.* Some proteins act as chemical messengers—regulating body processes; not all hormones are proteins.
- *Antibodies.* Proteins assist the body in maintaining its resistance to disease by acting against foreign disease-causing substances.
- *Fluid balance.* Proteins help regulate the quantity of fluids in body compartments.
- *Acid-Base Balance.* Proteins act as buffers to maintain the normal acid and base concentrations in body fluids.
- *Transportation.* Proteins move needed nutrients and other substances into and out of cells and around the body.
- *Body structures.* Proteins form vital parts of most body structures such as skin, nails, hair, membranes, muscles, teeth, bones, organs, ligaments, and tendons.
- *Energy.* Protein can be used to provide calories (4 calories per gram) to help meet the body's energy needs.

Growth and Maintenance

One function of dietary protein is to ensure the availability of amino acids to build the proteins of new tissue. The new tissue may be found in an embryo; in a growing child; in the blood that replaces that which has been lost in burns, hemorrhage, or surgery; in the scar tissue that heals wounds; or in new hair and nails. Not so obvious is the protein that helps replace wornout cells. The cells that line the digestive tract live for about three days and are constantly being shed and excreted. You have probably observed that the cells of your skin die, rub off, and are replaced from underneath. For this new growth, amino acids must constantly be resupplied by food.

Enzymes

All enzymes are proteins, and they are among the most important proteins formed in living cells. Enzymes are catalysts—biological spark plugs—that help chemical reactions take place. There are thousands of enzymes inside a single cell, each type facilitating a specific chemical reaction. Enzymes are involved in such processes as the digestion of food, the release of energy from the body's stored energy supplies, and tissue growth and repair.

A mystery that has been partially explained is how an enzyme can be specific for a particular reaction. The surface of the enzyme is contoured so that the enzyme can recognize the substances it works on and ignore others. The surface provides a site that attracts one or more specific chemical compounds and promotes a specific chemical reaction. For example, two substances might become attached to the enzyme and then to each other. The newly formed product is then expelled by the enzyme into the fluid of the cell (see Figure 5–4). Enzymes are the hands-on workers in the production and processing of all substances needed by the body.

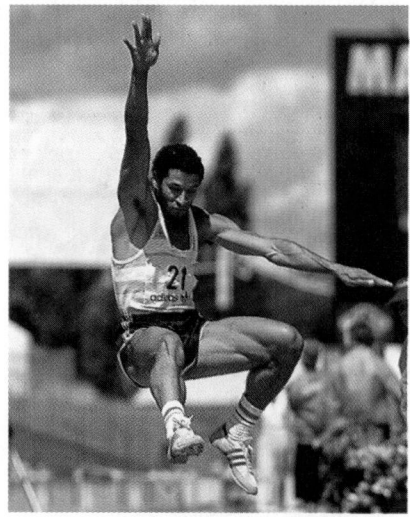

Proteins perform many different tasks in the body—for example, our muscles are made of protein.

Hormones

Similar to the enzymes in the profoundness of their effects are the **hormones.** However, these molecules differ from the enzymes. For one thing, not all of them are made of protein. For another, they don't catalyze chemical reactions directly but rather are messengers that elicit the appropriate responses to maintain a normal environment in the body. Hormones regulate overall body conditions, such as the blood glucose level (the hormones insulin and glucagon) and the metabolic rate (thyroid hormone).

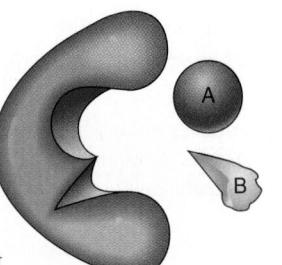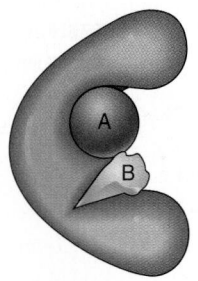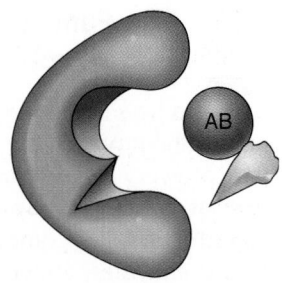

Enzyme plus two compounds, A and B.

Enzyme complexed with A and B.

Enzyme plus new compound AB.

FIGURE 5–4   ENZYME ACTION

Each enzyme facilitates a specific chemical reaction.

Antibodies

Of all the great variety of proteins in living organisms, the **antibodies** best demonstrate that proteins are specific for one organism. Antibodies are formed in response to the presence of **antigens** (foreign proteins or other large molecules) that invade the body. The foreign protein may be part of a bacterium, a virus, or a toxin, or it may be present in food that causes allergy. The body, after recognizing that it has been invaded, manufactures antibodies, which inactivate the foreign substance. Without sufficient protein to make antibodies, the body cannot maintain its resistance to disease.

One of the most fascinating aspects of this response is that each antibody is designed specifically to destroy one foreign substance. An antibody that has been manufactured to combat one strain of flu virus would be of no help in protecting a person against another strain. Once the body has learned to make a particular antibody, it never forgets, and the next time it encounters that same foreign substance, it will be equipped to destroy it even more rapidly (see Figure 5–5). In other words, it develops an **immunity.** This is the principle underlying the vaccines and antitoxins that have nearly eradicated most childhood diseases in the Western world.

Clearly, malnutrition injures the immune system. Without adequate protein in the diet, the immune system will not be able to make its specialized cells and other tools to function optimally. Often protein deficiency and immune incompetence appear together.

Resistance to Disease

Strong immune system

Feelings of well-being

Optimal nutrition status

Healthy appetite

Optimal Nutrition

An optimal diet helps to provide strength and support to the body's immune system.

HORMONES chemical messengers. Hormones are secreted by a variety of glands in the body in response to altered conditions. Each affects one or more target tissues or organs and elicits specific responses to restore normal conditions.

ANTIBODIES large proteins of the blood and body fluids, produced by one type of immune cell in response to invasion of the body by unfamiliar molecules (mostly foreign proteins). Antibodies inactivate the foreign substances and so protect the body. The foreign substances are called **antigens.**

anti = against
gen = producer

IMMUNITY specific disease resistance derived from the immune system's memory of prior exposure to specific disease agents and its ability to mount a swift response against them.

For this reason, measles in a malnourished child can be fatal. Protein deficiency also can put the malnourished person at risk for increased incidence of **opportunistic infections**—as is the case with many of those diagnosed with **acquired immune deficiency syndrome (AIDS).** Such infections are often the cause of death in the AIDS patient. While adequate protein cannot prevent infection with the AIDS virus, nutrition intervention can be important in preventing the weight loss and malnutrition seen in people with AIDS.

Many other nutrients besides proteins participate in conferring immunity, and many factors besides the antibodies are involved.[13] The immune system is extraordinarily sensitive to nutrition, and almost any nutrient deficit can impair its efficiency and reduce resistance to disease.

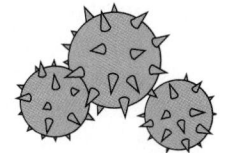

A. The body is challenged by foreign substances.

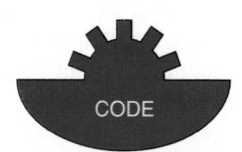

B. The body makes the code for manufacturing the antibody.

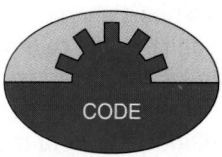

C. The code makes the antibody.

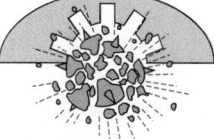

D. The antibody inactivates the foreign substance.

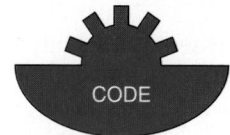

E. The code remains to make antibodies faster the next time this foreign substance attacks.

FIGURE 5–5   DEVELOPMENT OF IMMUNITY

Fluid Balance

Proteins help regulate the quantity of fluids in the compartments of the body to maintain the **fluid balance.** To remain alive, a cell must contain a constant amount of fluid. Too much might cause it to rupture, and too little would make it unable to function. Although water can diffuse freely into and out of the cell, proteins cannot—and proteins attract water. By maintaining a store of internal

OPPORTUNISTIC INFECTIONS infections produced by organisms that do not affect people whose immune systems are working normally. An example is the unusual form of pneumonia caused by *Pneumocystis carinii*, often seen in individuals with AIDS.

ACQUIRED IMMUNE DEFICIENCY SYNDROME (AIDS) an immune system disorder caused by the human immunodeficiency virus (HIV). Its attack on the individual's immune cells (T-cells) results in a decreased ability to fight foreign organisms, thus increasing the individual's susceptibility to a variety of opportunistic infections. AIDS is transmitted to a person through direct contact of the person's body fluids with contaminated body fluids. It is most often transmitted through sexual intercourse, contaminated needles, contaminated blood products, or from mother to infant during pregnancy or lactation. Since the early 1980s, AIDS has become a major public health problem.

FLUID BALANCE distribution of fluid among body compartments.

Fluid within cell (intracellular fluid)

Fluid between cells (intercellular or interstitial fluid)

Nucleus

Cell

Fluid within blood vessel (intravascular fluid)

Blood vessels

Shown here are the fluids within and surrounding a cell.

proteins, the cell retains the fluid it needs (it also uses minerals this way). Similarly, the cells secrete proteins (and minerals) into the spaces between them to keep the fluid volume constant in those spaces. The proteins secreted into the blood cannot cross the blood vessel walls, and thus they help to maintain the blood volume in the same way.

Acid-Base Balance

Normal processes of the body continually produce **acids** and their opposite, **bases,** which must be carried by the blood to the organs of excretion. The blood must do this without allowing its own **acid-base balance** to be affected. To accomplish this, some proteins act as **buffers** to maintain the blood's normal **pH.** They pick up hydrogens when there are too many in the blood (the more hydrogen, the more concentrated the acid). Likewise, protein buffers release hydrogens again when there are too few in the blood. The secret is that the negatively charged side chains of the amino acids can accommodate additional hydrogens (which are positively charged) when necessary.

The acid-base balance of the blood is one of the most accurately controlled conditions in the body. If it changes too much, the dangerous condition **acidosis** or the opposite, basic condition **alkalosis** can cause coma or death. The hazards of these conditions are a result of their effect on proteins. When the proteins' buffering capacity is exceeded—for example, when proteins have taken on board or released all the acid hydrogens they can—additional acid or base deranges their structure by pulling them out of shape; that is, it denatures them. Knowing how indispensable the structures of proteins are to their functions and how vital their functions are to life, you can imagine how many body processes would be halted by such a disturbance.

Transport Proteins

A specific group of the body's proteins specializes in moving nutrients and other molecules into and out of cells. Some of these act as pumps—picking up compounds on one side of the membrane and depositing them on the other—and thereby decide what substances the cell will take up or release. One such pump is the "sodium-potassium pump," which resides in the cell membrane and acts as a revolving door—picking up potassium from outside the cell and depositing it inside the cell, and picking up sodium from within the cell and depositing it outside the cell as necessary. The protein machinery of cell membranes can be switched on or off in response to the body's needs. Often hormones do the switching with a marvelous precision.

Other transport proteins move about in the body fluids, carrying nutrients and other molecules from one organ to another. Those that carry lipids in the lipoproteins are an example. Special proteins also can carry fat-soluble vitamins, water-soluble vitamins, and minerals. As a result, a protein deficiency can cause a vitamin A deficiency or a deficiency of whatever other nutrient is in need of a transport protein in order to reach its destination in the body.

This sampling of the major roles proteins play in the body should serve to illustrate their versatility, uniqueness, and importance. All the body's tissues and

ACIDS compounds that release hydrogens in a watery solution; acids have a low pH.

BASES compounds that accept hydrogens from solutions; bases have a high pH.

ACID-BASE BALANCE equilibrium between acid and base concentrations in the body fluids.

BUFFERS compounds that help keep a solution's acidity (amount of acid) or alkalinity (amount of base) constant.

pH the concentration of hydrogen ions. The lower the pH, the stronger the acid; pH 2 is a strong acid; pH 7 is neutral; and a pH above 7 is alkaline.

ACIDOSIS (a-sih-DOSE-iss) blood acidity above normal, indicating excess acid.

ALKALOSIS (al-kah-LOH-sis) blood alkalinity above normal.

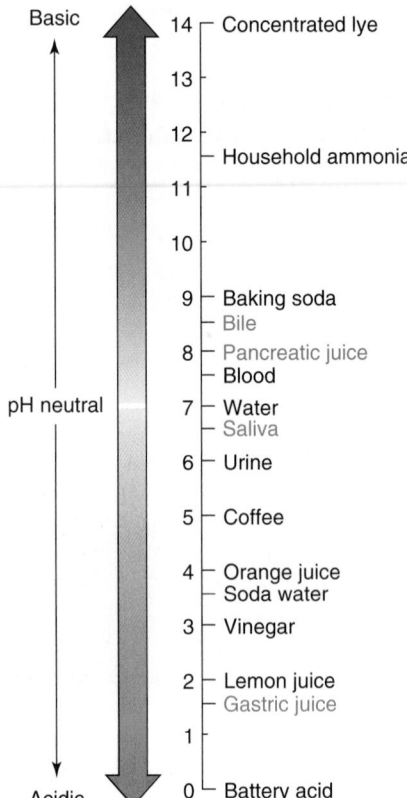

pH values of selected fluids. A fluid's acidity or alkalinity is measured in pH units.

organs—muscles, bones, blood, skin, and nerves—are made largely of proteins. No wonder proteins are said to be the primary material of life.

Protein as Energy

Only protein can perform all the functions previously described, but it will be sacrificed to provide needed energy if insufficient fat and carbohydrate are eaten. The body's number one need is for energy. All other needs have a lower priority.

When amino acids are degraded for energy, their amine groups are usually incorporated by the liver into **urea** and sent to the kidney for excretion in the urine. The remaining components are carbon, hydrogen, and oxygen, which are available for immediate energy use by the body.

Only if the **protein-sparing** calories from carbohydrate and fat are sufficient to power the cells will the amino acids be used for their most important function—making proteins. Thus, energy deficiency (starvation) is always accompanied by the symptoms of protein deficiency.

If amino acids are oversupplied, the body has no place to store them. It will remove and excrete their amine groups and then convert the fragments that remain to glucose and glycogen, or to fat, for energy storage. Amino acids are not stored in the body except in the sense that they are present in proteins in all the tissues. When there is a great shortage of amino acids, such tissues as the blood, muscle, and skin have to be broken down so that their amino acids can be used to maintain the heart, lungs, and brain.

How the Body Handles Protein

When a person eats a food protein, whether from cereals, vegetables, meats, or dairy products, the digestive system breaks the protein down and delivers the separated amino acids to the body cells. The cells then put the amino acids together in the order necessary to produce the particular proteins they need.

The stomach initiates protein digestion (see Figure 5–6). By the time proteins slip into the small intestine, they are already broken into different-sized pieces—some single amino acids and many strands of two, three, or more amino acids—**dipeptides, tripeptides,** and longer chains. Digestion continues until almost all pieces of protein

UREA (yoo-REE-uh) the principal nitrogen-excretion product of metabolism, generated mostly by the removal of amine groups from unneeded amino acids or from those amino acids being sacrificed to a need for energy.

PROTEIN-SPARING a description of the effect of carbohydrate and fat, which, by being available to yield energy, allow amino acids to be used to build body proteins.

DIPEPTIDES (dye-PEP-tides) protein fragments two amino acids long. A peptide is a strand of amino acids.

TRIPEPTIDES (try-PEP-tides) protein fragments three amino acids long.

In the **small intestine**, the fragments of protein are split into free amino acids, dipeptides, and tripeptides with the help of enzymes from the pancreas and small intestine. Enzymes on the surface of the small intestinal cells break these peptides into amino acids, and they are absorbed through the microvilli of the small intestine into the blood.

The **large intestine** carries any undigested protein residue out of the body. Normally, practically all the protein is digested and absorbed.

In the **mouth**, chewing crushes and softens protein-rich foods and mixes them with saliva.

Stomach acid works to uncoil protein strands and activate stomach enzymes. The enzyme pepsin breaks the protein strands into dipeptides, tripeptides, and polypeptides. A mucous coating on the stomach wall protects the stomach's own proteins from both the harsh stomach acid and the protein-digesting enzymes.

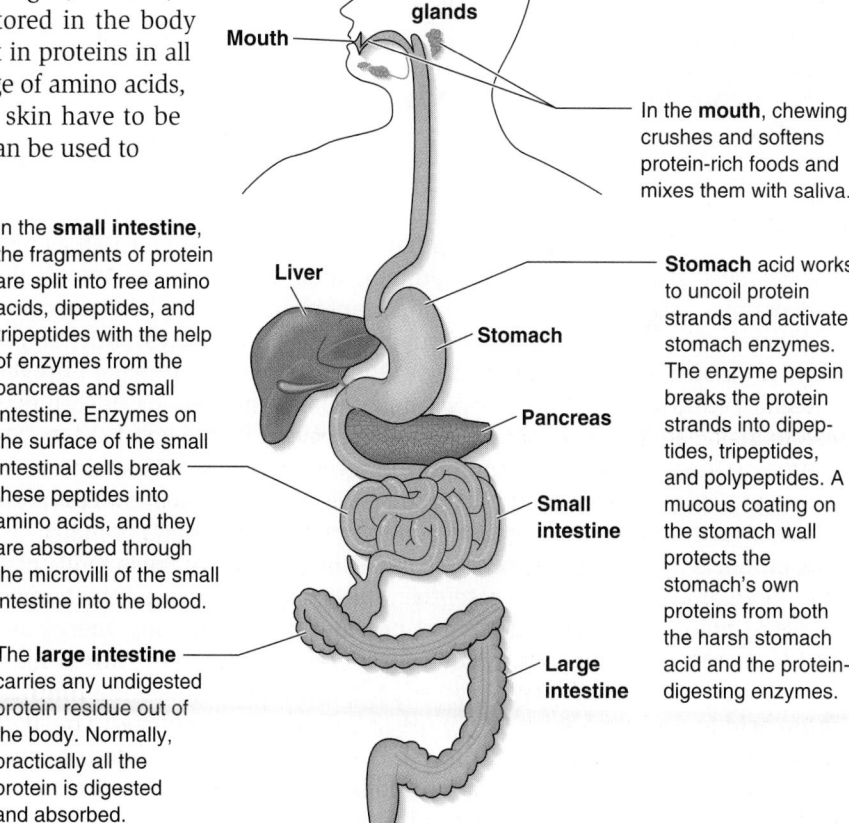

FIGURE 5–6   A SUMMARY OF PROTEIN DIGESTION AND ABSORPTION

are broken into dipeptides, tripeptides, and more free amino acids. Absorption of amino acids takes place all along the small intestine. As for dipeptides and tripeptides, the cells that line the small intestine capture them on their surfaces, split them into amino acids on the cell surfaces, absorb them, and then release them into the bloodstream.

To review the digestive and absorptive systems relevant to the body's handling of protein, turn to Appendix B.

Once they are circulating in the bloodstream, the amino acids are available to be taken up by any cell of the body. The cells can then make proteins, either for their own use or for secretion into the circulatory system for other uses.

If a *non*essential amino acid (that is, one the body can make for itself) is unavailable for a growing protein strand, the cell will make it and continue attaching amino acids to the strand. If, however, an essential amino acid (one the body cannot make) is missing, the building of the protein will halt. The cell cannot hold partially completed proteins to complete them later, for example, the next day. Rather, it has to dismantle the partial structures and return surplus amino acids to the circulation, making them available to other cells. If other cells do not soon pick up these amino acids and insert them into protein, the liver will remove their amine groups for the kidney to excrete. Other cells will then use the remaining fragments for other purposes. Whatever need prompted the calling for that particular protein will not be met.

Protein Quality of Foods

The role of protein in food, as already mentioned, is not to provide body proteins directly but to supply the amino acids from which the body can make its own proteins. Since body cells cannot store amino acids for future use, it follows that all the essential amino acids must be eaten as part of a balanced diet. To make body protein, then, a cell must have all the needed amino acids available. Three important characteristics of dietary protein, therefore, are (1) that it should supply at least the nine essential amino acids, (2) that it should supply enough other amino acids to make nitrogen available for the synthesis of whatever nonessential amino acids the cell may need to make, and (3) that it should be accompanied by enough food energy (preferably from carbohydrate and fat) to prevent sacrifice of its amino acids for energy. This presents no problem to people who regularly eat **complete proteins,** such as those of meat, fish, poultry, cheese, eggs, milk, or many soybean products, as part of balanced meals.[14] The proteins of these foods contain ample amounts of all the essential amino acids relative to our bodies' need for them, and the rest of the diet provides protein-sparing energy and needed vitamins and minerals. An equally sound choice is to eat two or more **incomplete protein** foods from plants, each of which supplies the **limiting amino acid** in the other—also, of course, as part of a balanced diet. The *quality* of plant proteins (legumes, grains, and vegetables) having different *limiting* amino acids can therefore be improved by combining different sources of plant proteins, either during a meal or over the course of a day, so that sufficient amounts of all the essential amino acids become available for protein synthesis. This strategy—using **complementary proteins**—is shown in Figure 5–7. Note that by combining a grain (whole-wheat bread) that is low in lysine

COMPLETE PROTEINS proteins containing all the essential amino acids in the right proportion relative to need. The *quality* of a food protein is judged by the proportions of essential amino acids that it contains relative to our needs. Animal proteins are the highest in quality.

INCOMPLETE PROTEIN a protein lacking or low in one or more of the essential amino acids.

LIMITING AMINO ACID a term given to the essential amino acid in shortest supply (relative to the body's need) in a food protein; it therefore *limits* the body's ability to make its own proteins.

COMPLEMENTARY PROTEINS two or more food proteins whose amino acid assortments complement each other in such a way that the essential amino acids limited in or missing from each are supplied by the others.

with a legume (peanut butter) that is low in methionine, the limiting amino acid disappears.

A person in good health can be expected to use dietary protein efficiently. However, malnutrition or infection can seriously impair digestion (by reducing enzyme secretion), absorption (by causing degeneration of the absorptive surface of the small intestine or losses from diarrhea), and the cells' use of protein (by forcing amino acids to meet other needs). In addition, infections cause the stepped-up production of antibodies made of protein. Malnutrition or infection can greatly increase protein needs while making it hard to meet them.

People usually eat many foods containing protein. Each food has its own characteristic amino acid balance, and together, a mixture of foods almost invariably supplies plenty of each individual amino acid. However, when food energy intake is limited, this is not the case (as dis-

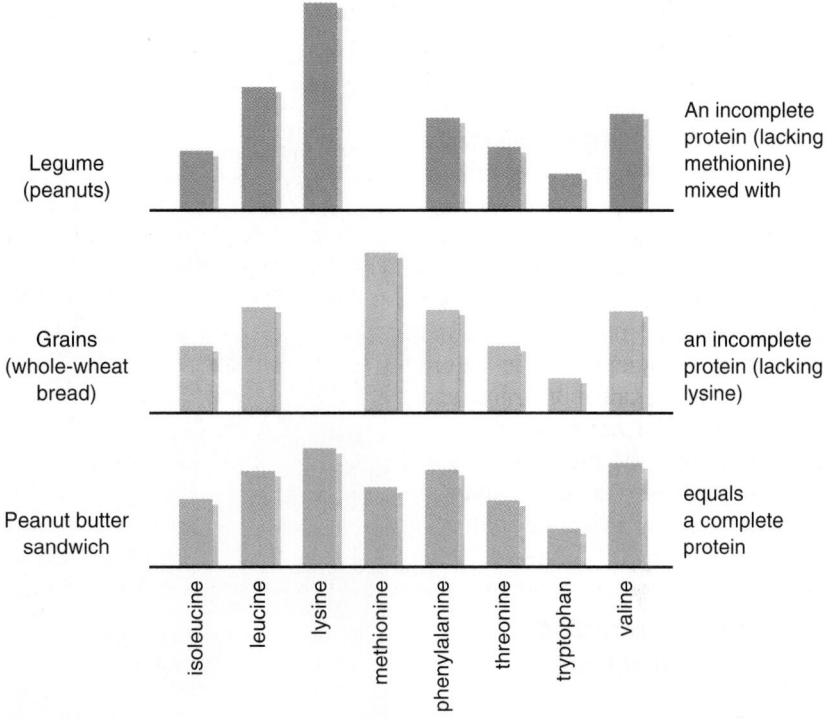

FIGURE 5–7
HOW TWO PLANT PROTEINS COMBINE TO YIELD A COMPLETE PROTEIN

cussed in the section titled "Protein-Energy Malnutrition," later in the chapter). Also, even if food energy intake is abundant, if the selection of foods available is severely limited (where, for example, a single food such as potatoes or rice provides 90 percent of the calories), protein intake may not be adequate. The primary food source of protein must be checked, for its protein quality is of great importance.

Researchers have studied many different individual foods as protein sources and have developed many different methods of evaluating their **protein quality.** In general, amino acids from animal proteins are the best absorbed (over 90 percent). Those from legumes follow (about 80 percent), and those from grains and other plant foods vary (from 60 percent to 90 percent).

When amino acids are wasted, their amine groups (which contain their nitrogen) cannot be stored. Therefore, the efficiency of a protein can be assessed experimentally by measuring the net loss of nitrogen from the body. The higher the amount of nitrogen retained, the higher the quality of the protein. This is the basis for determination of the **biological value (BV)** of proteins. A high-quality protein by this standard is egg white protein, which has been designated the **reference protein** and given a score of 100. Other proteins are compared with it.

Another method of evaluating the protein quality of foods is the **protein digestibility-corrected amino acid score,** or **PDCAAS.** The PDCAAS takes into account both the proportion of amino acids that a food provides and the relative digestibility of the protein. Foods are first assigned a score based on their amino acid composition. This score is then adjusted to reflect the food's

PROTEIN QUALITY a measure of the essential amino acid content of a protein relative to the essential amino acid needs of the body.

BIOLOGICAL VALUE (BV) a measure of protein quality, assessed by determining how well a given food or food mixture supports nitrogen retention.

REFERENCE PROTEIN egg white protein, the standard with which other proteins are compared to determine protein quality.

PROTEIN DIGESTIBILITY-CORRECTED AMINO ACID SCORE (PDCAAS) a measure of protein quality; the PDCAAS takes into account both the amino acid balance of a food and its digestibility.

digestibility. A sampling of the PDCAAS for selected foods is given in Table 5–3. The PDCAAS is used in determining the protein values listed on food labels.

Protein scores are of great importance in dealing with widespread malnutrition. However, perhaps the most relevant lesson to be learned from them by the average well-fed American is that although animal proteins tend to have slightly higher scores than plant proteins, the two overlap considerably (see Figure 5–8). The best guarantee of amino acid adequacy is to eat a variety of food containing protein in the presence of adequate amounts of vitamins, minerals, and energy from carbohydrate and fat.

Recommended Protein Intakes

Recommended protein intakes can be stated in one of two ways—as a percentage of total calories or as an absolute number (grams per day). It is recommended that protein provide about 12 percent of total caloric intake.

The committee on the RDA of the Food and Nutrition Board of the National Academy of Sciences states the RDA in grams per day. It considers that a generous protein allowance for a healthy adult would be 0.8 gram per kilogram (or 2.2 pounds) of desirable body weight per day. Protein RDA for people of average heights at all ages are presented in Table 5–4. If your height is not average, you can compute your own individualized RDA for protein. Suppose your desirable weight is 50 kilograms; your protein RDA would then be 0.8 times 50, or 40 grams of protein each day.

The committee uses the desirable, not the actual, weight for a given height because the desirable weight is proportional to the *lean* body mass of the average person. Lean body mass determines protein need. If you gain weight, your fat tissue increases in mass, but fat tissue is composed largely of fat and, as mentioned, does not require much protein for maintenance.

TABLE 5–3 RATING THE PROTEINS FOR QUALITY USING THE PDCAAS

FOOD PROTEIN	PDCAAS %
Egg white	100
Ground beef	100
Milk protein	100
Nonfat milk powder	100
Tuna	100
Soybean protein	94
Chick-peas	69
Kidney beans	68
Pinto beans	61
Rolled oats	57
Black beans	53
Lentils	52
Peanut meal	52
Whole wheat	40

SOURCE: G. Sarwar and F. E. McDonough, Evaluation of protein digestibility-corrected amino acid score method for assessing protein quality of foods, *Journal of the Association of Official Analytical Chemists* 73 (1990): 347–356.

TABLE 5–4 THE PROTEIN RDA

AGE (YR)	RDA (G/KG)*
0–½	2.2
½–1	1.6
1–3	1.2
4–6	1.1
7–14	1.0
15–18 (males)	0.9
15–18 (females)	0.8
19 and up	0.8

*The RDA is 10 g/day higher during pregnancy, 15 g/day higher during the first six months of lactation, and 12 g/day higher during the remainder of lactation.

To calculate the percentage of calories you derive from protein:

1. Use your total calories as the denominator (example: 1,900 cal).
2. Multiply your protein *grams* by 4 cal/g to obtain calories from protein as the numerator (example: 70 g protein × 4 cal/g = 280 cal).
3. Divide to obtain a decimal, multiply by 100, and round off (example: 280/1,900 × 100 = 15% cal from protein).

To figure your protein RDA:

1. Find the desirable weight for a person your height (on inside back cover). Assume this weight is appropriate for you.
2. Change pounds to kilograms (divide pounds by 2.2; one kilogram = 2.2 pounds).
3. Multiply kilograms by 0.8 g/kg.

Example (for a 5′8″ male):

1. Desirable weight: about 150 lb.
2. 150 lb ÷ 2.2 lb = 68 kg (rounded off).
3. 68 kg × 0.8 g/kg = 54 g protein (rounded off).

FIGURE 5–8

CHECKING OUT THE FOOD LABEL FOR PROTEIN INFORMATION

The Nutrition Facts panel lists the number of grams of protein per serving. This refers to the quantity of protein present and does not reflect protein quality. Listing the "% Daily Value" for protein is optional for manufacturers. When listed, the "% Daily Value" must be corrected to reflect protein quality. If the protein is of as high a quality as milk protein (casein) or higher, 50 grams a day is considered sufficient for an adult. Thus, the % Daily Value is calculated using 50 grams as the reference point. If the protein's quality is lower than that of milk protein, 65 grams a day is recommended.

According to these food labels, a serving of chili with meat contains 12 grams of protein; a serving of the vegetarian chili, 15 grams. To reflect differences in protein quality on the food labels, different protein standards exist for higher-quality protein (50 grams a day) and lower-quality protein (65 grams a day). Therefore, the "% Daily Value" when listed would by law have to reflect this difference in protein quality. For example, the "% Daily Value" for the vegetarian chili would be slightly lower (23%) than that for the chili with meat (24%)—even though the vegetarian chili contains more grams of protein per serving.

As you can see, these two chilis are about the same in terms of their contribution of needed protein to the diet. However, as a consumer, be sure to also check the fat information on the Nutrition Facts panel of the protein foods you eat. Note on the labels shown here that whereas the chili made with black beans contributes no fat to the diet, the chili with meat contains 15 grams of fat (135 calories from fat or 23 percent of the recommended Daily Value for fat for the day). You'll want to keep track of your total fat intake from all the foods in your diet that contribute fat. You can use this information about total fat and calories from fat to help you meet the dietary guideline that recommends that you get no more than 30 percent of your total calories from fat. Depending on the rest of your day's food intake, either of these chilis might fit within this recommended guideline.

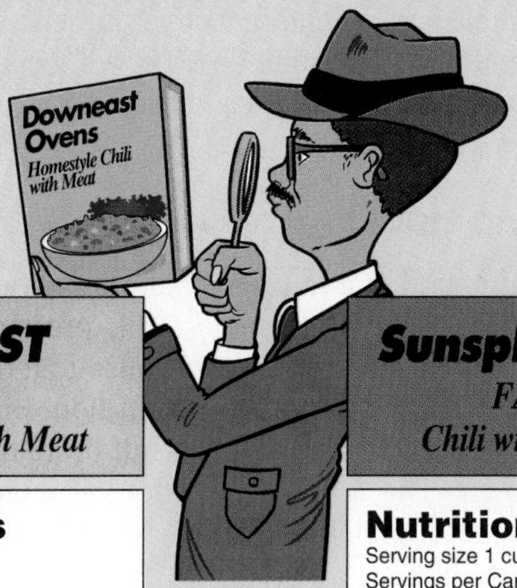

DOWNEAST OVENS
Homestyle Chili with Meat

Nutrition Facts
Serving size 1 cup (180g)
Servings per Can 2

Amount Per Serving	
Calories 303	Calories from Fat 135

	% Daily Value*
Total Fat 15g	23%
Saturated Fat 7g	35%
Cholesterol 55mg	18%
Sodium 1,030mg	43%
Total Carbohydrate 27g	9%
Dietary Fiber 8g	32%
Sugars 3g	
Protein 12g	

Vitamin A 6%	•	Vitamin C 5%
Calcium 9%	•	Iron 36%

* Percent Daily Values are based on a 2,000 calorie diet. Your Daily Values may be higher or lower depending on your calorie needs:

	Calories:	2,000	2,500
Total Fat	Less than	65g	80g
Sat Fat	Less than	20g	25g
Cholesterol	Less than	300mg	300mg
Sodium	Less than	2,400mg	2,400mg
Total Carbohydrate		300g	375g
Dietary Fiber		25g	30g

Calories per gram
Fat 9 • Carbohydrate 4 • Protein 4

Ingredients: Water, beans, beef, tomatoes, corn flour, chili powder, (chili peppers, flavoring), salt, modified food starch, sugar, natural flavoring.

Sunsplash Valley
FAT-FREE
Chili with Black Beans

Nutrition Facts
Serving size 1 cup (180g)
Servings per Can 2

Amount Per Serving	
Calories 140	Calories from Fat 0

	% Daily Value*
Total Fat 0g	0%
Saturated Fat 0g	0%
Cholesterol 0mg	0%
Sodium 360mg	15%
Total Carbohydrate 27g	9%
Dietary Fiber 14g	56%
Sugars 5g	
Protein 15g	

Vitamin A 80%	•	Vitamin C 8%
Calcium 12%	•	Iron 25%

* Percent Daily Values are based on a 2,000 calorie diet. Your Daily Values may be higher or lower depending on your calorie needs:

	Calories:	2,000	2,500
Total Fat	Less than	65g	80g
Sat Fat	Less than	20g	25g
Cholesterol	Less than	300mg	300mg
Sodium	Less than	2,400mg	2,400mg
Total Carbohydrate		300g	375g
Dietary Fiber		25g	30g

Calories per gram
Fat 9 • Carbohydrate 4 • Protein 4

Ingredients: Water, tomatoes, black beans, onions, pinto beans, carrots, tomato paste, green bell pepper, soy granules, chili pepper, honey, sea salt, unsulphured molasses, garlic powder, cumin, soy lecithin, potato flakes, paprika, ground bay leaves, sage, basil, oregano.

In setting the RDA, the committee assumes that the protein eaten would be a combination of plant and animal proteins, that it will be consumed with adequate calories from carbohydrate and fat, and that other nutrients in the diet will be adequate. The committee also assumes that the RDA will be applied only to healthy individuals with no unusual metabolic need for protein.

Protein and Health

With all the attention that has been paid to the health effects of starch, sugars, fibers, fats, oils, and cholesterol, protein has been slighted. Protein deficiency effects are well-known because together with energy deficiency, they are the world's main form of malnutrition. But the health effects of too much protein—and particularly the effects of proteins of different kinds—are far less well-known. The following sections discuss protein deficiency, excess protein, and types of protein.

Protein-Energy Malnutrition

Protein deficiency and energy deficiency go hand in hand so often that public health officials have given a nickname to the pair: **protein-energy malnutrition (PEM).** The two diseases and their symptoms overlap all along the spectrum, but the extremes have names of their own. Protein deficiency is **kwashiorkor,** and energy deficiency is **marasmus.**[15]

Kwashiorkor is the Ghanaian name for "the evil spirit that infects the first child when the second child is born." In countries where kwashiorkor is prevalent, parents customarily give their newly weaned children watery cereal rather than the food eaten by the rest of the family.* The child has been receiving the mother's breast milk, which contains high-quality protein designed beautifully to support growth. Suddenly the child receives only a weak drink with scant protein of very low quality. It is not surprising that the just-weaned child sickens when the new baby arrives.

The child who has been banished from its mother's breast faces this threat to life by engaging in as little activity as possible. Apathy is one of the earliest signs of protein deprivation. The body is collecting all its forces to meet the crisis and so cuts down on any expenditure of protein not needed for the heart, lungs, and brain. As the apathy increases, the child doesn't even cry for food. All growth ceases; the child is no larger at age four than at age two. New hair grows without the protein pigment that gives hair its color. The skin also loses its color, and open sores fail to heal. Digestive enzymes are in short supply, the digestive tract lining deteriorates, and absorption fails. The child can't assimilate what little food is eaten. Proteins and hormones that previously kept the fluids correctly distributed among the compartments of the

PROTEIN-ENERGY MALNUTRITION (PEM), also called **PROTEIN-CALORIE MALNUTRITION (PCM)** the world's most widespread malnutrition problem, including both kwashiorkor and marasmus as well as the states in which they overlap.

KWASHIORKOR (kwash-ee-OR-core) a deficiency disease caused by inadequate protein in the presence of adequate food energy.

MARASMUS (ma-RAZ-mus) an energy-deficiency disease; starvation.

---

*The exact cause of kwashiorkor remains uncertain. Some research suggests that kwashiorkor may involve more than protein deficiency and develops when malnourished children eat moldy grains or peanuts. The mold *Aspergillus flavus,* commonly found in hot, humid areas, produces a potent aflatoxin that inhibits protein synthesis. (R. G. Hendickse, Kwashiorkor: The hypothesis that incriminates aflatoxins, *Pediatrics* 88 (1991): 376–379.

body now are diminished, so that fluid leaks out of the blood (**edema**) and accumulates in the belly and legs. Blood proteins, including hemoglobin, are not synthesized, so the child becomes anemic; this increases the child's weakness and apathy. The kwashiorkor victim often develops a fatty liver, caused by a lack of the protein carriers that transport fat out of the liver. Antibodies to fight off invading bacteria are degraded to provide amino acids for other uses; the child becomes an easy target for any infection. Then **dysentery,** an infection of the digestive tract that causes diarrhea, further depletes the body of nutrients, especially minerals. Measles, which might make a healthy child sick for a week or two, kills the kwashiorkor child within two or three days. If the condition is caught in time, the starving child's life may be saved by careful nutrition therapy (see Figure 5–9).

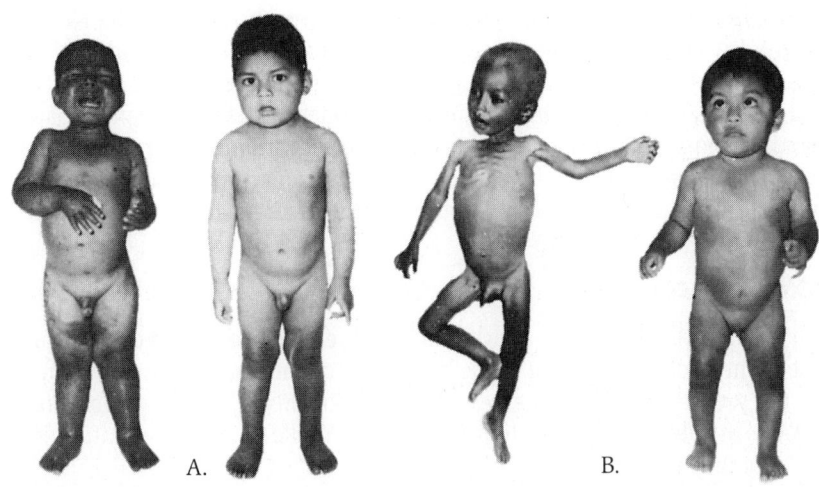

A. B.

FIGURE 5–9
KWASHIORKOR AND MARASMUS

A. Kwashiorkor. The child at the left has the characteristic "moon face" (edema), swollen belly, and patchy dermatitis (from zinc deficiency) often seen with kwashiorkor. At the right, the same child after nutritional therapy.
B. Marasmus. The child at the left is suffering from the extreme emaciation of marasmus. At the right is the same child after nutritional therapy.

Children with marasmus suffer symptoms similar to those of children with kwashiorkor, since both conditions cause loss of body protein tissue, but there are differences between the two conditions. Kwashiorkor children retain some of their stores of body fat (because they are still consuming calories), accumulate fat in their livers (because they can't make protein to carry it away), and develop edema (from protein deficiency). Marasmic children experience **ketosis** to conserve body protein, while kwashiorkor children do not, because they are receiving some carbohydrate.

A marasmic child looks like a wizened little old person—just skin and bones (see Figure 5–9). The child is often sick because his or her resistance to disease is low. All the muscles are wasted, including the heart muscle, and the heart is weak. Metabolism is so slow that body temperature is subnormal. There is little or no fat under the skin to insulate against cold. The experience of hospital workers with victims of this disease is that the victims' primary need is to be wrapped up and kept warm. Marasmic patients also need love because they have often been deprived of parental attention as well as food.

Unlike the kwashiorkor child, who is fed milk until weaning, the marasmic child may have been neglected from early infancy. The disease occurs most commonly in children from 6 months to 18 months of age in all the overpopulated city slums of the world. Since the brain normally grows to almost its full adult size within the first two years of life, marasmus impairs brain development and so may have a permanent effect on a child's learning ability.

EDEMA (eh-DEEM-uh) swelling of body tissue caused by leakage of fluid from the blood vessels, seen in (among other conditions) protein deficiency.

DYSENTERY (DISS-en-terry) an infection of the digestive tract that causes diarrhea.

KETOSIS (kee-TOE-sis) an adaptation of the body to prolonged (several days') fasting or carbohydrate restriction: body fat is converted to ketones, which can be used as fuel for some brain cells. (More about ketosis in Chapter 8.)

PEM is prevalent in Africa, Central America, South America, the Near East, and the Far East. Cases have also been reported on American Indian reservations and in the inner cities and impoverished rural areas of the United States.[16] PEM has also been recognized in many undernourished hospital patients, including those with anorexia nervosa, AIDS, cancer, and other wasting conditions. The extent and severity of malnutrition worldwide is a political and economic problem and is discussed further in the Spotlight feature in Chapter 11.

Too Much Protein

Many of the world's people struggle to obtain enough food and enough protein to keep themselves alive, but in the developed countries, protein is so abundant that the problems of protein *excess* are seen. For this reason, the committee on RDA has suggested an upper limit for protein intake of no more than twice the RDA amount when food energy is adequate.

Infants and children do not adjust well to diets containing large amounts of protein; their body composition is altered. Animals fed high-protein diets experience a protein overload effect, seen in the enlargement of their livers and kidneys. In human beings, high-protein diets eaten over a lifetime may cause problems in kidney function. Excess protein also creates an increased demand for vitamin B_6 in the diet so that the body can utilize the protein. As a result, a deficiency of this vitamin could result.

Animals experimentally fed high-protein diets similar to those that people typically eat in the United States experience loss of zinc from their tissues as they age. Increased zinc excretion is also seen in pregnant women and infants on protein supplements. The use of such supplements during pregnancy may do more harm than good, even to undernourished women. In infants, the use of protein supplements has been linked to deficits in cognitive development.

High dietary protein also increases the tendency to obesity, a finding in direct contrast to the popular belief that high-protein diets cause people to "burn off fat." Protein-rich foods are often high in saturated fat, cholesterol, and calories. The higher a person's intake of such protein-rich foods as meat and poultry, the more likely it is that fruits, vegetables, and grains will be crowded out of the diet, making the diet inadequate in other nutrients. Diets high in protein necessitate higher intakes of calcium as well, because such diets promote calcium excretion.[17]

Choose Your Protein Wisely

Misconceived notions abound regarding protein in the diet; the most obvious of these is that more is better. North Americans, on the average, consume more than 90 grams of protein daily, and about 70 percent of this protein comes from animal flesh and dairy products (see Figure 5–10). As you know, saturated fats can supply half or more of the calories in animal protein foods. You could better balance your food choices by selecting one-half or less of your protein from animal sources and the rest from plants.

Foods that supply protein in abundance can be found in the *Milk, Yogurt, and Cheese Group* and the *Meat, Poultry, Fish, Dry Beans, Eggs, and Nuts*

Group of the Food Guide Pyramid (refer to Figure 2–6 on page 45). Servings of vegetables and grain products from the *Vegetable Group* and the *Bread, Cereal, Rice, and Pasta Group* can also contribute significant amounts of protein to the diet. As the vegetarian knows, one can easily design a perfectly acceptable diet around plant foods alone by choosing a variety of them appropriately. Plant foods taken together will almost inevitably supply the complete spectrum of needed amino acids as long as energy intake is also adequate and not too many nutrient-empty foods are eaten.

Adequate protein in the diet is easy to obtain, as Table 5–5 illustrates. A breakfast of one egg, two slices of wheat bread, and a glass of milk provides close to 20 grams of protein. This meets about a third of an average man's recommended protein intake of 63 grams and about half of a woman's RDA for protein of 50 grams. The Protein Scorecard on page 185 shows you how to estimate your protein intake.

Many interesting sources of protein are available. One class of protein-rich foods other than meats has already been mentioned many times: the plant family known as **legumes** (see Figure 5–11 and the accompanying Miniglossary of Legumes on pages 186 and 187). The protein of legumes is of a quality almost comparable to that of meat. Legumes are also good sources of fiber, many B vitamins, iron, and other minerals. A cup of cooked legumes contains 25 percent of the protein recommended daily for an adult male. Like meats, though, legumes do not offer every nutrient, and they do not make a complete meal by themselves. Their balance of amino acids can be improved by using grains or other vegetables with them. This chapter's Spotlight feature discusses this concept further.

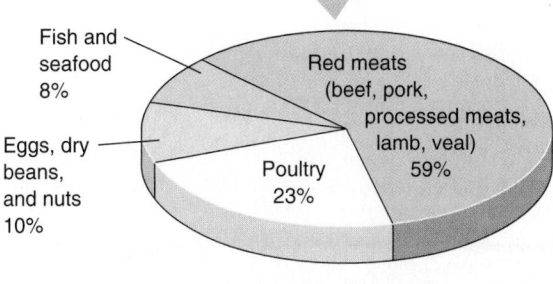

FIGURE 5–10

PROTEIN CONTRIBUTED BY THE FOOD GUIDE PYRAMID GROUPS IN THE AVERAGE AMERICAN DIET*

*The average protein consumption in the United States is 67.5 grams of protein per day, of which 37 grams (55%) come from the Meat Group. The Milk and Bread Groups are the next two largest contributors, providing 36% of the total daily protein.

SOURCE: Adapted from *Eating in America Today*, Edition II, © 1994 by the National Live Stock and Meat Board, p. 17.

LEGUMES (leg-GYOOMS) plants of the bean and pea family having roots with nodules that contain bacteria that can trap nitrogen from the air in the soil and make it into compounds that become part of the seed. The seeds are rich in high-quality protein compared with those of most other plant foods.

TABLE 5–5
PROTEIN SOURCES

FOOD	AMOUNT	GRAMS OF PROTEIN[a]	CALORIES
These are the foods people usually think of when they think of protein:			
Cheese			
Cheddar[b]	1 oz	7	115
Cottage (low- or nonfat)	½ c	14	85–130
Egg	1 large	7	80
Fish, light and dark, cooked	3 oz	21	125–175
Meat, cooked			
Ground beef[b]	3 oz	21	185–235
Beef roast (lean)	3 oz	21	160–215
Pork chop (lean)	3 oz	21	310
Poultry (without skin), light and dark, cooked	3 oz	21	145–175
Milk			
Nonfat	1 c	8	90
Whole[b]	1 c	8	160
Yogurt (nonfat)	1 c	8	90
These are other good sources of protein that you can use:			
Vegetables, cooked			
Broccoli	1 c	5	45
Brussels sprouts	1 c	6	55
Cauliflower	1 c	4	30
Greens	1 c	2–4	30–65
Legumes			
Dried, cooked	½ c	7–8	90–115
Mung sprouts, raw	½ c	2	20
Tofu (soybean curd)	4 oz	9	85
Cereal grain products			
Barley, whole-grain, cooked	½ c	4	135
Bran, unprocessed	½ c	4	55
Bran cereal (100% bran), uncooked	½ c	5	90
Breads	1 slice	2–3	60–80
Cornmeal, unrefined ground, uncooked	½ c	5	215
Millet, whole-grain, cooked	½ c	3	95
Oatmeal, cooked	1 c	5	155–200
Pasta, enriched, cooked	1 c	5–7	225–230
Rice, cooked	1 c	4–5	225
Tortilla	1 large	5–6	185
Wheat, bulgur, cooked	½ c	7	110
Wheat, cracked, cooked	½ c	4	110
Starchy vegetables			
Corn	1 medium ear or ½ c	3	70
Peas, fresh	1 c	9	115
Potato, baked	1 large	4	145
Winter squash, baked	1 c	4	130
Miscellaneous			
Nut butters[b]	1 tbsp	4	95
Nuts[b]	2 tbsp	2–5	80–115
Seeds[b]	2 tbsp	3–5	95–100
Brewer's yeast	2 tbsp	6	40–45

[a]The adult RDA is 46 grams for women aged 19 to 24 years and 58 grams for men aged 19 to 24 years. Different situations and stages of life can affect protein needs.
[b]These items are high in fat and should be used in moderation.
SOURCE: Adapted from Society for Nutrition Education materials.

PROTEIN SCORECARD

How to Estimate Protein Intake

Table 5–5 provides a way to estimate the amount of protein eaten at a meal or in a day. Using the values in Table 5–5 and Appendix I, let us estimate the amounts of protein in the meals shown here. Because the fats (butter) can be assumed to contain no protein, the only foods to inspect are the meats, milks, legumes, grains, fruits, and vegetables. Peas and beans contain more protein than other vegetables do. A 1-cup portion of legumes when used as a meat alternate has 14 grams of protein.

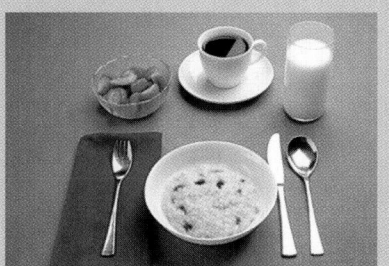

BREAKFAST	PROTEIN (G)
1 c oatmeal	5
¼ c raisins	1
1 c nonfat milk	8
1¼ c strawberries	1

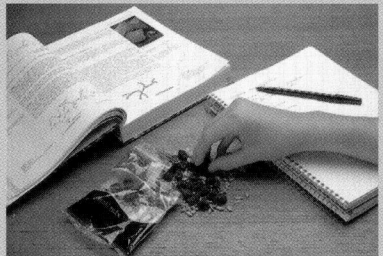

MORNING SNACK	
2 tbsp raisins	½
2 tbsp sunflower seeds	3

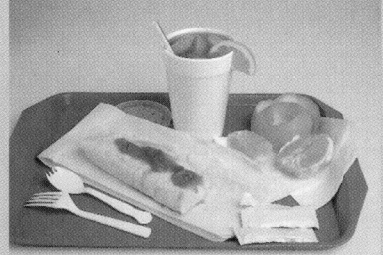

LUNCH	
1 beef and bean burrito	
(1 large tortilla	5
½ c beans	7
½ oz beef)	3½
1 packet sugar	—
1 orange	1

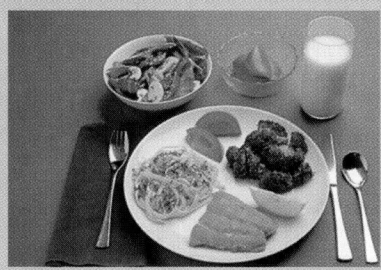

DINNER	
3 oz broiled salmon	21
1 c broccoli	5
½ c noodles	3
2 tsp butter	—
¼ tomato	½
¼ c mushrooms	½
¼ c water chestnuts	½
1 c fresh spinach	2
1 tbsp sesame seeds	2½
⅓ c chick-peas	3
1 tbsp vinaigrette dressing	—
1 c nonfat milk	8
½ c Italian ice	0
Day's totals	81 grams

The total calories for the meals shown here add up to 1,750. A total of 81 grams of protein multiplied by 4 calories per gram is 324 calories from protein, about 19 percent of the day's total 1,750 calories. This 81 grams is well above most people's RDA for protein.

MINIGLOSSARY OF LEGUMES

BLACK, CUBAN, or **TURTLE BEANS** These medium-size black-skinned ovals have a rich, sweet taste. They are best served in Mexican and Latin American dishes or thick soups and stews.

BLACK-EYED PEAS These are small and oval shaped, creamy white with a black spot. They have a vegetable flavor with mealy texture. Use in salads with rice and greens.

GARBANZO BEANS or **CHICK-PEAS** These legumes are large, round, and tan colored. They have a nutty flavor and crunchy texture. Use in soups and stews and puréed for dips.

GREAT NORTHERN BEANS This variety is medium white and kidney shaped. Enjoy the delicate flavor and firm texture in salads, soups, and main dishes.

KIDNEY BEANS These familiar beans are large, red, and kidney shaped (the white variety is called cannellini). They have a bland taste and soft texture but tough skins. Use in chili, bean stews, and Mexican dishes for red; Italian dishes for white.

LENTILS These legumes are small, flat, and round. Usually brown colored, lentils also can be green, pink, or red. They have a mild taste with firm texture. Best used when combined with grains or vegetables in salads, soups, or stews.

LIMA or **BUTTER BEANS** Limas are soft and mealy in texture. They are flat, oval shaped, and white tinged with green. The smaller variety has a milder taste. Use in soups and stews.

PINTO BEANS These medium ovals are mottled beige and brown with an earthy flavor. They are most often used in Mexican dishes, such as refried beans, stews, or dips.

RED BEANS This versatile bean is a medium-size, dark red oval. The taste and texture are similar to kidney beans. Use in soups and stews, and serve with rice.

SOYBEANS You can find these creamy white ovals in numerous food products, such as tofu, flour, grits, and milk. They have a firm texture and bland flavor. The fat content of soybeans is the highest of all legumes.

SPLIT PEAS Green or yellow, these small halved peas supply an earthy flavor with mealy texture. They are best used in soups and with rice or grains.

WHITE NAVY BEANS These beans are small, white ovals and are best used in soups and stews and as baked beans.

*All the legumes in this guide except lentils and split peas require at least 1 hour of soaking. After soaking, rinse and cover with fresh water. Then bring to a boil; simmer for 30 to 60 minutes or until soft. Canned varieties are available, too.

SOURCE: Adapted from K. Mangum, *Life's Simple Pleasures: Fine Vegetarian Cooking for Sharing and Celebration* (Boise, ID: Pacific Press Publishing, 1990), p. 149.

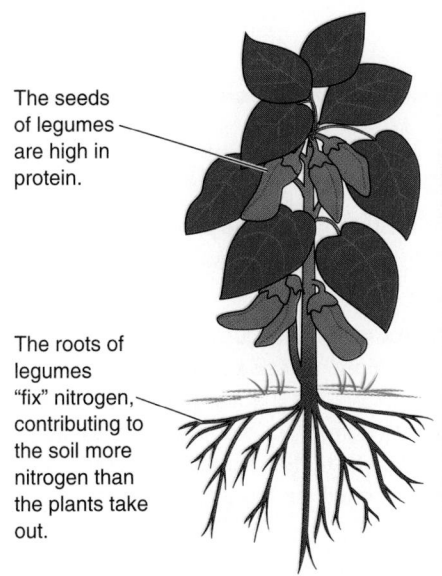

The seeds of legumes are high in protein.

The roots of legumes "fix" nitrogen, contributing to the soil more nitrogen than the plants take out.

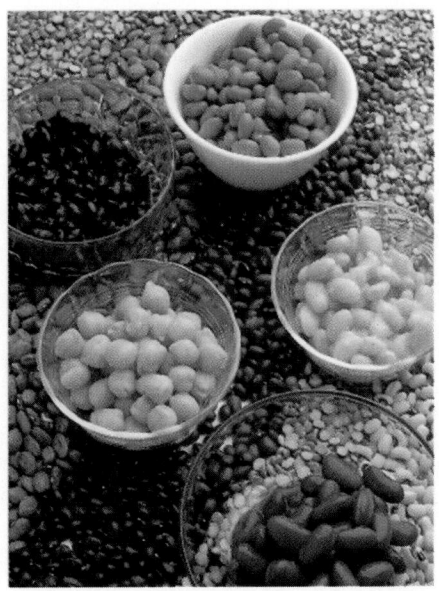

FIGURE 5–11
LEGUMES

Legumes have long been known as "the poor man's meat," but they are an inexpensive, health-promoting, land-sparing, nutritious food. Bacteria in the *root nodules* can "fix" nitrogen, contributing it to the *beans*. Ultimately, thanks to these bacteria, the plant leaves in the soil more nitrogen than it takes out. So efficient at trapping nitrogen are the legumes that farmers often grow them in rotation with other crops to fertilize fields. For a variety of legumes used in cooking, see the accompanying Miniglossary.

Another form in which the nutrients of soybeans are available is bean curd, or **tofu,** a staple used in many Asian dishes. Thanks to the way some types of tofu are made, tofu can be high in calcium and can serve as a milk substitute for people who are allergic to or cannot tolerate milk.

The protein-rich, high-fiber, nutrient-dense foods from plants are most often lower in fat than animal-derived foods. People who eat mostly the former can therefore enjoy a nutritious diet that is low in fat, but only if other high-fat foods such as nuts, olives, and butter are limited, too. The key to getting enough, but not too much, protein seems to be to consume a variety of foods in ample quantities, to deemphasize meats, and to emphasize vegetables, grains, and nonfat milk and nonfat milk products. The Consumer Tips feature shows you how to do this when packing bag lunches.

TOFU (TOE-foo) a curd made from soybeans, rich in protein and calcium (when a calcium salt is used as the curdling agent), used in many Asian and vegetarian dishes in place of meat. *Firm* tofu is dense and solid and holds up well in stir-fry dishes, soups, or on the grill—anywhere that you want the tofu to maintain its shape; *Soft* tofu is a better choice for recipes that call for blended tofu. *Silken* tofu is made by a different process that results in a creamy, custardlike product that works well in pureed or blended recipes.

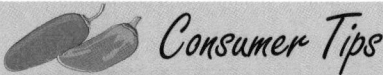

Consumer Tips

Advice on Brown-Bagging It

Whether you carry your lunch to work or school to save time and money, the following tips can help you pack nutritious meals and add variety to your noontime routine. Even if you don't carry your lunch regularly, you can use this advice when you take food on hikes, day trips, or picnics.

- Choose breads made with whole wheat, bran, or oatmeal to add fiber to your lunch.

- Get out of the peanut butter and jelly rut by filling sandwiches with water-packed tuna mixed with mandarin oranges, bean sprouts, and a bit of plain low-fat yogurt; chopped, cooked, skinless chicken combined with raw sliced vegetables and a little French dressing; cooked, mashed dried beans seasoned with chopped onion, garlic powder, rosemary, thyme, and pepper; or low-fat cottage cheese flavored with drained, chopped pineapple and a dash of cinnamon.

- Take a thermos filled with chili, vegetable soup, or a milk-based soup, such as cream of tomato, prepared with nonfat milk instead of a sandwich. Try cold lunches such as low-fat or nonfat yogurt and fruit, brown rice with cubes of skinless poultry or lean meat, or cooked pasta tossed with raw vegetables, low-fat cheese, and a bit of Italian dressing.

- Pack fresh fruit such as an apple, a banana, or grapes along with your sandwich or main dish.

- Substitute unsalted pretzels or air-popped popcorn for potato, corn, or tortilla chips.

- Replace Oreos and candy bars with lower fat treats, including fig bars, graham crackers, gingersnaps, or vanilla wafers.

- Drink low-fat or nonfat milk or fruit juice with your lunch instead of soft drinks. Freeze small cans or cartons of juice to take along. Put them in plastic wrap (they "sweat" as they defrost) and pack them into your lunch to help keep the other foods chilled. By lunchtime, the beverage will be thawed and ready to drink.

- Take along fresh cauliflower or broccoli florets, red or green pepper strips, cucumber or zucchini slices, or cherry tomatoes to munch on.

If you like the idea of packing a lunch every day but often feel too rushed in the morning to do so:

- Pack your lunch the night before and store it in the refrigerator; the food will be thoroughly chilled the following morning and will remain fresher longer.

- Make several sandwiches at one time and store them in the freezer. Pull one out to take with you in the morning, and it will be thawed by noon. Although sliced meats, sliced cheese, and mustard freeze well, egg salad, lettuce, tomatoes, jelly, and mayonnaise do not, and they will make a sandwich soggy.

SOURCE: Adapted from the U.S. Department of Agriculture, Human Nutrition Information Service, *Making Bag Lunches, Snacks & Desserts Using the Dietary Guidelines* (Home and Garden Bulletin No. 232-9), pp. 9–22.

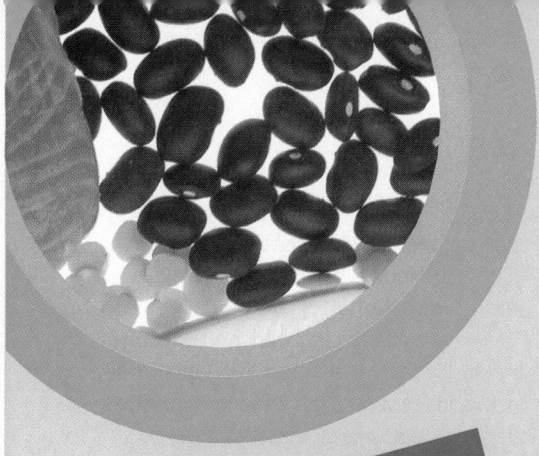

The Vegetarian Diet

More and more people are following vegetarian diets. Their reasons for becoming vegetarian vary widely. Some have religious reasons, while others have ethical reasons. Some believe that vegetarianism is ecologically sound and others, that it is less costly than the meat-eating alternative. In addition to the traditional types of vegetarians (see Table 5–6), there are people who eat seafood but not other meats, and those who include chicken and other poultry but not red meat. Whatever the particular reasons for choosing a vegetarian diet and regardless of the type of vegetarian diet followed, the vegetarian needs to be aware of the nutrition and health implications of such a diet.

I've been thinking about becoming a vegetarian, but I'm still not sure whether vegetarianism is nutritionally sound. Is it? The answer is yes if the vegetarian carefully plans his or her diet. Specifically, the goals for a vegetarian diet planner include the following:

- To obtain neither too few nor too many calories—that is, to maintain a healthful weight.
- To obtain adequate quantities of complete protein.
- To obtain the needed vitamins and minerals.

Balancing calories: that sounds familiar. How can the vegetarian adjust calories to maintain a healthful weight? The idea of balancing calories to maintain a healthful weight should be a familiar one.

You may recall from Chapters 1 and 2 that balancing calories is important in everyone's diet. The vegetarian can use the *Vegetarian Pyramid* (see Figure 5–12) to balance his or her diet. The base of this pyramid is made up of grains which should be consumed six to eleven times a day. The pyramid recommends at least three to five servings from the vegetable group and two to four servings from the fruit group. Milk products and milk substitutes are to be consumed two to three times daily, while meat and fish substitutes, which include dried beans, nuts, seeds, peanut butter, tofu, and eggs, should be consumed two to three times daily. At the tip of the pyramid are fats, oils, and sweets, which should be used sparingly.

Isn't it important, too, to obtain adequate amounts of complete protein? Yes, obtaining adequate amounts of all the essential amino acids is essential to life. Because proteins from animals contain ample amounts of the essential

---

TABLE 5–6
TYPES OF VEGETARIAN DIETS

SEMI-VEGETARIAN	Some but not all groups of animal-derived products, such as meat, poultry, fish, seafood, eggs, milk, and milk products, included in this diet.
LACTOVEGETARIAN	Milk and milk products included in this diet, but meat, poultry, fish, seafood, and eggs excluded. *possible limiting nutrient: iron*
LACTO-OVOVEGETARIAN	Milk and milk products and eggs included in this diet, but meat, poultry, fish, and seafood excluded. *possible limiting nutrient: iron*
OVOVEGETARIAN	Eggs included in this diet, but milk and milk products, meat, poultry, fish, and seafood excluded. *possible limiting nutrients: iron, vitamin D, calcium, riboflavin*
STRICT-VEGETARIAN/VEGAN	All animal-derived foods, including meat, poultry, fish, seafood, eggs, milk, and milk products excluded from this diet. *possible limiting nutrients: iron, vitamin D, calcium, riboflavin, vitamin B_{12}, high-quality protein*

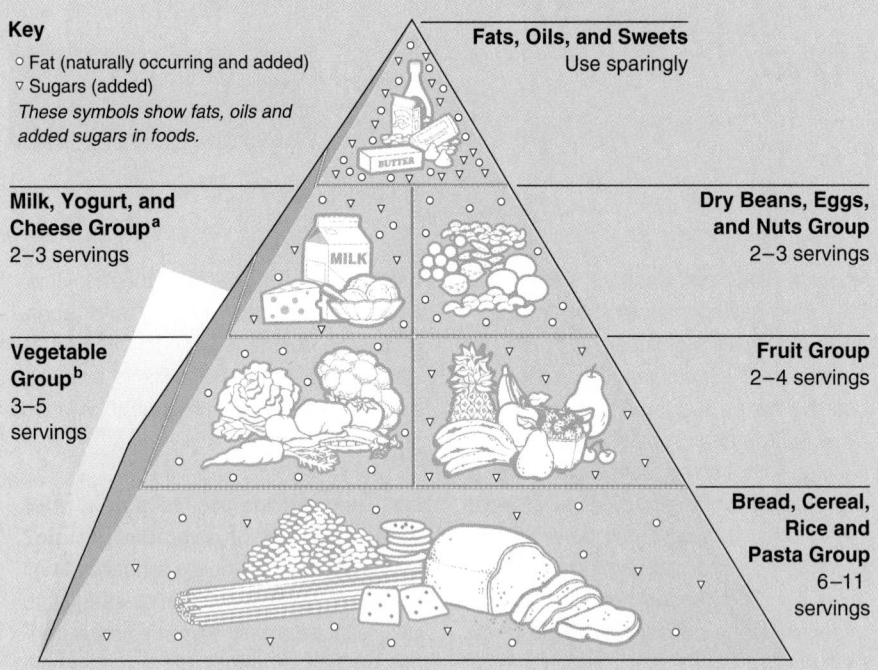

Key

○ Fat (naturally occurring and added)
▽ Sugars (added)
These symbols show fats, oils and added sugars in foods.

Fats, Oils, and Sweets
Use sparingly

Milk, Yogurt, and Cheese Group[a]
2–3 servings

Dry Beans, Eggs, and Nuts Group
2–3 servings

Vegetable Group[b]
3–5 servings

Fruit Group
2–4 servings

Bread, Cereal, Rice and Pasta Group
6–11 servings

**FIGURE 5–12
VEGETARIAN PYRAMID**

[a]People who do not use milk or milk products are advised to use soy milk fortified with calcium and vitamin B$_{12}$.

[b]Include 1 cup of dark green vegetables daily to help meet iron requirements.

amino acids, the lacto-ovovegetarian can get a head start on meeting protein needs by drinking two cups of milk daily or by consuming the equivalent in milk products in the day's diet.

Adequate amounts of amino acids can be obtained from a plant-based diet when a varied diet is routinely consumed on a daily basis. Mixtures of proteins from unrefined grains, vegetables, legumes, seeds, and nuts eaten over the course of a day complement one another in their amino acid profiles so that deficits in one are made up by another. Since the body is able to compensate for variations in amino acid intakes from day to day, researchers now believe that it is not necessary to include

complementary proteins within each meal, as proposed by the once popular theory of **mutual supplementation.**[18] Table 5–7 gives examples of how to combine nonmeat foods to form complete proteins.

Vegetarians should adopt a strategy of eating a wide variety of protein sources. In so doing, they can be virtually assured of an adequate protein intake.

If I go on a vegetarian diet, will I need to take vitamin supplements? That depends on the kind of vegetarian diet you follow. The lacto-ovo vegetarian diet can be adequate in all vitamins, but several vitamins may be a problem for the vegan. One such vitamin is vitamin B$_{12}$,

which doesn't occur in plant foods except in fortified foods, such as breakfast cereals or **nutritional** or **brewer's yeast,** grown in a vitamin B$_{12}$-enriched environment. Baker's yeast and live yeast are not good sources of this vitamin. The vegan needs a reliable B$_{12}$ source, such as vitamin B$_{12}$-fortified soy milk or **meat replacements.** Some vegetarians use seaweed, fermented soy, and other products in the belief that they provide vitamin B$_{12}$ in adequate amounts, but these products are not currently recommended as reliable sources. A pregnant or lactating woman who is eating a vegan diet should be aware that her infant can develop a vitamin B$_{12}$ deficiency that can damage the baby's nervous system, even if the mother remains healthy, because vitamin B$_{12}$ is stored in the body, and it may take years for a deficiency to develop.

What other vitamins might vegans lack? Another vitamin of concern is vitamin D.[19] The milk drinker is protected, provided the milk is fortified with vitamin

TABLE 5–7

NONMEAT MIXTURES THAT PROVIDE HIGH-QUALITY PROTEIN

COMBINE			EXAMPLES
For the Strict Vegetarian			

Cereal grains	+	Legumes	
Barley		Dried beans	Bean taco
Bulgur		Dried lentils	Chili and cornbread
Oats		Dried peas	Lentils or beans and rice
Rice		Peanuts	Peanut butter sandwich
Whole-grain breads		Soy products	Tofu and stir-fried vegetables with rice
Pasta			
Cornmeal			
Legumes	+	Seeds and nuts	
Dried beans		Sesame seeds	Hummus (chick-pea and sesame paste)
Dried lentils		Sunflower seeds	Split pea soup and sesame crackers
Dried peas		Walnuts	
Peanuts		Cashews	
Soy products		Nut butters	

Examples

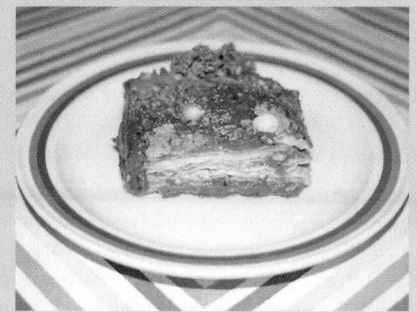

Black beans and rice

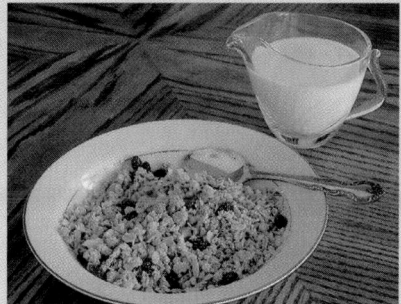

Peanut butter and wheat bread

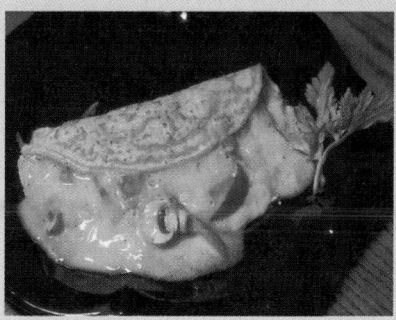

Tofu and stir-fried vegetables with rice

For the Lacto-Ovo Vegetarian			

Eggs or milk products[a]	+	Vegetable protein foods	
Eggs		Legumes	Macaroni and cheese
Milk		Nuts	Vegetable omelet
Yogurt		Seeds	Eggplant Parmesan
Cheese		Whole grains	Broccoli with cheese sauce
Cottage cheese		Vegetables	French toast
			Cereal with milk

Examples

Eggplant Parmesan

Cereal with milk

Vegetable omelet

[a]Choose low-fat or nonfat varieties of milk and other dairy products whenever possible.

D, but there is no practical source of vitamin D in plant foods. Fortified margarines and fortified breakfast cereals can supply some vitamin D. Regular exposure to the sun will prevent a deficiency, but a person confined indoors or a vegan living in a northern climate or smoggy city probably should take vitamin D supplements. Excesses of vitamin D are toxic; don't exceed the recommended dietary allowance of 5 micrograms.

Riboflavin, a B vitamin obtained from milk, is present in the diet of the vegan who eats ample servings of dark greens, whole and enriched grains, mushrooms, and legumes. The vegan who doesn't eat these foods, however, may not meet riboflavin needs. Nutritional yeast is a rich source of riboflavin for the vegetarian.

Can minerals be lacking in the vegetarian diet? Two minerals may be of concern for all vegetarians, not just for vegans: iron and zinc. Legumes, whole grains, dried fruit, nuts, and seeds are important sources of iron in the vegetarian diet. The iron in these foods, however, is not as easily absorbed by the body as that in meat. In fact, people absorb three times as much iron from a meal that includes meat as from one that does not (see Chapter 7). Because vitamin C in fruits and vegetables can triple iron absorption from other foods eaten at the same meal, vegetarian meals should be rich in foods offering vitamin C.

Zinc, too, may be a problem nutrient for vegetarians. It is widespread in plant foods, but its availability may be hindered by the fibers and other binders found in fruits, vegetables, and whole grains. The zinc needs of vegetarians and the effects of mineral binders remain the subjects of intensive study. While research continues, vegetarians

are advised to eat varied diets that include wheat germ, legumes, small amounts of nuts and seeds, and whole-grain breads well leavened with yeast. Yeast improves the availability of the minerals in the breads. Table 5–8 offers tips for easy-to-fix vegetarian meals and snacks.

Would low intakes of calcium be a problem for the strict vegetarian? Yes, special efforts are necessary to meet calcium needs. While the milk-drinking vegetarian is protected from calcium deficiency, the vegan must find other sources of calcium. Some good sources of calcium are *regular* servings of some fortified breakfast cereals, flours, and brands of orange juice; firm tofu (processed with calcium); calcium-fortified soy milk; some nuts, such as almonds; certain seeds, such as sesame seeds; and some vegetables, such as broccoli, collard greens, kale, mustard greens, turnip greens,

---

TABLE 5–8
EASY-TO-PREPARE VEGETARIAN MEALS AND SNACKS

BREAKFAST

- Cold cereal (preferably iron-enriched, as noted on the label): eat with nonfat or low-fat milk, yogurt, or soy milk.
- Hot cereals: add fresh fruit slices and nonfat yogurt and sprinkle with cinnamon.
- Toast, bagels: top with low-fat cheese, low-fat cottage cheese, or 1 to 2 tbsp of peanut butter.

SNACKS

- Assorted fresh fruits and vegetables with yogurt dip.
- Low-fat cheese or peanut butter on rice cakes or crackers.
- Nonfat or low-fat yogurt.
- English muffin pizza with part-skim mozzarella cheese.
- Hummus with pita bread wedges and crisp vegetables.*

LUNCH AND DINNER

- Salads: add tofu, chick-peas, three-bean salad, kidney beans, low-fat cottage cheese, sunflower seeds, and hard-cooked egg.
- Salad dressings: add salad seasonings to plain nonfat yogurt or blenderized tofu.
- Pasta: add diced tofu and/or canned kidney beans to tomato sauce; top with grated part-skim mozzarella.
- Baked potato: top it with canned beans, steamed vegetables, or low-fat cheese.
- Hearty soups: enjoy lentil, split pea, bean, and minestrone soups, either homemade or canned.
- Vegetarian pizza: top with nonfat or low-fat cheeses and steamed vegetables.

---

*To make hummus: Blend 1 cup cooked chick-peas, 2 tablespoons tahini (sesame seed paste), 2 tablespoons lemon juice, 1 minced clove garlic, and 1/4 cup chopped fresh parsley in food processor until smooth. Chill and serve with pita bread wedges, crackers, or crisp vegetables. (Makes 2 servings.)

okra, rutabaga, and Chinese cabbage (bok choy). The choices should be varied because the absorption of calcium from some of these foods is hindered by binders in them. The strict vegetarian is urged to drink two to four servings of *calcium-fortified* soy milk daily. This is especially important for children. Infant formula based on soy is fortified with calcium, and adults can easily use it in their cooking.

Are there any nutritional advantages to the vegetarian diet? Yes. Vegetarian foods are higher in fiber, richer in certain vitamins and minerals, and lower in fat than animal-derived foods.

Vegetarians can enjoy a nutritious diet very low in fat, provided they eat in moderation such high-fat foods as butter, oil, cheese, sour cream, and nuts. Vegetarians who follow the guidelines presented here and plan carefully can support their health as well as—or perhaps better than—nonvegetarians.

Are you saying that vegetarians may actually be healthier than meat eaters? Yes, abundant evidence supports that idea. Studies have found that people with vegetarian or near-vegetarian traditions, such as Seventh Day Adventists and the Chinese, have lower rates of heart disease, cancer, and obesity than those consuming the typical North American diet.[20] Informed vegetarians are more likely to be at the desired weight for their height and to have lower blood cholesterol levels, lower blood pressure, lower rates of certain types of cancer, and better digestive function.[21] Often vegetarianism goes with a healthful lifestyle (no smoking, abstinence from alcohol, emphasis on supportive family life, exercise, etc.), so it is unlikely that dietary practices *alone* account for all the aspects of improved health. Clearly, however, they contribute significantly to it.

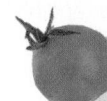

CHECK YOURSELF...

1. Name the element that appears exclusively in protein.

2. What will happen to protein synthesis if an essential amino acid is not in the diet?

3. On what does the quality of protein depend?

4. What is the recommendation regarding the percentage of calories in the diet that should come from protein?

5. Identify three roles of protein in the body.

6. What are the risks associated with using amino acid supplements?

7. Describe the concept of complementary proteins.

8. What are the health consequences of consuming too little (or too much) protein and too few (or too many) calories in the diet?

9. Can a vegetarian diet meet protein needs?

10. Which nutrients may be lacking in the strict vegetarian diet?

Answers to selected Check Yourself questions are found in Appendix H.

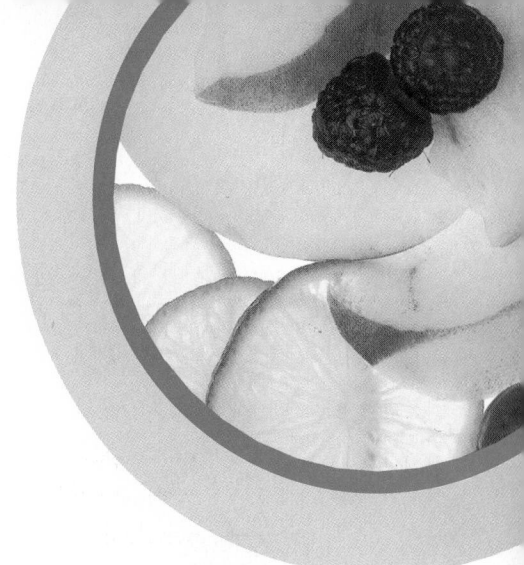

In France old Crainquebille
sold leeks from a cart, leeks called
"the asparagus of the poor." Now asparagus
sells for the asking, almost, in California markets,
and broccoli, that strong age-old green, leaps from
its lowly pot to the *Ritz's* copper saucepan.
Who determines, and for what strange reasons,
the social status of a vegetable?

M. F. K. Fisher
(1908–1992, U.S. food writer)

The Vitamins   SIX

Contents

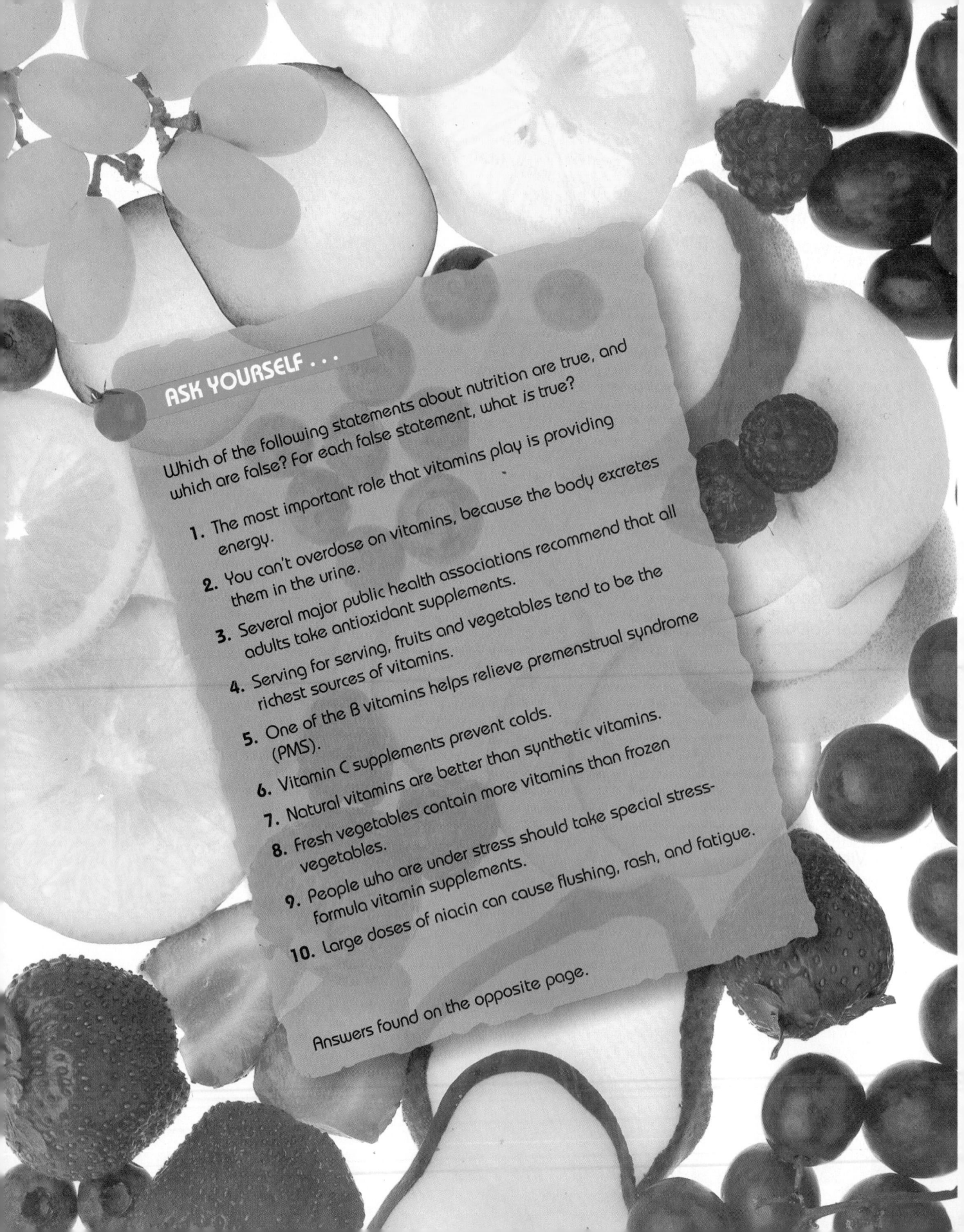

ASK YOURSELF . . .

Which of the following statements about nutrition are true, and which are false? For each false statement, what *is* true?

1. The most important role that vitamins play is providing energy.

2. You can't overdose on vitamins, because the body excretes them in the urine.

3. Several major public health associations recommend that all adults take antioxidant supplements.

4. Serving for serving, fruits and vegetables tend to be the richest sources of vitamins.

5. One of the β vitamins helps relieve premenstrual syndrome (PMS).

6. Vitamin C supplements prevent colds.

7. Natural vitamins are better than synthetic vitamins.

8. Fresh vegetables contain more vitamins than frozen vegetables.

9. People who are under stress should take special stress-formula vitamin supplements.

10. Large doses of niacin can cause flushing, rash, and fatigue.

Answers found on the opposite page.

Around the turn of the century, scientists ushered in a new era in the science of nutrition: the discovery of vitamins. They quickly realized that these substances, found in minute amounts in foods, were just as essential to health as fats, carbohydrates, and proteins. A diet lacking in one could cause a barrage of symptoms and, ultimately, death. Knowledge of the vital role played by vitamins quickly advanced, and today life-threatening vitamin deficiencies are rare in developed countries such as the United States.

Still, the vitamin research that has been conducted during the past decade or so has marked the beginning of yet another chapter in the annals of nutrition. Throughout the past ten years, more and more scientists have been investigating the possibility that large doses of certain vitamins will help stave off chronic diseases such as cancer and heart disease, problems that rank as major killers today. In fact, the study of vitamins, particularly a class known as the antioxidant vitamins, is one of the hottest, most widely publicized areas in nutrition research today. In addition, the pros and cons of taking vitamin supplements are the subject of heated debate among the scientific community. To help you sort through the steady stream of controversy regarding vitamins, this chapter explores the history, roles, and current thrust of research of the various vitamins and offers practical advice on how to incorporate the information into decisions about your own lifestyle.

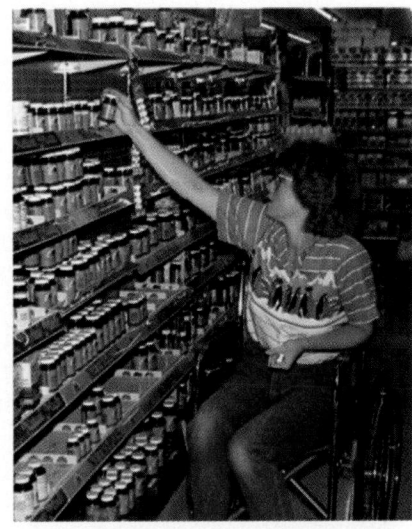

While vitamin deficiencies are rare in the United States and Canada, people are spending more money than ever on vitamin supplements.

Turning Back the Clock

Many of the vitamin-deficiency diseases that have been virtually eliminated today were first recognized in Greek and Roman times and ultimately led to the discovery of vitamins centuries later. One of the most prevalent was **scurvy,** a disease characterized by bleeding gums, tooth loss, and even death due to lack of vitamin C. The scourge of armies, sailors, and other travelers forced to do without vitamin C-rich foods for weeks on end, scurvy was recognized by Hippocrates, a Greek physician heralded today as the father of medicine.[1]

A cure for the disease was not recorded until the sixteenth century, however, when a beverage made of spruce needles or oranges and lemons was recommended. In 1753, a British physician named James Lind published a famous report recommending consumption of herbs, lettuce, endive, watercress, and summer fruits to prevent scurvy. By the early 1800s, sailors in the British navy had been dubbed "limeys" because they were required to drink lemon or lime

SCURVY the vitamin-deficiency disease characterized by bleeding gums, tooth loss, and even death in severe cases.

ASK YOURSELF ANSWERS: **1.** False. Vitamins do not provide energy, though they do play roles in energy-yielding reactions in the body. **2.** False. Excess doses of all of the vitamins can be toxic. **3.** False. No major health organization recommends that all adults take antioxidant pills. **4.** True. **5.** False. None of the B vitamins, or any other vitamin for that matter, has been shown to relieve PMS. **6.** False. Vitamin C has never been proved to prevent colds; at best, it may reduce the severity of cold symptoms. **7.** False. The chemical make-up of natural vitamins is identical to that of synthetic vitamins. **8.** False. Fresh vegetables do not necessarily contain more vitamins than their frozen counterparts, depending on such factors as how the fresh vegetable has been stored and how long since it has been harvested. **9.** False. People who are under stress need not worry about consuming extra vitamins. **10.** True.

juice daily.[2] While they still didn't know that vitamin C was the real antidote, they did recognize that certain foods prevented and cured the illness.

Similarly, a deficiency disease called **rickets** dates back to Roman times, when children frequently suffered skeletal deformities as a result of a lack of vitamin D. By the 1600s, rickets was known as the English disease because it afflicted so many English children. Some 200 years later, cod liver oil was finally recognized as a cure for the disease; no one knew at the time, however, that the "magic" ingredient in the oil was vitamin D.

Another deficiency disease, called **pellagra,** was not recognized until 1730, when a Spanish physician named Gaspar Casal first described the crusty, dry, scabby, blackish patches of skin symptomatic of the disease. In Italy, the disease was named pellagra, from the Italian *pelle agra,* meaning sour skin. Called *mal de la rosa* in Spanish, pellagra was thought to be incurable until Dr. Casal noticed that the people who developed the disease were typically poor and had inadequate diets made up of mostly corn and little meat.

By the nineteenth century, physicians had recognized that certain foods prevented or cured pellagra and other deficiency diseases. But they still hadn't determined exactly what it was in the various foods that worked as a remedy. By the middle of the nineteenth century, however, the science of chemistry had advanced to a point at which foods could be analyzed. Chemists had determined that foods consisted of fats, proteins, and carbohydrates along with minerals and water, and they assumed that they had identified all the nutritionally significant compounds.

Then, in the early twentieth century, scientists detected minute amounts of other substances that they found were essential in preventing disease and maintaining health. The substances were dubbed *vitamines,* a term coined in 1912 by a scientist named Dr. Casimir Funk to indicate that these substances were *vital* for survival and that they contained nitrogen—that is, they were *amines.* (The *e* was later dropped when scientists discovered that some of the vitamins were not amines.)

Over the next few decades, scientists identified the various **vitamins,** established their chemical formulas, and determined their functions in the body. They also measured the amount of vitamins in various foods and determined human and animal requirements for the compounds. Knowledge of vitamins constantly evolves as scientists continue to study their actions in the human body.

Today, scientists recognize that vitamins are potent compounds that perform many tasks in the body that promote growth and reproduction and maintain health and life. Vitamins constantly work to keep your nerves and skin healthy; build bone, teeth, and blood; and heal wounds, among other things. While they do not provide calories, they are essential to helping the body make use of the calories consumed via foods.

Vitamins fall into two categories: those that dissolve in water, or water-soluble, and those that dissolve in fat, or fat-soluble. To date, scientists have identified 13 vitamins, each with its own special roles to play (see Table 6–1).

The body requires various amounts of vitamins and minerals for health and well-being. Generally, a balanced diet supplies enough, but not too much, of each of the vitamins. An unbalanced diet, on the other hand, can be lacking in the right balance of vitamins. As Figure 6–1 shows, each of the major food

RICKETS a disease that occurs in children as a result of vitamin D deficiency and that is characterized by abnormal growth of bone, which in turn leads to bowed legs and an outward-bowed chest.

PELLAGRA (pell-AY-gra) niacin deficiency characterized by diarrhea, inflammation of the skin, and, in severe cases, mental disorders and death.

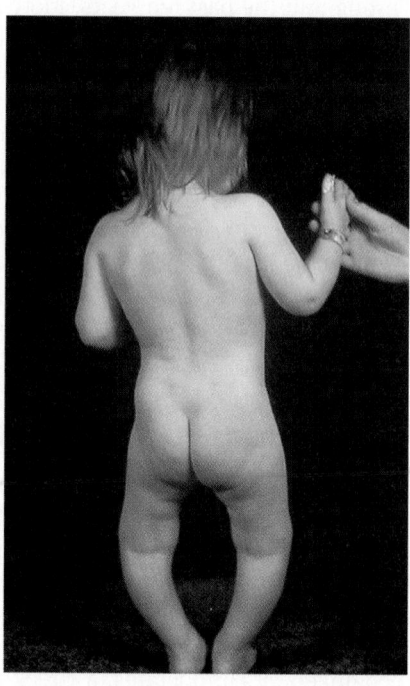

This child has the bowed legs characteristic of rickets. Worldwide, rickets afflicts many children who live in poverty and do not have access to sunlight or adequate foods containing vitamin D. (See vitamin D discussion starting on page 218.)

VITAMIN a potent, indispensable compound that performs various bodily functions that promote growth and reproduction and maintain health. Vitamins are **organic,** meaning that they contain or are related to carbon compounds. Contrary to popular belief, vitamins do not supply calories. **organic** of, related to, or containing carbon compounds.

TABLE 6–1
A GUIDE TO THE VITAMINS

VITAMIN (CHEMICAL NAME)	BEST SOURCES	CHIEF ROLES	DEFICIENCY SYMPTOMS	TOXICITY SYMPTOMS
WATER-SOLUBLE VITAMINS				
Thiamin	Meat, pork, liver, fish, poultry, whole-grain and enriched breads, cereals, pasta, nuts, legumes, wheat germ, oats.	Helps enzymes release energy from carbohydrate; supports normal appetite and nervous system function.	Beriberi: edema, heart irregularity, mental confusion, muscle weakness, low morale, impaired growth.	Rapid pulse, weakness, headaches, insomnia, irritability.
Riboflavin	Milk, dark green vegetables, yogurt, cottage cheese, liver, meat, whole-grain or enriched breads and cereals.	Helps enzymes release energy from carbohydrate, fat, and protein; promotes healthy skin and normal vision.	Eye problems, skin disorders around nose and mouth.	None reported, but an excess of any of the B vitamins could cause a deficiency of the others.
Niacin	Meat, eggs, poultry, fish, milk, whole-grain and enriched breads and cereals, nuts, legumes, peanuts, nutritional yeast, all protein foods.	Helps enzymes release energy from energy nutrients; promotes health of skin, nerves, and digestive system.	Pellagra: skin rash on parts exposed to sun, loss of appetite, dizziness, weakness, irritability, fatigue, mental confusion, indigestion.	Flushing, nausea, headaches, cramps, ulcer irritation, heartburn, abnormal liver function, low blood pressure.
Vitamin B_6 (pyridoxine)	Meat, poultry, fish, shellfish, legumes, whole-grain products, green leafy vegetables, bananas.	Protein and fat metabolism; formation of antibodies and red blood cells; helps convert tryptophan to niacin.	Nervous disorders, skin rash, muscle weakness, anemia, convulsions, kidney stones.	Depression, fatigue, irritability, headaches, numbness, damage to nerves, difficulty walking.
Folate	Green leafy vegetables, liver, legumes, seeds.	Red blood cell formation; protein metabolism; new cell division.	Anemia, heartburn, diarrhea, smooth tongue, depression, poor growth.	Diarrhea, insomnia, irritability, may mask a vitamin B_{12} deficiency.
Vitamin B_{12} (cobalamin)	Animal products: meat, fish, poultry, shellfish, milk, cheese, eggs; nutritional yeast.	Helps maintain nerve cells; red blood cell formation; synthesis of genetic material.	Anemia, smooth tongue, fatigue, nerve degeneration progressing to paralysis.	None reported.
Pantothenic acid	Widespread in foods.	Coenzyme in energy metabolism.	Rare; sleep disturbances, nausea, fatigue.	Occasional diarrhea.
Biotin	Widespread in foods.	Coenzyme in energy metabolism; fat synthesis; glycogen formation.	Loss of appetite, nausea, depression, muscle pain, weakness, fatigue, rash.	None reported.

continued

TABLE 6–1
continued

VITAMIN (CHEMICAL NAME)	BEST SOURCES	CHIEF ROLES	DEFICIENCY SYMPTOMS	TOXICITY SYMPTOMS
WATER-SOLUBLE VITAMINS				
Vitamin C (ascorbic acid)	Citrus fruits, cabbage-type vegetables, tomatoes, potatoes, dark green vegetables, peppers, lettuce, cantaloupe, strawberries, mangos, papayas.	Synthesis of collagen (helps heal wounds, maintains bone and teeth, strengthens blood vessels); antioxidant; strengthens resistance to infection; helps body absorb iron.	Scurvy: anemia, atherosclerotic plaques, depression, frequent infections, bleeding gums, loosened teeth, pinpoint hemorrhages, muscle degeneration, rough skin, bone fragility, poor wound healing, hysteria.	Nausea, abdominal cramps, diarrhea, nosebleeds, breakdown of red blood cells in persons with certain genetic disorders; deficiency symptoms may appear at first on withdrawal of high doses.
FAT-SOLUBLE VITAMINS				
Vitamin A	*Retinal:* fortified milk and margarine, cream, cheese, butter, eggs, liver. *Beta-carotene:* Spinach and other dark leafy greens, broccoli, deep orange fruits (apricots, peaches, cantaloupe), and vegetables (squash, carrots, sweet potatoes, pumpkin).	Vision; growth and repair of body tissues; reproduction; bone and tooth formation; immunity; hormone synthesis; antioxidant (in the form of beta-carotene only).	Night blindness, rough skin, susceptibility to infection, impaired bone growth, abnormal tooth and jaw alignment, eye problems leading to blindness, impaired growth.	Red blood cell breakage, nosebleeds, abdominal cramps, nausea, diarrhea, weight loss, blurred vision, irritability, loss of appetite, bone pain, dry skin, rashes, hair loss, cessation of menstruation, growth retardation; liver disease.
Vitamin D (cholecalciferol)	Self-synthesis with sunlight; fortified milk, fortified margarine, eggs, liver, fish.	Calcium and phosphorus metabolism (bone and tooth formation); aids body's absorption of calcium.	Rickets in children; osteomalacia in adults; abnormal growth, joint pain, soft bones.	Raised blood calcium, constipation, weight loss, irritability, weakness, nausea, kidney stones, mental and physical retardation.
Vitamin E	Vegetable oils, green leafy vegetables, wheat germ, whole-grain products, butter, liver, egg yolk, milk fat, nuts, seeds.	Protects red blood cells; antioxidant (protects fat-soluble vitamins); stabilization of cell membranes.	Muscle wasting, weakness, red blood cell breakage, anemia, hemorrhaging.	General discomfort.
Vitamin K	Bacterial synthesis in digestive tract, liver, green leafy and cabbage-type vegetables, milk.	Synthesis of blood-clotting proteins and a blood protein that regulates blood calcium.	Hemorrhaging.	May cause jaundice.

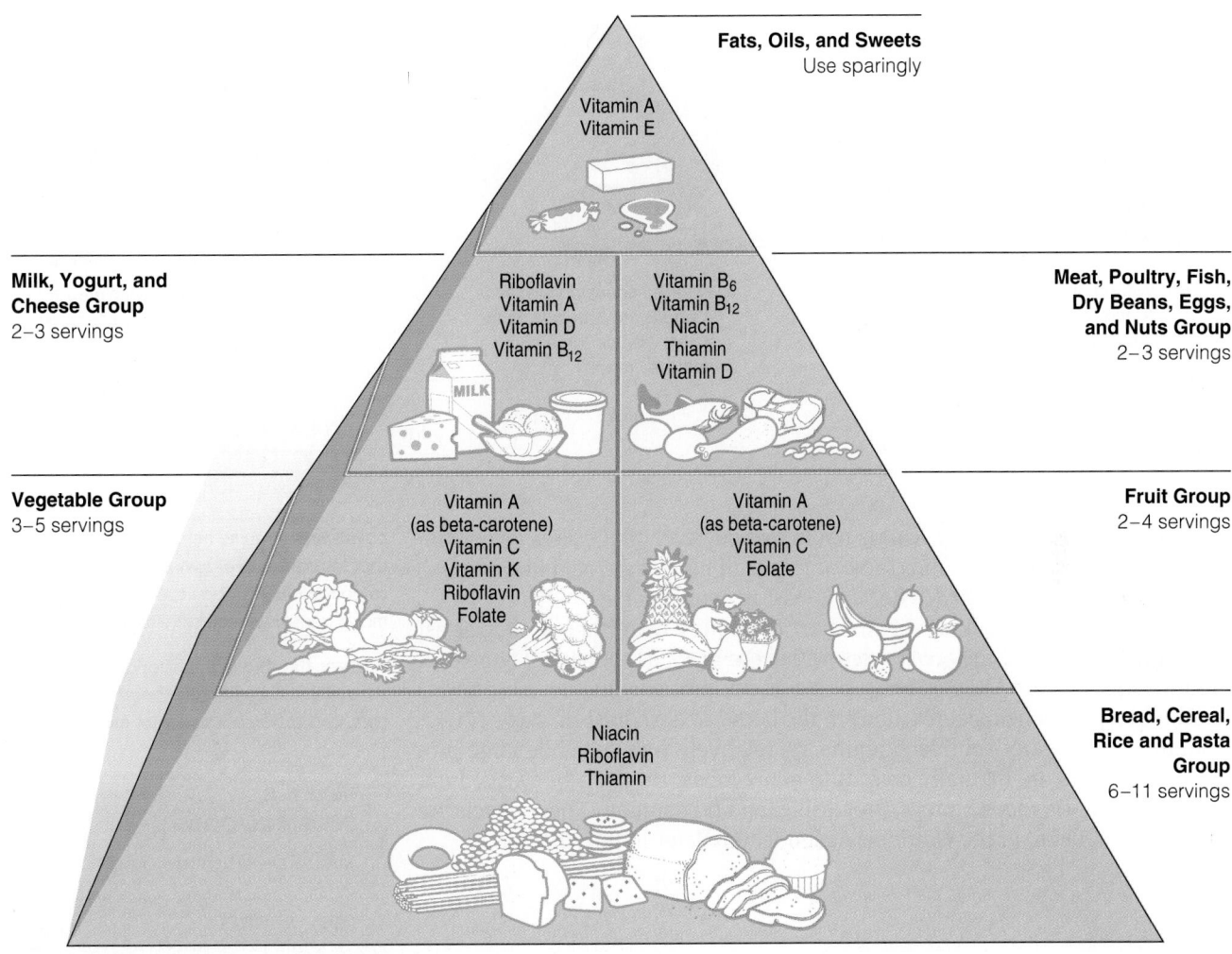

Milk, Yogurt, and Cheese Group
2–3 servings

Vegetable Group
3–5 servings

Fats, Oils, and Sweets
Use sparingly

Vitamin A
Vitamin E

Riboflavin
Vitamin A
Vitamin D
Vitamin B$_{12}$

Vitamin B$_6$
Vitamin B$_{12}$
Niacin
Thiamin
Vitamin D

MILK

Vitamin A
(as beta-carotene)
Vitamin C
Vitamin K
Riboflavin
Folate

Vitamin A
(as beta-carotene)
Vitamin C
Folate

Niacin
Riboflavin
Thiamin

Meat, Poultry, Fish, Dry Beans, Eggs, and Nuts Group
2–3 servings

Fruit Group
2–4 servings

Bread, Cereal, Rice and Pasta Group
6–11 servings

FIGURE 6–1
GOOD SOURCES OF VITAMINS IN THE FOOD GUIDE PYRAMID

groups in the Food Guide Pyramid supplies a number of vitamins. Eating plans that exclude entire food groups, or fail to include the minimum number of servings from each of the groups, may lead to vitamin deficiencies over time.

Water-Soluble Vitamins

There are nine water-soluble vitamins: eight B vitamins and vitamin C. Found in the watery compartments of foods, such as the juice of an orange, these vitamins are distributed into water-filled compartments of the body, including the fluid that surrounds the spinal cord. The body excretes water-soluble vitamins if the blood levels rise too high. As a result, they rarely

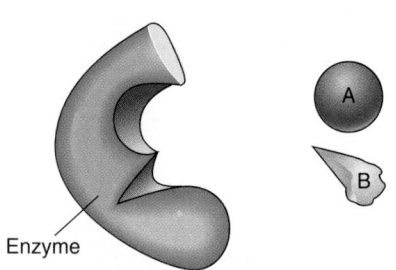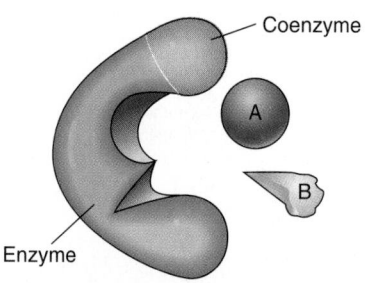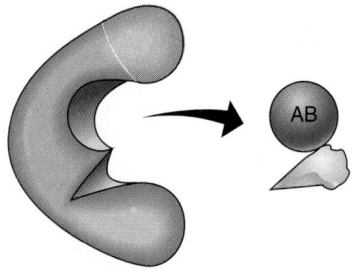

Without the coenzyme, compounds A and B don't respond to the enzyme.

With the coenzyme in place, A and B are attracted to the active side on the enzyme, and they react.

The reaction is completed. A new product, AB, has been formed.

FIGURE 6–2
HOW A COENZYME WORKS

reach toxic levels in the body. This is not to say, however, that excess levels cannot cause problems. Consuming large amounts of most water-soluble vitamins has been shown to have toxic effects, at least in some people.

In the body, water-soluble vitamins act as **coenzymes**—that is, they assist enzymes in doing their metabolic work within the body, as shown in Figure 6–2. (You may recall from Chapter 5 that enzymes are proteins that act as catalysts that help to boost chemical reactions in the body, as described on page 171.)

In foods, the water-soluble vitamins are relatively fragile. While large proportions of them are naturally present in many foods, they can be washed out or destroyed during food storage, processing, and preparation. These effects are spelled out in detail in the Nutrition Action feature later in this chapter.

Thiamin

One of the B vitamins, thiamin acts primarily as a coenzyme in reactions that release energy from carbohydrate. It also plays a crucial role in processes involving the nerves. So vital is thiamin to the functioning of the entire body that a deficiency affects the nerves, muscles, heart, and other organs. A severe deficiency, called **beriberi,** causes extreme wasting and loss of muscle tissue, swelling all over the body, enlargement of the heart, irregular heartbeat, and paralysis. Ultimately, the victim dies from heart failure. A mild thiamin deficiency, on the other hand, often mimics other conditions and typically manifests itself as vague, general symptoms such as stomachaches, headaches, fatigue, restlessness, sleep disturbances, chest pains, fevers, personality changes (aggressiveness and hostility), and neurosis.

Thiamin is found in a wide variety of foods, and virtually no single food will supply your daily needs in a single serving the way, say, an orange provides a plentiful supply of vitamin C. But people who eat a balanced diet that follows the framework of the Dietary Guidelines and/or the Food Guide Pyramid typically take in plenty of thiamin. As Table 6–2 shows, thiamin is found in a variety of meats, legumes, fruits, and vegetables.

COENZYMES enzyme helpers; small molecules that interact with enzymes and enable them to do their work. Many coenzymes are made from water-soluble vitamins.

BERIBERI the thiamin deficiency disease, characterized by irregular heartbeat, paralysis, and extreme wasting of muscle tissue.

TABLE 6–2
THIAMIN IN FOODS

Adult RDA is 1.0 to 1.5 mg.

(MG)	SOURCES
0.89	Ham, canned roasted (3 oz)
0.87	Pork chop (3 oz)
0.80	Sirloin steak (3 oz)
0.41	Sunflower seeds (2 tbsp)
0.39	Canadian bacon (2 pieces)
0.39	Watermelon (1" by 10" slice)
0.23	Green peas (½ c)
0.22	Baked potato (1)
0.21	Black beans (½ c)
0.21	Peanuts (⅓ c)
0.17	Black-eyed peas (½ c)
0.14	Kidney beans (½ c)
0.13	Oatmeal, cooked (½ c)
0.11	Asparagus, cooked (½ c)
0.11	Orange (1)
0.11	Whole-wheat bread (1 slice)
0.10	Cantaloupe (½)
0.09	Brown rice, cooked (½ c)
0.09	Nonfat milk (1 c)
0.05	Broccoli, cooked (½ c)

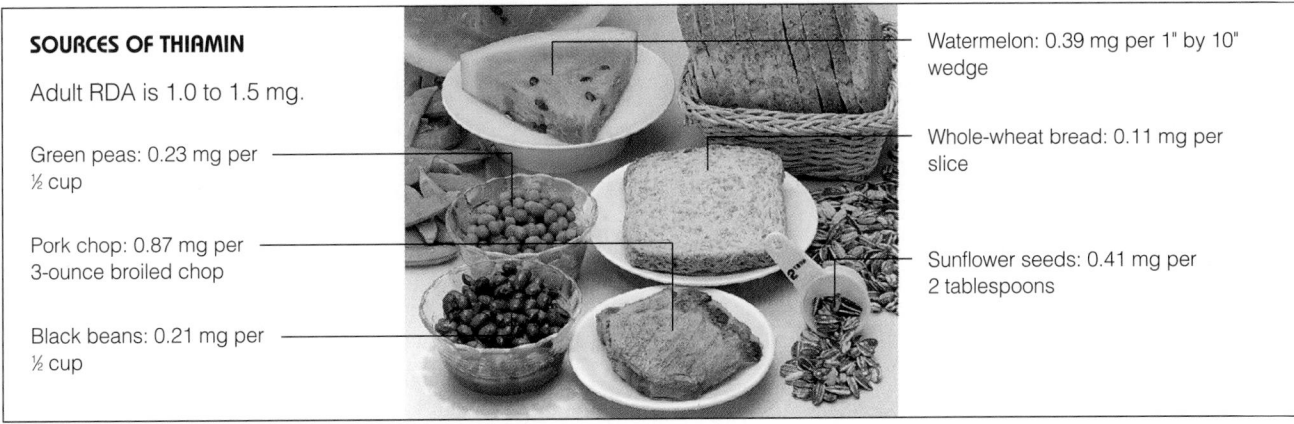

SOURCES OF THIAMIN

Adult RDA is 1.0 to 1.5 mg.

Green peas: 0.23 mg per ½ cup

Pork chop: 0.87 mg per 3-ounce broiled chop

Black beans: 0.21 mg per ½ cup

Watermelon: 0.39 mg per 1" by 10" wedge

Whole-wheat bread: 0.11 mg per slice

Sunflower seeds: 0.41 mg per 2 tablespoons

Riboflavin

Like thiamin, the B vitamin called riboflavin acts as a coenzyme in energy-releasing reactions in the body. In addition, riboflavin helps to prepare fatty acids and amino acids for breakdown. Deficiencies of the vitamin, which are rare, are characterized by severe skin problems, including painful cracks at the corners of the mouth; a red, swollen tongue; and teary or bloodshot eyes.

Table 6–3 shows the riboflavin content of foods. Milk and dairy products contribute a good deal of the riboflavin in most people's diet. Meats are another good source, as are dark green vegetables such as broccoli. Leafy green vegetables and whole-grain or enriched bread and cereal products also supply a generous amount of riboflavin in most people's diets.

Note that riboflavin can be destroyed by the ultraviolet rays of the sun or fluorescent lamps. That's why milk is usually sold in protective cardboard or opaque plastic containers rather than in transparent glass bottles.

Niacin

Like thiamin and riboflavin, the B vitamin niacin is part of a coenzyme vital to obtaining energy. Without niacin to form this coenzyme, energy-yielding reactions come to a halt. Over time, a deficiency of niacin leads to the disease pellagra, characterized by diarrhea, dermatitis, and, in severe cases, dementia—a progressive mental deterioration resulting in delirium, mania, or depression.

While niacin deficiency can be prevented by eating a diet rich in niacin itself, consuming plenty of protein also staves off the problem. That's because the essential amino acid tryptophan, which is a component of protein, can be converted to niacin in the body. In fact, 60 milligrams of tryptophan yield one milligram of niacin. Thus, the RDA for niacin is expressed in **niacin equivalents (NEs)**—that is, the amount of niacin present in food, including the amount that can be theoretically made from the tryptophan in the food.

TABLE 6–3
RIBOFLAVIN IN FOODS

Adult RDA is 1.2 to 1.7 mg.

(MG)	SOURCES
3.52	Beef liver (3 oz)
0.42	Low-fat cottage cheese (1 c)
0.37	Almonds (⅓ c)
0.34	Nonfat milk (1 c)
0.24	Pork chop (3 oz)
0.23	Mushroom pieces, ckd, (½ c)
0.23	Ricotta cheese, part-skim (½ c)
0.23	Sirloin steak (3 oz)
0.21	Beet greens, cooked (½ c)
0.21	Poached egg (1)
0.21	Spinach, cooked (½ c)
0.20	Ground beef (3 oz)
0.17	Cheddar cheese (1.5 oz)
0.16	Turkey (3 oz)
0.11	Asparagus, cooked (½ c)
0.10	Strawberries (1 c)
0.08	Broccoli, cooked (½ c)
0.08	Smoked salmon (3 oz)
0.08	Whole-wheat bread (1 slice)
0.05	Black-eyed peas (½ c)
0.05	Chicken breast (½)

NIACIN EQUIVALENTS (NEs) the amount of niacin present in food, including the niacin that can theoretically be made from tryptophan contained in the food.

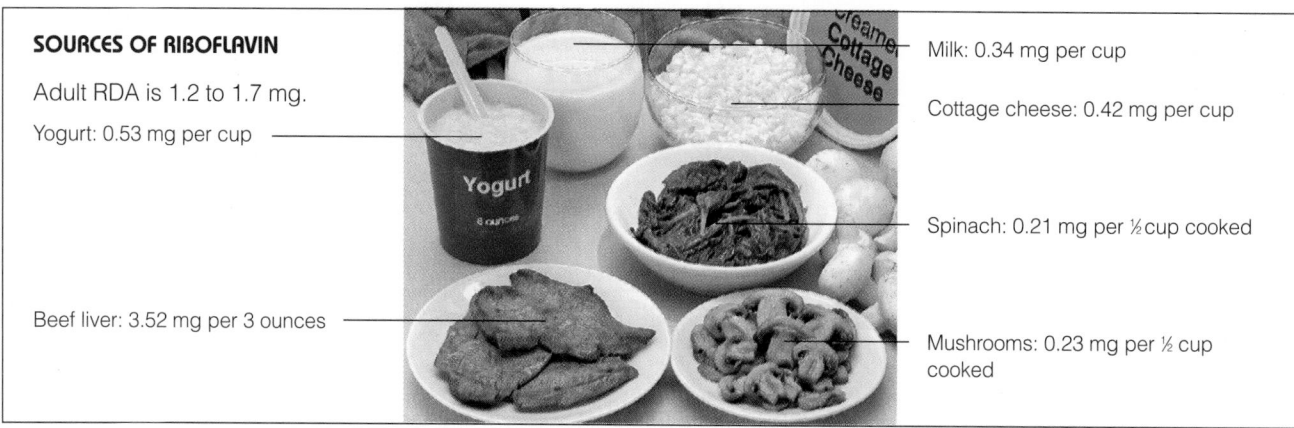

SOURCES OF RIBOFLAVIN

Adult RDA is 1.2 to 1.7 mg.

Yogurt: 0.53 mg per cup

Beef liver: 3.52 mg per 3 ounces

Milk: 0.34 mg per cup

Cottage cheese: 0.42 mg per cup

Spinach: 0.21 mg per ½ cup cooked

Mushrooms: 0.23 mg per ½ cup cooked

Milk, eggs, meat, poultry, and fish contribute most of the niacin equivalents consumed by most people, followed by enriched breads and cereals. Table 6–4 shows the niacin content of some common foods.

Diet aside, in recent years, niacin has been increasingly used as a druglike supplement to help lower cholesterol. Doses ranging from 10 to 15 times the RDA have been shown to reduce "bad" LDL-cholesterol and raise "good" HDL-cholesterol. The hitch, however, is that such high doses of niacin can lead to side effects such as nausea, flushing of the skin, rash, fatigue, and liver damage. Because of the side effects, many experts argue that niacin pills should be sold not as over-the-counter dietary supplements but rather as drugs prescribed and taken only while under a physician's supervision.[3]

Folate

Folate (also called folic acid or folacin*) is a coenzyme with many functions in the body. It is particularly important in the synthesis of DNA and the formation of red blood cells. A deficiency makes the red blood cells misshapen and unable to carry sufficient oxygen to all the body's other cells, thereby causing a certain kind of **anemia.** Thus, folate deficiency results in a kind of generalized malaise with many symptoms, including fatigue, diarrhea, irritability, forgetfulness, lack of appetite, and headache. Folate deficiency can easily be confused with general ill health, depressed mood, and senility in the elderly.

Folate deficiency tends to occur in people who eat few fresh vegetables, because folate is easily lost when foods are overcooked, canned, dehydrated, or otherwise processed. In addition, people who are growing rapidly run a high risk of folate deficiency because folate is needed to promote the rapid multiplication of cells that occurs during growth. That's why, for

---

*The folates are a group of chemically related compounds; folic acid is the biologically active form of the molecule, that is, the form used by the body to perform various functions. The term *folacin* is no longer widely used.

TABLE 6–4
NIACIN IN FOODS

Adult RDA is 13 to 19 mg NE.

(MG NE)	SOURCES
11.80	Chicken breast (½)
11.30	Tuna (3 oz)
6.57	Peanuts (⅓ c)
6.05	Halibut (3 oz)
5.57	Pink salmon (3 oz)
5.08	Ground beef (3 oz)
4.63	Turkey (3 oz)
4.37	Pork chop (3 oz)
3.31	Baked potato (1)
3.29	Sirloin steak (3 oz)
2.22	Shrimp (3 oz)
1.85	Flounder/sole (3 oz)
1.53	Cantaloupe (½)
1.49	Brown rice, cooked (½ c)
1.13	Whole-wheat bread (1 slice)
0.97	Asparagus, cooked (½ c)
0.89	Broccoli, cooked (½ c)
0.86	Peach (1)
0.59	Kidney beans (½ c)
0.44	Spinach, cooked (½ c)
0.15	Oatmeal, cooked (½ c)

ANEMIA any condition in which the blood is unable to deliver oxygen to the cells of the body. Examples include a shortage or abnormality of the red blood cells. Many nutrient deficiencies and diseases can cause anemia.

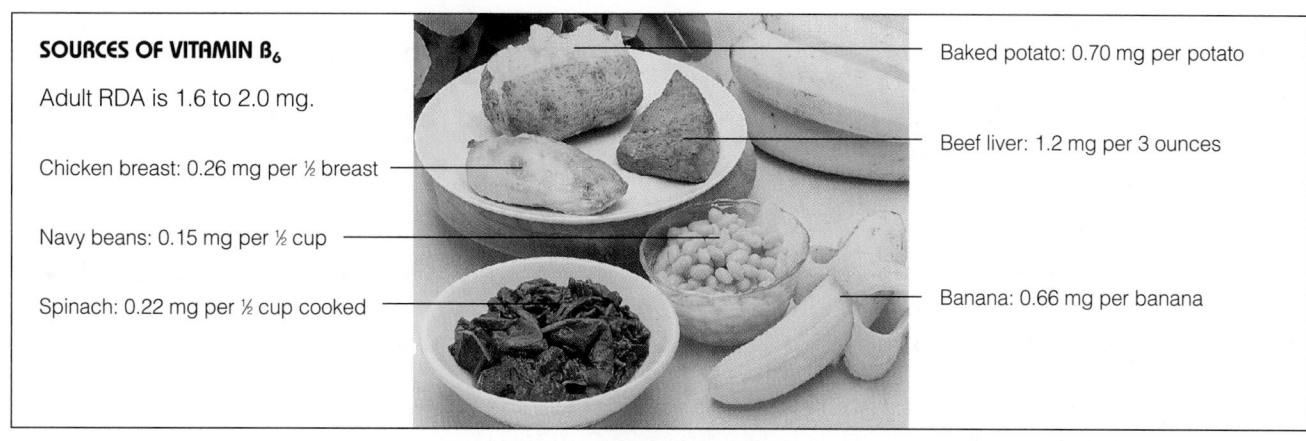

SOURCES OF VITAMIN B₆

Adult RDA is 1.6 to 2.0 mg.

Chicken breast: 0.26 mg per ½ breast

Navy beans: 0.15 mg per ½ cup

Spinach: 0.22 mg per ½ cup cooked

Baked potato: 0.70 mg per potato

Beef liver: 1.2 mg per 3 ounces

Banana: 0.66 mg per banana

Vitamin B_6 is also widely reputed as a cure for **premenstrual syndrome (PMS).** Some people have claimed that a deficiency of the vitamin goes hand in hand with imbalances of hormones, particularly estrogen, which cause the depression, mood swings, and other symptoms characteristic of PMS. Although this theory has never been proven to be scientifically sound, women have taken **megadoses** of B_6—as much as 2,000 times the RDA in some cases—in an effort to treat PMS. But in 1983, a number of these women began to experience symptoms associated with damage to the nervous system, such as loss of sensation in the hands and mouth.[6] Granted, not everyone is likely to suffer toxicity symptoms as a result of swallowing megadoses of vitamin B_6, because excess amounts are excreted in the urine. But the problems seen in women who take these megadoses underscore the potential hazards of taking megadoses of any vitamin or nutritional supplement.

Vitamin B_{12}

Vitamin B_{12} maintains the sheaths that surround and protect nerve fibers. The nutrient also works closely with folate, enabling it to manufacture red blood cells. When a B_{12} deficiency is present, folate is unable to do its work building red blood cells. As a result, a person suffering a lack of vitamin B_{12} ends up with the same sort of anemia seen in people with a folate deficiency and characterized by large, immature red blood cells. While extra folate will clear up the anemia, it will not take care of the other problems resulting from a B_{12} deficiency, namely a creeping paralysis of the nerves and muscles that can cause permanent nerve damage if left untreated. Thus, because excess folate can clear up the blood problems that signal an otherwise hard-to-diagnose vitamin B_{12} deficiency, the amount of folate in over-the-counter supplements is limited by law to an amount that is too low to cover up a B_{12} deficiency. Folate's ability to mask vitamin B_{12} deficiencies is another reason why experts are wary of advocating widespread fortification of foods with folic acid, as discussed earlier.

To be sure, dietary deficiencies of vitamin B_{12} are not likely to occur among people who eat animal foods such as meat, milk, cheese, and eggs, all of which supply generous amounts of the nutrient (see Table 6–7). Strict vegetarians who

PREMENSTRUAL SYNDROME (PMS) a cluster of physical, emotional, and psychological symptoms that some women experience seven to ten days before menstruating. Symptoms can include acne, anxiety, food cravings (especially for sweets), back pain, breast tenderness, cramps, depression, fatigue, headaches, irritability, moodiness, water retention, and weight gain. Because a clear-cut treatment for the symptoms of PMS has not been identified, women who suffer from the problem rank as prime targets for unproved nutritional remedies for the condition.

MEGADOSE a dose of ten or more times the amount normally recommended in the RDA. An overdose is an amount high enough to cause toxicity symptoms. Megadoses taken over a long period often result in an overdose.

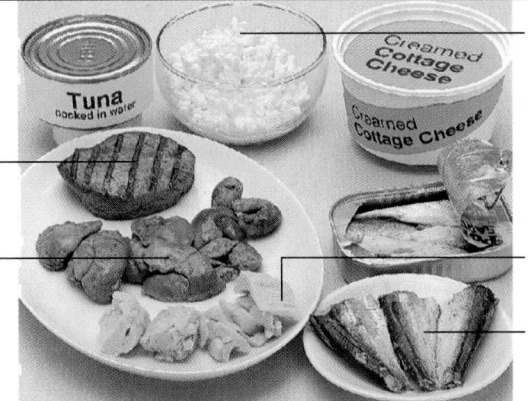

SOURCES OF VITAMIN B$_{12}$

Adult RDA is 2.0 μg.

Sirloin steak: 2.4 μg per 3 ounces

Chicken liver: 16.62 μg per 3 ounces

Cottage cheese: 1.43 μg per cup

Tuna (in water): 2.54 μg per 3 ounces

Sardines: 7.61 μg per 3 ounces

eschew meat, eggs, and dairy products, however, need to find alternative sources of the nutrient, such as vitamin B$_{12}$-fortified soy beverages or B$_{12}$ supplements.

Several other groups of people are also at high risk for vitamin B$_{12}$ deficiency, not because of a lack of the vitamin in their diets but because of physical conditions that hamper their body's ability to make use of the nutrient. One such group is people who inherit a genetic defect that leaves the body unable to make a compound known as **intrinsic factor.** Produced in the stomach, intrinsic factor enables the body to absorb and make use of vitamin B$_{12}$; without the compound, vitamin B$_{12}$ deficiency develops. In this instance or in the case of stomach damage that interferes with the production of intrinsic factor, people must get vitamin B$_{12}$ injections.

Another group likely to experience vitamin B$_{12}$ deficiencies is the elderly. An estimated 20 percent of seniors in their sixties and 40 percent in their eighties develop **atrophic gastritis,** an age-related condition characterized by the stomach's inability to produce enough acid, which in turn hampers the body's ability to use vitamin B$_{12}$. In severe cases, the condition also limits the stomach's ability to make intrinsic factor. Vitamin B$_{12}$ deficiencies resulting from atrophic gastritis appear to be easily treated with vitamin B$_{12}$ supplements or injections.[7]

Older adults whose diets lack not only vitamin B$_{12}$ but also vitamin B$_6$ and folate appear to suffer other serious health consequences. People with low blood levels of these B vitamins tend to have high blood levels of a chemical called **homocysteine,** which seems to raise the risk of suffering a

TABLE 6-7
VITAMIN B12 IN FOODS

Adult RDA is 2.0 μg.

(μG)	SOURCES
16.62	Chicken liver (3 oz)
7.61	Sardines (3 oz)
2.54	Tuna (3 oz)
2.01	Ground beef (3 oz)
1.43	Cottage cheese (1 c)
1.39	Plain nonfat yogurt (1 c)
1.27	Shrimp (3 oz)
1.18	Haddock (3 oz)
0.93	Nonfat milk (1 c)
0.50	Egg (1)
0.35	Cheddar cheese (1.5 oz)
0.29	Chicken breast (½)

INTRINSIC FACTOR a compound made in the stomach that is necessary for the body's absorption of vitamin B$_{12}$.

ATROPHIC GASTRITIS an age-related condition characterized by the stomach's inability to produce acid, which in turn leads to vitamin B$_{12}$ deficiencies. In severe cases, the condition limits the ability to make intrinsic factor as well.

HOMOCYSTEINE a chemical that appears to be toxic to the blood vessels of the heart. High blood levels of homocysteine have been associated with low blood levels of vitamin B$_{12}$, vitamin B$_6$, and folate.

heart attack or stroke as much as four-fold.[8] While still in its early stages, the research linking a vitamin B-poor diet with increased homocysteine levels highlights the importance of consuming generous amounts of these nutrients.

Finally, preliminary research suggests that some women have an inability to make sufficient amounts of a particular enzyme, called methionine synthase, after ingesting vitamin B_{12} and folic acid. This enzyme is needed to ensure proper development of fetuses and prevent neural tube defects. If confirmed by additional research, the evidence indicates that consumption of large amounts of both folic acid and vitamin B_{12} might boost enzyme levels and help stave off birth defects among women at risk.[9]

Pantothenic Acid and Biotin

Two other B vitamins—pantothenic acid and biotin—are needed for the synthesis of coenzymes that are active in a multitude of body systems. Biotin is also required for cell growth, synthesis of DNA (the genetic "blueprint" present in every cell), and maintenance of blood glucose (sugar) levels. Because both pantothenic acid and biotin are widespread in foods, people who eat a varied diet are not at risk for deficiencies.

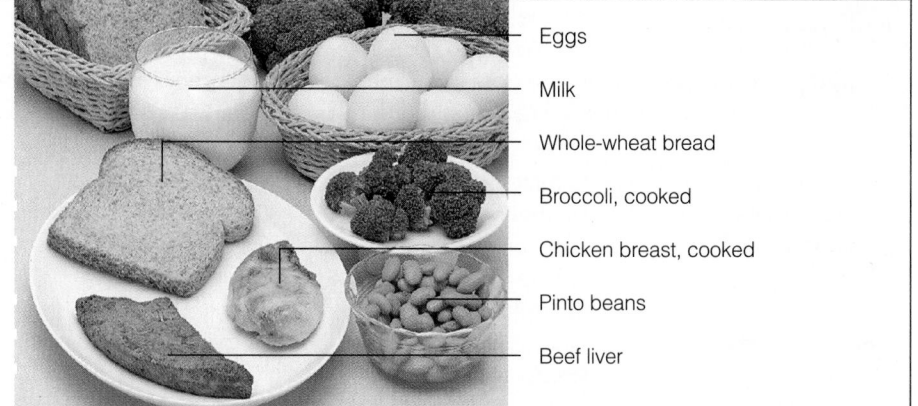

**SOURCES OF BIOTIN
AND PANTOTHENIC ACID***

Estimated safe and adequate
intake for adults:
    Biotin: 30–100 µg
    Pantothenic acid: 4–7 mg

*Information concerning biotin
and pantothenic acid in foods is
incomplete: deficiencies are rare.

Eggs
Milk
Whole-wheat bread
Broccoli, cooked
Chicken breast, cooked
Pinto beans
Beef liver

Vitamin C

Vitamin C is required for the production and maintenance of **collagen,**
the protein foundation material for the body's connective tissue, including
bones, teeth, skin, and tendons. Vitamin C also boosts the body's ability to
fight infections, and a growing body of research suggests that it may protect
against heart disease and certain types of cancer.[10] Vitamin C's potential role
as a chronic-disease fighter stems from its workings as an antioxidant,
described in detail in the Spotlight featuring antioxidants at the end of the
chapter.

COLLAGEN the characteristic protein of
connective tissue.
    kolla = glue
    gennan = to produce

Vitamin C has also been touted as a nutrient that can help fight stress. And
it's true that in times of stress, the body uses more vitamin C than usual
because the vitamin is involved in the release of stress hormones. Still, the
amount of extra vitamin C used as a result of, say, on-the-job
deadline stress or the stress of ending a significant relationship, is minuscule and is more than accounted for by a diet
that regularly includes vitamin C-rich foods. Special "stress
formula" vitamins are unnecessary, given that they contain
much more of those nutrients than are required. (For more
on stress, see the Nutrition Action feature in Chapter 9.)

Of course, vitamin C is most famous for its long-standing
notoriety as a cure for the common cold. Ever since the publication of the controversial book *Vitamin C and the
Common Cold* by the award-winning scientist Linus Pauling,
millions of Americans have followed Dr. Pauling's advice
and swallowed megadoses of vitamin C—sometimes exceeding 30 times the RDA for the nutrient.[11] Despite the popularity of vitamin C as a cold remedy, however, many carefully controlled studies have shown that it plays an
insignificant, if indeed it plays any, role in preventing colds.
At best, the nutrient may slightly reduce the severity of cold
symptoms in some people.

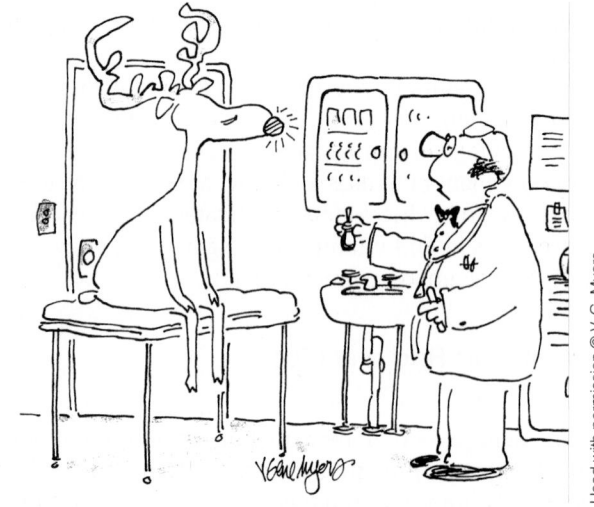

"A little vitamin C ought to clear that up in no time."

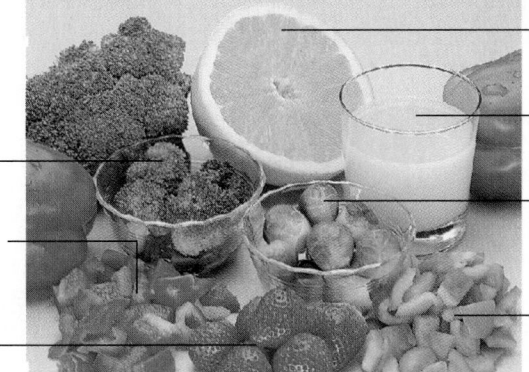

SOURCES OF VITAMIN C

Adult RDA is 60 mg.

Broccoli: 58 mg per ½ cup cooked

Sweet red pepper: 95 mg per ½ cup fresh

Strawberries: 42 mg per ½ cup

Grapefruit: 39 mg per ½ grapefruit

Orange juice: 93 mg per ¾ cup

Brussels sprouts: 48 mg per ½ cup cooked

Green pepper: 45 mg per ½ cup fresh

To be sure, many people swear by vitamin C, and it may be that their belief in the nutrient is so strong that they experience a placebo effect as a result of their faith in its curative powers. Still, people would be wise to take vitamin C with care. Cold sufferers who are not accustomed to taking megadoses of vitamin C and then do so when the sniffles begin may end up feeling worse. That's because large amounts of vitamin C can cause side effects such as nausea, abdominal cramps, diarrhea, and nosebleeds.[12]

Pills aside, vitamin C-rich foods are widely available in the United States and include not only oranges and other citrus fruits but also broccoli, Brussels sprouts, cantaloupe, and strawberries (see Table 6–8). A single serving of any of those foods provides more than half the RDA for the vitamin. Potatoes also contribute significant amounts of vitamin C to the American diet because they are eaten so often. Note that vitamins C and A are the only vitamins required to appear on the Nutrition Facts panel of the food label (see Figure 6–3).

Vitamin C is widespread in the food supply. Still, deficiencies occasionally arise both in infants not given a source of vitamin C (see Table 10–5 on page 380) and in the elderly, due to inadequate consumption of fruits and vegetables.

TABLE 6–8
VITAMIN C IN FOODS

Adult RDA is 60 mg.

(MG)	SOURCES
187	Papaya (1)
113	Cantaloupe (½)
93	Orange juice, fresh (¾ c)
71	Grapefruit juice (¾ c)
70	Orange (1)
66	Green pepper (1)
58	Broccoli, cooked (½ c)
57	Mango (1)
48	Brussels sprouts, ckd (½ c)
47	Pink/red Grapefruit (½)
46	Watermelon (1" by 10" slice)
42	Strawberries (½ c)
27	Cauliflower, cooked (½ c)
26	Baked potato (1)
22	Bok choy, cooked (½ c)
22	Cabbage, raw (1 c)
22	Tomato, fresh (1)
16	Raspberries (½ c)
12	Pineapple, fresh (½ c)
10	Asparagus, cooked (½ c)
9	Spinach, cooked (½ c)

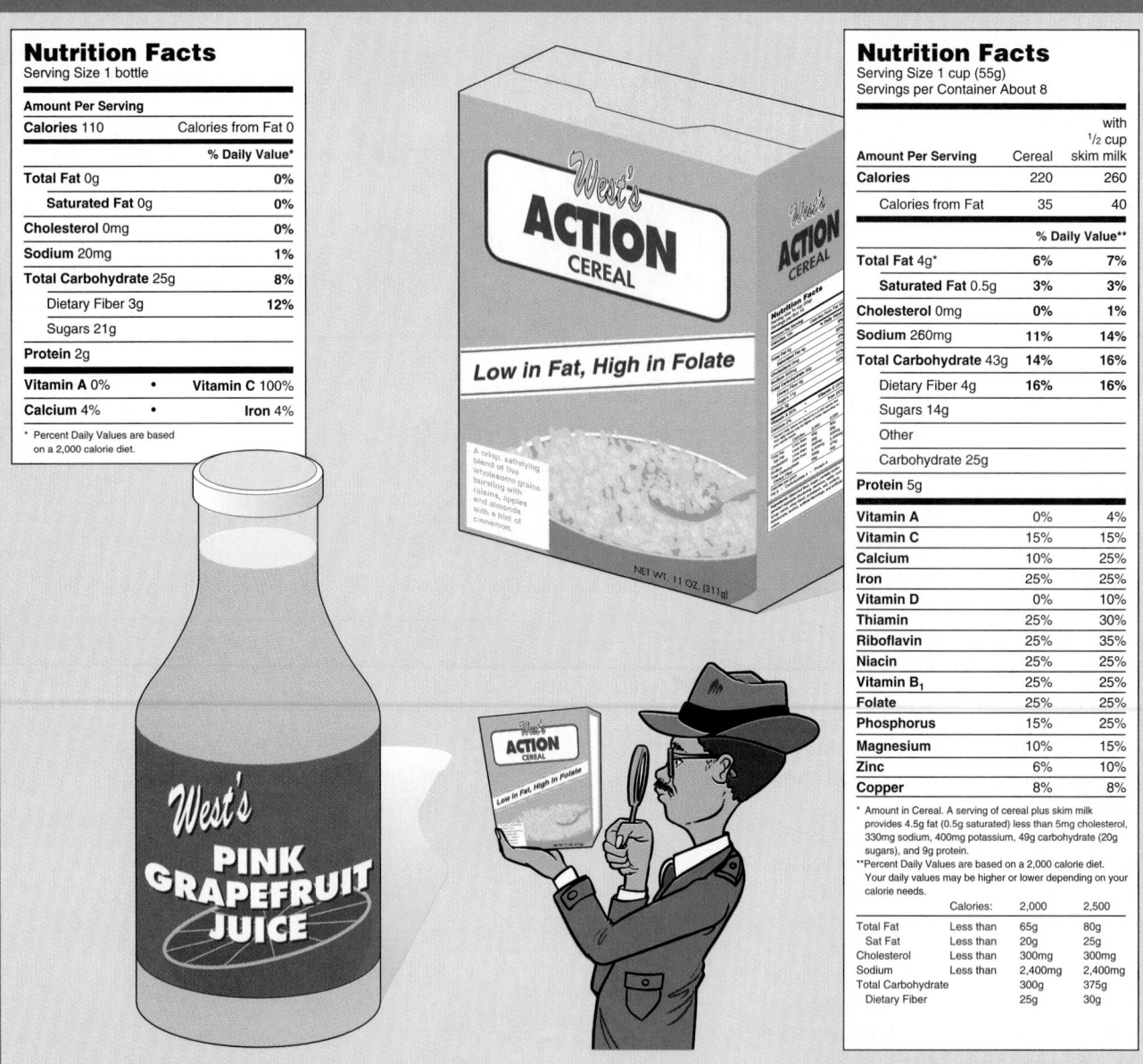

Nutrition Facts
Serving Size 1 bottle

Amount Per Serving

Calories 110	Calories from Fat 0

	% Daily Value*
Total Fat 0g	0%
Saturated Fat 0g	0%
Cholesterol 0mg	0%
Sodium 20mg	1%
Total Carbohydrate 25g	8%
Dietary Fiber 3g	12%
Sugars 21g	
Protein 2g	

Vitamin A 0%	•	Vitamin C 100%
Calcium 4%	•	Iron 4%

* Percent Daily Values are based on a 2,000 calorie diet.

Low in Fat, High in Folate

NET WT. 11 OZ. (311g)

Nutrition Facts
Serving Size 1 cup (55g)
Servings per Container About 8

Amount Per Serving	Cereal	with ½ cup skim milk
Calories	220	260
Calories from Fat	35	40
	% Daily Value**	
Total Fat 4g*	6%	7%
Saturated Fat 0.5g	3%	3%
Cholesterol 0mg	0%	1%
Sodium 260mg	11%	14%
Total Carbohydrate 43g	14%	16%
Dietary Fiber 4g	16%	16%
Sugars 14g		
Other		
Carbohydrate 25g		
Protein 5g		
Vitamin A	0%	4%
Vitamin C	15%	15%
Calcium	10%	25%
Iron	25%	25%
Vitamin D	0%	10%
Thiamin	25%	30%
Riboflavin	25%	35%
Niacin	25%	25%
Vitamin B₁	25%	25%
Folate	25%	25%
Phosphorus	15%	25%
Magnesium	10%	15%
Zinc	6%	10%
Copper	8%	8%

* Amount in Cereal. A serving of cereal plus skim milk provides 4.5g fat (0.5g saturated) less than 5mg cholesterol, 330mg sodium, 400mg potassium, 49g carbohydrate (20g sugars), and 9g protein.
**Percent Daily Values are based on a 2,000 calorie diet. Your daily values may be higher or lower depending on your calorie needs.

	Calories:	2,000	2,500
Total Fat	Less than	65g	80g
Sat Fat	Less than	20g	25g
Cholesterol	Less than	300mg	300mg
Sodium	Less than	2,400mg	2,400mg
Total Carbohydrate		300g	375g
Dietary Fiber		25g	30g

FIGURE 6–3
CHECKING OUT THE FOOD LABEL FOR VITAMINS

The only vitamins required to appear on the Nutrition Facts panel are vitamins A and C, as shown on the label of grapefruit juice. If a manufacturer makes a nutrition claim about another vitamin, however, the amount of that nutrient in a serving of the product must also be stated on the panel.

For instance, the cereal shown is touted as "High in Folate," so the percentage of the Reference Daily Intake for folate in a serving of the cereal (25 percent) is stated on the label. The manufacturer has the option of listing any other nutrients as well. (For more information about Reference Daily Intakes, review the discussion in the Spotlight on food labels in Chapter 2.)

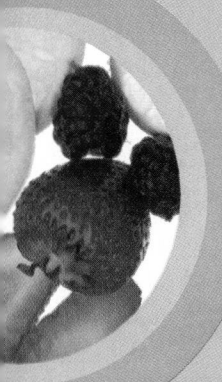

Vitamin Preservation

Buying vitamin-rich fruits and vegetables at the market is one of the first steps to obtaining plenty of those all-important nutrients in your diet. The next step is storing and cooking those foods in ways that minimize the loss of vitamins that can occur as a result of improper storage and preparation. To help get the most from the produce you buy, use the following tips on fruit and vegetable storage and preparation.

- Shop for produce at least once a week. The longer fruits and vegetables stay in your refrigerator before eating, the more nutrients that are likely to be lost. Table 6–9 shows the length of time that various fruits and vegetables can generally be refrigerated before their quality begins to deteriorate significantly.

- Store fruits and vegetables (other than bananas and potatoes) in your refrigerator rather than in a fruit bowl or on the kitchen counter. Chilling slows the metabolic rate of the cells of a fruit or vegetable, which in turn causes the cells to use less of the item's own nutrient supply. Thus, chilling prevents nutrient depletion.[13]

- Place potatoes in a basket or burlap or paper bag and store in a cool, dark place such as a cellar (the darkness will prevent the potatoes from greening). If you put potatoes in the refrigerator, do not keep them there for more than a day or two. Chilling causes the starch in the potato to turn to sugar, thereby altering its flavor and texture.[14]

- Store fruits and vegetables whole, peeling and cutting only what you need immediately before cooking or eating whenever possible. Once you cut into the skin of an item and expose it to air, vitamin loss begins. That's because the oxygen in the air causes a chemical reaction that "rusts" the produce (picture how brown an apple slice looks after an hour or two). After slicing, the vitamin C content of oranges, grapefruits, tomatoes, and strawberries begins to decline. If you do have leftover, cut produce, wrap it tightly in airtight plastic or store it in an airtight container inside the refrigerator. In addition, keep fruit juice in containers with tight-fitting lids; opened cans or bottles of fruit juice are susceptible to rapid vitamin loss.

- In the refrigerator, keep whole fruits and vegetables in perforated plastic bags. The perforated plastic allows some airflow while helping to maintain a moist environment, preventing produce from drying out. Thus, the bag creates an optimal environment for the preservation of the food's nutrients. Consider that water loss not only decreases the appeal of a fruit or vegetable but also may go hand in hand with nutrient loss.[15]

- Store frozen fruits and vegetables in a freezer kept at 0 degrees Fahrenheit (−17.7 degrees Centigrade) or less to ensure that they are solidly frozen

TABLE 6–9
RECOMMENDED STORAGE TIMES FOR REFRIGERATED FRUITS AND VEGETABLES

FRUITS	STORAGE TIME
Apples	3 to 8 months
Blueberries	2 weeks
Cherries	2 to 3 days
Lemons	3 weeks
Melons	3 to 5 days
Oranges	3 weeks
Peaches	3 to 5 days
Plums	3 to 5 days
Grapes	3 to 5 days
Strawberries	1 day

VEGETABLES	STORAGE TIME
Asparagus	2 to 3 days
Broccoli	3 to 5 days
Brussels sprouts	3 to 5 days
Celery	1 week
Cucumbers	1 week
Lettuce	1 week
Mushrooms	1 to 2 days
Peppers	1 week
Snap beans	7 days
Summer squash	3 to 5 days

*Times given are approximate. Note that the lower the refrigerator temperature, the longer the produce is likely to stay fresh.

SOURCE: Adapted from S. J. VanGarde and M. Woodburn, *Food Preservation and Safety: Principles and Practice* (Ames, Iowa: Iowa State University Press, 1994), p. 108.

and therefore retain their nutrients. To be sure, since the freezing process itself destroys few nutrients, the nutrient content of frozen foods is similar to that of fresh foods, provided they are stored properly. In fact, properly stored frozen foods often contain more nutrients by the time they reach the table than fresh fruits and vegetables that have been sitting in the supermarket for a day or two. Still, foods stored at temperatures higher than 0 degrees Fahrenheit may appear to be frozen on the exterior, but much of the interior may actually be partially thawed. In this unfrozen state, vitamin loss can occur quickly. To ensure that your freezer is sufficiently cold, buy a freezer thermometer and make sure its temperature is at or below 0 degrees Fahrenheit.

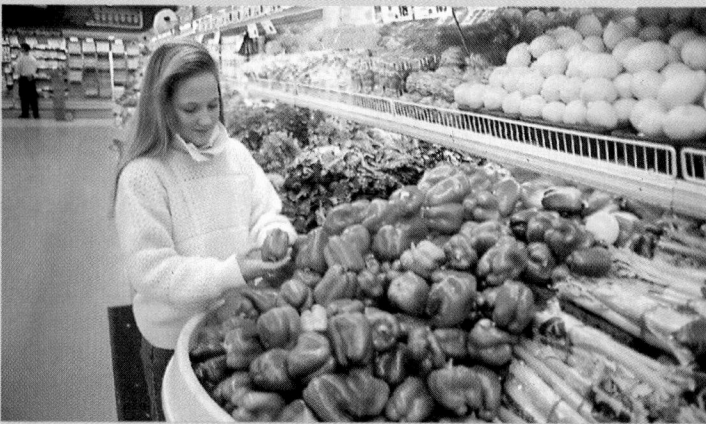

Once you've taken the time to select fresh, vitamin-rich vegetables, be sure to handle them with care when you get home.

- Try to eat frozen vegetables within a month or two of purchase. Although they will last in your freezer indefinitely, nutrient losses occur over time even in properly stored vegetables. For example, frozen vegetables such as snap beans, broccoli, cauliflower, and spinach can lose 60 percent to 75 percent of their vitamin C in a 0-degree Fahrenheit freezer over the course of a year.[16]

- If you prepare fresh vegetables for freezing at home, dip them in boiling water for a minute or two. This process, known as blanching, deactivates enzymes that would otherwise deplete the food's nutrients. Immediately dunk the vegetables in cold water to cool, place them in plastic containers with tight-fitting lids, and freeze.

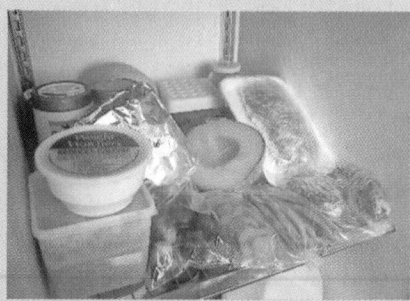

Wrap cut produce tightly to preserve its vitamin content.

- When it comes to freezing fruit, note that most varieties can be sliced and frozen in containers or freezer bags without any special preparation. However, light-colored varieties such as apples, bananas, pears, and peaches sometimes turn brown in the freezer. To help decrease the chances of discoloration, such fruits should be dipped in orange or lemon juice before freezing.[17]

- Don't throw away the liquid from canned vegetables. The liquid bathing the cut, canned vegetables leaches water-soluble vitamins as well as minerals such as calcium, iron, and phosphorus. Instead of getting rid of this nutrient-containing liquid, known as pot liquor, use it to make soups, cook rice, or moisten casseroles. The process used to can foods, incidentally, destroys some of the food's vitamins, such as thiamin, because during the canning process, when the food is heated to high temperatures to kill food-spoiling bacteria and yeast, heat-sensitive vitamins are also destroyed. This doesn't mean that canned foods have no place in the diet. Many vitamins hold up quite well under heat: riboflavin, niacin, vitamin D, and the vitamin A precursor, beta-carotene. Despite some nutrient losses, canned foods rank as convenient pantry stockers that provide essential nutrients year-round.[18]

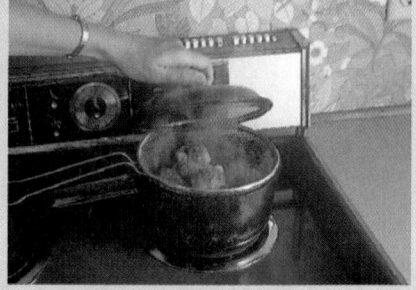

To preserve nutrients, don't boil vegetables. Instead, microwave cook them or steam them over small amounts of water.

- Cook vegetables in the least amount of water and for the shortest period of time possible. Water-soluble vitamins readily dissolve into cooking water, and heat destroys some as well. To minimize such losses, steam vegetables over water or boil or sauté them in very small amounts of water. Better yet, cook vegetables in a microwave oven for optimal nutrient retention. Because microwave cooking requires no water and a short heating period, few nutrient losses occur; the same goes for stir-frying. Table 6–10 compares nutrient retention in vegetables cooked using different methods, and Table 6–11 does the same for fruits.

- Plan to eat at least five servings of fruits and vegetables a day, regardless of the form in which you buy them. Remember that since the priority is to consume lots of fruits and vegetables, look for ways to do so that are realistic for your lifestyle and budget. In the best of all possible worlds, everyone would eat only vegetables purchased and prepared with optimal vitamin retention in mind. But that's not always possible. If you can't make it to the market every few days to buy fresh produce, don't give up fruits and vegetables altogether. Instead, keep canned, dried, and frozen alternatives on hand.

TABLE 6–10
COMPARISON OF NUTRIENT RETENTION IN VEGETABLES COOKED BY DIFFERENT METHODS

	% VITAMIN C	% BETA-CAROTENE	% FOLATE	% POTASSIUM
POTATOES				
Baked, broiled	80	90[a]	85	95
Microwave cooked[a]	100	95	100	95
TOMATOES				
Baked, broiled, or stewed	95	95	70	100
DARK GREEN LEAFY VEGETABLES				
Boiled	60	95	60	90
Microwave cooked[b]	25	100	100	80
ROOT, BULB, AND HIGH-STARCH VEGETABLES				
Boiled	70	90	70	90
Microwave cooked[c]	80	80	90	90
OTHER VEGETABLES				
Boiled	80	90	70	90

[a]Sweet potatoes.
[b]Spinach.
[c]Average retention values for carrots, green peas, lima beans, and squash.
SOURCE: Adapted from M. A. McCarthy and R. H. Matthews, *Conserving Nutrients in Foods*, Administrative Report No. 384 (Hyattsville, Md.: Nutrition Monitoring Division, Human Nutrition Information Service, U.S. Department of Agriculture, 1988), p. 17.

TABLE 6–11
COMPARISON OF NUTRIENT RETENTION IN FRUIT COOKED BY DIFFERENT METHODS

	% VITAMIN C	% THIAMIN	% PANTOTHENIC ACID	% FOLATE	% BETA-CAROTENE
BOILED OR STEWED	70	80	95	50	75
MICROWAVE COOKED[a]	90	100	75	100	90

[a]Apples.
SOURCE: Adapted from M. A. McCarthy and R. H. Matthews, *Conserving Nutrients in Foods*, Administrative Report No. 384 (Hyattsville, Md.: Nutrition Monitoring Division, Human Nutrition Information Service, U.S. Department of Agriculture, 1988), p. 18.

Fat-Soluble Vitamins

The four fat-soluble vitamins—A, D, E, and K—are generally found in the fats of foods and are absorbed from the digestive tract with the aid of fats in the diet and bile produced by the liver. Any disorder that interferes with fat digestion or absorption can precipitate a deficiency of the fat-soluble vitamins. Once in the bloodstream, these vitamins are escorted by protein carriers because they are insoluble in water. Since they are stored in the liver and in body fat, you need not consume them daily unless your intakes are typically marginal. It is possible for megadoses of the fat-soluble vitamins to build up to toxic levels in the body and cause undesirable side effects.

Vitamin A

Vitamin A has the distinction of being the first fat-soluble vitamin to be identified. It is one of the most versatile vitamins, playing roles in several important body processes.

The best known function of vitamin A is in vision. For a person to see, light reaching the eye must be transformed into nerve impulses that the brain interprets in producing visual images. The transformers are molecules of **pigment** in the cells of the **retina,** a paper-thin tissue lining the back of the eye. A portion of each pigment molecule is **retinal,** a compound the body can synthesize only if vitamin A is supplied by the diet in some form. Thus, when vitamin A is deficient, vision is impaired. Specifically, the eye has difficulty in adapting to changing light levels. A flash of bright light at night (after the eye has adapted to darkness) will be followed by a prolonged spell of **night blindness.** Because night blindness is easy to diagnose, it aids in the identification of vitamin A deficiency. Night blindness is only a symptom, however, and may indicate a condition other than vitamin A deficiency.

Vitamin A serves other roles in the body. It helps to maintain healthy skin and **epithelial tissue**—the cells (called epithelial cells) lining such body cavities as the small intestine. It is also involved in the production of sperm, the normal development of fetuses, the immune response, hearing, taste, and growth.

Up to a year's supply of vitamin A can be stored in the body, 90 percent of it in the liver. If you stop eating good food sources of vitamin A, deficiency symptoms will not begin to appear until after your stores are depleted. Then, however, the consequences are profound and include blindness and reduced resistance to infection. While vitamin A deficiency is rarely seen in developed countries such as the United States and Canada, it is one of the most serious public health problems in developing countries, where millions of children suffer from blindness and the other consequences of vitamin A deficiencies.

Vitamin A toxicity, on the other hand, is not nearly as widespread as deficiency. Nevertheless, it can lead to severe health consequences, including joint pain, dryness of skin, hair loss, irritability, fatigue, headaches, weakness, nausea, and liver damage. That's why it's especially important not to take megadoses of this nutrient.

While toxicity poses a hazard to people who take supplements of **preformed vitamin A,** toxicity poses virtually no risk to people who obtain vita-

PIGMENT a molecule capable of absorbing certain wavelengths of light. Pigments in the eye permit us to perceive different colors.

RETINA (RET-in-uh) the paper-thin layer of light-sensitive cells lining the back of the inside of the eye.

RETINAL (RET-in-al) one of the active forms of vitamin A that functions in the pigments of the eye. Other active forms of vitamin A include retinol.

NIGHT BLINDNESS slow recovery of vision following flashes of bright light at night; an early symptom of vitamin A deficiency.

EPITHELIAL (ep-ih-THEE-lee-ul) **TISSUE** those cells that form the outer surface of the body and line the body cavities and the principal passageways leading to the exterior. Examples include the cornea, digestive tract lining, respiratory tract lining, and skin.

PREFORMED VITAMIN A vitamin A in its active form.

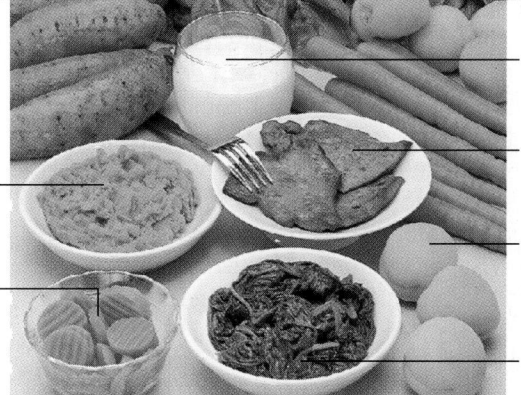

SOURCES OF VITAMIN A AND BETA-CAROTENE

Adult RDA is 800 to 1,000 RE.

Sweet potato: 1,017 RE[b] per 1/2 cup mashed

Carrots: 1,913 RE[b] per 1/2 cup cooked

[a]Preformed vitamin A.
[b]Beta-carotene.

Fortified milk: 149 RE[a] per cup

Beef liver: 9,124 RE[a] per 3 ounces

Apricots: 277 RE[b] per 3 fresh apricots

Spinach: 737 RE[b] per ½ cup cooked

min A in the form of **beta-carotene,** an orange plant pigment that is a vitamin A **precursor.** (Beta-carotene is also an antioxidant, and its role as such is described in the Spotlight later in the chapter.) Inside the body, beta-carotene is converted into vitamin A, but this happens so slowly that excess amounts are not stored as vitamin A, but rather are stored in fat deposits.

Because the body uses both the preformed vitamin A and the beta-carotene in foods to make **retinol,** the amount of vitamin A that comes from foods is usually expressed in **retinol equivalents (RE)**—a measure of the amount of retinol the body will derive from the food. Table 6–12 shows the amount of vitamin A, expressed in RE, that comes from various foods. Note that plant foods provide RE from beta-carotene, while animal foods such as milk and cheese provide RE via preformed vitamin A.

The major sources of vitamin A (in the form of beta-carotene) are almost all brightly colored in hues of green, yellow, orange, and red. Any plant food with significant vitamin A activity must have some color, since beta-carotene is a rich, deep yellow, almost orange color. (Preformed vitamin A is pale yellow.) The dark green leafy vegetables contain large amounts of the green pigment **chlorophyll,** which masks the carotene in them.

In the United States, about half of the vitamin A consumed in foods

TABLE 6–12
VITAMIN A IN FOODS

Adult RDA is 800 to 1,000 RE.

RE	SOURCES
9,124	Beef liver (3 oz)*
2,486	Sweet potato (1)
2,024	Carrot, fresh (1)
860	Cantaloupe (½)
805	Mango (1)
737	Spinach, cooked (½ c)
718	Butternut squash (½ c)
396	Turnip greens, cooked (½ c)
253	Apricot halves, dried (10)
219	Bok choy, cooked (½ c)
178	Watermelon (1" by 10" slice)
149	Nonfat milk (1 c)*
146	Romaine (1 c)
129	Cheddar cheese (1.5 oz)*
109	Broccoli, cooked (½ c)
89	Tomatoes, cooked (½ c)
85	Papaya (1)
76	Tomato, fresh (1)
54	Flounder/sole (3 oz)*
49	Asparagus, cooked (½ c)

*Preformed vitamin A. The rest of the items on the chart derive vitamin A from beta-carotene.

BETA-CAROTENE an orange pigment found in plants that is converted into vitamin A inside the body. Beta-carotene is also an antioxidant.

PRECURSOR a compound that can be converted into another compound. For example, beta-carotene is a precursor of vitamin A.

pre = before

cursor = runner, forerunner

RETINOL one of the active forms of vitamin A.

RETINOL EQUIVALENTS (RE) a measure of the amount of retinol the body will derive from a food containing preformed vitamin A or beta-carotene. Note that some tables list vitamin A in terms of *International Units (IU)*. See Appendix D for methods of converting from one measure to another.

CHLOROPHYLL the green pigment of plants that traps energy from sunlight and uses this energy in photosynthesis (the synthesis of carbohydrate by green plants).

comes from fruits and vegetables, and about half of that comes from *dark* leafy greens, such as broccoli and spinach (but not iceberg lettuce or green beans) and *rich* yellow or *deep* orange vegetables, such as winter squash, carrots, and sweet potatoes. The other half of the vitamin A comes from milk, cheese, butter, and other dairy products, eggs, and a few meats, such as liver. When whole milk is processed to produce nonfat milk, the vitamin is lost along with the fat that is skimmed. (Remember that vitamin A is found in the fat.) In the United States and Canada, nonfat milk is fortified with the nutrient to compensate for its loss. Likewise, margarine is fortified to provide the amount of vitamin A typically found in butter. (Milk and margarine are also fortified with vitamin D.)

One of the best and easiest ways of ensuring that you meet your vitamin A needs is to consume generous amounts of a variety of dark green and deep orange vegetables and fruits. Because these foods provide such an abundance of beta-carotene, along with other nutrients, most dietary guidelines advise eating at least five servings of fruits and vegetables daily, including at least one dark green or deep orange item every other day.

Vitamin D

Vitamin D is a member of a large bone-making and bone-maintenance team composed of several nutrients and other compounds, including vitamin C; hormones; the protein collagen; and the minerals calcium, phosphorus, magnesium, and fluoride. Vitamin D's special role involves assisting in the absorption of dietary calcium and helping to make calcium and phosphorus available in the blood that bathes the bones so that these minerals can be deposited as the bones harden. In addition, vitamin D acts very much like a hormone—a compound manufactured by one organ of the body that affects another. Indeed, vitamin D exerts an influence on a number of organs, including the kidneys and the intestines.

The precursor of vitamin D is made from cholesterol in the liver. This is one of the body's many good uses for cholesterol.

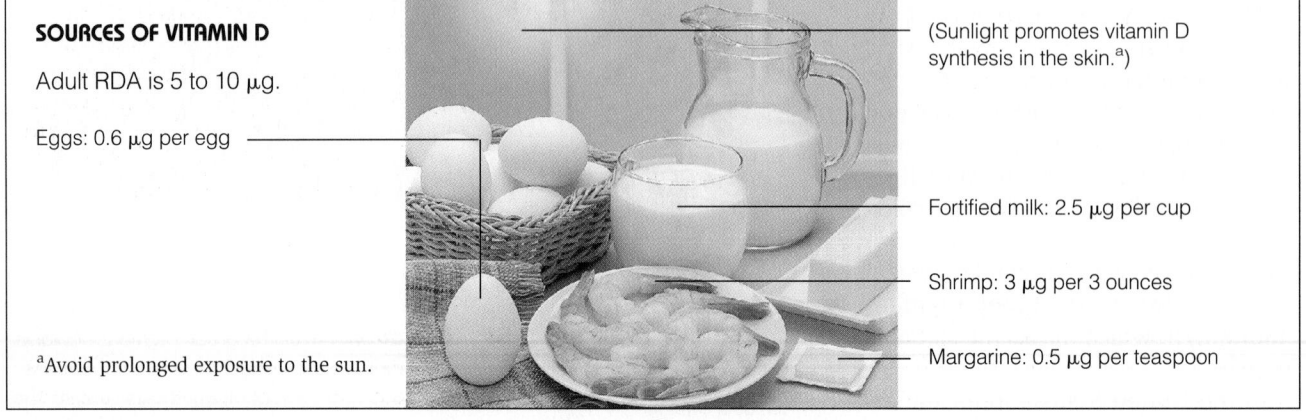

SOURCES OF VITAMIN D

Adult RDA is 5 to 10 μg.

Eggs: 0.6 μg per egg

(Sunlight promotes vitamin D synthesis in the skin.[a])

Fortified milk: 2.5 μg per cup

Shrimp: 3 μg per 3 ounces

Margarine: 0.5 μg per teaspoon

[a]Avoid prolonged exposure to the sun.

Another particularly unique feature of vitamin D is that the body can synthesize it with the help of sunlight, regardless of dietary consumption of the nutrient. Vitamin D is commonly called the sunshine vitamin because the liver makes a vitamin D precursor, which is converted to vitamin D with the help of the sun's ultraviolet rays. The liver alters the molecule, and the kidney alters it further to produce the active form of the vitamin. This is why diseases affecting either the liver or the kidney, which in turn upset vitamin production, may ultimately lead to bone deterioration.

Because the body can make vitamin D with the help of sunlight, you can meet your needs for the nutrient either via sun exposure or through diet. However, significant amounts of the nutrient come from only a few animal foods—notably eggs, liver, and some fish. And even in these, the vitamin D content varies greatly.[19] What's more, neither cow's milk nor human breast milk supplies enough vitamin D to reliably meet human needs. Hence, cow's milk is fortified with the nutrient, and infants require either vitamin D supplements, if breastfed, or fortified formula.

Although vitamin D is not prevalent in the diet, most adults, especially those living in sunny, southern regions, need not worry about the vitamin D content of the foods they eat because their bodies are getting plenty of the nutrient as a result of sun exposure. Sun exposure of the face, hands, and arms for just five to 15 minutes several times a week is usually all it takes. However, people who live in northern parts of the country—above an imaginary line drawn between Boston and the Oregon-California border—are not exposed from November through February to enough ultraviolet rays from the sun to synthesize vitamin D. The same holds true for housebound or institutionalized elderly people, who not only get outside less often than younger people but also tend to be much less efficient at producing vitamin D via the skin/sun.[20] For these people, eating vitamin D-rich foods, such as milk, fatty fish (including sardines, herring, mackerel, and swordfish), eggs, and some fortified cereals, is particularly important.

As discussed earlier in the chapter, children who fail to get enough vitamin D characteristically develop bowed legs, which are often the most obvious sign of the deficiency disease rickets (refer to the photograph on page 198). In adults, vitamin D deficiency causes **osteomalacia,** most often in women whose diets lack calcium, who get little exposure to the sun, and who go through several closely spaced pregnancies and prolonged periods of breast-feeding. Osteomalacia causes the bones, particularly the leg bones and spine, to become soft, porous, and weak.

While vitamin D deficiency depresses calcium absorption, resulting in low blood calcium levels and abnormal bone development, an excess of vitamin D does just the opposite. It increases calcium absorption, causing abnormally high concentrations of the mineral in the blood, which in turn tend to be deposited in the soft tissues. This is especially likely to happen in the kidneys, where calcium-containing stones may form as a result. Thus, vitamin D supplements should be taken only on the advice of a physician. Vitamin D is highly toxic, with as little as four to five times the RDA easily causing an overdose.

TABLE 6–13
VITAMIN D IN FOODS
Adult RDA is 5 to 10 μg.

μG	SOURCES
3	Shrimp (3 oz)
2.5	Nonfat milk (1 c)
1.3	Corn flakes (1 cup)
0.9	Cod liver oil (1 tbsp)
0.6	Egg (1)
0.5	Margarine (1 tsp)
0.3	Hot dog (1)

Sun exposure should always be moderate. It takes a minimum amount of exposure—five to 15 minutes on the hands, arms, and face—for the body to meet vitamin D needs. The rest of the time, body parts exposed to ultraviolet rays should be protected with a formula containing a sun protection factor of 15 or more to protect against skin cancer.

OSTEOMALACIA (os-tee-o-mal-AY-shuh) the disease resulting from vitamin D deficiency in adults. (Its counterpart in children is called rickets.) Osteomalacia can also be caused by calcium deficiency (see Chapter 7); it is characterized by bowed legs and a curved spine.

Vitamin E

Vitamin E is known as a vitamin in search of a disease.[21] That's because vitamin E is widespread in the food supply, and deficiencies of the nutrient are rare. The great majority of the nutrient in the diet comes from vegetable oils and products such as margarine, salad dressings, and shortenings (animal fats such as butter and lard contain negligible amounts of the nutrient). Soybean, cottonseed, corn, and safflower oils contain generous amounts of vitamin E, as do nuts and seeds. Smaller amounts come from fruits, vegetables, grains, and other foods. Wheat germ, for example, is an excellent source of vitamin E. Table 6–14 lists sources of vitamin E.

Despite the rarity of deficiency, however, vitamin E is one of the most popular vitamin supplements. For decades, people have swallowed all manner of extravagant claims reputing the power of the nutrient to improve athletic performance; increase sexual potency and performance; and prevent graying of the hair, wrinkling of the skin, development of age spots, and other signs of aging, to name just some of the claims. Vitamin E has never been proven to be a panacea for any of those problems. Vitamin E supplements are also often touted as a remedy for nighttime leg cramps. Again, the evidence to support that claim is limited, so the nutrient should not be self-prescribed as a treatment for the condition.[22]

A much more tangible link between vitamin E and heart disease and other chronic diseases is supported by accumulating scientific research. Because vitamin E performs a key role as an antioxidant in the body (as detailed in the Spotlight at the end of the chapter), scientists suspect it is involved in protecting the membranes of the lungs, heart, and other organs against damage from pollutants and other environmental hazards.

The role of antioxidants including vitamins C, E, and beta-carotene is the subject of the Spotlight at the end of the chapter.

The cell membranes harbor vitamin E, and a deficiency of the nutrient causes those membranes, particularly the red blood cells, to rupture and cause a type of anemia. While extremely rare in healthy adults, this scenario sometimes occurs in premature infants who are born before vitamin E is transferred

TABLE 6–14 VITAMIN E IN FOODS	
Adult RDA is 8 to 10 mg.	
MG	**SOURCES**
14.18	Sunflower seeds (1 oz)
4.6	Safflower oil (1 tbsp)
4.5	Sweet potato, mashed (½ c)
3.2	Shrimp (3 oz)
3.0	Peanut butter (2 tbsp)
2.9	Canola oil (1 tbsp)
2.32	Avocado (1)
2.32	Mango (1)
2.04	Wheat germ (2 tbsp)
1.9	Corn oil (1 tbsp)
1.67	Olive oil (1 tbsp)
1.60	Peanut oil (1 tbsp)
0.81	Apple (1)
0.66	Brussels sprouts, cooked (½ cup)
0.52	Spaghetti, cooked (½ c)
0.20	Sesame oil (1 tbsp)

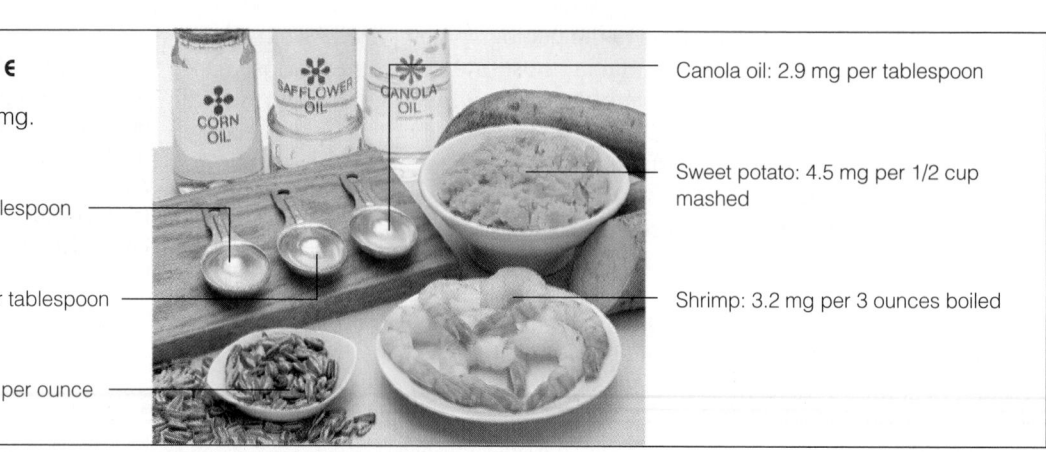

SOURCES OF VITAMIN E

Adult RDA is 8 to 10 mg.

Corn oil: 1.9 mg per tablespoon

Safflower oil: 4.6 mg per tablespoon

Sunflower seeds: 14.18 per ounce

Canola oil: 2.9 mg per tablespoon

Sweet potato: 4.5 mg per 1/2 cup mashed

Shrimp: 3.2 mg per 3 ounces boiled

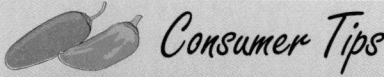 *Consumer Tips*

Choosing a Vitamin/Mineral Supplement

For years, health experts have been saying that most healthy people can meet their vitamin and mineral needs with a balanced diet. Nevertheless, about half of young adults and college students pop vitamin and mineral pills. And Americans overall spend some $3 billion annually on pills, powders, liquids, and other vitamin and mineral supplements, often in the mistaken belief that such preparations will ensure proper nutrition, help reduce stress, decrease fatigue, and increase pep and energy.[23]

But before you buy a supplement, remember that most major health organizations—from the American Dietetic Association to the American Medical Association to the American Academy of Pediatrics—essentially agree that healthy children and adults should be able to get all the nutrients they need by eating a variety of foods. However, those organizations and other experts say that taking a multivitamin/mineral supplement, under the guidance of a physician or dietitian, may be in order for particular groups of people:

- people following very-low-calorie diets
- people with certain diseases or those taking medications that interfere with appetite, digestion, absorption, or excretion of nutrients
- strict vegetarians, whose diets may fall short in vitamin B_{12}, calcium, iron, and zinc
- women who are pregnant or breastfeeding, phases that bolster the need for nutrients, including iron, folic acid, and calcium
- women with excessive menstrual bleeding, who may need iron supplements
- newborn infants, who are commonly given vitamin K shots (discussed on page 223)

If you decide to start taking a supplement, keep the following points in mind when choosing one:

- Remember that price is not an indication of quality. Generally, a 30-day supply of a multi-

vitamin/mineral supplement should cost no more than $10. Many products sold at major retail chains and drugstores are just as high in quality as pricier versions sold in health food stores.

- Look for a product that meets high standards for manufacturing. One way to do this is to check the label to see whether the product meets USP standards—manufacturing practices set forth by the U.S. Pharmacopeia, the organization that establishes drug standards. The organization's standards require that a supplement be able to disintegrate and dissolve thoroughly in the stomach within a certain period of time, thereby increasing the chances that the nutrients inside are absorbed and used by the body. If you're curious about a particular brand and don't see anything about USP approval on the label, call and ask the company (many have toll-free numbers).

- Look for a bottle or package that carries an expiration date. If it doesn't, you run the risk of buying a product that has been sitting on a shelf for an indefinite period of time. After a while, the product may lose its potency.

- Look for a supplement that contains both vitamins and minerals, with no more than 100 percent to 150 percent of the U.S. RDA for each. For the most part, nutrients work in concert with one another, promoting the body's ability to make use of them. Products that include a balanced mix of the essential vitamins and minerals are the best bet for most people.

- Choose a product that supplies most of the vitamin A in the form of beta-carotene rather than preformed vitamin A. Beta-carotene is highly unlikely to be toxic, because it is converted into vitamin A relatively slowly in the body. But excess preformed vitamin A is much more likely to cause harm over time. What's more, buying a product with beta-carotene allows you to reap its potential antioxi-

continued

Consumer Tips

(continued)

dant benefits. Note that some brands will state on the label what percentage of the vitamin A comes from beta-carotene. Again, if a certain supplement label doesn't have USP approval, try contacting the manufacturer.

- Steer clear of products containing extraneous substances such as PABA, hesperidin, inositol, and bee pollen. These nonvitamin substances have never been proved essential to humans and only add to the price of the supplement.

- Be wary of spurious claims, such as statements that suggest that expensive "natural" nutrients are preferable to synthetic versions. As far as the body is concerned, natural and synthetic nutrients are one in the same. Also, beware of products

touted as "stress" formulas—remember that everyday stress doesn't alter nutrient requirements significantly. Likewise, stay away from "energy-boosting" vitamins. As discussed earlier in the chapter, vitamins don't provide energy in and of themselves.

- Buy products sold in childproof bottles or packages if you have children around. Vitamins and minerals, especially iron, can be highly toxic to children. Every year, tens of thousands of children swallow excess vitamin/mineral supplements, and iron-tablet overdoses alone are one of the top causes of accidental death in youngsters (many multivitamin/mineral pills now carry warning labels about the risk of excess iron to children).

---

to them from their mothers. Other groups of people who run the risk of deficiency include those who cannot absorb fats as a result of diseases and those with certain blood disorders.

Vitamin E toxicity appears to be rare, occurring only in people who take extremely high doses. Suspected symptoms include alteration of the body's blood-clotting mechanisms and interference with the function of vitamin K.

Vitamin K

The key function of vitamin K is its role in the blood-clotting system of the body, where its presence can mean the difference between life and death. It is essential for the synthesis of at least four of the 13 proteins involved, along with calcium, in making the blood clot. When *any* of these blood-clotting factors is absent, blood cannot clot, leaving a person vulnerable to excessive bleeding upon injury. Vitamin K works with vitamin D in synthesizing a bone protein that helps to regulate the calcium levels in the blood.

Vitamin K can be synthesized by the **intestinal flora**—the bacteria that reside in the digestive tract. In addition, as Table 6–15 shows, many foods supply ample amounts of the vitamin, green leafy vegetables and members of the cabbage family in particular.

Because vitamin K is obtained both in the diet and via the intestinal bacteria, deficiencies are rare and occur only under unusual circumstances. Taking antibiotics for an extended period of time, for instance, could kill some of the intestinal bacteria and thereby prompt a deficiency.

K stands for the Danish word *koagulation* ("coagulation" or "clotting").

INTESTINAL FLORA the normal bacterial inhabitants of the digestive tract.

flora = plant inhabitants

SOURCES OF VITAMIN K

Adult RDA is 60 to 80 μg.

Nonfat milk: 10 μg per cup

Beef liver: 89 μg per 3 ounces

Cabbage: 104 μg per 1 cup raw

Spinach: 148 μg per 1 cup raw

Cauliflower: 96 μg per ½ cup raw

Eggs: 25 μg per egg

Garbanzo beans: 52 μg per ½ cup

Newborn babies are the one group that is commonly susceptible to a vitamin K deficiency because a baby's digestive tract is free of bacteria until birth. After birth, the infant's intestinal tract gradually becomes populated with bacteria, but this happens over time. What's more, the formula or breast milk fed to the baby generally doesn't contain adequate amounts of vitamin K. Thus, newborns are given a dose of vitamin K to prevent the possibility of a life-threatening hemorrhage in the case of injury.

Vitamin K toxicity is rare, but it can occur when supplemental doses are taken. Because the consequences of toxicity are extreme—red blood cell breakage, yellowing of the skin, and brain damage—vitamin K is available as a supplement only by prescription.

One group of adults who often have to keep on eye on the amount of vitamin K in their diet is people taking drugs designed to prevent the blood from clotting and causing, say, a stroke. People taking such medications (known as anticoagulants) are advised to keep their consumption of vitamin K fairly constant from day to day, because large fluctuations can limit the effectiveness of the anticlotting drugs.[24]

TABLE 6–15
VITAMIN K IN FOODS

Adult RDA is 60 to 80 μg.

μG	SOURCES
364	Turnip greens, raw (1 c)
148	Spinach, raw (1 c)
104	Cabbage, raw (1 c)
96	Cauliflower, raw (½ c)
89	Beef liver (3 oz)
58	Broccoli, raw (½ c)
52	Chick-peas (½ c)
25	Egg (1)
10	Nonfat milk (1 c)
10	Strawberries (½ c)

An RDA for vitamin K was established for the first time in 1989 (see RDA table on the inside front cover of the book).

Nonvitamins

A variety of substances have been mistaken for essential nutrients for human beings because bacteria or animals need them to live. Sometimes called nonvitamins, they include PABA (para-aminobenzoic acid), the bioflavonoids (vitamin P or hesperidin) and ubiquinone, vitamin B_{15} (a hoax), and vitamin B_{17} (laetrile, an unproven cancer "cure"). Some other substances sometimes classed as nonvitamins are nutrients that are essential for some animals but have never been shown to be required by humans.[25] They include choline, carnitine, taurine, and *myo*-inositol. Research into the role of these nutrients for humans is ongoing.

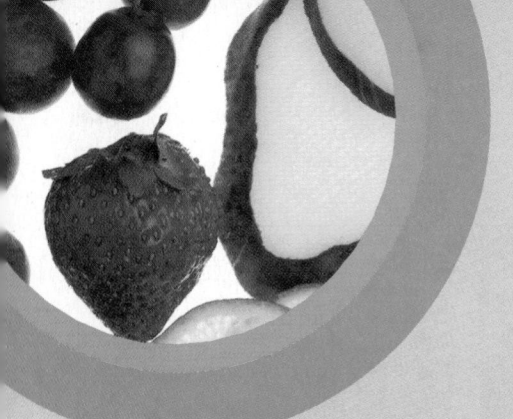

The Antioxidant Vitamins

Just ten years ago, few consumers had ever heard of **antioxidant** vitamins. Today, Americans spend some $5.7 million on antioxidant supplements—that is, supplements containing beta-carotene, vitamin C, and/or vitamin E.[26] The reason, of course, is that a large body of headline-making research suggests that those nutrients can help stave off heart disease, cancer, and other chronic diseases.

Although millions of people have jumped on the antioxidant bandwagon, no major health organization has recommended that the public at large swallow antioxidant pills and potions. Why isn't the nutrition community encouraging widespread consumption of antioxidant supplements? How do these antioxidants work? Why are they the subject of so much controversy? These are some of the questions explored in this Spotlight to help you make informed decisions about the role of these substances in your own diet.

What are antioxidants, and how do they work in the body? As their name suggests, antioxidants are "anti-oxygen"—they fight oxygen, in a manner of speaking. Consider that certain chemical reactions occur in the body that involve the use of oxygen. While these reactions are essential to the body's ability to function, they lead to the creation of highly toxic compounds called **free radicals.** Environmental pollutants such as cigarette smoke and ozone also prompt the formation of free radicals. Left unchecked, these compounds can cause severe cell injury and ultimately may contribute to the development of chronic diseases such as cancer and heart disease.

Fortunately, the body has a built-in defense system to protect against potential damage from free radicals. That defense system makes use of the antioxidant nutrients—beta-carotene as well as vitamins C and E. In addition, the body manufactures certain enzymes, one of which contains the mineral selenium, that help to fight free radicals.

How do the antioxidant nutrients work to fight free radicals? The nutrients all work in one way or another to squelch free radicals before they injure the body. For instance, vitamin E resides in the fatty cell membranes that surround cells, where it acts as a scavenger of free radicals that enter the area. When vitamin E is not around, the free radicals can attack the cell and start a chemical chain reaction that damages the cell membrane, making it leaky and ultimately causing it to break down completely. (A similar reaction can occur in fatty foods such as vegetable oils, causing rancidity.) A good deal of evidence suggests that large doses of vitamin E may protect against heart disease because it may thwart the free radicals that would otherwise damage the walls of blood vessels and contribute to hardening of the arteries.[27]

Like vitamin E, vitamin C helps to stop free radicals in their tracks, working with vitamin E to block damaging chain reactions that appear to promote heart dis-

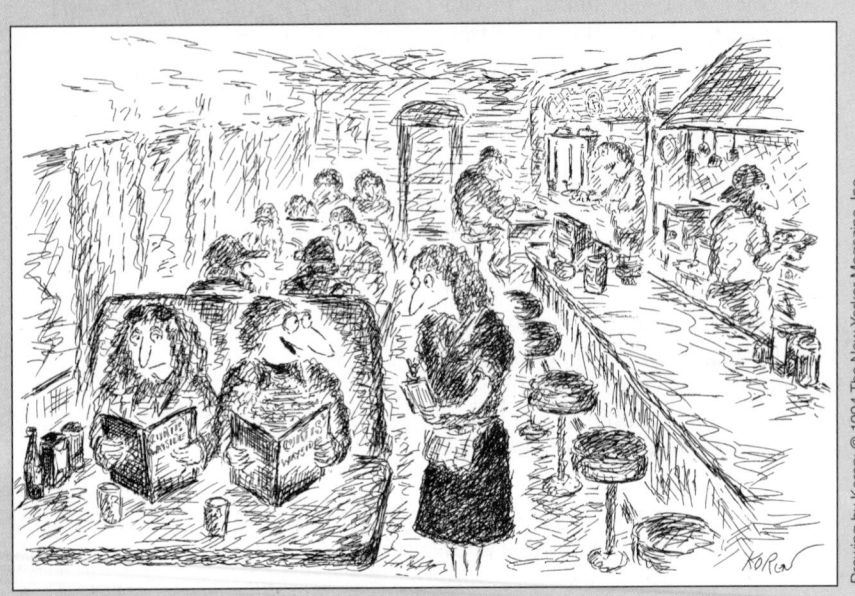

"What do you have that's rich in antioxidants?"

ease and cancer. In addition, vitamin C is a particularly powerful scavenger of environmental air pollutants. In fact, the National Academy of Sciences advises smokers to consume nearly twice as much vitamin C as nonsmokers. The more smoke a person inhales, the more free radicals that are produced and the more vitamin C that is needed to fight them.[28] Beta-carotene seems to work with vitamins E and C to protect against free radical damage that leads to diseases of the respiratory tract, such as lung cancer, as well as other chronic conditions.

It sounds like I'll lessen my chances of getting cancer and other diseases as long as I take enough antioxidants to fight free radicals. How much of the antioxidant nutrients do I need? More than the RDA? That's a good question. Unfortunately, there is no clear-cut answer. Theoretically, as you say, the more antioxidants you consume, the more able your defense system is to fight the millions of free radicals that are produced in the body every day. Many scientists speculate that people need several times the RDA of the antioxidant nutrients to help protect them against both natural free radical damage and the damage resulting from exposure to environmental pollutants. The problem is that no one knows just how much is enough to help prevent disease but not too much to cause potential long-term damage.

In addition, keep in mind that even if scientists were to pinpoint certain amounts of antioxidants that help to promote health, it doesn't mean that the vitamins are the magic bullet that will necessarily prevent disease. For instance, it's highly unlikely that simply swallowing antioxidant supplements could significantly protect a sedentary smoker against lung disease. In other words, even if large doses of antioxidants are shown to help stave off chronic disease to some extent, most scientists speculate that such doses

won't be able to undo the damage caused by a poor diet, obesity, smoking, and a sedentary lifestyle.

Still, it can't hurt to start taking antioxidant pills, can it? Again, the jury is still out on that question, which is why public health organizations are hesitant to recommend widespread consumption of antioxidant supplements. Granted, on the face of it, it sounds as if antioxidants would be harmless. But remember that vitamins are biologically active compounds, and taking large doses is akin to taking drugs and could bring about undesirable side effects. (You may recall that niacin is often used as a "drug" to lower cholesterol—refer to discussion on page 204.) Until scientists have carried out numerous large-scale studies in which people who take various doses of antioxidants are carefully monitored over time, there is no way of knowing whether large doses of antioxidants are safe to swallow for long periods of time or that their benefits outweigh their possible side effects.

Take vitamin C, the most popular vitamin supplement. As just discussed, the nutrient can be a powerful antioxidant in the body. But chemists and food scientists have long known that in a test-tube type of environment, vitamin C can exert a **pro-oxidant** effect when it is around iron or another metal. That is, vitamin C may *stimulate* free radical damage. Whether this occurs in the body is unclear, but it raises the concern that there may be a point at which too much vitamin C, or any other antioxidant for that matter, will do more harm than good.[29]

I see your point, but haven't scientists already conducted big studies using antioxidant supplements? I'm sure I've heard about them on TV. And isn't that how they came up with these theories in the first place? Yes, some large studies using vitamin supplements have been conducted, but those studies were begun

after scientists had gathered information using other kinds of research. Much of the interest in antioxidant nutrients has been generated by looking at the eating habits of people living in parts of the world where chronic disease rates have been historically low, such as the island of Crete (discussed in the Spotlight in Chapter 3). Time and again, scientists

MINIGLOSSARY

ALLYL SULFIDES compounds in garlic that may help lower blood cholesterol levels and protect against some types of cancer.

ANTIOXIDANT a substance, such as a vitamin, that is "anti-oxygen"—that is, it helps to prevent damage done to the body as a result of chemical reactions that involve the use of oxygen.

DESIGNER FOODS foods "fortified" with phytochemicals or plants bred to contain high levels of phytochemicals; also known as "future foods."

FREE RADICAL highly toxic compound created in the body as a result of chemical reactions that involve oxygen. Environmental pollutants such as cigarette smoke and ozone also prompt the formation of free radicals.

ISOFLAVONES compounds found in many fruits, vegetables, and soy-based foods that are thought to play a role in fighting breast cancer by blocking the action of the hormone estrogen.

PHYTOCHEMICALS chemicals found in plants that are not nutrients but that appear to help fight diseases such as cancer.

phyto = plant

PRO-OXIDANT a compound that stimulates free radical damage.

have seen that people who eat lots of fruits and vegetables seem to have the lowest rates of certain diseases, such as lung cancer. Observing this relationship, they have tried to identify what it is about fruits and vegetables that might be responsible for low lung-cancer rates. One way to do so has been to measure people's blood levels of, say, beta-carotene. If people with high levels are less likely to suffer lung cancer, then beta-carotene might be protective.

Scientists have also conducted animal experiments to see the effects of anti-oxdants on the health of the animals. Through these and other research studies, they try to keep honing in on the different factors that have an effect on disease. As you can imagine, however, it can take hundreds of studies before conclusions can be drawn.

In addition to all of this research, a number of studies in which large groups of people were given antioxidant supplements have been conducted, as you pointed out, and more research is currently underway. The reason the evidence can't be used to make public health recommendations is that there are too few studies, and the findings have not all pointed in the same direction. For example, in the spring of 1994, the results of a landmark study involving more than 29,000 people led to a flurry of disturbing headlines. After five to eight years of swallowing vitamin E and/or beta-carotene supplements, male smokers were no less likely to suffer lung cancer than men who hadn't swallowed the pills. What's more, the people taking the beta-carotene were more likely to suffer lung cancer than the nonsupplementers.[30]

What this study highlights is not that beta-carotene is dangerous—it would take more studies that came to the same conclusion to "prove" that—but rather that more research on supplementation is needed because so many questions remain: Would the outcome have been different in women smokers? What would happen if the smokers had taken supplements for 40 or 50 years instead of just five to eight years? What is the effect of beta-carotene in nonsmokers? What would have happened if the men had taken a different dose of beta-carotene? What if they had taken pills containing beta-carotene as well as vitamins C and E? and so forth.[31]

So basically, what you're saying is that antioxidant research is interesting, but I can't really apply it to my own diet, right? Not at all. To be sure, in our own view, more research needs to be conducted before we can endorse self-prescribing large doses of antioxidant supplements. But this is an individual decision that you have to make for yourself.

What we wholeheartedly recommend, however, is that you use your knowledge of antioxidants as an impetus to eat lots of fruits and vegetables—shoot for at least five servings a day. Produce is an excellent source of antioxidants as well as fiber and other vitamins and minerals so essential to good health. Indeed, while the FDA has not authorized any food label health claims linking antioxidants with health, it does allow health claims on fruits and vegetables that are a good source of fiber or vitamins A and C. The claim relates a diet low in fat and rich in fruits and vegetables to reduced cancer risk.

Another benefit of choosing fruits and vegetables rather than supplements is that the produce contains what are known as **phytochemicals**—chemicals found in plants (*phyto* is the Greek word for plant). While phytochemicals are not nutrients as are vitamins and minerals, they appear to play a definite role in helping to fight diseases such as cancer.

For example, compounds called **isoflavones** are found in many fruits and vegetables as well as soy-based foods such as tofu. Isoflavones are thought to play a role in fighting breast cancer by blocking the action of the hormone estrogen, which in large amounts can encourage the growth of cancerous tumors.

Other phytochemicals appear to confer protection against heart disease. Consider that certain phytochemicals in garlic, called **allyl sulfides,** may help lower blood cholesterol levels as well as protect against some types of cancer. (See the Spotlight in chapter 4 for more on garlic and heart disease.)

So far, scientists have identified hundreds of phytochemicals, and many appear to function as antioxidants that help to squelch free radicals. Research is currently underway to develop methods of creating **designer foods,** that is, plants bred to contain high levels of beneficial phytochemicals or foods "fortified" with phytochemicals. Table 6–16 lists some examples of phytochemicals and the effects they seem to have in the body. More and more emerging research indicates that these substances hold enormous potential to increase our understanding of why a plant-based diet that includes lots of fruits and vegetables is so beneficial to health. If you haven't already done so, try the Vegetable Variety Scorecard on page 209 to see how your vegetable-eating habits measure up.

TABLE 6–16
PHYTOCHEMICAL FOCUS

FOOD	PHYTOCHEMICAL(S)	EFFECT
Brassica Vegetables *(Includes broccoli, cauliflower, cabbage, Brussels sprouts, and kohlrabi)*	Sulforaphane and other isothiocyanates	Seem to stimulate the production of anticancer enzymes, bolstering the body's natural ability to ward off cancer.
	Indoles	Stimulate enzymes that make the hormone estrogen less effective, possibly reducing breast cancer risk.
Allium Vegetables *(Includes garlic, onions, leeks, and chives)*	Allyl sulfides	May block the action of cancer-causing chemicals. May help lower blood cholesterol levels.
Citrus Fruits	Limonene	Increases production of enzymes that may help the body dispose of carcinogens.
Soybeans and Legumes *(Dried beans)*	Protease inhibitors	Suppress enzyme production in cancer cells to slow tumor growth.
	Phytosterols	Hinder cell reproduction in the large intestine, possibly preventing colon cancer.
	Isoflavones	Block estrogen from entering cells, possibly reducing the risk of breast and ovarian cancer.
	Saponins	Interfere with DNA replication, preventing cancer cells from multiplying.
Fruits	Caffeic acid	Aids production of an enzyme that makes it easier for the body to get rid of carcinogens.
	Ferulic acid	Binds to nitrates, possibly preventing them from converting to cancer-causing nitrosamines.

SOURCE: Reprinted with permission from *American Institute for Cancer Research NEWSLETTER*, Winter 1995, Issue 46.

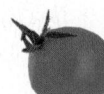

CHECK YOURSELF...

1. Name three water-soluble vitamins and their key functions in the body.

2. Explain the difference between beta-carotene and preformed vitamin A.

3. Name three groups of people who might need a multivitamin/mineral supplement.

4. Compare the nutrient losses likely to occur when cooking vegetables via boiling, steaming, and microwave cooking.

5. Explain why people need not obtain all their vitamin D from food.

6. Describe vitamin A's role in vision.

7. Explain why women of childbearing age are advised to consume generous amounts of folate.

8. Define phytochemical.

9. Name three reasons why major health organizations do not advise that everyone take antioxidant supplements.

10. Name three things to look for when purchasing a multivitamin/mineral supplement.

Answers to selected Check Yourself questions are found in Appendix H.

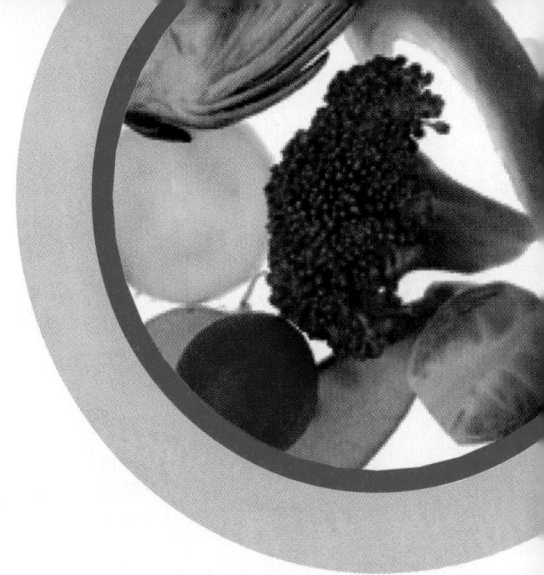

> The pleasure of eating . . . is of all times, all ages, all conditions. . . . Because it may be enjoyed with other enjoyments, and even console us for their absence. . . . Because its impressions are more durable and more dependent on our will. . . . Because in eating we experience a certain indescribably keen sensation of pleasure, by what we eat we repair the losses we have sustained, and prolong life.
>
> Anthelme Brillat-Savarin
> (1755–1826, French politician and gourmet; author of *Physiology of Taste*)

The Minerals and Water   SEVEN

Contents

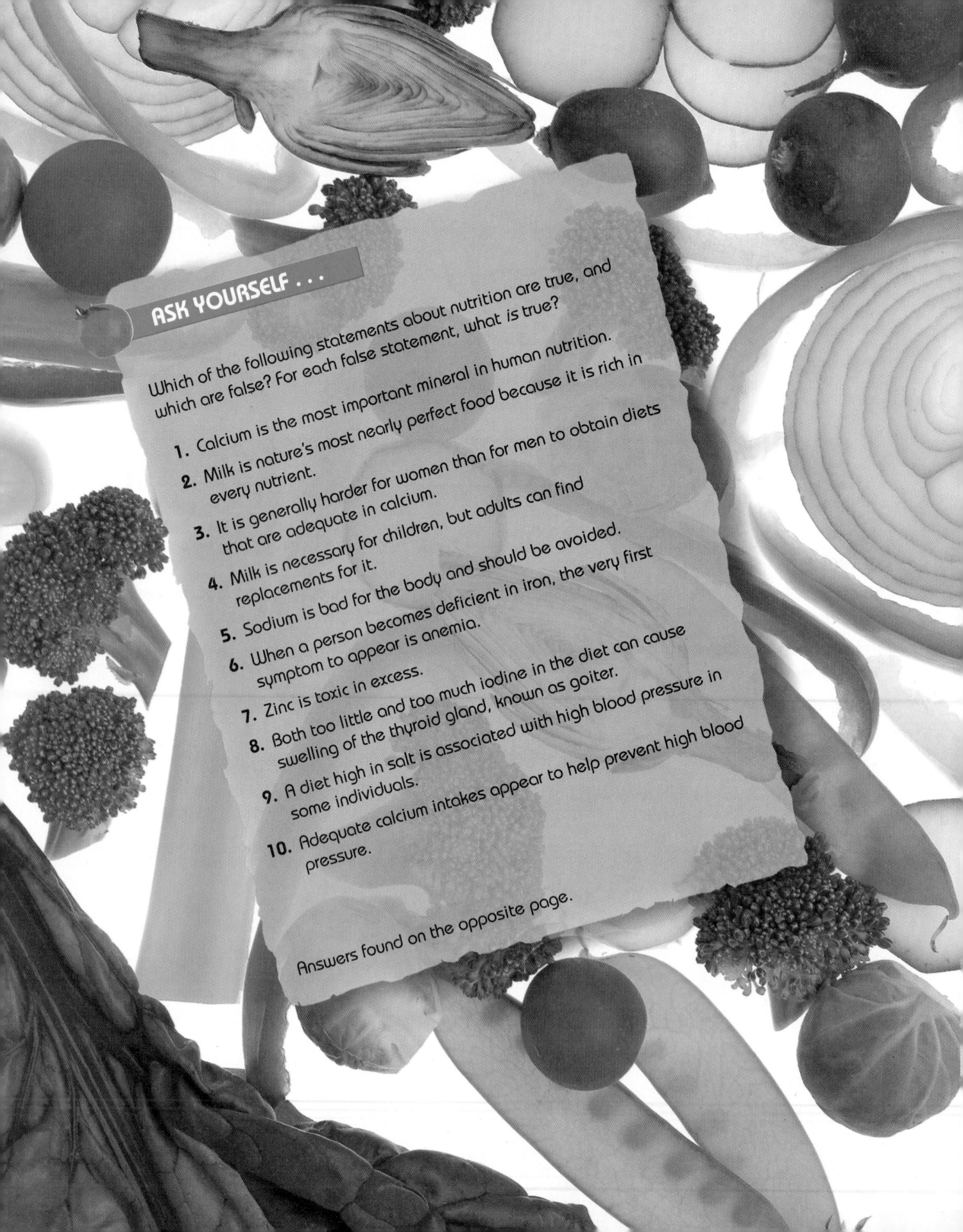

ASK YOURSELF . . .

Which of the following statements about nutrition are true, and which are false? For each false statement, what *is* true?

1. Calcium is the most important mineral in human nutrition.

2. Milk is nature's most nearly perfect food because it is rich in every nutrient.

3. It is generally harder for women than for men to obtain diets that are adequate in calcium.

4. Milk is necessary for children, but adults can find replacements for it.

5. Sodium is bad for the body and should be avoided.

6. When a person becomes deficient in iron, the very first symptom to appear is anemia.

7. Zinc is toxic in excess.

8. Both too little and too much iodine in the diet can cause swelling of the thyroid gland, known as goiter.

9. A diet high in salt is associated with high blood pressure in some individuals.

10. Adequate calcium intakes appear to help prevent high blood pressure.

Answers found on the opposite page.

For hundreds, if not thousands, of years, the physical and chemical properties of minerals such as gold, silver, lead, and copper, were known to metallurgists and alchemists. Even so, the role of some minerals in biological processes was recognized only within the past few hundred years. The discovery of iron in blood, for example, occurred in 1713. The identification of calcium in bone was made in 1771.[1] Not until the late nineteenth century was the role of minerals in human nutrition fully appreciated.

The previous chapter described the water-soluble and fat-soluble vitamins, their biological roles, food sources, and human requirements. This chapter discusses the minerals known to be important in human nutrition. In some respects, minerals are similar to vitamins. Like the vitamins, minerals do not themselves contribute energy (calories) to the diet. Of those known to be important in human nutrition, most minerals have diverse functions within the body and work with enzymes to facilitate chemical reactions. As with the vitamins, most minerals are required in the diet in very small amounts.

In other respects, minerals are different from vitamins. Whereas vitamins are organic compounds, **minerals** are **inorganic** compounds that occur naturally in the earth's crust. And unlike the vitamins, some minerals (such as calcium) contribute to the building of body structures (such as bone).

As with other areas of research in human nutrition, there are many unanswered questions related to mineral metabolism. Scientists are studying the biochemical functions of minerals, the mechanisms by which they activate enzymes, the factors that control their blood and tissue levels, and the ways in which the composition of the diet affects the body's ability to make use of these dietary components. The many complex metabolic interactions of minerals make this a challenging area of research.

MINERALS small, naturally occurring, inorganic, chemical elements; the minerals serve as structural components and in many vital processes in the body.

INORGANIC being or composed of matter other than plant or animal.

The Major Minerals

The minerals are traditionally divided into two large classes: the **major minerals** and the **trace minerals.** The distinction between them is that the major minerals occur in relatively large quantities in the body and are needed daily in relatively large amounts—on the order of a gram or so each. The trace minerals occur in the body in minute quantities and are needed in smaller amounts in the daily diet. Table 7–1 lists the minerals known to be essential in human nutrition and Table 7–2 offers tips for locating the minerals in the Food Guide Pyramid. The discussions that follow focus on the minerals that are of particular interest in human nutrition, primarily because people are known to suffer deficiencies of them.

MAJOR MINERAL an essential mineral nutrient found in the human body in amounts greater than 5 grams.

TRACE MINERAL an essential mineral nutrient found in the human body in amounts less than 5 grams.

ASK YOURSELF ANSWERS: 1. False. No one essential mineral is more important than any other. **2.** False. Milk is an excellent food, but it is poor in several nutrients, including iron. **3.** True. **4.** False. Strictly speaking, milk is not absolutely necessary in anyone's diet, but its nutrients are hard to obtain from other foods, and it is recommended for both children and adults. **5.** False. Sodium is an essential nutrient, but excesses should be avoided. **6.** False. When a person becomes deficient in iron, one of the last symptoms to appear is anemia; fatigue and weakness appear first. **7.** True. **8.** True. **9.** True. **10.** True.

TABLE 7–1
A GUIDE TO THE MINERALS

MINERAL	BEST SOURCES	CHIEF ROLES	DEFICIENCY SYMPTOMS	TOXICITY SYMPTOMS
MAJOR MINERALS				
Calcium	Milk and milk products, small fish (with bones), tofu, certain green vegetables, legumes.	Principal mineral of bones and teeth; involved in muscle contraction and relaxation, nerve function, blood clotting, blood pressure.	Stunted growth in children; bone loss (osteoporosis) in adults.	Excess calcium is excreted except in hormonal imbalance states.
Phosphorus	All animal tissues.	Part of every cell; involved in acid-base balance.	Unknown.	Can create relative deficiency of calcium.
Magnesium	Nuts, legumes, whole grains, dark green vegetables, seafoods, chocolate, cocoa.	Involved in bone mineralization, protein synthesis, enzyme action, normal muscular contraction, nerve transmission.	Weakness, confusion, depressed pancreatic hormone secretion, growth failure, behavioral disturbances, muscle spasms.	Not known.
Sodium	Salt, soy sauce; processed foods: cured, canned, pickled, and many boxed foods.	Helps maintain normal fluid and acid-base balance.	Muscle cramps, mental apathy, loss of appetite.	High blood pressure (in salt-sensitive persons).
Chloride	Salt, soy sauce; processed foods.	Part of stomach acid, necessary for proper digestion, fluid balance.	Growth failure in children, muscle cramps, mental apathy, loss of appetite.	Normally harmless (the gas chlorine is a poison but evaporates from water); disturbed acid-base balance; vomiting.
Potassium	All whole foods: meats, milk, fruits, vegetables, grains, legumes.	Facilitates many reactions, including protein synthesis, fluid balance, nerve transmission, and contraction of muscles.	Muscle weakness, paralysis, confusion; can cause death; accompanies dehydration.	Causes muscular weakness; triggers vomiting; if given into a vein, can stop the heart.
Sulfur	All protein-containing foods.	Component of certain amino acids; part of biotin, thiamin, and insulin.	None known; protein deficiency would occur first.	Would occur only if sulfur amino acids were eaten in excess; this (in animals) depresses growth.

continued

TABLE 7–1
continued

MINERAL	BEST SOURCES	CHIEF ROLES	DEFICIENCY SYMPTOMS	TOXICITY SYMPTOMS
TRACE MINERALS				
Iodine	Iodized salt, seafood, bread.	Part of thyroxine, which regulates metabolism.	Goiter, cretinism.	Very high intakes depress thyroid activity.
Iron	Beef, fish, poultry, shellfish, eggs, legumes, dried fruits, fortified cereals.	Hemoglobin formation; part of myoglobin; energy utilization.	Anemia: weakness, pallor, headaches, reduced immunity, inability to concentrate, cold intolerance.	Iron overload: infections, liver injury, possible increased risk of heart attack.
Zinc	Protein-containing foods: meats, fish, poultry, grains, vegetables.	Part of many enzymes; present in insulin; involved in making genetic material and proteins, immunity, vitamin A transport, taste, wound healing, making sperm, normal fetal development.	Growth failure in children, delayed development of sexual organs, loss of taste, poor wound healing.	Fever, nausea, vomiting, diarrhea.
Copper	Meats, drinking water.	Absorption of iron; part of several enzymes.	Anemia, bone changes (rare in human beings).	Unknown except as part of a rare hereditary disease (Wilson's disease).
Fluoride	Drinking water (if naturally fluoride containing or fluoridated), tea, seafood.	Formation of bones and teeth; helps make teeth resistant to decay and bones resistant to mineral loss.	Susceptibility to tooth decay and bone loss.	Fluorosis (discoloration of teeth).
Selenium	Seafood, meats, grains.	Helps protect body compounds from oxidation.	Anemia (rare).	Digestive system disorders.
Chromium	Meats, unrefined foods, fats, vegetable oils.	Associated with insulin and required for the release of energy from glucose.	Diabetes-like condition marked by inability to use glucose normally.	Unknown as a nutrition disorder. Occupational exposures damage skin and kidneys.
Molybdenum	Legumes, cereals, organ meats.	Facilitates, with enzymes, many cell processes.	Unknown.	Enzyme inhibition.
Manganese	Widely distributed in foods.	Facilitates, with enzymes, many cell processes.	In animals: poor growth, nervous system disorders, abnormal reproduction.	Poisoning, nervous system disorders.
Cobalt	Meats, milk, and milk products.	As part of vitamin B_{12}, involved in nerve function and blood formation.	Unknown except in vitamin B_{12} deficiency.	Unknown as a nutrition disorder.

TABLE 7–2
LOOKING FOR MINERALS IN THE FOOD GUIDE PYRAMID

FOOD GROUP/SERVING SIZE	MINERALS PROVIDED	SELECTION TIPS
Bread, Cereal, Rice, and Pasta (6 to 11 servings) ½ cup cooked cereal 1 ounce dry cereal 1 slice bread 2 cookies	Iron, Zinc, Magnesium	Choose foods made from whole grains, such as whole-wheat bread and whole-grain cereals. Choose most often foods that are made with little fat or sugars. Go easy on the fats and sugars you add as spreads, seasonings, or toppings.
Vegetables (3 to 5 servings) ½ cup cooked or raw chopped vegetables 1 cup raw leafy vegetables ¾ cup vegetable juice	Iron, Magnesium, Calcium	Different types of vegetables provide different nutrients—so, eat a variety. Include dark green leafy vegetables such as broccoli and spinach; deep yellow or orange vegetables like carrots and sweet potatoes; starchy vegetables like potatoes and corn; and legumes like kidney beans and chick-peas. Go easy on the fat you add to vegetables when cooking or at the table.
Fruit (2 to 4 servings) 1 medium apple, banana, or orange ½ cup chopped, cooked, or canned fruit ¾ cup fruit juice ¼ cup dried fruit	Potassium	Choose fresh fruits, fruit juices, and frozen or canned fruits without added sugar. Eat whole fruits most often—they are higher in fiber than juices. Only 100% fruit juice should be counted as fruit.
Milk, Yogurt, and Cheese (2 to 3 servings) 1 cup milk or yogurt 1½ ounces natural cheese 2 ounces process cheese 2 cups cottage cheese 1½ cups ice cream 1 cup frozen yogurt	Calcium, Phosphorus	Choose the nonfat varieties of milk and milk products like yogurt most often. Go easy on high-fat cheeses and ice cream; use the low-fat or fat-free varieties.
Meat, Poultry, Fish, Dry Beans, Eggs, and Nuts (2 to 3 servings) 2-3 ounces cooked lean meat, fish, or poultry 1 egg 2 tablespoons peanut butter } ½ cup cooked dry beans } equal to 1 ounce of meat ⅓ cup nuts	Iron, Copper, Zinc, Sulfur, Phosphorus, Magnesium, Chromium, Selenium	Choose lean meat, poultry without skin, fish, and dry beans and peas most often—they are the choices lowest in fat. Prepare meats in low-fat ways. For example, cook by broiling, roasting, grilling, or boiling. Limit egg yolks, which are high in cholesterol, and nuts and seeds, which are high in fat.
Fats, Oils, and Sweets (use sparingly) Butter, mayonnaise, salad dressing, cream cheese, sour cream, jam, jelly	——	These items are high in calories and low in nutrients. Select low-fat spreads and dressings.

Calcium

Calcium is the most abundant mineral in the body. Ninety-nine percent of the body's calcium is stored in the bones, which play two important roles. First, they support and protect the body's soft tissues. Second, they serve as a calcium bank, providing calcium to the body fluids whenever the supply is running low.

Although only a small part (about one percent) of the body's calcium is in the fluids, circulating calcium is vital to life. Calcium is required for the transmission of nerve impulses. It is essential for muscle contraction and so helps maintain the heartbeat. It appears to be essential for the integrity of cell membranes and for the maintenance of normal blood pressure. Calcium must also be present if blood clotting is to occur, and it is a **cofactor** for several enzymes.

Everyone knows that children need calcium daily to support the growth of their bones and teeth, but not everyone is aware of adults' needs for daily intakes of calcium. Abundant evidence now supports the importance of calcium for adults, especially women, who need at least as much calcium in their later years as they did when they were adolescents and young adults. A deficit of calcium during the growing years and in adulthood contributes to gradual bone loss, **osteoporosis,** which can totally cripple a person in later life.

Other nutrients are also important to bone growth and maintenance. Fluoride and vitamin D deficiencies, like calcium deficiencies, can cause loss of bone density. So can heredity, abnormal hormone levels, alcohol (even in moderate use), prescription medications, other drugs, and lack of exercise (especially weight-bearing exercises), but dietary calcium is one of the most important factors. This chapter's Nutrition Action feature discusses osteoporosis and its possible causes and prevention.

Table 7–3 shows that calcium appears almost exclusively in three classes of foods: milk and milk products, green vegetables such as broccoli, kale, bok choy, collards, and turnip greens, and a few fish and shellfish. Milk and milk products typically contain the most calcium per serving. Many greens are also good choices, but a complication enters in—

COFACTOR a mineral element that, like a coenzyme, works with an enzyme to facilitate a chemical reaction.

OSTEOPOROSIS (OSS-tee-oh-pore-OH-sis) also known as adult bone loss; a disease in which the bones become porous and fragile.

osteo = bones
poros = porous

TABLE 7–3
CALCIUM IN FOODS

Adult RDA is 800 to 1,200 mg.

(MG)	SOURCES
413	Yogurt, low-fat (1 c)
408	Swiss cheese (1.5 oz)
348	American cheese (2 oz)
345	Yogurt with fruit, low-fat (1 c)
325	Sardines (with bones) (3 oz)
316	Nonfat milk (1 c)
306	Cheddar cheese (1.5 oz)
275	Shrimp (3 oz)
248	Frozen yogurt (1 c)
186	Cream soup (1 c)
182	Salmon (with bones) (3 oz)
179	Collard greens, cooked (½ c)
154	Cottage cheese, low-fat (1 c)
144	Pudding, chocolate (½ c)
130*	Tofu (½ c)
126	Almonds (⅓ c)
124	Turnip greens, cooked (½ c)
91	Ice milk (½ c)
87	Ice cream (½ c)
80	Bok choy (½ c)
52	Tortilla, corn (1)
50	Dried beans, cooked (½ c)
36	Broccoli (½ c)

*The calcium content of tofu varies depending on processing methods. Look for tofu processed with calcium salts.

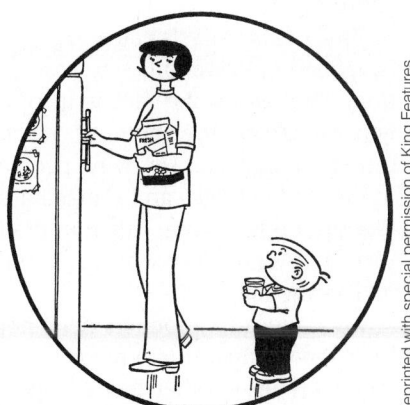

Reprinted with special permission of King Features Syndicate, Inc.

Guess what, Mommy—you were right! My teacher says milk is good for us."

absorption. It is not clear to what extent calcium is absorbed from certain green vegetables—notably, spinach—while calcium is known to be very well absorbed from milk.[2] Milk contains both vitamin D and lactose, which both enhance calcium absorption and promote bone health. Milk and milk products also normally supply about 40 percent of people's intake of riboflavin. Thus, experts recommend that everyone consume milk and milk products daily.[3] Figure 7–1 shows the current recommendations for calcium intakes.

Some foods contain **binders** that combine chemically with calcium and other minerals such as iron and zinc to prevent their absorption, carrying them out of the body with other wastes. For example, **phytic acid** renders the calcium, iron, and zinc in certain foods less available than they might be otherwise; **oxalic acid** also binds calcium and iron. Phytic acid is found in oatmeal and other whole-grain cereals; oxalic acid is found in beets, rhubarb, and spinach, among other foods. These binders seem to depress absorption of the calcium present in the food but not of calcium in other calcium-containing foods consumed at the same time. Since fiber in general seems to hinder calcium absorption, the higher the diet is in fiber (especially wheat bran), the higher it should be in calcium. This fact doesn't diminish the overall value of high-fiber foods; such foods are nutritious for many reasons, but they are not as useful as calcium sources.

Protein also affects calcium status by affecting excretion, not absorption. The higher the diet is in protein, the greater the amount of calcium excreted. This is why people in the United States and Canada are told to ingest more calcium than people in countries whose protein intakes are lower.

Milk and milk products need not be taken as such; there are ways to include them in other foods. Yogurt is an acceptable substitute for regular milk. Puddings, custards, and baked goods can be prepared in such a way that they also contain appreciable

BINDERS in foods, chemical compounds that can combine with nutrients (especially minerals) to form complexes the body cannot absorb. Examples of such binders are **phytic** (FIGHT-ic) **acid** and **oxalic** (ox-AL-ic) **acid.**

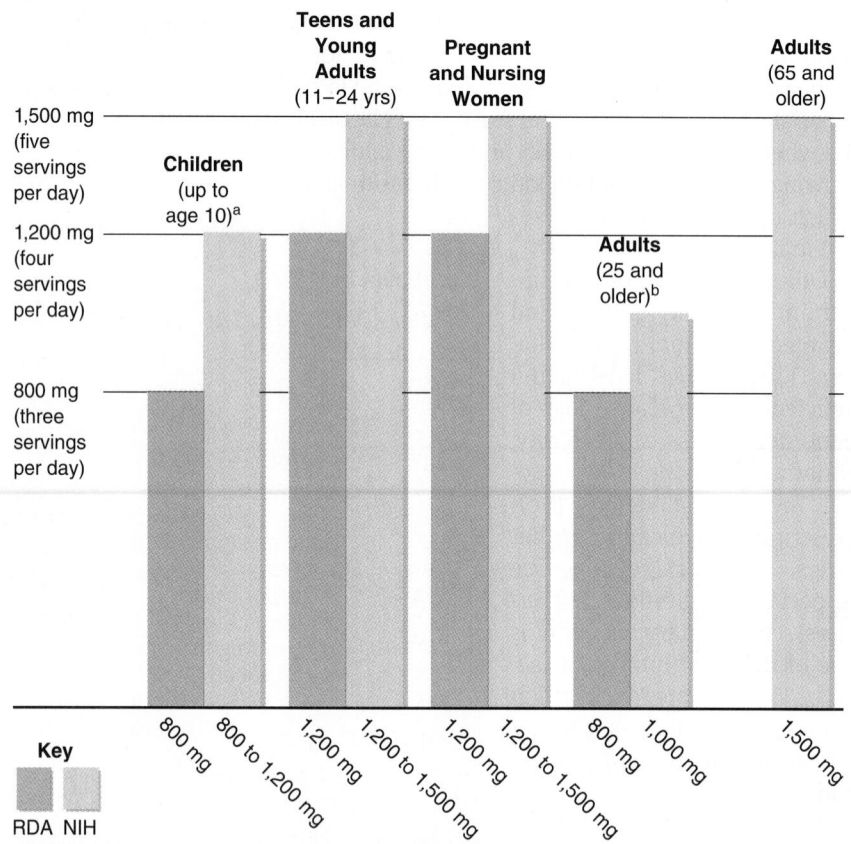

FIGURE 7–1
RECOMMENDED INTAKES OF CALCIUM

The RDA values shown here differ somewhat from the more recent 1994 National Institutes of Health (NIH) recommendations for optimal calcium requirements.

[a]The NIH recommendations for children are: 1 to 5 years........800 mg
                                                6 to 10 years.......800 to 1,200 mg

[b]The NIH recommendation for adults states that optimal calcium intake for women over age 50 years (postmenopausal) who are not taking estrogen is 1,500 mg.

SOURCE: NIH Consensus Statement: Optimal Calcium Intake, June 6–8, 1994, 12(4): 1–31.

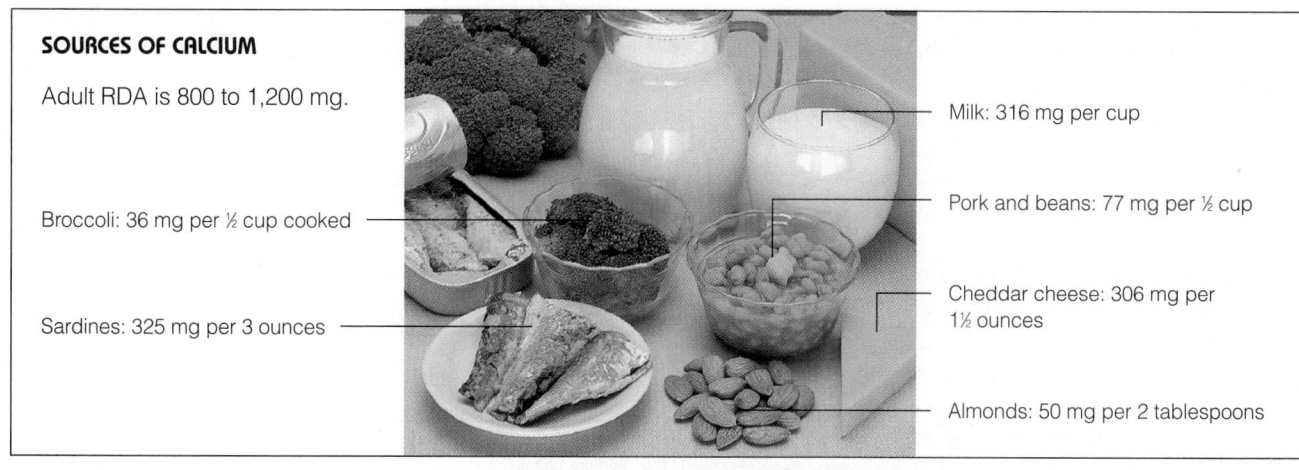

SOURCES OF CALCIUM

Adult RDA is 800 to 1,200 mg.

Broccoli: 36 mg per ½ cup cooked

Sardines: 325 mg per 3 ounces

Milk: 316 mg per cup

Pork and beans: 77 mg per ½ cup

Cheddar cheese: 306 mg per 1½ ounces

Almonds: 50 mg per 2 tablespoons

amounts of milk. Powdered nonfat milk, which is an excellent and inexpensive source of protein, calcium, and other nutrients, can be added to many foods (such as cookies, soups, casseroles, and meatloaf) during preparation. Nonfat yogurt fortified with extra milk solids is another excellent calcium source. Equal to milk and milk products in calcium richness are small fish such as sardines or herring or salmon with soft edible bones, or oysters.

A number of calcium-fortified foods are available, including calcium-fortified juices, fruit drinks, breads, and cereals. Many times, these foods are fortified to match the amount of calcium in a cup of milk; for example, an 8-ounce serving of fortified orange juice provides about 300 milligrams of calcium. Remember to check the Nutrition Facts panel on food labels for the amount of calcium contained in the foods you eat (see Figure 7–2).

The word *daily* should be stressed with respect to food sources of calcium. Because of the body's limited ability to absorb calcium, it cannot handle massive doses periodically but needs frequent opportunities to take in small amounts.

Milk Substitutes. Some people have **milk allergy** or **lactose intolerance** and can't drink milk. For them, calcium-rich substitutes must be found. Among the possible substitutes for persons with milk allergy are boiled milk, milk of goats or other species, calcium-fortified soy milk, nondairy foods containing the nutrients of milk, imitation milk, and calcium supplements. People with lactose intolerance can choose enzyme-treated milk, calcium-fortified soy milk, small amounts of milk products such as plain yogurt and aged cheese, as well as nondairy foods containing calcium, or calcium supplements.

In theory, it should be easy to choose the appropriate milk substitute. If the person is allergic to milk, in theory, the milk protein is the offending substance, and a substitute with altered or different proteins must be found—such as soy milk. If the person is intolerant to lactose, a lactose-free substitute is needed—such as enzyme-treated milk. It is often difficult, however, to determine why someone tolerates milk poorly. Both the kinds and the amounts of milk any

MILK ALLERGY the most common food allergy; caused by the protein in raw milk. Milk allergy is sometimes overcome by cooking the milk to denature the protein; it is sometimes alleviated by an abstinence from and a gradual reintroduction to milk.

LACTOSE INTOLERANCE as described in Chapter 3, an inherited or acquired inability to digest lactose as a result of a failure to produce the enzyme lactase. Lactose intolerance is prevalent in the majority of adult human populations.

FIGURE 7–2
CHECKING OUT THE FOOD LABEL FOR MINERALS

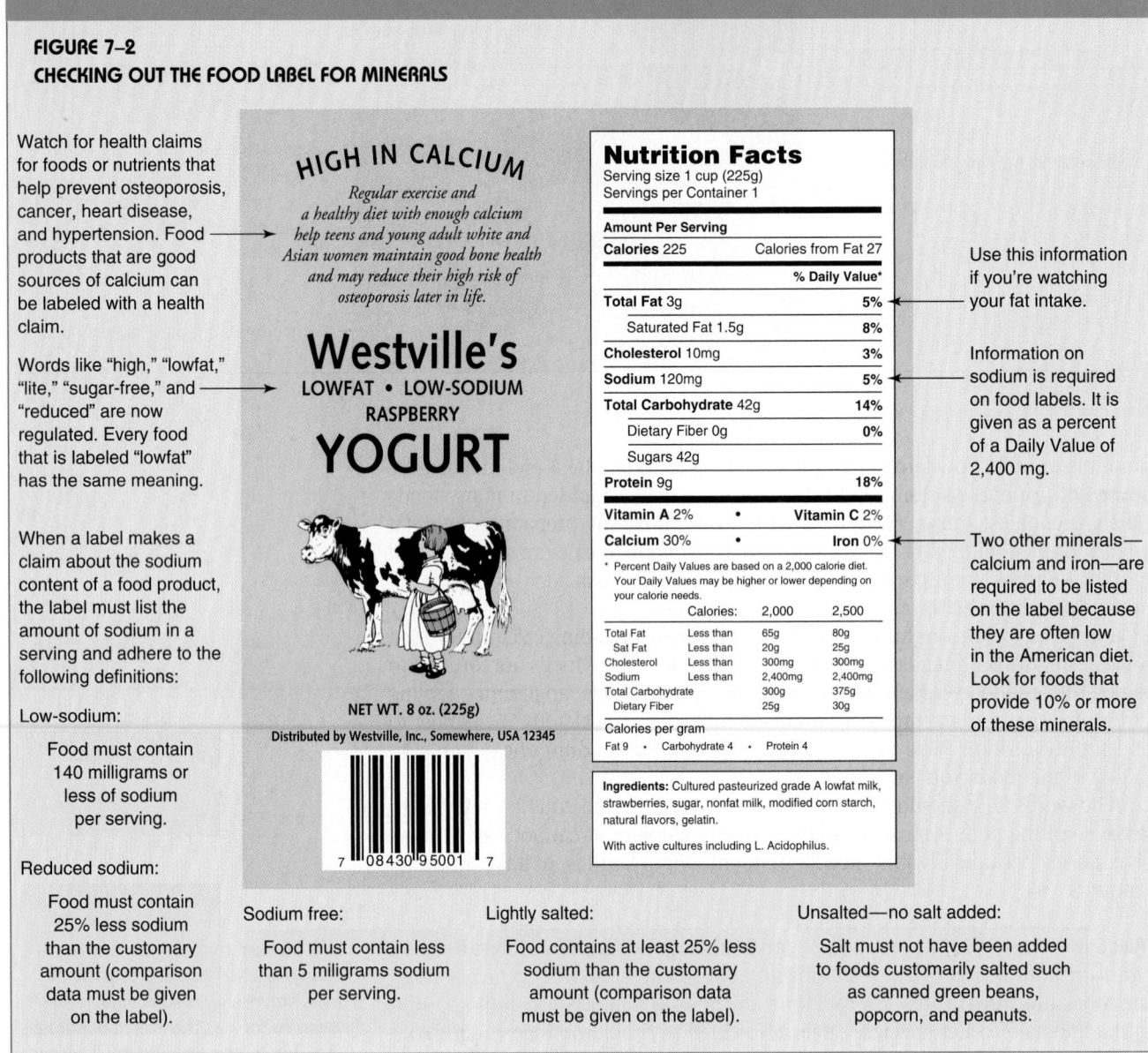

Watch for health claims for foods or nutrients that help prevent osteoporosis, cancer, heart disease, and hypertension. Food products that are good sources of calcium can be labeled with a health claim.

Words like "high," "lowfat," "lite," "sugar-free," and "reduced" are now regulated. Every food that is labeled "lowfat" has the same meaning.

When a label makes a claim about the sodium content of a food product, the label must list the amount of sodium in a serving and adhere to the following definitions:

Low-sodium:

Food must contain 140 milligrams or less of sodium per serving.

Reduced sodium:

Food must contain 25% less sodium than the customary amount (comparison data must be given on the label).

HIGH IN CALCIUM

Regular exercise and a healthy diet with enough calcium help teens and young adult white and Asian women maintain good bone health and may reduce their high risk of osteoporosis later in life.

Westville's
LOWFAT • LOW-SODIUM
RASPBERRY
YOGURT

NET WT. 8 oz. (225g)

Distributed by Westville, Inc., Somewhere, USA 12345

7 08430 95001 7

Nutrition Facts
Serving size 1 cup (225g)
Servings per Container 1

Amount Per Serving

Calories 225	Calories from Fat 27

	% Daily Value*
Total Fat 3g	**5%**
Saturated Fat 1.5g	**8%**
Cholesterol 10mg	**3%**
Sodium 120mg	**5%**
Total Carbohydrate 42g	**14%**
Dietary Fiber 0g	**0%**
Sugars 42g	
Protein 9g	**18%**

Vitamin A 2%	•	Vitamin C 2%
Calcium 30%	•	Iron 0%

* Percent Daily Values are based on a 2,000 calorie diet. Your Daily Values may be higher or lower depending on your calorie needs.

	Calories:	2,000	2,500
Total Fat	Less than	65g	80g
Sat Fat	Less than	20g	25g
Cholesterol	Less than	300mg	300mg
Sodium	Less than	2,400mg	2,400mg
Total Carbohydrate		300g	375g
Dietary Fiber		25g	30g

Calories per gram
Fat 9 • Carbohydrate 4 • Protein 4

Ingredients: Cultured pasteurized grade A lowfat milk, strawberries, sugar, nonfat milk, modified corn starch, natural flavors, gelatin.

With active cultures including L. Acidophilus.

Use this information if you're watching your fat intake.

Information on sodium is required on food labels. It is given as a percent of a Daily Value of 2,400 mg.

Two other minerals— calcium and iron—are required to be listed on the label because they are often low in the American diet. Look for foods that provide 10% or more of these minerals.

Sodium free:

Food must contain less than 5 miligrams sodium per serving.

Lightly salted:

Food contains at least 25% less sodium than the customary amount (comparison data must be given on the label).

Unsalted—no salt added:

Salt must not have been added to foods customarily salted such as canned green beans, popcorn, and peanuts.

given person can tolerate can be determined only by experimenting. The selection of a substitute may have to proceed by trial and error.

Milk protein is denatured when milk is boiled. Some cases of milk allergy can be solved by this simple means. Preboiled liquid or powdered milk can be cooked into foods such as custards and baked goods. Another alternative is goat's milk. The proteins in goat's milk differ somewhat from the proteins in cow's milk; thus, goat's milk may be tolerated by the person who can't tolerate cow's milk. Nutritionally, the two milks are similar in most respects. Both should be fortified with vitamins A and D, however, to properly complement the standard diet.

The treatment of milk with enzymes to digest its lactose offers a possible solution to the problem of lactose intolerance. An enzyme preparation (for example, LactAid) can be purchased over the counter and mixed with the milk before it's served. Or, you can take lactase tablets just before eating dairy products. Another possible alternative is low-lactose or lactose-free milk. Fermented dairy products, such as yogurt and aged cheeses, offer the same nutrients as milk but with a lower lactose content because in fermenting the milk, bacteria use the lactose as an energy source to do their work.[4] Table 7–4 shows the lactose contents of fermented dairy products compared with the lactose content of milk.

If foods are to be chosen to help replace milk in the diet, their calcium content should be the basis for making the choice because milk and milk products normally supply about 75 percent of people's intake of calcium. Foods to emphasize could be selected from Table 7–3 on page 235.

The alternatives offered for milk thus far have been superior in the sense that they are whole foods—milk dairy products—that offer many nutrients besides the ones listed in the tables. An inferior alternative is imitation milk. Since a milk substitute is satisfactory only if it provides high-quality protein, calcium, riboflavin, and vitamins A and D in quantities comparable to those in fortified fresh milk, the use of imitation milks in the diets of infants and children is generally undesirable.

Figure 7–3 is a decision tree for people seeking a milk substitute. Note that it recommends calcium supplements only as a last resort, simply because such supplements are not foods. Supplements do not offer the variety of nutrients that foods do, and their calcium is not, for the most part, absorbed as well as calcium from milk. Whenever possible, a person would do better to obtain calcium from suitable substitutes in some kind of food form. To evaluate your own diet for sources of calcium, see the Calcium Sources Scorecard on page 247.

Calcium Supplements. The demand for calcium supplements is on the rise. Sales of the supplement rose 30 percent between 1991 and 1994, accounting for $245 million in sales in the United States.[5] Calcium comes in a number of different salts, and the cost for a one-month supply of 1,000 milligrams per day can vary from $2 to almost $18 (see Table 7–5).[6] The organic salts include calcium lactate, calcium gluconate, and calcium citrate; the inorganic salts include, among others, calcium carbonate and calcium phosphate. Since calcium carbonate is 40 percent calcium and calcium gluconate is only 9 percent, fewer pills are necessary to get the needed calcium from calcium carbonate. On the other hand, an organic salt, such as calcium citrate is probably better absorbed, especially by older people, whose secretion of stomach acid—a factor known to enhance calcium absorption—tends to be reduced. A strategy to overcome this problem

TABLE 7–4
LACTOSE CONTENTS OF SELECTED DAIRY PRODUCTS

DAIRY PRODUCT	LACTOSE (GRAMS)
Whole milk (1 c)	11.0
2% low-fat milk (1 c)	9.0-13.0
Nonfat milk (1 c)	12.0-14.0
Chocolate milk (1 c)	10.0-12.0
Lactose-reduced low-fat milk (1 c)	3.3
Cultured buttermilk (1 c)	9.0-11.0
Low-fat yogurt (1 c)	11.0-15.0
Cheese (1 oz)	
Blue, cream, Parmesan, Colby	0.7-0.8
Camembert, Limburger	0.1
Cheddar, Gouda	0.4-0.6
Processed American	0.5
Processed Swiss	0.4-0.6
Cottage cheese, lowfat (1 c)	7.0-8.0
Butter (2 pats)	0.1
Ice cream/ice milk (1 c)	9.0-10.0

SOURCE: Adapted from K. Meister, *Much ado about milk,* American Council on Science and Health, July, 1993, p. 6.

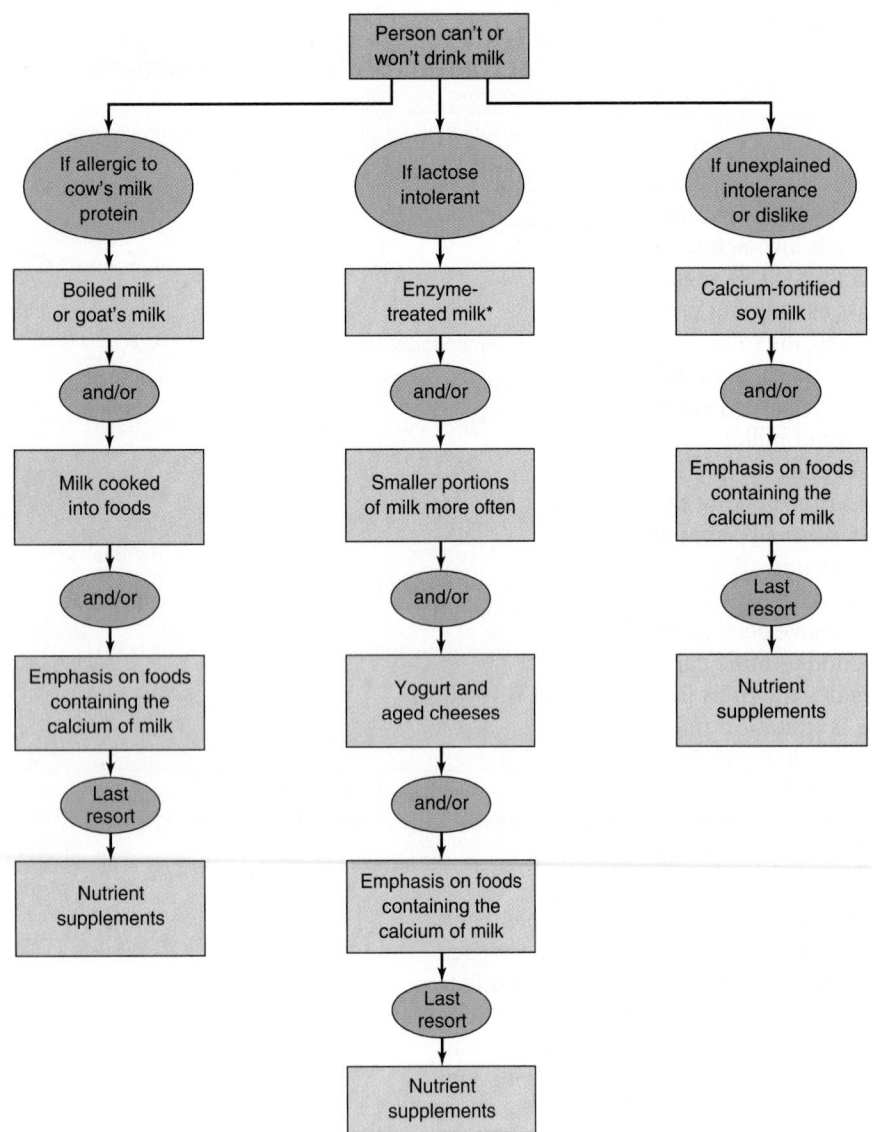

FIGURE 7–3
CHOOSING A MILK SUBSTITUTE

*You can buy milk already treated or add the enzyme (LactAid) yourself. Or, you can take lactase pills just before eating foods containing lactose. Enzyme treatment may not reduce lactose content sufficiently to relieve symptoms, and you may have to try the other alternatives.

is to take calcium carbonate two or three times a day in divided doses, with meals, to improve absorption.[7] Or, try a chewable tablet, or take the calcium carbonate pill with a glass of orange juice to aid its dissolving.

Since regular vitamin-mineral pills contain only small amounts of calcium, read the label carefully. Do not take dolomite, bonemeal, or oyster shell, as their

TABLE 7–5
TYPES OF CALCIUM SUPPLEMENTS

SUPPLEMENT	AMOUNT OF CALCIUM (MG)	COST PER MONTH ($)[a]
Calcium Carbonate (40% calcium)		
Rolaids™ Antacid tablets[b]	165	5.45
Tums™ Antacid, assorted flavors[b]	200	4.50
Os-Cal 500™	500	6.96
Schiff Natural Oyster Shell Calcium	500	4.00
Tums 500 Calcium[b]	500	4.80
Os-Cal 500 + D™[c]	500	6.72
Eckerd Naturalized Calcium™	600	5.25
Caltrate 600™	600	5.83
Walgreens Calcium 600™	600	2.00
AARP Formula 564 Calcium with Vitamin D™[c,d]	600	2.50
Kmart Calcium™	600	4.00
Calcium Citrate (21% calcium)		
Citracal 200™	200	10.05
Schiff Natural Calcium Citrate™	250	11.33
Calcium Lactate (13% calcium)		
AARP Formula 257™[d]	84	6.31
Solgar Calcium Lactate™	84	12.57
Calcium Gluconate (9% calcium)		
Solgar Calcium Gluconate™	60	18.00

[a]Prices reported in Calcium: How to get enough, *Consumer Reports*, August 1995, p. 513. Price based on a 30-grams-of-calcium-per-month supply—for people who supplement their diet with an average of 1,000 milligrams of calcium daily.

[b]Chewable.

[c]Tablet supplies 31% of Daily Value for vitamin D.

[d]Available by mail from the pharmacy service of the American Association of Retired Persons.

composition varies from one source to another, and some have been found to be contaminated with heavy metal poisons such as arsenic and lead.[8]

Supplements have the advantage of being easy to take, but they have the disadvantage of containing only calcium; they do not offer the other nutrients such as thiamin, riboflavin, niacin, potassium, phosphorus, vitamin A, and vitamin D found in milk. The person who omits milk and attempts to make up for it by taking supplements is still left with the task of obtaining these other nutrients. Milk drinking squares with the philosophy that using whole foods is preferable to taking supplements. In the final analysis, nutrition experts, including scientists participating in the Consensus Development Conference on Osteoporosis and members of the American Society for Bone and Mineral Research, strongly recommend that people use milk and milk products daily as a source of calcium.[9] There's an easy way to do this: Include them in meals.

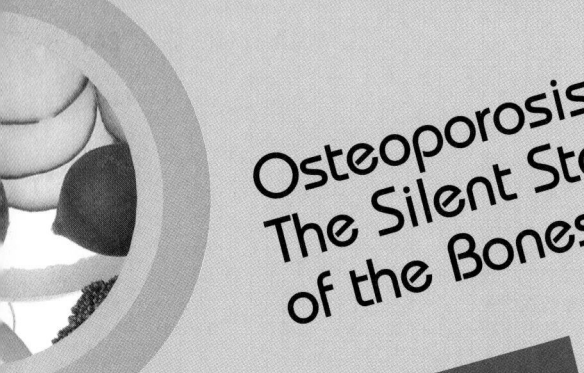

Osteoporosis— The Silent Stalker of the Bones

• As she waited in a grocery checkout line, Nancy Miller Friesen felt a stab of pain in her left hip. The 40-year-old Fort Worth woman had always been healthy and active—suddenly she could barely stand. When she went to her family doctor, she learned that several of her vertebrae had fractured. The radiologist studying her x-rays thought he was looking at the bones of a 70-year-old woman.

• Lila Rubin had just teed off at a New Jersey golf course. Putting down her club, the robust 63-year-old felt a searing back pain. When Rubin met with her orthopedic surgeon, she was told she'd suffered a serious compression fracture.

• Debra Epstein of New Haven, Connecticut, wasn't worried when her physician diagnosed a mild curvature of her upper spine seven years ago. She was only 31 and in otherwise excellent health. Then last year, her right wrist began aching and her back would tire easily. After tests, she learned that at age 37, she had the brittle bones of a woman twice her age.

The three women just described share the potentially crippling and sometimes deadly condition: osteoporosis.[10] Osteoporosis strikes some 25 million adults in the United States and threatens the integrity of the skeleton in at least one out of every three people over the age of 65 as well as 40 percent of women over age 45.[11] Osteoporosis strikes both sexes, although it is eight times more prevalent in women than in men after age 50 for several reasons:

• Women generally have less bone mass than men.

• Women typically have lower calcium intakes than men.

• Women more often use weight-reducing diets, which tend to be low in calcium.

• Bone loss begins earlier in women because of women's different hormonal make-up, and the loss is accelerated at **menopause,** when their protective **estrogen** secretion declines.

• Pregnancy and lactation decrease the calcium reserves in bones whenever calcium intake is inadequate.

• Women live longer than men, and bone loss continues with aging.

Adult bone loss affects the entire skeleton, but it occurs first in the pelvis and the spine. Unfortunately, osteoporosis establishes itself silently in its victims' lives. Symptoms do not usually occur until late in life. The disease often results in fractures of the hip, spine, and wrists—over one million such fractures a year—that occur with very little or no stress or pressure (see Figure 7–4). Often, it first becomes apparent when someone's hip suddenly gives way. People say, "She fell and broke her hip." The fact of the matter is that often the hip was so

MENOPAUSE the time of life at which a woman's menstrual cycle ceases, usually at about 45 to 50 years of age.

ESTROGEN a major female hormone—important in connection with nutrition because it maintains calcium balance and because its secretion abruptly declines at menopause.

fragile that it was already broken and caused the fall. Fewer than 50 percent of all women with hip fractures return to previous activity levels—many are confined to wheelchairs for the remainder of their lives. Approximately 30 percent of these women die of complications within the first year after hip fracture.

Figure 7–5 shows the effect of the loss of spinal bone on a woman's height and posture. It is not inevitable that people "grow shorter" as they age, but it does happen if they don't take the measures necessary to prevent bone loss.

Bones are made up of a complex matrix based on the protein collagen, into which the crystals of the bone minerals—principally calcium and phosphorus—are deposited. Bone tissue has two forms: **trabecular bone** and **cortical bone.** The thick ivorylike outer portion of a bone is the cortical bone. Cortical bone provides a covering for the inner trabecular bone—a lacy network of calcium-containing crystals, almost spongelike in appearance (see Figure 7–5). When calcium intakes are low, hormones call first upon the trabecular bone to release calcium into the blood for use by the rest of the body whenever levels fall too low.* Over time, the lacy network of bones becomes less dense and fragile as calcium deposits are withdrawn.

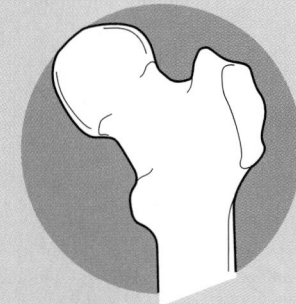

Broken Hips
- Most serious type of fracture
- 200,000 per year
- Most occur at 70 years or older
- 20% die within 4 months
- 50% become institutionalized

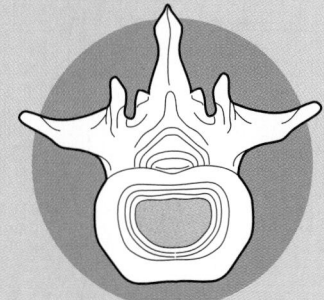

Spinal Vertebrae
- More likely at ages 55 to 75 years
- Fractures occur from bending or lifting, or can occur spontaneously
- Chronic back pain results from:
  - Several fractures which lead to loss of height
  - Spinal curvature

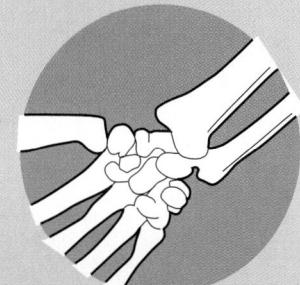

Broken Wrists
- Most occur at age 50 years or older
- Least severe type of fracture
- Early warning sign for osteoporosis

FIGURE 7–4
TYPES OF FRACTURES

Although bones undergo remodeling throughout life—adding and losing bone minerals—the total amount of bone mass in the human body reaches a peak in the mid-thirties. Afterwards, bones lose strength and density as bone minerals are lost. The principal determinant of bone health is peak bone mass. Think of bone mass as money in the bank: The larger the savings account, the easier it will be to withstand some loss of bone as one ages. To attain a healthful peak bone mass, it is necessary to have an optimal intake of calcium during

TRABECULAR (tra-BECK-you-lar) **BONE** the lacy inner network of calcium-containing crystals—spongelike in appearance—that supports the bone's structure.

CORTICAL BONE the dense outer ivorylike layer of bone that provides an exterior shell over trabecular bone.

---

*Vitamin D and parathyroid hormone circulate in the blood whenever the calcium concentration in the blood falls too low. These hormones cause the release of calcium from the bones, a decreased excretion of calcium from the kidneys, and an increased absorption of dietary calcium from the intestines. The hormone calcitonin is released from the thyroid gland when levels of blood calcium get too high; it acts to stop the release of calcium from bone and to slow intestinal absorption of the mineral.

FIGURE 7-5
BONE LOSS IN WOMEN

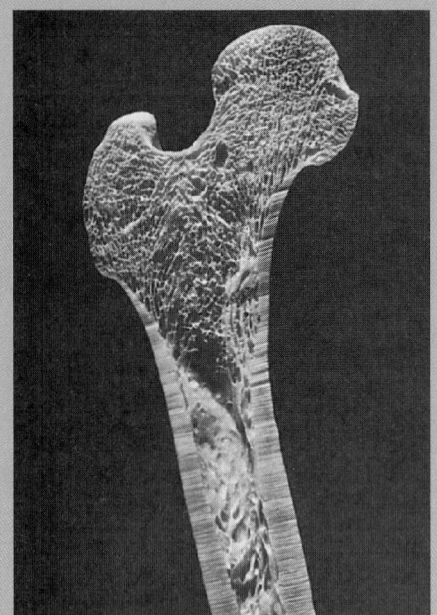

A. Cross section of bone. The lacy structural elements are trabeculae (tra-BECK-you-le), which can be drawn on to replenish blood calcium.

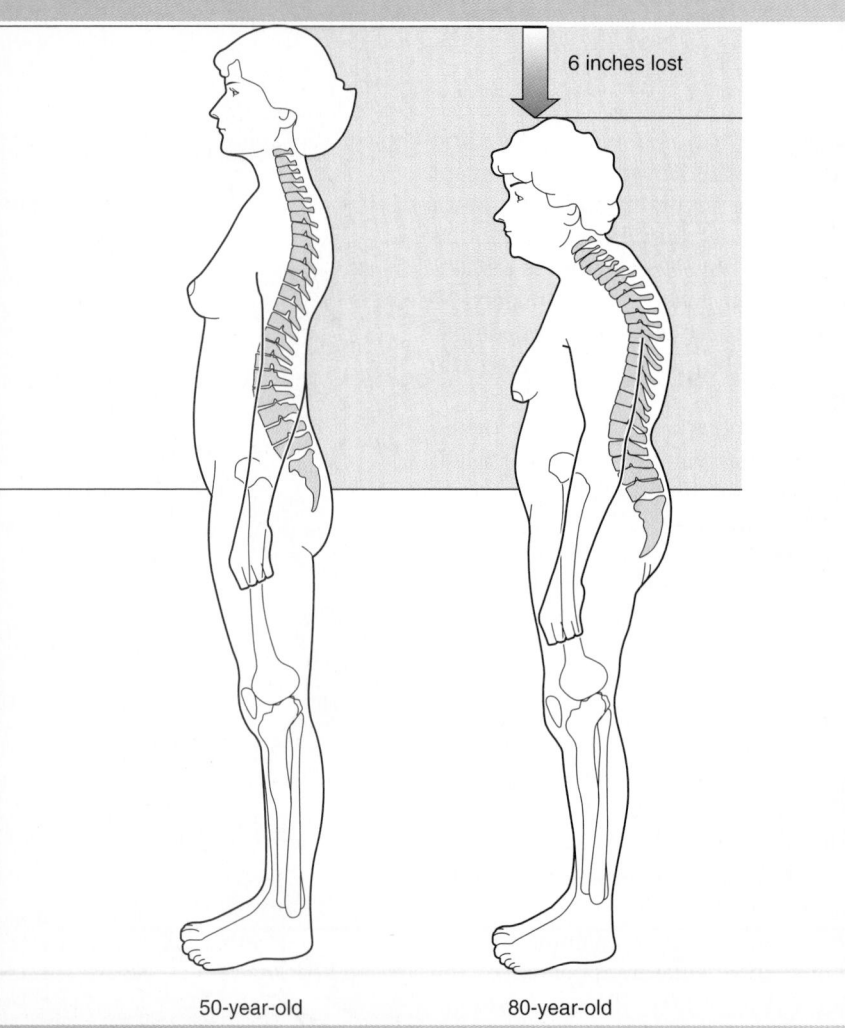

6 inches lost

50-year-old

80-year-old

C. Loss of height in a woman caused by adult bone loss. The woman on the left is about 50 years old. On the right, she is 80 years old. Her legs have not grown shorter; only her back has lost length as a result of collapse of her spinal bones (vertebrae). Collapsed vertebrae cannot protect the spinal nerves from pressure that causes excruciating pain.

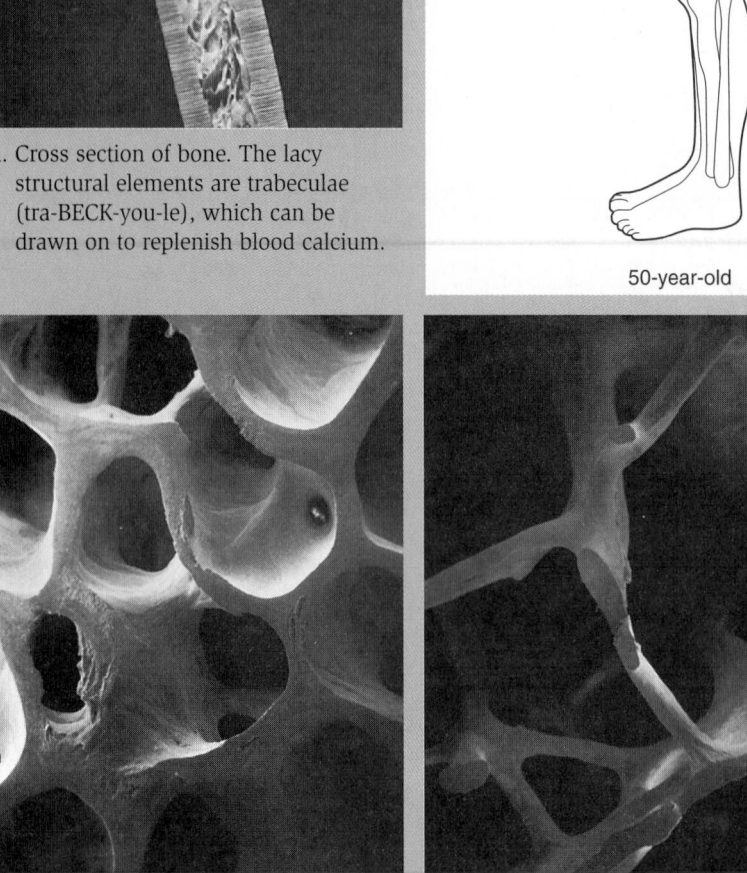

B. Electron micrograph of healthy trabecular bone.

Electron micrograph of trabecular bone affected by osteoporosis.

the years of bone growth—all through the growing years and on into the years of young adulthood.[12]

Although there is no cure for osteoporosis, the good news is that you can take steps to minimize your risk. First, determine your risk by considering the following list of factors that play a role in osteoporosis:

- *Age.* During childhood, adolescence, and the young adult years, the cells that build bone form more bone than the bone-dismantling cells take away. With aging, the bone-building cells become less active, while the bone dismantlers continue to work—causing bone tissue and strength to decline.

- *Gender.* Osteoporosis is eight times more common in women. Men achieve a higher peak bone mass than women do, and the rate of age-related bone loss is lower in men than in women.

- *Menopause and the hormone estrogen.* Menopause deprives women of the protective effects of estrogen. Estrogen improves calcium absorption from the intestines and reduces excretion of the mineral by the kidneys. Bone loss accelerates in women for the five to ten years following menopause. The earlier that menopause occurs, the greater a woman's risk of osteoporosis. Women who have ceased menstruating (a reliable indicator of reduced estrogen levels) comprise the largest segment of people with osteoporosis. Menopause occurs naturally in women typically between the ages of 45 and 55, but it can occur earlier in life with the removal of diseased ovaries. Estrogen replacement therapy slows the calcium losses from the bones of such women.[13] Menstruation can also cease in women who overexercise and are underweight, a condition called athletic amenorrhea (discussed in Chapter 9).

- *Family history.* The greater the history of skeletal fractures of the hips and vertebrae among elderly relatives, the greater your risk for osteoporosis.

- *Race and ethnic background.* People of British, Northern European, Chinese, Japanese, or Mexican-American background or Hispanic people from Central and South America are at the highest risk; African-American women tend to have denser bones and are at a low risk.[14]

- *Body build.* The smaller the frame and the thinner the person, the greater the risk. Petite women have less bone to lose than larger-boned women.

- *Sedentary lifestyle.* Inactivity leads to bone loss.

- *Smoking and alcohol.* Smoking and alcohol abuse increase the risk. Smokers tend to have lower body weights than nonsmokers. Some women who smoke have lower levels of estrogen in their blood compared to nonsmokers. Alcohol interferes with the absorption of calcium and may increase excretion of calcium from the kidneys. People who abuse alcohol also tend to have poor nutrition status, including low intakes of calcium.

- *Calcium and Vitamin D intakes.* Although data are incomplete, calcium intake early in life affects the attainment of peak bone mass, achieved by about age 35, which may be the most important determinant of the risk of a fracture in later life. Hence, ensuring an adequate calcium intake throughout life appears to be a sensible strategy. Adequate intake of Vitamin D is required for the absorption of calcium. In a multicountry study examining the relationship between the prevalence of osteoporosis in the population and customary levels of dietary calcium, Japan, with one of the lowest levels of calcium intake had the highest percentage of people with osteoporosis. Conversely, Finland, with the highest ranking for calcium intake had the lowest incidence of osteoporosis.[15]

The calcium intake of a sizeable portion of the U.S. population is estimated to be below the RDA for calcium—in the neighborhood of 400 to 600 milligrams—and some studies indicate the need for intakes higher than the current RDA for adolescents, and pre- and post-menopausal women.[16] Between the ages of 18 and 30 years—the time of the attainment of peak bone mass—more than two-thirds of all American women consume less than the RDA for calcium; after age 35, more than 75 percent of women have intakes lower than the RDA for calcium.[17] One explanation is the obsession—especially among adolescent girls—with dieting. Consumption of diet sodas increased 476 percent between the years 1960 and 1992, displacing milk as an accompanying beverage to meals.[18] To maximize peak bone mass and thereby guard against the debilitating effects of osteoporosis, the National Institutes of Health recently recommended increasing the recommended calcium intakes for young people ages 11 to 24 to 1,500 milligrams.[19]

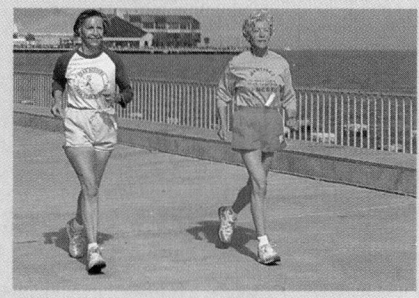

Incorporate regular sessions of weight-bearing exercise, such as brisk walking, into your weekly schedule to slow and possibly even prevent bone loss.

What can be done to prevent the debilitating effects of osteoporosis? Not surprisingly, the same recommendations have been made before for lowering risks for other chronic diseases: Eat a nutritious diet and exercise *throughout life.* Consider the following steps for building bone mass and lowering your risk for osteoporosis:

- Maximize peak bone mass and be vigilant about keeping the bones well supplied with calcium. To meet the recommended intakes of calcium, four servings of foods containing the amount of calcium found in a cup of milk are needed during childhood and adolescence and until 25 years of age; after that, two to three servings are recommended. According to researcher Robert Heaney of Omaha's Creighton University, only a few simple changes can add an extra 1,000 milligrams of calcium to an ordinary diet: Put a couple of heaping teaspoons of nonfat dried milk powder in each cup of coffee or tea, drink calcium-fortified orange juice, and eat one cup of low-fat yogurt, a dark green leafy vegetable, and a one-inch cube of hard cheese.[20]

Servings of foods providing about 300 milligrams of calcium (the amount found in 1 cup of milk) include ¾ cup plain, low-fat yogurt; 1 cup low-fat fruit yogurt; 1¼ ounces Swiss cheese; 1½ ounces cheddar cheese; 2 ounces American cheese; 1¼ cups pudding; 1¾ cups cream soup; 2 cups low-fat cottage cheese; and 1¼ cups frozen yogurt, or 2 cups ice cream. Keep in mind that the calories for these items vary from 90 calories for the cup of nonfat milk to 600 calories for the ice cream.

- Exercise regularly, since exercise can reduce the risk of developing osteoporosis by making bones stronger and increasing their ability to absorb calcium. Incorporate regular sessions of weight-bearing exercise, such as brisk walking, weight training, stair climbing, rope jumping, dancing, hiking, tennis, or aerobic dance classes, into your weekly schedule to slow and possibly even prevent bone loss.[21] Swimming and cycling are less effective at building bone mass, since they put less weight on the bones. Increase your exercise gradually up to 30- to 60-minute sessions three to five times a week. Exercises designed to strengthen the back muscles and improve posture are also recommended, since they will aid the skeleton in bearing its burden of weight.

For more about exercise, see Chapter 9.

- As a last resort, consider taking calcium supplements if you are unable to meet the RDA for calcium using foods. If you must use supplements, consider the perspective on calcium supplements offered earlier in the chapter.

CALCIUM SOURCES SCORECARD

We need at least 800 milligrams of calcium each day. Think about what you ate yesterday and answer the following questions:

1. Did you drink milk (nonfat, low-fat, or whole) yesterday? If so, give yourself 3 points for every 8-ounce glass (1 cup). _____

2. Did you eat yogurt? Give yourself 4 points for each 8-ounce serving (1 cup). _____

3. Did you eat (1 cup) calcium-fortified cereal with 1/2 cup of milk? Give yourself 4 points for every serving. _____

4. Did you eat 1 cup other type of cereal with 1/2 cup of milk? Give yourself 2 points for every serving. _____

5. Did you drink juice that is fortified with calcium? For every 6-ounce serving give yourself 2 points. _____

6. Did you eat canned salmon with bones or tofu (that's been processed with calcium) yesterday? Give yourself 3 points for each 3-ounce portion eaten (or ½ cup tofu). _____

7. Did you eat cheese yesterday? For every 1 ounce eaten, give yourself 2 points. _____

8. Did you eat cottage cheese? For each 1/2-cup serving give yourself 1 point. _____

9. Did you eat broccoli, kale, collards, or bok choy? For every 1 cup, raw or cooked, give yourself 1 point. _____

10. Did you have ice cream, pudding, or frozen yogurt yesterday? For a 1-cup serving give yourself 1 point. _____

Now add up all your points.

Total Points:_____

Multiply your total points × 100:_____

This gives you an idea of how many milligrams of calcium you are getting each day.

SOURCE: Adapted from *The Calcium Connection*, © 1994 Continental Baking Company.

Phosphorus

Phosphorus is second to calcium in abundance in the body. About 85 percent of it is found combined with calcium in the crystals of the bones and teeth as calcium phosphate, the chief compound that gives them strength and rigidity. Phosphorus is also a part of DNA and RNA, the genetic code material present in every cell. Phosphorus is thus necessary for all growth because DNA and RNA provide the instructions for new cells to be formed.

Phosphorus plays many key roles in the cells' use of energy nutrients. Many enzymes and the B vitamins become active only when a phosphate group is attached. The B vitamins, you will recall, play a major role in energy metabolism. Phosphorus is critical in energy exchange.

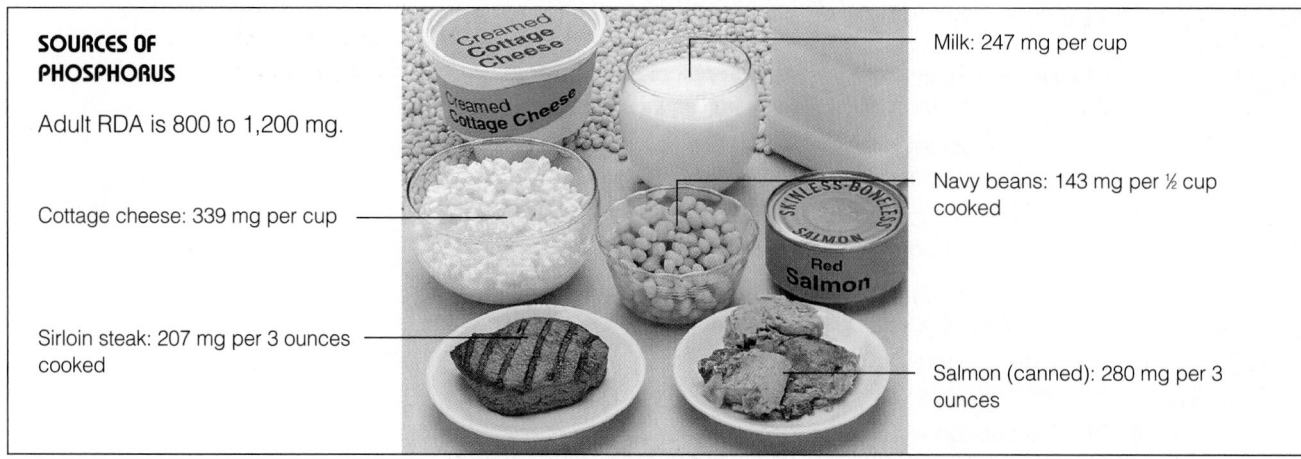

SOURCES OF PHOSPHORUS

Adult RDA is 800 to 1,200 mg.

Cottage cheese: 339 mg per cup

Sirloin steak: 207 mg per 3 ounces cooked

Milk: 247 mg per cup

Navy beans: 143 mg per ½ cup cooked

Salmon (canned): 280 mg per 3 ounces

Some lipids (phospholipids) contain phosphorus as part of their structure. They help to transport other lipids in the blood; they also form part of the structure of cell membranes, where they affect the transport of nutrients and wastes into and out of the cells.

Animal protein is the best source of phosphorus because phosphorus is so abundant in the energetic cells of animals. People who eat large amounts of animal protein have high phosphorus intakes. The intakes of phosphorus are also greater in people who regularly consume carbonated beverages because of their phosphoric acid content. Soft drink consumption is now estimated to be about 40 gallons per person each year. When soft drinks replace milk in the diet, fracture risks in both girls and women increase.[22]

The recommended intake of phosphorus is the same as for calcium so that a one-to-one ratio is maintained, a level believed to provide a sufficient intake of phosphorus and ensure adequate absorption and retention of calcium. Higher intakes of phosphorus can interfere with the absorption of calcium. People need not make a special effort to eat foods containing phosphorus, since phosphorus is present in virtually all foods (see Table 7–6).

Sodium and Potassium

Special conditions are needed to regulate the amounts of water inside and outside the cells so that the cells do not collapse from water leaving them or swell up under the stress of too much water entering them. The cells cannot manage this by pumping water across their membranes, because water slips back and forth freely. However, they can pump minerals across their membranes, and these minerals attract the water to come along with them. This is how the cells maintain water balance. Minerals are used for this purpose in a special form: as **ions** or **electrolytes.** In this form, as single, electrically charged particles, the minerals play many roles, including helping to maintain water balance and acid-base balance.

Sodium and potassium are examples of electrolytes—dissolved substances in blood and body fluids that carry electric charges. Sodium is the chief positively charged ion used to maintain the volume of fluid outside cells; potassium is the

	TABLE 7–6 **PHOSPHORUS IN FOODS**
	Adult RDA is 800 to 1,200 mg.
(MG)	**SOURCES**
422	American cheese (2 oz)
339	Cottage cheese (1 c)
325	Yogurt (1 c)
280	Salmon (canned) (3 oz)
247	Nonfat milk (1 c)
242	Pork (3 oz)
207	Sirloin steak (3 oz)
186	Turkey (3 oz)
174	Peanuts (⅓ c)
161	Hamburger (3 oz)
149	Shredded wheat (1 c)
143	Navy beans (½ c)
139	Tuna (3 oz)
127	Sunflower seeds (2 tbsp)
115	Potato (1)
104	Peanut butter (2 tbsp)
67	Corn (½ c)
51	Cola (12 oz)
46	Broccoli (½ c)
46	Whole-wheat bread (1 slice)
45	Diet cola (12 oz)

IONS (EYE-ons) electrically charged particles, such as sodium (positively charged) and chloride (negatively charged).

ELECTROLYTES compounds that partially dissociate in water to form ions; examples are sodium, potassium, and chloride.

chief positively charged ion inside body cells. Electrolytes influence the distribution of fluids among the various body compartments. As an example of how electrolytes affect fluid volume, let's consider the hypothetical case of a man given one tablespoon of salt (sodium chloride) to eat and no water (NOT something we recommend trying!). The salt would become distributed in the space outside of his body's cells and would be excluded from his cells. To counterbalance this sudden change in electrolyte concentration, water would move from the cells into the space outside of the cells. The result would be an increase in the man's fluid volume outside of his cells and a decrease in the fluid volume inside his cells. Under normal circumstances, many factors work together to keep the fluid volume fairly constant inside and outside of cells.

About 40 percent of the body's water weight is inside the cells, and about 15 percent bathes the outsides of the cells. The remainder is in the blood vessels.

Electrolytes also provide the environment in which the cells' work takes place—work such as nerve-to-nerve communication, heartbeats, and contraction of muscles. When a person's body loses fluid—whether it be sweat, blood, or urine—the person also loses electrolytes. The concentrations of electrolytes are crucial to the life-sustaining activities of the vital organs. When large amounts of body fluid are lost, as in heat stroke, infant diarrhea, or injury, their replacement is a task for a medical team.

People who exercise lose fluids and must replace them to avoid dehydration. Chapter 9 discusses fluid needs during and after exercise, including a discussion of popular sports drinks.

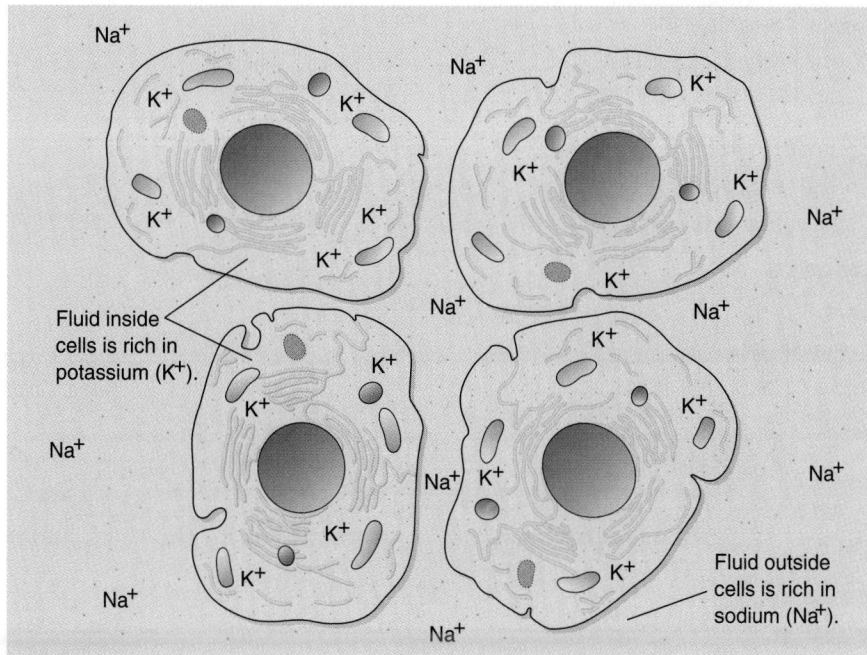

Fluid inside cells is rich in potassium (K⁺).

Fluid outside cells is rich in sodium (Na⁺).

Electrolytes

Sodium and potassium are examples of body electrolytes. Potassium, which is usually found in the fluids inside the cells, carries a positive charge; sodium, which is usually found in the fluids outside the cells, carries a positive charge.

Sodium is part of sodium chloride, ordinary table **salt,** a food seasoning and preservative. No recommendation is necessary for a minimum intake of sodium, since sodium is so abundant in the U.S. diet. For some people, however, a ceiling is suggested (see inside front cover), because the use of highly salted foods can contribute to high blood pressure (**hypertension**) in those who are genetically susceptible. (A discussion of the causes and prevention of hypertension appears in the Nutrition Action feature starting on page 255.)

If some members of your family have high blood pressure (and this is more likely if you are black than if you are white), you are advised to curtail your sodium consumption and make sure that your potassium and calcium intakes are ample. Table 7–7 shows a sampling of the sodium content of common foods and reveals that generally, the more processed a food is, the more sodium and the less potassium it contains. Whole, unprocessed foods, on the other hand, tend to be high in potassium and low in sodium.

Persons who wish to avoid salt need to know that what they pour from the salt shaker may be only a sixth of the total salt they consume. Up to 75 percent of the salt in the diet is that added to foods by food processors. Processed foods don't always taste salty. This makes eating something of a guessing game; remember to check food labels for sodium content. The serious sodium avoider must eat fresh rather than processed foods, or look for reduced-sodium processed foods. Reducing your salt intake doesn't have to be unpleasant. Many sodium-free flavoring agents such as lemons, onions, chilies, curries, and other spices excite the taste buds and enhance the flavors of traditional foods.

Potassium is critical to maintaining the heartbeat. The sudden deaths that occur during fasting, severe diarrhea, or severe vomiting are thought to be due to heart failure caused by potassium loss. As the principal positively charged ion inside body cells, potassium plays a major role in maintaining water balance and cell integrity.

See Consumer Tips on the next page for a list of foods that are high in sodium and for suggested ways to reduce salt intake.

SALT a pair of charged mineral particles, such as sodium ($Na+$) and chloride ($Cl-$), that associate together. In water, they dissociate and help to carry electric current—that is, they become electrolytes.

HYPERTENSION sustained high blood pressure.
 hyper = too much
 tension = pressure

TABLE 7–7
WHOLE UNPROCESSED FOODS VERSUS PROCESSED FOODS—POTASSIUM AND SODIUM CONTENT

FOOD	POTASSIUM (MG)[a]	SODIUM (MG)[a]	POTASSIUM-TO-SODIUM RATIO
MILK FOODS			
Milk, 1 c	370	120	3:1
Chocolate pudding (homemade), 1 c	424	268	3:1
Chocolate pudding (instant), 1 c	432	738	1:2
MEATS			
Beef roast, 3 oz	254	54	5:1
Corned beef (canned), 3 oz	116	855	1:7
Chipped beef, 3 oz	377	2,946	1:8
VEGETABLES			
Corn, 1 c	390	6	65:1
Creamed corn, 1 c	344	730	1:2
Sugar-coated cornflakes, 1 c	17	103	1:6
FRUITS			
Peaches (fresh), 1	171	0	171:1
Peaches (canned), 1	150	10	15:1
Peach pie, 1 piece	149	288	1:2
GRAINS			
Whole-wheat flour, 1 c	486	6	81:1
Whole-wheat bread, 1 slice	34	135	1:4
Wheat crackers, 4	17	69	1:4

[a]Data are taken from Appendix I

Seasoning Foods Without Excess Salt

You've decided to cut your salt intake. How do you know which foods to buy? How can you cook foods with less salt and good flavor? Fortunately, cutting some of the salt out of your diet isn't difficult. Here are a few basic principles.

At the supermarket

- Read labels! Look for the key words *salt* and *sodium* in the ingredients list. These are signals that the foods contain added sodium. Here is a short list of a few sodium-containing ingredients used in food processing: baking powder, baking soda, disodium phosphate, monosodium glutamate (MSG), salt, sodium benzoate, sodium hydroxide, sodium nitrite, sodium propionate, and sodium sulfite.
- Choose reduced-sodium products when possible. Many commercially prepared products are available in sodium-reduced versions. For example, most supermarkets carry reduced-sodium soy sauce, canned tuna, soups, and canned vegetables.
- Buy fresh, natural foods more frequently than processed foods, which tend to be high in salt. Here is a list of processed and convenience foods that are typically high in salt:

Meat, Poultry, Fish

- Cured meats: ham, bacon, luncheon meats
- Sausages
- Fish: canned in oil or brine
- Fish: commercially frozen, prebreaded
- Canned shellfish
- Hot dogs

Meat Substitutes

- Salted nuts or seeds
- Soy protein products
- Canned beans and peas

Main Dish Items

- Pizza, lasagna, macaroni and cheese
- Commercially prepared main course foods (e.g., frozen dinners)
- Tacos, enchiladas, burritos
- Canned or dehydrated soups or chowders

Dairy Products

- Cheeses
- Buttermilk
- Instant cocoa mixes
- Dutch process cocoa

Bread Products

- Salted snack foods (e.g., crackers, potato chips)
- Commercially baked goods (e.g., cakes, cookies)

Canned Vegetables and Vegetable Juices

Miscellaneous Products

- Catsup, chili sauce
- Salted gravies and sauces
- Olives, pickles, pickle relish
- Seasoning salts
- Bouillon cubes
- Commercial salad dressings
- Meat tenderizers (e.g., MSG, Accent)

At home—in the kitchen and at the table

- Put the salt shaker in the kitchen cabinet, not on the table, and use it only on rare occasions. It's surprising how much additional sodium is added to foods with just a few shakes of the salt shaker. Here's a handy guide for the sodium content of common kitchen measures of salt:

  ¼ tsp of salt = 575 mg of sodium
  ½ tsp of salt = 1,150 mg of sodium
  1 tsp of salt = 2,300 mg of sodium

- Flavor your foods with seasonings and spices, most of which are virtually salt and sodium free. Try some of the seasonings listed in your favorite dishes:

allspice	curry powder	onion (not onion salt)
basil	dill	paprika
bay leaves	garlic powder	parsley
caraway seeds	ginger	rosemary
chives	lemon juice	sage
cider vinegar	mustard (dry)	thyme
cinnamon	nutmeg	turmeric

- Make an herb mixture of your own. Combine garlic powder, basil, rosemary, oregano, and anise seed in equal amounts. Mix in a blender. Label your herb mix. Add a few grains of rice to prevent caking. Try this with other herb combinations, too!
- Salt substitutes can be used as a means of reducing sodium intake. They usually consist of a mineral base other than sodium and are compounded to give a taste sensation similar to sodium chloride. The most common components are potassium chloride, calcium chloride, and ammonium chloride. [**Caution:** Before using salt substitutes, check with your doctor. Some people, especially those with kidney problems or liver disease, should *not* use these products.] A few salt substitutes are Adolph's Salt Substitute, Diamond Crystal, Morton's Lite Salt, Morton's Salt Substitute, No Salt, and Nu-Salt.

SOURCES OF SODIUM Daily Value recommended for sodium is no more than 2,400 mg.

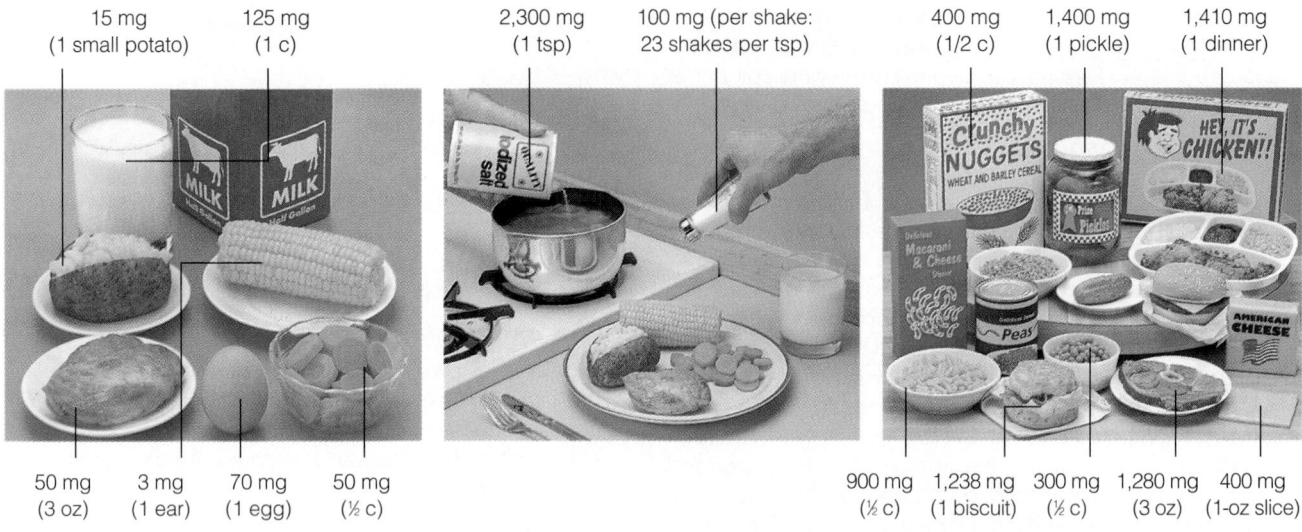

15 mg (1 small potato) 125 mg (1 c) 2,300 mg (1 tsp) 100 mg (per shake: 23 shakes per tsp) 400 mg (1/2 c) 1,400 mg (1 pickle) 1,410 mg (1 dinner)

50 mg (3 oz) 3 mg (1 ear) 70 mg (1 egg) 50 mg (½ c) 900 mg (½ c) 1,238 mg (1 biscuit) 300 mg (½ c) 1,280 mg (3 oz) 400 mg (1-oz slice)

Many whole, unprocessed foods are low in sodium. These foods contribute less than 10 percent of the sodium in the U.S. diet.

The salt added during cooking or at the table contributes about 15 percent of the sodium in the U.S. diet.

Most of the sodium (about 75 percent) in our diet is added by food manufacturers to processed foods such as these.

When sodium is lost with water from the body, the ultimate damage comes when potassium moves out of the cells with cell water and is excreted. This is especially dangerous because potassium deficiency affects the brain cells, making the victim unaware of the need for water. Adults are warned not to take **diuretics** (water pills), except under the direction of a physician, because some of them cause potassium excretion. Physicians prescribing such diuretics will tell their patients to eat potassium-rich foods to compensate for the losses and, depending on the diuretic, may also advise a lowered sodium intake.

DIURETICS (dye-you-RET-ics) medications causing increased water excretion.
dia = through
ouron = urine

SOURCES OF POTASSIUM

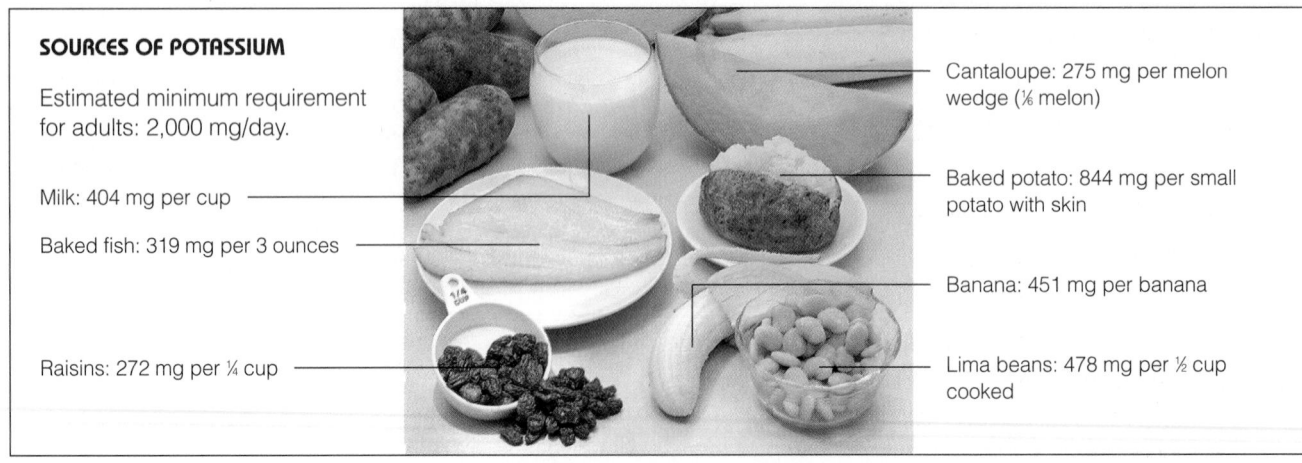

Estimated minimum requirement for adults: 2,000 mg/day.

Milk: 404 mg per cup

Baked fish: 319 mg per 3 ounces

Raisins: 272 mg per ¼ cup

Cantaloupe: 275 mg per melon wedge (⅙ melon)

Baked potato: 844 mg per small potato with skin

Banana: 451 mg per banana

Lima beans: 478 mg per ½ cup cooked

The relationship of potassium and sodium in maintaining the blood pressure is not entirely clear. Abundant evidence supports the simple view that the two minerals have opposite effects. In any case, it is clear that increasing the potassium in the diet can promote sodium excretion under most circumstances and thereby lower the blood pressure.[23] A lifelong intake of foods low in sodium and high in potassium protects against hypertension and is thought to play a role in the low blood pressure seen in vegetarians.[24]

A dietary deficiency of potassium is unlikely, but high-sodium, highly processed diets low in fresh fruits and vegetables can make it a possibility. Whole foods of all kinds, including fruits, vegetables, grains, meats, fish, and poultry, are among the richest sources of potassium. Potassium is also abundant in milk. Table 7–8 shows the potassium content of foods.

TABLE 7–8 POTASSIUM IN FOODS	
Suggested minimum intake: 2,000 mg.	
(MG)	**SOURCES**
844	Baked potato (1)
529	Yogurt (1 c)
478	Lima beans (½ c)
451	Banana (1 medium)
419	Spinach, cooked (½ c)
404	Nonfat milk (1 c)
400	Pinto beans (½ c)
355	Orange juice (¾ c)
329	Kidney beans (½ c)
319	Salmon (3 oz)
315	Bok choy, cooked (½ c)
299	Pork (3 oz)
297	Hamburger (3 oz)
275	Cantaloupe (⅙ melon)
273	Tomato (1 medium)
272	Raisins (¼ c)
254	Raisin bran (1 c)
237	Chicken (3 oz)
232	Carrots (½ c)
228	Broccoli (½ c)

Some people have medical reasons for needing potassium supplementation, but these people need to be medically supervised. For example, people on medically-supervised, very-low-calorie weight-loss diets may be advised to take a potassium supplement. A physician must monitor the potassium status of these people and order supplements commensurate with the degree of depletion.

Potassium supplements should never be self-prescribed. Potassium toxicity from potassium in supplement form is a greater concern than potassium deficiency. The body protects itself from this eventuality as best it can. If you consume more than you need, the kidneys accelerate their excretion and so maintain control. Should their limit be exceeded (if you ingest too much potassium too fast), a vomiting reflex is triggered. However, if the digestive tract is bypassed and potassium is injected into a vein at a high rate, the heart can stop.

Chloride, Sulfur, and Magnesium

The chloride ion is the major negatively charged ion of the fluids outside the cells, where it is found mostly in association with sodium. Chloride can move freely across membranes and so is also found inside the cells in association with potassium. In the blood, chloride helps in maintaining the acid-base balance. In the stomach, the chloride ion is part of hydrochloric acid, which maintains the strong acidity of the stomach. Nearly all dietary chloride comes from sodium chloride or salt.

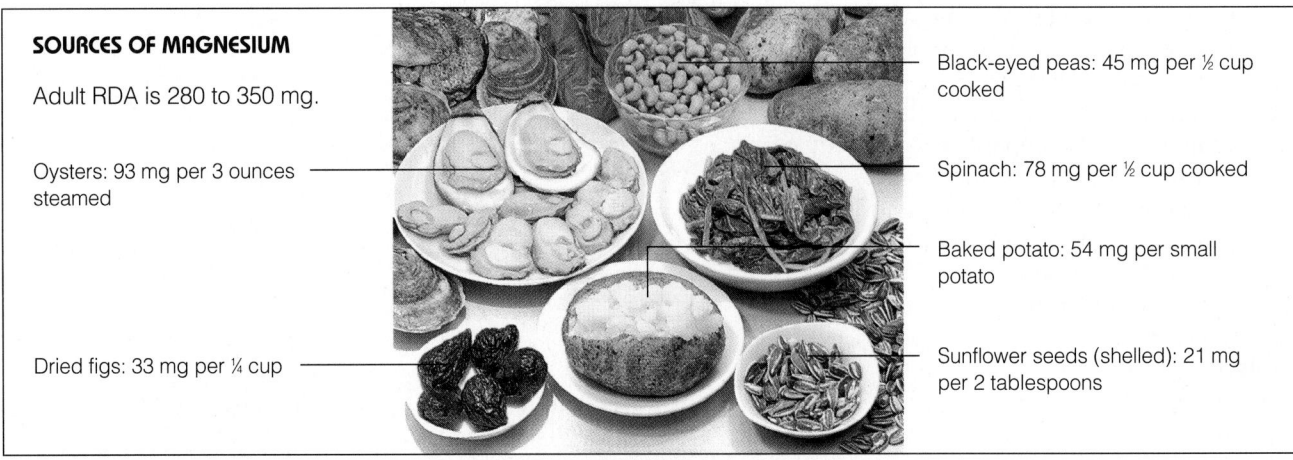

SOURCES OF MAGNESIUM

Adult RDA is 280 to 350 mg.

Oysters: 93 mg per 3 ounces steamed

Dried figs: 33 mg per ¼ cup

Black-eyed peas: 45 mg per ½ cup cooked

Spinach: 78 mg per ½ cup cooked

Baked potato: 54 mg per small potato

Sunflower seeds (shelled): 21 mg per 2 tablespoons

Sulfur is present in some amino acids and in all proteins. Its most important role is in helping strands of protein to assume and hold a particular shape, thus enabling them to do their specific jobs, such as enzyme work. Skin, hair, and nails contain some of the body's more rigid proteins, and these have a high sulfur content. There is no recommended intake for sulfur, and no deficiencies are known. Only a person who lacks dietary protein to the point of severe deficiency will lack the sulfur-containing amino acids.

Magnesium acts in all the cells of the muscles, heart, liver, and other soft tissues, where it forms part of the protein-making machinery and is necessary for the release of energy. Magnesium also helps to relax muscles after contraction and promotes resistance to tooth decay by helping to hold calcium in tooth enamel. Bone magnesium seems to be a reservoir to ensure that some will be on hand for vital reactions regardless of recent dietary intake. A dietary deficiency of magnesium is not likely but may occur as a result of vomiting, diarrhea, alcohol abuse, or protein malnutrition; in people who have been fed incomplete fluids into a vein for too long; or in people using diuretics. Good food sources of magnesium include nuts, legumes, cereal grains, dark green vegetables, seafoods, chocolate, and cocoa (see Table 7–9).

TABLE 7–9
MAGNESIUM IN FOODS

Adult RDA is 280 to 350 mg.

(MG)	SOURCES
140	Almonds (⅓ c)
126	Tofu (½ c)
119	Cashews (⅓ c)
95	Raisin bran (1 c)
93	Oysters (steamed) (3 oz)
85	Peanuts (⅓ c)
78	Spinach, cooked (½ c)
54	Baked potato (1)
45	Black-eyed peas (½ c)
42	Brown rice, cooked (½ c)
40	Lima beans (½ c)
36	Lentils, cooked (½ c)
35	Split peas, cooked (½ c)
33	Dried figs (¼ c)
28	Nonfat milk (1 c)
27	Chicken (3 oz)
21	Sunflower seeds (2 tbsp)
21	Hamburger (3 oz)
20	Pork (3 oz)
17	Milk chocolate (1 oz)

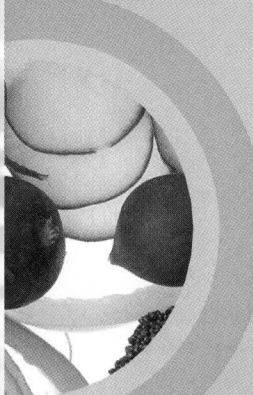

Diet and Blood Pressure—The Salt Shaker and Beyond

Think "diet" and "blood pressure," and the first thing that comes to mind is salt. Small wonder, given that experts have long emphasized that a diet high in salt—or more specifically, the sodium it contains—contributes to a public health problem known as hypertension (or high blood pressure).[25] Nevertheless, a number of other, albeit less notorious, dietary factors play a role in the unhealthful rise in blood pressure that afflicts some 60 million Americans.

Obesity, for instance, inarguably ranks as the number one dietary culprit linked to hypertension.[26] That's because excess weight forces the heart to work harder to supply the extra pounds of tissue with blood. High blood pressure occurs about twice as often among obese people as it does in thinner people. Fortunately, losing as little as 5 percent of the excess weight has been shown, in some cases, to lower blood pressure to a point at which taking antihypertensive medications may become unnecessary.[27] In other words, a little weight loss, regardless of sodium intake, can be enough to get a high blood pressure level back under control.

Another dietary factor that may lead to high blood pressure (not to mention poor compliance with drug regimens and other treatments for the problem) is drinking excessive amounts of alcohol. In fact, consuming more than a couple of ounces of alcohol daily has been blamed for leading to 5 percent to 11 percent of cases of hypertension among men.[28] The Joint National Committee on Detection, Evaluation, and Treatment of High Blood Pressure thus recommends that to control high blood pressure, those who drink should limit themselves to no more than one ounce of alcohol a day—an amount found in two ounces of 100-proof whiskey, an eight-ounce glass of wine, or two 12-ounce cans of beer.[29]

In addition to recommending that hypertensive people lose weight and drink alcohol in moderation, the Committee advises those with hypertension to limit the amount of sodium in their diet. Whether such advice is appropriate for the public at large, however, has been widely debated; some experts argue against the necessity of doing so in all but a few select cases. The controversy revolves around a growing body of evidence suggesting that not everyone's blood pressure rises as a result of eating a high-sodium diet. Only certain people, presumably because of their genetic make-up, appear to be **salt sensitive,** meaning that their blood pressure rises in proportion to the amount of sodium they consume. For them, of course, keeping dietary sodium to a minimum can help lower elevated blood pressure.

The problem is that it is difficult to identify who is salt sensitive and who is not. Thus, some experts argue that a call to the general public to reduce sodium consumption is unwarranted because it recommends that even people who are not salt sensitive avoid the seasoning. On the other side of the fence are experts and organizations, the National Research Council among them, whose position is that because lowering the amount of sodium in the diet does not pose any health hazard and may be beneficial to some people, it is still prudent for the

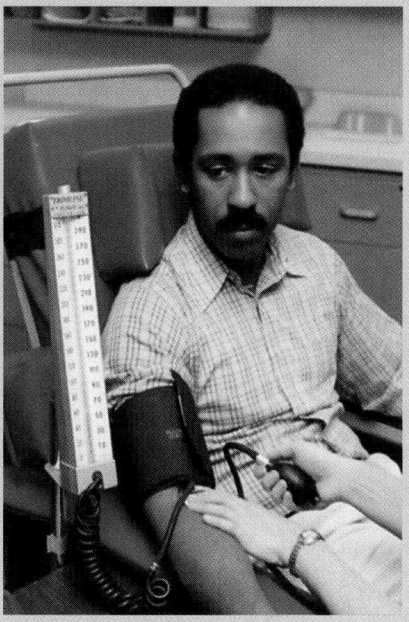

The most effective single measure you can take to protect yourself against high blood pressure is to know what your blood pressure is.

SALT SENSITIVE the tendency for blood pressure to rise in proportion to salt consumption that certain people seem to have from birth.

public as a whole to keep sodium intake in check.[30] And for those who take medication to control their blood pressure, the argument in favor of adhering to a low-sodium diet is stronger: Eating too much salt can limit the effectiveness of some antihypertensive medications.

In any case, it is clear that modest changes in lifestyle can add up to significant gains in controlling high blood pressure.[31] In addition, it appears that attention to a healthful lifestyle can help to prevent the problem from arising in the first place. Consider that researchers at Northwestern University Medical School in Chicago put one group of adults prone to elevations in blood pressure on a preventive program that included losing weight, lowering sodium intake, cutting down on alcohol, and exercising more and compared them to a similar group left to their own devices. The researchers found that over the course of five years, only one in eleven persons who changed their lifestyle wound up with full-blown hypertension. But of those who didn't alter their habits, one in five became hypertensive.[32]

Along with the factors just explained, scientists are exploring other nutrients that may influence blood pressure. Some researchers believe, for instance, that it is not dietary sodium per se that alters blood pressure, but rather the ratio between it and potassium, sodium's partner in regulating the body's water balance. In other words, the more potassium and less sodium in the diet, the greater the likelihood that the body will maintain a normal blood pressure. While the evidence is not strong enough to imply that people with high blood pressure need to take potassium supplements (such a practice can be dangerous), it's worth keeping in mind, particularly because diets rich in high-potassium foods such as fresh fruits and vegetables tend to go hand in hand with low sodium consumption.[33]

In addition, some studies indicate that people who eat high-calcium diets are less likely to have high blood pressure; conversely, people with inadequate calcium intakes are more likely to have hypertension.[34] It is recommended, therefore, that people with hypertension or at risk for hypertension eat a diet that contains two to three servings daily of calcium-rich foods such as milk and milk products.

Another nutrient under investigation for contributing to hypertension is chloride, the mineral found along with sodium in salt. (Salt is about 40 percent sodium and 60 percent chloride.) Some evidence has come to light that dietary sodium raises blood pressure only when accompanied by chloride. In other words, it may not be sodium in and of itself, but rather salt, that contributes to elevations in blood pressure. In the United States, incidentally, about 95 percent of sodium consumed comes from salt.[35]

Finally, some evidence suggests that eating a diet that includes monounsaturated or polyunsaturated fat and is low in saturated fat helps to lower blood pressure. Though the relationship remains tenuous, it certainly makes sense for those with high blood pressure to eat such a diet if for no other reason than to help prevent heart disease, a condition that hypertensives run a high risk of developing (refer to the Spotlight feature in Chapter 4).[36]

Risk factors for high blood pressure:

Obesity

Family history of high blood pressure

Race (black people are more likely than whites to develop hypertension)

Age (in the United States, blood pressure tends to rise with age)

Excess alcohol consumption

Sedentary lifestyle

ARE YOUR NUMBERS UP?

One of the characteristics of hypertension is that it has been called a silent killer that cannot be felt and may go undetected for years. This is why it is crucial to have your blood pressure checked on a regular basis. Diagnosis of hypertension requires at least two elevated readings. The first of the two numbers in a blood pressure reading—systolic pressure—represents the force exerted by the heart as it contracts to pump blood throughout the body, as measured by the number of millimeters that the pressure pushes a column of mercury up a tube. The second number—diastolic pressure—is a measure of the pressure the blood exerts on artery walls between heartbeats. A reading of up to 120 over 80 millimeters of mercury is considered "normal" for people aged 18 or under. Over the age of 18, measurements as high as 140 over 90 are normal. Beyond those levels, the risk of heart attack and stroke rises in direct proportion to increasing blood pressure.[37]

The Trace Minerals

If you could extract all of the trace minerals from the body, you would obtain only a bit of dust, hardly enough to fill a teaspoon. As tiny as their quantities are, though, each of the trace minerals performs several vital roles for which no substitute will do. A deficiency of any of them may be fatal, and an excess of many is equally deadly.

Iron

Iron is the body's oxygen carrier. Bound into the protein **hemoglobin** in the red blood cells, it helps transport oxygen from lungs to tissues and so permits the release of energy from fuels to do the cells' work. When the iron supply is too low, **iron-deficiency anemia** occurs, characterized by weakness, tiredness, apathy, headaches, and a paleness that reflects the reduction in the number and size of the red blood cells. A person with this anemia can do very little muscular work without disabling fatigue but can replenish iron status by eating iron-rich foods (see Table 7–10).

It is difficult to convey the extent and severity of iron deficiency among the world's people. Iron deficiency occurs in as many as half of all persons in some settings, even in developed countries—most predictably in the inner city and among the rural poor. People begin to feel iron deficiency's impact, without knowing it, long before anemia is diagnosed. They don't appear to have an obvious deficiency disease; they just appear unmotivated and apathetic. Because they work and play less, they are less physically fit. Prevalence rates for iron-deficiency anemia in developed countries range from 10 percent to 20 percent. Since rates are higher in the developing countries, the incidence of iron deficiency less severe than anemia must be higher still.[38] If this one worldwide malnutrition problem could be alleviated, millions of people would benefit.[39]

The cause of iron deficiency is usually malnutrition—that is, inadequate intake, either from limited access to food or from high consumption of foods low in iron. Among causes other than malnutrition, blood loss is the primary one, caused in many countries by parasitic infections of the digestive tract.

The subject of marginal deficiencies—deficiencies that exhibit few or none of the classic symptoms of severe deficiencies—is a touchy one with reputable dietitians because it is the stuff of which quackery is made. On the pretext that you have "subclinical deficiencies," quacks will try to sell you an arsenal of expensive and unneeded nutrition nostrums. The majority of subclinical deficiencies are fantasies created by such tricksters, who are clever at stating their claims in such a way that they are hard to either prove or disprove. This is one reason why they are so often successful. Another reason, unfortunately, is that sometimes they are right. Subclinical deficiencies do exist, they do make people miserable, and the relief that can be gained by having them properly diagnosed and treated can be enormous. The case of iron is a case in point. Published scientific research provides massive amounts of evidence that subclinical deficiencies are real and widespread. (Review Chapter 1 for approaches to evaluating nutrition and health claims.)

HEMOGLOBIN (HEEM-oh-globe-in) the oxygen-carrying protein of the blood; found in the red blood cells.
  hemo = blood
  globin = spherical protein

IRON-DEFICIENCY ANEMIA a reduction of the number and size of red blood cells and a loss of their color because of iron deficiency.

TABLE 7–10
IRON IN FOODS

Adult RDA is 10 to 15 mg.

(MG)	SOURCES
25.20	Clams, steamed (3 oz)
8.90	Raisin bran (1 c)
6.70	Tofu (½ c)
5.30	Beef liver (3 oz)
3.13	Beef pot roast (3 oz)
2.80	Sirloin steak (3 oz)
2.75	Baked potato (1)
2.65	Shrimp (3 oz)
2.48	Sardines (3 oz)
2.35	Hamburger (3 oz)
2.25	Lima beans (½ c)
2.25	Prune juice (¾ c)
2.20	Navy beans (½ c)
2.15	Black-eyed peas (½ c)
2.00	Swiss chard (½ c)
1.61	Kidney beans (½ c)
1.59	Oatmeal, cooked (1 c)
1.44	Spinach, cooked (½ c)
1.30	Tuna (3 oz)
1.30	Dried figs (¼ c) —*dried on iron sheets*
1.26	Green peas (½ c)
0.94	Whole-wheat bread (1 slice)
0.82	Apricot halves, dried (5)
0.76	Raisins (¼ c)
0.65	Broccoli, cooked (½ c)

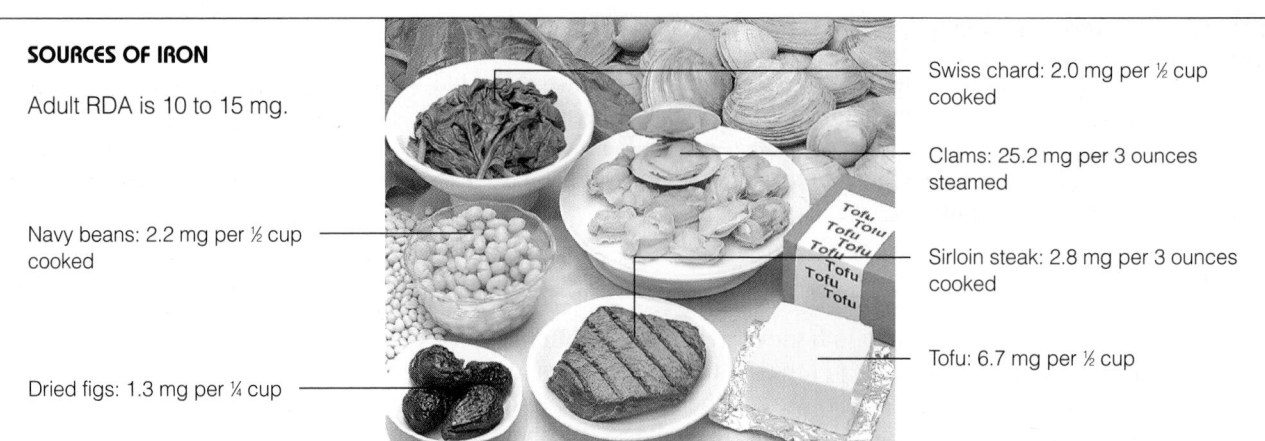

SOURCES OF IRON

Adult RDA is 10 to 15 mg.

Navy beans: 2.2 mg per ½ cup cooked

Dried figs: 1.3 mg per ¼ cup

Swiss chard: 2.0 mg per ½ cup cooked

Clams: 25.2 mg per 3 ounces steamed

Sirloin steak: 2.8 mg per 3 ounces cooked

Tofu: 6.7 mg per ½ cup

The usual Western mixed diet provides only about 5 to 6 milligrams of iron in every 1,000 calories. The recommended daily intake for an adult man is 10 milligrams. Because most men easily eat more than 2,000 calories, they can meet their iron needs without special effort.

The situation for women is different. Women may have normal blood cell counts or hemoglobin levels and yet may need more iron because their body stores may be depleted, a factor that doesn't show up in standard tests. Because most women typically eat less food than men, their iron intakes are lower. And because women menstruate, their iron losses are greater. These two factors may put women much closer to the borderline of deficiency.

The recommended intake for a woman before menopause is 15 milligrams per day; pregnant women need 30 milligrams daily. Because women typically consume fewer than 2,000 calories per day, they understandably have trouble achieving adequate iron intakes. A woman who wants to meet her iron needs from foods must increase the iron-to-calorie ratio of her diet so that she will receive about double the average amount of iron—about 10 milligrams per 1,000 calories. This means she must emphasize iron-rich foods in her daily diet.

Table 7–10 shows the amounts of iron in foods. Meats, fish, and poultry are superior sources on a per-serving basis. People must select foods carefully to obtain enough iron because it is present in such small quantities in most foods. The best meat sources are liver and other organ meats, red meats, poultry, fish, oysters, and clams. Among the grains, whole grains and enriched and fortified breads and cereals are best, and dried beans are a good source. Some fruits and vegetables contain appreciable amounts of iron, as shown in the table. Foods in the milk group are notoriously poor iron sources.

Ways to Enhance Iron Absorption.   Iron occurs in two forms in foods—as **heme iron,** bound into the iron-carrying proteins such as hemoglobin in meats, poultry, and fish, and as **nonheme iron** in both plant and animal foods. Heme iron is much more reliably absorbed than is nonheme iron. Nonheme iron's absorption is affected by many factors, including the amount of vitamin C consumed

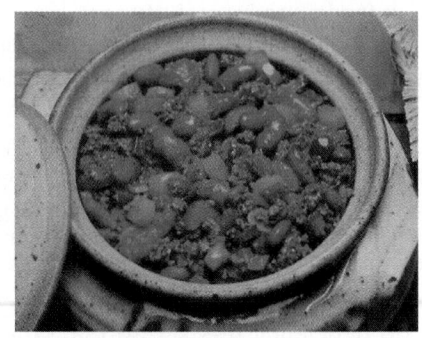

You can combine foods to achieve maximum iron absorption—the heme iron in the meat and the vitamin C in the tomatoes in this chili help you absorb the nonheme iron from the beans.

HEME (HEEM) **IRON** the iron-holding part of the hemoglobin protein, found in meat, fish, and poultry. About 40% of the iron in meat, fish, and poultry is bound into heme. Meat, fish, and poultry also contain a factor (MFP factor) other than heme that promotes the absorption of iron, even of the iron from other foods eaten at the same time as the meat.

NONHEME IRON the iron found in plant foods.

with meals.[40] Vitamin C promotes iron absorption and can triple the amount of nonheme iron absorbed from foods eaten at the same meal. Another factor—the **MFP factor**—also enhances the absorption of nonheme iron from other foods eaten with it.

Contamination iron—that is, iron obtained from cookware or soil—can also increase iron intake significantly. Consumers who cook their foods in iron cookware can contribute to their iron intake. For example, the iron content of a half-cup of spaghetti sauce simmered in a glass dish is 3 milligrams, but it is 87 milligrams when the sauce is cooked in an iron skillet. Similarly, the reason why dried apricots and raisins contain more iron than the fresh fruit is that they are dried in iron pans. Admittedly, this form of iron is not as well absorbed as the iron from meat, but every little bit helps.

Some food components interfere with iron absorption. Phytic acid is one example; it occurs in some fruits, vegetables, and whole grains, as mentioned earlier, as well as in nonherbal tea. Another example is tannic acid, which occurs in commercial black and pekoe teas, coffee, cola drinks, chocolate, and red wines. Fiber also can reduce iron absorption because it speeds up the transit of materials through the intestine.

Iron Toxicity.   Large amounts of iron can be toxic to the body. **Iron overload** is a condition in which the body absorbs excessive amounts of iron and is more common in men than in women. As a result, tissue damage occurs, especially in organs that store iron such as the liver. Infections are more likely to occur because bacteria thrive on iron-rich blood.

Researchers are currently investigating a possible link between excess iron stores in the body and increased risk of chronic conditions such as heart disease.[41] Researchers in Finland found that in a three-year study of 2,000 healthy men, the risk of heart attack was twice as great for men with the highest levels of stored iron in their bodies.[42] Although iron is an important essential nutrient in the body, it can also act as a powerful oxidizing agent in reactions that produce free radicals in the body. As noted in Chapter 4, free radicals can initiate the changes in LDL–cholesterol that eventually damage artery walls and lead to heart disease. Much more research is needed in this area before the relationship between iron and heart disease can be clarified. Until all the answers are in, avoid taking extra supplemental iron unless you have been diagnosed as deficient. Be sure to keep iron supplements out of the reach of children, too, who can fatally overdose on such tablets.

Zinc

Zinc plays a major role in association with the cellular machinery in every body organ. It is necessary for the normal metabolism of protein, carbohydrate, fat, and alcohol. Zinc is associated with the hormone insulin, which regulates the body's fuel supply. It is involved in cell multiplication, immune reactions, the utilization of vitamin A, taste perception, wound healing, the synthesis of sperm, and the development of the fetus. Because zinc is lost from the body daily in much the same way as protein is, it must be replenished daily.

MFP FACTOR a factor in **M**eat, **F**ish, and **P**oultry that promotes the absorption of nonheme iron present in the same foods or in other foods eaten at the same time.

CONTAMINATION IRON iron found in foods as the result of contamination by inorganic iron salts from iron cookware, iron-containing soils, and the like.

IRON OVERLOAD a condition in which the body contains more iron than it needs or can handle; excess iron is toxic and can damage the liver.

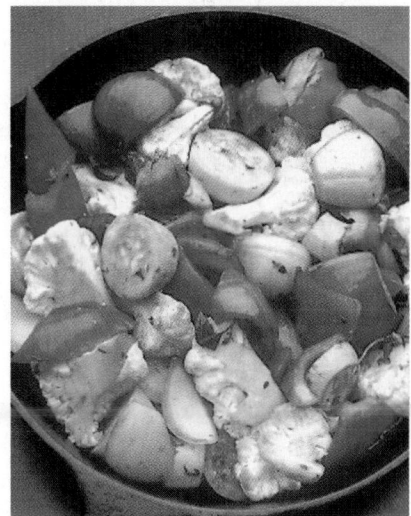

Iron cookware adds supplemental iron to foods.

Zinc deficiencies were first reported in the 1960s in the Middle East, where studies on adolescent boys revealed severe growth retardation and delayed sexual maturation—symptoms responsive to zinc supplementation. The native diets were typically low in animal protein and zinc and high in fiber and other compounds that bind minerals. The researchers learned that the binders were carrying zinc out of the boys' bodies, thus causing the deficiency.

Since then, cases of zinc deficiency have been discovered closer to home.[43] A number of Denver school children had poor growth, poor appetite, and decreased taste sensitivity from zinc deficiency. The children were described as picky eaters and ate less than an ounce of meat per day.

People who are building new tissue have the highest zinc needs—infants, children, teenagers, and pregnant women. The pregnant teenager is at particular risk because she needs zinc for her own growth as well as for her fetus's growth. Pregnant vegetarians are at risk, too, because their diets are high in fiber and zinc-binding factors. Dieters also need to be reminded that very-low-calorie diets cause not only a low zinc intake but also a loss of zinc from body tissues as they break down to release fuel.

Zinc is a relatively nontoxic element. However, it can be toxic if consumed in large enough quantities. Consumption of high levels of zinc can cause a host of symptoms, including vomiting, diarrhea, fever, and exhaustion.[44] The hazards of overconsumption are greatest when consumers dose themselves with supplements. Excess supplemental zinc can cause imbalances of both copper and iron in the body. Chronic consumption of zinc exceeding 15 milligrams per day is not recommended without close medical supervision.

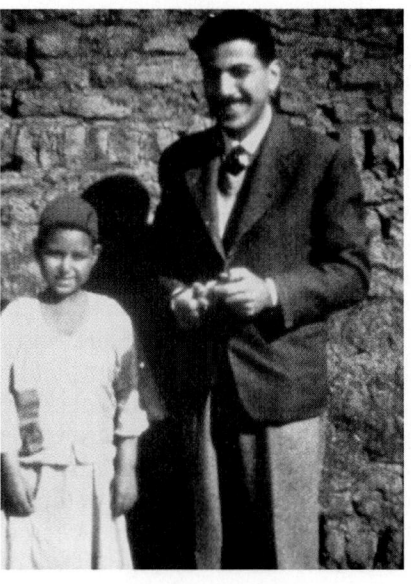

The Egyptian boy in the picture is 17 years old but is only 4 feet tall, the height of an average 7-year-old in the United States. His genitalia are like those of a 6-year-old. The retardation, known as dwarfism, is rightly ascribed to zinc deficiency because it is partially reversible when zinc is restored to the diet.

Table 7–11 shows the zinc amounts in foods. An average 1,500-calorie diet provides about 6.3 milligrams of zinc per day, or about 40 percent to 50 percent of the RDA. Zinc is highest in foods of high protein content, such as shellfish (especially oysters), meats, and liver. As a rule of thumb, two servings a day of animal protein will provide most of the zinc a healthy person needs. Eggs and whole-grain products are good sources of zinc if large quantities are eaten (the phytate in grains does not inhibit the absorption of zinc in people consuming ordinary diets). Cow's milk protein (casein) binds zinc avidly and seems to prevent its absorption somewhat; infants absorb zinc better from human breast milk. Fresh and canned vegetables vary in zinc content, depending on the soil in which they are grown. The zinc content of cooking water varies from region to region as well.

TABLE 7–11
ZINC IN FOODS

Adult RDA is 12 to 15 mg.

(MG)	SOURCES
77.00	Oysters, cooked (3 oz)
5.50	Sirloin steak (3 oz)
5.27	Ground beef (3 oz)
4.65	Beef pot roast (3 oz)
3.60	Crabmeat (3 oz)
2.97	Raisin bran (1 c)
2.20	Yogurt (1 c)
1.73	Turkey (3 oz)
1.66	Swiss cheese (1.5 oz)
1.61	Peanuts (⅓ c)
1.34	Shrimp (3 oz)
1.32	Cheddar cheese (1.5 oz)
1.10	Black-eyed peas (½ c)
1.00	Black beans (½ c)
1.00	Tofu (½ c)
0.98	Nonfat milk (1 c)
0.75	Green peas (½ c)
0.70	Kidney beans (½ c)
0.68	Spinach, cooked (½ c)
0.55	Whole-wheat bread (1 slice)

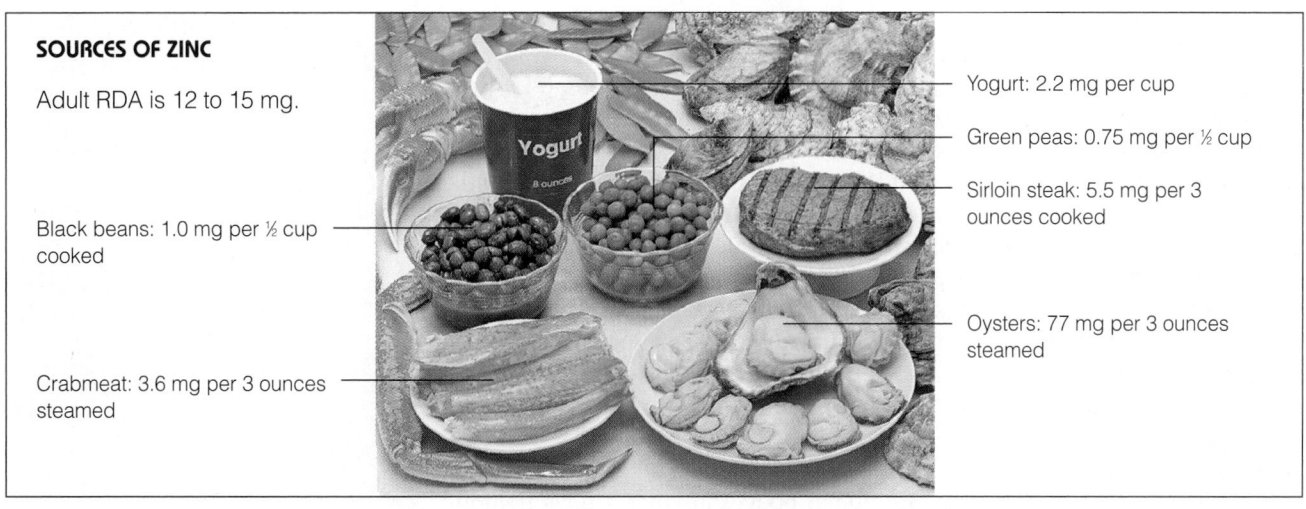

SOURCES OF ZINC

Adult RDA is 12 to 15 mg.

Yogurt: 2.2 mg per cup

Green peas: 0.75 mg per ½ cup

Sirloin steak: 5.5 mg per 3 ounces cooked

Black beans: 1.0 mg per ½ cup cooked

Oysters: 77 mg per 3 ounces steamed

Crabmeat: 3.6 mg per 3 ounces steamed

Iodine

very minute

Iodine occurs in the body in an infinitesimal quantity, but its principal role in human nutrition is well-known. It is part of the thyroid hormones, which regulate body temperature, metabolic rate, reproduction, and growth. The hormones enter every cell of the body to control the rate at which the cells use oxygen and release energy.

When the iodine level of the blood is low, the thyroid gland may enlarge until it causes swelling in the throat area—a condition called **goiter.** Goiter is estimated to affect 200 million people the world over.

In addition to causing sluggishness and weight gain, an iodine deficiency can have serious effects on fetal development. Severe thyroid undersecretion of a woman during pregnancy causes the extreme and irreversible mental and physical retardation of the child known as **cretinism.** A person with this condition has a face and body with many abnormalities, including mental retardation. Much of the mental retardation associated with cretinism can be averted by early diagnosis and treatment of the mother's iodine deficiency.

The amount of iodine in foods reflects the amount present in the soil in which plants are grown or on which animals graze. Soil iodine is greatest along the coastal regions. In the United States, in areas where the soil is low in iodine (most notably in the plains states and around the Great Lakes and St. Lawrence River areas and in the Willamette Valley of Oregon), widespread goiter and cretinism appeared in the local people during the 1930s. Iodized salt was introduced as a preventive measure, and these scourges disappeared.

People sometimes ask whether they should be sure to buy the *iodized* variety of salt in the grocery store to ensure adequate iodine intake. Usually it does not matter whether your salt is iodized, although it probably is a good idea for people living in noncoastal areas. Most consumers now have access to fruits and vegetables grown in other parts of the country, such as from coastal areas

GOITER (GOY-ter) enlargement of the thyroid gland caused by iodine deficiency.

CRETINISM (CREE-tin-ism) severe mental and physical retardation of an infant caused by iodine deficiency during pregnancy.

rich in iodine. Also, a dramatic increase in iodine intakes in the United States has occurred recently. The toxic level at which detectable harm results is thought to be only a few times higher than current average consumption levels.[45] Most of the excess iodine seems to be coming from iodates (dough conditioners used in the baking industry) and from milk produced by cows exposed to iodine-containing medications and disinfectants during the milk treatment process. Now that the problem has been identified, both the baking and the dairy industries have reduced their use of these compounds, but the sudden emergence of this problem points to a need for continued surveillance of the food supply. Excessive intakes of iodine can cause an enlargement of the thyroid gland resembling goiter; in infants it can be so severe as to block the airways and cause suffocation.[46]

Fluoride

Only a trace of fluoride occurs in the human body, but studies have demonstrated that where diets are high in fluoride, the crystalline deposits in teeth and bones are larger and more perfectly formed than where diets are low in it. Fluoride not only protects children's teeth from decay but also makes the bones of older people resistant to adult bone loss (osteoporosis). Its continuous presence in body fluids is desirable.

Drinking water is the usual source of fluoride. Where fluoride is lacking in the water supply, the incidence of dental decay is very high. Fluoridation of community water where needed to raise its fluoride concentration to one part per million (ppm) is thus an important public health measure (see Figure 7–6).

In some communities, the natural fluoride concentration in water is high (2 to 8 ppm), and children's teeth develop with mottled enamel. This condition, called **fluorosis,** may not be harmful (in fact, these children's teeth may be extraordinarily decay resistant), but it violates the prejudice that teeth should be white. Fluorosis does not occur in communities where fluoride is added to the water supply.

True toxicity from fluoride overdoses can occur, but only after years of chronic daily intakes of 20 to 80 times the amounts normally consumed from fluoridated water. Despite the value of fluoride, violent disagreement often surrounds the introduction of fluoridation to

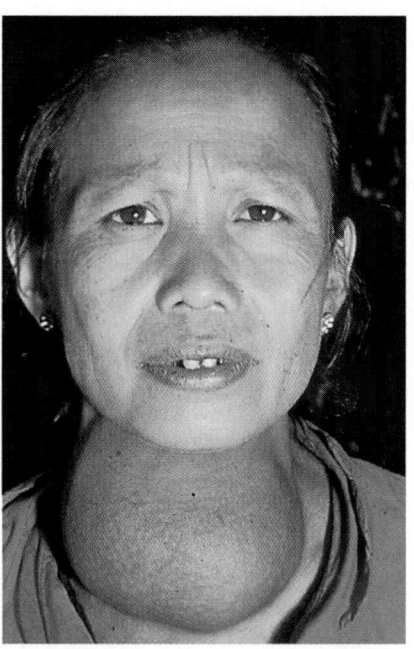

In iodine deficiency, the thyroid gland enlarges—a condition known as simple goiter.

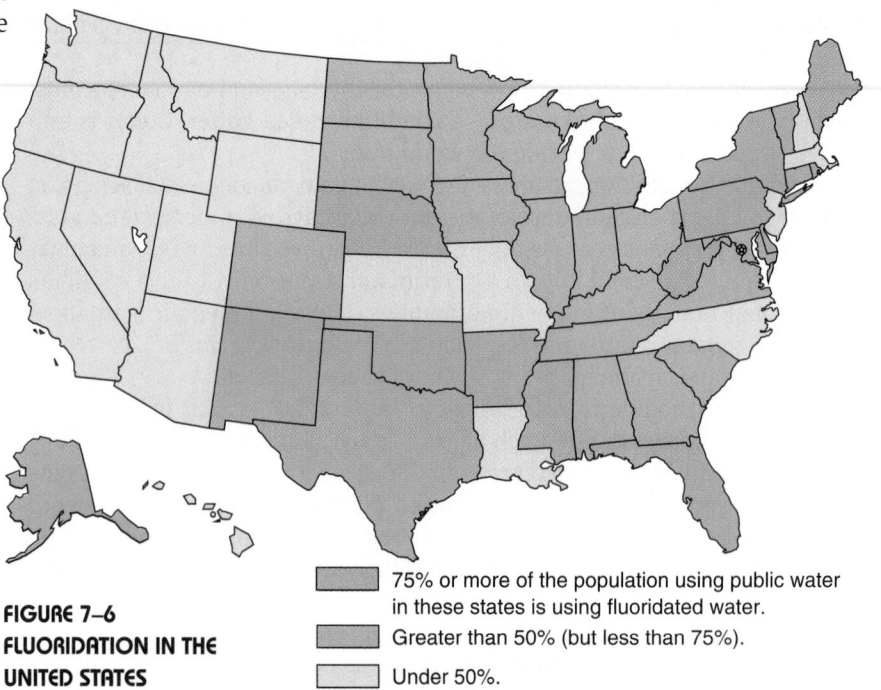

FIGURE 7–6
FLUORIDATION IN THE UNITED STATES

▨ 75% or more of the population using public water in these states is using fluoridated water.

▨ Greater than 50% (but less than 75%).

☐ Under 50%.

SOURCE: Fluoridation Census Summary, U.S. Department of Health and Human Services, Public Health Service, Centers for Disease Control and Prevention, National Center for Prevention Services, Division of Oral Health, Atlanta, Ga., April 1993.

a community's water. Additional coverage of the debate about the health effects of fluoride is given in the Spotlight at the end of this chapter.

Copper, Manganese, Chromium, Selenium, and Molybdenum

Several trace minerals have been found to have important roles in a variety of metabolic and physiologic processes. Copper, for example, is involved in making red blood cells, manufacturing collagen, healing wounds, and maintaining the sheaths around nerve fibers. Chromium works closely with the hormone insulin to help the cells take up glucose and break it down for energy.[47] Selenium functions as part of an antioxidant enzyme and can substitute for vitamin E in some of that vitamin's antioxidant activities. Manganese and molybdenum both function as working parts of several enzymes. (Refer to Table 7–1 on page 233 for a brief description and common food sources of each of these minerals.)

FLUOROSIS (floor-OH-sis) discoloration of the teeth from ingestion of too much fluoride during tooth development.

Alternatives to water fluoridation:

- Fluoride toothpastes
- Fluoride treatments for teeth
- Fluoride tablets and drops

See Chapter 6 for more discussion of the role of the antioxidants in health and disease.

Trace Minerals of Uncertain Status

None of the trace minerals has been known for very long, and some are extremely recent newcomers. Some researchers consider boron to be one factor that contributes to the risk of osteoporosis because of its effects on calcium metabolism.[48] Nickel is now recognized as important for the health of many body tissues; deficiencies harm the liver and other organs. Silicon is known to be involved in bone calcification, at least in animals. Tin is necessary for growth in animals and probably in humans. Vanadium, too, is necessary for growth and bone development as well as for normal reproduction. Cobalt is recognized as the mineral in the large vitamin B_{12} molecule; the alternative name for this vitamin—cobalamin—reflects the presence of cobalt. In the future, we may discover that many other trace minerals—for example, silver, mercury, lead, barium, and cadmium—also play key roles in human nutrition. Even arsenic, famous as the poisonous instrument of death in many murder mysteries and known to be a carcinogen, may turn out to be an essential nutrient in tiny quantities.

Water—The Most Essential Nutrient

Although we often take it for granted, water is by far the nutrient most needed by the body. While we can survive for months or even years without some vitamins and minerals, we can last only a few days without water. The discussion that follows will help you to understand why water is so vital and to recognize how the various sources of the nutrient may differ.

Why is water so important? A combination of hydrogen and oxygen, water makes up part of every cell, tissue, and organ in the body and accounts for about 60 percent of body weight (see Figure

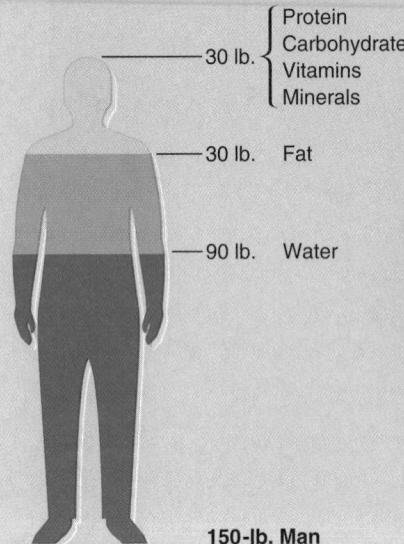

30 lb. { Protein
Carbohydrate
Vitamins
Minerals

30 lb. Fat

90 lb. Water

150-lb. Man

FIGURE 7–7
WATER—THE NUMBER ONE NUTRIENT

SOURCE: C. Lecos, Water: The Number One Nutrient, *FDA Consumer,* November 1983.

7–7), even contributing to body parts thought of as "dry." For example, bone is more than 20 percent water, muscle is three-quarters water, and teeth are about 10 percent water.

Inside the body, water performs many tasks vital to life. It helps to transport the nutrients needed to nourish the cells, for example. The blood is a river of water that flows through the arteries, capillaries, and veins, bringing each cell the exact substances and particles it requires. The same river carries away waste products formed during the reactions that take place in the cells. In addition, water acts as a shock absorber in joints and around the spinal cord, lubricates the digestive tract as well as all the tissues moistened with mucus, and surrounds and cushions an unborn child. Moreover, water plays a key role in maintaining body temperature. When water is changed from a liquid to a gas, a great deal of heat is used. Thus, when sweat evaporates, heat is released, leaving the body cooler.

How much water do we take in daily?
Adults consume and excrete some two and a half to three quarts of water a day. While most of the water we take in comes from juice, milk, soft drinks, and other beverages, foods also add considerable amounts of water to the diet. Fruits and vegetables, for instance, consist of 85 percent to 95 percent water.[49]

I often hear people talk about hard water and soft water. What do they mean? The make-up of water differs depending on where the water comes

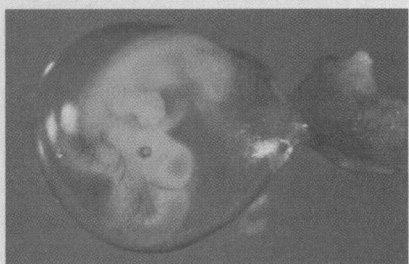

Life begins in water.

from and how it is processed, and these variations can have significant health implications. One of the most basic distinctions—hard versus soft water—is based on the concentrations of three minerals: calcium, magnesium, and sodium. Hard water usually comes from shallow ground and contains relatively high levels of minerals, primarily calcium and magnesium. Soft water, on the other hand, generally flows from deep in the earth and has a higher concentration of sodium.

How can I figure out which type of water I have in my home? While your water utility company can tell you whether your water is soft or hard, you can probably distinguish between the two based on your own experience. Soft water helps soap lather better than hard water and leaves less of a ring on the bathtub. Hard water, on the other hand, doesn't clean clothes as thoroughly as soft water and leaves a residue of rocklike crystals on the inside of the teakettle over time. That's why many consumers prefer soft water to hard water.

Which one is better to drink? From a health standpoint hard water seems to be the better alternative. One reason is that excess sodium carried in soft water, even in small amounts, adds more of the mineral to our already sodium-laden diets. More importantly, soft water can dissolve potentially toxic substances such as lead from pipes into the water. Thus, people who install water softeners in their homes for the purpose of getting cleaner laundry and better mileage from soap would do well to connect them only to their hot water lines for washing and bathing and use cold, hard water for drinking and cooking.

What about contamination? I've heard that some people's tap water isn't safe to drink. It's true that water taken from the earth contains different levels of bacteria, microorganisms, and heavy metals such as lead. Still, to ensure that the water that flows from the tap is safe to drink, the Environmental Protection Agency (EPA), the arm of the government responsible for monitoring municipal water supplies, sets limits for potential contaminants such as mercury, nitrate, and silver in drinking water. The EPA also mandates that tap water be disinfected if bacteria levels run high so as to prevent the spread of waterborne diseases such as typhoid and dysentery. Such precautionary measures go a long way in keeping our water supply one of the safest in the world.[50]

One potential contaminant that the federal government does not regulate is a parasite called *Cryptosporidium.* Found in lakes and rivers that have come into contact with sewage or animal waste, *Cryptosporidium* has emerged as a health threat to vulnerable people because it is highly resistant to chlorine and other disinfectants used in municipal water supplies. In healthy people, the parasite can cause diarrhea and other flu-like symptoms that typically subside within a week to 10 days. In people with

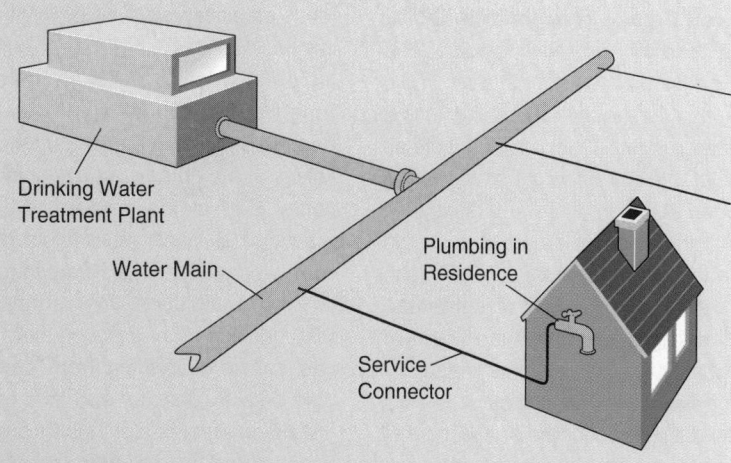

FIGURE 7–8
LEAD IN DRINKING WATER

Lead usually gets into water after the water leaves the local drinking-water treatment plant and makes its way through lead-containing plumbing systems.

weak immune systems, however, the parasite leads to severe, long-lasting gastrointestinal problems that can even cause death.

Because of the *Cryptosporidium* hazard, in 1995 the Environmental Protection Agency and the Centers for Disease Control and Prevention recommended special precautions for people with severely weakened immune systems—those with HIV infection, cancer and transplant patients taking immunosuppressive drugs, and people born with a weakened immune system. The public health groups advised those groups to talk to a healthcare provider about bringing tap water intended for drinking to a boil for one minute, which will destroy any *Cryptosporidium* present, buying a special water filter system*, or drinking distilled bottled water or bottled water that has been filtered by a technique called reverse osmosis.[51]

---

*To obtain a list of suitable filters, contact NSF International at 1-800-673-8010 and ask for a list of filters certified under a regulation called Standard 53.

Another potential health threat over which the EPA has little control is the level of lead that comes out of your faucet. Although the EPA has put a ceiling on the concentration of lead allowed in public water supplies, once the water leaves a reservoir, unhealthfully high levels of the metal may be dissolved into it (see Figure 7–8). That's because it may flow through pipes made of lead or joined by lead solder, which then can leach the metal into the water as it passes through. Granted, the government banned the use of lead-containing plumbing systems back in 1986, but dwellings built before that time may not have lead-free pipes.

The issue has generated a good deal of publicity and concern of late. Certainly, attention to the matter is warranted, given that once lead accumulates in the body, it begins to damage the nerves, kidneys, and liver along with the cardiovascular, reproductive, immunologic, and gastrointestinal systems. The metal is especially toxic to children and fetuses, in whom it can cause neurologic problems as severe as brain damage.

How can I make sure that my water doesn't contain too much lead? Lead levels can usually be kept to a minimum simply by flushing the tap, that is, letting the water run until it becomes as cold as possible, thereby ridding it of water that has been sitting in pipes and dissolving lead for any length of time. Pipes should be flushed with cold water only, because cold water is less likely to dissolve lead as it flows through them than warm or hot water. To be sure, in some instances, flushing is not enough to reduce harmful lead levels. Some homes or apartments may need special water treatment systems, the necessity of which can be determined only by subjecting tap water to a lead test. Most tests cost between $20 and $100; names of certified laboratories that analyze water can be obtained from a local branch of the EPA or by calling the EPA's Safe Drinking Water Hotline (800-426-4791).[52]

Another mineral in water that worries me is fluoride. A friend of mine told me not to drink water that contains fluoride because it can cause cancer. What do you think about that? As explained earlier in the chapter, drinking fluoridated water ranks as one of the most effective ways to prevent dental cavities. But despite the clear-cut benefits of fluoridation, some 40 percent of Americans continue to drink water not treated with the mineral, putting themselves at a high risk of developing tooth decay. Part of the problem is that the practice has been the subject of bitter controversy ever since it was introduced in 1945. Antifluoridation groups claim that drinking fluoride-containing water can cause everything from cancer to birth defects, despite reports to the contrary issued by major health organizations, including the American Medical Association and the American Dietetic Association.[53] In fact, a 1993 report from the National Research Council—based on hundreds of studies and the most comprehensive investigation of the health effects of fluoride to date—concluded that current levels of fluoride in drinking water are not associated with cancer, kidney disease, stomach and intestinal problems, infertility, birth defects, genetic mutations, or any other health problems for which fluoride has been blamed. Granted, fluoride in water combined with excess fluoride from toothpaste, mouth rinses, and other sources can lead to a condition known as fluorosis, a staining or pitting of tooth enamel. Still, cases of fluorosis tend to be mild as well as few and far between.[54]

You seem to be saying that our water supply is fine. Still, wouldn't it be better to play it safe and drink bottled water? Not necessarily. Granted, Americans drink nearly three times as much bottled water these days as a decade ago, totaling about 2.3 billion gallons annually.[55] And while the reasons for the trend are many, bottled water's perceived health benefits fall near the top of the list. Surveys have found that about 25 percent of bottled water drinkers choose the beverage for health and safety reasons; another quarter believe it is pure and free of contaminants.[56]

Regardless of its pristine image, bottled water is not necessarily purer or more healthful than what flows right out of the tap. Consider that the Food and Drug Administration (FDA)—the bottled-water industry watchdog—does not require that bottled water meet higher standards for quality, such as the maximum level of contaminants, than public water supplies regulated by the EPA. For the most part, the FDA simply follows the EPA's regulatory lead. Granted, bottled water is filtered to remove chemicals such as chlorine that may impart a certain taste. But that doesn't make it any safer. In fact, about 25 percent of bottled water comes from the same municipal water supplies as tap water.[57] Furthermore, some bottled waters do not contain any or enough of the fluoride needed to fight cavities.[58] The only way to determine whether a certain water contains the mineral is to check with the company that bottles it.

This is not to say that bottled water is necessarily any better or worse, from a health standpoint, than tap water. It's certainly preferable to tap water for those who like its taste. The problem is that many consumers pay 300 to 1,200 times

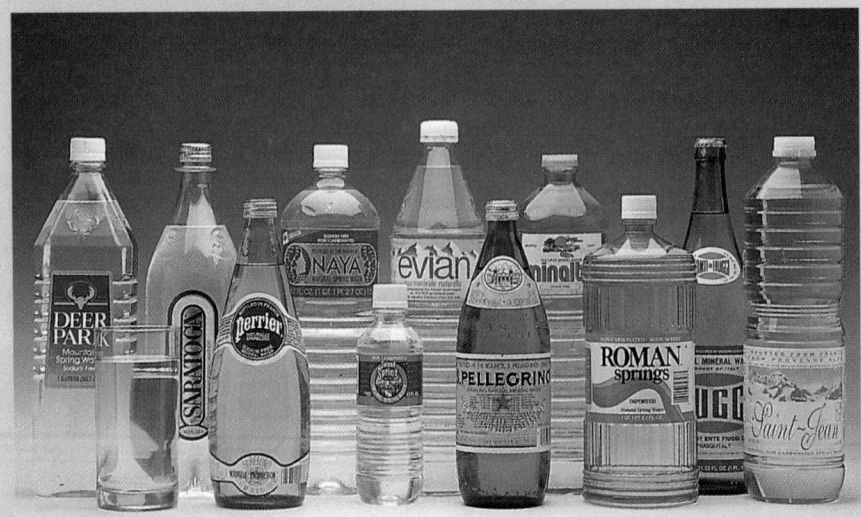

more per gallon for bottled water than tap water because they think bottled water is the more healthful of the two. Bottlers have long added to the confusion by sprinkling terms such as *pure, crystal pure,* and *premium* on labels illustrated with pictures of glaciers, mountain streams, and waterfalls, even when the water inside comes from a public reservoir. In 1995, however, the FDA set forth regulations mandating clear labeling of bottled waters. The Miniglossary of Bottled Waters explains what some of the terms used on bottles actually mean.

MINIGLOSSARY OF BOTTLED WATERS

ARTESIAN WATER or **ARTESIAN WELL WATER** water drawn from a well that taps a confined water-bearing rock or rock formation.

GROUND WATER water that comes from an underground body of water that does not come into contact with any surface water.

MINERAL WATER water that is drawn from an underground source and that contains at least 250 parts per million of dissolved solids. If the water contains between 250 and 500 parts per million total dissolved solids, the statement "low mineral content" must appear. If it contains more than 1,500 parts per million, the statement "high mineral content" must appear. If a cup of the water contains at least 20 milligrams of calcium, .36 milligrams of iron, or 5 milligrams of sodium, the product must carry nutrition labeling.

PURIFIED WATER (also know as **DEMINERALIZED WATER, DISTILLED WATER, DEIONIZED WATER,** or **REVERSE OSMOSIS WATER**) water from which all the minerals have been removed, thereby eliminating the possibility that the minerals might corrode, say, a steam iron.

SPARKLING BOTTLED WATER water whose carbon dioxide (the ingredient that makes soda pop bubbly) is naturally present. That is, carbonation is not added from an outside source.

SPRING WATER water derived from an underground formation from which water flows naturally to the surface of the earth and to which minerals have not been added or taken away. It may be collected either at the spring itself or through a hole tapping the underground formation feeding the spring.

WELL WATER water derived from a rock formation by way of a hole bored, drilled, or otherwise constructed in the ground.

FROM A COMMUNITY WATER SYSTEM or **FROM A MUNICIPAL SOURCE** statement that must appear on bottles containing water derived from a municipal water supply. The phrase must conspicuously precede or follow the name of the brand.

SELTZER* tap water injected with carbon dioxide and containing no added salts.

CLUB SODA* artificially carbonated water containing added salts and minerals.

---

*These are not considered bottled water in government parlance. The FDA defines bottled water as water that is sealed in bottles or other containers and is intended for human consumption, excluding soda, seltzer, flavored, and vended water products.

SOURCE: U. S. Department of Health and Human Services, Food and Drug Administration, Beverages: bottled water, *Federal Register* 60 (November 13, 1995): 57076–57130.

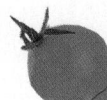

CHECK YOURSELF...

1. What do the terms *major* and *trace* mean when referring to the minerals found in the body?

2. State the major functions of chloride, potassium, magnesium, and sulfur in the body.

3. Which mineral is least likely to be deficient in the diet?

4. What affects the sodium-potassium ratio in foods?

5. When would the use of a calcium supplement be recommended; how would you go about selecting one?

6. Discuss the dietary factors that may affect blood pressure and describe the lifestyle changes recommended for reducing blood pressure.

7. Name the bone minerals.

8. State the function of iodine in the body and describe the two conditions that can result from an iodine deficiency.

9. List factors that enhance iron absorption; factors that inhibit iron absorption.

10. Iron deficiency results in _____. How is it diagnosed? What food has the most absorbable form of iron?

11. What are the deficiency symptoms of zinc in children? in adults?

12. List three functions of water in the body.

Answers to selected Check Yourself questions are found in Appendix H.

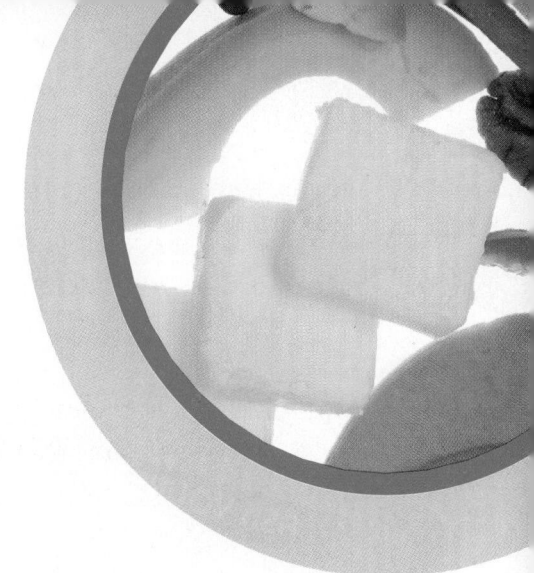

Before you begin a thing remind yourself that difficulties and delays quite impossible to foresee are ahead. . . . You can see only one thing clearly, and that is your goal. Form a mental vision of that and cling to it through thick and thin.

K. Norris

Weight Control

EIGHT

Contents

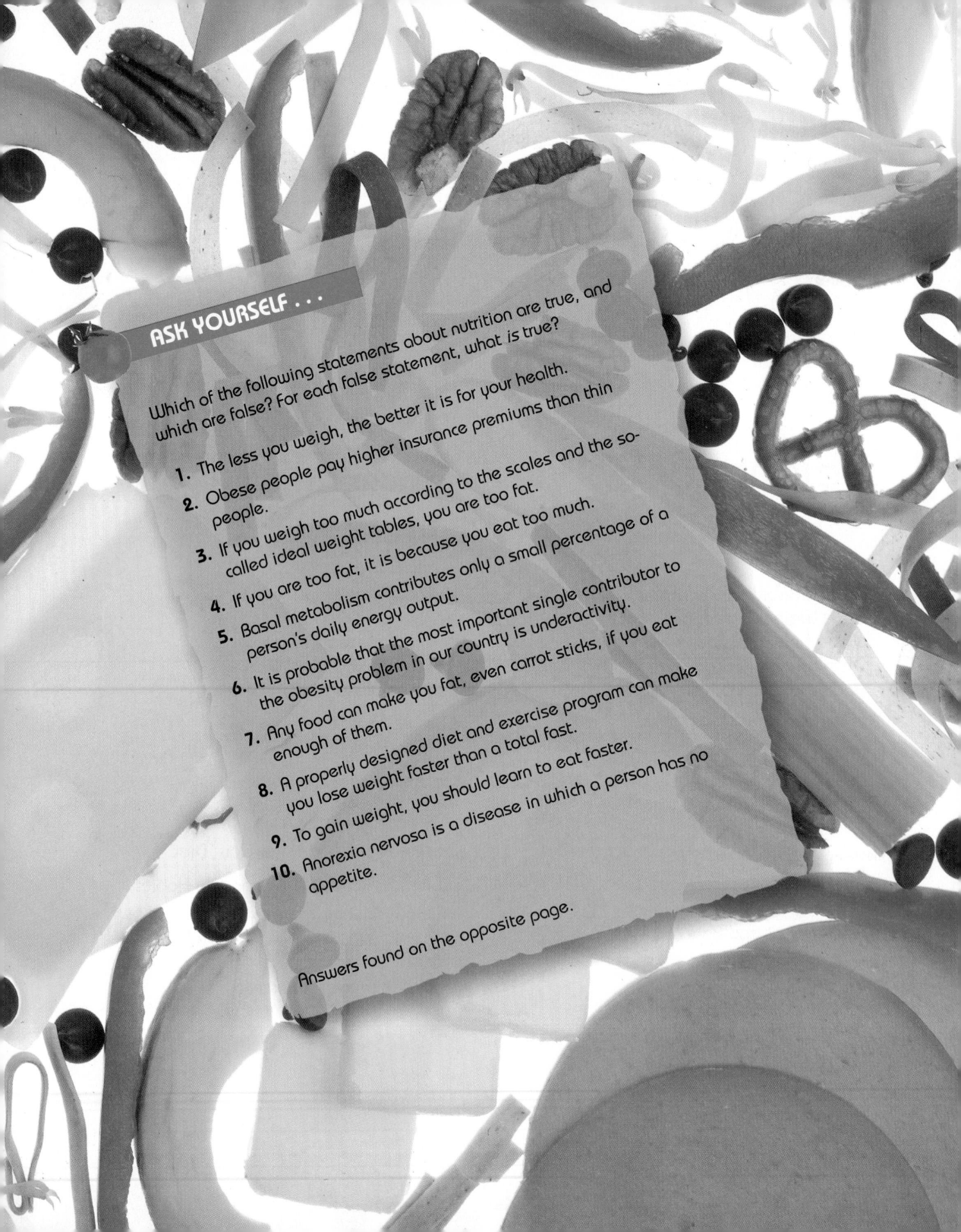

ASK YOURSELF . . .

Which of the following statements about nutrition are true, and which are false? For each false statement, what *is* true?

1. The less you weigh, the better it is for your health.

2. Obese people pay higher insurance premiums than thin people.

3. If you weigh too much according to the scales and the so-called ideal weight tables, you are too fat.

4. If you are too fat, it is because you eat too much.

5. Basal metabolism contributes only a small percentage of a person's daily energy output.

6. It is probable that the most important single contributor to the obesity problem in our country is underactivity.

7. Any food can make you fat, even carrot sticks, if you eat enough of them.

8. A properly designed diet and exercise program can make you lose weight faster than a total fast.

9. To gain weight, you should learn to eat faster.

10. Anorexia nervosa is a disease in which a person has no appetite.

Answers found on the opposite page.

How much should you weigh? At one time, you could look up the answer in the so-called ideal weight tables. Defining **overweight** and **underweight** was simple: If a person's weight was 10 percent or more above the ideal weight, the person was overweight; 20 percent or more meant the person was **obese.** If the person's weight was 10 percent or more below the ideal weight, the person was underweight. Now the term *ideal weight* is no longer in use, and defining overweight and underweight is no longer simple. But regardless of how you define it, obesity has become a major public health problem for both young and old in the United States today. Some 35 percent of women and 31 percent of men 20 years of age or older are considered obese, as are approximately one-fourth of all children and teenagers.[1]

Clearly, such a thing exists for each individual as a weight too low or a weight too high to be healthful. The too-thin person has minimal body fat stores with which to meet prolonged starvation and will be at a disadvantage in situations where energy reserves might be needed, such as a prolonged period of physiological stress or injury. A fact not always recognized, even by health-care providers, is that thin people are also at a disadvantage when hospitalized, where they may have to go for days without food while undergoing tests or surgery. Underweight also increases the risk for any person fighting a wasting disease such as cancer, tuberculosis, or AIDS. In fact, people with cancer die as often from starvation as from the cancer itself. Thus, underweight people are urged to learn how to nourish themselves optimally, not just to gain body fat—although even that is desirable—but to acquire healthful reserves of all the nutrients that can be stored.

The physical risks of obesity are greater for some people than for others, depending on inherited susceptibilities to conditions such as high blood pressure, high blood cholesterol, and diabetes.[2] High blood pressure is made worse by weight gain and can often be normalized merely by weight loss. Diabetes can be precipitated in genetically susceptible people if they become overweight. If any of these conditions run in your family, you are urgently in need of a sensible weight-control program to prevent obesity.

OVERWEIGHT conventionally defined as weight between 10% and 20% above the desirable weight for height.

UNDERWEIGHT weight 10% or more below the desirable weight for height.

OBESITY conventionally defined as weight 20% or more above the desirable weight for height, but see body mass index (BMI) on page 275 for a more accurate definition. Morbid obesity is a weight of at least 100 pounds above "ideal" weight for height.

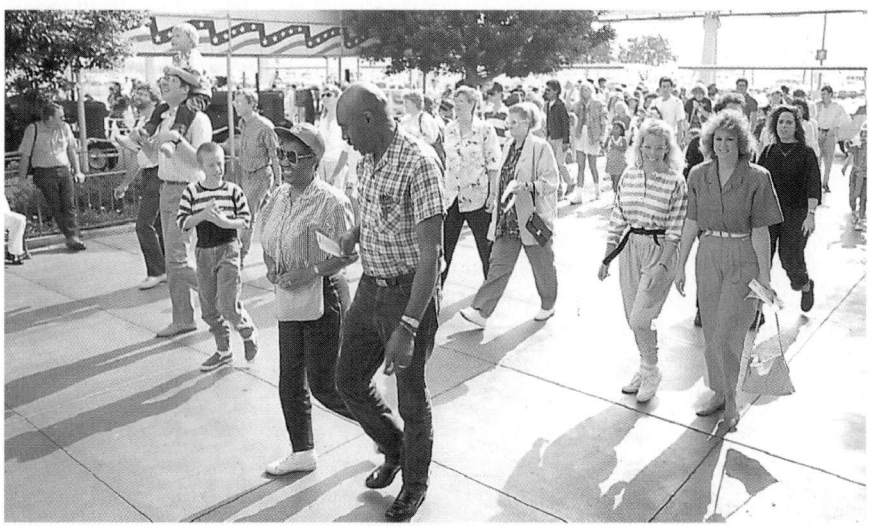

Bodies come in many shapes and sizes. Which are healthy?

ASK YOURSELF ANSWERS: 1. False. Being thin is good for health only to a point; being too thin is as risky as being too fat. **2.** True. **3.** False. A high weight according to the scales and the so-called ideal weight tables may reflect heavy bones and muscles rather than excess fatness. **4.** False. If you are too fat, it could be because you exercise too little. **5.** False. Basal metabolism contributes about 60 percent or more of the average person's daily energy output. **6.** True. **7.** True. **8.** True. **9.** True. **10.** False. Anorexia nervosa is misnamed; people with anorexia nervosa are constantly hungry but control their hunger.

Obesity also increases the risk of heart disease because excess fat pads crowd the heart muscle and the lungs within the body cavity. These fat pads encumber the heart as it beats, making it work hard to deliver oxygen and nutrients. The lungs, too, cannot expand fully, which limits the oxygen intake of each breath, causing the heart to work even harder to pump the needed amount of oxygen to the other body parts. Furthermore, since each extra pound of fat tissue demands to be fed by way of miles of capillaries, the heart in a fat person labors to pump its blood through a network of blood vessels vastly larger than that of a thin person. Even a healthy heart is strained by excess fatness. If a diseased heart finds itself in this bind, a sudden burst of exercise may be more of a workload than it can handle. Chapter 9 discusses precautions relevant to exercise.

Gallbladder disease, too, can be brought on in susceptible people merely by excess weight. Similarly, obesity increases a woman's risk of developing breast cancer. Table 8–1 shows other conditions brought on or made worse by obesity.

Besides being at risk for these health hazards, millions of obese people throughout much of their lives incur risks from ill-advised, misguided dieting. Some fad diets are more hazardous to health than is obesity itself. Many of the claims, treatments, devices, and gadgets for losing weight can be described as simply ineffective to truly dangerous to your health.[3] Over the centuries, "magical" weight-loss plans have been offered time and again, the success of which is in their popularity, not in their achievements.

Some people can be obese and suffer none of the risks of these physical health hazards, but there is one disadvantage of obesity that no one in our society quite escapes. Obesity in many parts of North America is a social and economic handicap.[4] Obese individuals suffer from discrimination in many areas, including social relationships and the job market. Psychologically, a body size that embarrasses or shames a person confers severe disadvantages. For people who cannot talk freely about their own self-doubt, a less-than-ideal body image becomes a private anguish. For people who perceive themselves as fat in a society that prizes thinness, real or imagined obesity can thrust them into withdrawal, shame, humiliation, and isolation.

How thin, then, is too thin—and how fat is too fat? Because the term *ideal weight* cannot be defined, the following section discusses the concept of a healthful weight.

What Is a Healthful Weight?

The problems of defining a healthful weight are many. Consider the question, Healthful for what? For long-distance runners, every unneeded pound is a disadvantage; the lowest amount of body fat that doesn't compromise hormonal balance and fuel availability is desirable. Weight matters less for swimmers, and fat contributes to their buoyancy and insulates them against the cold. In the case of swimmers, to a point, more is desirable. Dancers and models may value thinness so highly that to attain it, they compromise their health.

TABLE 8–1
PROBLEMS ASSOCIATED WITH OBESITY

- Abdominal hernias
- Accidents
- Arthritis (knees, hips, lower spine)
- Certain cancers
  In men: colon, rectum, prostate gland
  In women: breast, uterus, ovaries
- Complications during pregnancy
- Complications after surgery
- Decreased longevity
- Decreased quality of life
- Depression
- Diabetes
- Gallbladder and liver disease
- Gout
- Heart disease
- High blood cholesterol levels
- Hypertension
- Injury to weight-bearing joints
- Poor self-esteem
- Respiratory problems
- Varicose veins

Some societies value fatness, equating it with prosperity; others value thinness to the point of obsession (our own being an example). This chapter first asks what range of weights is compatible with wellness and long life and then suggests that personal preferences dictate the choice of a weight within that range.

Body Weight Versus Body Fat

The question of what weight is healthful is harder to answer than you might at first think. To think merely in terms of weight oversimplifies the issue of body fatness and health. Two people of the same sex, age, and height may both weigh the same, yet one may be too fat and the other too thin. The difference lies in their body composition. One may have small, light bones and minimally developed muscles, while the other has big, heavy bones and well-developed muscles. The first person could have too much body fat and the second person too little. For example, football players, body builders, and other athletes may weigh in as overweight for their height according to the weight tables. However, they probably will have less body fat than the amount that poses a risk to health. Likewise, many sedentary persons may weigh in as normal weight but be overly fat. This comparison points to the need to define obesity in terms of people's body fatness rather than in terms of their weight.

The health risks of obesity refer to people who are overfat. On the average, men having over 25 percent body fat and women having over 30 percent body fat are considered obese. More desirable measures are 12 percent to 18 percent body fat for most men and 20 percent to 28 percent body fat for most women (see Table 8–2).

Measuring Body Fat

Body fatness is hard to measure. One very accurate way is to obtain a measure of the body's density—that is, weight divided by volume. Weight is easy enough; just step on an accurate scale. But to obtain the body's volume, you have to immerse the whole body in a tank of water. Not many health professionals have space in their offices for the equipment needed for this procedure, known as **hydrostatic weighing** or **underwater weighing.** Most employ the **skinfold test,** using a caliper—a pinching device that measures the thickness of a fold of fat in such areas as the back of the arm, below the shoulder blade, and the side of the waist. About 50 percent of the body's fat lies beneath the skin, and its thickness at these locations can be compared with standard tables to give a fair approximation of total body fat, at least for most people.

An alternative method for assessing body fatness is **bioelectrical impedance,** in which electrodes are attached to a person's hand and foot. This method provides a measure of how much fat a person has by measuring the speed at which electrical current is conducted through the body (from the ankle to the wrist). Since fat is a poor conductor of electricity, the more fat one has, the more resistance this current encounters in the body.[5]

**TABLE 8–2
BODY-FAT STANDARDS**

	MEN	WOMEN
Average	15%–18%	20%–28%
Athletes	12%–15%	20%–25%
Elite athletes	7%–10%	12%–18%
Obesity	25% +	30% +

SOURCE: Adapted from S. Escott-Stump, *Nutrition and Diagnosis-Related Care* (Philadelphia: Lea & Febiger, 1988), p. 19.

HYDROSTATIC WEIGHING or **UNDERWATER WEIGHING** a weighing method in which the less a person weighs underwater compared to the person's out-of-water weight, the greater the proportion of body fat (fat is less dense or more buoyant than lean tissue).

SKINFOLD TEST a clinical test of body fatness in which the thickness of a fold of skin on the back of the arm (the triceps), below the shoulder blade (subscapular), or in other areas is measured with an instrument called a caliper. Obesity is defined by triceps skinfold thickness equal to or greater than 18–19 mm in adult men or 25–26 mm in women.

BIOELECTRICAL IMPEDANCE estimation of body fat content made by measuring how quickly electrical current is conducted through the body.

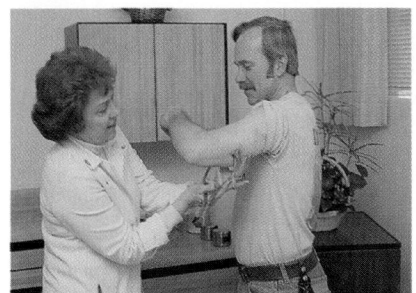

The fatfold test gives a fair approximation of total body fat.

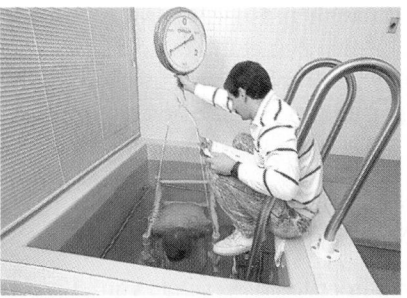

Hydrostatic (underwater) weighing.

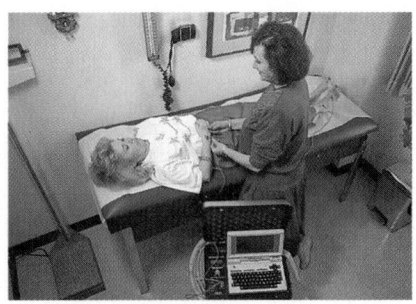

Electrical impedance measurement of body fat content.

Distribution of Fat

Not everyone carries his or her body fat distributed in the same way. To complicate matters still further, the distribution itself turns out to have health implications. Excess fat around the middle—**central obesity**—is associated with increased health hazards.[6] Body types are compared as being either apple-shaped or pear-shaped. One theory proposes that people who store most of their excess fat around the abdomen (typically men) are at a greater risk for developing diabetes, hypertension, elevated levels of blood cholesterol, and heart disease than are people who store excess fat elsewhere on the body—notably, hips, thighs, and buttocks (typically women).[7] A simple comparison of a person's waist-to-hip measurement can be used to assess abdominal fat.

CENTRAL OBESITY excess fat on the abdomen and around the trunk. Peripheral obesity is excess fat on the arms, thighs, hips, and buttocks.

Body Weight and Frame Size

Although the problem of how to define obesity has not been solved, everyone agrees that obesity presents one of the most serious health risks that people face—and one that people should, theoretically, be able to control. While the health experts argue, medical professionals are making do with a definition based temporarily on three measures. The first is the body weight

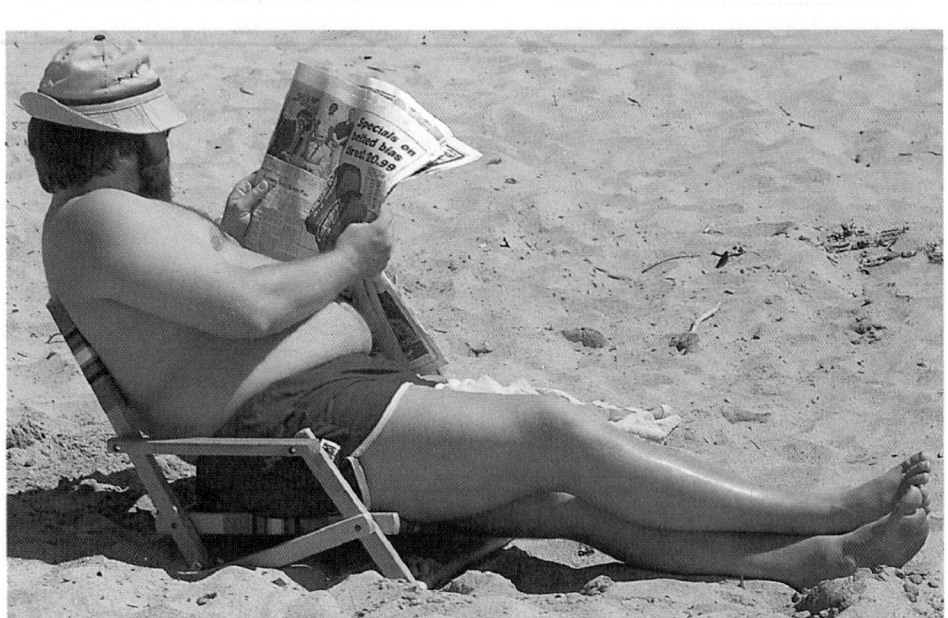

Central obesity, characterized by an "apple-shaped" body with large abdominal-type fat stores, is a strong risk factor for Type II diabetes.

TABLE 8–3
FRAME SIZE

To make a simple approximation of your frame size:

Extend your arm and bend the forearm upward at a 90-degree angle. Keep the fingers straight and turn the inside of your wrist away from your body. Place the thumb and index finger of your other hand on the two prominent bones on either side of your elbow. Measure the space between your fingers against a ruler or a tape measure.[a] Compare the measurements with the following standards. (These standards represent the elbow measurements for medium-framed men and women of various heights. Measurements smaller than those listed indicate you have a small frame, and larger measurements indicate a large frame.[b])

MEN Height in 1-in. Heels	Elbow Breadth	WOMEN Height in 1-in. Heels	Elbow Breadth
5 ft 2 in. to 5 ft 3 in.	2½ to 2⅞ in.	4 ft 10 in. to 4 ft 11 in.	2¼ to 2½ in.
5 ft 4 in. to 5 ft 7 in.	2⅝ to 2⅞ in.	5 ft 0 in. to 5 ft 3 in.	2¼ to 2½ in.
5 ft 8 in. to 5 ft 11 in.	2¾ to 3 in.	5 ft 4 in. to 5 ft 7 in.	2⅜ to 2⅝ in.
6 ft 0 in. to 6 ft 3 in.	2¾ to 3⅛ in.	5 ft 8 in. to 5 ft 11 in.	2⅜ to 3⅝ in.
6 ft 4 in. and over	2⅞ to 3¼ in.	6 ft 0 in. and over	2½ to 3¾ in.

[a]For the most accurate measurement, have your health-care provider measure your elbow breadth with a caliper.

[b]A simple estimate of frame size can be derived by circling your wrist with the thumb and middle finger of your other hand. If the thumb and finger do not meet, you most likely have a large frame. If the thumb and finger just meet, you most likely have a medium frame, and if the fingers overlap greatly, you may have a small frame.

taken on accurate scales and compared with **frame size,** determined by measuring the breadth of the elbow. Table 8–3 provides the information you need to determine your frame size. The second measure is the **body mass index (BMI),** which is an index of your weight in relation to your height. The third measure is the waist-to-hip circumference ratio referred to earlier. The accompanying Healthy Weight Scorecard guides your use of the new healthy weight tables, the body mass index, and the waist-to-hip circumference ratio to help you answer the question for yourself.

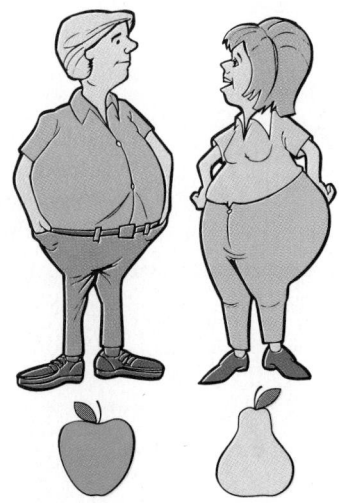

FRAME SIZE the size of a person's bones and musculature. A person with a large frame can weigh more than one the same height with a small frame without increased risks.

BODY MASS INDEX (BMI) an index of degree of obesity derived from the height and weight.

People (mostly men) storing excess fat in the chest and stomach areas (apple-shaped) are at a higher risk for diabetes, heart disease, and hypertension than people storing excess fat in the hips, thighs, and buttocks (pear-shaped).

A wide range of weights is compatible with good health. Within this range, the definition of desirable or healthful weight is up to the individual, depending on such factors as family history, occupation, physical and recreational activities, and personal preferences. To determine if your weight is a healthful weight for you:

- See if your weight is within the range suggested for persons of your height (see Table 8–4). The weights in the table apply to men and women of all ages. The health risks due to excess weight appear to be the same for older as for younger adults. Weights above this range are less healthy for most people. The higher you are above the healthy weight range for your height, the higher your weight-related risk (see Figure 8–1).

- Determine your frame size as previously shown in Table 8–3. The range in weights for a given height shown in Table 8–4 allows for differences in amount of muscle and bone. The higher weights in each range apply to people with more muscle and bone. What size frame do you have?

- Calculate your BMI using the following equation:

$$BMI = \frac{weight\ (lb)}{height\ (in)^2} \times 705$$

Compare your BMI to the standards:

TABLE 8–4
HEALTHY WEIGHT RANGES FOR MEN AND WOMEN

HEIGHT[a]	WEIGHT IN POUNDS[b]
4'8"	83–110
4'9"	87–115
4'10"	91–119
4'11"	94–124
5'0"	97–128
5'1"	101–132
5'2"	104–137
5'3"	107–141
5'4"	111–146
5'5"	114–150
5'6"	118–155
5'7"	121–160
5'8"	125–164
5'9"	129–169
5'10"	132–174
5'11"	136–179
6'0"	140–184
6'1"	144–189
6'2"	148–195
6'3"	152–200
6'4"	156–205
6'5"	160–211
6'6"	164–216

[a]without shoes
[b]without clothes

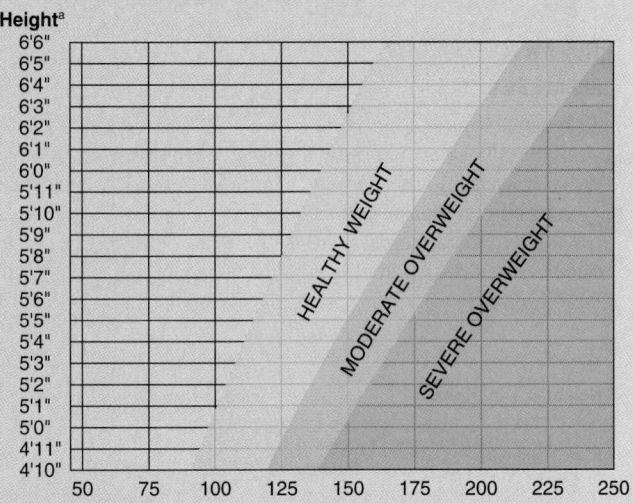

[a]Without shoes.

[b]Without clothes. The higher weights apply to people with more muscle and bone, such as many men.

FIGURE 8–1
RANGES FOR HEALTHFUL AND UNHEALTHFUL WEIGHTS

SOURCE: U.S. Department of Agriculture, U.S. Department of Health and Human Services, *Nutrition and Your Health: Dietary Guidelines for Americans* (Home and Garden Bulletin No. 232, 1995), p. 18.

- Determine if your fat distribution is associated with health risks. Excess fat in the abdomen is a greater health risk than excess fat in the hips and thighs. Calculate your waist-to-hip ratio by dividing the number of inches around your waistline by the number of inches around the widest part of your hips:

$$\frac{your\ waist\ in\ inches}{your\ hips\ in\ inches} = \frac{\boxed{}}{\boxed{}} = \boxed{}\ \text{waist-to-hip ratio}$$

A ratio above 0.80 for women and above 0.95 for men suggests an excess of abdominal fat, an increased risk of obesity-related health problems, and a need to reduce body fatness to reduce health risks.

- How does your current weight measure up to these considerations? If your current weight is within the healthful range for your height, if your BMI is acceptable for good health, and if your waist-to-hip ratio is not high, you will want to maintain this weight. If you need to lose weight or gain weight, consider the tips offered throughout this chapter for healthfully changing your weight.

	MEN	WOMEN
Underweight	<20.7	<19.1
Acceptable weight	20.7 to 27.8	19.1 to 27.3
Overweight	≥27.8	≥27.3
Severe overweight	≥31.1	≥32.3
Morbid obesity	≥45.4	≥44.8

Energy Balance

Suppose you decide that you are too fat or too thin. You got that way by having an unbalanced energy budget—that is, by eating either more or less food energy than you spent. Fatness and thinness are reflections of excessive or deficient energy stores. You store extra energy as fat only if you eat *more* food energy in a day than you use to fuel your metabolic and other activities. Similarly, you lose stored fat only if you eat *less* food energy in a day than you use as fuel. A day's energy balance can be stated like this:

Change in energy stores = Energy in − Energy out.

WEIGHT LOSS: calories eaten are less than calories burned.
WEIGHT GAIN: calories eaten are greater than calories burned.

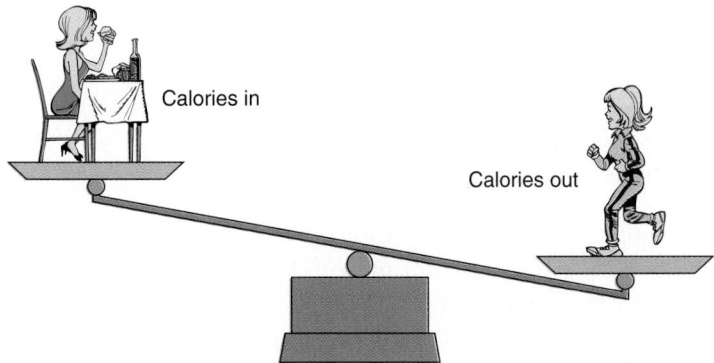

The balance between energy in and energy out determines whether a person stores or uses body fat.

You know about the "energy in" side of this equation. An apple brings you 100 calories; a candy bar, 290 calories.* You probably also know that for each 3,500 calories you eat in excess of need, you store one pound of body fat.

As for the "energy out" side, the body spends energy in two major ways: to fuel its metabolic activities and to fuel its muscle activities. You can change your activity level to spend more energy in a day, and if you do so consistently, your metabolic activities also will ultimately speed up somewhat. The following three sections discuss the body's needs for energy.

Basal Metabolism

About 60 percent or more of the energy the average person spends goes to support the ongoing metabolic work of the body's cells, the **basal metabolism.** This is the work that goes on all the time, without conscious awareness. The beating of the heart, the inhaling and exhaling of air, the maintenance of body temperature, and the sending of nerve and hormonal messages to direct these activities are the basal processes that maintain life. Basal metabolic needs are

BASAL METABOLISM the sum total of all the chemical activities of the cells necessary to sustain life, exclusive of voluntary activities—that is, the ongoing activities of the cells when the body is at rest.

*Calorie amounts for more than 1,900 foods are listed in Appendix I.

surprisingly large. A person whose total energy expenditure amounts to 2,000 calories per day spends as many as 1,200 to 1,400 of them to support basal metabolism.

The **basal metabolic rate** (often abbreviated **BMR**) is influenced by a number of factors (see Table 8–5). In general, the younger a person is, the higher the basal metabolic rate, partly because of the increased activity of cells undergoing division. The BMR is most pronounced during the growth spurts that take place during infancy, puberty, and pregnancy. Body composition also influences metabolic rate. Muscle tissue is highly active even when it is resting, whereas fat tissue is comparatively inactive. The more lean tissue in a body, the higher the BMR; the more fat tissue, the lower the BMR. Lean body mass decreases with age, and it is estimated that the BMR decreases by about 5 percent every ten years after age 50.

Gender correlates roughly with body composition. Men generally have a faster metabolic rate than women, and researchers believe that this is because of men's greater percentage of lean tissue. (A woman athlete has a greater percentage of lean tissue than a sedentary man of the same weight and so would have a higher metabolic rate.) Fever increases the energy needs of cells, whose increased activities to generate heat and fight off infection speed up the metabolic rate.

Fasting and constant malnutrition lower the metabolic rate because of the loss of lean tissue and the slowdown of activities the body can't afford to support fully. This slowing of metabolism seems to be a protective mechanism to conserve energy when there is a shortage, and it hampers weight loss in a person who fasts or undertakes a very-low-calorie diet.

Some hormones—the stress hormones, for example—influence metabolism. They increase the energy demands of every cell and thus raise the metabolic rate. This raised metabolism partly accounts for the weight loss sometimes seen in people experiencing extreme stress in their life, although other factors, such as upset digestion and loss of appetite, also enter in.

The activity of the thyroid gland also influences the basal metabolic rate. The less thyroid hormone secreted, the lower the energy requirement for maintenance of basal functions.

Voluntary Activities

Muscular activity does not make as big a contribution as basal metabolism does to most people's energy outputs. On the average, it amounts to only about 30

BASAL METABOLIC RATE (BMR) the rate at which the body spends energy to support its basal metabolism. The BMR accounts for the largest component of a person's daily energy (calorie) needs.

TABLE 8–5
FACTORS THAT INFLUENCE THE BASAL METABOLIC RATE

FACTORS THAT INCREASE BMR:

Fever

Growth (higher in children and pregnant women)

Height (higher in tall, thin people)

Male gender (more lean tissue)

Muscle mass (the more lean tissue, the higher the BMR)

Stress

Thyroid hormone

FACTORS THAT DECREASE BMR:

Age (slows down with age)

Reduced energy intake (fasting, starvation, low-calorie diets)

percent of the total. But unlike basal metabolism, which cannot be changed immediately, physical activity can be changed at will. If you want to tinker with your energy balance, this is the component—on the output side—that you can alter significantly in the short term. If you increase it consistently, you will also ultimately increase the energy your body spends on metabolic activity because you will have an increase in lean body mass.

The energy spent on physical activity is the energy spent moving the body's skeletal muscles—the muscles of the arms, back, abdomen, legs, and so forth—and the extra energy spent to speed up the heartbeat and respiration rate as needed. The number of calories spent depends on three factors: (1) the amount of muscle mass required, (2) the amount of weight being moved, and (3) the amount of time the activity takes. Thus, an activity involving both the arms and the legs requires more calories than an activity of the same intensity involving only the legs; an activity performed by a heavier person requires more energy than the same activity performed by a lighter person; and an activity performed for 40 minutes requires twice as much energy as that same activity performed for 20 minutes.

As disheartening as it may be for a college student to discover, mental activity requires little energy, even though it may be tiring. Studying for an exam may be hard work, but it won't burn body fat. People who are very, very busy—writing letters, making phone calls, riding in their cars from place to place—may wonder why they tend to gain weight, because they think of themselves as active people. They may be socially or intellectually active, but such activity involves few muscles and therefore little energy expenditure.

Total Energy Needs

A typical breakdown of the total energy spent by a lightly active person (for example, a student who walks back and forth to classes) might look like this:

Energy for basal metabolism:	1,400 calories
Energy for physical activity:	560 calories
	Total: 1,960 calories

The first component is larger, and you cannot change it much. You can, however, change the second component—physical activity—and so use more calories. If you want to increase your basal metabolic output, make exercise a daily habit. Your body composition will gradually change, and your basal energy output will pick up the pace as well. You can figure out roughly how much energy you spend in a day by using the Energy Output Scorecard.

In summary, the amount of fat stored in a person's body depends on the balance between the total food energy the person has taken in and the total energy the person has expended. Later in the chapter, you will learn how to alter both—with diet and exercise—to regulate body weight. But first: Why do so many people have excessive fat stores?

A. First figure the energy you spend on BMR.* It's about 10 calories per pound of your body weight if you are a woman or 11 calories per pound if you are a man (men generally have more muscle than women):

A. _____ cal

B. Now figure the energy you spend on activities:

If you are not very active (sedentary)—you sit down most of the day and drive or ride whenever possible—take 25% to 40% (men) or 25% to 35% (women) of your BMR calories in A.

If you are lightly active—you sit most of the day, but you move around two to four hours of the day as a teacher might—take 50% to 70% (men) or 40% to 60% (women) of A.

If you are moderately active—you do some amount of regular exercise four or five times a week or your job requires some physical labor—take 65% to 80% (men) or 50% to 70% (women) of A.

If you are very physically active—your job requires much physical labor or you are physically active four or more hours each day—and you do little standing or sitting, take 90% to 120% (men) or 80% to 100% (women) of A.

B. _____ cal

C. Total energy need = A + B = _____

C. _____ cal

*Note: Another way to estimate the energy spent on basal metabolism is to use the factor (for men) 1.0 cal/kg/hour (or for women 0.9 cal/kg/hr) for a 24-hour period. Then add an increment of this amount depending on how physically active you are.

Causes of Obesity

Some people eat more than they need or exercise less than they should to maintain their body weight, and they get fat. Some eat less or exercise more, and they get thin. Perhaps most amazingly, some people—most people, in fact—eat exactly what they need and stay at the same weight year after year. A single extra pat of butter each day would make them gain five pounds in a year, but if they overeat by that much one day, they undereat by the same amount the next. How do they do this—and, in contrast, why do some people fail to maintain their weight?

Genetics Versus Environment

In general, two schools of thought address the problem of obesity's causes.[8] One attributes it to inside-the-body causes; the other, to environmental factors. One popular inside-the-body theory is the so-called **set-point theory.** Noting that many people who lose weight on reducing diets subsequently return to their original weight, some researchers have suggested that the body "wants" to maintain a certain amount of fat and regulates eating behaviors and hormonal actions to defend its "set point." The theory implies that science should search inside obese people to find the causes of their problems—perhaps in their hunger-regulating mechanisms.

Recently, researchers identified a gene—named *ob* (for *obese*)—that appears to produce a hormone (called *leptin* after the Greek word for thin) that seems to tell the body to stop eating when it is activated in fat cells.[9] Researchers report that mice with a defective form of the gene can weigh as much as three times

SET-POINT THEORY the theory that the body tends to maintain a certain weight by adjusting hunger, appetite, and food energy intake on the one hand and metabolism (energy output) on the other so that a person's conscious efforts to alter weight may be foiled.

more than normal mice. Overweight people, too, may have a defective form of this gene (or may be unresponsive to its hormone), which fails to give an accurate report of the size of the fat cells to the brain, thus making the set point too high—resulting in weight gain. Much more research is needed to clarify this mechanism.

The other point of view is that obesity is environmentally determined. Proponents of this view hold that people overeat or underexercise because they are pushed to do so by factors in their surroundings—foremost among them, the availability of a multitude of delectable foods and the lack of opportunities for vigorous physical activity. The two views are not mutually exclusive, and they may both be operating, even within the same person.

Perhaps some people have inherited or learned a way of resisting external stimuli to eat, while others have not. Of interest in this connection is the report of a classic experiment with "cafeteria rats." Ordinary rats fed regular rat chow are of normal weight (for rats), but if those very same rats are offered free access to a wide variety of tempting, rich, highly palatable foods, they greatly overeat and become obese. Similarly, in one study, overweight people more often overconsumed the foods that they described as most palatable and ate these foods more quickly than lean subjects.[10] This is the basis of the **external cue theory**—the theory that, at least in some people, the internal regulatory systems are easily overridden by environmental influences. A question to ponder: Does this make obesity hereditary, environmental, or both?

It seems likely that both hereditary and environmental factors influence obesity in human beings. The tendency to obesity is probably inherited, but the environment is probably influential in the sense that it can prevent or permit the development of obesity when the potential is there.

The complexity of the situation is reflected in observations of the ways obesity develops from infancy on. Some fat infants become fat adults, but most grow out of their obesity in childhood. An overweight child, however, is more likely to remain overweight into adulthood.[11] Researchers propose the **fat cell theory**—that childhood obesity is persistent because early overfeeding (during the growing years) may cause fat cells to increase abnormally in *number* (**hyperplastic obesity**). The number of fat cells is thought to become fixed by adulthood; afterwards, a gain or loss of weight either increases or diminishes the *size* of the fat cells (**hypertrophic obesity**). Unfortunately, persons with greater than normal numbers of fat cells are least likely to lose weight successfully. Some researchers suggest that the body triggers hunger signals when the fat stored in these cells begins to decrease.

The theory that a hereditary, inside-the-body basis for obesity may exist is supported by the existence of animal strains that are genetically fat. Such animals tend to be fat in any environment—that is, they are fat regardless of the kind or variety of food offered. In humans, studies have shown that identical twins—whether raised together or apart, tend to have similar weight-gain patterns.[12] Also, twins raised by adoptive parents tend to have body shapes similar to their biological parents. Not all studies confirm this, however.[13] Moreover, pairs of twins purposefully overfed in clinical experiments tend to respond similarly to the extra calories. Some sets of twins gain considerable amounts of weight when fed a certain number of calories, whereas other pairs put on relatively few pounds even on the same diet.[14]

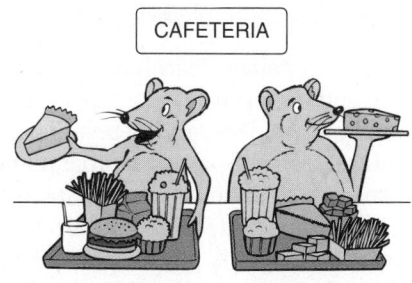

Given a wide variety of tempting foods, these laboratory animals become obese, just as human beings do.

EXTERNAL CUE THEORY the theory that some people eat in response to such external factors as the presence of food or the time of day rather than to such internal factors as hunger.

FAT CELL THEORY states that during the growing years, fat cells respond to overfeeding by producing additional fat cells (**hyperplastic obesity**); the number of fat cells eventually becomes fixed, and overfeeding from this point on causes the body to enlarge existing fat cells (**hypertrophic obesity**). Hypertropic obesity is the more common type and is usually seen in adults.

Environment and Behavior

In human beings, learning plays an important role. Although we have genetically inborn instincts, superimposed on these are learnings from our early childhood experiences, and depending on our environments, the two may differ. Thus, **hunger** is a drive programmed into us by our heredity, but learned responses to **appetite** can teach us to ignore or overrespond to our hunger. In contrast, appetite is more influenced by learning. Another way to say this is to say that hunger is physiological, while appetite is psychological, and the two don't always coincide. We have all experienced appetite without hunger: "I'm not hungry, but I'd love to have some." We also often experience the reverse, hunger without appetite: "I know I'm hungry, but I don't feel like eating." Hunger is a negative experience (and we may eat to avoid it); appetite is positive.

The ways people respond to hunger and appetite determine whether they eat too much, too little, or just enough to maintain their weight. A third factor enters in, too: satiety, which signals that it is time to stop eating. One view holds that eating behavior is turned on all the time, except when the satiety signal turns it off. But much remains to be learned about the ways in which hunger, appetite, and satiety regulate food intake.

In human physiology, research is beginning to find possible answers to what regulates food behavior. The stomach's nerves perceive stretching, and you stop eating when your stomach feels stretched full. Blood glucose level is thought to be involved: You get hungry when your blood glucose level falls—or perhaps when your liver glycogen is beginning to be exhausted. Blood lipids, and possibly amino acids and other molecules, also play a role. When you eat, you secrete hormones to regulate digestive activity; these hormones may also convey the message to the brain that it is time to stop eating.

This brings us to the question, Where in the brain are these messages received (whatever they are)? One brain area stands out as a regulator for food behavior—the **hypothalamus.** The hypothalamus is a center that communicates with both the hormonal and the nervous systems. It integrates many kinds of signals received from the rest of the body, including information about the blood's temperature, sodium content, and glucose content. We know it is important in regulating eating because damage to the hypothalamus produces derangements in eating behavior and body weight—in some cases causing severe weight loss; in others, vast overeating. In the person with a normal hypothalamus, however, appropriate eating behavior seems to be a response not to a single signal arriving at some one location in the hypothalamus but to a whole host of signals. Somehow these many inputs become integrated into a final common path—the act of eating.

A person who eats inappropriately may have established a habitual behavior pattern that wrongly links many different stimuli to the act of eating. In this connection, the study of behavior offers insight into the problem of overeating by viewing it as a conditioned response to a variety of stimuli. Sometimes eating behavior tends to get turned on by the wrong triggers. A crying child with a skinned knee who is offered a lollipop to help soothe the hurt may learn to associate food with comfort and so seek food inappropriately when experiencing emotional pain later in life.

HUNGER the physiological drive to find and eat food, experienced as an unpleasant sensation.

APPETITE the psychological desire to find and eat food, experienced as a pleasant sensation, often in the absence of hunger.

HYPOTHALAMUS (high-poh-THALL-ah-mus) a part of the brain that senses a variety of conditions in the blood, such as temperature, salt content, and glucose content, and then signals other parts of the brain or body to change those conditions when necessary.

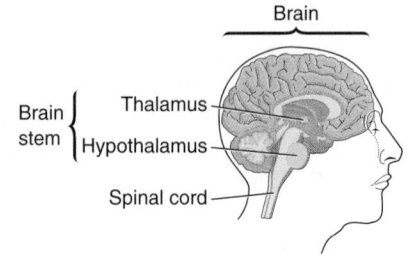

Researchers believe that the hypothalamus controls the sensations of hunger and satiety.

Eating behavior, then, may be a response not only to hunger or appetite but also to complex human sensations such as yearning, craving, addiction, or compulsion. For an emotionally insecure person, eating may be less threatening than calling a friend when lonely and risking rejection. Often, eating is used to relieve boredom or to ward off depression. Some people respond to anxiety—or, in fact, to any kind of **arousal**—by eating. Significantly, however, if they are able to give a name to their aroused condition and thereby gain a feeling that they have some control over it, they are not as likely to overeat.

AROUSAL as used in this context, heightened activity of certain brain centers associated with excitement and anxiety.

Stress may also directly promote the accumulation of body fat. The stress hormones favor the breakdown of energy stores (glycogen and fat) to glucose and fatty acids, which can be used to fuel the muscular activity of fight or flight. If a person fails to use the fuel in physical exertion, however, the body cannot turn these fragments back into glycogen. It has no alternative but to convert them to fat. Each time glucose is pulled out of storage in response to stress and then transformed into fat, the lowered glucose level or exhausted glycogen will signal hunger, and the person will eat again soon after.

Stress eating may appear in different patterns. Some people eat excessively at night, while others characteristically binge during emotional crises. The overly thin often react oppositely. Stress causes them to reject food and thus become thinner. It is not yet known why these behaviors occur, but research continues.

The many possible causes of obesity mentioned so far all relate to the input side of the energy equation. What about output? It is probable that the most important single contributor to the obesity problem in our country is underactivity.[15] The control of hunger and appetite works well in active people and fails only when activity falls below a certain minimum level. Some obese people eat less than lean people, but they are so extraordinarily inactive that they still manage to store surplus calories. Some people move more efficiently than others, too. Two people of the same age, height, and weight might use different amounts of calories walking five miles because of the different ways in which they move their muscles.

It is probable that the most important single contributor to the obesity problem in our country is underactivity.

No two people are alike, either physically or psychologically. No doubt, the causes of obesity are as varied as the obese people themselves. Many causes may contribute to the problem in a single person. Given this complexity, it is obvious that there is no panacea. The top priority should be prevention, but where prevention has failed, the treatment of obesity must involve a simultaneous attack on many fronts.[16]

Weight Gain and Loss

When you step on the scale and note that you weigh a pound more or less than you did the last time you weighed yourself, this doesn't necessarily mean you have gained or lost body fat. Changes in body weight reflect shifts in many different materials—not only fat but also fluid, bone minerals, and lean tissues such as muscles. This means that the loss of a pound does not always reflect the loss of fat. Similarly, the gain of a pound may not reflect gained fat; some of it may reflect gained muscle and bone and an overall shift toward a leaner body type. Because it is so important for people concerned with weight control to realize this, this section discusses the changes that take place with gains and losses of weight.

A healthy man or woman about 5 feet 10 inches tall who weighs 150 pounds carries about 90 of those pounds as water and 30 as fat. The other 30 pounds are the so-called lean tissues: muscles; organs such as the heart, brain, and liver; and the bones of the skeleton.* Stripped of water and fat, then, the person weighs only 30 pounds. This lean tissue is the body's vital machinery that maintains health and life. When a person who is too fat seeks to lose weight, it should be fat—not this precious lean tissue—that is lost. And for someone who wants to gain weight, it is desirable to gain weight in proportion—lean *and* fat, not just fat.

Weight is gained or lost in different body tissues, depending on how a person goes about it. To lose fluid, for example, one can take a diuretic ("water pill"), causing the kidneys to siphon extra water from the blood into the urine. Or one can engage in heavy exercise in the heat, losing abundant fluid in perspiration. (Both practices are dangerous, incidentally, and are NOT being recommended here.) To gain water weight, a person can overconsume salt and water; for a few hours the body will then retain water, until it manages to excrete the salt. (This, too, is not recommended.) Most quick-weight-loss diet schemes promote large losses of fluid that create large, temporary changes in the scale's weight with little or no real loss of body fat. The rest of this chapter underscores this distinction, and a later section on weight-loss strategy stresses exercise as a means of supporting lean tissue during weight loss.

Weight Gain

When you eat more calories than you need, where does this excess go in your body? The energy nutrients—carbohydrate, fat, and protein—contribute to body stores as follows:

- Carbohydrate is broken down to small units (sugars) for absorption. Inside the body, these sugars may be built up to glycogen or converted to fat and stored as such.

- Fat is broken down to its component parts (including fatty acids) for absorption. Inside the body, these components are most easily converted to storage fat.

- Protein, too, is broken down to its basic units (amino acids) for absorption. Inside the body, these units may be used to replace body proteins. Those amino acids that are not used cannot be stored as protein for later use. They lose their nitrogen and are converted to fat.

Notice in Figure 8–2 that although three kinds of materials enter the body, they are stored for later use in only two forms: glycogen and fat. Also notice that when protein is stored in the form of fat, it cannot be recovered later as protein. The amino acids lose their nitrogen—the nitrogen is actually excreted in the urine. It does not matter whether you are eating hamburgers, brownies, or carrot sticks; if you eat enough of the food, the excess will be turned to fat within

---

*For a healthy woman or man 5 feet tall who weighs 100 pounds, the comparable figures would be 60 pounds of water, 20 pounds of fat, and 20 pounds of lean tissue.

hours. (On the other hand, as Chapter 9 will make clear, a judicious program of eating well and exercising will help build muscle.)

Of the three energy nutrients, fat from food is especially easy for the body to store as fat tissue. This implies, then, that the calories from fat may be more fattening than those from carbohydrate or protein. Researchers have shown in both animals and humans that subjects who ate higher fat diets had higher body fat contents than those who ate diets high in carbohydrates and lower in fat, even though the two diets were similar in terms of total calories.[17] This suggests that obesity more easily develops from eating a high-fat diet.[18] If you choose to overeat, therefore, there may be some advantage to overeating carbohydrate-rich bread or potatoes than overeating fat-rich butter or sour cream—you may deposit less fat.

Weight Loss and Fasting

When the tables are turned and you stop eating altogether, your body has to draw on its stored supplies of nutrients to keep going. Nothing is wrong with this; in fact, it is a great advantage to you that you can eat periodically, store fuel, and then use up that fuel between meals. The between-meal interval is ideally about 4 to 6 hours—about the length of time it takes to use up most of the available liver glycogen—or 12 to 14 hours at night, when body systems are slowed down and the need for energy is lower. If a person doesn't eat for, say, three whole days or a week, the body makes one adjustment after another.

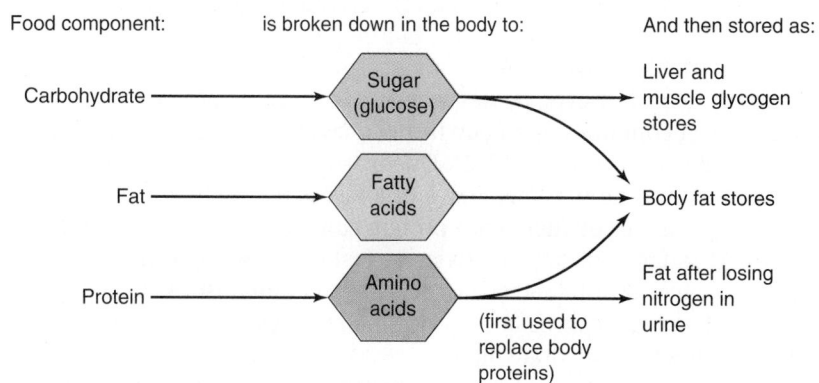

a. When a person overeats (feasting):

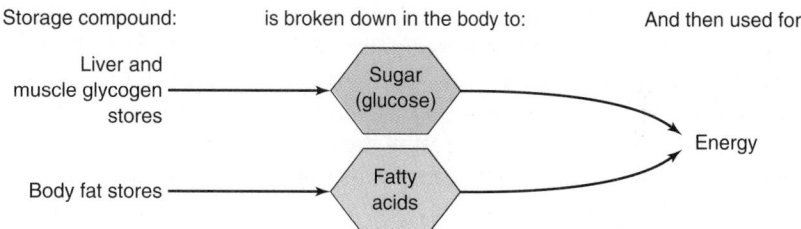

b. When a person draws on stores (fasting):

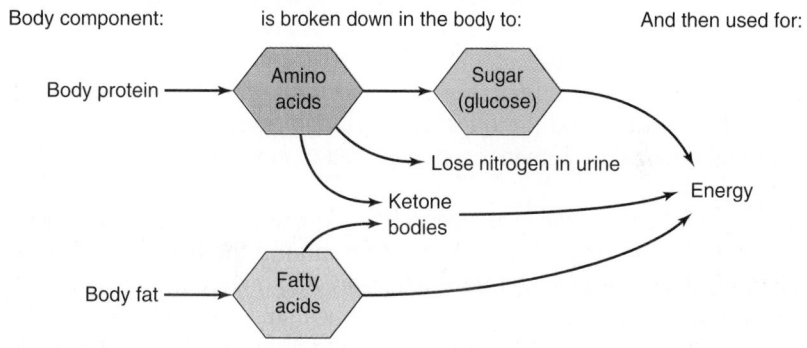

c. If the fast continues beyond glycogen depletion:

FIGURE 8–2
FEASTING AND FASTING

In A, the person is storing energy. In B, the person is drawing on stored energy. In C, the person is in ketosis.

The first adjustment is to use the liver's glycogen. (The muscles' glycogen is reserved for the muscles' own use—and they are using it.) The liver's glycogen, remember, is the body's source of blood glucose to fuel the brain's and nerves' activities. Ordinarily, the brain and nerves can use no other fuel. But after about a day, the primary supply is gone. Where, then, does the body turn to keep its nervous system going? Whatever it has to do, it will do, for the nervous system runs the body, and when it stops, the body dies.

An obvious alternative source of energy would be the abundant fat stores most people carry. At first, these are of no use to the nervous system. The muscles and other organs use fat as fuel, but the nervous system ordinarily cannot. Nor can the body convert this fat to glucose, because it possesses no enzymes to do so. It does, however, possess enzymes to convert protein to glucose.

As the fast continues, the body turns to its own lean tissues to keep up the supply of glucose (see Figure 8–2). One reason why people lose weight so dramatically within the first three days of a fast is that they are devouring their own protein tissues as fuel. Since protein contains only half as many calories per pound as fat, it disappears twice as fast. Also, with each pound of body protein, three or four pounds of associated water are lost. As you will see in a moment, the same reasons account for the rapid weight loss seen in the early stages of a low-carbohydrate diet.

If the body were to continue to consume itself at this rate, death would ensue within about ten days. After all, the liver, the heart and skeletal muscles, the lung tissue, and the blood—all vital tissues—are being burned as fuel. (In fact, fasting or starving people remain alive only until their body fat is gone or until half their lean tissue is gone, whichever comes first.) But now the body plays its last ace: It begins converting fat stores into a form it can use to help feed the nervous system and so forestall the end. This is known as **ketosis.**

Ketosis is an adaptation to prolonged fasting or carbohydrate deprivation. Instead of breaking down fat molecules all the way to carbon dioxide and water, as it normally does, the body takes partially broken down fat fragments, combines them into ketone bodies (compounds that are normally rare in the blood), and lets them circulate in the bloodstream. The advantage is that about half of the brain's cells can use these compounds for energy. Thus, indirectly, the nervous system begins to feed on the body's fat stores. This reduces the nervous system's need for glucose. It spares the muscle and other lean tissue from being devoured so quickly and prolongs the starving person's life. Because of ketosis, an initially healthy person totally deprived of food can live for as long as six to eight weeks.

KETOSIS (kee-TOE-sis) an adaptation of the body to prolonged (several days') fasting or carbohydrate restriction: body fat is converted to ketones, which can be used as fuel for some brain cells.

Fasting has been practiced as a periodic discipline by respected, wise people in many cultures. However, ketosis may be harmful to the body by upsetting the acid-base balance of the blood. For the person who merely wants to lose weight, then, fasting is usually not the best way. For one thing, even in ketosis, the body's lean tissue continues to be lost at a rapid rate to supply glucose to those nervous system cells that cannot use ketones as fuel. For another, the body becomes conservative during a fast and slows its metabolism so as to lose as little energy as it possibly can. A well-designed low-calorie diet, accompanied by the appropriate exercise program, has actually been observed to promote the same rate of *weight* loss as, and a faster rate of *fat* loss than, a total fast. Just how to design a low-calorie diet is the subject of a later section. But first the low-carbohydrate diet—an example of how *not* to design a diet—deserves attention.

The Low-Carbohydrate Diet

People are attracted to low-carbohydrate diets because of the dramatic weight loss that occurs within the first few days. Such people would be disillusioned if they realized that the major part of this weight loss is a loss of body protein, along with quantities of water and important minerals.

The low-carbohydrate diet is designed to make a person go into ketosis. The sales pitch is that "you'll never feel hungry" and that "you'll lose weight fast—faster than you would on any ordinary diet." Both claims are true, but knowledgeable consumers see through them. They know that the loss of appetite is common to any low-calorie diet. To the fast weight loss, they say, "Yes, but what kind of weight loss: water and lean tissue, or fat?"

The body responds to a low-carbohydrate diet as it does to a fast. It is receiving protein and fat (on a fast it draws on its own protein and fat), but it has used up its stored glycogen. It therefore turns to protein to make the needed glucose. Why should you give your body protein if it will only convert that protein to glucose? And why *not* give it carbohydrate if that is the very material it needs? Carbohydrate will sustain it and allow it to use up its stored fat at the maximal rate.

> To identify fraudulent low-carbohydrate diets for what they are, learn to add up the carbohydrate grams they supply: fewer than 100 to 125 grams a day is inadequate.

Protein, then, is inefficient fuel for a carbohydrate-deprived body. It has another disadvantage as well. On being converted to glucose, protein loses its nitrogen, and that nitrogen has to be excreted. This puts a burden on the kidneys. Advising the low-carbohydrate dieter to drink sufficient water is intended to prevent kidney damage that may result from the large amounts of nitrogen-containing waste materials and ketone bodies circulating in the blood. A multitude of other physiological hazards accompany these diets—metabolic abnormalities such as high blood cholesterol, hypoglycemia, and mineral imbalances. Legitimate practitioners never recommend these diets.

Low-carbohydrate diets come in many disguises with many different names: Air Force Diet, the Atkins Diet, the Calories Don't Count Diet, the Herbalife Diet, the Mayo Diet, the Protein-Sparing Fast, the Scarsdale Diet, and the Doctor's Quick Weight-Loss Diet. Some of these diets involve eating foods that are high in both protein and fat (abundant meats, for example); others allow only protein-rich foods (fish and chicken without the skin); and some offer no foods at all, but only powders or liquids that are supposed to "spare" body protein while the body burns its own fat as fuel. The latter are the most dangerous of all. Numerous deaths have been traced to them, many caused by abnormalities found in the heart muscle.

Bringing out new diet books and products every year is a profitable business, and it will continue to be successful as long as people are deceived by the initial rapid weight loss into thinking that the diets work. Before adopting any new diet plan, compare it to the guidelines presented in Table 8–6.

BLOOM COUNTY   by Berke Breathed

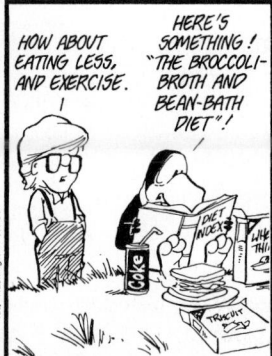
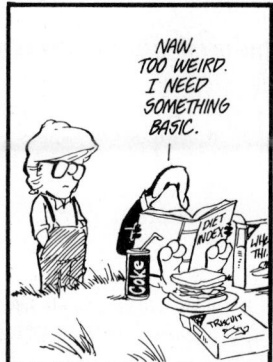
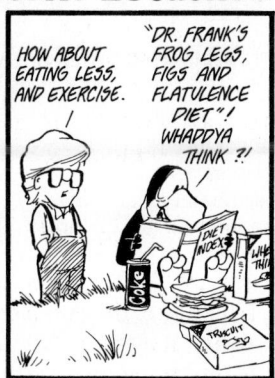

The Very-Low-Calorie Diets

Very-low-calorie diets (VLCDs) are mostly powdered formulas available by prescription, are usually medically supervised, and provide fewer than 800 calories. VLCDs consist of about 30 grams of carbohydrate (not enough to spare protein), and high-quality protein equivalent to about twice the RDI. Supplements of vitamins and minerals are provided.

For particular individuals, especially the morbidly obese, these diets may provide some benefit in that they promote rapid weight loss and free the individual from having to make decisions regarding food intake—dieters simply drink the prescribed formula. Because of the health risks that may accompany these diets, it is recommended that a VLCD be undertaken only when other more traditional approaches have failed and always under the supervision of a health team that includes both a physician and a registered dietitian. A significant loss of heart muscle can occur and lead to sudden death from heart attack if the client loses weight too rapidly on a VLCD.[19] Other risks are listed in Table 8–7. The more valid VLCD programs include exercise, nutrition education, behavior modification, and support groups to improve their long-term effectiveness.[20] Table 8–8 evaluates popular weight-loss diets, programs, and books.

TABLE 8–6
GUIDELINES FOR EVALUATING WEIGHT-LOSS PROMOTIONS

Beware of weight-loss programs that

1. Promise or imply dramatic, rapid weight loss (i.e., substantially more than 1% of total body weight per week).

2. Promote diets that are extremely low in calories (i.e., below 800 cal/day; 1,200-cal/day diets are preferred) unless under the supervision of competent medical experts.

3. Attempt to make clients dependent upon special products rather than teaching how to make good choices from the conventional food supply. (This does not condemn the marketing of low-calorie convenience foods that may be chosen by consumers.)

4. Do not encourage permanent, realistic lifestyle changes, including regular exercise and the behavioral aspects of eating wherein food may be used as a coping device (i.e., programs should focus on changing the causes of overweight rather than simply on the overweight itself).

5. Misrepresent salespeople as "counselors" supposedly qualified to give guidance in nutrition and/or general health. Even if adequately trained, such counselors would still be objectionable because of the obvious conflict of interest that exists when providers profit directly from products they recommend and sell.

6. Require large sums of money at the start or require that clients sign contracts for expensive, long-term programs. Such practices too often have been abused as salespeople focus attention upon signing up new people rather than delivering continuing, satisfactory service.

7. Fail to inform clients about the risks associated with weight loss in general or the specific program being promoted.

8. Promote unproven or spurious weight-loss aids, such as chromium picolinate, human chorionic gonadotropin (HCG) hormone, starch blockers, diuretics, sauna belts, body wraps, passive exercise, ear stapling, acupuncture, electric muscle stimulating (EMS) devices, spirulina, amino acid supplements (e.g., arginine or ornithine), and glucomannan.

9. Claim that cellulite exists in the body.

10. Claim that the use of an appetite suppressant or methylcellulose (a bulking agent) enables a person to lose body fat without restricting accustomed caloric intake.

TABLE 8–7   RISKS ASSOCIATED WITH THE VERY-LOW-CALORIE DIETS

• Blood sugar imbalance	• Emotional problems	• Kidney infection
• Cold intolerance	• Fatigue/weakness	• Loss of lean body tissue
• Constipation	• Gallstones and kidney stones	• Menstrual irregularity
• Decreased basal metabolic rate	• Headaches	• Mineral and electrolyte imbalances
• Dehydration	• Heart irregularity	• Sleeplessness
• Diarrhea	• Ketosis	• Sudden death

SOURCE: Adapted from ADA report: Position of The American Dietetic Association: Very-low-calorie weight loss diets, *Journal of the American Dietetic Association*, May 1990, p. 722.

TABLE 8-8 WEIGHT-LOSS DIETS, PROGRAMS, AND BOOKS COMPARED

With a balanced perspective on foods and a sense of what is important in diet planning and what is not, you can evaluate the many different available diets and decide which might be best for you. Here's a summary of the questions you might ask, followed by a comparison of some of the currently popular diets, programs, and books.

1. Is this a diet you could live with indefinitely?
2. What is the recommended rate of weight loss?
3. Does the program take individual differences into account to determine caloric needs?
4. To what extent does the plan educate the client about nutrition, behavior modification, and the importance of exercise?
5. Does the program put you in contact with professionals such as physicians or registered dietitians?
6. Does the program offer a maintenance plan once the weight is lost?
7. What is the nature of the advertisements and endorsements?
8. How much does the program cost (can you afford it)?

DIET/PROGRAM	ENTRY CRITERIA	COST	M.D. SUPERVISION?	EDUCATION?*	DESCRIPTION, COMMENTS
Health Management Resources (HMR)	20% above desirable body weight or 40 lb overweight for VLCD diet	$115/week for medically supervised program; $90/week for moderate program	Yes	Yes	Medically supervised VLCD (520–800 cal) program and moderate program with less intensive supervision (800–1,000 cal) available. Three phases: weight loss, refeeding, and maintenance. Use of liquid formula diet or HMR frozen entrees (150–230 cal).
Medifast	20% above desirable body weight	$62.50 to $75/week	Yes	Prescribed but not necessarily provided by professionals	Four-phase program: medical evaluation, weight reduction (450–480 cal), realimentation, and maintenance.
Optifast	30% above desirable body weight; 20% if medically at risk or 50 lb overweight	$100/week	Yes	Yes	Four-phase program: modified fast (420–800 cal liquid diet), refeeding, stabilization, and maintenance (optional).
Total fasting	Not appropriate for anyone	—	No	No	Not advised because of high loss of lean body mass, vitamin and mineral deficiencies, and other complications.
Diet Center	M.D. approval needed for people more than 40% or 50 lb overweight or who have preexisting health problems	$50/week for reducing phase; less for other phases	Varies	Prescribed but not necessarily provided by a multidisciplinary team of professionals	Four-phase program: conditioning (unlimited cal); reducing (minimum of 1,000 cal); stabilizing; and maintenance. Individual differences in caloric needs are considered. Vitamin/mineral supplement taken daily. 1,000 mg of vitamin C is recommended daily, which seems excessive.
Diet Workshop	M.D. approval needed for people with preexisting health problems	Registration fee of $14, $9/week	No	Prescribed but not provided by a multidisciplinary team of professionals	Based on system of food "units." Reducing phase (900–1,000 cal, increased gradually to 1,200 cal until goal is achieved) and maintenance. Vitamin/mineral supplement recommended.
Jenny Craig Weight Loss Centers	M.D. approval needed for people with preexisting medical conditions	$185 for membership, $60 to $70/week for food	No	Prescribed but not provided by a multidisciplinary team of professionals	Two phases: reducing (about 1,000–1,400 cal) and maintenance. Complete reliance on packaged foods initially.

*Education refers to a three-pronged approach to weight loss that includes nutrition education, behavior modification, and exercise.

continued

289

TABLE 8-8 continued

DIET/PROGRAM	ENTRY CRITERIA	COST	M.D. SUPERVISION?	EDUCATION?*	DESCRIPTION, COMMENTS
Nutri/System	M.D. approval needed for people with preexisting medical problems or more than 100 lb overweight	Variable; $60 to $69/week for food	No	Prescribed but not provided by a multidisciplinary team of professionals	Two phases: weight loss (1,000–1,200 cal) and maintenance. Reliance on packaged foods until maintenance; low-fat (14%) high-carbohydrate (61%) diet; special diets for medical conditions.
Weight Watchers	More than 10 lb overweight	$12 to $20 fee, $7 to $9/week	No	Prescribed but not provided by professionals	Based on system of food exchanges. Weight loss (1,040–1,910 cal) and maintenance.
Slim Fast/ Ultra Slim Fast	M.D. approval recommended for people who are pregnant, nursing, under 18 years old, have health problems, or want to lose more than 30 lb or more than 15% of their body weight	$8 to $12/week	No	Limited	Over-the-counter meal replacement is mixed with low-fat milk (Slim Fast) or water (Ultra Slim Fast). Slim Fast is 190 cal/serving, Ultra Slim Fast is 220 cal/serving. Two phases: weight loss (1,100–1,200 cal) and maintenance (1,450–1,520 cal). Frozen entrees also available. This diet can be dangerous if instructions are not followed properly.

DIET BOOK	ALL FOOD GROUPS?	EDUCATION?*	DESCRIPTION, COMMENTS
Hilton Head Over-35 Diet by Peter Miller. New York: Warner Books, 1989	No—low in milk and fruit/vegetable groups during low-calorie phase	Yes—but limited behavior modification	Three phases: Low calorie (rotates between 900 cal/day on weekdays and 1,200 cal/day on weekends); reentry (about halfway between low-calorie and maintenance phases); and maintenance (cal equal to resting metabolic rate plus activity factor). Varying energy intake in weight loss has not been proved to prevent drops in basal metabolic rate (BMR).
The New Pritikin Program by Robert Pritikin. New York: Simon and Schuster, 1990	Yes—heavy emphasis on fruit/vegetable and bread/cereal groups	Yes	Energy intakes of 1,000 cal/day for women, 1,200 cal/day for men on "maximum weight loss" plan. Does not take individual needs for weight loss into account. Low-fat (10%), high-carbohydrate (75% to 80%) diet that is also low in sodium and high in fiber. May be difficult to follow such a low-fat diet.
Dr. Berger's Immune Power Diet by Stewart Berger. New York: New American Library, 1985	No—low in milk and bread/cereal groups	Limited	Diet to improve immune system but includes weight loss as an added benefit based on unsupported claims that certain foods affect immune system and levels of energy, creativity, mood, and emotion. Three phases: elimination (about 1,050 cal/day); reintroduction (about 1,400 cal/day); and maintenance (about 1,650 cal/day). Individual differences in caloric needs for weight loss are not considered; recommends megadoses of supplements, which can be dangerous.

*Education refers to a three-pronged approach to weight loss that includes nutrition education, behavior modification, and exercise.

continued

TABLE 8–8 continued

DIET BOOK	ALL FOOD GROUPS?	EDUCATION?*	DESCRIPTION, COMMENTS
Rotation Diet by Martin Katahn. New York: Bantam Books, 1987	No—low in milk and bread/cereal groups for most phases	Yes	Energy intakes of 600 to 1,500 cal/day rotated over 4 weeks; maintenance level is 1,800 cal/day. Individual differences in caloric needs for weight loss are not considered. Varying energy intakes in weight loss has not been proved to prevent drops in BMR.
Fat Attack Plan by Annette Natow and Jo-Ann Hestin. New York: Pocket Books, 1990	May be low in meat or bread/cereal group, depending on what dieter chooses	Yes	Teaches dieter to count grams of fat in foods. Three phases: "super start" (about 1,350 cal/day); "getting ahead"—15 g fat (about 1,400 cal/day); and "in control"—45 g of fat for women (about 1,700 cal/day), 60 g of fat for men (about 1,900 cal/day). May be difficult to follow such a low-fat diet.
Fit or Fat Target Diet by Covert Bailey. Boston: Houghton Mifflin, 1984	Yes	Limited—more guidance may be needed for weight loss, focus is on long-term weight management	Emphasis on healthful balanced diet rather than weight loss. Recommended minimum calorie level to promote weight loss is 1,000 to 1,400 cal/day for women, 1,400 to 1,800 cal/day for men. Diet is based on basic food groups, with emphasis on low-fat, low-sugar, and high-fiber foods (about 1,500 cal/day).
Set Point Diet by Gilbert Leveille. New York: Ballantine Books, 1985	Yes	Yes	1,200 to 2,400 cal/day food plans. Maintenance adds 300 cal/day. More research is needed regarding the set-point theory of body weight being confined to narrow range, and whether diet can lower one's set-point weight.
T-Factor Diet by Martin Katahn. New York: WW Norton, 1989	Yes	Yes	Two diets provided. T-factor diet is relatively low in calories and involves counting fat grams (20 to 40 g fat for women or about 1,200 cal/day, 30 to 60 g fat or about 1,800 cal/day for men). "Quick Melt Diet" restricts women to 1,000 to 1,300 cal/day and men to 1,500 to 1,800 cal/day. Does not take individual caloric differences for weight control into account. May be difficult to follow such low-fat diet. Based on thermogenesis studies suggesting that dietary fat is more efficiently converted into body fat than carbohydrates.
Callaway Diet by Wayne Callaway. New York: Bantam Books, 1990	No—low in milk group	Yes—but limited advice on maintenance	1,400- to 2,000-cal/day menus. Geared toward dieters who are "starvers" (periodically fast or near fast with VLCD), "stuffers" (compulsive eaters), or "skippers" (skip meals).
Fit for Life by Harvey and Marilyn Diamond. New York: Warner Books, 1985	No—low in milk, meat, and bread/cereal groups; very high in fruit/vegetable groups	Yes—but little emphasis on behavior modification and weight maintenance	Based on unsupported claims that fat deposits are caused by improper food combinations. Diet is high in fat (41%) and lacks variety. Individual differences in caloric needs for weight control are not considered, and high bulk may make it difficult to consume adequate calories.

*Education refers to a three-pronged approach to weight loss that includes nutrition education, behavior modification, and exercise.

SOURCE: Adapted from J. T. Dwyer and D. Lu, Popular diets for weight loss from nutritionally hazardous to healthful, In A. J. Stunkard and T. A. Wadden, eds., *Obesity: Theory and Therapy*, 2nd ed. (New York: Raven Press, 1993), pp. 231–252.

Drugs and Weight Loss

The search is on to find a safe and effective drug solution to the problem of obesity. The ideal drug needs to be safe, free of undesirable side effects and abuse potential, and effective at reducing body fat. Thus far, only appetite–suppressant drugs are available, either as prescription or over–the–counter drugs.

Stimulant drugs such as the amphetamines Dexedrine and Benzedrine can suppress appetite and thereby cause a drop in food intake. However, their effects are usually short-lived, and a person's appetite returns to normal after a few weeks. The drugs can be addictive and leave the dieter with another problem—how to get off them without gaining more weight. Other side effects include nervousness, headache, dizziness, weakness, fatigue, and insomnia.[21]

Another class of drugs, chemically similar to the amphetamines, but generally non-addictive as drugs, are the agents that enhance or stimulate the release of the brain chemical (neurotransmitter) serotonin. Upon its release, serotonin then acts to curb the appetite, and thus reduces food intake. Such drugs—including dex-fenfluramine and fluoxetine—are the focus of current obesity research and the FDA's scrutiny. Both drugs show potential as safe weight-loss agents. However, as with the drug treatment of other chronic disorders (for example, high blood pressure), these drugs may be required for long-term use for the effective treatment of obesity.[22]

Other prescription drugs currently under testing include drugs that speed up energy metabolism in the obese person, thus causing the body to use more fat for fuel and expend more total calories. Thyroid hormone was once used for this purpose, but it is no longer recommended for use in the treatment of obesity because it can increase heartrate abnormally and have other undesirable effects on heart function.[23] The drugs currently under study in this area include agents such as phentermine, which mimics the effects of moderate levels of exercise, acting similarly to the brain chemical norepinephrine.

Only two over-the-counter (OTC) appetite-suppressant ingredients are currently approved for sale by FDA without prescription. The first—**phenylpropanolamine (PPA) hydrochloride**—is found in some cold remedies and in weight-loss products such as Dexatrim, AcuTrim, and Appedrine. PPA is a chemical relative of the amphetamines, and researchers report an extra half pound of weight loss for users of this drug compared to a placebo.[24] Misuse of the drug (for example, taking larger than recommended doses) can produce dizziness, high blood pressure, heart palpitations, and sleeplessness. The second approved OTC ingredient is the anesthetic—**benzocaine**—usually found in gum or candy form. Benzocaine acts by numbing the taste buds and other sensory signals, thereby reducing the desire for food. The safety and effectiveness of both of these drugs as well as a host of new weight–loss drugs is a matter of ongoing research and review by the Food and Drug Administration (FDA).

Fiber pills increase bulk in the stomach and could ideally lead to satiety, but they can also cause intestinal gas and blockage. Moreover, the fiber typically found in diet pills does not seem to be effective at producing satiety.[25]

Diuretics, or water pills, do nothing to solve an overweight problem, although they may bring about the loss of a few pounds on the scale for half a day and cause dehydration. Numerous other diet aids on the market include products with

PHENYLPROPANOLAMINE HYDROCHLORIDE (PPA) a stimulant of the central nervous system available in over–the–counter weight-loss products used to suppress appetite.

BENZOCAINE an anesthetic found in gum or candy form that numbs the taste buds and reduces the desire for food.

mysterious sounding ingredients, such as spirulina, ephedrine, inositol, chromium picolinate, ginseng and numerous other herbs. Manufacturers suggest such products can aid in weight loss, but their ingredients often serve as little more than fillers. To date, none have proven effective in aiding weight loss. For example, manufacturers of products that include chromium picolinate praise its drug–like abilities to reduce fat, build lean tissue, suppress appetite, and increase metabolism and imply that our diets lack chromium. However, chromium picolinate has not been approved for weight loss by the FDA, and its claims are not backed by scientific data.[26]

Surgery and Weight Loss

Sheer desperation prompts some obese people to request surgery. One operation—intestinal bypass surgery—involves removing or disconnecting a portion of the small intestine to reduce absorption. After bypass surgery, the person can continue overeating but will absorb fewer calories. Dangerous side effects from this procedure are many, including liver failure, massive and frequent diarrhea, urinary stones, intestinal infections, and malnutrition. Such surgery is seldom performed anymore because results have been so disappointing.

Another more common operation—**gastroplasty**—involves stapling the stomach to make it smaller, thus forcing the person to eat less (see Figure 8–3). Nausea and vomiting occur if the person continues to overeat following the procedure. Still, although the theory is pleasingly simple, stapling involves hazards in practice: stomach tissue is damaged, scars are formed, staples pull loose.[27] The person contemplating such surgery should think long and hard before submitting to it.

Another approach involves cosmetic surgery. One such procedure is **liposuction,** in which the surgeon uses a small hollow tube to suction out fatty tissue from beneath the skin (see Figure 8–3). People who wish to remove the fat from a particular area can elect this procedure, which sometimes brings pleasing results but sometimes produces a figure in which one part of the body is disproportionately thin relative to the others.

Surgery is appropriate in some instances. Cosmetic surgery can minimize disfigurements, improve self-confidence, and ease the way toward concentration on life issues more important than external appearances. But after surgery, the same person resides within the skin as before. A changed appearance does not guarantee changed eating habits, a better personality, reduced interpersonal conflicts, or any other improvements in the quality of one's life.

GASTROPLASTY surgery on the stomach (also called stomach stapling) that reduces its volume to less than two ounces (the size of a shot glass) to prevent overeating.

LIPOSUCTION a type of surgery (also called lipectomy) that vacuums out fat cells that have accumulated, typically in the buttocks and thighs. If the person continues to eat more calories than are expended through physical activity, fat will return to the fat cells that remain in those regions.

🍎 Weight-Loss Strategies

Given that so many approaches are likely to fail, what weight-loss strategies work? How can a person lose weight safely and permanently? The secret is a sensible (we didn't say *easy*) three-pronged approach involving healthful eating habits, exercise, and behavior change.[28] Such an approach takes tremendous dedication, especially at first, for a person whose habits have all promoted obesity to learn and make habits of the hundred or so new behaviors necessary to promote a healthful weight. Even the most effective weight-loss

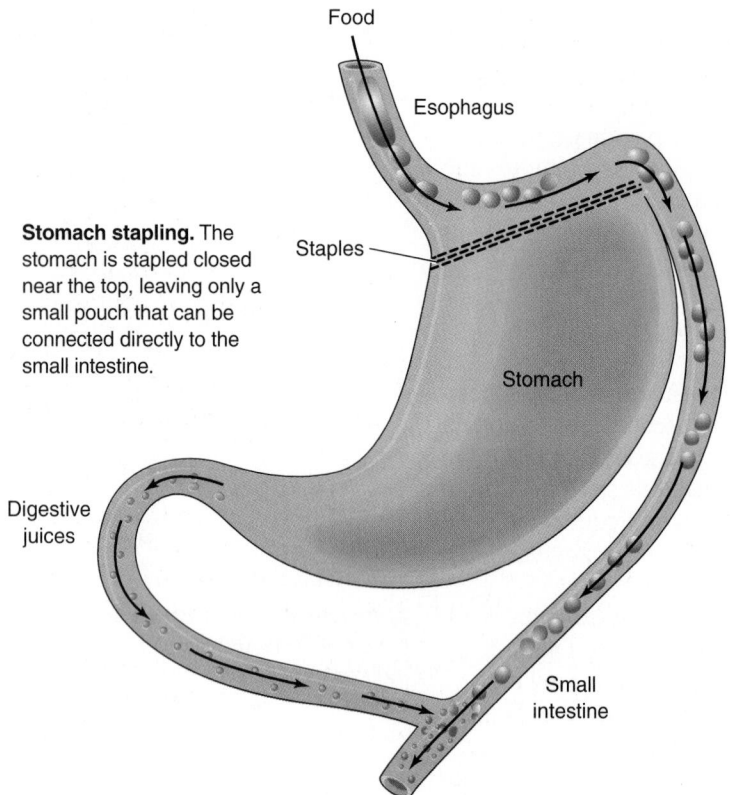

Stomach stapling. The stomach is stapled closed near the top, leaving only a small pouch that can be connected directly to the small intestine.

Food

Esophagus

Staples

Stomach

Digestive juices

Small intestine

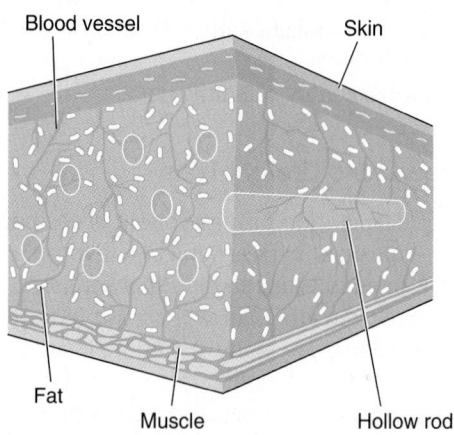

Blood vessel

Skin

Fat

Muscle

Hollow rod

Liposuction. In this fat-suctioning procedure, a thin, hollow rod is inserted into an incision. A powerful vacuum hose is attached to the other end of the rod and suctions out fat cells. The diagram shows a cross-section of tissue revealing the horizontal tunnels made by suctioning the fat out.

FIGURE 8–3
SURGICAL PROCEDURES FOR OBESITY: GASTROPLASTY AND LIPOSUCTION

programs reveal a grim pattern: Those who complete weight-loss programs lose about 10 percent of their body weight, only to regain two-thirds of it back within one year and almost all of it back within five years.[29] But when people succeed, they typically do so because they have employed many of the techniques described in this chapter.

The way a particular person loses weight is a highly individual matter. Two weight-loss plans may both be successful and yet have little or nothing in common. To emphasize the personal nature of weight-loss plans, the following sections are written in terms of advice to "you." This is intended not to put you under pressure to take it personally but to give you the illusion of listening in on a conversation in which a person with, say, anywhere from 10 to 200 pounds to lose is being competently counseled by someone familiar with the techniques known to be effective. Notes in the margin highlight the principles involved.

Meal Planning

No particular diet is magical, and no particular food must be either included or avoided. Since you are the one who will have to live with the eating plan, you had better be involved in its planning. Don't think of it as a diet you are going

Eating Plan Strategies

1. Get involved personally.
2. Adopt a realistic plan, and then keep track of calories—especially those from fat.
3. Make the eating plan adequate.
4. Emphasize high nutrient density.
5. Individualize. Eat foods you like.
6. Stress dos, not don'ts.
7. Eat regular meals, at least three a day—no skipping.
8. Take a positive view of yourself.
9. Visualize a changed future self.
10. Take well-spaced weighings to avoid discouragement.

"on"—because then you may be tempted to go "off" it. Lifestyle changes can be called successful only if the pounds do not return. Think of it as an eating plan that you will adopt for life. The diet must consist of foods that you like or can learn to like, that are available to you, and that are within your means.

For the person wanting to lose weight, a deficit of 500 calories a day for seven days (3,500 calories a week) is enough to lose a pound of body fat a week. If you were to spend an extra 500 calories a day in some form of exercise, you could double this energy deficit.

Choose a calorie level you can live with. The 10-calorie rule will enable you to lose a pound or two a week while supporting your basal metabolism: Allow 10 calories a day for each pound of your present body weight. As you lose weight, you can gradually adjust calories downward to keep losing at this rate. Thus, a person who starts at 220 pounds should eat 2,200 calories a day at first; one who starts at 150 should eat 1,500 calories.

Put nutritional adequacy high on your list of priorities. This is a way of putting yourself first. "I like me, and I'm going to take good care of me" is the attitude to adopt. This means including foods that are rich in valuable nutrients—vegetables and fruits; whole-grain breads and cereals; and a reasonable amount of protein-rich foods such as lean meats, skinless poultry, fish, eggs, low-fat cheeses, and nonfat milk. Within these categories, learn what foods you like, and eat them often. If you resolve to include a certain number of servings of food from each of these groups each day, you may be so busy making sure you get what you need that you will have little time or appetite left for high-calorie or empty-calorie foods. Researchers have shown that reducing the intake of fat alone can promote significant weight loss, especially when coupled with a high complex-carbohydrate diet.[30]

A small amount of fat should be included in each meal to make it satisfying and keep you from getting hungry again too soon. You don't have to use pure fat—butter, margarine, or oil. Rather, most of the fat should come from protein-rich foods, such as lean meats, eggs, poultry, fish, and low-fat cheeses. Add any pure fat with extra caution. A slip of the butter knife adds more calories than a slip of the sugar spoon. Keep concentrated sweets to a minimum, and let your carbohydrate come from starchy foods. Table 8–9 shows a suitable pattern for a weight-loss eating plan, Table 8–10 offers more tips on cutting back on fat and calories, and the Consumer Tips on page 297 gives suggestions for defensive dining.

If you include alcohol or other empty-calorie items in your eating plan, limit it to no more than 150 calories a day. Budget this amount into your chosen calorie level, and reconcile yourself to a slower rate of weight loss.

Three meals a day is standard for our society, but no law says you shouldn't have four or five meals—only be sure that they are smaller, of course. What is important is to eat regularly and, if at all possible, to eat before you become very hungry.

Keep a record of what you have eaten each day for at least a week or two until your habits are automatic. Resume record keeping whenever you need to.

At first it may seem as if you have to spend all your waking hours thinking about and planning your meals. Such a massive effort is always required when a new skill is being learned. But after about three weeks, it will be much easier. Your new eating pattern will become a habit. Some of the characteristics of successful dieters are listed in the margin.[31]

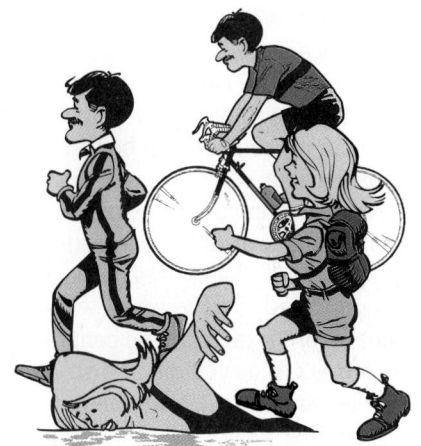

To burn 250 extra calories a day (equal to half a pound of fat loss per week), you could add one of these activities to your daily routine: Walk (briskly) for 45 minutes (5.5 cal/min). Bike (moderate pace) for 36 minutes (7.0 cal/min). Swim (fast) for 23 minutes (11 cal/min). Run (moderate pace) for 18 minutes (14 cal/min).

Profile of Successful Dieters

They know their weight.

They know what they eat (they keep records).

They engage in regular exercise.

They have social support (relationships/groups).

They control their intake of alcohol, fat, and sugar.

They follow an individualized diet plan—one that they can enjoy permanently.

Do not weigh yourself more than once a week, at most. Although 3,500 calories roughly equals a pound of body fat, there is no simple relationship between calorie balance and weight loss over short intervals. Gains or losses of a pound or more in a matter of days reverse themselves quickly; the smoothed-out average is what is real. Don't expect to lose continuously as fast as you did at first. A sizable water loss is common during the first week, but it will not happen again.

Many dieters experience a temporary plateau after about three weeks—not because they are slipping but because they have gained water weight temporarily while they are still losing body fat. The fat they are hoping to lose must be used for energy. To use it, the body must combine it with oxygen (oxidize it) to make carbon dioxide and water. These compounds are heavier than the fat they are made from because oxygen has been added to them.* The carbon dioxide will be exhaled quickly, but the water stays in the body for a longer time. The water takes a while to leave the cells, then makes its way into the spaces between them, and finally enters the bloodstream. Only after the water has arrived in the blood do the kidneys "see" it and send it to the bladder for excretion. Meanwhile, the dieter has a weight gain, but one day the plateau will break. The signal that this is happening is frequent urination.

If you have been working out lately, successive weighings may show an occasional gain when you

TABLE 8–9

A SAMPLE BALANCED WEIGHT-LOSS DIET USING THE FOOD GUIDE PYRAMID

FOOD GROUP	NUMBER OF SERVINGS FOR A 1,200-CAL DIET[a, b]	SERVING SIZE
Bread, Cereal, Rice, and Pasta	6[c]	1 slice bread, ½ c rice, 1 small potato
Vegetable	3	½ c (carrots, broccoli, etc.)
Fruit	2	1 small orange, ¾ c juice
Milk, Yogurt, and Cheese	2[d]	1 c nonfat milk
Meat, Poultry, Fish, Dry Beans, Eggs, and Nuts	2[e]	2 oz meat, poultry, fish

[a]Not recommended for pregnant or lactating women, children (depending on age), or those who have special dietary needs. At or below this low level of calorie intake, it may not be possible to obtain recommended amounts of all nutrients from foods; therefore, it is important to make careful food choices, and the need for dietary supplements should be evaluated.

[b]This plan allows up to 1 teaspoon of added sugar and 5 grams (1 teaspoon) of added fat.

[c]For maximum nutritional value, make whole-grain, high-fiber choices.

[d]Choose nonfat milk products. The discretionary 5 grams of added fat can be used here to select low- or reduced-fat dairy products.

[e]Select lean meat and use cooking methods that do not require added fat.

TABLE 8–10

HEALTHFUL EATING TIPS: CUTTING BACK ON FAT AND CALORIES

- Watch out for second helpings of higher calorie foods.
- Choose low-calorie versions of foods you like.
- Go easy on foods that are high in fat or sugar.
- Limit alcoholic beverages.
- Roast, broil, boil, steam, or poach foods rather than fry them.
- Select lean cuts of meat and trim visible fat.
- Eat poultry and fish without skin.
- Use spices and herbs instead of sauces, butter, or other fats.
- Consume low-fat or nonfat dairy products.
- Try fresh fruit for dessert or baked products made with less fat and sugar (for example, angel food cake).
- Use alternatives to foods as rewards (for example, long walks, relaxing baths, a visit with a friend, a hobby, gardening, a good book).

---

*Water weight accumulates during fat oxidation because one fatty acid weighing 284 units leaves behind water weighing 324 units—14 percent more.

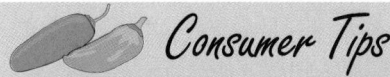

Consumer Tips

Defensive Dining

Dining out can be a pleasant time to relax, socialize, and provide a break from your usual schedule, and it does not have to involve overindulgence in high-calorie, low-nutrient foods. With practice, you can maximize the benefits of eating out by adopting some of the following strategies:

- Make specific requests: "I'd like to have this sandwich with only half the cheese and just a teaspoon of mayonnaise served on the side."

- Ask for salad dressings, sauces, or gravies *on the side*. This puts you in control of the portions.

- Request fresh fruit for dessert. It will give you the sweetness you want without the calories of fat and sugar.

- Order low-fat or nonfat milk instead of whole milk. If a restaurant doesn't have low-fat milk, your requests might make a difference.

- At fast-food windows, ask that they hold the sauce on your sandwich and give you extra tomato and lettuce or other vegetables instead.

- Order mineral water or club soda with a twist, alcoholic drinks with just the mix and not the alcohol (e.g., Bloody Marys without the vodka), or a wine spritzer. Remember, alcohol supplies empty calories.

- When ordering, inquire about preparation. Ask for entrees to be broiled, baked, grilled, poached, boiled, or roasted, with only a minimal amount of fat (or none at all).

- Cut down on overall portion sizes. Order à la carte: one or two nutritious low-fat appetizers like steamed shrimp or raw vegetables and a low-fat dip along with a salad and bread instead of a huge main meal.

- Request a plain baked potato or one with plain nonfat yogurt and chives instead of butter and sour cream. Order your vegetables steamed or stir-fried without added butter or sauces.

- Request a vegetable-based sauce for your pasta rather than the traditional meat sauces.

- Order a special omelet. Instead of the usual three-egg version, ask for one made with egg substitutes, or with one egg plus extra egg whites with no salt, filled with plenty of vegetables.

- Watch out for the all-you-can-eat restaurants and those that specialize in fried foods. Overindulgence is easy at these places.

- Finally, take time to enjoy your meal, along with the company and conversation. Eating slowly gives your body time to digest the food and feel satisfied.

expect a loss. This may reflect a welcome development: the gain of lean body mass—just what you want if you want to be healthy. In fact, weight loss without exercise can have a negative effect on body composition. No doubt you've heard someone say as a joke, "I've lost 200 pounds, but I've never been more than 20 pounds overweight." This person expects to diet, lose weight, regain the weight, and diet again throughout life, without exercising.

This pattern of losing, gaining, and then losing weight again may set the stage for a lifetime of weight fluctuations that may have a lasting impact on the make-up of the body and the way it burns calories. Dubbed the *yo-yo effect*, the up-and-down movement of the needle on the scales may cause the body to accumulate a greater percentage of fat and less lean muscle with each round of dieting.[32]

If you cut back drastically the number of calories you consume without exercising for, say, a month or two, each week you'll probably lose a great deal of weight in the form of not only fat but also lean muscle. The problem is that if you later put the weight back on, the regained pounds may be primarily fat—not muscle. Thus, you may end up weighing the same as you did when you began the diet, but your body will now be composed of more fat and less muscle. Because muscle burns more calories just to sustain itself than fat does, your body will need fewer calories to maintain its weight than it did before. If you go back to eating the way you used to, chances are you will gain even more weight.

In addition to the risk of altering the body's overall composition during repeated bouts of weight loss, consider that each unsuccessful attempt to keep weight off is often viewed by the dieter as a personal failure, which can erode the person's self-esteem and trigger painful feelings of guilt and depression.[33] Despite these possible consequences of repeated bouts of dieting, a recent Task Force on the Prevention and Treatment of Obesity states that "obese individuals should not allow concerns about weight cycling to deter them from efforts to control their body weight," since evidence of the adverse effects of weight cycling in humans is insufficient.[34] As the Nutrition Action feature on page 301 points out, a more healthful alternative to crash dieting is to gradually develop healthful, permanent lifestyle habits that will help you to lose weight and keep it off.

Exercise

The physical contributions exercise makes to a weight-control program are threefold: exercise increases one's calorie expenditure, it alters body composition in a desirable direction, and it alters metabolism. It also offers the psychological benefits of looking and feeling healthy and the increased self-esteem that accompanies these benefits, which can enhance the motivation to maintain a healthful lifestyle for the long run.

Compared with lean tissue, fat tissue is relatively inactive metabolically. Metabolic activity burns calories—lots of them. Thus, the more lean tissue you develop, the faster your metabolism becomes, the more calories you spend, and the more you can afford to eat. This brings you both pleasure and nutrients. Exercise, by shifting body composition toward more lean tissue, speeds up the metabolism *permanently*—that is, for as long as you keep your body conditioned. Furthermore, the more muscle and lean tissue you have, the more fat you will burn—all day long, even when you are resting.

The next chapter offers many pointers about becoming fit, but a few notes on strategy are in order here. For one thing, keep in mind that if exercise is to help with weight loss, it must be active exercise—voluntary moving of muscles. Being moved passively, such as by a machine at a health spa or by a massage, does not increase calorie expenditure. The more muscles you move, the more calories you spend (see Table 8–11).

People sometimes ask about spot reducing. Can you lose fat in particular locations? Unfortunately, muscles don't "own" the fat that surrounds them.

Examples of easy-paced to moderate exercise:

Walking at about 3 miles per hour.

Bicycling on level ground at about 9 miles per hour.

You can tell that the exercise is moderate if you are breathing a little faster than normal but can still easily carry on a conversation.

Strategies for Using Exercise for Weight Control

1. Make it active exercise; move your muscles.

2. Think in terms of quantity, not speed.

3. Exercise informally, in daily routines.

TABLE 8-11 CALORIES SPENT DURING VARIOUS ACTIVITIES

To calculate the exercise calories you expend per hour, find your "exercise" in the left column and your "weight" in the right column. In the place where they intersect is the figure indicating the calories burned **per hour.** For example, if you aerobic dance for 1 hour and weigh 125 pounds, you will expend 285 calories.

WEIGHT (IN POUNDS): EXERCISE	110	125	150	175	200
	CALORIES EXPENDED PER HOUR				
Aerobic Dancing	250	285	340	395	450
Archery	225	255	305	360	410
Baseball	225	255	305	360	410
Basketball	415	470	565	660	750
Bowling	180	205	245	285	325
Calisthenics (vigorous)	225	255	305	360	410
Cross-country skiing					
moderately hilly	595	675	810	945	1080
indoor machine (11 mph)	330	375	450	525	600
Cycling					
outdoor (5.5 mph)	195	220	260	305	350
outdoor (9.4 mph)	300	340	410	475	545
outdoor racing (19 mph)	505	575	690	805	920
Schwinn Aerodyne	510	580	695	810	925
stationary (moderate tension)	330	375	450	525	600
Golf					
with cart (90-120 minutes)	145	165	200	230	265
no cart (90-120 minutes)	185	210	255	295	340
Handball/Squash	635	725	870	1015	1155
Hiking 4 mph, 20-lb pack	355	405	490	570	650
Horseback Riding	225	255	305	360	410
Ice Skating	275	300	350	390	425
Nordic Ski Machine					
heavy (18 mph)	1100	1250	1500	1750	2000
medium (11 mph)	330	375	450	525	600
light (6 mph)	225	255	305	360	410
Racquetball	550	625	750	875	1000
Roller Skating/Blading	275	300	350	390	425
Rope Skipping (100 skips/min)	560	640	765	895	1020
Rowing (sculling or machine)	620	705	845	990	1130
Running (Jogging)					
6 min/mile (10 mph)	755	860	1030	1200	1375
7 min/mile (8.5 mph)	685	780	935	1090	1245
8 min/mile (7.5 mph)	625	710	850	990	1135

WEIGHT (IN POUNDS): EXERCISE	110	125	150	175	200
	CALORIES EXPENDED PER HOUR				
Running (Jogging)					
9 min/mile (6.5 mph)	580	660	790	920	1050
10 min/mile (6 mph)	535	605	730	850	970
11 min/mile (5.5 mph)	470	530	640	745	850
12 min/mile (5 mph)	375	425	510	600	680
Scuba Diving	355	405	490	570	650
Snow Skiing - Downhill	300	340	410	480	545
Softball	225	255	305	360	410
Stair Climbing (moderate)	515	600	750	850	960
Stairmaster (machine)	595	675	810	945	1080
Step Aerobics - 120 steps/min	550	625	750	875	1000
Swimming					
45 min/mile	385	435	525	610	700
60 min/mile	300	335	405	475	540
Table Tennis (moderate)	200	225	270	315	360
Tennis					
doubles	225	255	305	360	410
singles	325	370	445	520	600
Treadmill					
12 min/mile	375	425	510	600	680
13.5 min/mile	330	375	450	525	600
Volleyball					
competitive	435	495	595	700	800
recreational	165	185	225	260	300
Walking/Race Walking					
12 min/mile (5 mph)	435	495	595	700	800
Walk/Jog Combination					
13:30 min/mile (4.5 mph)	330	375	450	525	600
Walking					
15:00 min/mile (4 mph)	300	345	415	480	550
17:00 min/mile (3.5 mph)	250	285	345	400	450
20:00 min/mile (3 mph)	225	255	310	360	410
30:00 min/mile (2 mph)	145	165	200	230	265
Weight Training/Lifting (Light)	270	310	370	430	500

SOURCE: G. Kostas, M.P.H., R.D., *The Balancing Act Nutrition and Weight Guide*, Dallas, TX, 1993.

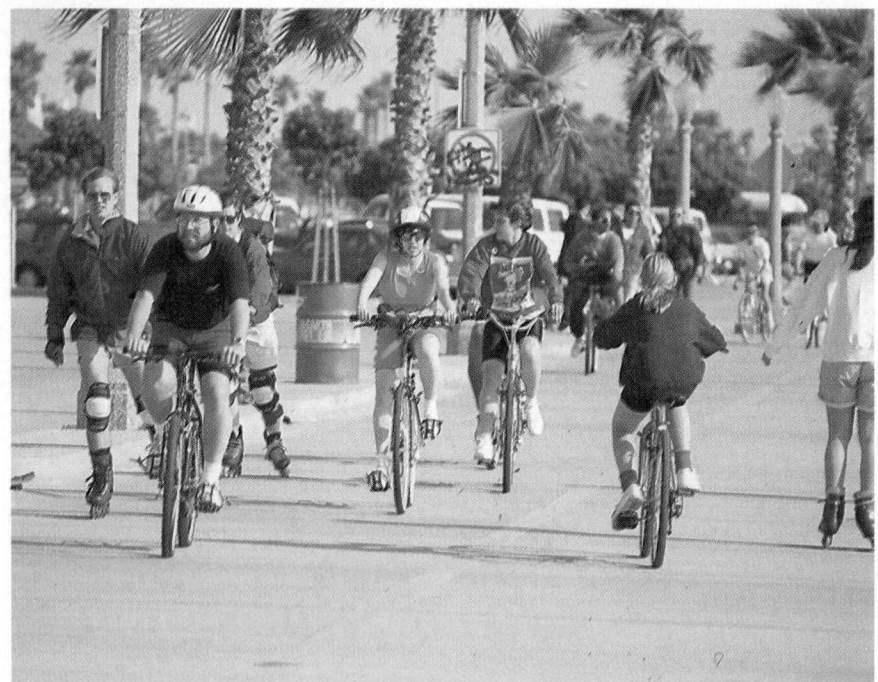

Exercise is essential for weight control.

Since all body fat is shared by all the muscles and organs, spot-reducing exercises that work only the flabby parts won't help reduce the fat located there. There is some good news, though: Tightening muscles in trouble spots by way of a balanced, all-over exercise program may improve the appearance of the fatty areas.

Another thing to keep in mind is that the number of calories spent in an activity depends more upon how much a person weighs than on how fast the person can do the exercise (see Table 8–11). For example, a person who weighs 125 pounds burns off 85 calories by running a 12-minute mile. That same person, walking a mile in 15 minutes, burns almost the same amount—86 calories. Similarly, a 200-pound person spends 136 calories on the 12-minute mile, and a similar amount—138 calories—on the 15-minute walk. The rule seems to be that you don't have to work fast to use up calories effectively. If you choose to walk rather than run the distance, you will use up about the same energy; it will just take you longer.

You may have heard the suggestion to incorporate more exercise into your daily schedule in many simple, small-scale ways. Park the car at the far end of the parking lot; use the stairs instead of the elevator; do a round of sit-ups before you get up in the morning. If you also incorporate both regular aerobic exercise and strength-training into your schedule, your heart and lungs as well as your skeletal muscles will be fit (see Chapter 9).

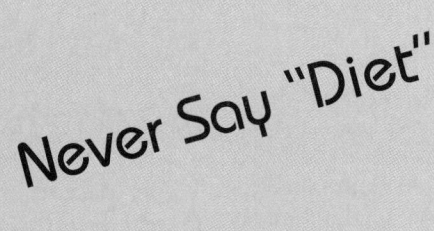

Never Say "Diet"

Say the word *diet,* and most people think "starvation," "deprivation," "hunger," and something to go "on" and "off." But this kind of thinking can be unrealistic and self-defeating. Strict, temporary diets—and the attitudes that go with them—don't work for the great majority of overweight people, as history has borne out. In fact, while Americans spend more than $30 billion a year on programs and products aimed at weight loss, obesity rates are higher than ever.[35]

The problem with going on a rigid diet with a goal of, say, a 15-pound weight loss in three weeks is that it's a quick fix—the dieter attempts to gain a temporary solution to what is typically a chronic problem. Often, the dieter tries to rigidly restrict eating by, for example, skipping meals or eating salads all day. But trying not to eat is like trying not to breathe, as one group of psychologists put it.[36] After a while, the body and mind rebel and, like a person gasping for air, the dieter loses control and binges. In fact, experts believe that rigid diets play a strong role in the development of binge-eating problems.[37] As a result of the binge, the person feels that he has failed, gives up the diet altogether, eats more to make himself feel better, puts on some weight, feels even worse, gains even more weight, decides to try another restrictive diet, and begins the whole cycle all over again.

The solution, say many experts, is not to focus on losing a certain amount of weight within a set period of time. A more healthful alternative is to gradually develop habits that you can live with permanently and that will help you shed pounds and keep them off over the long run. Instead of measuring your success by the needle on the scale, gauge your progress by the strides you make in adopting good eating and exercise habits as well as healthful attitudes about yourself and your body.

While most people recognize the importance of the eating and exercise habits discussed in this chapter in helping to achieve and maintain a healthy weight, few recognize the attitude problems that often go hand in hand with restrictive dieting and can stand in the way of long-term weight loss. One of the most common is "all-or-nothing," or "on-or-off," thinking. People with all-or-nothing attitudes tend to view the world as either black or white, right or wrong, good or bad, and so forth. When it comes to food, the attitude translates into good or bad, on or off limits, diet or junk food.[38] Often, a person who thinks this way sets the stage for failure by trying to live up to extremely rigid, unrealistic goals: "Ice cream is bad, so I must never eat it," "I will jog three miles every day," or "I will never order anything but a salad when I go out to eat."

Typically, a person who has an all-or-nothing attitude might go several days without, say, ice cream, which she views as "bad junk food," and then splurge one day on a double-dip cone. Instead of recognizing that ice cream isn't "bad" and that indulging in some every now and then won't undo all her previous efforts, she tells herself, "I've blown my diet completely—I have no willpower."

Consequently, she feels guilty and depressed, and because she's "blown it" anyway, she decides she might as well eat another pint of ice cream and some cookies to make herself feel better. If she had looked at her situation with a different attitude—"I've been eating lots of fruits and vegetables and bicycling several times a week, so one ice cream cone won't hurt me"—she may have avoided a bout of despair and binging.

Another type of attitude that can thwart efforts to achieve a healthy weight is the "lookist" attitude—that is, the notion that weight and appearance are the determinants of a person's worth and happiness.[39] Just about everyone holds lookist attitudes in one form or another and wishes that he could change something about his appearance in the hopes that it would make life more enjoyable. But in our "thin-is-in" society, overweight people suffer tremendous prejudice and tend to be painfully self-conscious about their bodies. As a result, they may mistakenly believe that all their dreams will come true once they lose weight and their problems will be lost with the pounds. By pinning all their hopes for happiness on losing weight, they put themselves under enormous pressure to shed pounds. In addition, people who hold this type of attitude often put off living in the present because they are so caught up in fantasizing about what they think life will be like once they lose weight.

Using weight and appearance as a measure of self-worth and happiness can be extremely destructive, however. Consider that the person who does so may desperately try to lose weight with restrictive, unrealistic diets or unhealthfully strenuous exercise regimens. Each "slip-up" whittles away at the person's self-esteem, which in turn may lead to feelings of rejection, depression, and social isolation, which in turn may prompt a binge, and so forth. And even a person who drops a desired number of pounds may then realize that she still has many of the same problems as before, which can lead to depression and loss of self-esteem.

The way around lookist thinking is to try to focus on health, both mental and physical, rather than appearance. Table 8–12 lists some common characteristics of the obese self (which holds lookist attitudes) and the healthy self. While it can be difficult to overcome society's prejudices about weight, striving to adopt the ideals of the healthy self, regardless of your weight, can be a major step in helping you take care of your mental and physical health.

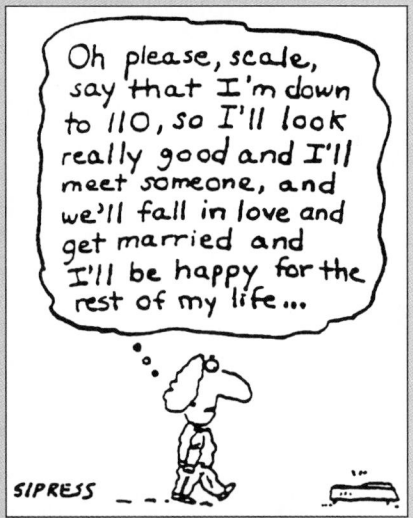

Brownell K. D. *The LEARN Program for Weight Control*, 1994. Reproduced with permission. All rights reserved. Dallas: American Health Publishing Company.

TABLE 8–12   THE OBESE SELF VERSUS THE HEALTHY SELF

THE OBESE SELF	THE HEALTHY SELF
Uses appearance as measure of self-worth	Uses caring for others/self as measure of self-worth
Is socially isolated	Is socially involved
Rejects self	Accepts self
Goes on and off extreme diets	Eats healthfully
Rarely exercises (or overdoes it and quits)	Exercises regularly and sensibly
Focuses on mistakes; feels like a failure	Views mistakes as learning experiences and recognizes that nobody is perfect
Uses obesity as excuse for failures in life	Doesn't allow obesity to interfere with life
Focuses on past	Focuses on present
Allows negative emotions to reduce self-control	Uses positive attitude to enhance self-control
Focuses on appearance	Focuses on health
Wants to improve appearance to get love/affection	Wants to be healthy to participate fully in loving relationships

SOURCE: Adapted from J. P. Foreyt and G. K. Goodrick, *Living Without Dieting* (New York: Warner Books, 1992), p. 55.

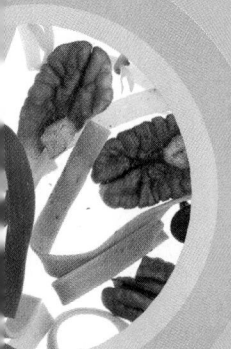

Breaking Old Habits

"Just do it," urge the makers of Nike sportswear on billboards, in magazines, and wherever else they promote their products, implying that adhering to a fitness program is just a matter of donning sneakers and heading for the track or gym. But as most of us know from experience, sticking to a regular exercise program for the first time or changing eating habits isn't always easy. The majority of people who successfully quit smoking make three or four attempts before they finally kick the habit. And most people make the same New Year's resolution at least five years in a row before they stick to it permanently.[40] That's because breaking old patterns of behavior and developing new ones involves going through a number of stages before reaching the point at which you're able to change for good.

First, you must be aware that you could change. "I could lose some weight and try to become more physically fit," you might tell yourself. Then you must be inspired to *want* to change, which in turn will help to motivate you to find out how to do so, say, by talking to a registered dietitian about strategies for cutting back on fat and calories in your diet and by reading about various forms of exercise. After you've gone through those steps, you will be ready to take action—that is, to "just do it." Once you've taken these initial steps, you need to maintain your behavior change by creating a game plan that will help you handle the inevitable slips and lapses that will occur over time. After you've done so and have stuck with your plan for a good deal of time, you're home free.

Of course, as you go through those steps, making lasting changes in behavior poses ongoing challenges. That's where a process known as **behavior modification** can help. Developed by psychologists to help people change their habits, behavior modification uses techniques similar to mapping out a game plan.

To start, identify your goals. You might decide, for example, that you want to lower the fat and calorie content of your diet. Once you've chosen your goals, record your present pattern of behavior along with the reasons behind it. Keep a food diary by writing down everything you eat for five days as well as how you feel at the time you eat (see Table 8–13 for a sample food diary). This technique can help you understand why you behave the way you do in certain situations. You might find, for instance, that every time you are angry at your significant other or get a bad grade you eat a candy bar or two to comfort yourself. Or perhaps without even thinking about it, you nibble on whatever happens to be handy while watching television.

Once you've identified your goals and current patterns of behavior, determine some new strategies that will help you meet these goals and set yourself

Elements of behavior change:[41]

1. *Precontemplation:* You need to change, but you're not yet ready to accept that fact.

2. *Contemplation:* You want to change, but you're not sure how.

3. *Preparation:* You gain knowledge to set up a plan of action for change.

4. *Action:* You jump in and "just do it."

5. *Maintenance:* You work on sticking to your plan of action.

6. *Termination:* You have achieved lasting change and experience few, if any, temptations or relapses.

BEHAVIOR MODIFICATION a process developed by psychologists for helping people make lasting behavior changes.

TABLE 8–13
SAMPLE ENTRIES IN FOOD DIARY

FOOD EATEN	TIME AND PLACE	WITH WHOM	MOOD	OTHER ACTIVITY
1 large blueberry muffin 1 cup coffee with 1 oz cream and 1 tsp sugar	7:30 a.m., donut shop	alone	stressed—late for class	skimming notes for upcoming class
1 hot dog with 2 tbsp ketchup 1 small bag potato chips 12-oz can diet soda	12:45 p.m., cafeteria	2 friends	relaxed	talking with friends
1 candy bar	2:35 p.m., bedroom	alone	angry about argument with significant other	watching TV

some rewards for sticking to them. If you talk to a friend instead of heading to the kitchen cupboard or vending machine when you're angry, for instance, you'll save hundreds of calories and probably experience the relief of getting your feelings off your chest. After you've pinpointed behaviors you want to alter, commit yourself to make the changes and try to envision the healthier person you'll become as a result.

The next step is to divide the behavioral goals into small portions that can be achieved one at a time. While you may have come up with 20 behaviors that you want to change to meet your overall goals, trying to accomplish all 20 in a week or two is asking a great deal of yourself and may be setting the stage for disappointment and failure. Instead, pick one or two, see whether you can stick to them for, say, two weeks, and then reward yourself for doing so before going on to try more.

As you meet your goals, remind yourself of the progress you're making as well as the benefits you're gaining—weight loss, increased energy, better health. Give yourself a tangible reward, such as a night out at the movies or a new item of clothing. This step is key because behavior research indicates that once you have instituted a change in your life, you will maintain it only by positive reinforcement. Along with rewarding yourself, feel free to modify your goals if you think that those you initially set were too difficult or too simple to achieve, and evaluate your progress on a regular basis.

While you're working on modifying your behavior, it is critical to keep in mind that you're only human and there will be days when you slip and revert back to an old pattern of behavior. Instead of dwelling on it or berating yourself, realize that relapses are par for the course, forgive yourself, and simply move on. Keep in mind that even though you may feel a setback, you're still moving forward if you learn from your mistakes and get right back on track again. That's why some experts prefer the term *recycle* to *relapse;* people who

Behavior modification steps:

1. Identify the goal.

2. Record your present behavior pattern. Identify the reasons you practice these behaviors.

3. Identify the behaviors that will lead to the goal and the rewards of those behaviors.

4. Commit yourself to changing. Face what you'll have to give up or change to make the desired behavior a reality. Envision your changed future self.

5. Plan. Divide the behavior into manageable portions. Set small, achievable goals and plan periodic rewards.

6. Try out the plan. Modify the plan, if necessary, in ways that will help you succeed.

7. Evaluate your progress on a regular basis.

cathy®   **by Cathy Guisewite**

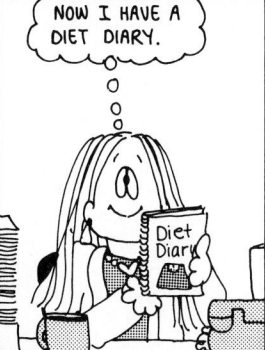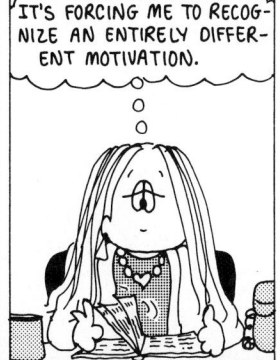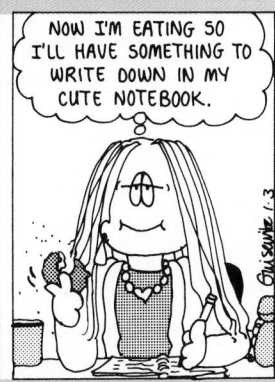

make a mistake and then learn from it can reuse, or recycle, their new knowledge.

In addition, set priorities to ensure that you adopt one or two behaviors that you make it a point to stick to all the time. Furthermore, be aware of how other areas of your life are affecting your readiness to make changes and meet your goals. Many people waste a great deal of time and energy trying to change when the timing isn't right for them. Someone who is going through the breakup of a long-term relationship or having difficulties at work or school, for example, may be under too much stress to deal with making a change in behavior on top of everything else. Realizing that you have limits and waiting until the timing is right can stave off additional frustration and guilt brought about by feeling like a failure if you aren't able to change.

Another point to keep in mind is that you might need to try new behaviors more than once before you begin to like them. Dietitians sometimes use a "rule of three" in counseling. Try nonfat milk once, and you may not like it. Try it a second time, and you may be able to tolerate drinking it, even though it doesn't taste as good as whole milk. Try it a third time, and you may conclude that while it's not as good as whole milk, you don't really mind drinking it. Then you'll be able to maintain your new habit more easily.

Strategies for Changing the Way You Eat

This section covers the steps designed specifically to help with weight control (Chapter 9 includes strategies for modifying exercise behavior.) To begin with, keep a record of your present eating behavior that you can compare with your future progress and use to determine situations that trigger your reaching for food. In this way, you can see how far you've come in changing your eating habits.

Next, try to identify cues that prompt you to eat when you're not hungry, such as watching television, talking on the telephone, and walking by a convenience store or vending machine. Then resolve to stop responding to those cues, and try to eat only in one place in a certain room, such as at the table in

Continued motivation:

- Persist long enough to experience the rewards, such as improved self-image and enhanced self-esteem.
- Remember the price of the old behavior.
- Keep in mind where you started.
- Tune in to the benefits of the new behavior.

the dining room. In addition, try the following tips to eliminate the temptation to eat when you really don't want to:

- Don't buy hard-to-resist foods such as cakes, cookies, and ice cream.
- Don't shop when you're hungry and thereby more likely to buy tempting foods.
- Create obstacles to eating tempting foods. Make it necessary to unwrap, cook, and serve each one separately, for example, or store the food in a hard-to-reach cupboard or in the back of the refrigerator.
- Don't leave large amounts of food within easy reach. Keep serving dishes off the table, for instance, and put the cookie jar out of sight.
- Make small portions of food look large by spreading food out and putting it on smaller plates. Garnish empty space with low-calorie vegetables.
- Try to eat regular meals and snacks instead of skipping them, thereby reducing the likelihood of becoming uncomfortably hungry and then overeating later.
- Ask your family and friends to encourage you to eat a healthful diet and not to criticize you if you splurge occasionally.

Third, make it easy for yourself to eat the way you want to eat.

- Keep a variety of nutritious foods such as fruits and vegetables readily available.
- If you like to eat between meals, plan snacks that fit easily into your diet, such as low-fat yogurt and fruit.
- Prepare attractive meals for yourself.

Fourth, take a look at and then, if necessary, alter the manner in which you eat. If you eat quickly, slow down by chewing food thoroughly, pausing between bites, putting down your utensils and swallowing before reloading your fork or spoon. Eating slowly will give your body a chance to feel full and satisfied.

Finally, reward yourself for positive behaviors.

- Plan to buy something new to wear or do something you enjoy, such as attending a favorite sporting event or a concert, each time you meet your goals.
- Ask your friends and family to support and encourage you as you change.

Weight-Gain Strategies

It is as hard for a person who tends to be thin to gain a pound as it is for a person who tends to be fat to lose one. The person who wants to gain weight is faced with some of the same challenges as the one who wants to lose weight—learning new habits, learning to like new foods, and establishing discipline related to meals and mealtimes. But there are major differences.

Knowing that vigorous physical activity costs calories, an active person may wonder whether it is advisable to curtail activity. The answer is no, not unless the underweight condition is so extreme as to be life-threatening. The healthful way to gain weight is to build yourself up by patient and consistent training and at the same time to eat enough calories (of nutritious foods) to support the weight gain. If you add a big snack of high-calorie, nutritious foods (for example, a bowl of chili and rice and a milkshake) between meals, you can eat 700 to 800 extra calories a day, and achieve a healthful weight gain of 1 to 1 1/2 pounds per week.

A person wanting to gain weight often has to learn to eat different foods. No matter how many helpings of carrots you consume, you won't gain weight very fast because carrots simply don't offer enough calories. The person who can't eat much volume is encouraged to use calorie-dense foods at meals (the very ones the dieter is trying to stay away from). Choose a milkshake instead of milk, peanut butter instead of lean meat, avocado instead of cucumber, blueberry bran muffin instead of whole-wheat bread. When you do eat carrots, put margarine on them; use creamy dressings on salads, yogurt on fruit, sour cream on potatoes, and the like. (Because fat contains twice as many calories per teaspoon as sugar, it adds calories without adding bulk.) These dietary recommendations may not apply to everyone trying to gain weight. If you have a history of heart disease, a diet low in saturated fat is recommended (consult a registered dietitian).

Eat more frequently. Make three sandwiches in the morning, and eat them between classes in addition to the day's three regular meals. Spend more time eating each meal: If you fill up fast, eat the highest-calorie items first. Don't start with soup or salad; start with the main course. Always finish with dessert. Many an underweight person has simply been too busy (for months) to eat enough to gain or maintain weight. These strategies will help you change this behavior pattern.

Whether you need to gain, lose, or maintain weight, attention to what you eat can pay off in long-term wellness benefits. This chapter has emphasized the relationship of food and eating to body weight and has come to the same conclusion reached earlier in the book: To support wellness, you should eat regular, balanced meals composed of a wide variety of foods you enjoy.

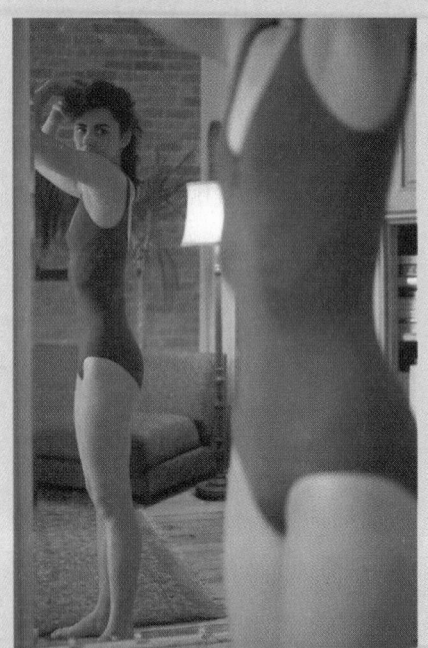

The Eating Disorders

For an estimated 8 million American teens and adults, the relentless pursuit of thinness and fear of being fat are a haunting nightmare that drives them to starve, vomit, or purge.[42] The illness of **anorexia nervosa**—self-starvation—has been recognized as a psychiatric syndrome since the 1870s. Its companion disease **bulimia nervosa**—gorging on food and then purging—was not recognized as a separate eating disorder until the 1960s and 1970s. Some researchers suspect that a complex interplay between environmental, social, and perhaps genetic factors triggers the disorder in victims, mostly women. Others

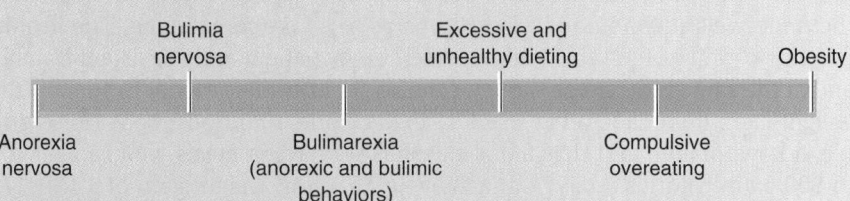

Bulimia nervosa | Excessive and unhealthy dieting | Obesity

Anorexia nervosa | Bulimarexia (anorexic and bulimic behaviors) | Compulsive overeating

FIGURE 8–4
THE CONTINUUM OF EATING DISORDERS

The spectrum of eating disorders includes anorexia nervosa, bulimia nervosa, anorexic and bulimic behaviors, excessive and unhealthy dieting, compulsive or uncontrolled binge eating, and obesity.

SOURCE: Adapted from D. Neumark-Sztainer, Excessive weight preoccupation: Normative but not harmless, *Nutrition Today* 30 (1995): 68.

question whether or not the fear of fatness isn't a mask for underlying emotional problems. Experts speculate that focusing on the body diverts these people's attention away from and suppresses the painful emotion of anger, feelings of low self-esteem, the inability to express their feelings, or poor family relationships. The acute focus on the body develops into an intense fear of fatness, a characteristic intrinsically linked with food.[43] As a result, food is seen only as a source of body fat and so becomes carefully controlled. But why food? Why not use some other method of coping with stress?

Enter the societal link. In a society where thinness is equated with material success and even self-worth, especially for women, becoming thin appears to be the yellow brick road that leads to happiness. Unfortunately, as victims of eating disorders come to learn, practicing self-starvation or gorging and purging leads instead to physical and emotional pain.

What conditions are referred to by the term *eating disorder*? The term **eating disorder** comprises a wide spectrum of conditions from **anorexia nervosa** and **bulimia nervosa** to **compulsive overeating** to **binge-eating disorder** to obesity and excessive dieting (see Figure 8–4).[44] Although the various conditions differ in their origin and consequences, they appear to have similarities among them—all of the conditions exhibit an excessive preoccupation with body weight, a fear of body fatness, and a distorted body image. Many times the person with an eating disorder falls short of the diagnostic criteria shown in Table 8–14 for anorexia nervosa or bulimia nervosa. Some of these people are described as having an **unspecified eating disorder** and can include people who:[45]

Anorexia nervosa.

- Meet all the criteria for anorexia nervosa except irregular menses.

- Meet all the criteria for anorexia nervosa except that their weight remains within a normal range.

- Meet all the criteria for bulimia nervosa except that their binges are less frequent.

- Have recurrent episodes of binge eating but do not compensate using the methods of those with bulimia nervosa.

What are the symptoms of anorexia nervosa? Anorexics deprive themselves of food except for controlled amounts of very-low-calorie foods such as unbuttered toast or popcorn, apples, and green beans. And even these foods are painstakingly limited. After three to four days of eating very small amounts of food, hunger pangs subside. Once their appetite is suppressed, anorexics report feeling quite energetic, as if on a high, making the strict fast easier to stick to. But the body needs fuel to run. To compensate for the lack of fuel from food, the

---

TABLE 8–14
DIAGNOSIS OF EATING DISORDERS

ANOREXIA NERVOSA	BULIMIA NERVOSA
A person with anorexia nervosa demonstrates the following: 1. Refusal to maintain body weight at or above a minimal normal weight for age and height, e.g., weight loss leading to maintenance of body weight less than 85% of that expected, or failure to make expected weight gain during period of growth, leading to body weight less than 85% of that expected. 2. Intense fear of gaining weight or becoming fat, even though underweight. 3. Disturbance in the way in which one's body weight or shape is experienced, undue influence of body weight or shape on self-evaluation, or denial of the seriousness of the current low body weight. 4. In females past puberty, amenorrhea, i.e., the absence of at least three consecutive menstrual cycles. (A woman is considered to have amenorrhea if her periods occur only following administration of hormones, such as estrogen.) Two types: *Restricting type:* During the episode of anorexia nervosa, the person does not regularly engage in binge eating or purging behavior (i.e., self-induced vomiting or the misuse of laxatives or diuretics). *Binge eating/purging type:* During the episode of anorexia nervosa, the person regularly engages in binge eating or purging behavior (i.e., self-induced vomiting or the misuse of laxatives or diuretics).	A person with bulimia nervosa demonstrates the following: 1. Recurrent episodes of binge eating. An episode of binge eating is characterized by both of the following: a. eating in a discrete period of time an amount of food that is definitely larger than most people would eat during a similar period of time and under similar circumstances. b. a sense of lack of control over eating during the episode (e.g., a feeling that one cannot stop eating or control what or how much one is eating). 2. Recurrent inappropriate compensatory behavior to prevent weight gain, such as self-induced vomiting; misuse of laxatives, diuretics, or other medications; fasting; or excessive exercise. 3. Binge eating and inappropriate compensatory behaviors that both occur, on an average, at least twice a week for three months. 4. Self-evaluation unduly influenced by body shape and weight. 5. The disturbance does not occur exclusively during episodes of anorexia nervosa. Two types: *Purging type:* the person regularly engages in self-induced vomiting or the misuse of laxatives or diuretics. *Nonpurging type:* the person uses other inappropriate compensatory behaviors, such as fasting or excessive exercise, but does not regularly engage in self-induced vomiting or the misuse of laxatives or diuretics.

SOURCE: Adapted from American Psychiatric Association, *Diagnostic and Statistical Manual of Mental Disorders* (DSM-IV) (Washington, D.C.: American Psychological Association, 1994), used with permission.

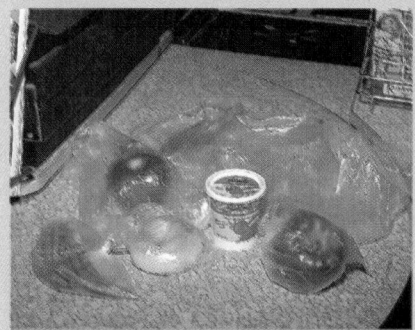

For many people with anorexia nervosa, a full day's diet may consist of no more than three or four items.

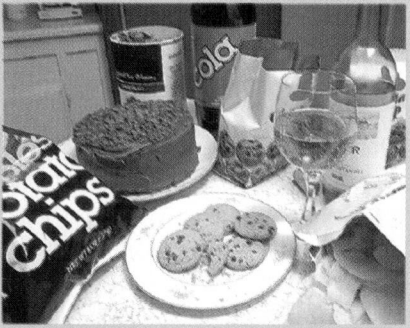

For many people with bulimia, guilt, depression, and self-condemnation follow a binge-eating episode.

body turns inward for its fuel and begins to slowly destroy muscle and fat tissue for energy. The following are some of the physical symptoms associated with starvation seen in anorexics:

- Wasting of the whole body, including muscle tissue and bones.
- Arresting of sexual development and stopping of menstruation due to loss of body fat.
- Drying and yellowing of the skin from an accumulation of a stored vitamin A compound released from body fat.
- Intolerance to cold weather due to loss of subcutaneous fat.
- Growth of hair on the body, perhaps in response to a decrease in body temperature.
- Loss of health and texture of hair.
- Pain on touch.
- Lowered blood pressure and metabolic rate.
- Anemia.
- Severe sleep disturbance.[46]

Simultaneously, bizarre mental symptoms develop. Looking in the mirror, the anorexic does not see the emaciated body others see but continues to see someone who is too fat. A preoccupation with death develops, accompanied by a frantic pursuit of physical fitness by means of stringent exercise routines. The person deals with parents and family in a manipulative way so as to become the center of attention. Diet becomes so all-engrossing that the person may be quite isolated socially except from friends who stick close by and worry without knowing how to help.

By this time, the anorexic has reached absolute minimum body weight—for example, 65 to 70 pounds for a woman of average height. The person is on the verge of incurring permanent brain damage and chronic debilitation or death. The National Association of Anorexia Nervosa and Associated Disorders (ANAD) estimates that of those with severe eating disorders, 6 percent die, usually because major organs—heart and kidneys—fail.

What are the symptoms of bulimia? Unlike anorexics, bulimics don't shrink to skeleton-like proportions. They usually are of healthy body weight or even slightly overweight. Bulimics also follow rigid rules of dietary restraint, but their routine is not as rigorous as the anorexic's starvation routine, and occasionally, they break their rigid rules.

Quickly, and usually privately, bulimics gorge on foods that are often sweet, starchy, and high in fat or calories and require little chewing. The binge ends when it would hurt to eat any more, when they are interrupted, or when they go to sleep or induce vomiting to expel the food just eaten.

Bulimics often feel controlled by the vicious circle that develops: anxiety about being "fat" leads to rigid dietary restraint. Mounting hunger from not eating and an increased preoccupation with food lead to a break in the rules—binging. After gorging, an intense fear of fatness overtakes the person, who then vomits to get rid of the food and release the fear of becoming "fatter." Feelings of guilt and shame follow the purge, building a new level of anxiety over the body, and the cycle begins again. Each binge reinforces the idea that additional rigidity of dietary restraint is required to prevent weight gain. Excessive use of laxatives or diuretics or bouts of vigorous exercise replace vomiting in some cases.

Binge eating is seldom life-threatening, but at the extreme, it can be physically damaging, causing lacerations of the stomach, tearing or irritation of the esophagus (in those who vomit frequently), dental caries (from acidic vomit attacking the teeth), electrolyte imbalances and malnutrition (in vomiters and laxative takers).

Bulimics also suffer from distorted body image. They see themselves as fat and needing to restrict food, even though they usually have a healthy body weight. Bulimics prefer a body size somewhat smaller than normal.

How are anorexia nervosa and bulimia treated? There are several philosophies regarding the treatment of eating disorders. The four major approaches include individual psychotherapy, hospitalization, family therapy, and behavior modification therapy. Some therapists use more than one approach. Most treatment methods focus on identifying the societal and environmental pressures that triggered the eating disorder and on exposing the emotions masked by it. An interdisciplinary team made up of a psychologist, a social worker, a family therapy counselor, and a dietitian work with the family and the patient to reestablish emotional and nutritional health.[47] Length of treatment varies from two months to two to three years, depending on the patient's readiness for change and the type of treatment. American researcher Hilde Bruche, M.D., focuses on the problems of low self-esteem, guilt, anxiety, depression, and a sense of helplessness. In addition, family therapy focuses on changing patterns of family interaction.

Normal nutrition must be restored in the anorexic. After some progress is made in counseling, the dietitian can help the patient gain a new understanding of a healthful eating pattern, and clear up some earlier misconceptions about food and nutrition.[48]

Are there any early warning signs to watch for regarding eating disorders? Families and friends can be alerted to several key symptoms of eating disorders (see Table 8–14). A diet often precedes the illness. Anorexics develop an exaggerated interest in food but at the same time deny their hunger and stop eating. A distorted body image makes them feel fat even as weight loss continues. The anorexic begins to have sleep problems, shows unusual devotion to schoolwork, and often undertakes a program of unrelenting exercise. Bulimics may binge and self-induce vomiting or use excessive amounts of laxatives. Reduced food intake usually causes sufficient weight loss to stop menstrual cycles in women. People with eating disorders were usually good children who did not indulge in rebellion. Not all anorexics and bulimics exhibit all symptoms. Early detection is vital. Use the Eating Attitudes Scorecard that follows to see if your own eating attitudes and behaviors are within a normal range.

For more information regarding anorexia and bulimia and a list of qualified professionals to treat these diseases, write to the National Association of Anorexia Nervosa and Associated Disorders, Box 7, Highland Park, IL 60035, or call 708-831-3438. Other resources are listed in Appendix A.

MINIGLOSSARY

ANOREXIA NERVOSA literally "nervous lack of appetite," a disorder (usually seen in teenage girls) involving self-starvation to the extreme.

  an = without   *orexis* = appetite

COMPULSIVE OVEREATING an eating disorder characterized by uncontrolled chronic episodes of overeating (binge eating) without other symptoms of eating disorders. If the episodes of binge eating occur at least twice a week on average for a period of six months or more, the behavior is referred to as **binge-eating disorder**.

BULIMIA NERVOSA, BULIMAREXIA (byoo-LEE-me-uh, byoo-lee-ma-REX-ee-uh) binge eating (literally, "eating like an ox"), known popularly as pigging out. Combined with an intense fear of becoming fat and sometimes followed by self-induced vomiting or the taking of laxatives, this form of eating behavior has also been called the **binge-purge syndrome.**

  buli = ox

EATING DISORDER general term for several conditions (anorexia nervosa, bulimia nervosa, bulimarexia, compulsive overeating, obesity, and excessive dieting) that exhibit an excessive preoccupation with body weight, a fear of body fatness, and a distorted body image.

UNSPECIFIED EATING DISORDERS some people suffer from unspecified eating disorders; that is, they exhibit some but not all of the criteria for specific eating disorders.

EATING ATTITUDES SCORECARD

 Answer the following questions to evaluate your own eating attitudes and behaviors. Do they fall within a normal range?

Answer the following questions using these responses:

A = always   S = sometimes
U = usually   R = rarely
O = often   N = never

_____ 1. I am terrified about being overweight.

_____ 2. I avoid eating when I am hungry.

_____ 3. I find myself preoccupied with food.

_____ 4. I have gone on eating binges where I feel that I may not be able to stop.

_____ 5. I cut my food into very small pieces.

_____ 6. I am aware of the calorie content of the foods I eat.

_____ 7. I particularly avoid foods with a high carbohydrate content.

_____ 8. I feel that others would prefer that I ate more.

_____ 9. I vomit after I have eaten.

_____ 10. I feel extremely guilty after eating.

_____ 11. I am preoccupied with a desire to be thinner.

_____ 12. I think about burning up calories when I exercise.

_____ 13. Other people think I am too thin.

_____ 14. I am preoccupied with the thought of having fat on my body.

_____ 15. I take longer than other people to eat my meals.

_____ 16. I avoid foods with sugar in them.

_____ 17. I eat diet foods.

_____ 18. I feel that food controls my life.

_____ 19. I display self-control around food.

_____ 20. I feel that others pressure me to eat.

_____ 21. I give too much time and thought to food.

_____ 22. I feel uncomfortable after eating sweets.

_____ 23. I engage in dieting behavior.

_____ 24. I like my stomach to be empty.

_____ 25. I enjoy trying new rich foods.

_____ 26. I have the impulse to vomit after meals.

Scoring: Never = 3
Rarely = 2
Sometimes = 1
Always, usually, and often = 0

A total score under 20 points may indicate abnormal eating behavior and the risk of having or developing an eating disorder. Share your results with a health professional for further evaluation.

SOURCE: J. A. McSherry, Progress in the diagnosis of anorexia nervosa, *Journal of the Royal Society of Health* 106 (1986): 8–9; *Eating Attitudes Test* and scoring developed by Dr. P. Garfinkel.

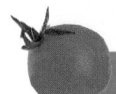

CHECK YOURSELF...

1. What is the primary factor that determines BMR (basal metabolic rate)?

2. Name the two major components of energy expenditure.

3. What does the fatfold test tell us?

4. What are the possible risk factors associated with obesity?

5. What is the most likely cause of obesity in this country?

6. List the four components recommended for a successful weight-loss program.

7. What is the recommended rate for weekly weight loss (in pounds)?

8. List three examples of behavior modification techniques.

9. What are the advantages of exercise in a weight-control program?

10. What is central obesity, and what are the risks associated with it?

11. What is the measure of a successful weight-loss program?

12. What are the characteristics of anorexia nervosa and bulimia?

Answers to selected Check Yourself questions are found in Appendix H.

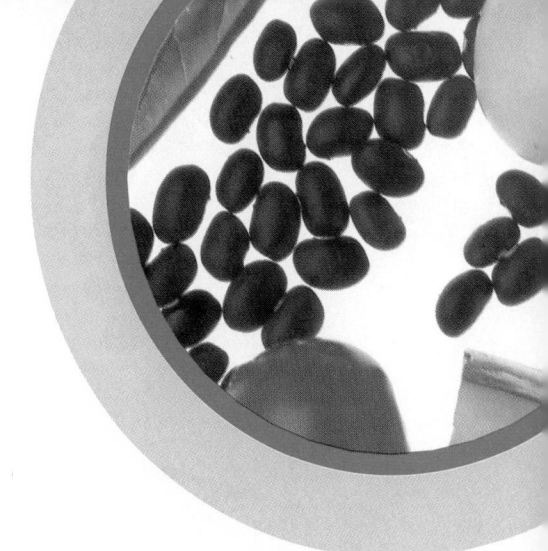

> Get health. No labor, effort, nor exercise that can gain it must be grudged.
>
> R. W. Emerson
> (1803–1882, American essayist and poet)

Nutrition and Fitness   NINE

Contents

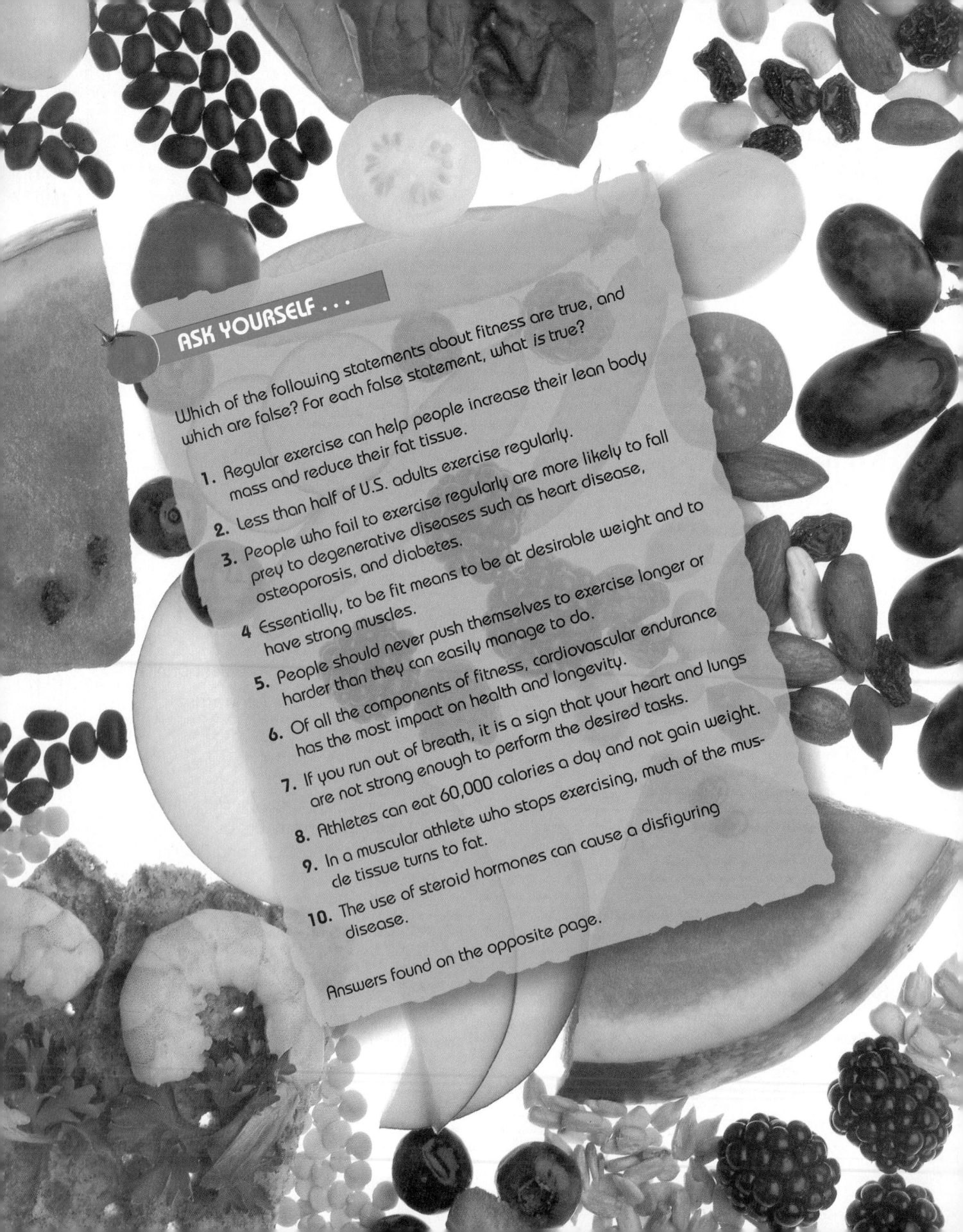

ASK YOURSELF . . .

Which of the following statements about fitness are true, and which are false? For each false statement, what *is* true?

1. Regular exercise can help people increase their lean body mass and reduce their fat tissue.

2. Less than half of U.S. adults exercise regularly.

3. People who fail to exercise regularly are more likely to fall prey to degenerative diseases such as heart disease, osteoporosis, and diabetes.

4. Essentially, to be fit means to be at desirable weight and to have strong muscles.

5. People should never push themselves to exercise longer or harder than they can easily manage to do.

6. Of all the components of fitness, cardiovascular endurance has the most impact on health and longevity.

7. If you run out of breath, it is a sign that your heart and lungs are not strong enough to perform the desired tasks.

8. Athletes can eat 60,000 calories a day and not gain weight.

9. In a muscular athlete who stops exercising, much of the muscle tissue turns to fat.

10. The use of steroid hormones can cause a disfiguring disease.

Answers found on the opposite page.

Fitness is in! Never before has our culture been so focused on fitness. That's good news, because people who are fit not only look good but also feel good. They can perform the activities they must and still have energy left over to do the things they want to do. In a general sense, then, fitness is a state of physical well-being that lets you lead a higher quality of life.

In addition, mounting evidence suggests that our bodies need regular, moderate exercise that gets our hearts beating and forces our muscles to work harder than they usually do to stay healthy. Physiologically speaking, overall fitness is a balance between different body systems. With respect to the joints, flexibility is important. With respect to muscles, strength and endurance are important. Endurance is also important to the heart and lungs (this type of endurance is called cardiovascular endurance, discussed later in the chapter).

This chapter illustrates the effects of nutrition on fitness—and vice versa, for a two-way relationship exists. Optimal nutrition contributes to athletic performance; and conversely, regular exercise contributes to a person's ability to use and store nutrients optimally. The two together are indispensable to a high quality of life; **fitness,** like good nutrition, is an essential component of good health.

FITNESS the body's ability to meet physical demands, composed of four components: flexibility, strength, muscle endurance, and cardiovascular endurance.

Reasons to Exercise

The benefits of regular exercise make up an impressive list, which is growing longer as new discoveries are made. Through regular exercise, people can gain energy and confidence, increase their lean body tissue, reduce their body fatness, improve the health of their skin and their muscle tone, improve their sleeping habits, reduce their risk of heart disease and diabetes, reduce their blood cholesterol levels, reduce their blood pressure, build bones that remain strong into old age, and live a more enjoyable, perhaps even longer, life.[1]

No one can promise that you will receive all of these benefits if you exercise, but almost everyone who exercises reaps at least some of them. Despite evidence of the benefits, less than a quarter of U.S. adults are adequately active.[2] Perhaps this is because an unworked body requires some time to adapt—and creating a new habit takes time. However, one of the greatest benefits derived from physical activity is moving from a sedentary to a moderate level of activity.[3] *Moderate* means 30 minutes of brisk walking (3 to 4 miles per hour), walking up stairs, calisthenics, dancing, bicycling—any activity that will expend approximately 200 calories a day (refer to Table 8–11 on page 299). Once a routine of physical activity is established, the felt benefits far outweigh any inconveniences. People may begin a fitness program to trim fat or add muscle, but

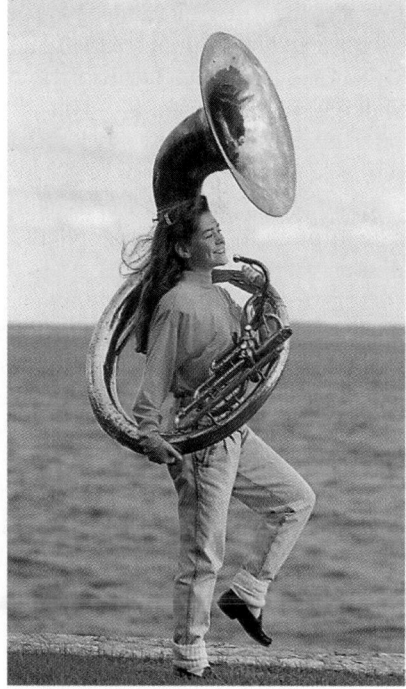

Being fit is more than being free of disease; it is feeling full of vitality and enthusiasm for life.

ASK YOURSELF ANSWERS: 1. True. **2.** True. **3.** True. **4.** False. To be fit means not only to be at desirable weight and to have strong muscles but also to be flexible and, most importantly, to have muscular and cardiovascular endurance. **5.** False. The overload principle states that people *should* push themselves to exercise longer or harder than they can easily manage to do—although not, of course, to the point of strain. **6.** True. **7.** False. If you run out of breath, it is not a sign that your heart and lungs are weak but a sign that you are going into oxygen debt. **8.** False. No one can eat 60,000 calories a day, but many football players can eat 6,000 calories a day and not gain weight. **9.** False. Muscle tissue does not turn to fat, but in a muscular athlete who stops exercising, muscle tissue is lost and fat is gained. **10.** True.

soon they are pleasantly surprised to find that they have more energy, feel less tense, sleep better, and feel healthier, and so they keep it up.

People can get in the habit of doing things that are good for them, just as they can get hooked on things that are not good for them, such as alcohol and other drugs, including nicotine. You can cultivate the habit of engaging in regular physical activity if you:

Choose an activity that you can do without a great deal of mental effort.

Choose an activity that doesn't depend on other people's presence—that is, one you can do alone when a partner is not available.

Believe that it has physical, mental, or spiritual value for you.

Enjoy the activity or some aspect of it (even just enjoying the knowledge that you do it).

Can experience progress through doing it.

Can do the activity without criticizing yourself.[4]

There is no RDA for physical activity, although there probably should be. The notion that a certain minimum daily average amount of activity is indispensable to health is just now reaching public consciousness. A consequence of sedentary living is accelerated development of the diseases associated with a sedentary lifestyle—cardiovascular disease, some forms of cancer, stroke, diabetes, osteoporosis, and hypertension.[5] The Centers for Disease Control and Prevention and the American College of Sports Medicine recommend that we spend an accumulated total of at *least* 30 minutes on most days of the week engaged in any one of numerous forms of physical activities (for example, bicycling, brisk walking, using the stairs).[6] This 30 minutes can be accumulated in relatively brief sessions of activity—just mix and match your preferred activities in periods as short as 8 to 10 minutes that total 30 minutes by the end of the day. For example, walk your dog for 12 minutes in the morning, enjoy a 10-minute bike ride through the neighborhood after classes, and take an 8-minute walk after dinner. The new guidelines stress the value of moderate activity and suggest that the total *amount* of activity is more important than the manner in which it is carried out. See this chapter's Consumer Tips feature on page 320 for suggestions on adding physical activities to your daily routines.

Fitness is not restricted to the seasoned athlete. With a basic understanding of the concept of total fitness and a personal commitment to a physically active lifestyle, anyone can become fit (see Figure 9–1). To be fit, you don't have to be able to finish the local marathon, nor do you have to develop the muscles of a Mr. Universe or Miss Olympia. Rather, what you need is a reasonable weight (refer to Chapter 8) and enough flexibility, muscle strength, muscle endurance, and cardiovascular endurance to meet the everyday demands that life places on you, plus some to spare.

Physical Conditioning

It seems obvious that people's bodies are shaped by what they do, but this fact is often overlooked. Physical conditioning refers to a planned program of exercise directed toward improving the function of a particular body system. Placing

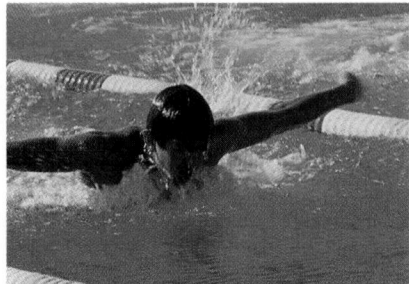

People's bodies are shaped by what they do.

If you are generally *inactive*, increase daily activities at the base of the Activity Pyramid by:
- taking the stairs
- hiding the TV remote control
- making extra trips around the house or yard
- stretching while standing in line
- walking whenever you can

If your activity routines are *sporadic* (active in summer, but not in the winter), become consistent with activity by increasing activity in the middle of the Pyramid by:
- finding activities you enjoy
- planning activities in your day
- setting realistic goals

If your physical activity is *consistent* (at least 4 times per week), think about the long term as you move throughout the Pyramid by:
- changing your routine if you start to get bored
- exploring new activities

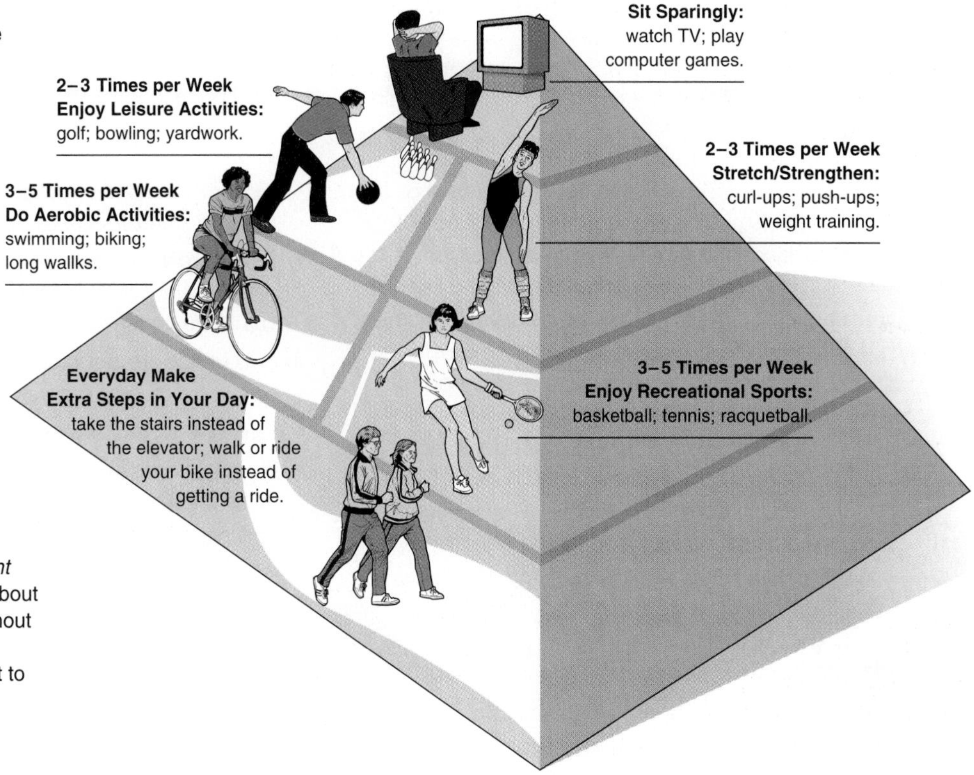

Sit Sparingly: watch TV; play computer games.

**2–3 Times per Week
Enjoy Leisure Activities:** golf; bowling; yardwork.

**2–3 Times per Week
Stretch/Strengthen:** curl-ups; push-ups; weight training.

**3–5 Times per Week
Do Aerobic Activities:** swimming; biking; long walks.

**Everyday Make
Extra Steps in Your Day:** take the stairs instead of the elevator; walk or ride your bike instead of getting a ride.

**3–5 Times per Week
Enjoy Recreational Sports:** basketball; tennis; racquetball.

**FIGURE 9–1
THE ACTIVITY PYRAMID**

SOURCE: Adapted from J. Norstrom, Ten Tips to Healthy Eating and Physical Activity for You, © 1995 The American Dietetic Association National Center for Nutrition and Dietetics, International Food Information Council, and President's Council on Physical Fitness and Sports.

regular, physical demand on the body and forcing the body to do more than it usually does will cause it to adapt and function more efficiently. This is called **overload.** Muscles respond to the overload of exercise by gaining strength and ability to endure. Strength gains may not be visible in all cases. But in some, such as with male bodybuilders, muscles increase in strength and size, a response called **hypertrophy.** The converse is also true: muscles, if not called on to perform, decrease in size, a response called **atrophy.** For example, an arm that is in a cast for six weeks will gradually become smaller in size because the arm muscles are not being used.

Runners often have well-developed strong legs; a tennis player may have one arm that is stronger than the other. Swimmers usually develop in a balanced way—all limbs, chest, back, and so forth are called on to perform and so develop uniformly. This doesn't mean that everyone should give up tennis and running and take up swimming; it only means that a variety of exercises will produce the most uniform overall fitness. This is why people are told to use different muscle groups in their exercise from day to day.

OVERLOAD an extra physical demand placed on the body. A principle of training is that for a body system to improve, its workload must be increased by increments over time.

HYPERTROPHY an increase in size in response to use.

ATROPHY a decrease in size in response to disuse.

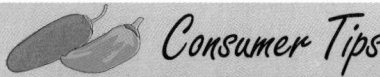

Consumer Tips

Ways to Include Physical Activity in Your Day

Physical activity can add years to your life as well as life to your years. It helps you feel and perform at your best. The key to sticking with a regular exercise program is to choose activities that you enjoy. For example, if you love birdwatching, plan time for nature hikes or early-morning walks. If you prefer to exercise with a group, consider joining a health club or gym. If you like mall shopping, plan to do a few laps of brisk walking around the mall first before you actually shop. Be flexible. Remember that you don't always have to spend 30 consecutive minutes engaged in physical activity—a few minutes here and a few minutes there add to the benefits of moderate exercise. Keep in mind that *any* activity is good (for example, "Just do something"), but *more* is better. The goal is to have a *physically active* lifestyle. Consider the following tips to help you be more active and do what you enjoy as often as possible:

- Register for community or college classes in dancing, adult fitness, strength training, tennis, or swimming.
- Take your dog on frequent walks; teach him to play frisbee.
- Find a workout partner to help you stay on track.
- Sign up to play a community sport such as softball, volleyball, or soccer.
- Tie exercise to social opportunities—run at the local track and get to know the regulars, join a tennis or

racquet club and sign up regularly for doubles, or take an aerobics class.

- If you prefer to exercise alone, designate a certain area where you live for exercise and invest in some stationary exercise equipment.
- Add variety to your routine to avoid boredom—walk a new route or try cross-country skiing.
- Plan ahead for weekend hikes or bike rides.
- Plant a flower or vegetable garden and stay busy with its cultivation and weeding.
- Choose the stairs instead of taking the elevator or escalator.
- Find the parking space farthest away from your destination when shopping or doing errands.
- Carry your own luggage, grocery bags, laundry, and books.
- Forget the car and walk or bike to campus or nearby stores and offices.
- Mow the lawn using the old-fashioned push type of mower rather than a power mower.
- Seek convenience—look for exercise classes held on campus or near your home or workplace.
- Focus on your achievements and reward yourself along the way as you meet your fitness goals step by step.
- Be creative and have fun!

The overload principle applies equally to all aspects of fitness: flexibility, muscle strength, muscle endurance, and cardiovascular endurance. It also applies to the skeleton. To develop a strong, dense skeletal system, you must start by demanding that the bones bear slightly more stress (through weight-bearing exercises such as walking, running, weightlifting, or aerobic dance) than they are used to. The bones respond by depositing more minerals. Eventually, a maximum is reached. People can develop an amazing fitness level by progressively increasing overload.

You can apply overload in several ways. You can do the activity more often—that is, increase its **frequency;** you can do the activity more strenuously—that is, increase its **intensity;** or you can do it for longer periods of **time**—that is, increase its duration. All three strategies work well, and you can pick one or a combination, depending on your fitness goals.

For *fitness*, remember the *FIT* principle:

F—FREQUENCY number of exercise sessions per week; at least 3 or 4 sessions per week are recommended.

I—INTENSITY how hard you exercise (for example, the degree of exertion while exercising); it is recommended that you exercise at 60% to 85% of your maximum heart rate per minute—known as your target heart rate.

T—TIME duration or length of time that you exercise with your heart rate elevated into your target heart rate zone (the minimum amount is thought to be 20 to 30 minutes per session).

The Four Components of Fitness

Strength

Strength is the ability of the muscles to work against resistance: pulling yourself up and out of a swimming pool, carrying a backpack full of large books, or opening a jar of pickles. The purpose of strength training is to build well-toned muscles that let you accomplish daily activities at work and during recreation as well as to prevent injury. As muscles get stronger, individual fibers thicken and enlarge. Our ability to respond to strength training continues to a very old age.[7] The connective tissues making up muscles, tendons, and ligaments also strengthen and become more efficient at using energy. The benefit: Strong muscles, tendons, and ligaments play a key role in preventing injury. For example, strong quadriceps—muscles on the front of the thigh—stabilize your knee as you bike. Strong calf muscles and ankle ligaments decrease the risk of an ankle sprain when walking briskly or jogging.

Many of today's mechanical aids invented to make life easier rob us of the opportunity to develop strength—for example, the strength we would gain from chopping firewood instead of turning up a thermostat. Today, we must put forth conscious effort to develop strength. The kind of equipment you use is largely a matter of availability and personal preference. If you belong to a health club, you probably have access to weight-training equipment. If not, you can use equipment you have at home, such as plastic gallon milk jugs filled with water or sand or store-bought ankle weights and dumbbells (see Figure 9–2). No matter what method you choose, safety in strength training is essential. Get proper instruction. Before you set up a strength-training program, consult an exercise physiologist or physical therapist or enroll in a college class.

The American College of Sports Medicine now recommends strength training as an integral part of a good overall exercise program.[8] To reap the benefits of strength training, consider the following tips:

- Aim for two to three sessions a week.
- Choose an intensity—the amount of weight you lift—that allows you to perform 8 to 12 repetitions; adjust the amount of weight upwards as your strength improves so that you are still able to perform in the 8 to 12 repetitions range.
- Perform each repetition slowly—allowing six to nine seconds per repetition.
- Remember to breathe! Inhale before you lift, exhale as you lift, and breathe in slowly as you lower the weight to the starting position; pause and breathe fully between repetitions.
- Warm up before lifting weights and cool down afterwards—you can begin and end each session with several repetitions without using weights or by doing some stretching exercises.
- Allow your muscles time to recover between sessions; do not strength train the same muscle groups on consecutive days.

Because many women mistakenly think they will develop enlarged muscles, which they view as undesirable and unattractive, they don't participate in strength-training programs. Testosterone—a male hormone—is responsible for muscle overdevelopment. Women only have 10 percent of the amount of testosterone that men do. Because of their lower testosterone levels, it is unlikely that

STRENGTH the ability of muscles to work against resistance.

Choose a chair that has a firm seat and back and no arms. The seat should be high enough so that when you sit in it your feet barely touch the floor. It should also be long enough to reach the back of your knees. And the back of the chair should be high enough for you to hold onto while standing behind it.

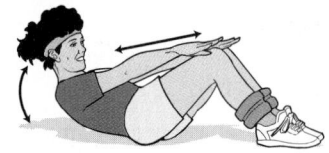

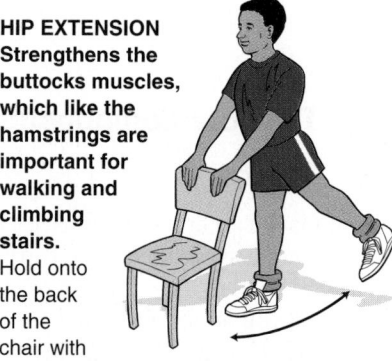

**HIP EXTENSION
Strengthens the buttocks muscles, which like the hamstrings are important for walking and climbing stairs.**
Hold onto the back of the chair with weights around the ankles and bend forward about 45 degrees at the waist. Lock the knee and lift one leg straight out behind you as high as possible without moving your upper body. (The movement should be smooth and controlled.) Slowly lower your leg to the starting position. Alternate with the other leg until you have completed 8 to 12 repetitions on *both* sides.

**SIDE SHOULDER RAISE
Helps improve the flexibility and strength of the shoulder muscles (deltoids) as well as muscles in the upper back.** Sit forward on the chair (not resting against the back) with a straight back and relaxed shoulders. Feet should be flat on the ground, shoulder-width apart. With weights in both hands and your arms straight down at your sides, slowly raise your arms, keeping them straight out, to just above shoulder level. Do not lean forward or backward while performing the lifts. Your back and shoulders should remain fixed (but not hunched) throughout.

BENT-KNEE SITUP Works the abdominal muscles. Lie on your back with your knees bent and your feet flat on the floor, about 12 inches apart. Keep your palms down on your thighs. Gently tuck in your chin and lift your shoulders off the floor while sliding your palms up toward your knees. Stop about halfway up, at the point where it would be a struggle to continue. Hold for a moment, then go slowly back down. When it becomes too easy to do 8 to 12 repetitions at a time, increase the number of repetitions. Do not add weight for this exercise.

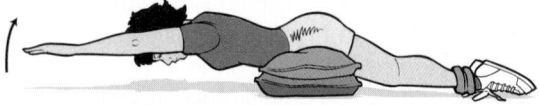

BACK EXTENSION Works the lower back muscles. Lie on your stomach with two pillows under your pelvis (hips). Leave ankle weights on to anchor your feet to the ground. With your arms straight out in front of your head, slowly lift your back 4 to 5 inches off the floor (straight, not arching). Hold, then slowly lower your back. When it becomes too easy to do 8 to 12 repetitions at a time, increase the number of repetitions. Do not add weight for this exercise.

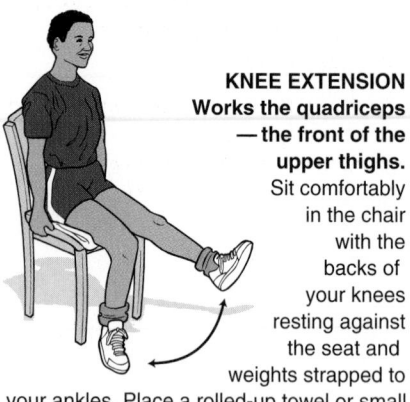

**KNEE EXTENSION
Works the quadriceps — the front of the upper thighs.**
Sit comfortably in the chair with the backs of your knees resting against the seat and weights strapped to your ankles. Place a rolled-up towel or small cushion under your knees to lift them slightly so that just the balls of your feet touch the floor. Extend one leg out in front of you until your leg is as straight as possible. Do not grip the chair as you lift, but you may gently hold onto the seat of the chair to help stabilize you. Slowly lower your leg until your foot is resting on the floor. Alternate legs from lift to lift. One set equals 8 to 12 repetitions on *both* sides.

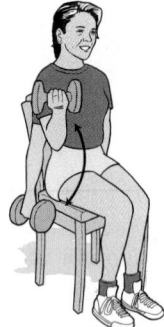

**BICEPS CURL
Strengthens the biceps muscles at the front of the upper arm, needed for carrying and lifting.**
Sit straight in the chair with feet shoulder-width apart. Place your lifting arm straight down to the side of the chair with your palm facing your body. Bring the hand with the weight three-quarters of the way up toward your shoulder (bend from the elbow). While lifting, slowly rotate your hand around so that at the end of your lift, your palm is facing your shoulder. Slowly lower the hand. After lifting 8 to 12 times with one arm, proceed to the other. It takes 8 to 12 repetitions on *both* sides to equal one set.

**KNEE FLEXION
Strengthens the hamstring muscles at the back of the upper thigh, important for walking and climbing stairs.**
Stand behind the chair with weights strapped to your ankles. Place one foot slightly farther back than the other. Then, without moving your upper leg at all, bend (at the knee) the leg that is slightly back so that your heel comes as close to the back of your thigh as possible. Slowly lower your leg to the starting position. Do the same with the other leg. Eight to 12 repetitions on *both* sides make a set.

**FIGURE 9–2
EXERCISES FOR ADDED STRENGTH**

SOURCE: Reprinted with permission from *Tufts University Diet & Nutrition Letter* 13(1), March 1995, p. 5.

women would develop bulging or overdeveloped muscles as a result of two or three weekly sessions of weight training. What will occur, though, is improved muscle strength, shape, and tone.[9]

A final note: Only muscle can be shaped and toned, skin and fat can't. So even with regular strength training, "flabby" regions may not look toned until the fat is reduced. Aerobic exercise (explained in another section) is the best way to burn excess body fat.

Flexibility

Keeping your muscles and joints pliable is critical for developing a fit body. A flexible body can move as it was designed to move and will bend rather than tear or break in response to sudden stress. **Flexibility** (range of motion) depends upon the condition and interrelationships of bones, ligaments, muscles, and tendons.

Stretching exercises improve flexibility by increasing muscle and tendon elasticity and length. Stretching should be done slowly—called **static stretches.** When you feel a slight strain in the muscle, hold the position for 10 to 30 seconds. Bouncy, rapid stretches—known as **ballistic stretches**—can cause minute tears in the muscle and also set up a reaction in the muscle that makes it resist the stretch. Avoid painful stretches. They are clearly excessive.

Flexibility tends to decrease as you age but improves in response to stretching, and it can be maintained in most people by doing frequent stretching exercises. While regular exercise will increase muscle tone and strength, some types of exercise can also make muscles stiffer—making them more prone to strain and injury. For example, jogging and dancing can reduce flexibility of the lower back, front of thighs, and calves. Joggers and dancers should emphasize flexibility exercises for these areas. When beginning an exercise program, stretching is especially critical for previously sedentary people whose muscles are short and tight.

Stretching routines are commonly done as part of a warm-up routine before exercise. Low-intensity preliminary exercise allows your heart—also a muscle—to slowly accelerate and make adjustments in bloodflow and oxygen supply, preparing for the work it is about to perform. Using calisthenics as a warm-up, such as walking, marching in place, or doing some other moderate rhythmic activity, prepares your heart muscle for action. After your light warm-up, stretch the muscles that you will be using in your main exercise activity.

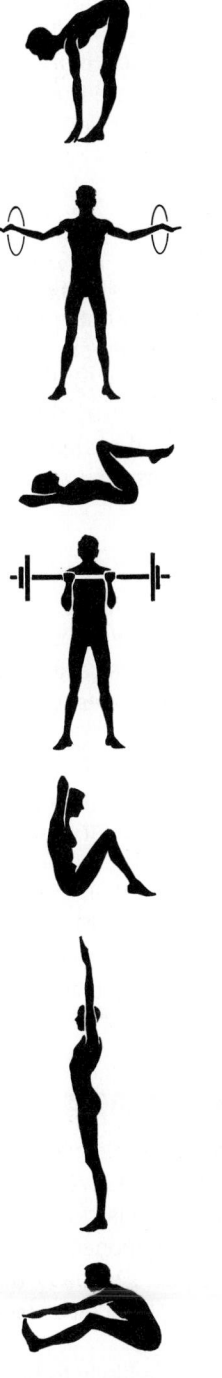

Flexibility and strength

FLEXIBILITY the ability to bend or extend without injury; flexibility depends on the elasticity of the muscles, tendons, and ligaments and on the condition of the joints.

STATIC STRETCHES stretches that lengthen tissues without injury; characterized by long-lasting, painless, pleasurable stretches.

BALLISTIC STRETCHES stretches characterized by short, choppy, sometimes painful movements that often pull connective tissues beyond their elastic limits.

Waiting to stretch until after your warm-up allows blood to move into the muscles, making them easier to stretch. Doing stretches after your exercise session gives your heart a chance to gradually slow its pace. It also allows you to lengthen those muscles that have become tight and tense from the exercise. You can make greater gains in flexibility by stretching after your workout because muscles are warm and easier to stretch.

Muscle Endurance

Muscle endurance, the third component of fitness, is the power of a muscle to keep on going for long periods. Your muscle endurance influences your performance in the last set of a tennis match, your swing on the eighteenth hole of a golf game, or your ability to pedal during the last 10 miles of a 100-mile bike tour. Endurance of certain muscles can be tested by the number of situps or pushups you can accomplish in a certain period of time. But remember, these tests evaluate only the abdominal and upper arm muscles.

ENDURANCE the ability to sustain an effort for a long time. One type, **muscle endurance,** is the ability of a muscle to contract repeatedly within a given time without becoming exhausted. Another type, **cardiovascular endurance,** is the ability of the cardiovascular system to sustain effort over a period of time.

Cardiovascular Endurance

Another realm in which endurance is important is the length of time that you can keep going with an elevated heart rate—that is, how long your heart can endure a given demand. This kind of endurance is **cardiovascular endurance.** The heart is a muscle, and it, like your other muscles, can respond to repeated demands by becoming larger and stronger.

Exercises that promote cardiovascular endurance are the best for making short-term fitness gains and long-term health improvements as well as for weight control. The best exercises to develop cardiovascular endurance are those that repetitively use large muscle groups—arms and legs—and that last for a continuous 20 to 30 minutes. Examples include brisk walking, aerobic dance, running, cycling, cross-country skiing, and rowing. The American College of Sports Medicine recommends that people participate in cardiovascular conditioning activities at least three times a week for a continuous 20 to 30 minutes.[10]

To develop cardiovascular fitness, choose an activity that

- Is steady and constant.
- Uses large muscle groups, such as the arms, legs, and buttocks. If you move 50 percent of your muscle mass, the activity is aerobic.
- Is uninterrupted, lasts for more than 20 minutes, and is done at least 3 times a week.

Getting Started on Lifetime Fitness

For total fitness, an exercise program that incorporates strength training, stretching, and cardiovascular endurance activity is best. If you are just beginning a fitness program, though, it makes sense to begin with cardiovascular endurance, which is the most basic of all components to health and long life. Cardiovascular fitness is discussed in a separate section of this chapter. You can get an indirect estimate of your current fitness level by answering the questions in the Physical Activity Scorecard.

The more active you are, the more fit you are likely to be. Tests that measure your ability to perform various physical activities reveal more, and if you were to have an **exercise stress test** or other such measurement taken by a professional, you would obtain an accurate estimate of your fitness.

In proceeding with a fitness program, it is important to keep your own goals in mind, since they can carry you through periods of discouragement and help

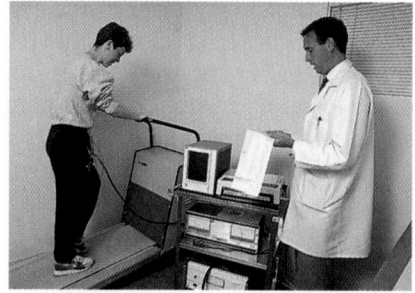

The exercise stress test measures heart function during exercise.

EXERCISE STRESS TEST a test that monitors heart function during exercise to detect abnormalities that may not show up under ordinary conditions; exercise physiologists and trained physicians or health-care professionals can administer the test.

How physically active are you? For each question answered yes, give yourself the number of points indicated. Then total your points to determine your score.

A. Vigorous Exercise Routines

1. I participate in active recreational sports such as tennis or racquetball for an hour or more:
   a. About once a week. (*2 points*)
   b. About twice a week. (*4 points*)
   c. Three times a week. (*6 points*)
   d. Four times a week. (*8 points*)

2. I participate in vigorous fitness activities like aerobic dancing, roller blading, jogging, or swimming (at least 20 minutes each session):
   a. About once a week. (*3 points*)
   b. About twice a week. (*6 points*)
   c. Three times a week. (*9 points*)
   d. Four times a week. (*12 points*)

B. Other Exercise Routines

3. At least two times a week, I work out with weights for at least ten minutes:
   a. Two sessions a week. (*2 points*)
   b. Three sessions a week. (*3 points*)
   c. Four or more sessions a week. (*4 points*)

4. At least two times a week, I perform floor workouts (sit-ups, push-ups) for at least ten minutes:
   a. Two sessions a week. (*2 points*)
   b. Three sessions a week. (*3 points*)
   c. Four or more sessions a week. (*4 points*)

5. At least two times a week, I participate in yoga or perform stretching exercises for at least ten minutes:
   a. Two sessions a week. (*2 points*)
   b. Three sessions a week. (*3 points*)
   c. Four or more sessions a week. (*4 points*)

C. Occupation and Daily Activities

6. I walk to and from school, work, and shopping (½ mile or more each way), two or three times a week or more. (*1 point*)

7. I climb stairs rather than using elevators or escalators, every other day or more. (*1 point*)

8. My school, job, or household routine involves physical activity that fits the following description:
   a. Most of my day is spent in desk work or light physical activity. (*0 points*)
   b. Most of my day is spent in farm activities, moderate physical activity, brisk walking, or comparable activities. (*4 points*)
   c. My typical day includes several hours of heavy physical activity (shoveling, lifting, etc.). (*2 points per day*)

D. Leisure Activities

9. I do several hours of gardening, lawn work, or similar hobby work each week. (*1 point*)

10. At least once a week I dance vigorously (folk or line dancing) for an hour or more. (*1 point*)

11. In season, I play 9 to 18 holes of golf at least once a week, and I do not use a power cart. (*2 points*)

12. I walk for exercise or recreation.
    a. One to two hours a week. (*1 point*)
    b. Three to four hours a week. (*2 points*)
    c. Five hours or more a week. (*3 points*)

13. In *addition* to the above, I engage in other forms of physical activity:
    a. One to two hours a week. (*1 point*)
    b. Three to four hours a week. (*2 points*)
    c. Five hours or more a week. (*3 points*)

Scoring:
Record your point scores here

Category	Score
A. Vigorous Exercise Routines	___
B. Other Exercise Routines	___
C. Occupation and Daily Activities	___
D. Leisure Activities	___
	Total: ___

Evaluation of total score (circle one):

- Inactive (0 to 5 points).
- Moderately active (6 to 11 points).
- Active (12 to 20 points).
- Very active (21 points or over).

If your score categorized you as inactive or only moderately active, think of activities that you could realistically engage in on a regular basis to raise your score to "active" (12 points).

SOURCE: Adapted with permission of Russell Pate (University of South Carolina, Human Performance Laboratory).

you to choose the activities that best meet your needs. Keep in mind that fitness builds slowly, and so activity should increase gradually. Don't rush things by taking on too much, too soon. View your exercise time as a lifelong commitment.

A few cautions on getting started: If you are an apparently healthy male older than 40 years of age or an apparently healthy female older than 50 years of age, the American College of Sports Medicine recommends that you have a medical examination and diagnostic exercise test before you start a *vigorous* exercise program. Beginning a *moderate* program, such as walking, however, would not require the physicians's exam.[11]

For most people, physical activity should not pose any problem or hazard. The Physical Activity Readiness Questionnaire was designed to identify the small number of adults for whom physical activity might be inappropriate or those who should have medical advice concerning suitable type of activity.[12] If you answer yes to any of the following questions, seek advice from a health-care provider before you begin a *vigorous* exercise program.

1. Has your doctor ever said you have heart trouble?
2. Do you frequently suffer from pains in your chest?
3. Do you often feel faint or have spells of dizziness?
4. Has a doctor ever said your blood pressure was too high?
5. Has a doctor ever told you that you have a bone or joint problem such as arthritis that might be made worse with exercise?
6. Is there a good physical reason not mentioned here why you should not follow an activity program even if you wanted to?
7. Are you over age 65 and not accustomed to vigorous exercise?

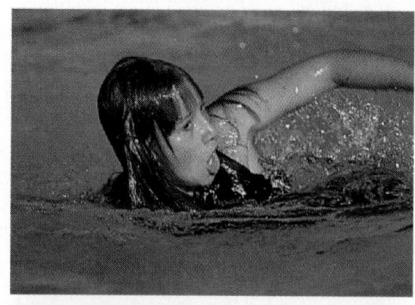

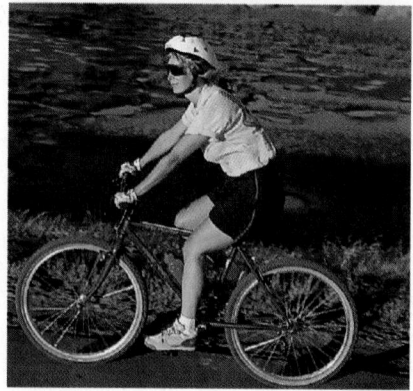

Make exercise a habit: Choose an activity you enjoy.

Energy for Exercise

Your body runs on water, oxygen, and food—primarily carbohydrate and fat. The chemical reactions that use these substances to make energy are called metabolism. Your body has two interrelated energy-producing systems—one dependent on oxygen—**aerobic** metabolism—and the other able to function without oxygen—**anaerobic** metabolism. An understanding of how the two systems work is important because it explains why you choose certain exercises over others to strengthen your heart, why you eat what you do, and what factors influence your performance during sporting events.

AEROBIC requiring oxygen.

ANAEROBIC not requiring oxygen.

Aerobic and Anaerobic Metabolism

At rest, your muscles burn mostly fat and some carbohydrate for energy. During exercise, though, the amounts the muscles use depend on an interplay between fuel availability and oxygen availability. To an exercising muscle, oxygen is everything. With ample oxygen, muscles can extract all available energy from carbohydrate and fat by means of aerobic metabolism. During moderate exercise, your lungs and circulatory system have no trouble keeping up with the muscles' need for oxygen. You breathe deeply and easily, and your heart beats steadily—the exercise is aerobic. But the heart and lungs can supply only so much oxygen so fast.

When the muscles' exertion is great enough that their energy demand outstrips their oxygen supply, they must also rely on anaerobic metabolism to make energy. Since the anaerobic metabolic pathway can burn only carbohydrate for fuel, it draws heavily on your limited body stores of carbohydrate. Nevertheless, this system does provide an immediate source of energy without relying on oxygen. Because of this system, you can dash out of the way of an oncoming car or sprint ahead of your competitor at the finish line. Unfortunately, this energy-yielding system is extremely inefficient. Only 5 percent of carbohydrate's energy-producing potential is harnessed by this pathway.[13]

Because the anaerobic metabolic pathway only partially burns your carbohydrate, it litters your muscle with partly broken down portions of glucose. You may have heard the name for these partly broken down products: lactic acid. The buildup of lactic acid causes burning pain in the muscles and can lead to muscle exhaustion within seconds if it is not drained away. A strategy for dealing with lactic acid buildup is to relax the muscles at every opportunity so that the circulating blood can carry it away and bring oxygen to support aerobic metabolism. Fortunately, lactic acid is not a waste product. When oxygen reaches your muscles, lactic acid is ushered to your liver, which converts it back to glucose.

Neither the aerobic nor the anaerobic metabolic pathway functions exclusively to supply energy to your body. The two work together, complementing and supporting each other. Keep in mind, however, that carbohydrate is absolutely essential for exercise. Without it, your muscles can't perform. You want to exercise aerobically because muscles burn fat and extract energy from carbohydrate more efficiently in the presence of oxygen, thereby conserving your body's limited store of carbohydrate. Thus, you want to exercise at an intensity that allows your heart and lungs to keep pace with your working muscles' oxygen needs.

Aerobic Exercise—Exercise for the Heart

To meet your body's increased oxygen needs during aerobic exercise, your heart must pump oxygen-rich blood to muscles at a faster pace than normal. This increased demand on the heart makes the heart stronger and increases its endurance. In addition, aerobic exercise improves the endurance of the lungs and the muscles along the arteries and in the walls of the digestive tract and, of course, the muscles directly involved in the activity. These all-over improvements are called **cardiovascular conditioning** or the **training effect.** In cardiovascular conditioning, the total blood volume increases so that the blood can carry more oxygen. The heart muscle becomes stronger and larger. Since each beat of the heart pumps more blood, it needs to pump less often. The muscles that work the lungs gain strength and endurance, and breathing becomes more efficient. Circulation through the body's arteries and veins improves. Blood moves easily, and the blood pressure falls. Muscles throughout the body become firmer. Figure 9–3 shows the major relationships between the heart, circulatory system, and lungs.

To make these gains in cardiovascular conditioning, you must work up to a point where you can continuously exercise aerobically for 20 minutes or longer. This means you must elevate your heart rate (pulse). This heart rate—called your **target heart rate**—must be considerably faster than the resting rate to push (overload) the heart but not so fast as to strain it.

Aerobic exercises:

Aerobic dancing	Roller skating
Bench stepping	Rope jumping
Bicycling	Rowing
Cross-country skiing	Running
Fast walking	Speed skating
Jogging	Stair climbing
Mini-trampoline jumping	Swimming
Roller blading	Treadmill walking or running

Sports:

Sports add fun to your exercise routine, but because of frequent starts and stops, they don't allow for a continuous 20-minute bout of aerobic exercise. Aerobic training, however, will help you perform these sports:

Baseball	Ice hockey
Basketball	Lacrosse
Downhill skiing	Racquetball
Fencing	Soccer
Football	Squash
Frisbee	Softball
Golf	Tennis
Handball	Volleyball
Horseback riding	

CARDIOVASCULAR CONDITIONING or **TRAINING EFFECT** the effect of regular exercise on the cardiovascular system—including improvements in heart, lung, and muscle function and increased blood volume.

TARGET HEART RATE the heartbeat rate that will achieve a cardiovascular conditioning effect for a given person—fast enough to push the heart but not so fast as to strain it.

An informal pulse check can give you some indication of how conditioned your heart is to start with. As a rule of thumb, the average resting pulse rate for adults is around 70 beats per minute, but the rate can be higher or lower. Active people can have resting pulse rates of 50 or even lower. Figure 9–4 gives instructions for taking your pulse.

For cardiovascular conditioning, your target heart rate can be calculated from your age. The older you are, the lower your maximum heart rate. As your heart gets stronger, more intense exercise will be required to reach the same target rate. For example, at first, walking at a pace of three miles per hour may cause you to reach your target heart rate. After six to eight weeks of walking at this pace, you may notice you no longer reach your target heart rate. That's because your heart is stronger. It now needs more of a challenge to beat faster. Increasing the intensity of your workout by walking faster can provide this challenge.

To calculate your target heart rate range, take the following steps:

1. *Estimate your maximum heart rate (MHR).* Subtract your age from 220. This provides an estimate of the absolute maximum heart rate possible for a person your age. You should never exercise at this rate, of course.
2. *Determine your target heart rate range.* Multiply your MHR by 60 percent and 85 percent to find your upper and lower limits.

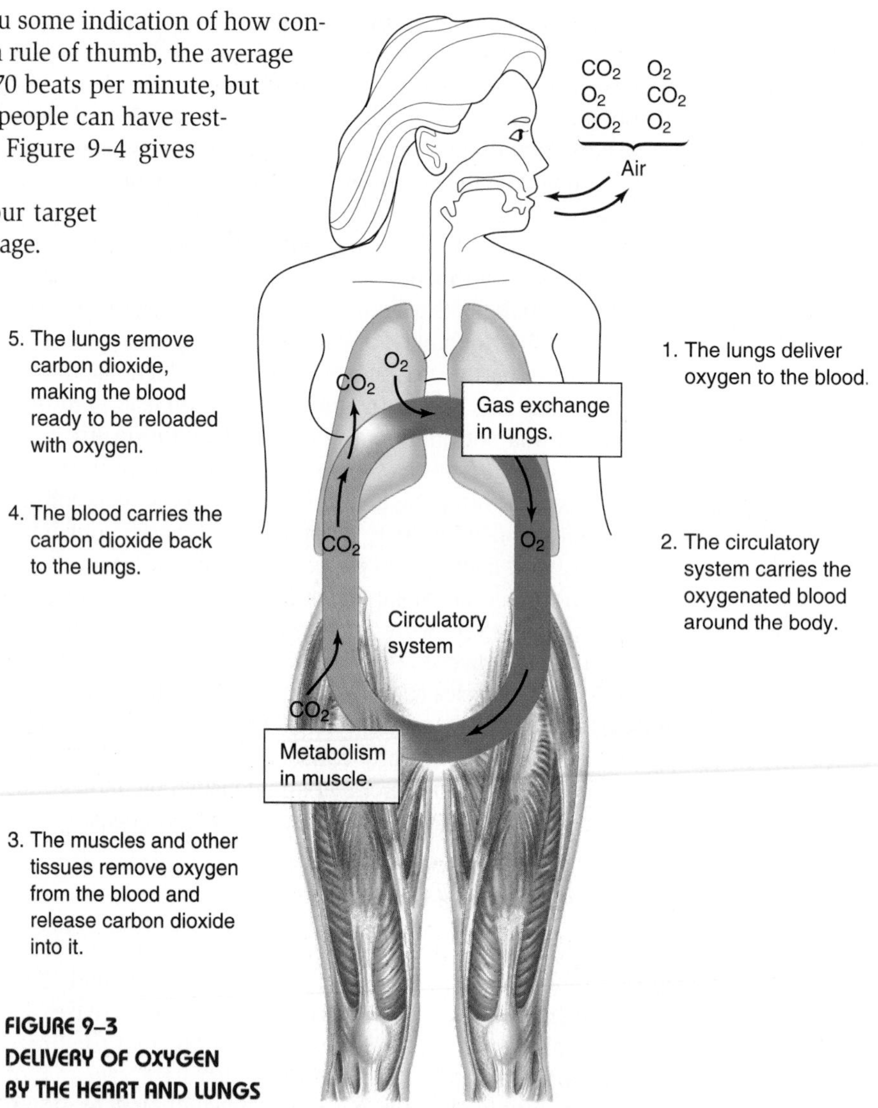

When you can work out at your target heart rate for 20 to 30 minutes, you know that you have arrived at your cardiovascular fitness goal. In the building-up stage, a pattern used to make progress is called **fartlek** training. To use it, a jogger might run at the target heart rate for two minutes before tiring, then rest by walking until ready to jog again, run another two minutes, then rest by walking, and so on for 20 minutes. At each session, the jogger can make the running periods longer and the resting periods shorter. Eventually, in about two months or so, the rest periods will no longer be needed at all. Once you have worked up to that, you can maintain

5. The lungs remove carbon dioxide, making the blood ready to be reloaded with oxygen.

4. The blood carries the carbon dioxide back to the lungs.

3. The muscles and other tissues remove oxygen from the blood and release carbon dioxide into it.

1. The lungs deliver oxygen to the blood.

2. The circulatory system carries the oxygenated blood around the body.

FIGURE 9–3
DELIVERY OF OXYGEN BY THE HEART AND LUNGS TO THE MUSCLES

The more fit a muscle is, the more oxygen it draws from the blood. That oxygen is drawn from the lungs, so the person with more fit muscles extracts more oxygen from the inhaled air than a person with less fit muscles. The cardiovascular system responds to the demand for oxygen by building up its capacity to deliver oxygen. Researchers can measure cardiovascular fitness by measuring the amount of oxygen a person consumes per minute while working out, a measure called VO_2 max.

FARTLEK speed play; alternating periods of fast and slow exercise.

your level of fitness by repeating the workout about every other day. The American College of Sports Medicine recommends that to maintain your cardiovascular endurance, you should exercise within your target heart rate range at least three times a week for 20 to 60 minutes. Activities of lower intensity should be performed for longer periods of time.

Fuels for Exercise

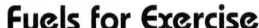

Most of what we know about fuel use during exercise comes from research on athletes, but you do not have to be an athlete to make use of this knowledge. As mentioned before, your energy-producing pathways require oxygen and the two muscle fuels: glucose and fatty acids. As Figure 9–3 showed, the oxygen comes from the lungs, which pass it to the blood, which carries it to the muscles. Your muscles, and to some extent your liver, supply carbohydrate to your muscles from their carbohydrate supply (see Figure 9–5). The fatty acids come mostly from fat inside the muscles but partly from fat that is released from the body's fat stores, and the blood delivers these fatty acids to the muscles.

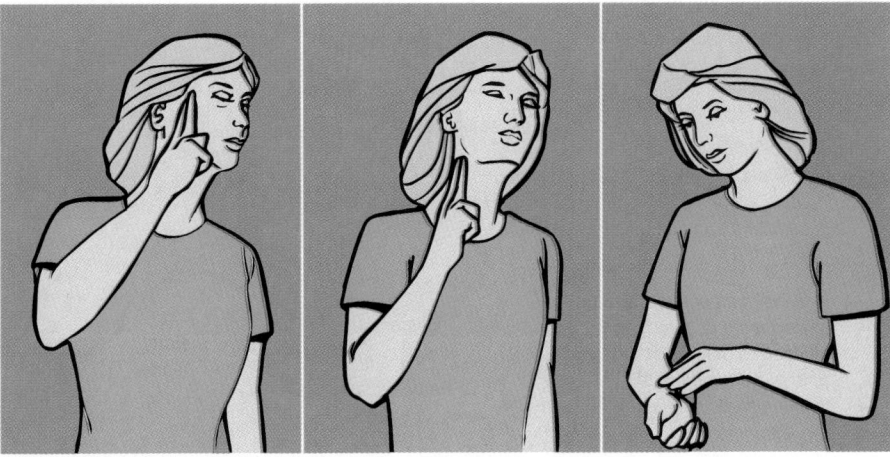

FIGURE 9–4
HOW TO TAKE YOUR PULSE

Use a watch or a clock with a second hand. Rest a few minutes for a resting pulse; for an exercising pulse, take the reading immediately after stopping the workout. Convenient places to feel the pulsations of your heartbeat are (a) the temporal arteries, (b) the carotid arteries, next to your trachea (windpipe), and (c) the radial artery (on the thumb side of the wrist). Start counting your pulse at a convenient second and continue counting for 10 seconds. Multiply by 6 to obtain your heart rate per minute. To ensure a true count:

- Use only fingers, not your thumb, on the pulse point (the thumb has a pulse of its own).
- Press just firmly enough to feel the pulse. Too much pressure can interfere with the pulse rhythm.

Exercise and Glucose

Glucose comes from carbohydrate-rich foods—breads, pasta, rice, legumes, fruits, vegetables, milk, and yogurt. Your body stores glucose in your liver and muscles as glycogen, a long chain of glucose molecules linked together.

During exercise, the body supplies glucose to the muscles from the stores of glycogen in the liver and in the muscles themselves. Interestingly, only the glycogen stores of active muscles are reduced. Because the body can't transfer glycogen between muscles, the other muscles not involved in the exercise retain their glycogen stores. The longer the exercise lasts or the more intense it is, the more glucose a person uses. Recall that exercise done at an intensity that outstrips the ability of the heart and lungs to supply oxygen to working muscles relies primarily on glucose for fuel. Thus, activities such as sprinting quickly deplete the body's stores of glycogen. Other activities, such as jogging or brisk walking, where the body can meet the muscles' oxygen demands, are more conservative of glycogen. Nonetheless, joggers and walkers still use it, and eventually they can run out of it.

Training can increase the amount of glycogen a muscle can conserve during exercise. The more fit a muscle is, the more fat it can burn for energy when oxygen is present—sparing the valuable glycogen.

Glycogen
↓
Glucose

Liver

Blood

Glucose

Triglycerides
↓
Fatty acids

Body fat

Fatty acids

Muscle

4. The muscle can convert its own limited supply of glycogen to glucose for use as energy.

Muscle Glycogen
↓
Glucose

1. The liver can convert its limited store of glycogen to glucose to help meet the energy demands of the working muscles.

2. The body can also help meet the energy demands of the working muscles by breaking down its unlimited supply of body fat (triglycerides) to fatty acids.

3. The circulatory system carries fuel (glucose and fatty acids) to the muscle.

Energy

5. The working muscles can pick up circulating glucose and fatty acids from the blood and metabolize them for energy. Since the trained muscle is better equipped to use fat for energy, it can use more fat for energy than the untrained muscle and can thereby conserve its limited glycogen supply for a longer period of time.

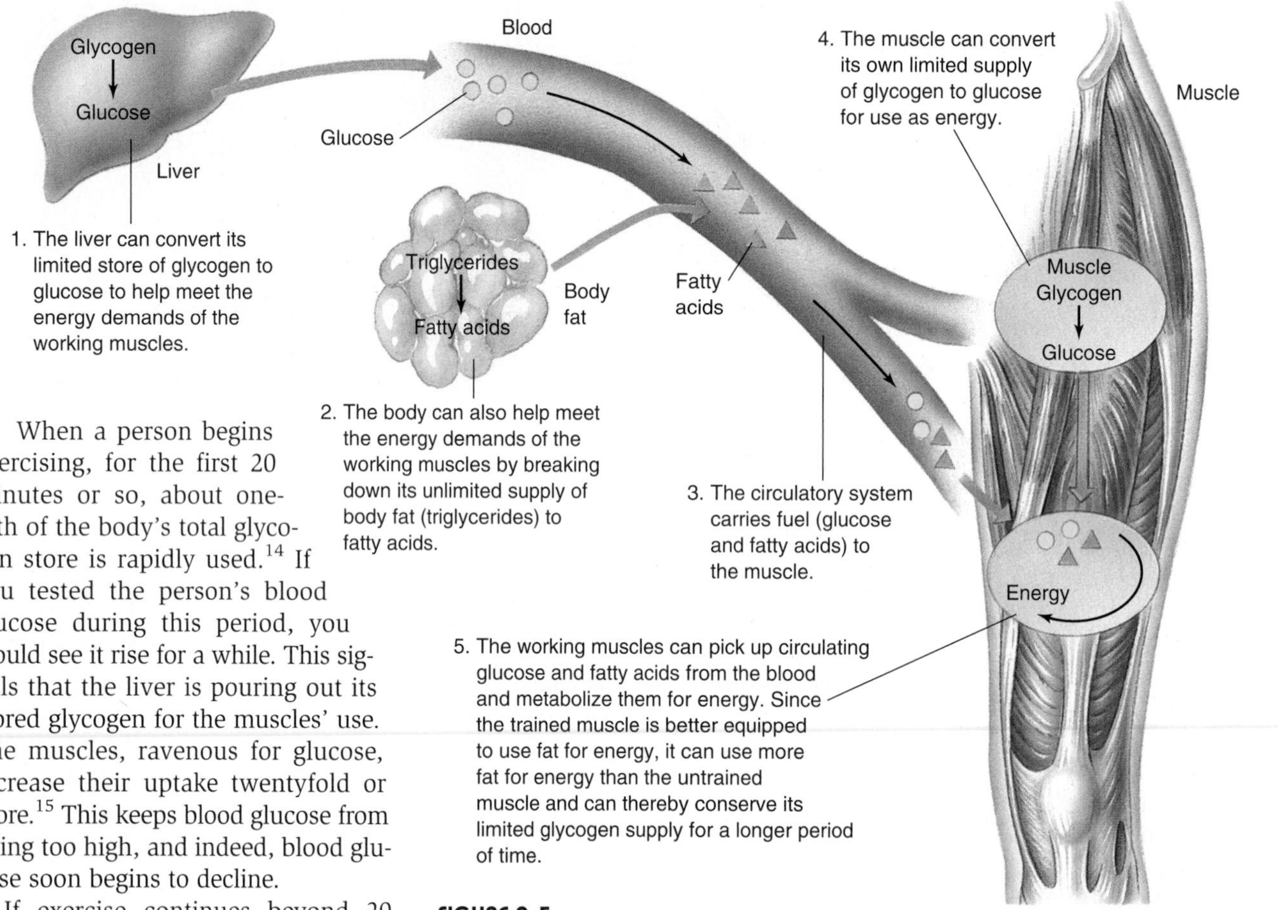

FIGURE 9–5

THE USE OF GLYCOGEN AND BODY FAT FOR ENERGY DURING EXERCISE

Training can increase the amount of glycogen a muscle can conserve during exercise. The more fit a muscle is, the more fat it can burn for energy when oxygen is present—sparing the valuable glycogen.

When a person begins exercising, for the first 20 minutes or so, about one-fifth of the body's total glycogen store is rapidly used.[14] If you tested the person's blood glucose during this period, you would see it rise for a while. This signals that the liver is pouring out its stored glycogen for the muscles' use. The muscles, ravenous for glucose, increase their uptake twentyfold or more.[15] This keeps blood glucose from rising too high, and indeed, blood glucose soon begins to decline.

If exercise continues beyond 20 minutes, glycogen use slows down (see Figure 9–6). To conserve the remaining glycogen supply, the body begins to rely more on fat for fuel. It protects its glycogen supply because without it, muscles simply can't run. Also, without glucose, fat can't be used for energy either. At some point, if exercise continues long enough, glycogen will run out almost completely. People who run out of muscle glycogen during an event (for example, before the finish line in a marathon) "hit the wall"—they have to slow down their pace since muscle glycogen is no longer available to fuel their activity. Exercise can continue for a short time after that, only because the liver scrambles to produce the minimum amount of glucose needed to briefly forestall body shutdown. When blood sugars dip too low, the nervous system function comes almost to a halt, making exercise difficult, if not impossible, although there is still plenty of fat left to burn.

Another factor that influences how much glycogen a person uses during exercise is how well trained the person is to do the particular exercise. When first

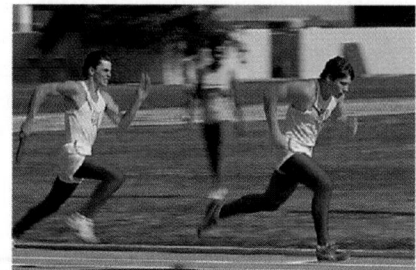

Anaerobic exercise. Glucose is the principal source of energy for activities of high intensity.

attempting an activity, a person uses more glucose than a trained athlete. This is because the muscles can quickly and easily extract energy from glucose. Extracting energy from fat takes longer and requires that the muscle cells contain abundant fat-burning metabolic enzymes. Untrained muscle cells must rely heavily on the quick energy source, glucose; with training, the muscles adapt, packing their cells with more fat-burning enzymes. As a result, trained muscles use more fat and conserve their glucose. Training has another effect: It moderates the initial hormonal response to exercise, so the rate of glucose released from the liver is slower. This, too, conserves glycogen. Finally, the amount of glycogen present in the muscles before exercise influences glycogen use. A later section shows how to store a maximum of glycogen in the muscles (see page 345).

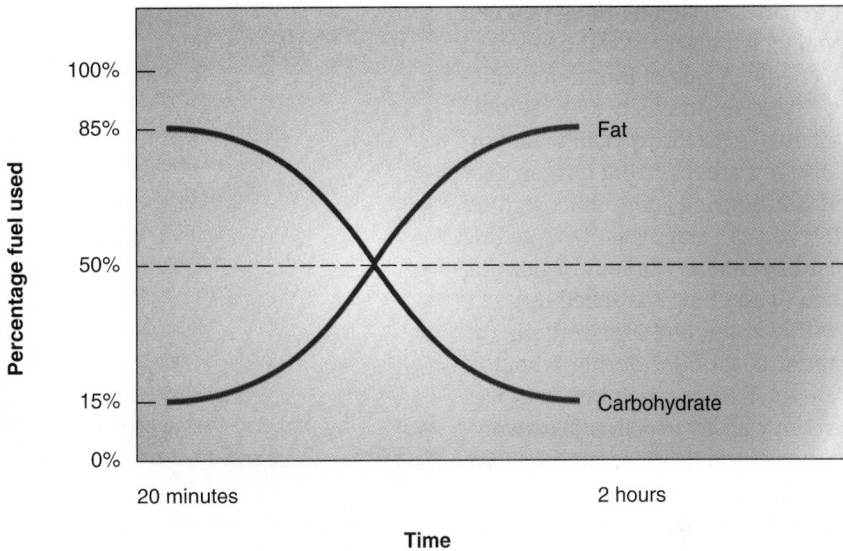

FIGURE 9–6
FUEL USE AND DURATION OF EXERCISE

For most people, fat isn't used much as a fuel for exercise until you've been working out aerobically for at least 20 minutes, and it is not used as a primary fuel until after two hours.

Exercise and Fatty Acids

When you exercise, the fat your muscles burn comes from the fatty deposits all over the body, especially from those with the greatest amounts of fat to spare, such as the abdomen and buttocks. That is why physically fit people look trim all over—they reduce their fat stores all over the body, not just those overlaying the working muscles.

The body can store lots of fat but very little carbohydrate in the form of glycogen. A person who is of desirable body weight may store 25 to 30 pounds of body fat but only about one pound of carbohydrate. Each pound of fat contains about 3,500 calories—more than twice as much as one pound of carbohydrate. You may wonder why body fat can't be used exclusively for energy if fat is such a concentrated source of energy and your body has virtually an unlimited amount. Although your supply of fat is almost unlimited, the ability of your muscles to use fat for energy is not. Fat use depends on a simultaneous supply of glucose from glycogen. An old saying, "Fat burns in the flame of carbohydrate," is true. That's why exercise duration is limited by the supply of carbohydrate, not body fat.

The intensity of the activity also matters.[16] Recall that for a working muscle to burn fat, oxygen must be present. If you work out at a rate that allows your heart to supply ample oxygen to working muscles, the muscles will draw heavily on fat stores for fuel. When exercise intensity outstrips your oxygen supply, fat still contributes as much energy as ever, but glucose pitches in and is burned by the anaerobic pathway. Thus, the percentage of the total energy supplied by

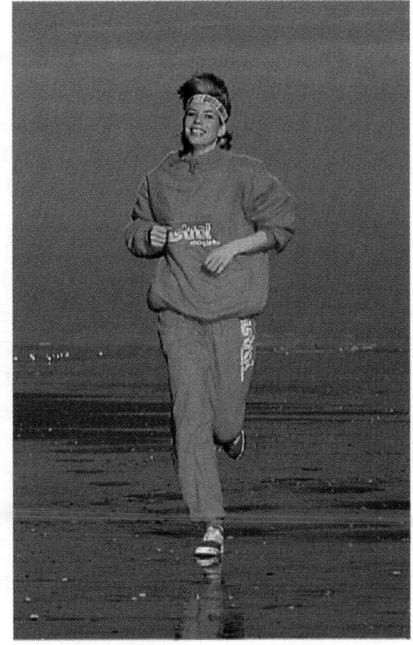

Aerobic exercise. Fats are the main source of energy for activities of low- to moderate-intensity.

fat declines. Your breathing rate can signal which fuel is providing most of the energy. A rule of thumb for gauging exercise intensity for aerobic workouts is this: If you can't talk normally, you are incurring oxygen debt and are burning more glucose than fat; if you can sing, you aren't getting a cardiovascular workout or burning much of anything (so speed up).

Athletic training also controls the amount of fat used during a bout of exercise. Exercise training improves the body's ability to deliver fat to working muscles, and trained muscles have an increased ability to use the fat.

Much attention has been focused on the type of fuel used for varying exercise intensities and duration. Research shows that when athletes exercise at a moderate intensity, they initially use more carbohydrate than fat for fuel.[17] Gradually, as exercise continues for more than 20 minutes, the fuel ratio shifts, and the athletes

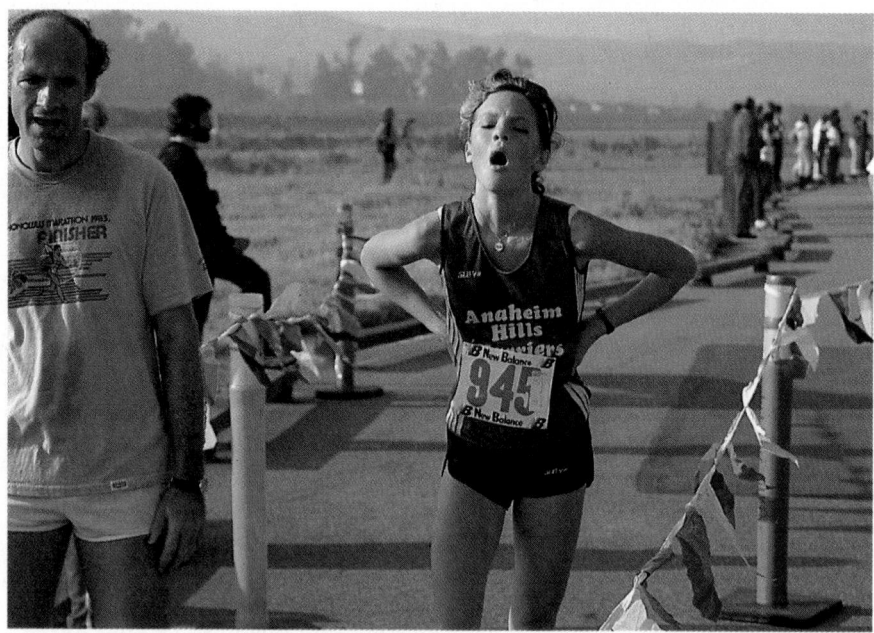

People who participate in endurance events know to build up their reserves of muscle glycogen before an event, so that they do not run out of glycogen—"hit the wall"—before the finish line.

use more fat. For athletes participating in endurance sports, such as marathon runners and long-distance cyclists, who want to conserve their limited supply of carbohydrate, switching to a fat-burning energy system is crucial. However, for people who want to lose weight—body fat—it doesn't matter whether they burn body fat or carbohydrate for energy during exercise. For people trying to lose weight, a calorie burned is a calorie burned, regardless of whether it came from carbohydrate or from fat.

A commonly held misbelief is that you must exercise for at least 20 minutes before you will burn body fat. Recall that your body is always using a combination of glucose and fat for fuel. While it's true that glucose is the primary fuel source during the first 20 minutes or so of exercise, body fat is being burned, too. After 20 minutes, your fuel mixture changes, and you burn more fat than glucose. Body fat stores will shrink and weight will be lost when you expend more energy than you eat, and body fat must be burned to make up for the lack of energy intake. There appears to be no scientific evidence that the type of fuel used for exercise influences weight loss.[18]

Protein Needs for Fitness

Fit people have more muscle than fat; exercise involves muscles; muscles are made largely of protein. It would seem logical, then, that to become or stay fit, an athlete might need more protein. While it's true that fat and glucose are the primary fuels for working muscles, 5 percent to 15 percent of energy needs of weightlifters and athletes competing in endurance sports comes from muscle protein. So, do athletes need more protein?

The body of an athlete may use slightly more protein, especially during the initial stages of training. Initial increases in muscle mass, numbers of red blood cells to carry oxygen, and amounts of aerobic enzymes in muscles to use fuel efficiently may elevate an athlete's protein needs. In addition, hormonal changes during exercise can temporarily slow the amount of protein the muscle makes and can encourage the muscle to break down its protein stores.[19] This combination of using fewer amino acids and breaking down muscle, thereby releasing amino acids, builds up a pool of available amino acids. The circulating blood can then transport some liberated amino acids to the liver, where some can be converted into glucose. The blood then ushers the glucose back to working muscles to feed them. How much protein an athlete uses for fuel during hard exercise (endurance exercise and heavy weightlifting) depends on exercise intensity and duration, the athlete's fitness level, and the glycogen stores in the athlete's muscles. When glycogen stores are well stocked, protein contributes only 5 percent of fuel needs.

Although muscle protein breakdown dominates during exercise, muscle growth escalates after exercise. Muscles use the available amino acids to repair and build. The net effect of these changes is muscle protein buildup. Training enhances muscle protein buildup after exercise.

The American Dietetic Association recommends that athletes consume 1 to 1.5 grams of protein per kilogram of ideal body weight.[20] Some athletes involved in prolonged heavy endurance training may need more than 1.5 grams of protein per kilogram.[21] The recommendation of one gram per kilogram is not much more than the 0.8 gram per kilogram recommended for nonathletes. This is nothing for most athletes to be concerned about, given that the average American eats twice the protein needed.

You might ask whether eating even more protein would help build muscle. Muscles won't respond to excess protein by helplessly accepting it. They respond to the hormones that regulate them and to the demands put upon them. So the way to make muscle cells grow is to put a demand on them—that is, to make them work. They will respond by taking up nutrients—amino acids included—so that they can grow.

In summary, don't push protein at your muscles. Exercise your muscles so that they demand and pull protein in for themselves. Then just eat a healthful diet. (Since athletes generally eat considerably more food than nonathletes eat, their diets may contain three to four times the recommended amount of protein.)

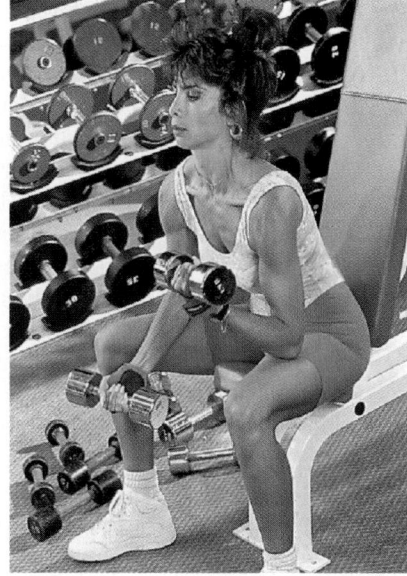

Muscles grow in response to work, not to eating protein.

Energy Needs and Weight Control

Depending on the sport or exercise, a person in active training and competition may have extraordinarily high energy needs. Football players, for example, seem to average close to 6,000 calories a day during the football season, with intakes on some days topping 10,000 calories. Along with the increased energy expenditure goes an increased need for the B vitamins used to generate energy in metabolism. The increased intake, therefore, shouldn't be just any high-calorie food but should be food rich in B vitamins—breads, cereals, fruits, and vegetables. It is a rare individual who can eat more than 5,000 calories of nutritious food in only three meals during a day; eating five to six meals makes the task easier. Food sufficient to provide this much energy will also supply the vitamins and minerals needed to go with it—provided the selection is balanced and varied.

Chapter 8 was devoted to weight control for everyone, but a few words especially for the athlete are appropriate here. First of all, the recommended weight for an athlete is whatever weight and body composition let the athlete perform the best. When the muscles are in top condition for performance of the chosen sport, the amount of body fat and total body weight should be whatever the muscles can carry most easily. Too little fat can make the body susceptible to too-rapid heat loss; too much creates a drag on motion.

Great variation in body composition exists among athletes of various sports (see Table 9–1). Body fat content of world-class male runners ranges from 4 percent to 9 percent—the less fat a runner has, the less he or she has to transport while running. Some professional football defensive backs have been measured with body fat levels as low as one percent of body weight.

Sometimes seasonal sports or competitions require that an athlete gain or lose weight. The healthful way to gain weight is to build oneself up by patient and consistent training while eating nutritious foods containing enough extra calories to support the weight gain. A pound of muscle mass contains about 2,500 to 3,000 calories' worth of material. To gain a pound of muscle requires about a week of hard workouts along with an energy intake 3,000 calories above the amount sufficient to support that work. Eating two or three snacks of complex carbohydrate-rich, low-fat foods between meals can add 700 to 800 extra calories to a person's daily intake. This, together with strength-training workouts, will support a weight gain of one to one and a half pounds, mostly muscle, in a week. A later section in this chapter, Food for Fitness, illustrates how to plan meals and snacks for exercisers.

Athletes need to remember to cut down on calories between and after training periods. Otherwise, these calories will be stored as fat unless they are expended in activity. It should be no surprise, then, that a heavily muscled 20-year-old who stops working out but keeps on eating like a football player in training can become flabby and obese at age 30. It is not literally true that the person's muscle has turned to fat, but it is true that muscle has been lost and fat has been gained.

Losing weight, like gaining it, can be done wisely or unwisely. The goal is to lose primarily body fat. All people, including athletes, should be wary of techniques such as sauna bathing, using diuretics or laxatives, or inducing vomiting, all of which achieve fast weight loss by causing dehydration. As athletes know, dehydration seriously impairs performance. The hazards of fasts and fad diets were described in Chapter 8, but a reminder should be repeated here. What is achieved by quick weight-loss dieting is loss of lean tissue, glycogen, bone minerals, and fluids—all materials vital to healthy body functioning. Abnormal heart rhythms have been seen in healthy adults after only ten days of

TABLE 9–1
AVERAGE PERCENTAGE OF BODY FAT

	MALES	FEMALES
NONATHLETES		
Lean	<8%	<13%
Optimal	8–15%	13–20%
Slightly overfat	16–20%	21–25%
Fat	21–24%	26–32%
Obese (overfat)	>25%	>32%
ATHLETES		
Long-distance runners	4–9%	6–15%
Wrestlers	4–10%	—
Gymnasts	4–10%	10–17%
Elite bodybuilders	6–10%	10–17%
Swimmers	5–11%	14–24%
Basketball players	7–11%	18–27%
Tennis players	14–17%	19–22%

SOURCE: Adapted from D. C. Nieman, *Fitness and Sports Medicine: An Introduction* (Palo Alto, Calif.: Bull, 1990), p. 126.

fasting. Weight loss of about two pounds per week achieved by calorie control and exercise will encourage fat loss. The American College of Sports Medicine's exercise prescription for weight loss is similar to the one for cardiovascular conditioning.[22] It recommends participating in aerobic exercise (such as brisk walking, jogging, bicycling, swimming, aerobic dance) three to five times a week at a moderate intensity (60 percent to 85 percent of maximum heart rate) for 20 to 60 minutes. Strength training also helps with weight loss by increasing lean muscle mass and thus increasing a person's resting metabolic rate.[23]

Before leaving the issue of energy expenditure, let's look at the issues surrounding elevated calorie burning after exercise and elevated resting metabolic rate. Regular exercise can cause a relatively permanent increase in resting metabolic rate.[24] Researchers have shown that fit individuals do expend more calories at rest. Such expenditure is most likely because of their having a greater portion of muscle than fat; muscle burns more calories than fat.[25] Once again, the benefits of exercise come from doing it.

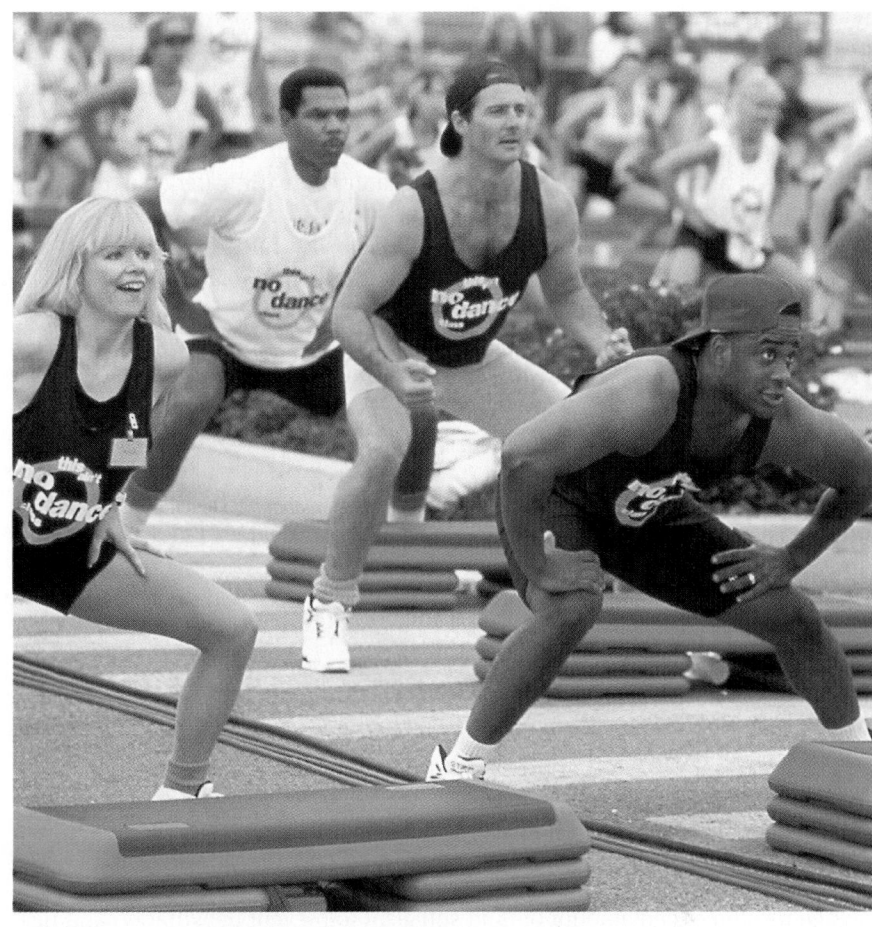

Aerobic exercise burns body fat and contributes to weight control.

Fluid Needs and Exercise

Replenishing fluid lost during exercise is easily accomplished by drinking fluid before, during, and after exercise. Yet many athletes and fitness enthusiasts either don't drink enough or don't drink at all.[26] Ignoring body fluid needs can hinder performance and increase risk of heat-related injury.[27] This section reviews both why your body needs fluids during exercise and how much and what to drink.

Water and Exercise

The water in your blood—known as plasma volume, or just plasma—serves a similar function as the water in the radiator of your car. It continually circulates throughout your body, picking up the tremendous amount of heat generated by working muscles. The plasma then transports this heat to your skin, through which the heat is expelled from the body primarily by evaporation of sweat. Think of sweating as your body's air-conditioning system. As sweat evaporates from your skin, it expels large amounts of heat, helping to keep your body cool. However, sweating works only when the sweat is evaporated from your skin. If the sweat simply rolls down your face or down your back, body heat is not released. On a humid day, the air is already saturated with water, which impairs evaporation of sweat from your skin. Hot, humid days, then, are doubly dangerous: You continue to sweat and lose precious body water, but your body temperature doesn't fall. You need to pay particular attention to your fluid needs on humid days.

Sweat is the primary way your body loses water during exercise. How much sweat you lose depends on the intensity and duration of the activity. The more intense the exercise, the more heat you generate and the more sweat you will lose. If you don't replace the water you lose from sweat, your plasma volume decreases. In an attempt to maintain plasma volume, your body will pull water from your muscles and organs. Since approximately 45 percent of total body water is stored in muscle, muscle contributes the greatest amount of water to maintain plasma volume.[28] As water is pulled from muscles, cramps may occur, along with premature fatigue. The complex reactions that produce energy in muscles must occur in a water medium. Thus, a lack of water compromises the muscles' ability to fuel the activity and results in noticeable decline in performance.

Lower plasma levels also force your heart to beat faster. Since the heart pumps less blood with each beat, it must beat more often to supply oxygen to your muscles. Finally, with less plasma available to transport the heat to your skin, the heat builds, and your body's internal temperature continues to rise. All these changes force your body to work at a higher intensity level, leading to early exhaustion. A water loss equal to 5 percent of body weight can reduce muscular work capacity by 20 percent to 30 percent.

The recommended amount of fluid sufficient to prevent dehydration and **heat stroke** can be quite a bit. Athletes can lose two to four quarts of fluid during every hour of heavy exercise and must rehydrate before, during, and after exercise to replace the lost fluid. Even casual exercisers must drink some fluids while exercising. Thirst is unreliable as an indicator of how much to drink—it signals too late, after fluid stores are depleted.[29] If you wait to drink until you are thirsty, you've waited too long! Table 9–2 presents one schedule of hydration before, during, and after exercise. To know how much water is needed to replenish fluid losses after a workout, weigh yourself before and after—the difference is all water. One pound equals roughly two cups of fluid.

Water and Fluid-Replacement Drinks

For fitness enthusiasts, the choice between water and a sports drink (a properly balanced carbohydrate-electrolyte fluid-replacement drink) is more a matter of personal taste and desired performance abilities. But for endurance events (continuous exercise for longer than 90 minutes), mounting evidence indicates that consuming a properly balanced sports drink during exercise enhances energy status and endurance and maintains plasma volume levels better than drinking water does.[30]

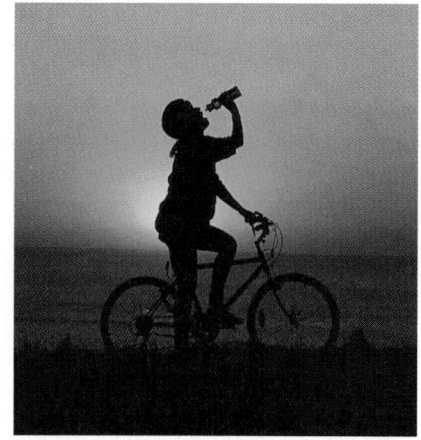

Plan to drink fluids before, during, and after exercise.

HEAT STROKE an acute and dangerous reaction to heat buildup in the body.

TABLE 9–2
SCHEDULE OF HYDRATION BEFORE, DURING, AND AFTER EXERCISE

WHEN TO DRINK	AMOUNT OF FLUID
2 hours before exercise	About 3 c
10 to 15 minutes before exercise	About 2 c
Every 15 minutes during exercise	1 c (about 1 qt per hour)
After exercise	2 c fluid for each pound of body weight lost

SOURCE: A. L. Hecker, "Nutrition and Physical Performance," in *Drugs and Performance in Sports*, R. H. Strauss ed. (Philadelphia: W. B. Saunders, 1987), pp. 23–52.

TABLE 9–3
FLUID-REPLACEMENT DRINKS

SPORTS DRINK	CALORIES/CUP	CARBOHYDRATE PERCENTAGE	CARBOHYDRATE TYPE	SODIUM
Body Fuel	70	7.0%	Glucose polymer, fructose	70 mg
Exceed	70	7.0%	Glucose polymer, fructose	50 mg
Gatorade	70	6.0%	Sucrose, glucose	110 mg
10-K Thirst Quencher	60	6.5%	Sucrose, fructose, and glucose	54 mg
Powerade	70	7.0%	High fructose corn syrup	55 mg

How the body manages water and carbohydrate use during exercise determines how well it performs. Sports drinks are designed to enhance the body's use of carbohydrate and water (see Table 9–3). The carbohydrate in a sports beverage serves three purposes during exercise: (1) it becomes an energy source for working muscles; (2) it helps maintain blood glucose at an optimum level; and (3) it helps increase the rate of water absorption from the small intestine, helping to better maintain plasma volume. In addition, the drink can supply water and minerals lost from sweating.[31]

There are many factors to consider when choosing a sports drink. The ideal beverage should leave the digestive tract rapidly and enter circulation, where it is needed. Carbohydrate solutions don't all empty from the stomach at the same rate. The drink should contain at least 5 percent but no more than 7 percent carbohydrate by volume (50 grams of carbohydrate per quart). Drinks containing more than 10 percent carbohydrate, such as sodas, fruit juice, Kool-Aid types of drinks, and some sports drinks, take longer to absorb. They also can cause cramps, nausea, bloating, and diarrhea. Drinks with less than 5 percent carbohydrate may not offer an endurance-enhancing effect. Drinks using a blend of glucose polymers—short chains of carbohydrate—and fructose leave the stomach at the same rate as water, speeding the availability of the carbohydrate and water to working muscles.[32]

Sodium is another ingredient to pay attention to. Since most people eat enough salt in their regular diet to replace the sodium they lose during exercise, it's not essential that the fluid-replacement drink provide large amounts of sodium. In fact, too much sodium can delay muscles' receipt of water.

Research shows that about 50 milligrams of sodium per cup will help stimulate water absorption from your gut. Other studies have found that people who drink a beverage with some sodium drink more of it. If the drink tastes good, athletes and exercisers will want to drink it and so meet their fluid needs.[33]

There are several practical considerations to keep in mind when using an energy drink. The drink should be consumed cold, in 4-ounce to 8-ounce portions, and frequently (every 15 to 20 minutes *once exercise begins*). Cooled beverages leave the digestive tract quickly to supply water to muscles and cool the body. Competitive athletes should establish fluid consumption patterns during practice. An athletic event is not the time to try a new product or employ a new system of drinking.

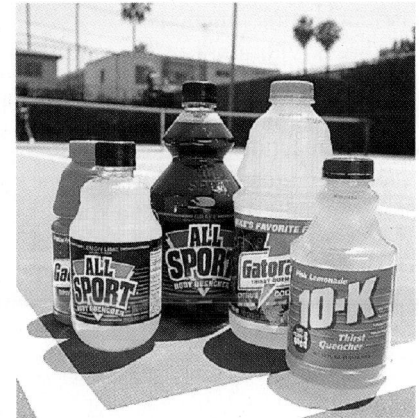

Sports drinks can enhance energy status during endurance events.

In summary, water is always an adequate fluid-replacement beverage. However, if a proper sports drink is available, endurance athletes should consider it as a fluid-replacement beverage particularly if they prefer the taste. For people who are exercising to lose weight, however, drinking a quart of a sports drink to meet fluid needs may supply the amount of calories they expended during a 40-minute aerobic class or in 30 minutes of continuous swimming or biking. The choice to drink a sports drink or water is, of course, up to the individual.

As for salt loss, when the exercise is over, eating regular food can make it up. Salt tablets are not recommended because they increase potassium losses and can irritate the stomach. After exercise, the replacement of magnesium and potassium may be more important than the replacement of sodium. Potassium is abundant in fruits, fruit juices, and fresh vegetables; unprocessed foods of all kinds are especially good sources of both potassium and magnesium.

Vitamins and Minerals for Exercise

Your muscles burn food and oxygen to make energy. How well they burn these fuels depends, however, on your supply of vitamins and minerals. Without small amounts of these potent substances, your muscles' ability to work is compromised.

The Vitamins

Vitamins are the links and regulators of energy-producing and muscle-building pathways. Without them, your muscles' ability to convert food energy to body energy is hindered and muscle protein formation is slowed. Table 9–4 shows a few vitamins and minerals and their exercise-supporting functions.

The B vitamins are of special interest to athletes and exercisers because they govern the energy-producing reactions of metabolism. Needs for these vitamins increase proportionally with energy expenditure. A person who expends 4,000 calories per day needs twice as much of the B vitamins as someone who expends 2,000 calories.

Many athletes have been falsely led to believe that they can enhance energy production by taking supplements of B vitamins. No experimental evidence exists to support this theory.[34] Once the system that uses B

TABLE 9–4
EXERCISE-RELATED FUNCTIONS OF VITAMINS AND MINERALS

VITAMIN OR MINERAL	FUNCTION
Thiamin, riboflavin, niacin, magnesium	Energy-releasing reactions.
Vitamin B_6, zinc	Building of muscle protein.
Folate, vitamin B_{12}	Building of red blood cells to carry oxygen.
Vitamin C	Collagen formation for joint and other tissue integrity; hormone synthesis.
Vitamin E	Protect cell membranes from oxidative damage.
Iron	Transport of oxygen in blood and in muscle tissue; energy transformation reactions.
Calcium, vitamin D, vitamin A, phosphorus	Building of bone structure; muscle contractions; nerve transmissions.
Sodium, potassium, chloride	Maintenance of fluid balance; transmission of nerve impulses for muscle contraction.
Chromium	Assistance in insulin's energy-storage function.
Magnesium	Cardiac and other muscle contraction.

NOTE: This is just a sampling. All vitamins and minerals play indispensable roles in exercise.

vitamins is full, generally the extra vitamins will be washed away through the urine. A well-balanced diet that meets athletes' energy needs and that features complex carbohydrate-rich foods will ensure B vitamin intakes proportional to energy intake.

Researchers are presently studying the protective effects of antioxidants on recovery from exercise and performance. Since the body uses oxygen at a higher rate during exercise, the generation of free radicals and the potential for exercise-induced tissue damage increase in the body. Although more research is needed, preliminary studies support a role for the antioxidant nutrients—particularly vitamin E—in enhancing recovery from exercise by reducing exercise-induced oxidative injury.[35] The evidence for any role of the antioxidants in improving performance is inconsistent thus far.[36]

The Minerals

Iron is a core component of the body's oxygen taxi service: hemoglobin and myoglobin. A lack of oxygen compromises the muscles' ability to perform. Iron deficiency has not been reported to be a problem for fitness enthusiasts who exercise moderately.[37] Male and female endurance athletes, though, may be prone to developing mild iron deficiency, diagnosed by low blood ferritin levels, a measure of the body's store of iron. Menstruating female athletes are at particular risk—growth and menstruation combined with strenuous training can take a toll on a woman's iron stores.[38]

A combination of factors increases an athlete's chances of depleting his or her iron stores. Inadequate dietary intakes of iron-rich foods combined with iron losses aggravated by physical activity compromise iron status. Physical activity may cause increased iron losses in sweat, feces, and urine, plus increased destruction of red blood cells that occurs during exercise. Preparing meals with adequate iron requires careful planning. Iron-rich meals include meats, legumes, and dark green vegetables combined with absorption-enhancing factors such as (again) meats and foods rich in vitamin C. Chapter 7 contains numerous suggestions for obtaining sufficient iron from foods.

Sometimes iron deficiencies can be corrected only with iron supplements. If you are concerned about your iron level, see a physician. Iron supplements should not be taken without medical supervision. High iron intakes can induce deficiencies of trace minerals, such as copper and zinc, and produce an iron overload in some people.

An apparent anemia—sometimes called "sports anemia"—also can occur in athletes that reflects no reduction in the blood's iron supply, but rather an increase in the blood plasma volume.[39] This occurs because athletic training causes the kidneys to conserve sodium and water. In other words, the extra blood volume dilutes the concentration of iron, thereby making it seem as if the blood does not contain enough of the mineral. The causes of sports anemia have not yet been determined, but this temporary state probably reflects a normal adaptation to physical training.

Adequate electrolytes are essential for fluid balance, a crucial factor in athletic performance. When sodium is retained, potassium is lost. There has been some concern that potassium depletion might occur in people who engage in vigorous activity day after day, particularly if the activity involves sweating. The ordinary nutritious diet can easily supply enough potassium to cover the athlete's needs. (Chapter 7 offers more on this subject.)

This brief treatment of vitamins and minerals for the athlete is intended to show the importance of proper nutrition for athletes. It is not meant to imply that special supplements are needed, except for diagnosed medical conditions (the upcoming Nutrition Action feature provides more information about supplements that athletes sometimes use). A diet composed of a variety of nutritious foods offers the best support for athletic performance.

The Bones and Exercise

Bones absorb great stresses during exercise, and like the muscles, they respond by growing thicker and stronger. Weight-bearing exercises—running, walking, dancing, rope skipping, or activities such as strength training in which significant muscular force can be generated against the long bones of the body—encourage bone development. A bone not strong enough to withstand the strain placed on it by athletic exertion can break in what has become known as a **stress fracture.** When a person suffers such a break, there are three probable causes. One is unbalanced muscle development, which allows strong muscles to pull against the bone opposed only by weaker, undeveloped muscles, thereby leaving the bone susceptible to fractures. Another is bone weakness caused by inadequate calcium intake. A possible third cause, which occurs in women, is reduced estrogen concentration, which leads to bone mineral loss and therefore to fragile bones in women who have ceased menstruating.

STRESS FRACTURE bone damage or breakage caused by stress on bone surfaces during exercise.

Balanced muscle development can protect the bones from undue stresses. Each set of muscles pulling against bone should be kept in check by an equally strong set of opposing muscles. You should not work a set of muscles in training without working the opposing muscles. So if you work your back and leg muscles a lot (by jogging or walking, for example), work your abdominal muscles too (do situps). Bones, like muscles, take time to develop strength. Giving bones and muscles plenty of time to build up to one level of performance before moving up to the next level can also prevent stress fractures.

Eating an adequate amount of calcium throughout life may be one of the primary defenses against developing weak bones.[40] The ideal sources of dietary calcium are milk and milk products and other calcium-containing foods, not calcium supplements. (Refer to Chapter 7 for more information.)

Some women who exercise strenuously cease to menstruate, a condition called **athletic amenorrhea.** Such women have lower than normal amounts of estrogen, a hormone essential for maintaining the integrity of the bones. With low estrogen levels, the mineral structures of the bones are rapidly dismantled, weakening the skeleton. Women who have athletic amenorrhea are at risk for stress fractures now and adult bone loss later in life.[41] To reverse the condition, they should not stop exercising altogether, for reasonable amounts of exercise may be a key defense against bone depletion. They should, however, seek evaluation from a health-care provider who specializes in sports medicine to find the cause of and receive treatment for their amenorrhea.

ATHLETIC AMENORRHEA cessation of menstruation associated with strenuous athletic training.

Eating disorders are sometimes related to athletic amenorrhea, and a logical part of diagnosis is to look carefully at the woman's diet for adequacy.[42] It could be that a diet too low in calories, coupled with low body fat stores and strenuous exercise, sets the stage for athletic amenorrhea to develop. In such cases, calcium intakes between 1,000 and 1,500 milligrams per day may help to protect the bones somewhat.[43]

Athletes and Supplements: Help or Hype?

Competitors in the ancient Greek Olympiad reportedly used mushrooms and herbs.[44] Since then, virtually every food has at one time or another been touted as the "magic bullet" that will enhance performance. Athletes have been known to swallow everything from bee pollen to brewer's yeast to kelp to wheat germ in their quest to gain the competitive edge.

Nutritional Supplements as Ergogenic Aids

Seductive as the idea of using pills and potions to achieve peak performance may be, the scientific evidence to support claims that special supplements will make an athlete run farther or jump higher is sorely lacking.[45] Most so-called **ergogenic aids,** that is, substances that increase the ability to exercise harder, are costly versions of vitamins, minerals, sugar, and other nutrients provided easily by a balanced diet.[46]

Take bee pollen, a mixture of protein, carbohydrate, a bit of fat, and a few vitamins and minerals.[47] Though touted by one manufacturer as a "natural and balanced source of extra energy" appreciated by "athletes worldwide," it has been tested at Louisiana State University among both runners and swimmers and found to confer no benefit whatsoever on an athlete's training or performance abilities.[48] The same goes for chromium picolinate, touted to increase lean body mass and delay fatigue due to its role in glucose utilization. While chromium is necessary for muscle function by transfering glucose from the blood to the muscle cells, true chromium deficiencies are rare to nonexistent. To date, there is no evidence that chromium supplements improve athletic performance in healthy individuals without a chromium deficiency.

Surveys of athletes have found that between 53 percent and 80 percent use a vitamin or mineral supplement, although no evidence exists that doing so improves performance.[49] More than 40 years of research has provided no strong evidence that popping vitamins and minerals increases energy or athletic prowess

ERGOGENIC AIDS anything that helps to increase the capacity to work or exercise.
ergo = work
genic = give rise to

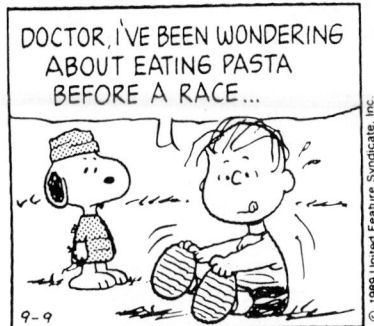
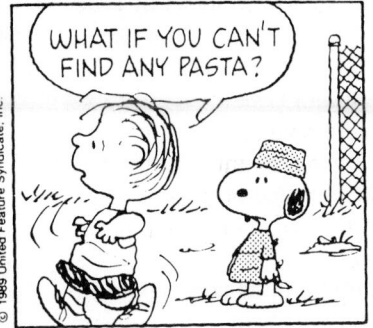
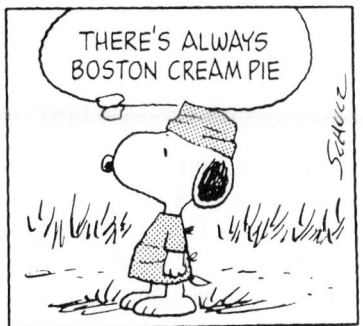

PEANUTS reprinted by permission of UFS, Inc.

of adequately nourished people. Except for iron, vitamin and mineral deficiencies are rare among athletes. Since most athletes eat more food than nonathletes eat to meet their increased energy demands, they usually get the additional vitamins and minerals they need, provided they eat a well-balanced diet.

An ordinary multivitamin and mineral supplement might be prudent in one instance: when an athlete's need for energy outstrips the ability to eat the quantity of food required to supply it. Then, many athletes must turn to concentrated energy sources, such as sugars and fats. While such foods supply abundant energy, they are practically devoid of vitamins and minerals—thus, they are commonly referred to as empty-calorie foods. The energy they supply, though, requires processing by vitamin- and mineral-containing enzymes. For a short time, say, during the heaviest training, a supplement may be appropriate. It's best to choose one based on the Consumer Tips feature on page 221 in Chapter 6. Don't be led astray by the word *athlete* or *fitness* on a label.

Of course, when athletes firmly hold that one or another ergogenic aid does indeed improve performance, convincing them otherwise can be extremely difficult. One reason is that the profound belief that a substance will help can actually produce a psychological benefit, known as the **placebo effect.**

Anabolic Steroids: Use and Abuse

Psychological impact aside, pill popping may be harmful in some cases. Taking large doses of vitamin A or D, for example, can cause liver damage over time. Swallowing supplements known as **anabolic steroids**—synthetic hormones that appear to help build muscle—can be even more dangerous.

A particularly popular practice among weightlifters and bodybuilders, steroid abuse often begins around the age of 18 years.[51] But while steroids may help to increase muscular size and strength in some people, they can bring about numerous side effects, including acne, liver abnormalities, temporary infertility, and offensive outbursts, often referred to as roid rages.

Among adults, many effects of steroid use are reversible. Unfortunately, adolescents aren't so lucky. Several studies show that adolescent steroid users may suffer serious consequences of premature skeletal maturation, decreased spermatogenesis, and elevated risk of injury.[52]

Along with being unhealthful, steroid use is considered unethical by domestic and international sports organizations such as the American College of Sports Medicine and the International Olympic Committee. As a case in point, track star Ben Johnson lost his Olympic gold medal for the 100-meter sprint in 1988 after officials discovered he had been using steroids.[53]

Amino Acid Supplements and the Athlete

Many athletes also swallow amino acid supplements in hopes of building larger muscles. These supplements are advertised as "pre-digested protein" and so supposedly are easily absorbed and readily available to encourage muscle growth brought on by training. Let's look at the facts.

Your intestinal tract is better prepared to handle protein in its complex form of di- and tripeptides (refer to Chapter 5). You absorb 85 percent to 99 percent

PLACEBO EFFECT an improvement in a person's sense of well-being or physical health in response to the use of a placebo (a substance having no medicinal properties or medicinal effects).

ANABOLIC STEROIDS synthetic male hormones with a chemical structure similar to that of cholesterol; such hormones have wide-ranging effects on body functioning.

Side effects of steroids:[50]

acne
anxiety
blood clots
blood poisoning
cancer
diarrhea
dizziness
fatigue
heart disease
hypertension
irreversible baldness in women
jaundice
kidney damage
liver disease
male pattern baldness
mood swings
nausea
oily skin
prostate enlargement
psychotic depression
shrunken testicles
sterility (reversible)
stroke
stunted growth in adolescents
swelling of feet or lower legs
yellowing of the eyes or skin

of the animal protein you eat and 90 percent of protein from vegetable sources. Amino acid solutions, on the other hand, will draw water into your gut, and their digestion can cause cramping and diarrhea.

In addition, your body can't store extra amino acids, whether they come from food you eat or from supplements. Your body converts the excess into fat. This conversion of amino acids to fat generates urea, which increases your body's need for water. Both diarrhea and increased urination of urea can lead to dehydration, impeding training and performance.

There is no benefit to rapid absorption of amino acids. It takes your body hours, not minutes, to rebuild muscle protein damaged by exercise. And as mentioned before, most athletes already eat more protein than they need.

Caffeine, Alcohol, and Performance

Some athletes look to other dietary means besides pill popping to promote athletic prowess. For instance, many exercisers drink caffeine-containing beverages such as coffee, tea, or cola to enhance performance and endurance. Caffeine apparently stimulates the release of fats into the blood that the body can then use instead of glycogen as a source of energy. Thus, the glycogen is "spared," or saved, for later use, and the amount of time an exerciser can endure physical activity before running out of fuel is prolonged.

The glycogen-sparing effect of caffeine, however, is beneficial only for athletes who exercise for more than one and a half to two hours at a time. As we said earlier, the muscles generally store enough glycogen to fuel as many as 90 minutes of activity. Moreover, even endurance athletes can experience certain downsides to consuming caffeine. A diuretic, the drug promotes frequent urination and fluid loss that can lead to dehydration. In addition, caffeine can induce rapid heart rate and jitters, which can interfere with performance. Athletes would also do well to remember that caffeine is a drug that neither the American College of Sports Medicine nor the International Olympic Committee condones for use among athletes.

Along with caffeinated beverages, alcoholic drinks are often touted as choice fluids for athletes. Beer, for example, is sometimes portrayed as the perfect carbohydrate-containing complement to both before- and after-competition meals. Despite such images, alcoholic drinks rank as poor sources of fluid and energy for several reasons. For one, alcohol is a diuretic that can bring about fluid loss and dehydration. More importantly, the amount of alcohol in just one beer or glass of wine depresses the nervous system, thereby slowing an athlete's reaction time and interfering with reflexes and coordination. Also, one can of beer provides only 50 carbohydrate calories. The rest of the calories come from alcohol, which must be metabolized by your liver, not your muscles. The American College of Sports Medicine and the American Dietetic Association both conclude that use of alcohol hinders performance. (The Spotlight feature later in the chapter presents a detailed explanation of how alcohol affects the body.)

The special supplements and drinks discussed here are just a sampling of the many "magic" pills and potions promoted to athletes. If you're in doubt about a particular product you see boasted as an ergogenic aid, use the Fitness Quackery Scorecard to separate legitimate claims from bogus ones.

Here are a few questions to ask yourself about any health gimmick, product, or device that you see advertised or that someone tries to sell you. Every yes answer gets one point:

1. Is the promised action of the product based on magical thinking? ("Eat all you want and lose weight." "Develop a trim body with no exercise.")

2. Does the promotion claim that "doctors agree" or "research has determined," without clarification? (Which doctors? What research?)

3. Does the promotion state that hormones, drugs, or nutrient doses useful in correcting an abnormal condition are needed to make the normal, healthy person more fit?

4. Does the promoter use scare tactics to pressure you into buying the product? ("It's the only one available without poisons.")

5. Is the product being sold or promoted by a crusading organization, a faith-healing group, or a self-styled health adviser who has no acceptable credentials?

6. Is the product advertised as having a multitude of different beneficial effects? ("Makes bigger muscles; gives that pumped-up feeling, improves digestion, coordination, and breathing.")

7. Does the sponsor claim persecution by the medical community and the government because they do not accept this wonderful discovery?

8. Is the product available only from the sponsor by mail order and with payment in advance?

9. Does the promoter use many case histories or testimonials from grateful users?

10. Is the product a special or "secret" formula not available from any other source?

Scoring: Even 1 point is a point against the claimant: it's your warning signal that you are dealing with misinformation. Three or more points is a sure sign of quackery.

Food for Fitness

The best nutrition prescription for peak performance is a well-balanced diet. Although no one eating plan meets every athlete's needs, certain fundamental components are common to all well-balanced diets. For athletes, the diet should account for increased energy needs, vitamin/mineral needs, the relative efficiency of various foods as fuels, and current knowledge about long-term health. An eating plan that supplies 60 percent of calories from complex carbohydrate, 15 percent of calories from protein, and 25 percent of calories from fat will enable both athletes and fitness enthusiasts to supply muscles with a proper fuel mix and maintain health.[54] Two critical nutrition periods for the athlete are the training diet and the precompetition diet.

Planning the Diet

A diet rich in complex carbohydrate and low in fat not only provides the best balance of nutrients for health but also supports physical activity best, as Figure 9–7 shows. Athletes should consume a significant proportion of their day's calories before beginning physical activities. This will assure that muscle fuel needs are met during exercise.

Following the diet prescription in Figure 9–7 will provide athletes' muscles with enough glycogen to support exercise. For the casual exerciser who participates in low- to moderate-intensity activities (walking, bicycling, dancing), the activity is rarely sufficient to totally deplete glycogen stores. Carbohydrate loading—a practice endurance athletes follow to trick their muscles into storing extra glycogen—may not be beneficial for people who exercise less than 90 minutes per workout at a low intensity, although competitive athletes who exercise at a high intensity for more than 90 minutes at a time may benefit from carbohydrate loading. Muscles typically have enough glycogen to fuel one-and-a-half to two-hour bouts of activity.

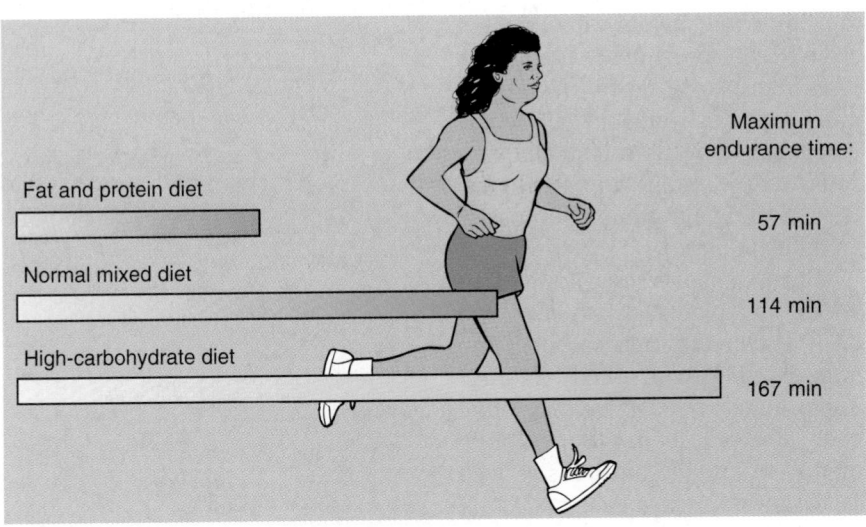

FIGURE 9–7   THE EFFECT OF DIET ON PHYSICAL ENDURANCE
A high-carbohydrate diet can increase an athlete's endurance. In this study, the fat and protein diet provided 94 percent of calories from fat and 6 percent from protein; the normal mixed diet provided 55 percent of calories from carbohydrate; and the high-carbohydrate diet provided 83 percent of calories from carbohydrate.

Fat and protein diet — 57 min
Normal mixed diet — 114 min
High-carbohydrate diet — 167 min
Maximum endurance time:

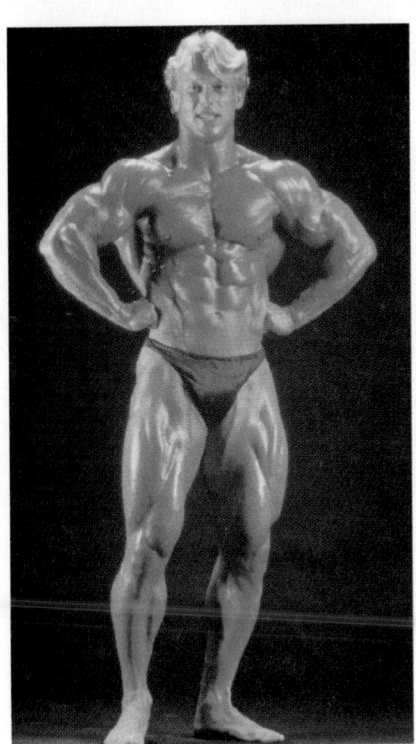

This is a body that vegetable foods maintain: Andreas Cahling, a vegetarian.

An athlete who follows the glycogen-loading technique in preparation for an upcoming event will first exercise intensely without restricting carbohydrates, then gradually cut back on exercise the week before the competition, rest completely the day before, and eat a very-high-carbohydrate diet.

Endurance athletes who follow this plan can keep going longer than their competitors without ill effects.[55] In a hot climate, extra glycogen offers an additional advantage. As glycogen breaks down, it releases water, which helps to meet the athlete's fluid needs.

For people who exercise less than 90 minutes per session, such extremes in glycogen storage are unnecessary. Glycogen isn't likely to run out in short exercise sessions, no matter how intense. All that is necessary to provide consistently full glycogen stores for workouts is to eat a balanced diet based on the Food Guide Pyramid and allow muscle groups to recover fully before working them again. Full recovery of glycogen stores takes from 24 to 48 hours. This doesn't mean you can work out only every other day. It means you should vary your exercise routine from day to day to work different groups of muscles on different days.

Table 9–5 shows some sample balanced diet plans for athletes who wish to increase their carbohydrate intake along with their calories. These plans are effective only if the user chooses foods (not supplements) to provide nutrients as well as calories—extra milk for calcium and riboflavin, many vegetables for B vitamins, meat or alternates for iron and other vitamins and minerals, and whole grains for magnesium and chromium. In addition, these foods provide plenty of sodium, potassium, and chloride. The photos in Figure 9–8 provide examples of high-carbohydrate meals for the athlete.

TABLE 9–5

HIGH-CARBOHYDRATE EATING PATTERNS FOR VARIOUS ENERGY LEVELS

Use the number of portions indicated to arrive at the specified energy levels.[a]

FOOD GROUP	CALORIE LEVEL					
	1,500	2,000	2,500	3,000	3,500	4,000
Milk	3	3	4	4	4	4
Fruit	5	6	7	9	10	12
Vegetable	3	3	3	5	6	7
Grain	7	11	16	18	20	24
Fat[b]	2	3	5	6	8	10
Meat[c]	5	5	5	5	6	6
Percentage of carbohydrate:	58%	58%	63%	64%	60%	62%

[a]Refer to Chapter 2, Figure 2-7 for portion sizes.
[b]A serving of fat is equivalent to 1 tsp butter, margarine, or oil.
[c]Meat portions are given as total ounces of meat; a typical serving includes 2 to 3 ounces.
NOTE: These plans supply 58% to 64% of calories as carbohydrate and less than 30% as fat. To increase the carbohydrate content to over 64%, substitute ½-c servings of legumes for the meats. People who cannot eat these quantities of whole foods may have to replace some of them with milkshakes or liquid-meal replacements to meet their energy needs.

Up to a point, adding more carbohydrate-rich foods is a sound and reasonable option for increasing calories. The point at which it becomes unreasonable is when the calories needed by the individual outstrip the ability to eat that much food. At that point, the person must find ways of adding calories to the diet. After the athlete has met the required number of servings from fruits, vegetables, grains, and dairy products, extra sugars and even some fat may be used to make up the caloric need. A homemade milkshake made with nonfat milk, ice milk, malted milk powder, and half a cup of fresh or frozen fruit can add 300 or more calories to the day's intake. High-carbohydrate liquid nutritional supplements also are available on the market.

An athlete may be able to eat more food by consuming it in six or eight meals each day rather than in three or four meals. Large snacks of milkshakes, dried fruits, peanut butter sandwiches, or cheese and crackers can add substantial calories and nutrients.

In summary, the diet that supports performance is similar to the diet recommended for good health. Both for health promotion and for fitness, the diet should consist mostly of whole, minimally processed foods low in fat, sugar, and salt and high in complex carbohydrates and vitamins and minerals.

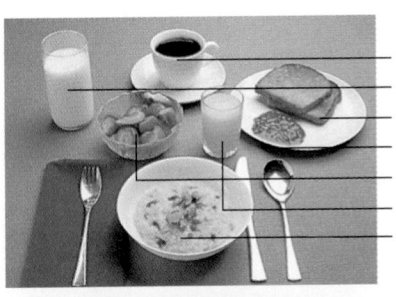

Breakfast

1 c coffee
8 oz low-fat milk
2 pieces whole-wheat toast
4 tsp jelly
½ c strawberries
½ c orange juice
1 c oatmeal and raisins with 2 tsp brown sugar

Breakfast

1 c coffee
½ c strawberries
8 oz nonfat milk

1 c oatmeal and raisins

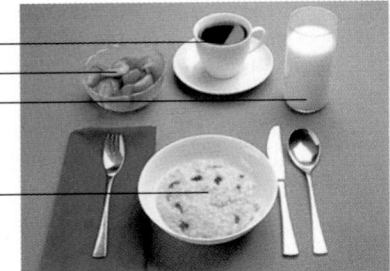

Morning Snack

4 tsp trail mix

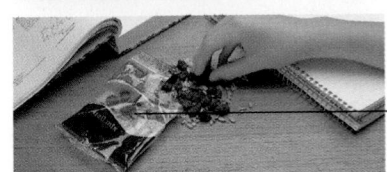

Lunch

12 oz iced tea with sugar
1 orange
1 banana
2 beef and bean burritos

Morning Snack

4 tsp trail mix

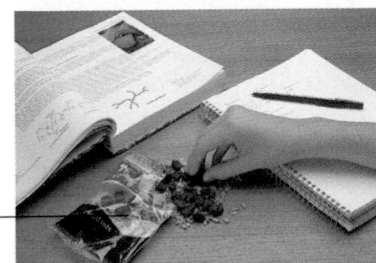

Afternoon Snack

A smoothie made from
 12 oz nonfat milk
 1 frozen banana
1 apple
4 rye wafers with 1 oz low-fat cheese

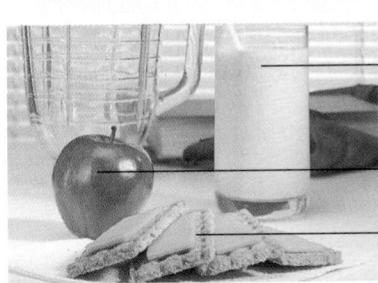

Lunch

12 oz iced tea with sugar

1 orange

1 beef and bean burrito

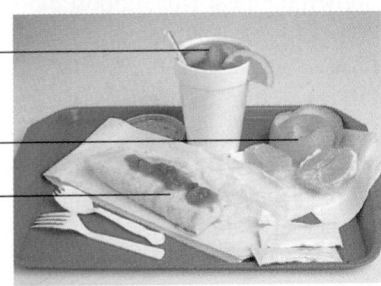

Dinner

8 oz low-fat milk
1 c sherbet
1 c spinich salad with 1 tbsp dressing
1 dinner roll with 2 tsp butter
1/4 tomato
1 c broccoli
4 oz salmon
¾ c noodles with parsley and 2 tsp butter

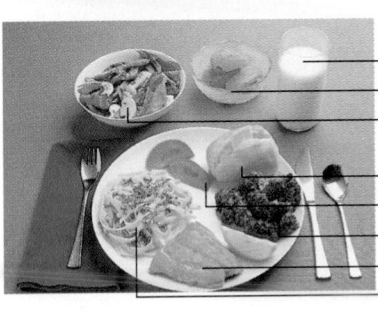

Dinner

½ c sherbet
1 c spinich salad with 1 tbsp dressing
8 oz nonfat milk
1/4 tomato
1 c broccoli
½ c noodles with parsley and 2 tsp butter
4 oz salmon

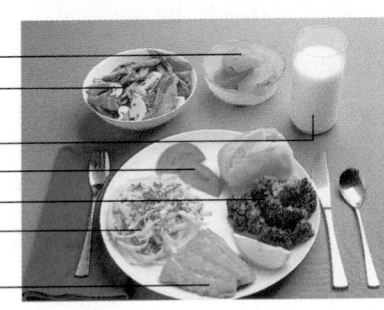

Total Calories: 3,119
61% cal from carbohydrates, 24% cal from fat, 15% cal from protein

Total Calories: 1,759
57% cal from carbohydrates, 24% cal from fat, 19% cal from protein

FIGURE 9–8
SAMPLE MEALS FOR HIGH-CARBOHYDRATE INTAKES FOR THE EXERCISE ENTHUSIAST AT TWO CALORIE LEVELS

The Pregame Meal

The meal before a competitive event can be an issue of heated debate. Many coaches and athletes believe intensely in special food rituals. For example, a bicyclist takes two tablespoons of honey before the race to give her "an energy boost" as she pedals away. Do rituals work?

Scientifically, no particular food confers a special benefit before an athletic contest. Honey demands water from the blood to dilute it and, depending on the individual, may or may not handicap the cyclist during exertion.[56] In short, some rituals have a neutral effect, and some can actually impair performance. However, if neutral practices give competitors a morale boost or extra confidence, they should be respected. People may have special personal meanings associated with certain foods, and their faith in rituals can make the difference between winning and losing a game.

This is not to say that it doesn't matter what the meal before an event consists of. The best choices are foods that are high in carbohydrate and low in fat, protein, and fiber. Fat and protein slow the stomach's emptying, and the protein's waste products generated during metabolism require that too much water be excreted with them. Fiber is not desirable right before physical exertion because it stays in the digestive tract too long and attracts water out of the blood. A high-carbohydrate meal will support blood glucose levels during competition. Olympic training tables are laden with foods such as breads, whole-grain cereals, pasta, rice, potatoes, and fruit juices. Competitors eat as much of these foods as they comfortably can because the foods supply energy without burdening the body. And they know it's especially important to include plenty of fluids—two or more 8-ounce glasses of water or juice per meal—to ensure adequate hydration.

For pregame meals and snacks, choose:

grape juice, apricot nectar, pineapple juice, jello, sherbet, popsicles, raisins, apricots, figs, dates, jams and toast, pancakes with syrup, honey, pasta, baked white or sweet potatoes, steamed vegetables, low-fat frozen yogurt, angel food or sponge cake with fresh fruit, gingersnaps, and graham crackers. Stay away from higher-fat foods such as meats, cheese, nuts, gravies, cream, French fries, muffins, croissants, biscuits, butter, potato chips, pies, and ice cream.

Any meal should be finished a good two to four hours before the event because digestion requires routing the blood supply to the digestive tract to pick up nutrients. By the time the contest begins, the circulating blood should be freed from that task and should be available instead to carry oxygen and fuel to the muscles. Liquid nutritional products can be consumed closer to the event (one to two hours) because they are emptied relatively rapidly from the stomach.[57] In addition, they supply an effective way to assure hydration.

A person who eats a snack closer to competition time should choose a food that is mostly carbohydrate because it is quickly digested. Better yet, just fill your fluid banks with beverages lacking sugar, such as water.

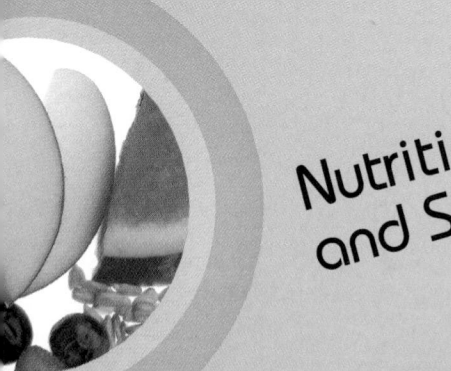

Nutrition and Stress

NUTRITION ACTION

Do you get the "munchies" when you are stressed out? Or does **stress** take away your appetite, making it just about impossible for you to eat or drink? Whatever your reaction to stress may be, it is virtually certain that your eating behavior is one of the many things that stress affects.

Stress can be loosely described as anything that pushes your body out of balance. For example, when you walk outside into the cold air, the low temperature becomes a source of stress, and in response, your body shivers in an effort to warm up. Similarly, when you eat a candy bar, your blood sugar rises, causing your pancreas to secrete insulin in an attempt to restore the blood sugar level to normal. But while your body likes to maintain the status quo, both physical and psychological stress regularly intrude upon your steady state and trigger your body's **stress response.**

Major physical stresses include pain, illness, surgery, wounds, burns, infections, dramatic changes in climate, toxic compounds, radiation, and pollution, to name just a few. Psychological stresses include, among other events, losing a job, moving, and becoming divorced or widowed. Even happy life events, such as getting married, can create stress. Of course, these stress-inducing events differ for every person. One person may not be affected at all by a situation because he or she previously handled a similar scenario successfully. For a person experiencing a situation for the first time, however, the event can be pressure packed!

One criterion for judging the stressfulness of an event is the amount of change in daily activities the event demands and how many coping behaviors are necessary to deal with it. The scale in Table 9–6 rates life events from the most to the least stressful. You can use this scale to see how you rate.

While many of the stresses we experience today are psychological, the body responds physically with what is called the fight-or-flight reaction. Your body mobilizes its defenses to either fight the enemy (stress) or run away whenever your equilibrium is disrupted. The sight of a car hurtling toward you, the fear that an intruder is present, the excitement of planning for a party, the feeling of pain, the anxiety of a mid-term exam, or any other event that alters your body's or mind's usual state signals your stress alarm to go off.

When the body is subject to stress, a chain of events ensues through both nerves and hormones to prepare for battle. The pupils of your eyes widen to allow more light to enter; your muscles tense up so that you can jump, run, or struggle with maximum strength; your breathing quickens to bring more oxygen into your lungs; and your heart races to rush this oxygen to your muscles so they can burn the fuel they need for energy. The liver pours forth the needed fuels—glucose and ketone bodies—from its stored supply, and the fat cells release fatty acids as alternative fuels. Body protein tissues break down to supply amino acids to back up the glucose supply and to be ready to heal wounds, if necessary. The muscles' blood vessels expand to feed the muscles better, while the vessels of the

STRESS any threat, be it physical or psychological, to a person's well-being.

STRESS RESPONSE the body's response to stress, initially mediated by both nerves and hormones. It begins with an alarm reaction, proceeds through a stage of resistance, and ends with recovery or, if prolonged, exhaustion.

349

TABLE 9–6

HOW STRESSED OUT ARE YOU?

People ranked these events according to how stressful they perceived them to be, on a scale from 1 to 100. Note that some "happy" events are included here. Individual people may score these events higher or lower than they are here. We have added in parentheses events that might be comparable to these in the lives of students.

LIFE EVENT	STRESS POINTS	LIFE EVENT	STRESS POINTS
Death of spouse	100	Change in responsibilities at work	
Divorce	73	(change in course demands)	29
Marital separation		Son or daughter leaving home	29
(breakup with boyfriend/girlfriend)	65	Trouble with in-laws (trouble with parents)	29
Jail term	63	Outstanding personal achievement	28
Death of close family member (except spouse)	63	Spouse beginning or stopping work	26
Major personal injury or illness	53	School beginning or ending (final exams)	26
Marriage	50	Change in living conditions	25
Being fired from a job (expulsion from school)	47	Revision of personal habits (self or family)	24
Marital reconciliation	45	Trouble with boss (trouble with professor)	23
Retirement	45	Change in work (or school) hours or conditions	20
Change in health of a family member (not self)	44	Change in residence	
Pregnancy	40	(moving to school, moving home)	20
Sex difficulties	39	Change in schools	20
Gain of new family member (change of roommate)	39	Change in recreation	19
Business readjustment	39	Change in church activities	19
Change in financial state	38	Change in social activities (joining a new group)	18
Death of a close friend	37	Taking on a small mortgage or loan	17
Change to different line of work		Change in sleeping habits	16
(change of major)	36	Change in number of family get-togethers	15
Change in number of arguments with spouse	35	Change in eating habits	13
Taking on a large mortgage		Vacation	13
(taking on financial aid)	31	Christmas	12
Foreclose of a mortgage or loan	30	Minor violations of the law	11

Check the list and identify the events that have happened to you in the past year or that you expect within the next year. Use the number system to determine how many stress points you are experiencing in this period of your life. Then score yourself as follows: over 200—urgent need of intelligent stress management; 150 to 199—careful stress management indicated; 100 to 149—stressful life, keep tabs on your mental health; under 100—no present cause for concern about stress.

SOURCE: Adapted from Lifescore: Holmes scale, *Family Health*, January 1979, p.32.

digestive tract constrict (digestion becomes a low priority in time of danger). Less blood flows to the kidneys to help conserve fluid, and less blood flows to the skin to help minimize blood loss at any wound site. In addition, more clotting factors form to allow the blood to clot faster, if need be. Hearing sharpens, and the brain produces local opium-like substances that dull its sensation of pain, which during an emergency might distract you from taking the needed action. And your hair stands on end—a reminder that there was a time when your ancestors had enough hair to bristle, look bigger, and frighten off their enemies.

This tightly synchronized, adaptive reaction to stress provides superb support for emergency physical action. You probably remember having had to take such action. You may have performed an amazing feat of strength or speed for a few minutes, and only after it was over did you notice that your heart was pounding, your breathing was fast, your fingers were cold, your skin was tingling, your mouth was dry, and the sensation of pain or exhaustion was just beginning to come through.

To be sure, many of the stresses that you deal with every day don't require you to engage in a fistfight or to run away. Navigating traffic jams, studying for final exams, and searching for employment all require calm, rational thought. Nevertheless, since your body prepares for heavy physical activity, over the long run, the cumulative stress can cause health problems in people who bottle it up.

To help your body "let off steam" when you are under stress, you should try to dance, run, jump rope, rollerblade, swim, walk, run up and down a flight of steps, or engage in any type of physical activity. Avoid the use of drugs (including alcohol and tranquilizers) that would discourage activity and exercise. If the stress is prolonged—and especially if you don't work it off—it can drain the body of its reserves. Indeed, many of the biochemical pathways used during the stress response rely on nutrients to run.

Consider that in preparation for potential blood loss that might occur with a physical injury, your body conserves water during stress. It does so by retaining sodium, because water clings to this mineral in your body. But to retain sodium, your kidneys must expel potassium. Thus, you need ample stores of potassium to be able to afford losses of this mineral.

All three calorie-containing nutrients—carbohydrates, fat, and protein—are drawn upon in increased quantities if the stress requires vigorous physical action or if there is injury. While the body is busy responding and not eating, say, during a serious illness, its fuels must be drawn from internal sources. Initially, carbohydrate is taken from the liver's stores, but that supply lasts only about a day. Thereafter, your muscles and some of your organs—heart, liver, and lungs—are broken down to supply protein that your body converts into carbohydrate for fuel. The breakdown of muscles also provides your body with available protein that it can use to make scar tissue to heal wounds.

Granted, some tissues can burn fat for fuel. In a normally nourished person, fat stores are adequate to meet energy needs for many days. (Chapter 8 described these processes as they occur during the stress of fasting.) Still, in times of stress, the body uses not only dispensable supplies (those that are stored for time of need, such as body fat)) but also vital tissue—such as muscle tissue—that your body can ill afford to lose.

The best nutritional preparation for stress is a balanced and varied diet as part of a lifestyle in which exercise plays a constant part. Notice that nothing is said here about supplements or gimmicks. Just eat well to obtain the nutrients and exercise regularly to promote overall good health.

How much you should eat and what you should eat during a stressful time depends in part on what your stomach can tolerate. During severe stress, the appetite is suppressed. This is an adaptive reaction to a physical threat. Energy at such a time is needed to fight off the threat. It would be wasteful and risky to spend energy looking for or eating food. The blood supply has been diverted to the muscles to maximize strength and speed, so even if you swallow food, you may not be able to digest or absorb it efficiently. (In a severe upset, the stomach and intestines will even reject solid food. Vomiting and diarrhea are their way of disposing of a burden they can't handle.) All of this means that it

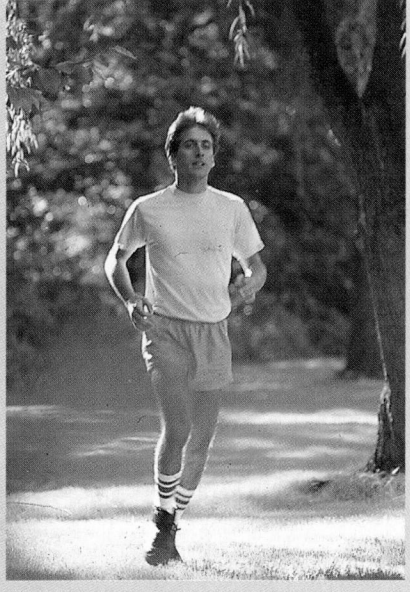

The stress response needs to be worked off physically.

is poor advice to tell someone under severe stress to eat. He or she can't. And a person who forces him or herself to eat often cannot assimilate what he or she has eaten. On the other hand, fasting is itself a stress on the body, and the longer a person goes without eating, the harder it can be to get started again. Thus, fasting can be a no-win situation. People often get into a downward spiral once they have let stress affect them to the point where they cannot eat, and not eating makes it harder for them to handle the stress. At this point, managing stress may require the help of a counselor.

If you can eat, do so, of course. Take only a little, if that is all you can handle, and eat more often to keep meeting your energy and nutrient needs. Choose a variety of foods. Drink fluids, too, but not too much with meals. Drinking too much water with your meals can make you feel full faster and cause you to cut back on the amount of food you eat. Try to drink water and other fluids between meals.

If you choose not to eat at all while under stress, you will deplete your body of vital nutrients. Aside from the protein and potassium already mentioned, the nutrients most susceptible to this depletion are the vitamins and minerals that are not stored in substantial quantities. You may already be aware that the water-soluble vitamins (B vitamins and vitamin C) fall into this category. But when the question arises whether you should take nutrient supplements during periods of extreme stress, the answer is probably yes, under the care of a physician, if you can't eat for a prolonged period of time.

Of course, while some people can't eat under stress, others get the munchies. One possible explanation is that as carbohydrate is drawn from body stores and the body fails to use it up by exercising, it becomes stored as body fat. The net effect is that body carbohydrate stores are used up. When your blood glucose (sugar) levels fall, you get hungry. If stress empties your body stores of carbohydrate and your blood glucose levels fall, you will get hungrier sooner than you should.

Another possibility is that the behavior of eating helps to relieve stress by occupying the nervous system with a familiar activity that discharges its nerves without doing them harm, as fighting might do. It may be that eating—or the food eaten—leads to the release of substances in the brain that are experienced as soothing. Much remains to be learned about stress-induced eating. The person who is caught up in this behavior and who is prone to obesity because of it would be well advised to find an alternative behavior with which to respond to stress—exercising, strolling, window shopping, gardening, listening to music, talking with others, or other relaxing, non-food related activities.

Finally, remember that stress is defined as anything you *perceive* as a threat to your status quo. Psychological counselors urge that you learn stress management techniques to help get you through the disruptive changes in your life. They suggest the following:

- *Change how you perceive the event.* View the event as one you can handle and as a learning opportunity rather than a disaster with which you can't cope.
- *Express yourself.* Air your feelings so that you will be less tense.
- *Take time out.* Meet your need for relief from pain, sadness, anxiety, or anger by exercising or using relaxation techniques.
- *Expand your social support system.* Much that is exhausting and painful to handle alone is easier to manage when you have understanding from a circle of supportive friends and helpers.

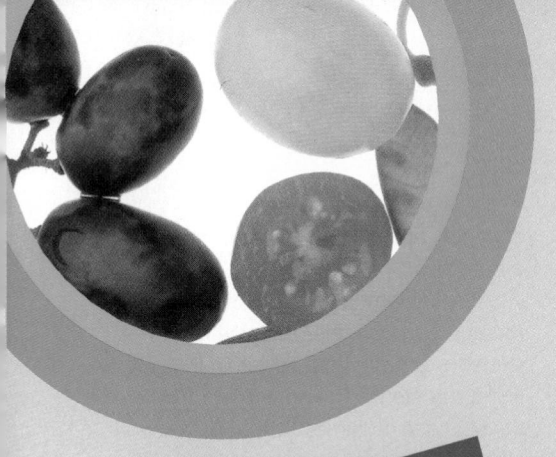

Alcohol and Nutrition

One of the many drugs— and usually the most common one—that enters people's lives as they arrive at their teen and adult years is alcohol. The National Institute on Alcohol Abuse and Alcoholism has estimated that about two-thirds of all adults in the United States drink alcohol. Of these, 33 percent are classified as light drinkers (3 drinks or less per week), about 24 percent are moderate drinkers (2 drinks or less per day), and 9 percent are heavy drinkers (5 or more drinks per day). Some 15.3 million people in the United States meet the criteria for alcohol abuse, alcohol addiction, or both.[58]

Even though people in the 20- to 40-year-old age group have the greatest alcohol consumption, many teen-agers are regular alcohol users. One survey showed that two–thirds of the high school seniors interviewed reported that they had consumed alcohol within the past month and 5 percent indicated that they drank alcohol every day. In addition, men are more likely than women to consume alcohol and to drink more heavily.[59]

Alcohol abuse and alcohol addiction are recognized as major public health problems in the United States today.[60] Approximately 100,000 excess deaths per year are associated with alcohol-related causes—including traffic accidents, homicides, suicides, cirrhosis, and hemorrhagic stroke—while the annual health cost to the nation associated with alcohol abuse and dependence is more than $98 billion.[61] Whether an individual is a social drinker, an alcohol abuser, or an alcoholic, the common element is managing the physiological, psychological, and social consequences of alcohol consumption. The difference between the alcohol abuser and the alcoholic is generally one of degree, with the alcoholic experiencing more difficulties in terms of illness, dependence on alcohol, loss-of-control symptoms, and disruption of family and work life than the alcohol abuser. As we will see, alcohol has a profound effect on all aspects of metabolism and health.[62]

Alcohol abuse refers to patterns of alcohol use that result in health problems, social problems, or both. *Alcohol addiction* (sometimes called *dependence*) refers to the disease—**alcoholism**—that is characterized by abnormal alcohol-seeking behaviors and a lack of control over drinking. Many of the harmful health effects of alcohol consumption are seen in both alcohol abusers and those with alcoholism. However, the disease—alcoholism—has four distinguishing features:[63]

- *tolerance*—more and more alcohol is needed to produce the desired effects.
- *physical dependence*—when the person refrains from using alcohol, a characteristic withdrawal syndrome appears that can be relieved by consuming alcohol.
- *impaired control over drinking*—the person cannot regulate alcohol intake once a drink has been taken.
- *discomfort of abstinence*—strong "cravings" for alcohol pervade the person addicted to alcohol during periods of abstinence and can lead to relapse.

Why doesn't everyone who drinks alcohol become an alcoholic? As the concept grew that alcoholism is a disease and not a mental illness or a lack of self-discipline, it also became apparent that alcoholism tends to run in families. Studies have shown that the natural children of alcoholics are three to four times more likely to be alcoholic themselves than are the biological children of nonalcoholic parents. This observation tends to hold true whether the child was raised by its natural parent or by an adoptive parent.[64] Research is underway to understand this process in greater detail and develop biochemical markers that will identify individuals who are at risk of becoming alcoholic.

How does alcohol affect the body? Alcohol (specifically, ethanol, the form found in alcoholic beverages) affects every organ, but the most dramatic evidence of its disruptive behavior appears in the liver—the only organ whose cells can oxidize alcohol for fuel to any great extent. All other cells are affected by the presence of alcohol but can do practically nothing about getting rid of it. Ethanol, like the other alcohols, is toxic—but less so than some. Sufficiently diluted and taken in small enough doses, it produces **euphoria**—an effect that people seek—not with zero risk but with a low enough risk (if the doses are low enough) to be tolerable. Used to achieve this effect, alcohol is a **drug**—that is, a substance that can modify one or more of the body's functions. Like all drugs, alcohol offers some benefits; it also has tremendous abuse potential.

What are the benefits offered by alcohol? The beneficial effects of alcohol have long been appreciated and praised.

Wine, beer, and other fermented beverages have given pleasure and relaxation to people for more than 5,000 years. Only recently have we begun to learn exactly how the ethanol molecule acts in our bodies, but people have always known that it affects their mood, sensations, and behavior. Because it alters mood, alcohol has many uses. Taken in moderation, alcohol relaxes people, reduces their inhibitions, and encourages desirable social interactions. The regular and moderate consumption of alcohol, especially wine, by elderly people results in better sleep patterns, improved mood, a lower heart rate, and reduced anxiety levels.[65] Alcohol may even lower an individual's susceptibility to heart disease, possibly by increasing the blood HDL level (see the Spotlight feature in Chapter 4).[66]

What do you mean by *moderation*?
We can't name an exact amount of alcohol per day that would be appropriate for everyone, because people differ in their tolerance levels. Still, authorities have attempted to set a limit that is appropriate for most healthy people. Moderate drinking is defined as no more than one **drink** a day for the average-sized woman, and no more than two drinks a day for the average-sized man. A drink is any alcoholic beverage that delivers ½ ounce of *pure ethanol*: 5 ounces of wine, 10 ounces of wine cooler, 12 ounces of beer, 1½ ounces of hard liquor (whiskey, gin, scotch, vodka, brandy, or rum). This amount is supposed to be enough to produce euphoria without incurring any long-term harm to health. Doubtless some people could consume slightly more; others could definitely not handle nearly so much without significant risk.

Since moderate alcohol intakes may be beneficial to heart disease, are scientists now recommending that everyone drink in moderation? No. Re-searchers warn that caution is needed in recommending moderate alcohol consumption to the public.[67] Many people need to refrain from alcohol consumption altogether (pregnant women, recovering alcoholics, people under age 21, persons on certain medications, and those intending to drive a vehicle). Alcohol can have profoundly negative effects on the body, and it is associated with five of the ten leading causes of death in this country—namely certain types of cancer, cirrhosis of the liver, motor vehicle and other accidents, suicides, and homicides.

In addition, the impact (positive or negative) of alcohol use varies with age and gender.[68] For example, the leading cause of death for middle-aged men is heart disease. For this group, there may be an advantage to moderate alcohol use, since the evidence with regards to alcohol and blood lipids points to a possible protective mechanism between moderate alcohol consumption and heart disease risk factors.[69] For younger men, however, the leading causes of death are accidents or violence—and both are often alcohol-related. An increase in alcohol consumption among this group is not encouraged. For premenopausal-aged women, the risk of death from breast cancer is greater than that for heart disease. Some re-searchers now point to a possible association between alcohol use (one, two, or three drinks per day) and breast cancer.[70] Therefore, any protection against heart disease derived from moderate consumption of alcohol in these women would be negated by the deleterious effects of the alcohol on breast cancer.

How does the body handle alcohol?
From the moment alcohol enters the body in a beverage, it is treated as if it has special privileges. Foods sit around in the stomach for a while, but not alcohol. The tiny alcohol molecules need no digestion; they can diffuse as soon as they arrive, right through the walls of the stomach, and they reach the brain within a minute.

A small amount of alcohol can be metabolized by the enzyme **alcohol dehydrogenase** housed within the cells lining the stomach. The extent to which the stomach cells metabolize this alcohol differs between women and men. The observation that "women can't seem to hold their liquor" compared with men is explained in part by a woman's lower alcohol dehydrogenase activity in the stomach. Women's inability to handle this alcohol holds true even when adjustments are made for the differences in body size between women and men.[71]

Regardless of your gender, you can feel euphoric right away when you drink, especially if your stomach is empty. When your stomach is full of food, the molecules of alcohol have less chance of touching the walls and diffusing through, so you don't feel the effects of alcohol as quickly. But when the stomach contents are emptied into the duodenum, it doesn't matter that plenty of food is mixed with the alcohol. The alcohol is absorbed rapidly anyway and transported to the liver "as if it were a V.I.P. (Very Important Person)."[72]

What does the alcohol do once it arrives at the liver? Although a small amount of alcohol can be metabolized by stomach cells, liver cells are the only cells in the body that can make enough alcohol dehydrogenase to oxidize alcohol at an appreciable rate. However, there is a limit to the amount of alcohol anyone can process in a given time. This limit is set by the number of molecules of the alcohol-processing enzymes in the liver. If more molecules of alcohol arrive at the liver cells than the enzymes can handle, the extra alcohol must wait. It enters the general circulation and moves on past the liver. From the liver, it is carried to all parts of the body, circulating again and again through the liver until enzymes are available to convert it to

acetaldehyde. The rate at which the liver enzymes can work limits the rate of the body's handling of alcohol.

How fast do the liver enzymes work? That depends on many individual factors. For example, the amount of enzymes present depends on when you last ate a good meal. Fasting causes degradation of the enzyme (protein) within the cells and can reduce the rate of alcohol metabolism by half. Drinking on an empty stomach thus not only lets the drinker feel the effects more promptly but also brings about higher blood alcohol levels for longer periods of time and increases the effect of alcohol in anesthetizing the brain.

What if you drink too fast? If you drink so fast that your liver enzymes can't keep up with the load, metabolic products of alcohol's metabolism accumulate in the blood and body organs. One is acid—dangerous for all body processes. Another is acetaldehyde, already mentioned, which is toxic to the brain and other organs. Another is fat, which accumulates in the liver itself and can't be moved out until the body is free of alcohol.

Alcohol also causes loss of body water by excretion, and that leads to thirst. Many people have observed the increase in urination that accompanies drinking, but they may not realize that they can easily get into a vicious cycle as a result. Loss of body water leads to thirst. Thirst leads to more drinking—but drinking of what? The only fluid that will relieve dehydration is water, but the thirsty person welcomes any cold fluid—even concentrated alcohol—that relieves the dry mouth associated with thirst. If a person tries to quench thirst with concentrated alcoholic beverages, the thirst only becomes worse.

What are the nutritional consequences of drinking alcohol regularly? If you are a light drinker in good health and oth-

TABLE 9–7
CALORIES IN ALCOHOLIC BEVERAGES AND MIXERS

BEVERAGE	AMOUNT (OZ)	CALORIES
Beer	12	150
Light beer	12	100
Nonalcoholic beer	12	32
Gin, rum, vodka, whisky (80 proof)	1½	100
Dessert wine	3½	160
Table wine (red, rosé, white)	3½	75
Wine cooler	12	150
Liqueurs	1½	155-185
Tonic, ginger ale	12	125
Cola	12	150
Fruit juice	8	110
Club soda, plain seltzer, diet soda pop	12	0

erwise well nourished, the occasional consumption of alcohol will probably have little effect on your nutritional status. The biggest risk to you will come most likely from the additional calories provided by alcohol; these extra calories may contribute to unwanted weight gain (see Table 9–7).[73] This is not to say that alcohol has *no effect* on your nutritional status, for it does. Alcohol causes fundamental changes in metabolism that occur whenever you consume alcohol. The extent to which alcohol affects your nutritional status depends on how much alcohol you consume and your current nutritional and health status.

If you drink excessively on a regular basis, your nutritional status will become compromised. Protein deficiency can develop, both from the depression of protein synthesis in the cells and, in the drinker who substitutes alcohol for food, from poor diet. Eating well does not protect the drinker from protein depletion. One has to stop drinking alcohol for complete protection.

Alcohol affects every tissue's metabolism of nutrients in other ways. Stomach cells become inflamed and vulnerable to ulcer formation. Intestinal cells fail to absorb thiamin, folate, and vitamin B_{12}. Liver cells lose efficiency in activating vitamin D, and they alter their production and excretion of bile. Rod cells in the retina, which normally process vitamin A alcohol (retinol) to the form needed in vision (retinal), find themselves processing drinking alcohol instead. The kidney excretes increased quantities of magnesium, calcium, potassium, and zinc.

Acetaldehyde interferes with metabolism, too. It dislodges vitamin B_6 from its protective binding protein so that it is destroyed, causing a vitamin B_6 deficiency and thereby lowered production of red blood cells.

Do alcoholics have special nutritional problems? Definitely. Some alcoholics tend to substitute alcohol for food and can consume more than 50 percent of their calories from alcohol. Because of the metabolic derangements that occur with alcohol consumption, the chronic alcoholic tends to develop hyperlipidemia (a high blood triglyceride level), a **fatty liver** that ultimately leads to **cirrhosis** of the liver, and impaired kidney function. Over time, a high level of alcohol intake may also damage the lining of the stomach, produce low blood sugar and high blood concentrations of uric acid, and cause metabolic bone disease. Even fairly young men in their 30s and 40s can develop osteoporosis from consuming excessive alcohol over the course of 10 to 15 years.[74] In addition, alcoholics have an increased risk of hypertension, stroke, and a variety of cancers, particularly cancers of the tongue, mouth, pharynx, esophagus, larynx, and liver, the latter occurring because of cirrhosis.

I've heard that alcohol and other drugs interact in a dangerous way. Is this true? Yes, they do. The liver's VIP treatment of alcohol is reflected in its altered handling of other drugs as well as nutrients. The liver possesses an enzyme system in addition to the enzyme alcohol dehydrogenase that metabolizes *both* alcohol *and* other drugs (any compounds that have certain chemical features in common). Called the **MEOS (microsomal ethanol-oxidizing system),** this system handles only about one-fifth of the total alcohol a person consumes, but the MEOS enlarges if repeatedly exposed to alcohol. This may not make the drinker able to handle much more alcohol at a time than before, because the total alcohol-metabolizing ability of the MEOS is small, but the effect on the ability to metabolize other drugs is considerable.

When the MEOS enlarges, it makes the body able to metabolize other drugs much faster than before. This can make it confusing and tricky to work out the correct doses of medications. The physician who prescribes sedatives to be taken every four hours, for example, assumes that the MEOS will dispose of the drug at a certain predicted rate. Well and good; but in a client who is a heavy drinker, the MEOS is adapted to metabolizing large quantities of alcohol. It therefore metabolizes the other drug extra fast. The drug's effects wear off unexpectedly fast, leaving the client undersedated. Imagine a surgeon's alarm if a client wakes up on the table during an operation! A skilled anesthesiologist always asks clients about their drinking patterns before putting them to sleep.

An enlarged MEOS will oxidize drugs *faster* than expected, but only as long as there is no alcohol in the system. If the person drinks and uses the drug at the same time, the drug will be metabolized more *slowly* and so will be much more potent. Since the MEOS is busy disposing of alcohol, the other drug can't be handled until later, and the dose may build up to where it greatly oversedates, or even kills, the user.

What does alcohol do to the brain? Alcohol acts as a **narcotic.** It was used for centuries as an anesthetic because of its ability to deaden pain. But it wasn't a very good anesthetic because one could never be sure how much a person would need and how much would be a lethal dose. As new, more predictable anesthetics were discovered, they quickly replaced alcohol. However, alcohol continues to be used today as a kind of

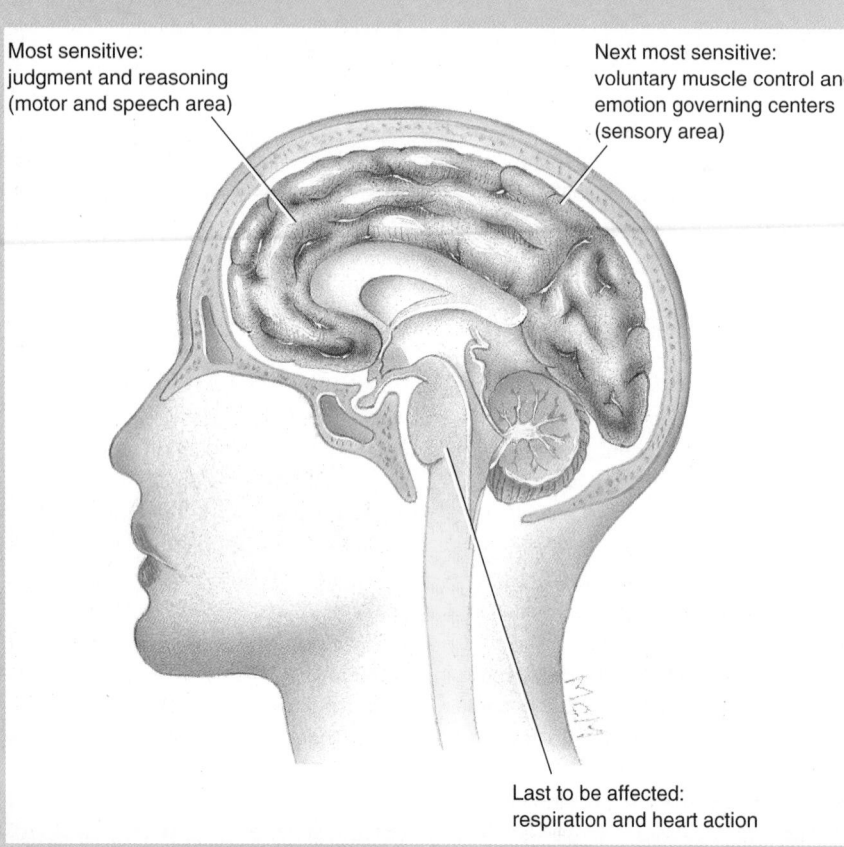

Most sensitive:
judgment and reasoning
(motor and speech area)

Next most sensitive:
voluntary muscle control and
emotion governing centers
(sensory area)

Last to be affected:
respiration and heart action

Alcohol is rightly termed an anesthetic because it puts brain centers to sleep in order: first the cortex, then the emotion-governing centers, then the centers that govern muscular control, and finally the deep centers that control respiration and heartbeat.

TABLE 9–8
ALCOHOL DOSES AND BRAIN RESPONSES

NUMBER OF DRINKS[a]	BLOOD ALCOHOL LEVEL (%)[b]	BRAIN RESPONSE
2	0.05	Judgment impaired
4	0.10[c]	Emotional control impaired
6	0.15	Muscle coordination and reflexes impaired
8	0.20	Vision impaired
12	0.30	Drunk, totally out of control
14	0.35	Stupor
More than 14	0.50–0.60	Total loss of consciousness; finally, death

[a]Taken within an hour or so.
[b]Percentage of blood alcohol in a 150-pound person.
[c]The legal limit for intoxication according to most states' highway safety ordinances.

anesthetic on social occasions, to help people relax or to relieve anxiety. People think that alcohol is a stimulant because it seems to make them lively and uninhibited at first. Actually, though, the way it does this is by sedating *inhibitory* nerves, which are more numerous than excitatory nerves. Ultimately, alcohol acts as a depressant because it affects all the nerve cells.

When alcohol flows to the brain, it first sedates the frontal lobe, the reasoning part. As the alcohol molecules diffuse into the cells of this lobe, they interfere with reasoning and judgment. If the drinker drinks faster than the rate at which the liver can oxidize the alcohol, the speech center of the brain becomes narcotized, and the area that governs reasoning becomes more incapacitated. Later, the cells of the brain responsible for large-muscle control are affected; at this point, people under the influence stagger or weave when they try to walk. Finally, the conscious brain is completely subdued, and the person passes out. Now, luckily, the person can drink no more. This is fortunate because a higher dose's anesthetic effect could reach

the deepest brain centers that control breathing and heartbeat, and the person could die. Table 9–8 shows the blood alcohol levels that correspond with progressively greater intoxication.

Why, then, don't people die from drinking alcohol? Since the brain centers respond to alcohol in the order just described, people pass out before they can drink enough to kill them. It is possible, though, to drink fast enough that the effects of alcohol continue to accelerate after one has fallen asleep. The occasional death that takes place during a drinking contest is attributed to this effect. The drinker drinks fast enough before passing out to receive a lethal dose.

The lack of glucose for the brain's function (once again, because of the body's VIP treatment of alcohol) and the length of time needed to clear the blood of alcohol account for some diverse consequences of drinking. Responsible aircraft pilots know that they must allow 24 hours for their bodies to clear alcohol completely, and they refuse to fly any sooner. Major airlines enforce this rule.

Women who might become pregnant are warned to abstain from the use of alcohol (see Chapter 10). One of the effects of an acute dose in experimental animals is to collapse the umbilical cord temporarily, depriving the developing fetus of oxygen. This can occur even before a woman knows that she is pregnant.

Does alcohol cause brain damage? Yes, and the damage is permanent in both the drinker and the child born to a pregnant woman who drinks. When liver cells have died, other cells may later multiply to replace them, but there is no regeneration of brain cells.

Suppose I want to drink but not get drunk. How can I go about drinking in moderation? If you want to drink socially, you should drink slowly, and you should sip, not gulp, your drinks. You should eat available snacks or a light meal along with the alcoholic beverages. With this strategy, the alcohol molecules should dribble slowly enough into the liver cells, allowing the enzymes to handle the load. Spacing of drinks is important, too. It takes about an hour and a half to metabolize one drink, depending on your body size, previous drinking experience, how recently you have eaten, and how you are feeling at the time.

Finally, you might elect to dilute your alcoholic beverages over the course of your drinking period. For example, after you've drunk half a glass of wine, fill up the glass with a non-cola soft drink to make a wine cooler. If you choose a low-calorie carbonated drink, you eliminate extra calories and alcohol. Or choose a low-alcohol beer or wine cooler.

What can I do to help a friend who has drunk too much? Does it help to walk my friend around? No, don't wear yourself out walking your friend around the block (and never allow your friend to drive a vehicle while under the influence of alcohol). The muscles have to work harder, but since they can't metabolize alcohol, they can't help clear it from the blood. Time is the only thing that will do the job; each person has a particular level of the enzyme alcohol dehydrogenase, and it clears the blood at a steady rate. This is not true for most nutrients. If you bring in more of a nutrient, generally the body can promptly step up the rate at which it metabolizes that nutrient. But not with alcohol.

Nor will it help to give your friend a cup of coffee. Caffeine is a stimulant, but it won't speed up the metabolism of alcohol. The police say ruefully, "If you give a cup of coffee to a drunk, you'll just have a wide-awake drunk on your hands."

How can you know whether you or a friend has or is developing a problem with alcohol? Sometimes, a person's judgment may tell him that he should limit himself to two drinks at a party, but the first drink may take his judgment away, so he has many more. The failure to stop drinking as planned, on repeated occasions, is a danger sign that indicates that the person should not drink at all.

If you answer yes to one or more of the following questions, it is suggestive of an alcohol problem and you may want to seek a professional evaluation:[75]

● Have you ever felt you ought to cut down on drinking?

● Have people annoyed you by criticizing your drinking?

● Have you ever felt bad or guilty about your drinking?

● Have you ever had a drink first thing in the morning to steady your nerves or get rid of a hangover?

Early identification and intervention—involving abstinence from alcohol—are

MINIGLOSSARY

ACETALDEHYDE (ass-et-AL-duh-hide) a substance to which drinking alcohol (ethanol) is metabolized.

ALCOHOL DEHYDROGENASE a liver enzyme that converts ethanol to acetaldehyde. The MEOS also oxidizes alcohol.

ALCOHOLISM a dependency on alcohol marked by compulsive uncontrollable drinking with negative effects on physical health, family relationships, and social health.

CIRRHOSIS (seer-OH-sis) advanced liver disease, often associated with alcoholism, in which liver cells have died and hardened and have permanently lost their function.

DRINK a dose of any alcoholic beverage that delivers one-half ounce of pure ethanol:
   5 ounces of wine
   12 ounces of beer
   1½ ounces of hard liquor (whiskey, gin, rum, or vodka)

DRUGS substances that can modify one or more of the body's functions.

EUPHORIA (you-FORE-ee-uh) a feeling of great well-being that people often seek through the use of drugs such as alcohol.
   eu = good
   phoria = bearing

FATTY LIVER an early stage of liver disease seen in several conditions (kwashiorkor, alcoholic liver disease), characterized by accumulation of fat in the liver cells.

MEOS (MICROSOMAL ETHANOL-OXIDIZING SYSTEM) a system of enzymes in the liver that oxidize not only alcohol but also several classes of drugs. (The **microsomes** are tiny particles of membranes with associated enzymes that can be collected from broken-up cells.)
   micro = tiny
   soma = body

NARCOTIC (nar-KOT-ic) any drug that dulls the senses, induces sleep, and becomes addictive with prolonged use.

critical to the successful treatment of alcoholism. If you think your own drinking patterns are not normal or beyond moderate, if your drinking has caused problems in your life, or if the alcohol abuse of a friend or relative is of concern to you, contact the National Clearinghouse for Alcohol and Drug Information (1-800-729-6686) for more information.

CHECK YOURSELF...

1. Name and describe the four components of fitness. Which has top priority?

2. What are the benefits of exercise?

3. Compare aerobic versus anaerobic exercise. Give examples.

4. Define target heart rate and calculate your own target heart rate.

5. What is the recommended prescription for cardiovascular fitness?

6. What is the training effect of cardiovascular exercise?

7. Define anabolic steroids; what are the potential side effects associated with steroid use?

8. How much protein is recommended for the diet of the athlete?

9. What is the best fluid replacement for exercise?

10. Describe the components of a healthful diet for athletic performance.

11. Describe the cascade of events that occur in the body during the stress response.

12. Describe the benefits and risks associated with alcohol consumption.

Answers to selected Check Yourself questions are found in Appendix H.

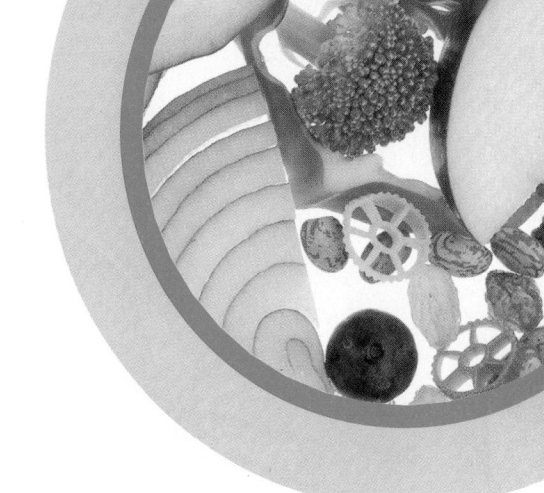

> How far you go in life depends on your being tender with the young, compassionate with the aged, sympathetic with the striving, and tolerant of the weak and the strong. Because someday in life you will have been all of these.
>
> George Washington Carver
> (1864–1943, American botanist)

The Life Cycle: Conception Through the Later Years

TEN

Contents

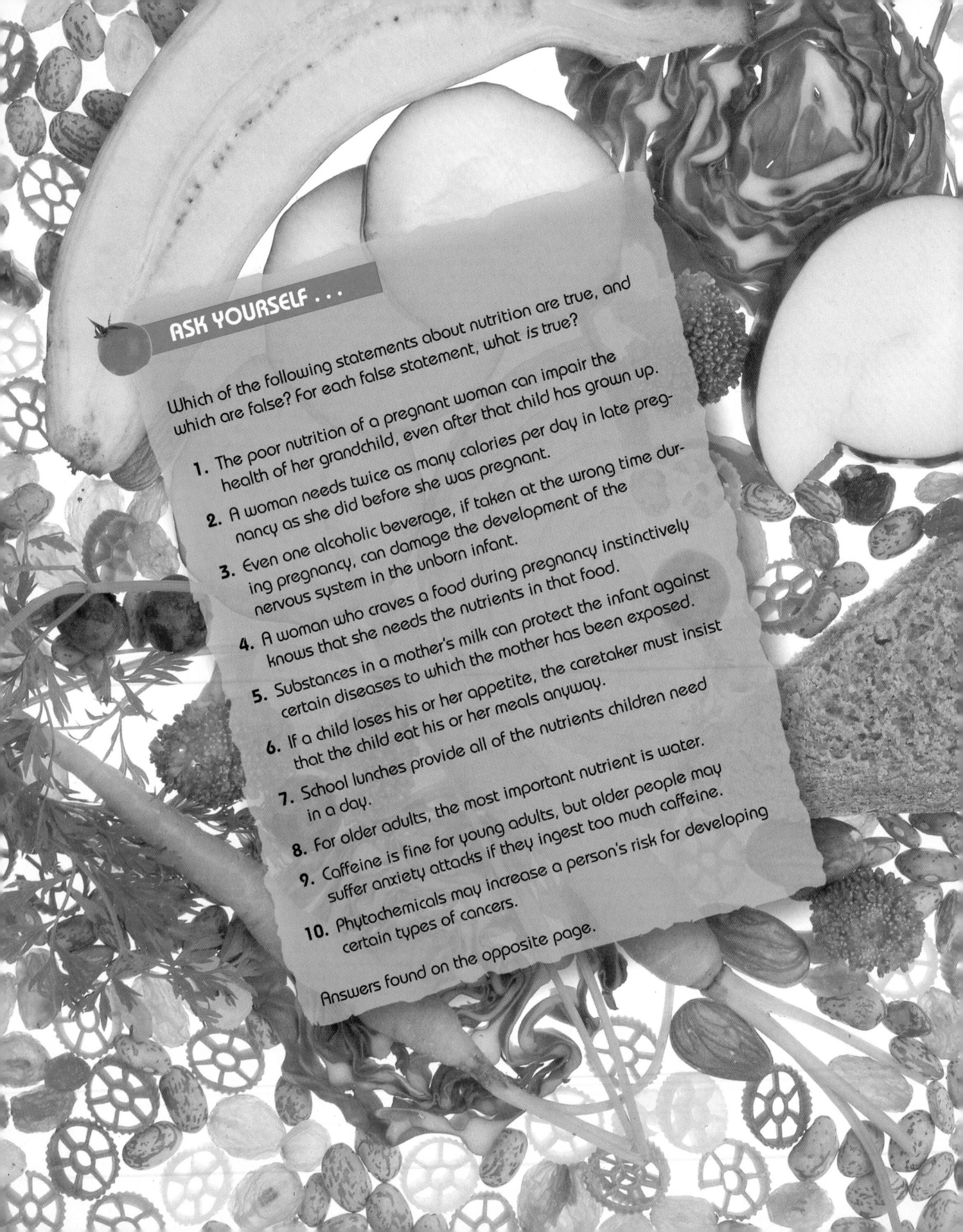

Which of the following statements about nutrition are true, and which are false? For each false statement, what *is* true?

1. The poor nutrition of a pregnant woman can impair the health of her grandchild, even after that child has grown up.

2. A woman needs twice as many calories per day in late pregnancy as she did before she was pregnant.

3. Even one alcoholic beverage, if taken at the wrong time during pregnancy, can damage the development of the nervous system in the unborn infant.

4. A woman who craves a food during pregnancy instinctively knows that she needs the nutrients in that food.

5. Substances in a mother's milk can protect the infant against certain diseases to which the mother has been exposed.

6. If a child loses his or her appetite, the caretaker must insist that the child eat his or her meals anyway.

7. School lunches provide all of the nutrients children need in a day.

8. For older adults, the most important nutrient is water.

9. Caffeine is fine for young adults, but older people may suffer anxiety attacks if they ingest too much caffeine.

10. Phytochemicals may increase a person's risk for developing certain types of cancers.

Answers found on the opposite page.

By the time you are 65 years old, you will have eaten about 100,000 pounds of food. Each bite may or may not have brought with it the nutrients you needed. The impact of the food you have eaten, together with your lifestyle habits, accumulates over a lifetime, and people who have lived and eaten differently all their lives are in widely different states of health by the time they reach 65.

Nutrition shares with other lifestyle factors the responsibility for maintaining good health. The complete prescription for good health presented in Chapter 1 reads as follows: avoid excess alcohol, don't smoke, maintain a desirable weight, exercise regularly, get regular sleep, and eat nutritious, regular meals. Nutrition is represented by three of the six items on this list—one-half of the total. A person who abides by all six practices can expect by later midlife to be physiologically 30 years younger than a person who abides by few or none of them.[1] If you subscribe to the view that your job is to accept the things you can't control and control the things you can, your nutritional health falls into the second category and deserves your conscientious attention.

The effects of nutrition extend from one generation to the next, and this is particularly evident during pregnancy. Research has demonstrated that the poor nutrition of a woman during her early pregnancy can impair the health of her *grandchild,* even after that child has become an adult. A woman should attend to her nutrition even before she becomes pregnant. If she needs supplementation, she should be taking a supplement; if she is underweight or overweight, she should try to gain or lose weight before she becomes pregnant to maximize her chances of having a healthy baby.

Similarly—to give but two of dozens of possible examples—the nutrition of a girl in her teens will help to determine the soundness of her skeleton when she is 80, and the nutrition of a boy in his teens will affect his chances of developing heart disease decades later. This chapter follows people through the life cycle and attends to their special nutritional needs at each stage.

Pregnancy: Nutrition for the Future

The only way nutrients can reach the developing fetus in the uterus is through the **placenta,** the special organ that grows inside the uterus to support the new life (see Figure 10–1). If the mother's nutrient stores are inadequate early in pregnancy when the placenta is developing, the fetus will develop poorly, no matter how well the mother eats later. After getting such a poor start on life, a female child may grow up poorly equipped to support a normal pregnancy, and she, too, may bear a poorly developed infant.

PLACENTA (pla-SEN-tuh) the organ inside the uterus in which the mother's and fetus's circulatory systems intertwine and in which exchange of materials between maternal and fetal blood takes place. The fetus receives nutrients and oxygen across the placenta; the mother's blood picks up carbon dioxide and other waste materials to be excreted via her lungs and kidneys.

ASK YOURSELF ANSWERS: **1.** True. **2.** False. A woman needs only 15 percent more calories per day during pregnancy than she did before. **3.** True. **4.** False. A woman's cravings during pregnancy do not seem to reflect real physiological needs. **5.** True. **6.** False. A child's appetite regulates food intake to meet need; caretakers should not force food on children because this will only create conflict. **7.** False. School lunch is designed to provide one-third of the nutrients schoolchildren need in a day. **8.** True. **9.** False. Too much caffeine can cause anxiety attacks in individuals of any age, even children. **10.** False. Phytochemicals found in fruits, vegetables, and other foods may decrease one's cancer risk.

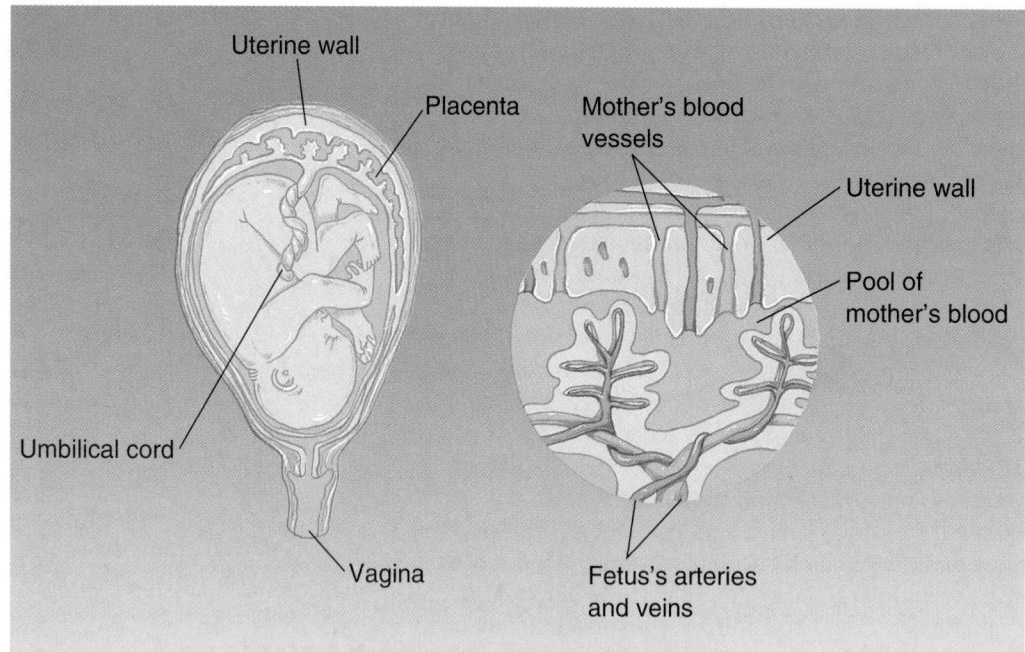

FIGURE 10–1
THE PLACENTA

The placenta is a sort of pillow or tissue in which maternal blood vessels lie side by side with fetal blood vessels entering it through the umbilical cord. This close association between the two circulatory systems permits the mother's bloodstream to deliver nutrients and oxygen to the fetus and to carry away fetal waste products.

Infants born of malnourished mothers are more likely than healthy women's infants to become ill, to have birth defects, and to suffer retarded mental or physical development. This remains true even if they later receive abundant, nourishing food. For example, among the many growth-retarded Korean orphans adopted by U.S. families after the Korean war, several years of catch-up growth occurred but did not completely remedy the growth deficits caused by early malnutrition.[2] Malnutrition in the **prenatal** and early **postnatal** periods also affects learning ability and behavior. Clearly, it is critical to provide the best nutrition at the early stages of life.

A number of factors contribute to maternal and infant health. Genetic, environmental, and behavioral factors affect risk and the outcome of pregnancy. A woman's nutrition prior to and throughout pregnancy is crucial both to her health and to the growth, development, and health of the infant she conceives. Ideally, a woman will start pregnancy at a healthful weight, with filled nutrient stores, and with the firmly established habit of eating a balanced and varied diet. The Pregnancy Readiness Scorecard permits women to evaluate their nutritional readiness for pregnancy and to identify the eating habits that might need improvement.

PRENATAL prior to birth.
POSTNATAL after birth.

Most critical risk factors for malnutrition in pregnancy:
Age 15 or under.
Unwanted pregnancy.
Many pregnancies close together.
History of poor pregnancy outcome.
Poverty.
Food faddism (strict dieting).
Heavy smoking.
Drug addiction.
Alcohol abuse.
Chronic disease requiring special diet (diabetes).
More than 15% underweight.
More than 15% overweight.

These factors at the start of pregnancy indicate that poor nutrition is very likely to be present and to adversely affect the pregnancy.

Are you nutritionally ready for pregnancy? Score each question as shown. A score of 21 is perfect; scores below 3 per question identify areas that need improvement.

1. My body weight is desirable for my height, according to the standards given in this book.

  a. Right on target. — 3 points

  b. Within 10%. — 2 points

  c. 10% to 20% above. — 1 point

  d. More than 20% above or 20% below. — 0 points

2. I drink milk and use milk products every day.

  a. Equivalent of 3 c or more a day. — 3 points

  b. About 2 c a day. — 2 points

  c. About 1 c a day. — 1 point

  d. No milk or milk products. — 0 points

3. I eat vegetables daily.

  a. Five servings a day. — 3 points

  b. Four servings a day. — 2 points

  c. Three servings a day. — 1 point

  d. Two or fewer servings a day. — 0 points

4. I eat fruits daily.

  a. Four servings a day. — 3 points

  b. Three servings a day. — 2 points

  c. Two servings a day. — 1 point

  d. One or fewer servings a day. — 0 points

5. I eat folate-rich foods, such as green leafy vegetables, orange juice, cantaloupe, legumes, and fortified breakfast cereals, daily.

  a. Three to four servings, or enough to provide 400 μg daily. — 3 points

  b. Two to three servings, or enough to meet the current RDA. — 1 point

  c. One or fewer servings, or less than half the RDA. — 0 points

6. I eat iron-rich foods, such as meats or legumes, daily.

  a. Two servings, or enough to meet the RDA. — 3 points

  b. One serving, or enough to meet about half the RDA. — 1 point

  c. Less than one serving, or less than half the RDA. — 0 points

7. I am physically fit because I have a well-established habit of exercising daily or every other day, and I will be able to continue exercising during pregnancy.

  a. I am as fit as I can be. — 3 points

  b. I am fairly fit. — 2 points

  c. I am not fit. — 0 points

Nutritional Needs of Pregnant Women

For most women, nutrient needs during pregnancy and lactation are higher than at any other time in their adult life and are greater for certain nutrients than for others (see Figure 10–2). Notice that although nutrient needs are much higher than usual, energy needs are not. An increase of only 15 percent of maintenance calories is recommended to support the metabolic demands of pregnancy and fetal development. The RDA is an additional 300 calories per day during the second and third **trimesters.**

Nearly all nutrients are recommended in increased amounts during pregnancy and lactation.[3] The Subcommittee on Dietary Intake and Nutrient Supplementation of the Institute of Medicine believes that the nutrient needs of pregnancy are best met by the routine intake of a variety of foods (see Table 10–1 on page 367) and advises against routine supplementation of all pregnant women with the exception of iron.[4] The advice is based in part on two observations:[5]

- Food supplies energy and other essential nutrients not necessarily provided by supplements.

- Nutrient supplements have the potential for inadvertent overuse, which may compromise nutrition status and be toxic to the fetus—especially early in pregnancy.

TRIMESTER one-third of the normal duration of pregnancy; the first trimester is 0 to 13 weeks, the second is 13 to 26 weeks, and the third trimester is 26 to 40 weeks.

Based on a review of several studies, the subcommittee concluded that protein, folate, iron, zinc, and calcium, as well as vitamins known to be toxic in excess amounts deserved special attention in the diets of pregnant women.[6]

The pregnancy RDA for protein is 60 grams—an additional 10 to 16 grams per day over nonpregnant requirements. Most women are already eating enough protein to cover the increased demand of pregnancy.

The pregnant woman's recommended folate intake is more than twice that of the nonpregnant woman because of the large increase in her blood volume and the rapid growth of the fetus. Certain studies have shown that folate supplements given around the time of conception reduce the recurrence of neural tube defects, such as spina bifida in the infants of women who previously have had such births.[7] To lower the risk of neural tube birth defects, women are advised to get the recommended 400 micrograms of folate a day for pregnancy—especially *before* becoming pregnant and during the first trimester of pregnancy.[8] It is possible to obtain the recommended amount of folate without supplements by following a diet that includes fresh fruits, juices, whole-grain or fortified cereals, legumes, and green vegetables. The routine use of a folate supplement thus is not recommended unless the pregnant woman's folate intake is low. In such instances, a supplement of 300 micrograms of folate per day is recommended.[9]

The body conserves iron even more than usual during pregnancy. Menstruation ceases, and absorption of iron increases up to threefold. However, the developing fetus draws on its mother's iron stores to create stores of its own to carry it through the first three to six months of life. This drain on the mother's supply can precipitate a deficiency; furthermore, the mother loses blood when she gives birth.

The RDA for iron during pregnancy is an additional 15 milligrams per day to meet maternal and fetal needs. Iron-deficiency anemia is a common problem among nonpregnant women, and as a result, many women begin pregnancy with diminished iron stores.

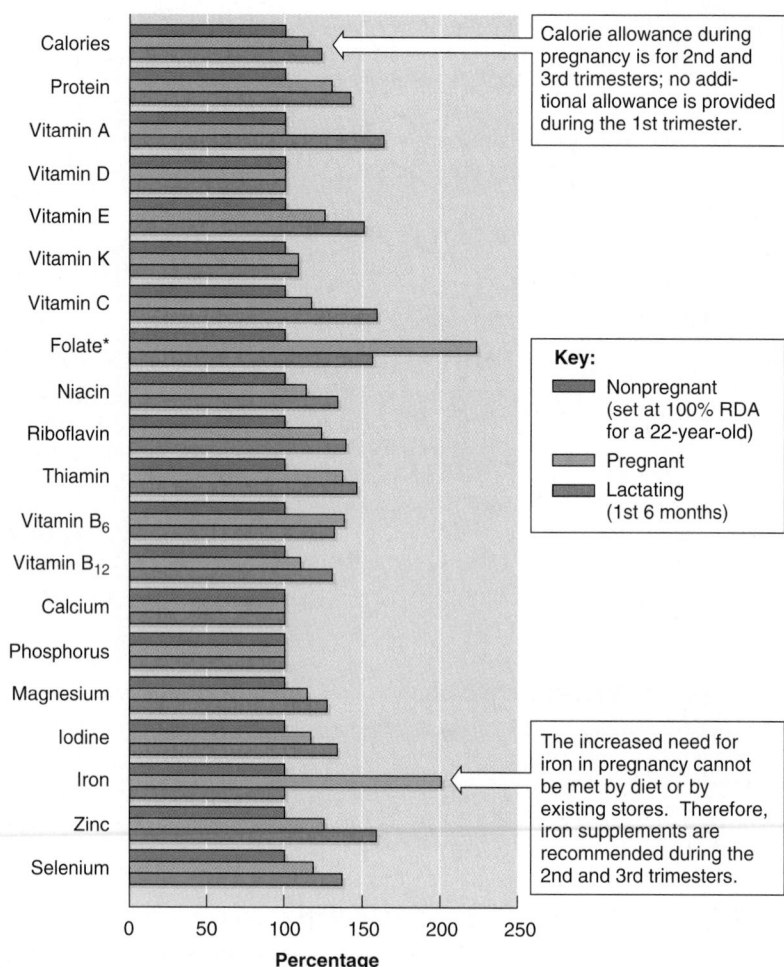

> Calorie allowance during pregnancy is for 2nd and 3rd trimesters; no additional allowance is provided during the 1st trimester.

Key:
- Nonpregnant (set at 100% RDA for a 22-year-old)
- Pregnant
- Lactating (1st 6 months)

> The increased need for iron in pregnancy cannot be met by diet or by existing stores. Therefore, iron supplements are recommended during the 2nd and 3rd trimesters.

FIGURE 10–2

COMPARISON OF NUTRIENT NEEDS OF NONPREGNANT, PREGNANT, AND LACTATING WOMEN

*The U.S. Public Health Service now recommends that all women of child-bearing age consume 400 μg of folic acid daily to reduce the risk of neural tube birth defects. To reduce risk, adequate folic acid consumption must begin before pregnancy because the defects occur within the first month after conception—generally before a woman is aware she is pregnant.

Neural tube defects include any of a number of birth defects in the orderly formation of the neural tube during early gestation. Both the brain and the spinal cord develop from the neural tube; defects result in various central nervous system disorders. The two main types are *spina bifida* (incomplete closure of the bony casing around the spinal cord) and *anencephaly* (a partially or completely missing brain). Since the neural tube closes by the fourth week of pregnancy, women are advised to consume adequate folate from as early as three months prior to conception and through at least the first three months of pregnancy.

For this reason, an iron supplement of 30 milligrams ferrous iron daily during the second and third trimesters is recommended. To facilitate absorption from the supplement, iron should be taken between meals with vitamin C-rich fruit juices or at bedtime. Since supplemental doses of iron greater than 30 milligrams can interfere with zinc absorption, pregnant women are encouraged to include good sources of zinc in their daily diets.

The RDA for calcium during pregnancy is 1,200 milligrams, a 50 percent increase over adult values and the same amount recommended for females up to the age of 24 years. Intestinal absorption of calcium doubles early in pregnancy, and the mineral is stored in the mother's bones. Later, during the last trimester of pregnancy when fetal skeletal growth is maximum and teeth are being formed, the fetus draws approximately 300 milligrams per day from the maternal blood supply.[10] Dairy products are recommended because they are also sources of vitamin D and riboflavin. However, in cases where lactose intolerance is a problem, a calcium supplement should be considered. This is particularly important for women under 25 years of age whose bone mineral density is still increasing. In such cases, a 600-milligram supplement of calcium per day during pregnancy is recommended if the woman normally consumes less than 600 milligrams of calcium a day.

Routine supplementation with vitamins during pregnancy is not advised, and excess intakes of certain vitamins, notably vitamins A and D, can cause fetal malformations.[11] Supplements should not contain more than one to two times the RDA levels. More than 10,000 International Units (more than two times the RDA) of vitamin A taken per day early in pregnancy may cause malformations of the newborn, for example.[12]

Nutrient supplementation may be appropriate in certain circumstances, however. For example, supplements of vitamin D (10 micrograms per day) and vitamin B_{12} (2 micrograms per day) may be recommended for vegans, or a multi-vitamin-mineral supplement (providing 100 percent of the RDA) beginning in the second trimester for women who do not ordinarily consume an adequate diet or are in high-risk categories, such as women carrying more than one fetus, heavy cigarette smokers, and alcohol and other drug abusers.[13] A summary of the Food and Nutrition Board's Guidelines on nutrient supplementation in pregnancy is provided in the box on the following page.

Because calorie needs increase less than nutrient needs, the pregnant woman must select foods of high nutrient density. A woman who already eats well can simply increase her servings of nutritious foods to meet her increasing nutrient

TABLE 10–1
FOOD GUIDE FOR PREGNANT AND LACTATING WOMEN

FOOD	NUMBER OF SERVINGS[a]	
	Nonpregnant Woman	Pregnant or Lactating Woman[b]
Breads/cereals	6 to 11	7 to 11 (7+)
Vegetables	3 to 5	4 to 5 (5+)
Fruits	2 to 4	3 to 4 (4+)
Meat/meat alternates	2 to 3	3 (3+)
Milk/milk products	2	3 to 4 (4+)

[a]Refer to Figures 2–6 and 2–7 in Chapter 2 for a summary of foods in each group and serving sizes.
[b]Numbers in parentheses indicate numbers of servings recommended for the pregnant teenager.

Foods containing folate:
green, leafy vegetables
legumes (dried beans, peas, and lima beans)
orange juice and cantaloupe
other vegetables
whole-grain and fortified breads and cereals

400 μg of folate can be obtained over the course of the day by consuming 1 c orange juice (75 μg), 2 slices whole wheat bread (22 μg), 1½ c Romaine lettuce (113 μg), ½ c kidney beans (65 μg), and ½ c asparagus, cooked (131 μg).

Foods containing iron:
red meat, fish, and other meat
dried fruits
legumes
whole-grain and fortified breads and cereals
dark green vegetables

Foods containing zinc:
lean meats and shellfish
legumes
fortified cereals
nuts and seeds
milk and milk products

Foods containing calcium:
milk (4 c per day will supply 1,200 mg of calcium)
other dairy products (yogurt, cheese)
green leafy vegetables (kale, broccoli, collard greens)
legumes
fortified soy milk
certain brands of tofu

needs. For most women, appropriate choices include such foods as nonfat milk, cottage cheese, lean meats, legumes, eggs, dark green vegetables, and whole-grain or fortified breads and cereals along with generous quantities of vitamin C-rich foods (refer to Table 10–1).

If the pregnant woman does not receive adequate nourishment and does not gain the recommended amount of weight, she might give birth to a baby of **low birthweight (LBW)**. Not all small babies are unhealthy, but birthweight and length of gestation are the primary indicators of an infant's future health status. A low-birthweight baby is more likely than a normal-weight baby to experience complications during delivery and has a statistically greater chance of having physical and mental birth defects, developing diseases, and dying early in life.

Low birthweight in full-term infants is a major contributing factor to infant mortality.[14] Clearly, a key to reducing infant mortality is reducing the incidence of low-birthweight babies. A host of factors need to be addressed to do so: low socioeconomic status, the lack of access to health care, inadequate prenatal care, poor nutrition, low level of educational achievement, unsanitary living conditions, and unhealthful habits such as smoking, drinking, and other drug use.[15]

Maternal Weight Gain

Normal weight gain and adequate nutrition support the health of the mother and the development of the fetus. The National Academy of Sciences Committee recommendations for weight gain take into account a mother's prepregnancy weight for height or body mass index (BMI), as shown in Table 10–2. The Committee recommends that a woman who begins pregnancy at a healthful weight should gain between 25 and 35 pounds. Women pregnant with twins need to gain 35 to 45 pounds. An underweight woman needs to gain between 28 and 40 pounds; an obese woman, between 16 and 25 pounds. Weight gains at the upper end of the range are recommended for pregnant teenagers because of their increased risk of low weight gains and delivery of low-birthweight infants.

Low weight gain in pregnancy is associated with increased risk of delivering a low-birthweight infant; such infants have high mortality rates. Excessive weight

---

NUTRIENT SUPPLEMENTATION IN PREGNANCY

- Dietary supplements should not replace dietary counseling or a well-balanced diet; improvement of diet quality through use of nutritious foods is preferred to supplementation.
- To meet the increased need for iron during the second and third trimesters of pregnancy, a low-dose iron supplement (30 milligrams of ferrous iron daily) is advised.
- If therapeutic levels of iron (more than 30 milligrams daily) are given to treat anemia, supplementation with 15 milligrams of zinc and 2 milligrams of copper is recommended because the iron may interfere with the absorption and utilization of these trace elements.
- With careful planning, pregnant women can meet the physiologic requirements for folate from diet; it is prudent to supplement the diet with low doses (300 micrograms a day) of folate if there is any question about the adequacy of intake of this nutrient.
- Because of accumulating data that excessive vitamin A consumption poses a risk of birth defects, supplementation with preformed vitamin A should be avoided during the first trimester unless there is specific evidence of a deficiency. Beta-carotene intake need not be restricted.
- For pregnant women who do not ordinarily consume an adequate diet and for those in high-risk categories, such as women carrying more than one fetus, heavy cigarette smokers, and alcohol and other drug abusers, a multivitamin-mineral supplement is recommended. The supplement should be taken between meals or at bedtime to facilitate absorption and should contain:

30 mg iron	2 mg vitamin B_6
15 mg zinc	300 μg folate
2 mg copper	50 mg vitamin C
250 mg calcium	5 μg vitamin D

- A 10-microgram (400 IU) supplement of vitamin D is recommended for vegans and others with a low intake of vitamin D-fortified milk. A vitamin B_{12} supplement of 2 micrograms daily is recommended for vegans.
- A calcium supplement of 600 milligrams daily is recommended for women under age 25 whose daily dietary calcium intake is less than 600 milligrams. To enhance absorption and limit interaction with iron supplements, the calcium should be taken with meals.

SOURCE: Food and Nutrition Board, Institute of Medicine, National Academy of Sciences, *Nutrition During Pregnancy* (Washington, D.C.: National Academy Press, 1990).

LOW BIRTHWEIGHT (LBW) a birthweight of 5½ lb (2,500 g) or less, used as a predictor of poor health in the newborn and as a probable indicator of poor nutrition status of the mother during and/or before pregnancy. Normal birthweight for a full-term baby is 6½ to 8¾ lb (about 3,000 to 4,000 g). LBW infants are of two different types. Some are premature (they are born early). Others have suffered growth failure in the uterus; they may or may not be born early, but they are small.

gain in pregnancy increases the risk of complications during labor and delivery as well as postpartum obesity.[16] Obese women also have an increased risk for complications during pregnancy, including hypertension and gestational diabetes.

The infant at birth will weigh only about 6 1/2 to 8 pounds, but the body tissues the mother builds (blood, blood vessels, muscle, fat stores, and others) to provide a healthful environment for the fetus's development weigh more than 20 pounds (see Table 10–3). Weight gain should be lowest during the first trimester—two to four pounds for the entire trimester—followed by a steady gain of about a pound per week thereafter. If a woman gains more than the recommended amount of weight early in pregnancy, however, she should not try to diet in the last weeks. Dieting during pregnancy is not recommended. A *sudden* large weight gain may indicate the onset of pregnancy-induced hypertension (discussed later). A woman experiencing this type of weight gain should see her health-care provider.

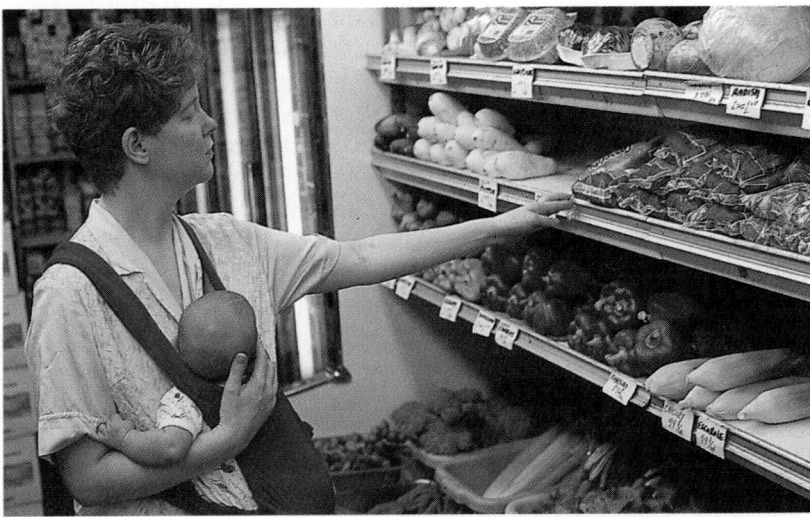

A nutritious diet supports pregnancy and successful lactation, which offers many health advantages to the newborn infant.

Some of the weight a woman gains in pregnancy is lost at delivery. For the woman who has gained the recommended 25 to 35 pounds, the remainder is generally lost within a few months as her blood volume returns to normal and she loses the fluids she has accumulated.

Practices to Avoid

Optimal pregnancy outcome is influenced by maternal nutrient intake but can also be affected by maternal use of nonfood substances, excess caffeine, low-calorie diets, megadoses of certain vitamins, tobacco, alcohol, and illicit drugs. **Pica** refers to the craving of nonfood items having little or no nutritional value. Pica of pregnancy typically involves the consumption of dirt, clay, or laundry starch, but episodes of pica have included compulsive ingestion of such things as ice, paper, and coffee grounds.[17] The medical consequences of pica can include malnutrition as nonfood items replace nutritious foods in the diet, obesity from overconsumption of items such as starch, the ingestion of toxic compounds, or intestinal obstruction by consuming large amounts of clay or starch.[18]

The Food and Drug Administration has advised pregnant women to avoid unnecessary consumption of caffeine because of animal studies suggesting that it causes birth defects.[19] Studies in humans have generally failed to show that caffeine use has a negative effect on pregnancy outcome, although limited evidence has shown that moderate to heavy use may contribute to lower infant birthweight.[20] Women who choose to use caffeine during pregnancy are generally advised to do so in moderation (the equivalent of one cup of coffee or two 12-ounce cola beverages a day) if at all (see the Nutrition Action feature starting on page 373).

TABLE 10–2
RECOMMENDED WEIGHT GAIN FOR PREGNANT WOMEN BASED ON BODY MASS INDEX (BMI)

BMI	RECOMMENDED GAIN (LB)[a]
<19.8	28–40
19.8–26.0	25–35
26.0–29.0	16–25

[a]Teens should strive to gain the maximum pounds in their ranges; short women (less than 62 inches tall) should strive for the minimum. Weight gain varies widely, and these values are suggested only as guidelines for identifying individuals whose weights may be too high or low for health.

SOURCE: National Academy of Sciences, Food and Nutrition Board, *Nutrition During Pregnancy* (Washington D.C.: National Academy Press, 1990).

PICA the craving of nonfood items such as clay, ice, and laundry starch. Pica does not appear to be limited to any particular geographic area, race, sex, culture, or social status.

Some practices are truly harmful, and their potential impact on pregnancy outcome is too great to risk. Low-carbohydrate or low-calorie diets that cause ketosis deprive the fetus's brain of needed glucose and cause congenital deformity. Most serious may be the invisible effects. For example, carbohydrate metabolism may be rendered permanently defective, or the infant's brain may be permanently damaged. Protein deprivation can cause children's height and head circumference to diminish markedly and irreversibly.

Another harmful maternal practice is smoking, which restricts the blood supply to the growing fetus, thereby limiting the delivery of nutrients and removal of wastes. Smoking stunts growth, thus increasing the risk of premature delivery, low infant birthweight, retarded development, and spontaneous abortions (fetal deaths).[21] Smoking is responsible for 20 percent to 30 percent of all low-birthweight deliveries in the United States.[22] Sudden infant death syndrome (SIDS) has also been linked to a mother's smoking during pregnancy.[23]

During the past 15 years, research has confirmed that consumption of alcohol adversely affects fetal development.[24] Even as few as one or two drinks daily can cause **fetal alcohol syndrome (FAS)**—irreversible brain damage and mental and physical retardation in the fetus. The most severe impact of maternal drinking is likely to occur in the first month, before the woman even is sure she is pregnant. This preventable condition (FAS) is estimated to occur in approximately one to two infants per 1,000 live births and is the leading known cause of mental retardation in the United States.[25] Birth defects, low birthweight, and spontaneous abortions occur more often in pregnancies of women who drink even as little as two ounces of alcohol daily during pregnancy. Accumulating evidence that even one drink may be too much has led the surgeon general to take the position that women should stop drinking as soon as they *plan* to become pregnant.[26]

Drugs other than alcohol taken during pregnancy can also cause birth defects. A particularly dramatic example is the acne medication Accutane (isotretinoin), which causes major deformities during fetal development. Pregnant women should avoid taking all drugs except on the advice of their physician.

Common Nutrition-Related Problems of Pregnancy

Common physical problems in pregnancy include morning sickness and, later, constipation. The nausea of morning sickness seems unavoidable because it arises from the hormonal changes taking place early in pregnancy, but it can sometimes be alleviated. Suggested strategies to alleviate the nausea and vomiting of morning sickness include:

- Eat small, frequent meals alternating dry and fluid feedings.
- Before getting up in the morning, eat saltines, hard candies, or other dry starchy foods.
- Eat as soon as you feel hungry.
- Avoid fatty foods.
- Avoid highly seasoned foods.
- Avoid any specific food (especially foods with strong odors) causing nausea or vomiting.[27]

Later, as the hormones of pregnancy alter her muscle tone and the growing fetus crowds her intestinal organs, an expectant mother may complain of con-

TABLE 10–3
AN EXAMPLE OF THE PREGNANT WOMAN'S WEIGHT GAIN

DEVELOPMENT	WEIGHT GAIN (LB)
Infant at birth	7–8
Placenta	1
Increase in mother's blood volume to supply placenta	4
Increase in mother's fluid volume	4
Increase in size of mother's uterus and the muscles to support it	2
Increase in size of mother's breasts	2
Fluid to surround infant in amniotic sac	2
Mother's fat stores (varies)	3–12
Total	25–35

Note: The pattern of gain should be about a pound a month for the first three months and a pound a week thereafter. Different patterns of weight gain are suggested for underweight, normal-weight, and overweight women.

FETAL ALCOHOL SYNDROME (FAS) the cluster of symptoms seen in an infant or child whose mother consumed excess alcohol during pregnancy, including retarded growth, impaired development of the central nervous system, and facial malformations.

stipation. A high-fiber diet, plentiful fluid intake, and moderate exercise will help to relieve this condition.

Pregnancy for many women is a time of adjustment to major changes. The woman who is expecting a baby is a growing person in more ways than one. Not only her physical needs but also her emotional needs are changing. If it is her first baby, she senses that her lifestyle will change as she takes on the new responsibility of caring for a child. Ideally, she will be encouraged to develop this sense of responsibility by caring for herself during pregnancy. The expectant mother needs support in thinking of herself as a thoroughly worthwhile and important person with a new and challenging task that she can and will perform well. Oftentimes, as a young adult, she is still working out her relationship with her mate, and they both know that the coming of a first baby will affect that relationship profoundly. A need exists for sensitive communication and understanding by both parties in this time of transition.

Women's cravings during pregnancy do not seem to reflect real physiological needs. People should not laugh at women going through this major experience and should recognize the validity of these women's feelings. If a woman craves pickles and chocolate sauce at two o'clock in the morning, for example, it is probably not because she lacks a combination of nutrients uniquely supplied by these foods. The woman is, however, expressing a need as real and as important as her need for nutrients—the need for support, understanding, and love. More serious problems needing control during pregnancy include hypertension and diabetes, described briefly in the following paragraphs.

Pregnancy-Induced Hypertension (PIH). **Preeclampsia** and **eclampsia** are hypertensive conditions induced by pregnancy. Preeclampsia is characterized by high blood pressure, protein in the urine, and generalized edema that may cause sudden, large weight gain from retained water. Fluid retention alone, which is quite common in pregnant women, is not sufficient to diagnose preeclampsia.[28] Warning signs of preeclampsia include severe and constant headaches, sudden weight gain (1 lb/day), swelling, dizziness, and blurred vision. Eclampsia, the more severe form of this pregnancy-induced hypertension (PIH), is characterized by convulsions that can lead to coma. Both conditions present serious health risks to mother and fetus. PIH can retard fetal growth and cause the placenta to separate from the uterus, resulting in stillbirth. The former practice of restricting salt and prescribing diuretics for the edema of PIH is not recommended, and pregnant women are advised to use salt to taste. Pregnant women who consume calcium supplements of 1,500 to 2,000 mg per day may be at lower risk of PIH.[29]

Diabetes. Infants born to women with diabetes are at greater risk for prematurity, congenital defects, excessively high birthweight, and respiratory distress syndrome.[30] Metabolic control of diabetes before and throughout pregnancy is critical. In some women, pregnancy can alter carbohydrate metabolism and precipitate a condition known as **gestational diabetes.** The abnormal blood glucose levels seen during pregnancy return to normal after pregnancy for about two-thirds of women diagnosed with the condition. Risk factors include age 35 or older, previous history of gestational diabetes, obesity, and a family history of diabetes.

Some women with gestational diabetes have the classic symptoms of diabetes—increased thirst, hunger, urination, weakness—but other women have

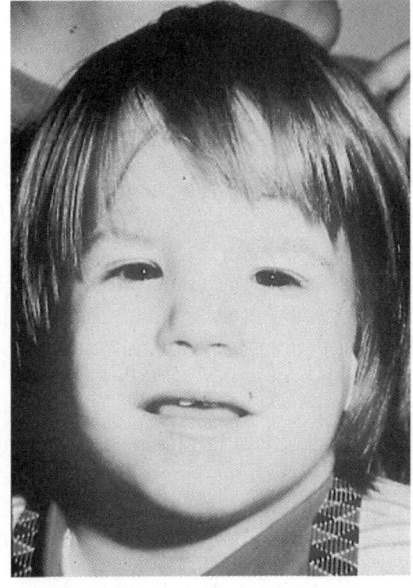

These facial traits (low nasal bridge, short eyelid opening, small head circumference, undeveloped groove in center of upper lip) are typical of fetal alcohol syndrome, caused by drinking alcohol during pregnancy. Irreversible abnormalities of the brain and other organs accompany these facial features.

PREGNANCY-INDUCED HYPERTENSION (PIH) high blood pressure that develops during the second half of pregnancy.

PREECLAMPSIA a condition characterized by hypertension, fluid retention, and protein in the urine.

ECLAMPSIA a severe extension of preeclampsia characterized by convulsions.

GESTATIONAL DIABETES the appearance of abnormal glucose tolerance during pregnancy, with a return to normal following pregnancy.

no warning signs of the condition. For this reason, all pregnant women today are screened for gestational diabetes during the twenty-fourth and twenty-eighth weeks of gestation.[31]

Adolescent Pregnancy

More than a million teenagers become pregnant in the United States each year—one out of every five babies is born to a teenager—and more than a tenth of these mothers are under age 15. The complexity of social, emotional, and physical factors makes teen pregnancy one of the most challenging situations for meeting nutritional needs. According to a position paper from the American Dietetic Association, pregnant adolescents are nutritionally at risk and require intervention early in and throughout pregnancy.[32] Medical and nutritional risks are particularly high when the teenager is within two years of menarche (usually 15 years of age or younger).[33] Risks include higher rates among pregnant teens than in older women of PIH, iron-deficiency anemia, premature birth, stillbirths, low-birthweight infants, and prolonged labor. In addition, mothers under 15 years of age bear more babies who die within the first year than do any other age group.[34]

Pregnancy places adolescent girls, who are already at risk for nutrition problems, at even greater risk because of the increased energy and nutrient demands of pregnancy. To support the needs of both mother and infant, adolescents are encouraged to strive for pregnancy weight gains at the upper end of the ranges recommended for pregnant women (refer to Table 10–2). Those who gain between 30 and 35 pounds during pregnancy have lower risks of delivering low-birthweight infants.[35] Adequate nutrition can substantially improve the course and outcome of adolescent pregnancy.[36]

Emphasis on preparing young girls for future pregnancy is needed in public schools and public health programs. A model program for giving nutritional help to teenage mothers is, among others, the WIC (Women's, Infants' and Children's) program, a federally funded program that provides nutrition education and low-cost nutritious foods to low-income pregnant women, mothers, and their children.

Nutrition of the Breastfeeding Mother

Adequate nutrition of the mother makes a highly significant contribution to successful lactation; without it, lactation is likely to falter or fail. The mother should continue to eat high-quality foods until the end of her pregnancy, not attempt to restrict her weight gain unduly, and plan to enjoy ample food and fluid at frequent intervals.

A nursing mother produces 30 ounces of milk a day, on the average, with wide variations possible. The RDA table suggests that 500 calories to support this milk production come from added food and that the rest come from the stores of fat the mother's body has accumulated during pregnancy for this purpose. (Table 10–1 showed a food pattern that would meet the lactating woman's nutrient needs.)

The period of lactation is the natural time for a woman to lose the extra body fat she accumulated during pregnancy. Once lactation has been established, if her choice of foods is judicious, a nursing mother can tolerate a calorie deficit and a gradual loss of weight (one pound per week) without any effect on her milk output. Fat can only be mobilized slowly, however, and too large an energy deficit will inhibit lactation. On the other hand, if a mother does not breastfeed, she may not as easily lose the fat she gained during pregnancy.

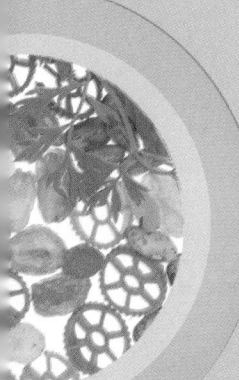

Not for Coffee Drinkers Only

NUTRITION ACTION

In 1657, when merchants first introduced Londoners to a Middle Eastern brew known as coffee, they boasted it to be a "wholesome and physical drink," an elixir of health suitable for treating colds, coughs, gout, and many other ills.[37] Modern-day coffee drinkers have heard otherwise. During the past decade, the "coffee generation" has been subject to a barrage of reports linking coffee and other **caffeine**-containing products such as colas and tea with more than 100 diseases. Fingers have repeatedly pointed at caffeine as the culprit behind breast disease, cancer, heart disease, birth defects, and high blood pressure, to name just a few.

Despite the brouhaha over the substance, the jury is still out as to whether caffeine is truly to blame. Scientists have yet to confirm long-standing suspicions that caffeine contributes to any health problems other than jitteriness. One reason for all the controversy is that much of the evidence linking the substance with different diseases has been clouded by a number of issues. Some studies do not measure sources of caffeine other than coffee and tea, such as soft drinks, chocolate, and certain medications. In addition, the amount of caffeine and other substances in coffee or tea can vary considerably depending on how the beverage is brewed, a fact most studies fail to take into account.

Consider the widely debated question of whether drinking coffee raises blood cholesterol. Granted, a great deal of strong evidence suggests that the beverage does contribute to high blood cholesterol and therefore to heart disease. The hitch is that most of the evidence comes from Scandinavia, where coffee is boiled rather than brewed in automatic drip coffeemakers or electric percolators. Subsequent research has found that whereas boiled coffee appears to boost blood cholesterol levels, filtered coffee does not, most likely because substances in boiled coffee other than caffeine may be the cholesterol-raising culprits.[38]

Another issue that most research has not filtered out is that while coffee drinking may not contribute to ill health in and of itself, it seems to be part of a lifestyle that does. After questioning some 2,600 men and women about their health habits, a group of Boston-based researchers found that women who opted for decaffeinated coffee exclusively were more likely than regular-coffee drinkers to, among other things, eat vegetables frequently and exercise regularly. Male decaf drinkers also tended to have adopted more healthful habits, such as eating low-fat diets, than did their regular-coffee-drinking counterparts. Thus, it may not be the coffee but rather the poor health habits that often go along with it that contribute to health problems.[39]

None of this is to say that caffeine is necessarily good for people. As anyone who can't get going in the morning without a cup of coffee or can of caffeinated soda is well aware, consuming caffeine day in and day out can be habit form-

CAFFEINE a type of compound, called a methylxanthine, found in coffee beans, cola nuts, cocoa beans, and tea leaves. A central nervous system stimulant, caffeine's effects include increasing the heart rate, boosting urine production, and raising the metabolic rate.

At least 8 out of 10 Americans consume caffeine, the most widely used behaviorally active drug in the world.

Contrary to popular belief, black coffee will not sober up a person who has had too many beers or other alcoholic drinks.

ing. In fact, some researchers have identified a condition called **caffeine dependence syndrome,** characterized by at least three of the four following criteria: withdrawal symptoms such as headache and fatigue; caffeine consumption despite knowledge that it may be causing harm; repeated, unsuccessful attempts to cut back on caffeine; and tolerance to caffeine.[40]

Along with people who are dependent on caffeine, people with certain medical conditions would do well to consume caffeine in moderation or avoid it completely. Pregnant women, for example, should limit the amount of caffeine they take in. While the substance has never been proven to cause birth defects, it does cross the placenta and enter the fetus, where large amounts can affect the unborn baby's heart rate and breathing.[41] Some research also suggests that the amount of caffeine in three or four cups of coffee could raise the risk of suffering a miscarriage, perhaps by decreasing bloodflow through the placenta.[42] In addition, those with ulcers should steer clear of caffeinated *and* decaffeinated coffee, both of which stimulate the secretion of acid, which can irritate the stomach's lining.

For a healthy person, drinking one or two cups of coffee, tea, or cola a day does not seem to pose any hazard. Only those who are particularly sensitive to caffeine and suffer symptoms such as headaches, nervousness, and insomnia after consuming it really need to consider avoiding—or at least cutting back on—it. (See Table 10–4 to figure out how much caffeine you're taking in each day.)

If you drink coffee or a can or two of cola every day and decide to quit, make sure you do it gradually. Even moderate caffeine users who try to stop cold turkey often suffer from withdrawal symptoms, such as splitting headaches, fatigue, moodiness, and nausea. Try instead to cut back gradually by, say, no more than a cup or so every couple of days. You can do that by substituting decaffeinated coffee for some of the regular roast in your morning brew and gradually using more and more decaf and less regular coffee. Likewise, you can drink a glass of decaffeinated rather than caffeinated soda here and there until you've weaned yourself off the caffeinated version.

Smokers, incidentally, metabolize the caffeine in their bloodstreams more quickly than nonsmokers, thereby needing more of the substance to obtain its stimulating effect. When smokers try to give up cigarettes, however, the caffeine stays in the bloodstream longer, giving them a stronger than usual dose and possibly causing jitteriness and irritability on top of the jitters already occurring as a result of giving up nicotine. Thus, smokers who kick the cigarette habit may want to try to cut back on caffeine at the same time to avoid that problem.[43]

TABLE 10–4
CAFFEINE COUNTDOWN

DRINKS AND FOODS	AVERAGE (MG)
Coffee (6-oz cup)	
Brewed	103
Instant	57
Decaffeinated, brewed or instant	2
Tea (6-oz cup)	
Brewed, black, steeped for 3 minutes	36
Instant iced tea (12-oz glass)	31
Soft drinks (12-oz can)	
Dr. Pepper	41
Colas:	
Regular	38–46
Diet	36–50
Caffeine free	0
Mountain Dew, Mello Yello	52–54
7-Up	46
Cocoa beverage (6-oz cup)	3–5
Chocolate milk beverage (8 oz)	5–8
Milk chocolate candy (1 oz)	7–18
Dark chocolate, semisweet (1 oz)	21
Baker's chocolate (1 oz)	25
Chocolate-flavored syrup (1 oz)	5

DRUGS[a]	AVERAGE (MG)
Pain relievers (standard dose)	
Excedrin Extra Strength	130
Bayer Select Headache Pain Relief Formula	130
Maximum Strength Multi-Symptom Formula Midol	120
Stimulants	
NoDoz, Vivarin	200

[a]Because products change, contact the manufacturer for an update on products you use regularly.

SOURCES: J. A. T. Pennington, *Bowes & Church's Food Values of Portions Commonly Used, 16th ed.* (Philadelphia: J. B. Lippincott Company, 1994), pp. 381–383; *Physicians' Desk Reference for Nonprescription Drugs, 15th ed.* (Montvale, N.J.: Medical Economics Data Production Company, 1994), pp. 522, 526, 721, 733, 738.

CAFFEINE DEPENDENCE SYNDROME dependence on caffeine characterized by at least three of the four following criteria: withdrawal symptoms such as headache and fatigue; caffeine consumption despite knowledge that it may be causing harm; repeated, unsuccessful attempts to cut back on caffeine; and tolerance to caffeine.

Chapter 9 discusses caffeine's effect on physical performance.

Healthy Infants

The growth of infants directly reflects their nutritional well-being and is the major indicator of their nutrition status. A baby grows faster during the first year of life than ever again, doubling its birthweight during the first four to six months, and tripling its birthweight by the end of the first year (see Figure 10–3). Adequate nutrition during infancy is critical to support this rapid rate of growth and development. Clearly, from the point of view of nutrition, the first year is the most important year of a person's life. This section provides an overview of nutrient requirements, current recommendations for feeding healthy infants, and the relationship between infant feeding and selected pediatric nutrition issues.

Milk for the Infant: Breastfeeding

Toward the end of her pregnancy, a woman needs to decide whether to breast-feed her baby or not. If she plans to breastfeed, she should begin to prepare so that she can get started smoothly. It is wise, ahead of time, to read a handbook on breastfeeding, talk with other women who have successfully breastfed their babies, and seek family and medical support. Ideally, before the baby is born, the mother and a partner can attend classes together to obtain basic information regarding breastfeeding.

Breastfeeding has both emotional and physical health advantages. Emotional bonding is facilitated by many events and behaviors of mother and infant during the early months and years; one of the first can be breastfeeding.

During the first two or three days of lactation, the breasts produce **colostrum,** a premilk substance containing antibodies and white cells from the mother's blood. Because it contains immunity factors, colostrum helps to protect the newborn infant from those infections against which the mother has developed an immunity—precisely those in the environment against which the infant needs protection. Entering the infant's body with the milk, these antibodies inactivate bacteria within the digestive tract, where they could otherwise cause intestinal infections.

Breast milk also contains antibodies, although not as much as colostrum. Colostrum and breast milk both contain the **bifidus factor** that favors the growth of the "friendly" bacteria *Lactobacillus bifidus* in the infant's digestive tract so that other, harmful bacteria cannot grow there. Breast milk also contains the powerful antibacterial agent **lactoferrin,** as well as other factors, including several enzymes, several hormones (including thyroid hormone and prostaglandins), and lipids that help to protect the infant against infection. Breast-fed infants have lower rates of hospital admissions, ear infections, diarrhea, rashes, allergies, and other health problems than bottle-fed infants.[44]

Breast milk is tailor-made to meet the nutrient needs of the young infant. It offers its carbohydrate in the easy-to-assimilate form of lactose; its fat contains a generous proportion of the essential fatty acid linoleic acid; and its protein, alpha-lactalbumin, is one that the infant can easily digest. With the exception of vitamin D, its vitamin contents are ample. As for minerals, calcium, phosphorus, and magnesium are present in amounts appropriate for the rate of growth expected in a human infant, and breast milk is low in sodium. Its iron

COLOSTRUM (co-LAHS-trum) a milklike secretion from the breast, rich in protective factors, present during the first day or so after delivery and before milk appears.

BIFIDUS FACTOR (BIFF-id-us) a factor in colostrum and breast milk that favors the growth in the infant's intestinal tract of the "friendly" bacteria *Lactobacillus bifidus* so that other, less desirable intestinal inhabitants will not flourish.

LACTOFERRIN (lak-toe-FERR-in) a factor in breast milk that binds iron and keeps it from supporting the growth of the infant's intestinal bacteria.

is highly absorbable, and the presence of a zinc-binding protein favors the absorption of the zinc it contains.

Breastfeeding provides other benefits as well. It protects a newborn against allergy development during the vulnerable first few weeks of life, the act of suckling favors a baby's normal tooth and jaw alignment, and breastfed babies are less likely to be obese because they are less likely to be overfed. A woman who wants to breastfeed can derive justification and satisfaction from all these advantages.

These attributes, along with the convenience and lower cost of breastfeeding, have led many organizations and medical experts to encourage breastfeeding for all normal full-term infants.[45] Despite the health benefits, however, the incidence of breastfeeding has declined since the early 1980s.[46] Analysis of data from a survey of mothers indicates that breastfeeding rates continue to be the highest among women who are older, are well-educated, are relatively affluent, and/or live in the western United States. Among those least likely to breastfeed are women who are low-income, are black, are less than age 20, and/or live in the southeastern United States.[47]

A number of barriers to achieving the nation's health objective for increasing the incidence of breastfeeding have been noted. They include lack of knowledge, an absence of work policies and facilities that support lactating women (e.g., extended maternity leave, part-time employment, facilities for pumping breast milk or breastfeeding, and on-site child care), the portrayal of bottle feeding rather than breastfeeding as the norm in the American society, the lack of breastfeeding incentives, and lack of support for low-income women.

Under most circumstances, a woman can freely choose to feed her baby breast milk or formula, knowing that the two modes of feeding are beneficial to the infant. However, if the infant is premature or if other factors act to the baby's disadvantage, breastfeeding becomes the pre-

FIGURE 10–3   GROWTH AND DEVELOPMENTAL CHARACTERISTICS FROM BIRTH THROUGH ONE YEAR

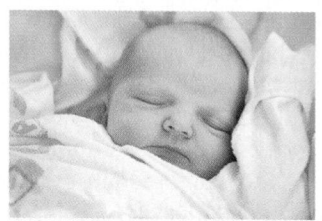

First Days of Life
Generally weighs from 7 to 9 pounds; length is 19 to 21 inches. Head is relatively large and has soft spot on top. Startles and sneezes easily. Jaw may tremble. May hiccup and spit up.

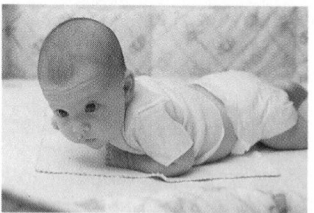

One Month
Has regained weight lost after birth and more. Lifts head briefly when placed on stomach. Whole body moves when infant is touched or lifted. Eats every two to four hours.

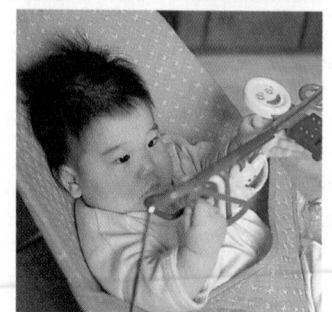

Four Months
Weight nearly doubled. Has grown three to four inches. Follows objects with eyes. Reaches toward objects with both hands; plays with fingers; puts fingers and objects into mouth. Holds head up steadily though back needs support. Attempts to roll over. Awake longer at feeding time. Eats seven or eight times per day. Sleeps six to seven hours at night.

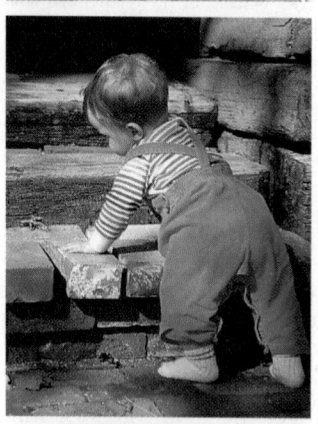

Eight Months
Gains in weight and height are less rapid, appetite has decreased. Rolls over; stands up with help; sits up; hitches self along the floor. Reaches for, grasps, and examines objects with hands, eyes, and mouth. Has one or two teeth. Takes two naps a day. Can feed self from bottle.

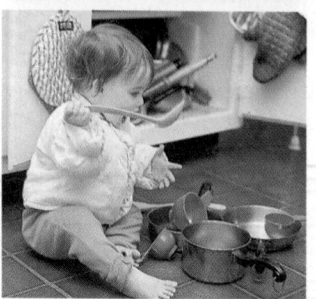

Twelve Months
Usually has tripled birthweight and increased length by 50%. Grasps and releases objects with fingers. Holds spoon, but uses it poorly.

SOURCE: Reprinted with permission from J. Brown, *Nutrition Now* (St. Paul, MN: West Publishing Company, 1994) p. 29–20.

ferred choice. The composition of the milk from a premature infant's mother is ideal for the premature infant. Even when separation prevents the mother from breastfeeding, she can express (pump) her milk to be given to the infant by bottle. Breastfeeding manuals show how to use manual massage or breast pumps to obtain milk. If the mother chooses not to breastfeed, a premature baby can, however, be successfully nourished on special formula for premature infants.

If a woman has a communicable disease such as AIDS, tuberculosis, or hepatitis or if she must take a medication that is secreted in breast milk and is known to affect the infant, she must not breastfeed. Drug addicts—including alcohol abusers—are capable of ingesting such high doses of their drug that their infants can become addicts by way of breast milk. In such cases, breastfeeding is also contraindicated.

Most prescription drugs do not reach nursing infants in sufficiently large quantities to affect them adversely. As a precaution, a nursing mother should consult with the prescribing physician before taking any drug. Minimal use of alcohol is compatible with breastfeeding. Smoking between feedings is permissible, although it is important not to expose the infant to secondhand smoke in the air. Coffee drinking is fine in moderation (two to three cups of coffee a day), as is the eating of foods such as garlic and spices. A particular food might affect the baby's liking for the mother's milk; this is a matter that requires individual detective work. (Examples are chocolate for some babies, excess caffeine for others, and foods that cause gas in the mother for still others.) If a woman has an ordinary cold, she can go on nursing without worry. The infant may well catch it from her anyway but may actually be less susceptible than a bottle-fed baby would be, thanks to the immunologic protection offered by breast milk.

A woman sometimes hesitates to breastfeed because she has heard that environmental contaminants may enter her milk and harm her baby. The decision whether to breastfeed on this basis might best be made after consulting with a physician or dietitian familiar with the local environment or with the state health department.

Feeding Formula

Like the breastfeeding mother, the mother who offers formula to her baby has reasons for making her choice, and her feelings should be honored. Infant formulas are manufactured to approximate the nutrient composition of breast milk. The immunologic protection of breast milk, however, cannot be duplicated, but the high level of preventive med-

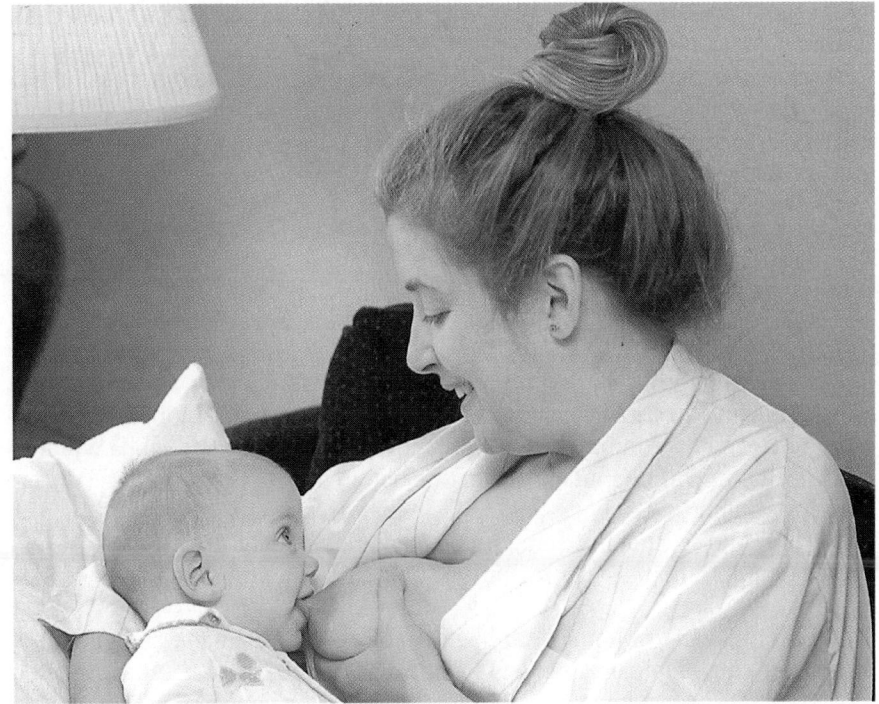

Breast milk is a very special substance.

ical care (vaccinations) and public health measures achieved in the developed countries, especially in the United States and Canada, make this consideration less important than it was in the past. Safety and sanitation can be achieved with either mode of feeding by the educated mother whose drinking water supply is reliable.

One of the major advantages of formula feeding is that gained by the mother whose attempts at breastfeeding have met with frustration. Formula provides adequate nourishment for the infant, and a mother can choose this alternative with confidence. Other aspects of formula feeding include the following:

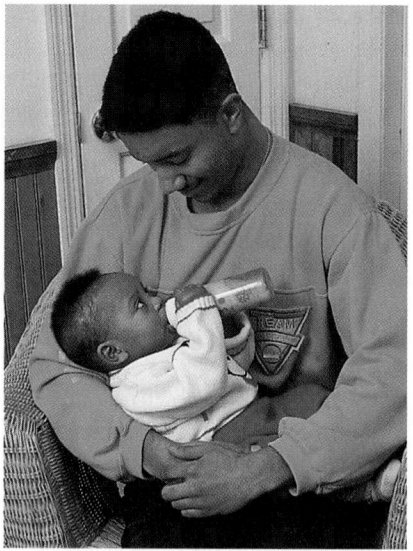

Formula feeding allows other family members to enjoy feeding the infant.

- The parents can see that the baby is getting enough milk during feedings.
- The mother can offer similar closeness, warmth, and stimulation during feedings as the breastfeeding mother does.
- Other family members can get close to the baby and develop a warm relationship in feeding sessions.

Many mothers breastfeed at first and then wean the baby within the first one to six months. When a woman chooses to wean her infant during the first six months of life, it is imperative that she shift to *infant formula*, not to plain cow's milk of any kind—whole, low-fat, or nonfat. Only formula contains enough iron (to name but one of many factors) to support normal development in the baby's first months of life. National and international standards have been set for the nutrient content of infant formulas.

For infants with special problems, many variations of infant formulas are available. Special formulas based on soy protein are available for infants allergic to milk protein, and formulas with the lactose replaced can be used for infants with lactose intolerance.

Cow's milk, both whole and reduced-fat, is not recommended during the first year of life, according to the American Academy of Pediatrics (AAP).[48] Cow's milk is an inappropriate replacement for breast milk or infant formula because it provides insufficient vitamin C and iron and excessive sodium and protein. Feeding cow's milk to infants may increase the risk of iron-deficiency anemia and cow's milk protein allergy.

Supplements for the Infant

Breast milk or formula and the infant's own internal stores will meet most nutrient needs for the first four to six months, except for vitamin D and fluoride. Thereafter, the introduction of properly chosen juices and foods will normally keep up with the infant's changing requirements. But if the time during which an infant is receiving only milk (either breast milk or formula) is prolonged beyond six months, some supplementation may be appropriate. At four to six months, infants may require an iron supplement, depending on food intake.

Breast milk does not provide enough vitamin D for the infant, and vitamin D deficiency causes impaired bone mineralization in children. Manufacturers fortify infant formulas with vitamin D, but due to the low concentration of vitamin D in breast milk, pediatricians routinely prescribe a vitamin D supplement for breastfed infants.

Supplemental fluoride may also be needed by the breastfed infant. The pediatrician should prescribe it, if appropriate. Fluoride does not appear to be secreted into breast milk even if the mother's fluoride supply is ample. As for iron, breast milk makes it easily absorbable. When breast milk ceases to be the infant's main food, iron-fortified cereals become important.

For the formula-fed infant, the make-up of the formula determines what further supplementation may be necessary. The pediatrician is the expert to consult on individual needs. In a baby's first six months, the choice of formula is important because whatever is chosen must supply the nutrients of human milk in similar forms and proportions.

Food for the Infant

The infant's rapid growth and metabolism demand an adequate supply of all essential nutrients. Because of their small size, infants need smaller total amounts of the nutrients than adults do, but when comparisons are made based on body weight, infants need over twice as much of many of the nutrients. Figure 10–4 compares a five-month-old baby's needs with those of an adult man. As you can see, some of the differences are extraordinary. After six months, calorie needs increase less rapidly as the growth rate begins to slow down, but some of the energy saved by slower growth is spent on increased activity.

The most important nutrient of all—for infants as for everyone—is the one easiest to forget: water. The younger a child, the greater the percentage of the body weight is water and the more rapid the turnover. Since proportionately more of the infant's body water than the adult's is between the cells and in the vascular spaces, this water is easy to lose. Conditions that cause fluid loss, such as vomiting, diarrhea, sweating, or normal urinary loss without replacement, can rapidly propel an infant into life-threatening dehydration. Fluid and electrolyte imbalances caused by diarrhea and infection kill more of the world's children than any disease or disaster. Because infants can only cry and cannot tell you what they are crying for, it is important to remember

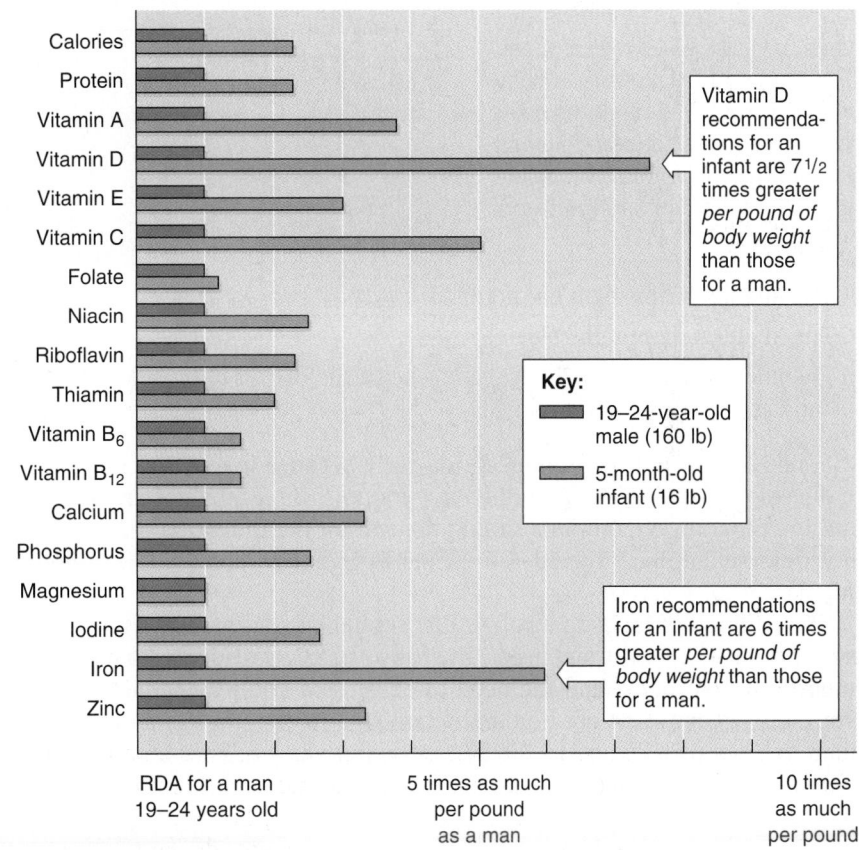

FIGURE 10–4

NUTRIENT RDA OF A FIVE-MONTH-OLD INFANT AND AN ADULT MALE COMPARED ON THE BASIS OF BODY WEIGHT

SOURCE: Reprinted by permission from *Understanding Nutrition*, 6th ed., by E. N. Whitney and S. R. Rolfes. Copyright © 1993 by West Publishing Company. All rights reserved.

that they may need fluid and to let them drink it until their thirst is quenched.

Iron is the nutrient hardest to provide for infants after weaning from breast milk or formula because its concentration in milk, the infant's major food, is low. By the end of the first year, half or more of all infants are receiving less than the RDA for iron, and one-fourth are receiving less than two-thirds of the RDA. Iron may be the nutrient most needing attention in infant nutrition.

Solid foods may normally be added to a breastfed baby's diet when the baby is between four and six months old. Likewise, a baby who is formula fed might be started on solid foods between four and six months, depending on readiness. The following are indicators of readiness:

TABLE 10–5
FIRST FOODS FOR THE INFANT

AGE (MONTHS)	ADDITION
4 to 6	Iron-fortified rice cereal, followed by other cereals (for iron; baby can swallow and can digest starch now)[a] Pureed vegetables and/or fruits and their juices, one by one (perhaps vegetables before fruits so that the baby will learn to like their less sweet flavors)[b]
6 to 8	Mashed vegetables and fruits and their juices, infant breads and crackers
8 to 10	Protein foods (soft cheeses, yogurt, tofu, mashed cooked beans, finely chopped meat, fish, chicken, egg yolk), toast, teething crackers (for emerging teeth), soft-cooked vegetables and fruit
10 to 12	Whole egg (allergies are less likely now), whole milk (at 1 year)

[a]Later, other cereals can be introduced, but they should still be iron-fortified varieties.

[b]All baby juices are fortified with vitamin C. Orange juice may cause allergies; apple juice may be a better juice to feed first. Dilute juices with water and offer in a cup to prevent nursing bottle syndrome.

SOURCE: Adapted from Committee on Nutrition, American Academy of Pediatrics, *Pediatric Nutrition Handbook,* 3rd ed., ed. L.A. Barness (Elk Grove Village, IL: American Academy of Pediatrics, 1993), pp. 23–33.

- The infant's birthweight has doubled.
- The infant is six months old.
- The infant is developmentally ready—he or she can sit upright with support and can control head movements.

Solids should not be introduced too early because infants are more likely to develop allergies to them in the early months. But all babies are different, and the program of additions should depend on the individual baby, not on any rigid schedule. Table 10–5 presents a suggested sequence for feeding infants.

The addition of foods to a baby's diet should be governed by three considerations: the baby's nutrient needs, the baby's physical readiness to handle different forms of foods, and the need to detect and control allergic reactions. Nutrients needed early are iron and vitamin C. Juices and fruits that contain vitamin C are usually among the first foods introduced. Since a baby's stored iron supply from before birth runs out after the birthweight doubles, formula with iron, iron-fortified cereals, and, later, meat or meat alternates such as legumes are recommended.

It has been suggested that the early introduction of sweet fruits to a baby's diet might favor the baby's developing a preference for sweets and lessen the baby's liking for vegetables introduced later. To prevent this, the order can perhaps be vegetables first, fruits later. This practice now has a wide following. As for other types of sweets (soda pop, candy, rich pies, and cakes), there is little room in the baby's diet for these empty-calorie foods. In contrast, naturally

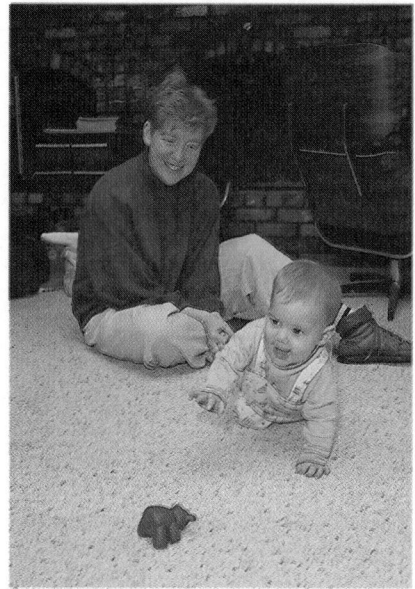

Energy saved by slower growth is spent in increased activity.

sweetened fruits supply not only calories, but also needed nutrients to support normal growth and development.

Physical readiness to handle foods develops in many small steps. For example, the ability to swallow solid food develops at around four to six months, and experience with solid food at that time helps to develop swallowing ability by desensitizing the gag reflex. Later still, when a baby can sit up, can handle finger foods, and is teething, hard crackers and other hard finger foods may be introduced. Such foods promote the development of manual dexterity and control of the jaw muscles. (An infant can choke on these foods, however, so an adult should keep a watchful eye on the learning process.)

Some parents want to feed solids at an earlier age on the theory that "stuffing the baby" at bedtime promotes sleeping through the night. There is no proof for this theory. On the average, babies start to sleep through the night at about the same age regardless of when solid foods are introduced. By three months, 75 percent are sleeping through the night whether or not they are receiving any solid foods.

As for the choice of foods, baby foods commercially prepared in the United States and Canada are safe, and except for mixed dinners and heavily sweetened desserts, are generally nutritious, and of high quality. In response to consumer demand, baby food companies have removed much of the added salt and sugar that many of their products contained in the past. Baby foods generally have high nutrient density, except for mixed dinners (which contain little meat) and desserts (which are heavily sweetened and which, as mentioned earlier, have no place in a baby's diet).

An alternative for parents who want the baby to have family foods is to "blenderize" a small portion of the table food at each meal. This necessitates cooking without salt, however, since foods that adults prepare for themselves often contain much more salt than commercial baby foods. The adults can salt their own food, if desired, after the baby's portion has been taken. Canned vegetables are inappropriate for infants; their sodium content is often too high. It is also important to take precautions against food poisoning. Honey should *never* be fed to infants because of the risk of botulism. Babies and even young children have difficulty swallowing certain foods—popcorn, whole grapes, bite-size hot dogs, and nuts, for instance. An infant can easily choke on these foods; it is not worth the risk to give such foods to infants.

At one year of age, the obvious food to supply most of the nutrients the baby needs is still milk; two to three and a half cups a day are now sufficient. More milk than this would displace foods necessary to provide iron and would cause the iron-deficiency anemia known as **milk anemia.** Infants under two years should drink whole milk and not low-fat or nonfat milk; they need the fat and vitamins A and D of fortified whole milk until two years of age. The other foods—meat, iron-fortified cereal, enriched or whole-grain bread, fruit, and vegetables—should be supplied in variety and in amounts sufficient to round out total calorie needs. Ideally, the one-year-old is sitting at the table and eating many of the same foods everyone else eats. A meal plan that meets the requirements for the one-year-old is shown in Table 10–6.

The wise parent of a one-year-old offers nutrition and love together. Both promote growth. It is literally true that "feeding with love" produces better growth in both weight and height of children than feeding the same food in an emo-

TABLE 10–6
MEAL PLAN FOR A ONE-YEAR-OLD

BREAKFAST
½ c whole milk
3 tbsp cereal
1–2 tbsp fruit
Teething crackers

SNACK
½ c whole milk
Teething crackers
1–2 tbsp fruit

LUNCH
1 c whole milk
2 to 3 tbsp vegetables
2 tbsp chopped meat or well-cooked, mashed legumes

SNACK
½ c whole milk
Teething crackers
1 tbsp peanut butter

SUPPER
1 c whole milk
1 egg
2 tbsp cereal or potato
2 to 3 tbsp vegetables
2 to 3 tbsp fruit

MILK ANEMIA iron-deficiency anemia caused by drinking so much milk that iron-rich foods are displaced from the diet.

tionally negative climate. It also promotes better brain development. The formation of nerve-to-nerve connections in the brain depends both on nutrients and on environmental stimulation.

The person feeding a one-year-old should keep in mind that the baby is also developing eating habits that will persist throughout life. Mealtimes should be relaxed and leisurely. Children should learn to eat slowly, pause and enjoy their table companions, and stop eating when they are full. The "clean your plate" dictum should be stamped out for all time, and in its place, parents who wish to avoid waste should learn to serve smaller portions or teach their children to serve themselves as much as they truly want to eat. Physical activity should be encouraged on a daily basis to promote strong skeletal and muscular development and to establish habits that will undergird good health throughout life.

Nutrition-Related Problems of Infancy

Iron deficiency and food allergies are two of the most significant nutrition-related problems of infants.

Iron Deficiency. Iron deficiency remains a prevalent nutritional problem in infancy, although it has declined in recent years in large part because of the increasing use of iron-fortified formulas. The use of cow's milk earlier than recommended in infancy can cause iron deficiency as a result of its poor iron content and the potential to cause gastrointestinal blood loss in susceptible infants.[49] Other factors contributing to iron deficiency in infancy include breastfeeding for more than six months without providing supplemental iron, intake of infant formula not fortified with iron, the infant's rapid rate of growth, low birthweight, and low socioeconomic status.[50] To prevent iron deficiency, the American Academy of Pediatrics recommends that infants be fed breast milk or iron-fortified formula for the first year of life, with appropriate foods added between the ages of four and six months as shown in Table 10–5.

Food Allergies. Genetics is probably the most significant factor affecting an infant's susceptibility to food allergies.[51] At-risk infants can be identified by means of careful skin testing and by a family history. Breast milk is recommended for those infants allergic to cow's milk protein and is preferable to soy or goat's milk formulas, since infants are sometimes allergic to these proteins as well. To reduce the risk of food sensitivity or allergic reactions to other foods, new foods should be introduced one at a time to facilitate prompt detection of allergies. For example, when cereals are introduced, try rice cereal first for five to seven days; it causes allergy least often. Try wheat cereal last; it is the most common offender. If a cereal causes irritability from skin rash, digestive upset, or respiratory discomfort, discontinue its use before going on to the next food. About nine times out of ten, the allergy won't be evident immediately but will manifest itself in vague symptoms occurring up to five days after the offending food is eaten, so it isn't easy to detect. Several days should elapse between the introduction of each new food to allow time for clinical symptoms to appear, so that the offending food may be identified.

Early and Middle Childhood

Childhood is a critical time in human development. Children typically grow taller by two to three inches and heavier by five or more pounds each year between the age of one and adolescence. They master fine motor skills (including those related to eating and drinking), become increasingly independent, and learn to express themselves appropriately. Nutrition plays a critical role in the development and growth of children. This section describes the nutrient requirements of children and the primary nutritional problems of this population.

Growth and Nutrient Needs of Children

After age one, a child's growth rate slows, but the body continues to change dramatically. At one, most babies have just learned to stand and toddle; by two, they can take long strides with solid confidence and are learning to run, jump, and climb. The internal change that makes these new accomplishments possible is the accumulation of a larger mass and greater density of bone and muscle tissue. The changes are obvious in Figure 10–5.

Children generally become leaner between the ages of six months and six years, after which time there is a gradual increase in fat thickness in both males and females until puberty is reached. Females have a greater body fat content than males at all stages of development.[52] The energy requirements of children are determined by their individual basal metabolic rates, activity patterns, and rates of growth. Toddlers (ages one to three years) need about 1,300 calories per day. By the age of 10, children need about 2,000 calories per day. Appetite decreases markedly around the age of one year, in line with the great reduction in growth rate. Thereafter, the appetite fluctuates; a child will need and demand much more food during periods of rapid growth than during slow periods.

The gradually increasing needs for all nutrients during the growing years are evident from the RDA table and the RNI for Canadians, which list separate averages for each span of three years. To provide these nutrients, the Food Guide Pyramid recommends a balance among milk and milk products; meats and meat alternates; fruits; vegetables; and breads and cereals (see Figure 10–6). Because the serving sizes adjust as the child grows older, these recommendations are good from age two to the teen years.

After the crucial first year, there is still much a parent can do to foster the development of healthful eating habits. Table 10–7 on page 385 offers tips to make feeding times enjoyable for both parent and child. The goal is to teach children to like nutritious foods in all food categories.

Candy, cola, and other concentrated sweets must be limited in a child's diet if the needed nutrients are to be supplied. If such foods are permitted in large quantities, there are only three possible outcomes: nutrient deficiencies, obesity, or both. A child can't be expected to choose nutritious foods on the basis of taste alone; the preference for sweets is innate. On the other hand, an active child can enjoy the higher-calorie nutritious foods in each category: ice cream or pudding in the milk group and whole-grain cookies and crackers in the bread group. These foods, made from milk and grain, carry valuable nutrients and encourage a child to learn, appropriately, that eating is fun.

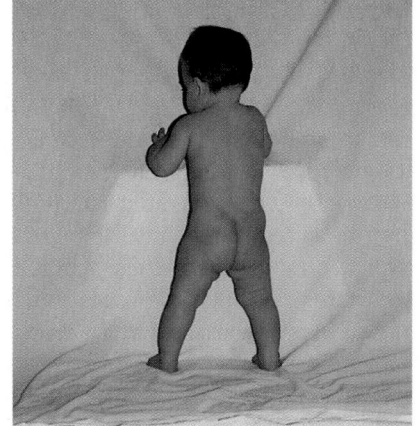

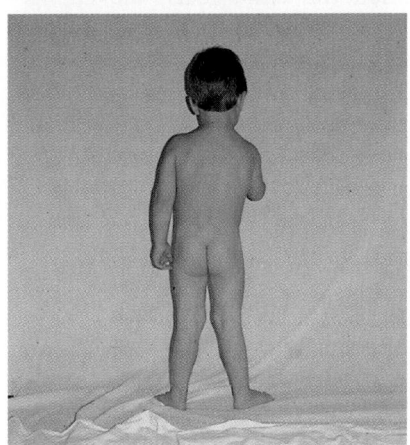

FIGURE 10–5
ONE-YEAR-OLD AND TWO-YEAR-OLD

The two-year-old has lost much of the baby fat; the muscles (especially in the back, buttocks, and legs) have firmed and strengthened, and the leg bones have lengthened and increased in density.

Nutrient intake recommendations for children are given in the RDA table on the inside front cover.

Children sometimes seem to lose their appetites for a while; this is nothing to worry about. The perfection of appetite regulation in children of normal weight guarantees that such children's calorie intakes will be right for each stage of growth.[53] As long as the food energy they do consume is from nutritious foods, they are well provided for. An overzealous parent, unaware that a one-year-old is supposed to slow down, may begin a lifelong conflict over food by trying to force more food on the child than the child feels like eating. Keep in mind that parents are responsible only for *what* the child is given to eat and where and when it is presented. The child is responsible for *how much*, if anything, is eaten.[54]

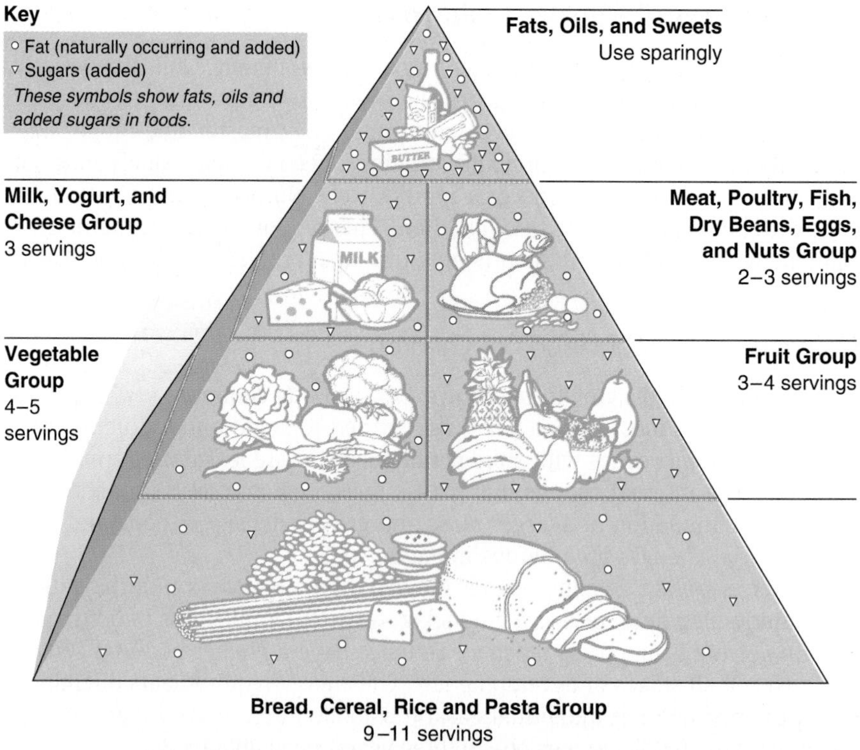

Other Factors That Influence Childhood Nutrition

While parents are doing what they can to establish favorable eating behaviors during the transition from infancy to childhood, children in preschool or grade school are encountering foods prepared and served by outsiders. The U.S. government funds several programs to provide nutritious, high-quality meals for children at school. School lunches are designed to meet certain requirements. They must include specified servings of milk, protein-rich foods (meat, cheese, eggs, legumes, or peanut butter), vegetables, fruits, and bread or other grain foods (see Table 10–8 on page 386). They are intended to follow the recommendations of the *Dietary Guidelines for Americans* and to provide at least a third of the RDA for protein, vitamins A and C, iron, calcium, and calories.[55] In addition, they are split into several patterns to provide for the nutritional needs of different ages. Along with the school lunch program is a program of nutrition education and training (NET program) in all the public schools. The NET program is designed to help children learn to apply the basic principles of healthful eating and good nutrition to their daily lives and

Key
○ Fat (naturally occurring and added)
▽ Sugars (added)
These symbols show fats, oils and added sugars in foods.

Fats, Oils, and Sweets
Use sparingly

Milk, Yogurt, and Cheese Group
3 servings

Meat, Poultry, Fish, Dry Beans, Eggs, and Nuts Group
2–3 servings

Vegetable Group
4–5 servings

Fruit Group
3–4 servings

Bread, Cereal, Rice and Pasta Group
9–11 servings

	SERVING SIZES BY AGE GROUP		
	1 to 3 years	**4 to 6 years**	**7 to 12 years**
Bread Group	½ slice	1 slice	1 to 2 slices
Fruit Group	2–4 tbsp or ½ c juice	¼–½ c or ½ c juice	½–¾ c or ½ c juice
Vegetable Group	2–4 tbsp or ½ c juice	¼–½ c or ½ c juice	½–¾ c or ½ c juice
Meat Group	1–2 oz	1–2 oz	2–3 oz
Milk Group	½–¾ c	¾ c	¾–1 c

FIGURE 10–6
EATING PATTERN FOR CHILDREN BASED ON THE FOOD GUIDE PYRAMID

to acquire a firm understanding of the relationship of good nutrition to good health. Children growing up today need not only to be fed well in the interest of their growth and development but also to learn enough about nutrition to become able to make adaptive food choices when the choices become theirs to make.

It is desirable for children to learn to like nutritious foods in all of the food groups. With one exception, this liking usually develops naturally. The exception is vegetables, which young children sometimes dislike and refuse. Even a tiny serving of spinach, cooked carrots, or squash may elicit an expression of disgust. Since most youngsters need to eat more vegetables, parents need to know how to make them appealing to children. Children prefer vegetables that are slightly undercooked and crunchy, attractive in color and shape, and easy to eat. They should be warm, not hot, because a child's mouth is much more sensitive than an adult's. The flavor should be mild (a child has more taste buds),

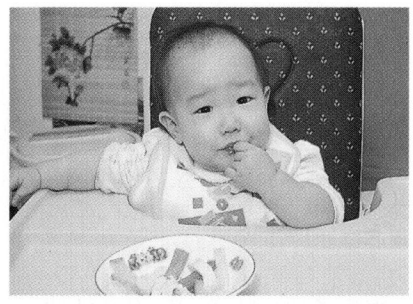

Let infants handle food as they become ready.

TABLE 10–7
STRATEGIES TO FOSTER HEALTHFUL EATING HABITS AND HAPPY MEALTIMES

These tips may make feeding time easier and more relaxing for both parent and child:

- Schedule regular meals and snacks for toddlers since they require frequent feeding to ensure adequate intake of calories and nutrients.
- Always try to offer at least one food that the child likes.
- Remain calm if the child leaves an entire meal untouched.
- Do not be concerned about short food jags, stretches of time when the child wants the same food over and over. If this behavior continues for a long period and eliminates entire food groups, consult with your pediatrician or registered dietitian.
- Teach and reinforce good table manners.
- Allow the child to eat slowly.

Offer healthy food in a relaxed manner and children will eat what they need. Try these suggestions for healthful snacking:

- Stock up on carbohydrates—bagels, pretzels, whole-grain breads and rolls, low-fat crackers, and English muffins.
- Keep plenty of washed and cut raw vegetables in the refrigerator. Team up with a yogurt or bean dip.
- Have an assortment of bread spreads handy, like peanut butter, smooth cottage cheese, reduced-fat cream cheese, jams, jellies, and preserves.
- Top frozen waffles and pancakes with fresh fruit for a tasty and refreshing snack.
- Serve canned soups—they are easy for a child to make for an after-school winter warmer.
- Make your own frozen juice pops in an ice cube tray, or freeze grapes, strawberries, or chunks of banana, pineapple, or melon.
- Bake your own oatmeal cookies. You can cut the shortening (margarine, butter, oil) and sugar in many recipes by at least one third without affecting quality.
- Put together a large batch of cereal, pretzel and nut mix. Divide into individual plastic bags.
- Serve healthy party foods—try serving carrot cake cupcakes, bobbing for apples, making fresh fruit kabobs.
- Prepare air-popped popcorn and sprinkle with grated parmesan cheese.

SOURCE: Adapted from M. G. Hermann, *The ABCs of Children's Nutrition* (Chicago: The American Dietetic Association, 1991), pp. 3–7.

TABLE 10–8
SCHOOL LUNCH PATTERNS FOR DIFFERENT AGES

FOOD GROUP	PRESCHOOL (AGE)		GRADE SCHOOL THROUGH HIGH SCHOOL (GRADE)		
	1 to 2	3 to 4	K to 3	4 to 6	7 to 12
Meat or meat alternate 1 serving:					
Lean meat, poultry, or fish	1 oz	1½ oz	1½ oz	2 oz	3 oz
Cheese	1 oz	1½ oz	1½ oz	2 oz	3 oz
Large egg(s)	½	¾	¾	1	1½
Cooked dry beans or peas	¼ c	⅜ c	⅜ c	½ c	¾ c
Peanut butter	2 tbsp	3 tbsp	3 tbsp	4 tbsp	6 tbsp
Vegetable and/or fruit					
2 or more servings, both to total	½ c	½ c	½ c	¾ c	¾ c
Bread or bread alternate					
Servings[a]	5 per week	8 per week	8 per week	8 per week	10 per week
Milk					
1 serving of fluid milk	¾ c	¾ c	1 c	1 c	1 c

[a]A serving is 1 slice bread; 1 biscuit, roll, or muffin; 1/2 c cooked rice, pasta, or cereal grain.
SOURCE: U.S. Department of Agriculture, *Food Program Facts—National School Lunch Program*, 1992.

and smooth foods like mashed potatoes or pea soup should have no lumps in them (a child wonders, with some disgust, what the lumps might be).

Little children like to eat at little tables and to be served little portions of food. They also love to eat with other children and have been observed to stay at the table longer and eat much more when in the company of their peers. A bright, unhurried atmosphere free of conflict is also conducive to good appetite.

Ideally, each meal is preceded, not followed, by the activity the child looks forward to the most. A number of schools have discovered that children eat a much better lunch if recess occurs before rather than after the meal. With recess after, children are likely to hurry out to play, leaving food on their plates that they were hungry for and would otherwise have eaten. Before sitting down to eat, small children should be helped to wash their hands and faces to decrease likelihood of contaminating the food with bacteria.

Many little children, both boys and girls, enjoy helping in the kitchen. Their participation provides many opportunities to encourage good food habits. Vegetables are pretty, especially when fresh, and provide opportunities to learn about color, about growing things and their seeds, about shapes and textures— all of which are fascinating to young children. Measuring, stirring, decorating, cutting, and arranging vegetables are skills even a very small child can practice with enjoyment and pride.

When introducing new foods at the table, parents are advised to offer them one at a time—and only a small amount at first. Whenever possible, the new food should be presented at the beginning of the meal, when the child is hungry. If the child is cross, irritable, or feeling sick, don't insist, but withdraw the new food and try it again a few days later. Remember, parents have inclinations and dislikes to which they feel entitled; children should be accorded the same privilege.

Never make an issue of food acceptance; a power struggle almost invariably results in a permanently closed mind on the child's part. Rather, let children participate in the planning and preparation of meals. If the beginnings are right, children will grow up with positive feelings toward themselves and the ways they relate to food. Remember, too, that parents can act as good role models—enjoying healthful meals and keeping in good physical shape themselves.

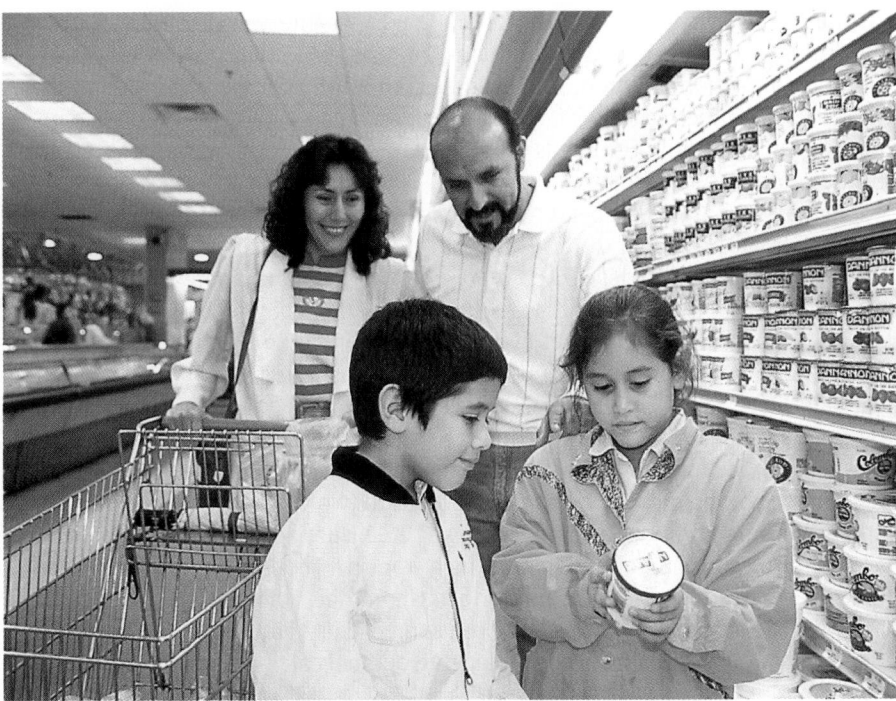

Make learning about nutrition fun. Read food labels together at the grocery store, checking for the supply of vitamins and minerals and the amounts of sugar, salt, and fat.

Nutrition-Related Problems of Childhood

Although most children in the United States are well nourished, malnutrition does occur in this population. Undernutrition, which occurs when children do not eat enough food or energy, is a problem for some children in the United States, especially those from low-income and migrant families or certain ethnic and racial minority groups (e.g., African-Americans, Asians).[56] Children in foster care, many of whom live in poverty, and young homeless children are also at risk for undernutrition.[57] More than 20 percent of U.S. children are considered poor.[58] The most common nutrition-related problems occurring among U.S. children include obesity, iron-deficiency anemia, and high blood cholesterol levels.

Obesity. The problem of overnutrition is one of the most widespread nutrition disorders among children in the United States. Obesity affects as many as 27 percent of children in the United States, and the prevalence of obesity among 6- to 11-year-old children has increased some 54 percent in the last 20 years.[59] Childhood obesity is associated with high blood insulin levels, high triglyceride levels, and reduced HDL-cholesterol concentrations and is considered a risk factor for obesity in adulthood.[60] According to recent studies, second to prior obesity, the strongest predictor of subsequent obesity in children is television viewing.[61]

Children also hear a great deal about foods via the television set. Many authorities are concerned that television commercials may have a less than desirable impact on children. It is estimated that the average child sees more than 21,000 commercials a year, of which approximately half are for foods high in fat, sugar, and salt.[62] Hundreds of millions of dollars are spent in the effort to sell these foods to children.

The more time children spend watching television, the less time they have for physical activity. Research results show that children who watch television more often had lower activity levels and were less likely to participate in organized sports or community activities.[63] Parents can encourage physical activity in children to help prevent overweight by participating in activities such as cycling, swimming, rollerblading, skating, or hiking with their children.

Iron-Deficiency Anemia.   Of all nutritional disorders other than obesity found in U.S. children, the most common is iron-deficiency anemia. It is most prevalent in low-birthweight infants, babies from six months to two years of age, and children and adolescents from low-income families.[64] To ensure adequate iron nutrition, parents should offer an abundance of such iron-rich foods as lean meats, fish, poultry, eggs, and legumes. Grain products should be whole-grain or enriched only. Milk, beneficial as it is, is a poor iron source; dairy products should be consumed only in the amounts needed to ensure optimal calcium intakes.

High Blood Cholesterol.   Considerable evidence exists that atherosclerosis begins in childhood and that this process is related to high blood cholesterol levels. Children and adolescents in the United States have higher blood cholesterol levels and higher dietary intakes of saturated fat and cholesterol than children in other countries.[65] A panel of experts representing 42 major U.S. health and professional organizations has recommended that children age two and older eat diets containing no more than 30 percent of total calories from fat, less than 10 percent of total calories from saturated fat, and no more than 300 milligrams of cholesterol daily. However, from birth to two years of age, a child's fat consumption should not be restricted because fat is a concentrated source of the calories needed to ensure proper physical development.

 The panel also advised that youngsters and teens should have their blood cholesterol measured if they have one parent with a high blood cholesterol level. For children and adolescents, a total of 200 milligrams per deciliter of blood or more is considered high; 170 to 199 is borderline high; and less than 170 is acceptable. In addition, youngsters born to families with a history of premature heart disease should have both total blood cholesterol and HDL-cholesterol checked.[66]

The Importance of Teen Nutrition

 Adolescence is a time of change. Between the ages of about 10 and 18 years in girls and 12 and 20 years in boys, marked changes take place in physical, intellectual, and emotional growth and development. The maturation process is initiated and controlled by a variety of hormones, including, among others, growth hormone, prolactin, estrogen, testosterone, and the thyroid hormones.[67] Many aspects of the maturation process are influenced by dietary intake and nutritional status. This section reviews the nutrient requirements and special nutrition-related problems of teenagers.

Nutrient Needs of Adolescents

The dramatic changes in body composition and the rate of growth that occur during early adolescence give rise to the familiar phrase "the adolescent growth spurt." The magnitude of these changes is such that the linear growth increments during adolescence can contribute about 15 percent to 25 percent of adult stature. The rate of weight gain can contribute anywhere from 40 percent to 50 percent of the adult body mass. This remarkable growth rate requires adequate intakes of energy and nutrients.[68]

No universally applicable formula exists for expressing the calorie demands of adolescents. The individual teenager's energy need is influenced by body size, activity levels, and biological factors affecting growth. For many nutrients, especially vitamins and minerals, few data are based specifically on measurements in adolescents. Recommended nutrient intakes for adolescents are based on extrapolations from studies conducted among either adults or children, with a safety factor built in.[69]

There is tremendous variation in the rates and patterns of individual teenagers in terms of growth.[70] Growth charts used for children cannot be used any longer when the signs of puberty begin to appear. The only way to be sure teenagers are growing normally is to compare their heights and weights with previous measures taken at intervals and note whether reasonably smooth progress is being made. Teenagers who want to know what they should weigh should be reassured that any of a wide range of weights is considered normal at this time in life. A rule of thumb can be applied to teenage girls (see margin); the result can be considered a weight to aim at, but weights well in excess of these are normal, too. Teenage boys can be told that when they have finished growing, they should expect to weigh what the adult charts show, but that while they are growing, it is not unusual for their weights to be quite different from the adult standards.

> Consult the RDA table shown on the inside front cover for the nutrient intake recommendations for adolescents.

> **Rule of thumb for teens:**
>
> For 5 ft, consider 100 lb a reasonable weight for girls (110 lb for boys).
>
> For each inch over 5 ft, add 5 lb.
>
> For each year under 25 (down to 18), subtract 1 lb.

Nutrition-Related Problems of Adolescents

Most adolescents in the United States are perceived as "healthy." However, many U.S. adolescents experience a variety of health and nutrition problems, some related to their risk-seeking behaviors and an inability to deal with abstract notions such as "good health" and the link between current behaviors and long-term health. In general, the nutritional health of U.S. teenagers is better today than ever before. Overt nutrient deficiencies, with the exception of iron deficiency, are not the public health problems they once were. Specific nutrition-related problems among U.S. adolescents include undernutrition, obesity, iron-deficiency anemia, low dietary calcium intakes, high blood cholesterol levels, dental caries, and eating disorders.

Undernutrition.   Some groups of adolescents are at risk for reduced energy and food intakes. Adolescents from low-income families and those who have run away from home or abuse alcohol or other drugs are at risk nutritionally. Approximately 16 percent of youth ages 14 to 21 are estimated to be living below the poverty line. African-American and Hispanic teenagers are nearly three times more likely to live in poverty than are white youth. Juveniles who live on the street tend to have a host of health problems, including substance abuse and malnutrition. Irregular meal patterns, combined with a high rate of use of substances such as alcohol, marijuana, cocaine, and amphetamines, contribute to low nutrient and energy intakes among street youth.[71] Chronic dieters are also at risk. Thirteen percent of the 17,354 females in grades 7 through 12 who were interviewed in the Minnesota Adolescent Survey reported being chronic dieters, defined as always on a diet or having been on a diet for 10 of the previous 12 months.[72]

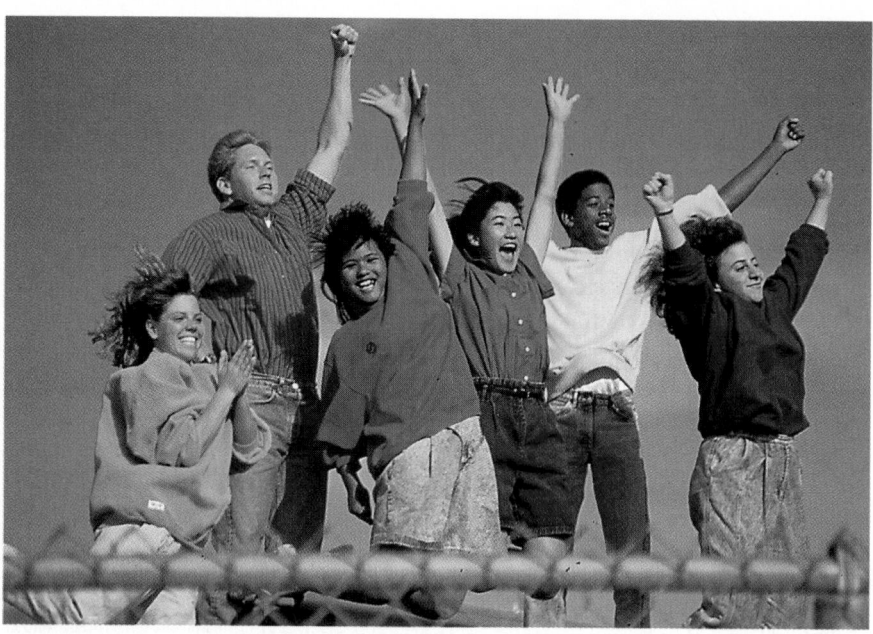

Successful nutrition education activities for teenagers focus on their interests and the relationship of good eating and physical activity to health.

Obesity. An analysis of recent survey data revealed that the prevalence of obesity among 12- to 17-year-olds in the United States increased by 39 percent in the past 15 to 20 years.[73] Given that childhood obesity can lead to adult obesity and that approximately 25 percent to 30 percent of the adult population is overweight, obesity among teenagers is cause for concern. Genetic susceptibility to obesity, lifestyle, family eating patterns, lack of positive role models, and physical inactivity all contribute to overweight and obesity in this population. Obese teenagers are also at risk for hypertension and diabetes mellitus, among other disorders.[74]

Iron-Deficiency Anemia. Iron needs increase during adolescence, especially for females as they start to menstruate. In boys, the requirements for absorbed iron increase because of an expanding blood volume and rise in hemoglobin concentration that accompanies the development of larger muscles and sexual maturation. (After the adolescent growth spurt, the need for iron falls off.[75]) Whereas most males have an adequate iron intake during adolescence, many females between 12 and 22 years of age have iron intakes below the current RDA. Girls typically consume fewer total calories and less meat than boys do. Moreover, a recent analysis of iron requirements in menstruating women suggests that 95 percent of menstruating teenage girls need 19 milligrams of iron to replace menstrual losses—more than the current RDA of 15 milligrams for menstruating women and more than most girls could normally consume without the use of fortified foods such as breakfast cereals or iron supplements.[76]

Low Calcium Intakes.   Another problem nutrient during the teen years is calcium. Low intakes of calcium-rich foods during adolescence compromise peak bone mass development and increase risk of osteoporosis later in life. Adolescents need a minimum of 1,200 milligrams of calcium each day in order to achieve an optimal peak bone mass and healthy bones. However, many teens, especially teenage girls, have calcium intakes below the RDA.[77] Adolescent girls following low-calorie diets and drinking diet soft drinks in place of milk are at particular risk for age-related bone loss and subsequent fractures.[78]

High Blood Cholesterol Levels.   Teenagers have many of the same risk factors for high blood cholesterol as adults: family history of coronary heart disease; diets high in total fat, saturated fat, and cholesterol; hypertension; low activity levels; and smoking. Although the process of atherosclerosis is not completely understood, it is believed that the fatty streaks that develop in young people progress to the fibrous plaques of adulthood.[79]

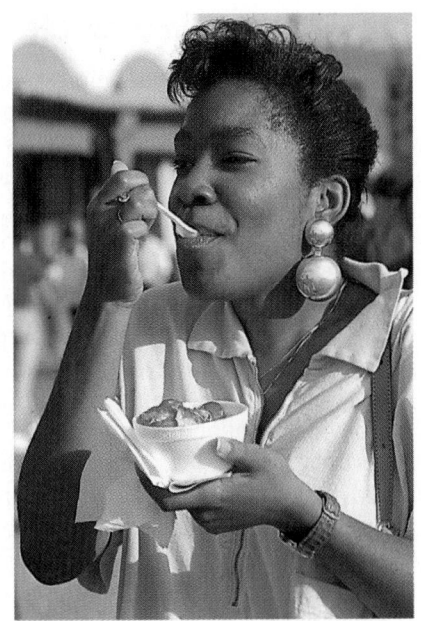

Nutritious snacks can supply added nutrients to the active teenager's diet.

Dental Caries.   Dental caries are a significant public health problem among teenagers, with about 78 percent of adolescents having one or more caries in permanent or primary teeth.[80] Dental caries are more prevalent among adolescents than among children. A National Dental Research Survey found that only 22 percent of 15-year-olds were caries free, compared with 56 percent of 10-year-olds.[81] Fortunately, the incidence of dental caries has decreased by as much as 30 percent to 50 percent over the past two decades, partly because of fluoridation of public drinking water, improved dental hygiene, and the use of fluoride in toothpastes and mouthwashes.[82] Some population subgroups, such as American Indians, Alaskan Natives, African-Americans, and Hispanics, are at greater risk of dental caries than other groups because they lack access to or do not avail themselves of dental services.

Eating Disorders.   Eating disorders have become serious health problems in recent years. The most common eating disorders are anorexia nervosa and bulimia nervosa. A constellation of individual, familial, sociocultural, and biological factors contribute to these disorders, which threaten physical health and psychological well-being.

Some individuals are more predisposed to developing an eating disorder than others. For example, about 90 percent of people with eating disorders are female. Most are Caucasian, with few cases seen among blacks and other minority groups. Most individuals who develop eating disorders are adolescents or young adults who typically began experiencing food-related and self-image problems between the ages of 14 and 30 years.

Because these syndromes are surrounded by secrecy, their prevalence is not known with certainty, although it has increased dramatically within the past two decades. Estimates of the prevalence in the general population range from one percent for anorexia nervosa to 1 to 5 percent for bulimia nervosa. These two types of eating disorders are also sometimes seen in adolescent athletes, many of whom compete in sports such as gymnastics, wrestling, distance running, diving, horse racing, and swimming, which demand a rigid control of body weight.[83]

Nutrition in Later Life

It is easy to get the impression from mortality statistics that people are living longer and longer lives, but this is not the case. Certainly the *average* age at death (life expectancy) has changed dramatically. Life expectancy at birth is now 74.8 years—most men die at a little past 72, and most women die at a little past 79.[84] On the other hand, the *maximum* age at which people die— that is the *maximum life span*—has changed very little. It seems that the aging phenomenon cuts off life at a rather fixed point in time.

To what extent is aging inevitable? Apparently, aging is an inevitable, natural process programmed into our genes at conception. Nevertheless, we can adopt lifestyle habits, such as consuming a healthful diet, exercising, and paying attention to our work and recreational environments, that will slow the process within the natural limits set by heredity. Clearly, good nutrition can retard and ease the aging process in many significant ways. However, no potions, foods, or pills will prolong youth. People who claim to have found the fountain of youth have been selling its waters for centuries, but products advertised to prevent aging profit only the sellers, not the buyers.

Technically, the life span is the oldest documented age to which a member of a given species is known to have survived. For humans, this is about 115 years.

One approach to the prevention of aging has been to study other cultures in the hope of finding an extremely long-lived race of people and then learning their secrets of long life. The views of the experts can best be summed up by saying that disease can *shorten* people's lives and poor nutrition practices make diseases more likely to occur. Thus, by postponing and slowing disease processes, optimal nutrition can help to prolong life up to the maximum life span—but cannot extend it further.[85] This section focuses on the nutrient requirements of older adults, the diseases that seem to come with age, their risk factors, and the relevance of nutrition to them. Test your own knowledge of the aging process with the Aging Scorecard found on the following page.

Demographic Trends and Aging

The number of elderly (aged 65 years and older) in the United States will double by 2030 to more than 65 million people. In 1988, the elderly accounted for 12.4 percent of the population, and this proportion is expected to rise to approximately 14 percent in 2010 and increase to nearly 22 percent by 2030. Nearly 12 percent of the population will be over age 74 by 2030. The increased growth in the elderly population in the United States is illustrated in Figure 10–7.[86]

Both the baby boom that took place between 1946 and 1964 and improved life expectancy are important contributors to the growing elderly population in the United States. Baby boomers will increase the numbers of the older middle-aged (ages 46 through 63) until 2010, when they will begin to swell the ranks of the retired population.[87]

Improved life expectancy has resulted from better prenatal and postnatal care and improved means of combating disease in older adults. For example, the death rate from heart disease began to decline in the 1960s and continues to fall today. Over half of the drop is attributed to a decline in smoking and fewer people with high blood pressure or high blood cholesterol.

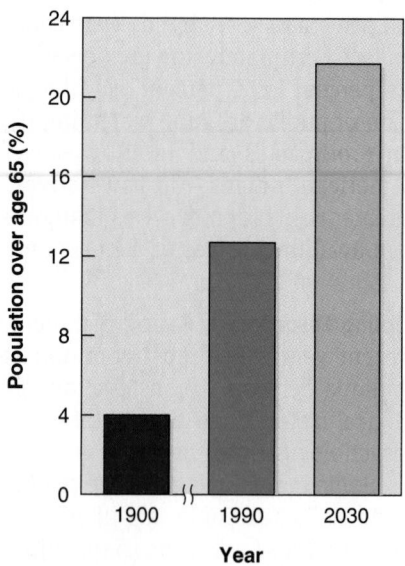

FIGURE 10–7
THE AGING OF THE POPULATION

In 1900, 4 percent of the U.S. population were over 65 years of age; in 1990, 12.7 percent were over 65; by 2030, 22 percent will have reached age 65.

SOURCE: Data from R. Chernoff, *Geriatric Nutrition: The Health Professional's Handbook* (Gaithersburg, MD: Aspen Publishers, 1991), p. 4.

AGING SCORECARD

	True	False	
	☐	☐	**1.** Everyone becomes "senile" sooner or later if he or she lives long enough.
	☐	☐	**2.** American families have by and large abandoned their older members.
	☐	☐	**3.** Depression is a serious problem for older people.
	☐	☐	**4.** The numbers of older people are growing.
	☐	☐	**5.** The vast majority of older people are self-sufficient.
	☐	☐	**6.** Mental confusion is an inevitable, incurable consequence of old age.
	☐	☐	**7.** Intelligence declines with age.
	☐	☐	**8.** Sexual urges and activity normally cease around age 55 to 60.
	☐	☐	**9.** If a person has been smoking for 30 or 40 years, it does no good to quit.
	☐	☐	**10.** Older people should stop exercising and rest.
	☐	☐	**11.** As you grow older, you need more calories, but fewer vitamins and minerals, to stay healthy.
	☐	☐	**12.** Only children need to be concerned about calcium for strong bones and teeth.
	☐	☐	**13.** Extremes of heat and cold can be particularly dangerous to older people.
	☐	☐	**14.** Many older people are hurt in accidents that could have been prevented.
	☐	☐	**15.** More men than women survive to old age.
	☐	☐	**16.** Deaths from stroke and heart disease are declining.
	☐	☐	**17.** Older people on the average take more medications than younger people.
	☐	☐	**18.** Snake oil salesmen are as common today as they were on the frontier.
	☐	☐	**19.** Personality changes with age, just like hair color and skin texture.
	☐	☐	**20.** Sight declines with age.

Answers

1. False. Even among those who live to be 80 or older, only 20 percent to 25 percent develop Alzheimer's disease or some other incurable form of brain disease. "Senility" is a meaningless term that should be discarded.

2. False. The American family is still the number one caretaker of older Americans. Most older people live close to their children and see them often; many live with their spouses. In all, 8 out of 10 men and 6 out of 10 women live in family settings.

3. True. Depression, loss of self-esteem, loneliness, and anxiety can become more common as older people face retirement, the deaths of relatives and friends, and other such crises—often at the same time. Fortunately, depression is treatable.

4. True. Today, 12 percent of the U.S. population are 65 or older. By the year 2030, 22 percent of the population will be over 65 years of age.

5. True. Only 6 percent of people over age 65 live in nursing homes; the rest are basically healthy and self-sufficient.

6. False. Mental confusion and serious forgetfulness in old age can be caused by Alzheimer's disease or other conditions that cause incurable damage to the brain, but some 100 other problems can cause the same symptoms. A minor head injury, a high fever, poor nutrition, adverse drug reactions, and depression can all be treated, and the confusion will be cured.

7. False. Intelligence per se does not decline without reason. Most people maintain their intellect or improve as they grow older.

8. False. Most older people can lead an active, satisfying sex life.

9. False. Stopping smoking at any age not only reduces the risk of cancer and heart disease but also leads to healthier lungs.

10. False. Many older people enjoy—and benefit from—exercises such as walking, swimming, bicycle riding, and strength training. Exercise at any age can help to strengthen the heart and lungs and lower blood pressure. See your physician before beginning a new exercise program.

11. False. Older people need fewer calories (due to lower basal metabolic rates) but the same amounts of most vitamins and minerals as younger people. Some authorities recommend higher intakes of certain nutrients (calcium, vitamin D, antioxidants, B vitamins) for older adults.

12. False. Older people require fewer calories, but adequate intake of calcium for strong bones can become more important as you grow older. This is particularly true for women, whose risk of osteoporosis increases after menopause.

13. True. The body's thermostat tends to function less efficiently with age, and the older person's body may be less able to adapt to heat or cold.

14. True. Falls are the most common cause of injuries among the elderly. Good safety precautions, including proper lighting, nonskid carpets, and living areas free of obstacles, can help to prevent serious accidents.

15. False. Women tend to outlive men by an average of 8 years. There are 150 women for every 100 men over age 65, and nearly 250 women for every 100 men over 85.

16. True. Fewer men and women are dying of stroke or heart disease. This has been a major factor in the increase in life expectancy.

17. True. The elderly consume 25 percent of all medications and as a result have many more problems with adverse drug reactions.

18. True. Medical quackery is a 10-billion-dollar business in the United States. People of all ages are commonly duped into "quick cures" for aging, arthritis, and cancer.

19. False. Personality doesn't change with age. Therefore, old people can't all be described as rigid and cantankerous. You are what you are for as long as you live, unless you *choose* to make a change (for example, to be more outgoing or more flexible).

20. False. Although changes in vision become more common with age, any change in vision, regardless of age, is related to a specific disease. If you are having problems with your vision, see your doctor.

SOURCE: Adapted from *What Is Your Aging I.Q.?* U.S. Department of Health and Human Services, Public Health Service, National Institutes of Health (Washington, D.C.: U.S. Government Printing Office).

Nutrition and Disease

An individual's current health profile is substantially determined by behavioral risk factors. The leading causes of death for adults ages 25 through 64 are cancer, heart disease, stroke, injuries, chronic lung disease, and liver disease, all of which have been associated with behavioral risk factors. To what extent can nutrition prevent or retard the development of these diseases?

Many of the health problems associated with the later years are preventable or can be controlled.[88] For example, changing certain risk behaviors into healthy ones can improve the quality of life for older persons and lessen their risk of disability. For example, incorporating exercise and a balanced, low-fat diet into one's lifestyle can contribute to weight loss and to controlling three important risk factors for heart disease: high fat intake, overweight, and a sedentary lifestyle. The *Surgeon General's Report on Nutrition and Health* demonstrates how the same set of dietary recommendations can both promote general health and help to prevent a broad spectrum of chronic diseases.[89] As Figure 10–8 shows, these basic dietary recommendations reduce the risk of a variety of chronic diseases or their complications.

Figure 10–9 puts nutrition (a factor you *can* control) in perspective with respect to heredity (a factor you can't control). It illustrates the point that some diseases are much more responsive to nutrition than others and that some are not responsive at all. At one extreme are diseases that can be completely cured by supplying missing nutrients, and at the other extreme are certain genetic, or inherited, dis-

Change diet →	Reduce fats	Control calories	Increase starch[a] & fiber	Reduce sodium	Control alcohol
Reduce risk ↓					
Heart disease	🍎	🍎		🍎	
Cancer	🍎	🍎	🍎		🍎
Stroke	🍎	🍎		🍎	🍎
Diabetes	🍎	🍎	🍎		
Gastrointestinal diseases[b]	🍎	🍎	🍎		🍎

[a] Starch refers to complex carbohydrates provided by fruits, vegetables, and whole-grain products.

[b] Gastrointestinal diseases affected by dietary factors are primarily gallbladder disease (fat and calories), diverticular disease (fiber), and cirrhosis of the liver (alcohol).

FIGURE 10–8   CONSISTENCY OF RECOMMENDATIONS FOR REDUCING THE RISK OF CHRONIC DISEASES OR THEIR COMPLICATIONS

SOURCE: J. M. McGinnis and M. Nestle, The Surgeon General's Report on Nutrition and Health: Policy implications and implementation strategies, *American Journal of Clinical Nutrition* 49 (1989): 26. © American Society for Clinical Nutrition.

Nutrition-unresponsive (genetic) diseases

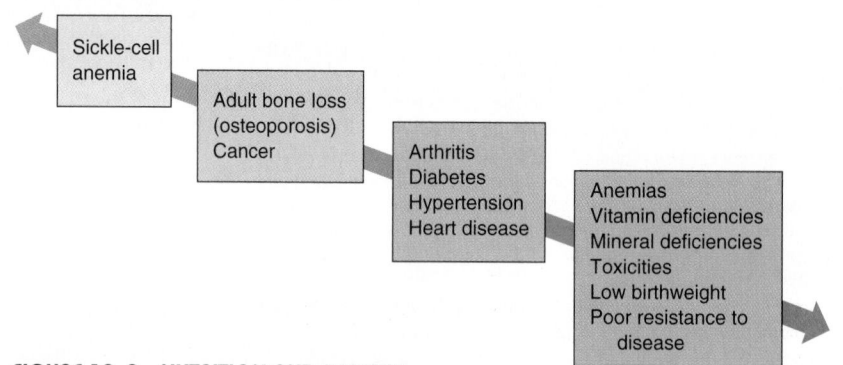

Nutrition-responsive diseases

FIGURE 10–9   NUTRITION AND DISEASE
Not all diseases are equally influenced by diet. Some are purely hereditary, like sickle-cell anemia. Some may be inherited (or the tendency to develop them may be inherited) but may be influenced by diet, like some forms of diabetes. Some are purely dietary, like the vitamin and mineral deficiency diseases. Some authorities are concerned that the offering of dietary advice to the public may seem to exaggerate the power of nutrition in preventing disease. Nutrition alone is certainly not enough to prevent many diseases, but it helps.

eases that are completely unaltered by nutrition. Most fall in between, being influenced by inherited susceptibility but responsive to dietary manipulations that help to normalize metabolism and counteract the disease process. Thus, diabetes may be controlled by means of a diet low in fat and high in complex carbohydrate; arthritis may be somewhat relieved by weight reduction, and cardiovascular disease may respond favorably to a diet low in saturated fat and cholesterol.

These scientific approaches differ markedly from nutrition quackery aimed at the aging population. Nutrition quackery is largely based on the notion that certain foods and nutrients have almost miraculous powers to promote health. People with cancer or AIDS, particularly those who feel they can't be helped by traditional therapy, are easy targets for peddlers of nutrition "cures." They may take massive doses of vitamins and/or minerals, some of which may be toxic. Although Figure 10–8 displays an impressive list of health-promoting effects of good nutrition, there is a difference. It does not advocate the use of specific foods—and certainly not of nutrient supplements—nor does it imply that even the most scrupulous attention to nutrition will guarantee freedom from disease. Taken together, the recommendations of the figure simply add up to an adequate, balanced, and varied diet composed of nutritious foods—a quiet, sensible prescription for good nutritional health.

Aging and Nutrition Status

Growing old is often associated with frailty, sickness, and a loss of vitality. Although chronic illness and associated disabilities are experienced by the aging in our society, there is great heterogeneity among this population—that is, older people vary greatly in their social, economic, and lifestyle situations, functional capacity, and physical conditions.[90] Each person ages at a different rate, sometimes making chronologic age different from biologic age. Most older persons live at home, are fully independent, and have lives of good quality.[91] Only 5 percent to 6 percent of older adults live in nursing homes.[92] Older persons who have problems with the **activities of daily living (ADL)** are known as the frail elderly. Because they depend on others to perform these essential activities, they are likely to be at risk for malnutrition.[93]

ACTIVITIES OF DAILY LIVING (ADL) include bathing, dressing, grooming, transferring from bed to chair, going to the bathroom, and feeding oneself.

Nutritional Needs and Intakes

Many of the nutrient needs of the elderly are the same as for younger persons, but some special considerations deserve emphasis. Calorie needs decline with age because of a decrease in basal metabolism related to loss of lean tissue and a decrease in physical activity. The RDA for energy intake is lower for older adults beginning at age 51. Given their limited energy allowances, older adults are advised to select mostly nutrient-dense foods.

On one side of the energy budget, energy is taken in; on the other side, it is spent. If you are motivated to maintain your good health into the later years, you should plan regular exercise into your days. Ideally, the exercise should be intense enough to increase the heartbeat and respiration rate and to prevent the atrophy of all muscles (not only the heart) that otherwise takes place. Many older people believe that they can't participate in strenuous exercise, but studies have shown that they can do more than they think they can. Any exercise—even a ten-minute walk each day—is better than none, and with persistence, one can achieve great improvement. Modest endurance training can improve cardiovascular and respiratory function and promote good muscle tone while controlling the accumulation of body fat.

The older person who has never worked out hard before may be encouraged to learn that the trainability of older people does not depend on their physical prowess in their youth. Improvement during training is due not only to improvement in muscles but also to the increased bloodflow to the brain engendered by the exercise. A major benefit is that with an increased energy output, a person can afford to eat more food and so obtain more nutrients.

Perhaps the most important nutrient of all is *water*. Older adults need to be reminded to take in fluids because they are likely to be somewhat insensitive to their own thirst signals.[94] They should consume six to eight glasses of fluid a day.

At present, the Committee on Dietary Allowances does not provide separate RDAs for the various categories of older adults. Rather, all people over 50 are grouped together. Some nutritionists think the recommended intakes of some of the vitamins—vitamins D, B_6, and B_{12}—are too low for the over-65 group.[95] The elderly absorb vitamins B_6 and B_{12} less efficiently and therefore may need to increase their intake. People's needs for these and other nutrients may change as aging progresses.[96]

Some practitioners recommend supplements, particularly for the water-soluble vitamins. Other nutritionists, however, say that until more appropriate age-specific RDAs are established, the current RDAs should continue to be used as standards for healthy older persons.[97] These nutritionists argue that recommending supplements often makes the elderly vulnerable to exploitation by quacks and that their money is better spent on nutrient-dense foods.

Surveys designed to find out what kinds of nutrient supplements older people are using tend to support the view that in many cases, older people are wasting their money. A recent study in a retirement community showed that about half of the subjects were taking nutrient supplements— mostly of vitamins C and E—but that these choices were not related to the users' dietary intakes; that is, the subjects had adequate dietary intakes of these nutrients, and therefore the supplements were not appropriate.[98] The older person would probably be wise to follow the rule of thumb that if food energy intake is below about 1,500 calories, a vitamin-mineral supplement—a once-daily type of supplement, not the megavitamin kind—is recommended.

Table 10–9 shows a recommended eating pattern that would supply the amounts of calories recommended by the RDA tables. Because overweight is recognized as a shortener of the life span, these recommendations seem to be life-sustaining. Clearly, an adequate intake of nutrients and fiber from a variety of foods throughout life, together with moderate intakes of calories and fat, helps immensely to promote good health in the later years.

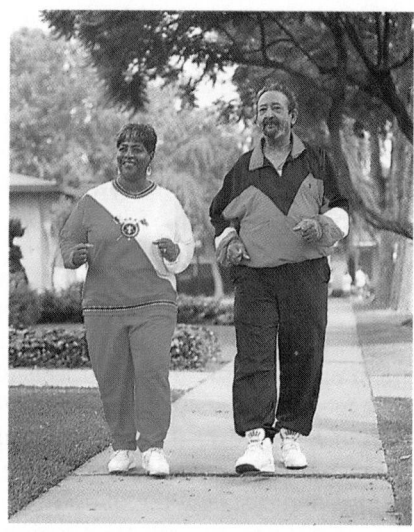

Any form of physical activity—even a 10-minute walk around the block—is better than nothing.

The RDA for older adults are shown inside the front cover. The Canadian RNI divide older people into two age groups: 50 to 74, and 75 and older.

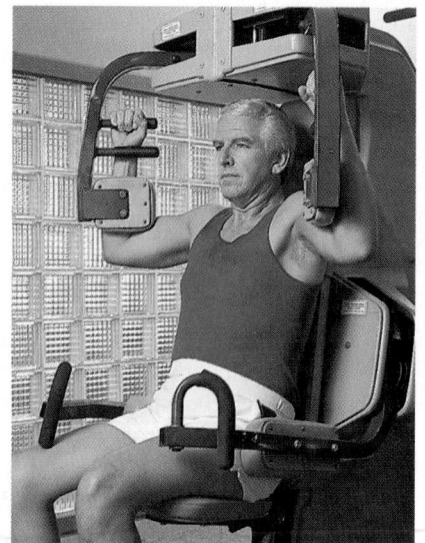

Strength training promotes healthy bones and muscles at any age.

TABLE 10–9
RECOMMENDED EATING PATTERN FOR OLDER PEOPLE

FOOD GROUP/ SERVINGS PER DAY	EQUIVALENT SERVING SIZES
Milk 2–3+*	1 c milk, yogurt, custard, pudding, soft-serve ice cream, or frozen yogurt; 1½ oz cheese; 1½ c creamed soup made with milk; 2 c cottage cheese, regular ice cream, or ice milk
Meat/substitute 2–3*	2–3 oz lean meat or fish (a piece the size of a deck of cards) or 2 eggs; 1 chicken breast or leg and thigh; ½–¾ c tuna, other flaked meat or fish; 1–1½ c dried beans or peas; 4–6 tbsp peanut butter; 2–3 slices low-fat cold cuts
Fruit 2–4+	½–¾ c (1 piece) citrus or other vitamin C-source fruit
Vegetables 3–5+	½–1 c dark green/deep yellow vegetables
Bread/cereals 6+	1 slice whole-grain or enriched bread; ½ bun, bagel, English muffin; ½ c rice, pasta, cooked cereal; 1 c cold cereal; 3–6 crackers*
Fats/sweets as needed for calories	not applicable
Alcohol in moderation	not applicable

*Lower-fat, lower-calorie items are recommended; women should aim for 3 servings of milk, cheese, or yogurt.

SOURCE: Reprinted with permission by the Nutrition Screening Initiative, a project of the American Academy of Family Physicians, The American Dietetic Association, and the National Council on Aging, Inc., and funded in part by a grant from Ross Laboratories, a division of Abbott Laboratories.

Nutrition-Related Problems of Older Adults

Although aging is not completely understood, we know that it involves progressive changes in every body tissue and organ: the brain, heart, lungs, digestive tract, and bones (see Table 10–10). After age 35, functional capacity declines in almost every organ system. Such changes affect nutrition status. Some, including oral problems, interfere with nutrient intake; others affect absorption, storage, and utilization of nutrients; and still others increase the excretion of and need for specific nutrients.[99] Examples of various conditions associated with aging that can affect nutritional status include sensory impairments, altered endocrine, gastrointestinal, and cardiovascular functions, and changes in the renal and musculoskeletal systems. Both genetic and environmental factors contribute to these declines.[100] Many of the changes are inevitable, but a healthful lifestyle that combines moderation with adequate intakes of all essential nutrients can forestall degeneration and improve the quality of life into the later years.

As a person gets older, the chances of suffering a chronic illness or functional impairment become greater. Among the diseases that befall some people in later life are heart disease, hypertension, cancer, diverticulosis, osteoporosis, dementia, diabetes, and gum disease. More than 60 percent of people over age 65 have high blood pressure, and approximately 30 percent have heart disease. Chronic conditions contributing to **disability** include arthritis, heart disease, strokes, disorders of vision and hearing, nutritional deficiencies, and oral-dental problems (see Figure 10–10). Dementia (especially Alzheimer's disease) is a major contributor to disability and nursing home placement for those over age 75.[101] As noted in Table 10–11, malnutrition can occur secondary to these conditions, many of which require special diets that can further compromise nutrition status in the older adult.[102]

TABLE 10–10
BIOLOGIC FUNCTION CHANGES BETWEEN THE AGES OF 30 AND 70

BIOLOGIC FUNCTION	CHANGE
Work capacity of heart (%)	↓25–30
Maximum heart rate	↓24
Blood pressure (mm Hg)	
Systolic	↑10–40
Diastolic	↑ 5–10
Maximum breathing capacity (%)	↓40–50
Basal metabolic rate (%)	↓ 8–12
Musculature (%)	
Muscle mass	↓25–30
Hand grip strength	↓25–30
Nerve conduction velocity (%)	↓10–15
Flexibility (%)	↓20–30
Bone (%)	
Women	↓25–30
Men	↓15–20
Kidney function (%)	↓30–50

SOURCE: Adapted from R. R. Watson, *Handbook of Nutrition in the Aged,* 2nd ed. (Boca Raton, FL: CRC Press, 1994), pp. 11–73.

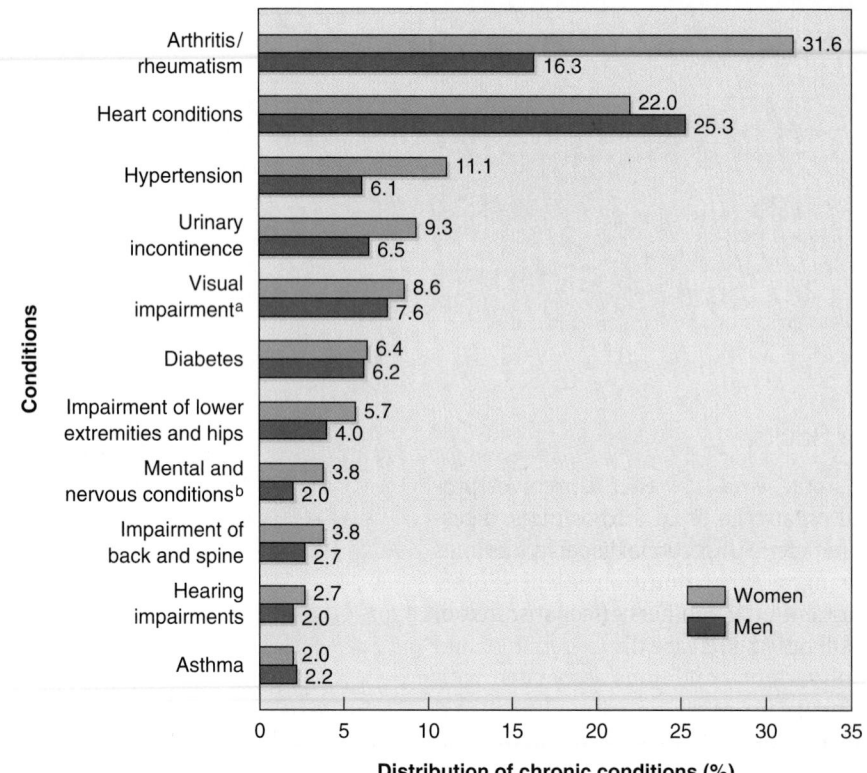

DISABILITY any restriction on or impairment in performing an activity in the manner or within the range considered normal for a human being.

FIGURE 10–10
DISTRIBUTION OF CHRONIC CONDITIONS THAT CAUSE DISABILITY IN PEOPLE OVER AGE 65

[a]Cataracts.

[b]Rate for depression: 147/1000. Rate for Alzheimer's disease: 112/1000 (5% to 10% > age 65 years; 35% > age 85 years).

SOURCE: Reprinted from R. Chernoff, *Geriatric Nutrition: The Health Professional's Handbook* (Gaithersburg, MD: Aspen Publishers, 1991), p. 457. Reproduced with permission of Aspen Publishers, Inc.,© 1991.

TABLE 10–11
MALNUTRITION THAT IS SECONDARY TO DISEASE OR PHYSIOLOGIC STATE

DISEASE OR CONDITION	EFFECTS ON NUTRITION STATUS
Atherosclerosis	May increase difficulties in regulating fluid balances if caused by congestive heart failure. If the individual is incapacitated, calorie needs decrease.
Cancer	Weight loss, lack of appetite, and secondary malnutrition are common.
Dental and oral disease	May alter the ability to chew and thus reduce dietary intake. Increased likelihood of choking and aspiration.
Depression and dementia	Increased or decreased food intakes are common. A person with dementia may have decreased ability to get food, or the appetite may be very small or very great. Judgment and balance in meal planning are generally absent.
Diabetes mellitus (Type I)	If untreated, increased risk of undernutrition results; increased risk of other diet-related diseases.
Diabetes mellitus (Type II)	Increased risk of other diet-related diseases; weight loss is needed if obesity is present.
End-stage kidney disease	Alters fluid and electrolyte needs. Infections and low-grade fever may increase energy output and weight loss.
Gastrointestinal disorders	Increased risk of malabsorption of nutrients and consequent undernutrition.
High blood pressure	Weight gain may exacerbate high blood pressure.
Osteoarthritis	Makes motion difficult, including those activities related to purchasing, serving, eating, and cleaning up after meals. Predisposes people to a sedentary lifestyle and may give rise to obesity. Drug-nutrient relationships are common.
Osteoporosis	Limits the ability to purchase and prepare food if mobility is affected. If severe scoliosis is present, the appetite may be altered.
Smoking	May alter weight status. Alters serum levels of some nutrients, such as ascorbic acid and beta-carotene. Chronic smoking gives rise to emphysema, which makes it difficult to eat because of breathing problems.
Stroke	May alter abilities in the cognitive and motor realms related to food and eating. If the individual is incapacitated, his or her energy needs decrease.

SOURCE: Adapted from Institute of Medicine, *The Second Fifty Years: Promoting Health and Preventing Disability* (Washington, D.C.: National Academy Press, 1992), pp. 168–69.

Polypharmacy, or the use of multiple drugs, is problematic for many older adults. The average older person receives more than 13 prescriptions a year and may take as many as six drugs at a time.[103] Cardiac drugs are most widely used by the elderly, followed by drugs to treat arthritis, psychiatric disorders, and respiratory and gastrointestinal conditions. Long-term use of a variety of drugs increases the risk of drug-nutrient interactions. Individuals with impaired nutrition status and poor dietary intakes are at the highest risk.[104]

POLYPHARMACY the taking of three or more medications regularly; occurs in one-third of those over 65 years.

Factors Affecting Nutrition Status of Older Adults

Individually or in combination, the social, economic, psychological, cultural, and environmental factors associated with aging may interact with the physiological changes and further affect nutrition status in older adults. These interactions are illustrated in Figure 10–11.[105]

Up to one-quarter of all elderly patients and one-half of all hospitalized elderly may be suffering from malnutrition.[106] In addition, a national survey in 1990 showed that one-third of noninstitutionalized Americans over the age of 65 live alone, 45 percent take multiple prescription drugs that can interfere with appetite and nutrient absorption, 30 percent skip meals almost daily, and 25 percent have annual incomes under $10,000—all factors placing elderly people at potential for nutritional risk.[107] Identifying older adults at nutritional risk is an important first step in maintaining quality of life and functional status.[108]

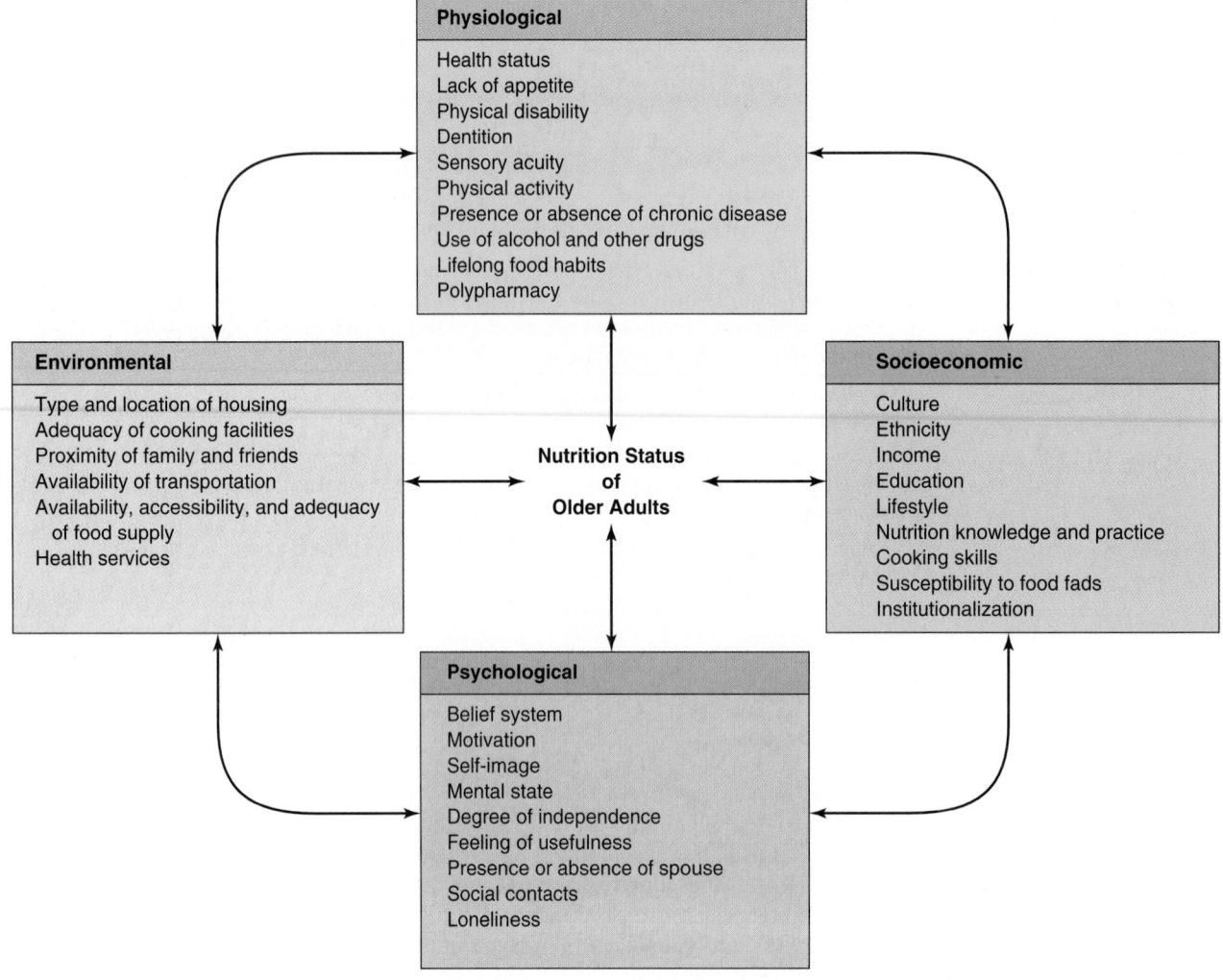

FIGURE 10–11

FACTORS INFLUENCING NUTRITION STATUS OF OLDER ADULTS

SOURCE: Adapted from H. T. Philips and S. H. Gaylord, eds., *Aging and Public Health* (New York: Springer Publishing, 1985), p. 80.

The American Dietetic Association, the American Academy of Family Physicians, and the National Council on Aging have collaborated on an effort —called the Nutrition Screening Initiative—to promote nutrition screening and early intervention as part of routine health care. A key premise to the Nutrition Screening Initiative is that nutrition status is a "vital sign"—as vital to health assessment as blood pressure and pulse rate.[109] The Nutrition Screening Initiative has developed a ten-question self-assessment "Checklist" (see Figure 10–12) to help individuals identify and score factors placing them at nutritional risk. This checklist addresses disease, eating status, tooth loss or mouth pain, economic hardship, reduced social contact, multiple medications, involuntary weight loss or gain, and need for assistance with self-care. The word *DETERMINE* is used as a mnemonic device with the checklist and helps to provide basic nutrition information (see Figure 10–13). Each letter in DETERMINE begins a word or phrase that describes a risk factor.[110]

Financial resources, living arrangements, and a social support network, including availability of caregivers, can also directly impact a person's nutrition status. Poverty (e.g., annual income of less than $6,000 per person) and social isolation particularly impair the nutrition status of many older adults, as noted perceptively by a professor of psychiatry:[111]

> It is not what the older person eats but with whom that will be the deciding factor in proper care for him. The oft-repeated complaint of the older patient that he has little incentive to prepare food for only himself is not merely a statement of fact but also a rebuke to the questioner for failing to perceive his isolation and aloneness and to realize that food . . . for one's self lacks the condiment of another's presence which can transform the simplest fare to the ceremonial act with all its shared meaning.

FIGURE 10–12

CHECKLIST TO DETERMINE YOUR NUTRITIONAL HEALTH

The warning signs of poor nutritional health are often overlooked. To see whether you (or people you know) are at nutritional risk, take this simple quiz. Read the statements above. Circle the number in the "yes" column for those that apply. To find your total nutritional score, add up all of the numbers you circled.

	Yes
I have an illness or condition that made me change the kind and/or amount of food I eat.	2
I eat fewer than two meals per day.	3
I eat few fruits, vegetables, or milk products.	2
I have three or more drinks of beer, liquor, or wine almost every day.	2
I have tooth or mouth problems that make it hard for me to eat.	2
I don't always have enough money to buy the food I need.	4
I eat alone most of the time.	1
I take three or more different prescribed or over-the-counter drugs a day.	1
Without wanting to, I have lost or gained 10 pounds in the past six months.	2
I am not always physically able to shop, cook, and/or feed myself.	2
Total nutritional score:	[ ]

If your total nutritional score is:

0–2—Good! Recheck your nutritional score in six months.

3–5—You are at a moderate nutritional risk. See what can be done to improve your eating habits and lifestyle. A local office on aging, senior nutrition program, senior citizens center, or health department can help. Recheck your nutritional score in three months.

6 or more—You are at a high nutritional risk. Bring this checklist next time you see your doctor, dietitian, or other qualified health or social service professional. Talk with him or her about any problems you have experienced. Ask for nutrition counseling.

SOURCE: Reprinted with permission by the Nutrition Screening Initiative, a project of the American Academy of Family Physicians, The American Dietetic Association, and The National Council on Aging, Inc. and funded in part by a grant from Ross Laboratories, a division of Abbott Laboratories.

FIGURE 10–13
THE NUTRITION CHECKLIST WARNING SIGNS

Use the word *DETERMINE* to remind you of the warning signs.

DISEASE

Any disease, illness, or chronic condition that causes you to change the way you eat, or makes it hard for you to eat, puts your nutritional health at risk. Four out of five adults have chronic diseases that are affected by diet. Confusion or memory loss that keeps getting worse is estimated to affect one out of five or more of older adults. This can make it hard to remember what, when, or if you've eaten. Feeling sad or depressed, which happens to about one in eight older adults, can cause big changes in appetite, digestion, energy level, weight, and well-being.

EATING POORLY

Eating too little and eating too much both lead to poor health. Eating the same foods day after day or not eating fruit, vegetables, and milk products daily will also cause poor nutritional health. One in five adults skip meals daily. Only 13% of adults eat the minimum amount of fruit and vegetables needed. One in four older adults drink too much alcohol. Many health problems become worse if you drink more than one or two alcoholic beverages per day.

TOOTH LOSS/MOUTH PAIN

A healthy mouth, teeth, and gums are needed to eat. Missing, loose, or rotten teeth or dentures that don't fit well or cause mouth sores make it hard to eat.

ECONOMIC HARDSHIP

As many as 40% of older Americans have incomes of less than $6,000 per year. Having less—or choosing to spend less—than $25–$30 per week for food makes it very hard to get the foods you need to stay healthy.

REDUCED SOCIAL CONTACT

One-third of all older people live alone. Being with people daily has a positive effect on morale, well-being, and eating.

MULTIPLE MEDICINES

Many older Americans must take medicines for health problems. Almost half of older Americans take multiple medicines daily. Growing old may change the way we respond to drugs. The more medicines you take, the greater chance for side effects such as increased or decreased appetite, change in taste, constipation, weakness, drowsiness, diarrhea, nausea, and others. Vitamins or minerals taken in large doses act like drugs and can cause harm. Alert your doctor to everything you take.

INVOLUNTARY WEIGHT LOSS/GAIN

Losing or gaining a lot of weight when you are not trying to do so is an important warning sign that must not be ignored. Being overweight or underweight also increases your chance of poor health.

NEEDS ASSISTANCE IN SELF-CARE

Although most older people are able to eat, one of every five has trouble walking, shopping, buying and cooking food, especially as they get older.

ELDER YEARS ABOVE AGE 80

Most older people lead full and productive lives. But as age increases, risk of frailty and health problems increase. Checking your nutritional health regularly makes good sense.

SOURCE: Reprinted with permission by the Nutrition Screening Initiative, a project of the American Academy of Family Physicians, The American Dietetic Association, and the National Council on Aging, Inc. and funded in part by a grant from Ross Laboratories, a division of Abbott Laboratories.

Sources of Nutritional Assistance

In response to the socioeconomic problems—low income, inadequate facilities for preparing food, lack of transportation, and inability to afford dental care, among others—that trouble many older adults and may lead to malnutrition, federal, state, and local agencies have mandated nutrition programs for the elderly.

Two programs are helpful to older people with nutrition problems, although they are not designed specifically for older people but are designed for the poor of all ages. The Food Stamp program enables people who qualify to obtain stamps with which to buy food. The Supplemental Security Income (SSI) program is aimed at directly improving the financial plight of the very poor by increasing a person's or family's income to the defined poverty level. This sometimes helps older people retain their independence.

In several areas, food banks enable older people on limited incomes to buy good food for less money. A food bank project buys industry "irregulars"—products that have been mislabeled, underweighted, redesigned, or mispackaged and would therefore ordinarily be thrown away. Nothing is wrong with this food; the industry can credit it as a donation, and the buyer (often a food-preparing site) can obtain the food for a small handling fee and make it available at a greatly reduced price.

The federal Nutrition Program for Older Americans (NPOA) is intended to improve older people's nutrition status and enable them to avoid medical problems, continue living in communities of their own choice, and stay out of institutions. Its specific goals are to provide

- Low-cost, nutritious meals.
- Opportunities for social interaction.
- Nutrition education and shopping assistance.
- Counseling and referral to other social and rehabilitation services.
- Transportation services.

The current Title III legislation makes one hot noon meal available five days a week, supplying a third of the RDA. There is no cost for meals, but participants sometimes make voluntary contributions.

A part of Title III is the congregate meal program. Administrators try to select sites for congregate meals so as to feed as many of the eligible elderly as possible. The congregate meal sites are often community centers, senior citizen centers, religious facilities, schools, extended care facilities, or elderly housing complexes. Volunteers may also deliver meals to those who are homebound either permanently or temporarily; these efforts are known as the Home-Delivered Meals Program. The home-delivery program ensures nutrition, but its recipients miss out on the social benefit of the congregate meal sites. Every effort is made to persuade recipients to attend the shared meals if they can.

Evaluations of the programs for congregate and home-delivered meals generally show that the programs improve the dietary intake and nutrition status of their clients.[112] Participants generally have greater diversity in their diets and higher intakes of essential nutrients and are less likely to report food insecurity than nonparticipants.[113] Other benefits come as a result of screening and the referrals generated by such programs. Additional benefits are derived from the

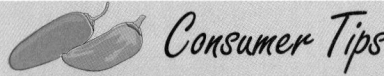

Consumer Tips

Meals for One

Planning nourishing meals for one that offer variety and optimal nutrition can be particularly challenging. The following tips help to solve some of the problems that singles of any age face concerning buying and preparing foods.

- Buy only what you will use: The individual-sized containers may be expensive, but it is also expensive to let the unused portion of a large-sized container spoil before you are ready to use it. Don't be timid about asking the grocer to break up a package of meat, eggs, fresh fruits, or vegetables and wrap a smaller quantity for you.

- Buy a loaf of bread and store half in the freezer. The freezer keeps it fresher than the refrigerator.

- Think up a variety of ways to use a vegetable when you buy it in a large quantity. For example, you can divide a head of broccoli into thirds. Cook one-third and eat it as a hot vegetable. Put one-third in a soup, and use one-third as an appetizer or in a salad. Buy large quantities of frozen vegetables if you have sufficient freezer space. You can take out the exact amount you need at mealtime.

- Buy large packages of meat such as pork chops, ground meat, or chicken when they are on special sale. Divide the package into individual servings and freeze them separately.

- Get the maximum nutritive value out of what you cook. Steam vegetables over water rather than boiling them. Broil meats rather than frying them. Experiment with stir-fried foods. A variety of vegetables and meats can be enjoyed this way; inexpensive vegetables such as cabbage and celery are delicious when crisp-cooked in a little oil with soy sauce and lemon or ginger added. Cooked, leftover vegetables can be dropped in at the last minute.

- Get the maximum value out of the time you spend cooking. Cook for several meals at a time. For example, boil three potatoes with skins. Eat one hot, with butter or margarine and herbs. When the others have cooled, use one to make a potato-cheese casserole ready to be put into the oven for the next evening's meal. Slice the third one and pour your favorite salad dressing over it. The potato will keep several days in the refrigerator and can be used in a salad.

- Make twice as much as you need of a recipe that takes time to prepare: spaghetti sauce, a casserole, vegetable pie, chili, or meat loaf. Label and store the extra servings in the freezer. Be sure to date these so that you will use the oldest first.

- Make mixtures of leftovers you have on hand: a thick stew prepared from leftover green beans, carrots, cauliflower, broccoli, and any beans or meat with some added fresh herbs, onion, pepper, celery, and potatoes makes a complete and balanced meal—except for milk.

- Set aside a place in your kitchen for rows of shelf staple items that you can't buy in single-serving quantities—rice, tapioca, lentils or other dried beans, flour, cornmeal, dry nonfat milk, pasta, or cereal, to name only a few possibilities. Place each jar, tightly sealed, in the freezer for a few days to kill any eggs or organisms before storing it on the shelf. The jars make an attractive display and will remind you of possibilities for variety in your menus. Include the directions-for-use labels from the packages in the jars.

- Cook for yourself with the idea that you are cooking for special guests. Invite guests when you can and make enough food so that you will have enough for a later meal.

activities associated with the congregate meals services: diet counseling, exercise, adult education, and other classes and activities. Participants benefit, too, from the opportunity for improved socialization.[114]

The *Meals-on-Wheels America* program is separate from but similar to the federal home-delivered meals program. Meals-on-Wheels is a national project operated under the auspices of local volunteer groups. Its purpose is to help fill gaps in services provided by the federal meals programs by reaching older adults in communities not serviced by the NPOA.[115]

Sometimes assistance programs are not enough to meet the needs of older people, some of whom require institutional care. A variety of options exist. A familiar alternative is the nursing home, which is a medical solution to what, in many cases, is a social problem, although it may be necessary for people who need constant medical care.

The relative inquiring into retirement centers or nursing homes should ask the director or dietitian some questions about the food service. Does the resident have a choice in the selection of food? How often are the menus repeated (is the cycle monotonous)? How often are fresh fruits and vegetables served? Does the staff keep track of each person's weight? Does good communication exist between the nursing staff and the dietitian so that the dietitian will know whether someone is not eating? Is the resident encouraged and helped to go to the dining room to eat so that some socializing will occur? Is the dining room attractive? Does someone help those who can't manage feeding themselves? Are religious dietary restrictions honored? Other questions that the investigator will want to ask have to do with the general atmosphere of the retirement center or nursing home in recognition of the effect of social climate on a person's appetite. A facility that views residents as people, not as patients, gets a mark in its favor.

In the nursing home, the dietitian, nutritionist, or nurse responsible for the residents' care should keep in mind the special needs associated with the residents' time in life. The average age of a nursing home resident is 81, and many residents have problems or habits that can affect their nutrition status:

- At least one chronic disease.
- Constipation or incontinence.
- Confusion due to the change in environment or dementia.
- Poor eyesight or hearing.
- Ill-fitting or missing dentures.
- Inability to feed themselves because of arthritis or stroke.
- Psychological problems, especially depression.
- Anorexia and loss of interest in eating.
- Lack of opportunity to socialize at mealtimes.
- Long-established food preferences.
- Slowed reactions (seeing, holding utensils, chewing, swallowing).

Looking Ahead: Growing Seasoned

As a nation, we tend to value the future more than the present, putting off enjoying today so that we will have money, prestige, or time to have fun tomorrow. The elderly feel this loss of future. The present is their time for leisure and enjoyment, but they often have no experience in using leisure time.

The solution is to begin to prepare for old age early in life, both psychologically and nutritionally. Preparation for this period should, of course, include financial planning, but other lifelong habits should be developed as well. Each adult needs to learn to reach out to others to forestall the loneliness that will otherwise ensue. Adults need to develop some skills or activities— volunteer work with organizations, reading, games, hobbies, or intellectual pursuits—that they can continue into their later years and will give meaning to their lives. Every adult needs to develop the habit of adjusting to change, especially when it comes without consent, so that it will not be seen as a loss of control over his or her life. The goal is to arrive at maturity with as healthy a mind and body as possible; this means cultivating good nutrition status and maintaining a program of daily exercise.

In general, the ability of the elderly to function well varies from person to person and depends on several factors. The following "life advantages" seem to contribute to good physical and mental health in later years:[116]

- Genetic potential for extended longevity. Some persons seem to have inherited a reduced susceptibility to degenerative diseases.

- A continued desire for new knowledge and new experiences. Some studies suggest that active minds, ever involved in learning new things, may be more resistant to decline.

- Socialization, intimacy, and family integrity. Older persons thrive in situations in which love, understanding, shared responsibility, and mutual respect are nurtured.

- Adherence to a prudent diet while avoiding excesses of food energy, fat, cholesterol, and sodium. A prudent diet with adequate intakes of all essential nutrients has a positive impact on health and weight management.

- Avoidance of substance abuse.

- Acceptable living arrangements.

- Financial independence.

- Access to health care—to include a family physician, health clinic, public health nursing service providing home health care, dentist, podiatrist, physical therapist, pharmacist, and registered dietitian.

Everyone knows older people who have maintained many contacts—through relatives, friends, church, synagogue, or fraternal orders—and have not allowed themselves to drift into isolation. Upon analysis, you will find that their favorable environment came through a lifetime of effort. These people spent their entire lives reaching out to others and practicing the art of weaving others into their own lives. Likewise, a lifetime of effort is required for good nutrition status in the later years. A person who has eaten a wide variety of foods, stayed trim, and remained physically active will be best able to withstand the assaults of change.

GROWING SEASONED

- Choose nutrient-dense foods.
- Maintain a healthful body weight.
- Reduce stress.
- For postmenopausal women, see a physician about possible hormone replacement against osteoporosis.
- For people who smoke, quit.
- Expect to enjoy sex and learn new ways of enhancing it.
- Use alcohol only moderately, if at all; use other drugs only as prescribed.
- Take care to prevent accidents; wear your seatbelt.
- Expect good vision and hearing throughout life; obtain glasses and hearing aids if necessary.
- Be alert to confusion as a disease symptom and seek diagnosis.
- Control depression through activities and friendships.
- Drink 8 glasses of water every day.
- Practice mental skills. Keep on solving math problems and crossword puzzles, playing cards or other games, reading, writing, imagining, and creating.
- Make financial plans early to ensure security.
- Accept change. Work at recovering from losses; make new friends.
- Cultivate spiritual health. Cherish personal values. Make life meaningful.
- Go outside for sunshine and fresh air as often as possible.
- Be physically active. Walk, run, dance, swim, bike, row, or climb for aerobic activity. Lift weights, do calisthenics, or pursue some other activity to tone, firm, and strengthen muscles.
- Be socially active—play bridge, join an exercise group, take a class, teach a class, eat with friends, or volunteer time to help others.
- Stay interested in life—pursue a hobby, spend time with grandchildren, take a trip, read, grow a garden, or go to the movies.
- Enjoy life.

SOURCE: Adapted by permission from *Understanding Nutrition.* 6th ed. by E. N. Whitney and S. R. Rolfes. Copyright © 1993 by West Publishing Company. All rights reserved.

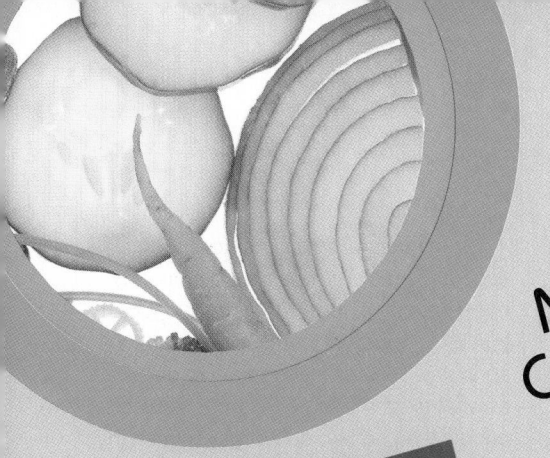

Nutrition and Cancer Prevention

You probably know someone who has cancer or who has recovered from it or who has died of it. After heart disease, cancer is our most prevalent disease and can be expected, in one form or another, to affect one out of every three Americans living today (see Figure 10–14). Given what is known now about the link between diet and cancer, you are well advised to learn about this connection. Unlike so many factors in our environment, the food you choose to eat is a factor you can control to a great extent. This discussion attempts to answer questions about the connection between diet and cancer.

How is diet associated with cancer?

Numerous studies conducted in both laboratory animals and humans over the past two decades have shown that many connections exist between diet and cancer.[117] Constituents in foods may be responsible for starting the cancer (a process called *initiation*) or for speeding its development (a two-step process that includes tumor *promotion* and *progression*), or they may protect against cancer. Also, for the person who has cancer, diet can make a crucial difference to recovery by helping to restore body weight and improve nutritional status.

Not all studies have shown a firm relationship between cancer and food and nutrient intake. In particular, some epidemiologic studies—that is, studies of disease rates and food patterns of groups of people—have failed to demonstrate such a link. Where a positive association has been found, caution should be used in interpreting data linking dietary components with cancer or other chronic diseases. Remember, an increase in one component of the diet can cause increases or decreases in others. If a close correlation is shown between cancer and, say, the consumption of animal protein by a human population, how can we be sure that the critical factor is the animal protein? It may be increased fat consumption, because fat goes with animal protein in foods. Or the cancer may occur because of what is crowded out: vitamins, minerals, fiber, or nonnutrients contained in the missing fruits, vegetables, and cereals.

These issues must be considered when examining the results of studies describing a connection between diet and cancer. Our diets are complex and diverse, making it difficult to separate the effect of a single dietary component from the hundreds of other constituents found in foods. In addition, the difficulty of evalu-

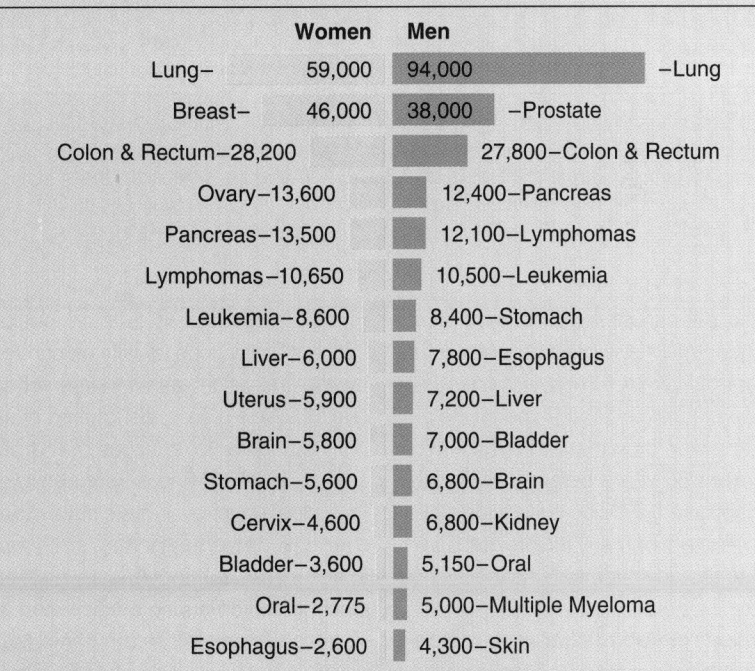

FIGURE 10–14
CANCER DEATHS

SOURCE: American Cancer Society, *Cancer Facts & Figures*—1994.

TABLE 10–12
DIET AND CANCER

CANCER SITE	ASSOCIATED WITH THESE DIETARY RISK FACTORS
Breast	High intakes of calories, fat, and alcohol; low fruit and vegetable intake
Colon or rectum	High-fat diets (particularly saturated fat) and alcohol; low-fiber diets
Esophagus	Excessive alcohol intake, low intakes of vitamins and minerals
Lung	Low beta-carotene intake; low fruit and vegetable intake
Ovary and endometrium	High-fat diets; obesity; low fruit and vegetable intake
Prostate	High-fat diets may promote tumor growth
Pancreas	Low fruit and vegetable intake
Stomach	Regular consumption of smoked foods and foods cured with salt or nitrite compounds; low fruit and vegetable intake
Liver	Ingestion of *aflatoxin*-contaminated grains; regular consumption of smoked foods and foods cured with salt or nitrite compounds; alcohol abuse
Mouth and throat	Excessive alcohol intake; low fruit and vegetable intake

SOURCES: Committee on Diet and Health (Food and Nutrition Board; National Research Council); *Diet and Health: Implications for Reducing Chronic Disease Risk* (Washington, D.C.: National Academy Press, 1989); and J. H. Weisburger, Nutritional approach to cancer prevention with emphasis on vitamins, antioxidants, and carotenoids, *American Journal of Clinical Nutrition* 53 (1991): 226S–237S; R. G. Ziegler, Vegetables, fruits, and carotenoids and the risk of cancer, *American Journal of Clinical Nutrition* 53 (1991): 251S–259S.

ating the diet-cancer link is compounded by the fact that many cancers take up to 20 years to develop. Thus, assessing a cancer patient's diet today is not as helpful as knowing how that patient ate 10, 20, or even 30 years before the cancer was diagnosed. Finally, our eating pattern is only one of many factors that contribute to the development of cancer.

Is nutrition related to cancer causation the way other environmental factors are—such as smoking or air pollution?
Yes. The National Cancer Institute estimates that 90 percent of all cancers are associated with lifestyle and environ-mental factors, including nutrition. Lifestyle factors can usually be controlled by the individual and include tobacco use, diet, exercise, consumption of alcohol, exposure to sunlight, patterns of sexual behavior, and personal hygiene. Individuals typically have little control over environmental factors, such as the exposure to carcinogens in the work-place, radiation during medical and dental procedures, or contaminants (either naturally occurring or artificially created) present in the soil, air, and water. Of course, we have no control over the genetic factors that contribute to the development of cancer.

Nutrition is a lifestyle factor that may account for as much as a third of all can-cer deaths. Thus, researchers have taken the study of nutrition and cancer seriously. They are attempting to discov-er what dietary differences exist between people who do and do not get cancer. In the process, they are trying to identify the various dietary factors that may con-tribute to or protect against many differ-ent types of cancer, including cancer of the esophagus, stomach, liver, pancreas, colon, rectum, breast, ovary, prostate, and lung (see Table 10–12).

What is some of the evidence linking diet and cancer? Studies of the eating habits of different population groups pro-vide some of the knowledge we have about the diet-cancer connection. Particularly telling is research involving Seventh-Day Adventists, a group of peo-ple with a remarkably low death rate from cancers of all kinds. This religious group has rules against smoking and using alcohol, discourages the use of hot condiments and spices, and encourages a meatless diet. After cancers linked to smoking and alcohol are discounted, these people still have a cancer mortali-ty rate about one-half to two-thirds that of the rest of the population. This may be due to a low consumption of meat (and therefore *fat*) and to a high consumption of fruits, vegetables, and cereal grains.

When it comes to colon cancer, stud-ies lend weight to the theory that colon cancer is associated with indicators of affluence, such as a high-fat diet rich in animal protein.[118] In one study, people with colon cancer were compared with a carefully matched set of people without cancer. Those with cancer were found to have a strikingly higher consumption of meat, especially red meat.[119] Another study showed fiber consumption to be lower in colon cancer victims than in comparable people who did not have cancer. Still another showed colon cancer victims to be eating less fiber and more saturated fat than people without cancer. Furthermore, among U.S. women between the ages of 34 and 59, the risk of colon cancer was related to their intake of animal (but not vegetable) fat, according to researchers at Harvard Medical School.[120] These examples are just a few of the many studies that have led researchers to the view that a diet high in total fat, especially animal fat, and low in fiber is associated with cancer of the colon.[121] Other results suggest that beta-carotene and vitamin C, or possibly other components of the foods that contain them, can help reduce the risk of colon cancer.[122]

So, diet is associated with the development of colon cancer. What about breast cancer? The case of the connection between diet and breast cancer is a good example of the difficulty of interpreting study results. Laboratory animals, particularly rodents, consistently develop mammary or breast tumors when fed diets high in either vegetable oils (omega-6 fatty acids) or animal fats.[123] Despite the strength of this link in the animal model, similar results have not been seen consistently in human studies.[124]

A group of researchers in Athens, Greece, who studied 120 women with breast cancer and 120 women without cancer, have reported no association between breast cancer and the consumption of fats and oils.[125] By comparison, a research group in China reported that women with a high intake of fat and calories and a low intake of vegetables and dietary fiber had an increased risk of breast cancer.[126] Several studies from Canada and the United States have also supported a link between breast cancer and fat intake.[127] Despite these apparently conflicting study results, the National Cancer Institute has determined that the bulk of the evidence suggests a link between fat intake and breast cancer.

What should consumers do? The American Cancer Society and the National Cancer Institute have reviewed the evidence independently and have pointed out to consumers the following specific concerns:

● *Total calorie intake.* Studies on animals show that reduced food intakes reduce cancer incidence at any age, but the evidence is less clear for human beings. Obesity, however, does increase risks for some cancers in both animals and people (refer to Chapter 8).

● *Fat.* Both animal studies and population studies support the view that high-fat intakes increase the incidence of cancers of the breast, ovaries, colon, and prostate. Evidence on the relationship between cholesterol and cancer is unclear at this point.

● *Protein.* High protein intakes may be associated with increased risks of certain kinds of cancer, but the evidence is not yet firm enough to permit a definitive statement.

● *Carbohydrate.* There is little evidence that carbohydrates as such play a role in cancer development.

● *Beta-carotene.* Inadequate intakes of beta-carotene correlate with a high incidence of cancers of the lung, bladder, and larynx; by inference, adequate intakes must help protect against these cancers.

● *Vitamin C.* Vitamin C may help prevent the formation of cancer-causing agents and thereby protect against cancers of the esophagus and stomach.[128]

● *Other vitamins and minerals.* Bits of evidence suggest that other nutrients may protect against certain types of cancer, but no firm conclusions can yet be made. The effect of the antioxidant nutrients—vitamin C, beta-carotene, and vitamin E, and selenium—on cancer risk is an area of active research (refer to the Spotlight feature in Chapter 6). The trace mineral, selenium, used in the body's

production of its own antioxidants, is believed to have a protective effect against cancer of the esophagus, stomach, colon, and rectum. Likewise, vitamin E may protect against cancer, particularly cancer of the gastrointestinal tract.[129]

● *Beta-carotene-rich and cruciferous vegetables.* The consumption of beta-carotene-rich and cruciferous vegetables is associated with a reduced incidence of cancer at several sites. Cruciferous vegetables, a group of vegetables named for their cross-shaped blossoms, have been shown to protect against cancer in laboratory animals. Examples of cruciferous vegetables are cauliflower, cabbage, Brussels sprouts, broccoli, kohlrabi, and rutabagas.

● *Calcium.* Low calcium intakes have been associated with increased colon cancer. Conversely, people consuming more calcium tend to develop less colon cancer.[130]

What about fiber? Wherever the diet is high in fat-rich foods, it is usually low in vegetable fiber. This raises the question of whether the absence of fiber may pro-

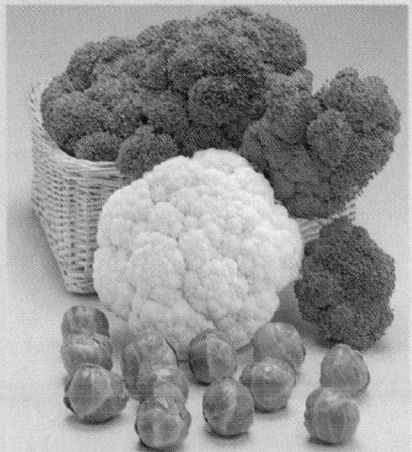

Cruciferous vegetables, such as cauliflower, broccoli, and Brussels sprouts, contain nutrients and nonnutrients that protect against cancer.

mote cancer independently of the presence of fat. The answer is difficult to discern, but the association of cancer with fat is stronger than with the lack of fiber. Still, fiber might help to protect against some cancers by, for example, speeding up the passage of all materials through the colon so that its walls are not exposed for long to cancer-causing substances.

Evidence from Finland supports fiber's independent protective effect. The Finns eat a high-fat diet, but unlike other such diets, theirs is very high in fiber as well. Their colon cancer rate is low, suggesting that fiber has a protective effect even in the presence of a high-fat diet.

Fat is linked to certain cancers, and fiber is associated with cancer prevention. Do vegetarians have a lower incidence of those cancers? Yes, they do. The Seventh-Day Adventists have already been mentioned. Vegetarian women also have less breast cancer than do women who eat meat.

A number of studies have examined the relationship between cancer and vegetable consumption. Many of them have shown that people with colon cancer eat vegetables less frequently than do others; one study revealed that colon cancer victims specifically consumed less cabbage, broccoli, and Brussels sprouts than did people free of cancer. Similarly, comparisons of stomach cancer victims' diets with those of carefully matched people without cancer showed lower consumption of vegetables in the cancer group—in one case, vegetables in general; in another, fresh vegetables; in others, lettuce and other fresh greens or vegetables containing vitamin C. Some of the suspects for the causation of stomach cancer are the chemicals known as nitrosamines, produced in the stomach and intestines from nitrites found in foods. Vegetables may help in cancer prevention by contributing vitamin C, which inhibits the conversion of nitrites to nitrosamines.[131]

What about alcohol. Is it connected with cancer? Yes. Environmental causes of head, neck, and esophageal cancer have been studied, and the major factor appears to be the combination of alcohol and tobacco use. However, dietary factors have turned up, pointing to a low intake of fruits and raw vegetables, specifically of the fruits and vegetables that contribute the orange pigment beta-carotene (which converts to vitamin A in the body) and the vitamin riboflavin. Beta-carotene—noted for giving carrots, winter squash, sweet potatoes, apricots, cantaloupe, oranges, and other fruits and vegetables their familiar colors—and its relatives (known as the retinoids, which are found in milk, cheese, butter, ice cream, and certain fish) may also be important in reducing the risk of skin cancer.

Researchers are currently probing the possible association of alcohol consumption with increased risk of breast cancer.[132] Although some studies have shown a modest but significant increase in risk of breast cancer for women who were classified as heavy drinkers (more than 40 grams of alcohol or more than 4 drinks per day), other studies have found no relationship.[133] More research is needed to clarify this issue. However, if a causal relationship between relatively heavy drinking and increased risk of breast cancer is confirmed, such evidence would lend support to the societal benefits derived from not consuming excessive amounts of alcohol.

What is the association between beta-carotene and cancer? Among the known actions of vitamin A (beta-carotene) are the important roles it plays in maintaining immune function. A strong immune system may be able to prevent cancers from gaining control even after they have gotten started in the body.

Although smoking is the predominant cause of lung cancer in all parts of the world, dietary factors, including beta-carotene intake, may also influence risk. A study conducted in India has shown lung cancer rates to be 20 percent to 30 percent lower in smokers who ate yellow or green vegetables daily than in those who did not.[134] In ex-smokers who ingested yellow or green vegetables daily, the reduction was much greater, indicating that the *repair* of damage done by smoking might be enhanced by something in the vegetables.

Would that "something" in the vegetables be beta-carotene? Not necessarily. Both fruits and vegetables appear to have a protective effect beyond those already discussed for beta-carotene, vitamin C, and fiber. Researchers have identified substances known as *phytochemicals*—naturally occurring plant compounds—in fruits and vegetables that may play a role in decreasing cancer risk and strengthening the immune system.[135] (Refer to Table 6–16 on page 227 in Chapter 6 for a sampling of these compounds.) These vegetables also contain folate, a vitamin, which is involved in cell multiplication, and may prove to play an important role in cervical cancer prevention.[136] The effects of the members of the cabbage family may be due to their containing substances known as indoles—a type of phytochemical—which may act by inducing an enzyme in the host that destroys cancer-causing agents.

Do these findings have any implications for the way a person should eat right now, today? Although clearly there is still much to learn, many experts believe that enough is known to take the first preventive steps. The following recommendations are commonly offered:

● Reduce total fat and maintain a healthful weight.

● Ingest more complex carbohydrates, both starch and fiber.

● Eat plenty of green, orange, and yellow vegetables and fruits, including generous servings from the cabbage family.

● Vary your choices. Don't let your diet become monotonous.

The National Cancer Institute has added three other recommendations: 1) maintain a desirable body weight; 2) consume alcoholic beverages in moderation, if at all; and 3) eat salt-cured, smoked, and nitrite-preserved foods sparingly.[137] Taken together, this advice agrees with most recommendations made to the public for helping prevent heart disease, diabetes, and many other ills as well as cancer.

Public efforts are now underway to reduce the major risk factors for cancer.[138] The National Cancer Institute (NCI) designed its *National 5 a Day for Better Health* program to increase per capita fruit and vegetable consumption. The NCI's 5 a Day program promotes a simple nutrition message: *Eat five or more servings of fruits and vegetables every day for better health.*[139]

Does it make a difference whether I choose to take supplements instead of eating vegetables? Yes. Fiber, vitamin C, beta-carotene, riboflavin, indoles, and other components found in *foods* appear to have preventive effects on cancer development. And because it is obvious that researchers do not have *the* answer—just many partial answers—it is best to stick with foods.

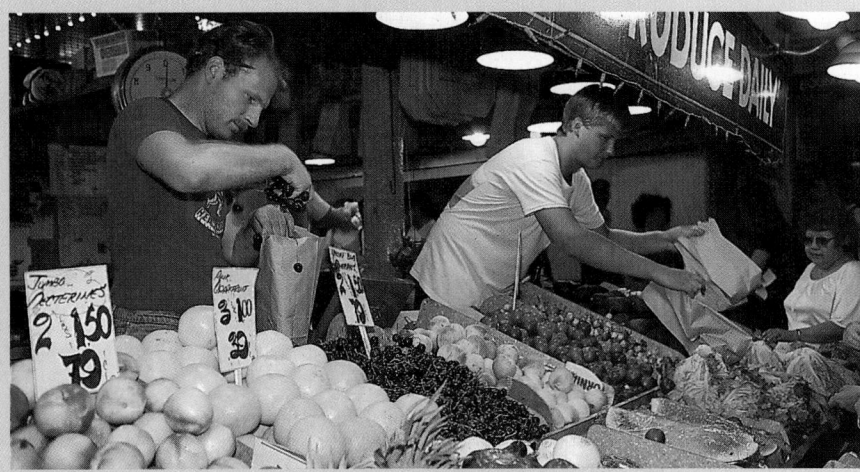

The National Cancer Institute's *National 5 a Day for Better Health* program urges consumers to eat five or more servings of fruits and vegetables every day for better health.

Supplements may not contain some as yet unidentified components found in foods that may help to protect against cancer. Also, with vitamin/mineral supplementation, there is always the risk of an excessively high intake; recall that vitamin A, selenium, and other vitamins and minerals can be toxic at high doses. *It is best to rely on foods.* Fruits and vegetables will add vitamins, minerals, and fiber to your diet—and color and flavor as well.

Why should I vary my diet? The recommendation to eat a varied diet is based on an important cancer-prevention strategy—dilution. The standard advice to eat a variety of foods takes on new meaning in this quote: "The wider the variety of food intake, the greater the number of different chemical substances consumed, and the less is the chance that any one chemical will reach a hazardous level in the diet."[140] In other words, whenever you add new foods to

the diet, you are diluting whatever is in one food with what is in another.

The variety principle has traditionally meant to eat foods from each of the various food groups. This principle needs to be applied within each of the food groups as well. Don't alternate just between corn and potatoes. Select different vegetables each time you go to the store—broccoli, peas, green beans, squash, and many others.

Although there are many cancer-causing factors that you cannot control, you can decide which food habits you will keep and which ones you will change. By using these guidelines in making your choices, you will have every reason to feel confident that you are providing your body with the best nutrition at the lowest possible risk. Remember that in the final analysis, your risk of developing cancer can be reduced significantly by not smoking, consuming alcohol in moderation, and by adopting healthful eating and exercise habits.

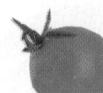

CHECK YOURSELF...

1. State which nutrients are needed in increased amounts in pregnancy; what supplements are needed?

2. State the recommended weight gain for pregnancy; list the components that this weight gain comprises.

3. Name the most potent indicator of an infant's future health status.

4. List practices that should be eliminated during pregnancy and provide a reason why.

5. Name three advantages of breastfeeding derived by the infant.

6. Describe the recommended infant feeding practices—when to introduce solid foods, whole milk, nonfat milk. Why is it recommended that items be introduced one at a time?

7. State why infants are at risk of dehydration.

8. State the importance of adequate intakes of calcium during preadolescence.

9. State food habits to be encouraged in children to avoid nutrient deficiencies, obesity, and dental caries.

10. Differentiate between adolescent growth patterns of males and females.

11. Describe three of the nutrition-related problems common among teenagers.

12. List physiological changes associated with aging.

13. Compare and contrast energy and nutrient requirements of older adults with those of young adults.

14. List factors contributing to nutrient deficiencies in older adults.

15. List nutrients thought to be protective of cancer formation and nutrients associated with increased risk of developing cancer.

Answers to selected Check Yourself questions are found in Appendix H.

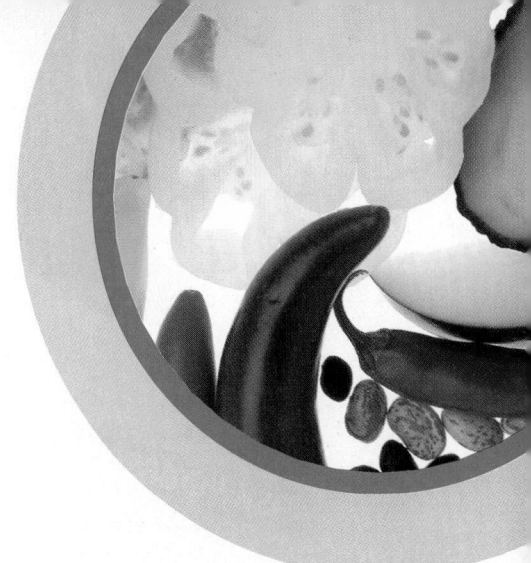

> **The role of the infinitely small is infinitely large.**
>
> Louis Pasteur
> (1822–1895, French chemist and microbiologist
> who developed the pasteurization process)

Food Safety and the Global Food Supply　　ELEVEN

Contents

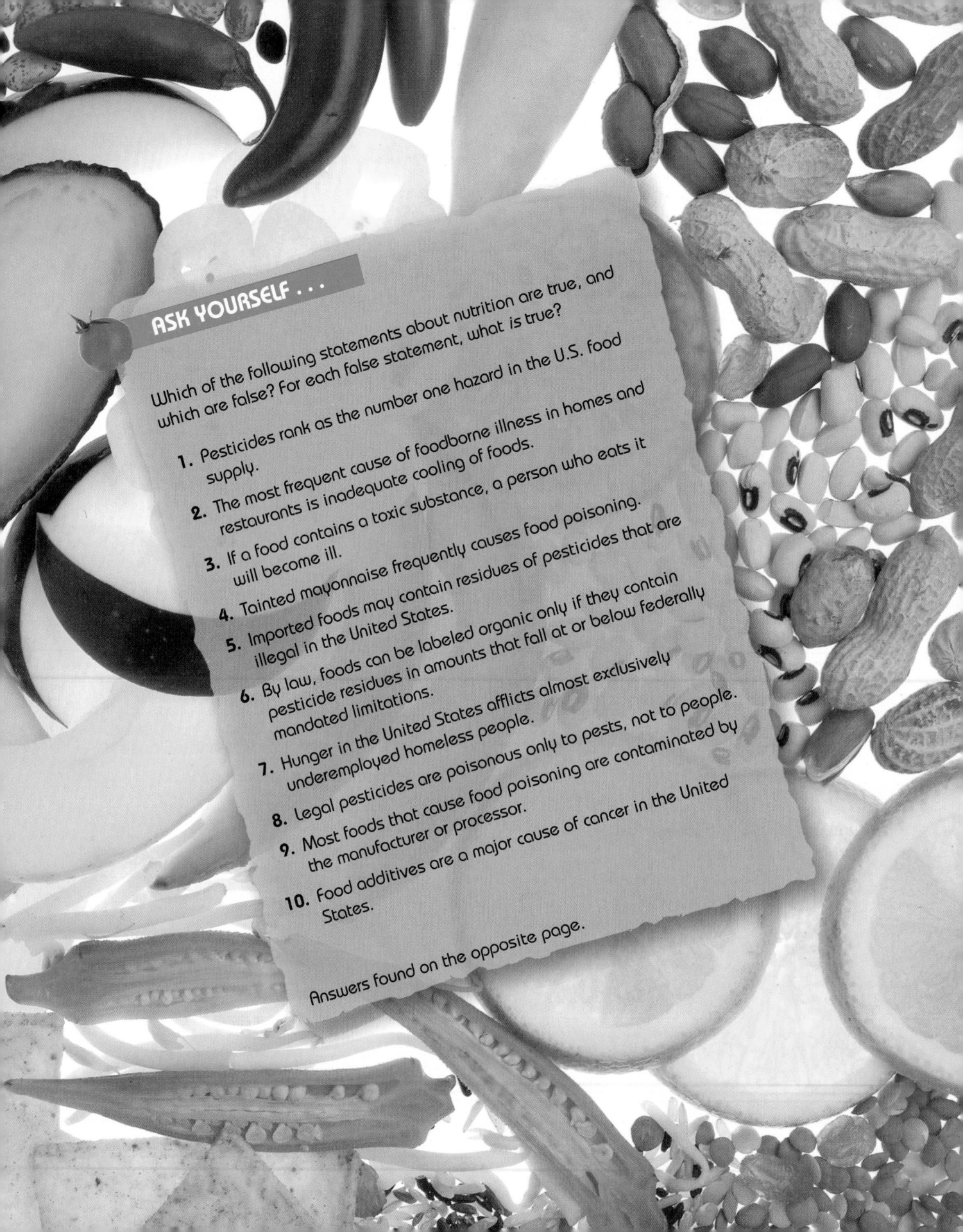

Which of the following statements about nutrition are true, and which are false? For each false statement, what *is* true?

1. Pesticides rank as the number one hazard in the U.S. food supply.

2. The most frequent cause of foodborne illness in homes and restaurants is inadequate cooling of foods.

3. If a food contains a toxic substance, a person who eats it will become ill.

4. Tainted mayonnaise frequently causes food poisoning.

5. Imported foods may contain residues of pesticides that are illegal in the United States.

6. By law, foods can be labeled organic only if they contain pesticide residues in amounts that fall at or below federally mandated limitations.

7. Hunger in the United States afflicts almost exclusively underemployed homeless people.

8. Legal pesticides are poisonous only to pests, not to people.

9. Most foods that cause food poisoning are contaminated by the manufacturer or processor.

10. Food additives are a major cause of cancer in the United States.

Answers found on the opposite page.

So far this book has dealt primarily with the nutrients and how your body handles them. This chapter takes the study of nutrition one step further and examines some nonnutrient components of food— bacteria, additives, and pesticides, to name a few—and how they affect the food supply. In addition, the chapter takes a global view of the science of nutrition, looking at how foodways in different countries influence each other as well as how some of our food habits affect the environment.

What sorts of additives do foods contain, and what are the effects of those additives? Are foods ever contaminated? How can you reduce your risk of food poisoning? What potential do new food technologies, such as irradiation and genetic engineering, hold for our lives and for the health of the environment? This chapter addresses these and other questions.

Foodborne Illnesses and the Agents That Cause Them

North America has the safest, most plentiful food supply in the world, thanks to the concerted efforts of food suppliers, food processors, and federal, state, and local governments, all of which are concerned with food safety. North Americans also enjoy the most diverse food supply in the world, consisting of an incredible array of fresh and processed foods. Most American supermarkets stock a variety of foods from other countries—cookies and crackers from Denmark and the United Kingdom, Belgian chocolates, Italian cheeses, beef and veal products from New Zealand and Australia, goose liver paté from France, and specialty foods from Japan, Mexico, and even China. Our international bent can be seen in the produce section as well, where exotic star fruit, papaya, and mango from overseas markets are widely available. Still, the diverse mix of fresh and processed foods coming from local, national, and international markets underscores the need to understand where the culprits behind foodborne illnesses originate.

Foodborne illness, or **food poisoning,** is one of the greatest concerns of public health experts and the food industry. Each year, as many as 33 million Americans experience foodborne illness, and an estimated 9,000 deaths are linked to tainted foods. Medical expenses and lost productivity cost $5 billion to $6 billion annually.[1] Incredible as these figures are, they probably represent only a fraction of the whole picture. Many mild cases of food poisoning are never reported for a number of reasons: The victims pass off the symptoms as flu and

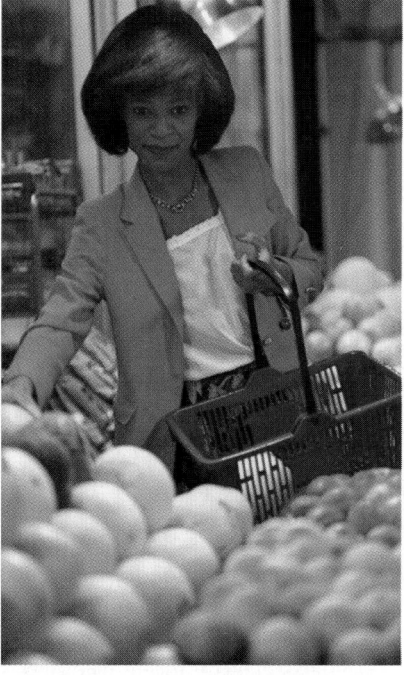

Americans enjoy the safest, most diverse food supply in the world.

FOODBORNE ILLNESS or **FOOD POISONING** illness occurring as a result of eating food contaminated with disease-producing microorganisms, such as bacteria, viruses, or parasites, or toxic substances such as chemicals.

ASK YOURSELF ANSWERS: 1. False. The greatest hazard present in the U.S. food supply today is not pesticides but bacteria, viruses, mold, and other microorganisms that cause food poisoning. **2.** True. **3.** False. If a food contains a toxic substance, a person who eats it *may* become ill, depending on whether enough of the toxin to cause illness is present. **4.** False. Mayonnaise rarely carries high levels of the bacteria that cause illness. **5.** True. **6.** False. The federal government has not set forth a legal definition of the word *organic* for use on food labels. **7.** False. Hunger in the United States affects not only the unemployed homeless but also homeowners and the working poor. **8.** False. Legal pesticides can be poisonous to people, animals, and plants, depending on the amount of the pesticide. **9.** False. Most cases of food poisoning are the result of improper handling of food *after* it leaves the processor or manufacturer. **10.** False. Food additives, which pose minimal health risks, are not a major cause of cancer.

do not seek medical attention, the illness is misdiagnosed as another problem with similar symptoms, the victim fails to recognize food as the source of the illness, or the physician doesn't report the food poisoning to local health agencies.

That more people aren't afflicted with foodborne illness is surprising because disease-producing microorganisms proliferate in our environment. Consider that all raw foods contain microbes, and foods often pick up more during production, processing, packaging, transport, storage, or preparation. That's why the food industry uses different types of control measures to limit the risk of foodborne illness to consumers. Destruction or inactivation of bacteria or their spores is accomplished through the use of heat treatments such as **pasteurization** and canning. Freezing, dehydrating, and refrigerating food also halts or slows down bacterial growth. In addition, special packaging techniques and antimicrobial preservatives help to control food-related pathogens.

What causes most cases of foodborne illness? Many people believe that chemical additives and pesticide residues added during the growing and processing of food pose the greatest risk. But contrary to popular belief, most foodborne disease is caused by mishandling of food, either in food-service establishments such as restaurants or in homes. In fact, food eaten in restaurants, cafeterias, and other food-service establishments accounts for about half of all reported outbreaks of foodborne illness, and food eaten at home, about a quarter.[2] Most cases of foodborne disease are caused by faulty handling, cooking, and storing of food long after it has left the manufacturer or processor. Table 11–1 ranks the most common food hazards.

Experts classify foodborne diseases into two types: intoxications and infections. **Food intoxications** occur when a chemical or toxin transmitted by way of food causes the body to malfunction. An example of food intoxication is the vomiting, nausea, abdominal cramping, sweating, and chills that result from eating food contaminated with a strain of bacteria called *Staphylococcus aureus*. This bacterium produces what is known as an **enterotoxin,** a toxin that causes severe gastrointestinal distress. Other types of bacteria can produce **neurotoxins,** or toxins that afflict the nervous system. Food intoxication can also be caused by eating food that has been contaminated with a chemical, such as lead or some other heavy metal.

Foodborne infections, on the other hand, occur as a result of eating a food that contains living microorganisms, such as bacteria, viruses, or parasites, capable of multiplying and thriving in the body. Ingested in large amounts, the microorganisms can wreak havoc in the digestive tract or other areas of the body. An example of this type of foodborne illness is infection with *Vibrio* bacteria, which often reside in raw

Diarrhea, nausea, abdominal pain, or vomiting without fever or upper respiratory distress is often taken to be flu, but people who experience such symptoms are highly likely to be suffering from food poisoning. If you suspect you've eaten tainted food, especially from a restaurant or other place where many people may have been infected, be sure to alert your local health department.

PASTEURIZATION the process of sterilizing food via heat treatment.

FOOD INTOXICATION illness caused by eating food that contains a harmful toxin.

ENTEROTOXIN a toxic compound, produced by microorganisms, that harms the gastrointestinal tract.
entero = intestine

NEUROTOXIN a poisonous compound that disrupts the nervous system.
neuro = nerve

FOODBORNE INFECTION illness caused by eating a food containing bacteria or other microorganisms capable of growing and thriving in a person's tissues.

TABLE 11–1
RANK OF HEALTH HAZARDS FROM FOOD

While most people think that chemicals such as pesticides and additives rank as the most dangerous, illness-producing substances in our food supply, the real hazard comes from naturally occurring bacteria and other microbes.

Most dangerous:	1. Microbial contamination
	2. Naturally occurring toxicants
	3. Environmental contaminants, such as metals
	4. Malnutrition, including overnutrition
	5. Pesticide residues
Least dangerous:	6. Food additives

SOURCE: D. O. Cliver, *Eating Safely* (New York, NY: American Council on Science and Health, 1993), p. 3.

seafood such as oysters and clams. Inside the body, the bacteria settle in quickly and cause abrupt onset of chills, fever, or prostration.

The following section provides an overview of the various agents that can cause a foodborne illness—be it an intoxication or infection.

Microbial Agents

When we scan a restaurant menu or reach for an egg or glass of milk from the refrigerator at home, we aren't usually thinking about the microorganisms that might be lurking in the foods or their potential to cause illness. We tend to assume that the foods and beverages we consume are safe to eat or drink. Granted, most of the time we don't need to worry. Typically, a food must harbor thousands of microorganisms before it causes nausea, diarrhea, cramps, or other symptoms of foodborne illness. What's more, a healthy body can usually defend itself against small amounts of the "bad bugs."

But when proper food-handling procedures are not followed carefully, the risk of food poisoning from bacteria or other microbial agents soars. Mishandled food, such as items cooked or stored improperly, provides the perfect medium in which microorganisms can flourish. In children, the elderly, people whose immune systems are compromised, or other vulnerable people, it might only take small amounts of the offending microorganisms to cause trouble. For these fragile people, proper handling of food rates as a particularly high priority.

In the United States, the many microorganisms responsible for most cases of foodborne illness range from *Salmonella* to *Clostridium botulinum* to *E. coli* 0157:H7. Table 11–2 summarizes the common food sources of these and other microbial agents responsible for most outbreaks of foodborne illness.

Of the microbial pathogens, *Salmonella* ranks as the leading cause of foodborne illness in the United States, and it appears to be growing more widespread.[3] Symptoms of the illness it causes, called salmonellosis, usually begin within 6 to 48 hours of eating the contaminated food and last for one to eight days. Many cases of salmonellosis probably go unreported because the illness's characteristic nausea, diarrhea, and abdominal pain mimic flulike gastrointestinal ills.

In the past, egg products were a major source of salmonellosis in the United States, but this is no longer the case as a result of mandatory pasteurization of eggs used in the commercial preparation of ice cream, baked goods, and other egg-containing food products. Raw eggs, however, have been implicated in outbreaks of salmonellosis, as has raw, unpasteurized milk. (Because of this health concern, the sale of raw milk has been banned in most states.) Today, most outbreaks of salmonellosis are caused by faulty handling of raw meat and poultry.

Staphylococcus aureus is another strain of bacteria responsible for many of the reported cases of foodborne illnesses that occur in the United States. The bacterium, found in the nose and throat and on the skin of most people, can be transmitted to food when an individual with an infected wound or boil or a respiratory infection handles food improperly. The bacterium itself isn't directly responsible for the illness, however. Rather, it produces staphylococcal enterotoxin,

(continued on page 420)

"I need 148 get-well cards."

TABLE 11–2
MICROBIAL FOOD AGENTS: ORGANISMS THAT CAN BUG YOU

DISEASE AND ORGANISM THAT CAUSES IT	SOURCE OF ILLNESS	USUAL ONSET AFTER EATING	SYMPTOMS
BACTERIA			
Botulism (*Botulinum* toxin produced by *Clostridium botulinum* bacteria)	Spores of these bacteria are widespread. But these bacteria produce toxin only in an anerobic (oxygenless) environment of little acidity. Found in low-acid canned foods such as corn, green beans, soups, beets, asparagus, mushrooms, tuna, and liver paté. Also in luncheon meats, ham, sausage, stuffed eggplant, lobster, smoked and salted fish and homemade, unrefrigerated garlic-in-oil preparations.	4–36 hours	Neurotoxic symptoms, including double vision, inability to swallow, speech difficulty, and progressive paralysis of the respiratory system. **Get medical help immediately. Botulism can be fatal.**
Campylobacteriosis (*Campylobacter jejuni*)	Raw poultry, meat, and unpasteurized milk.	2–5 days	Diarrhea, abdominal cramping, fever, and sometimes bloody stools. Lasts 7–10 days.
Listeriosis (*Listeria monocytogenes*)	Found in soft cheese, unpasteurized milk, imported seafood products, frozen cooked crab meat, cooked shrimp, and cooked surimi (imitation shellfish). *Listeria* bacteria resist heat, salt, nitrite, and acidity better than many other microorganisms.	48–72 hours (though symptoms can strike 7–30 days after eating)	Fever, headache, nausea, and vomiting.
Perfringens food poisoning (*Clostridium perfringens*)	In most instances, caused by failure to keep food hot. A few organisms are often present after cooking and multiply to toxic levels during cool-down and storage of prepared foods. Meats and meat products are the foods most frequently implicated.	8–12 hours	Abdominal pain and diarrhea and sometimes nausea and vomiting. Symptoms last a day or less and are usually mild.
Salmonellosis (*Salmonella* bacteria)	Raw meats, poultry, milk and other dairy products, shrimp, frog legs, yeast, coconut, pasta, and chocolate are most frequently involved.	6–48 hours	Nausea, abdominal cramps, diarrhea, fever, and headache.
E. coli 0157:H7 infection (Toxin released by *Escherichia coli* 0157:H7)	Undercooked hamburger and roast beef, raw milk, raw apple cider, contaminated water and mayonnaise, and vegetables grown in cow manure.	4–9 days	Abdominal cramps, vomiting, nausea, watery diarrhea that often turns bloody, low-grade fever, and, in severe cases, kidney failure, strokes, and seizures.

continued

TABLE 11–2
continued

DISEASE AND ORGANISM THAT CAUSES IT	SOURCE OF ILLNESS	USUAL ONSET AFTER EATING	SYMPTOMS
Shigellosis (*Shigella* bacteria)	Found in milk and dairy products, poultry, and potato salad. Food becomes contaminated when a human carrier does not wash hands and then handles liquid or moist food that is not cooked thoroughly. Organisms multiply in food left at room temperature.	1–7 days	Abdominal cramps, diarrhea, fever, sometimes vomiting, and blood, pus, or mucus in stools.
Staphylococcal food poisoning (Staphylococcal enterotoxin produced by *Staphylococcus aureus* bacteria)	Toxin produced when food contaminated with the bacteria is left too long at room temperature. Meats, poultry, egg products, tuna, potato and macaroni salads, and cream-filled pastries are good environments for these bacteria to produce toxin.	30 minutes–8 hours	Diarrhea, vomiting, nausea, abdominal pain, cramps, and prostration. Lasts 24–48 hours. Rarely fatal.
Vibrio infection (*Vibrio vulnificus*)	The bacteria live in coastal waters and can infect humans either through open wounds or through consumption of contaminated seafood. The bacteria are most numerous in warm weather.	Abrupt	Chills, fever, and/or prostration. At high risk are people with liver conditions, low gastric (stomach) acid, and weakened immune systems.
PROTOZOA			
Amebiasis (*Entamoeba histolytica*)	Exist in the intestinal tract of humans and are expelled in feces. Polluted water and vegetables grown in polluted soil spread the infection.	3–10 days	Severe crampy pain, tenderness over the colon or liver, loose morning stools, recurrent diarrhea, loss of weight, fatigue and sometimes anemia.
Giardiasis (*Giardia lamblia*)	Most frequently associated with consumption of contaminated water. May be transmitted by uncooked foods that become contaminated while growing or after cooking by infected food handlers. Cool, moist conditions favor organism's survival.	1–3 days	Sudden onset of explosive watery stools, abdominal cramps, anorexia, nausea, and vomiting.
VIRUS			
(Hepatitis A virus)	Mollusks (oysters, clams, mussels, scallops, and cockles) become carriers when their beds are polluted by untreated sewage. Raw shellfish are especially potent carriers, although cooking does not always kill the virus.	3–10 days	Begins with malaise, appetite loss, nausea, vomiting, and fever. After 3–10 days, patient develops jaundice with darkened urine. Severe cases can cause liver damage and death.

SOURCES: Adapted from A. Hecht, *The Unwelcome Dinner Guest: Preventing Food-borne Illness* (Washington, D.C.: U.S. Government Printing Office, DHHS Publication No. (FDA) 91-2244; U.S. Department of Agriculture Food Safety and Inspection Service, *E. coli* 0157:H7 at a glance, *Food News for Consumers* 10 (1993): 5.

which causes food poisoning within one half hour to eight hours of eating a contaminated food. The foods typically implicated in *S. aureus* intoxication include meat and poultry products, egg products, tuna, potato and macaroni salads, and cream-filled pastries. Proper food-handling and sanitation procedures, shown in Table 11–3, help to prevent food poisoning by this bacterium as well as from *Salmonella.*

Another particularly deadly foodborne pathogen is *Clostridium botulinum,* the agent that causes the nausea, vomiting, dizziness, and muscle paralysis known as botulism. This severe illness results from eating food in which the bacterium has flourished and produced a neurotoxin. The toxin binds irreversibly to nerve endings and causes paralysis, which makes swallowing and breathing difficult. Botulism typically develops within 4 to 36 hours of eating the contaminated food. Because it can be fatal, botulism warrants immediate medical attention.

Spores of *C. botulinum* are ubiquitous, having been detected in everything from shellfish to fruits and vegetables to honey to corn syrup. But the *botulinum* bacteria only produce the deadly neurotoxin if they are in a warm, oxygen-free, low-acid environment. That's why improperly sterilized low-acid canned goods are the most common culprits in botulism. Table 11–3 outlines some safety precautions for avoiding *C. botulinum* in canned goods. Note that trendy garlic-in-oil preparations can also harbor *C. botulinum.* While manufacturers of such mixtures must add antibacterial agents to their preparations, people who make their own should be sure to store them in the refrigerator; covered, bottled garlic-in-oil left at room temperature provides the perfect warm, oxygen-free, low-acid environment for the toxin-releasing spores.[4]

Another especially virulent pathogen that is emerging as a major public health concern is *Escherichia coli* 0157:H7.* First recognized as a cause of foodborne illness in 1982, *E. coli* garnered national attention about a decade later, when it caused a major outbreak of foodborne illness in the northwest part of the United States. Undercooked, contaminated hamburgers sold at a major fast-food chain prompted the 1993 scare, which ultimately led to more than 500 reported cases of illness, some 150 hospitalizations, and three deaths. The outbreak sparked a national debate about the safety of the U.S. meat and poultry supply.[5]

Found in the intestinal tracts of mammals, *E. coli* is usually transmitted via animal feces. It appears to be proliferating in the food supply and poses special concern because it is so dangerous. Unlike most other illness-producing microorganisms, *E. coli* need not be present in large numbers to make a person sick; just a few bacteria seem to do the trick. Once ingested, the bacteria clings to the intestinal wall, where it releases an enterotoxin that causes abdominal pain, watery diarrhea that often turns bloody, and, in vulnerable groups such as children and the elderly, serious complications, including kidney failure.[6]

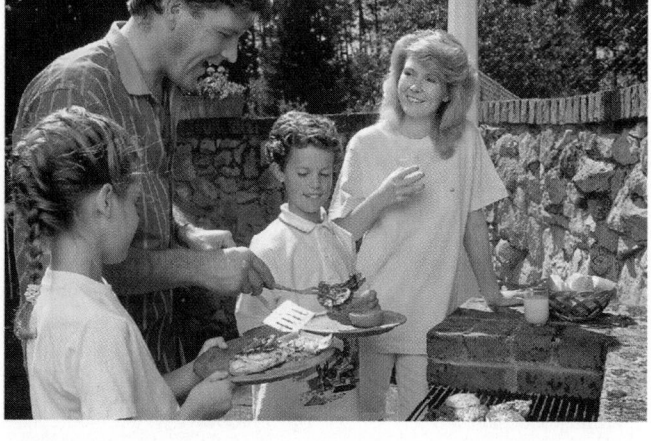

Handle raw meat and poultry with care and cook it thoroughly to destroy any bacteria present.

Honey has been found to contain dormant bacterial spores, which can awaken in the human body to produce botulism. In adults, this is not a hazard, but infants under one year of age should *never* be fed honey. Honey has been implicated in several cases of sudden infant death.

Escherichia coli 0157:H7 is a particular strain of *E. coli* bacteria. When *E. coli* is mentioned throughout the rest of the chapter, it refers to the 0157:H7 strain.

TABLE 11–3
HOW TO PREVENT FOOD POISONING

To prevent illness from *Salmonella* and *Staphylococcus aureus* varieties:

- Avoid cross-contamination: Wash hands with hot, soapy water before reusing utensils, cutting boards, or countertops that have been in contact with raw meats, poultry, or eggs.

- Thaw meats or poultry in the refrigerator, not at room temperature. If you must hasten the thawing, use cool running water or a microwave oven.

- Cook stuffing separately or stuff poultry just prior to cooking. Use a meat thermometer to avoid undercooking. Insert the thermometer between the thigh and the body of a turkey or in the thickest part of other meats, making sure the tip is not in contact with bone. Cook to the temperature shown for that meat on the thermometer.

- Refrigerate leftovers promptly and heat them thoroughly to at least 140° F before serving.

- Use clean eggs with intact shells and cook eggs before eating them (soft-boiled for 7 minutes, poached for 5, or fried for 3 minutes on each side).

- Keep susceptible foods at temperatures colder or hotter than room temperature. Keep hot foods at 140° F or more. Keep cold foods at 40° F or less.

- Mix foods with utensils, not hands; keep hands and utensils away from mouth, nose, and hair.

- Do not prepare food if you have a skin infection or infectious disease. Anyone, though, may be a carrier of bacteria and should avoid coughing or sneezing over food.

To prevent poisoning from *Clostridium botulinum*:

- Before canning anything, seek professional advice. The U.S. Department of Agriculture Extension Service provides such information free of charge.

- Throw out food with off odors. (An off odor, however, is not necessarily detectable in a food containing toxins.)

- Do not even taste food that is suspect.

- Discard food from cans that leak or bulge. Dispose of the food in a manner that will protect other people and animals from its accidental use.

To prevent illness from *Escherichia coli* 0157:H7:

- Cook all meat and poultry to 160° F—until the flesh is no longer pink and all the juices run clear.

- Avoid cross-contamination: Wash hands, utensils, cutting boards, or countertops that have come into contact with raw meat or poultry with hot, soapy water.

- Order hamburgers and other beef items well-done when eating out. Return any undercooked food.

- Do not drink raw milk or potentially contaminated water.

- Wash fruits and vegetables thoroughly before eating.

- Steer clear of fresh unpasteurized apple cider, particularly if you're serving it to a high-risk person such as a child, the elderly, or anyone with a compromised immune system. As an alternative, buy pasteurized cider or heat fresh cider to a temperature of 160° F (a slow simmer) before serving.

In general:

- Buy only those foods stored below the frost line in store freezers.

- Do not buy or use items that appear to have been opened or tampered with.

- When running errands, make the grocery store your last stop. When you get home, refrigerate perishables immediately.

- Follow label instructions for storing and preparing packaged and frozen foods.

- Immediately refrigerate cooked foods that are not to be served right away. Use shallow, not deep, containers—the foods will cool faster.

- Maintain a clean, dry kitchen that is free of flies and insects. Wash or replace dirty sponges and towels; clean up food spills and crumb-filled crevices. Use hot, soapy water for countertops as well as for dirty dishes. Hot water and soap will immobilize bacteria and wash them away; cold water will not.

Most *E. coli* outbreaks have been linked to undercooked beef, particularly hamburger. Fresh apple cider, presumably made from apples exposed to tainted animal manure, has also been implicated in some outbreaks.[7] As with all illness-causing microorganisms, the best defense against *E. coli* is careful food handling. Table 11–3 gives some tips for reducing your risk of exposure to the bacteria.

Mold is another potential microbial food contaminant. Certain molds produce poisonous compounds called **aflatoxins.** The compounds are powerful liver toxins in animals, are known to be carcinogenic in some species, and can be lethal if consumed in large doses. Aflatoxins have been found on peanuts, wheat, corn, meat pies, dry beans, and even refrigerated and frozen pastries. Molds that produce the aflatoxins typically flourish when foods such as corn and peanuts get wet and are then stored in a warm place, such as a grain silo or railroad boxcar. Controlling aflatoxins in food is difficult, but it is given high priority by the food industry and regulatory agencies.

To be sure, not all microorganisms are bad. A mold called *Penicillium roquefortii* imparts the special, pungent flavor of Roquefort cheese. Another mold strain, *P. camembertii,* lends flavor to Camembert cheese. Likewise, a strain of mold called *Bacteria aceti* causes the alcohol in wine and hard cider to turn to vinegar.[8] What's more, yogurt owes its existence to active cultures of bacteria added during processing, and some research suggests that the "good bugs" in the yogurt may help fight "bad bugs" that cause yeast infections and other ills.[9]

Natural Toxins

Most people assume that products derived from plants are safe because they are "natural." But natural food **toxicants** in plants—especially herbs—are sometimes to blame for poisonings. Even familiar foods that are generally safe sometimes harbor potential toxicants. For example, potatoes contain a substance called solanine, a powerful inhibitor of nerve impulses. The substance accumulates just beneath the vegetable's skin, usually in harmless amounts. When potatoes are exposed to light, however, they sometimes develop excess solanine and should be discarded.

When plants are transformed into powders and potions, their components become more concentrated, as do their potentially harmful effects. Nevertheless, people often assume that because they come from plants, these substances must be safe. Unlike the chemical composition of standard drugs, however, that of herbal products is not regulated by the government. This lack of safety standards for herbal pills, powders, teas, and other potions, which have become increasingly popular in recent years, ranks as a major concern among public health officials. The potential risks are amplified when an herb is mislabeled, misidentified, or mixed with another potentially toxic substance.

Consider that in 1993, several children and adults suffered life-threatening respiratory problems and liver malfunction as a result of taking a Chinese herb called Jin Bu Huan. When investigators looked into the matter, they found, among other problems, that the plant from which the product had been derived was misidentified and that the product carried false and misleading medical claims.[10] Along the same lines, in 1995, the FDA issued a warning about a product containing caffeine and a plant derivative called ma huang—an amphetamine-like substance often used in weight-loss concoctions. Together, the two substances make a deadly combination that has been linked to more than 100 injuries and several deaths.[11]

These are just a few of the herb-related problems that continue to surface. They highlight the need to be cautious about using herbs of any sort. Adults

AFLATOXIN a poisonous toxin produced by molds.

TOXICANTS poisons, that is, agents that cause physical harm or death when present in large amounts.

should not take large amounts of a particular herbal product or take more than one at a time without consulting a competent professional regarding the product's various effects. Pregnant and breastfeeding women should be especially careful because they can expose a fetus or an infant to a toxic dose. In addition, people with any type of liver disease or condition should be wary of herbal products; liver failure is one of the hallmarks of an herbal overdose, because toxins accumulate in that organ.

Like plants, other types of food, notably seafood, often harbor natural toxicants. For example, a type of fish called puffers, long considered a delicacy in Japan, serves as host to a potent poison—tetrodotoxin—which doesn't harm the fish but can be lethal to people and other animals. Tetrodotoxin, which is 275 times deadlier than cyanide, works by blocking nerve impulses; over a period of several hours, it will eventually close down a person's entire nervous system. The toxin is so deadly that sale of puffers is illegal in the United States.[13]

Puffer poisoning is just one example of a foodborne disease traced to eating a toxic sea creature. Others also exist. For instance, scombroid fish poisoning—which involves the scombroid fish family, including tuna, bonito, mackerel, and skipjack—results from ingesting a toxin produced by the action of bacteria on the dark meat in the fish. Fish contaminated with the scombroid toxin have a honeycombed look and a sharp, peppery taste. Another type, called ciguatera fish poisoning, results from eating certain fish that inhabit warm waters near coral reefs: grouper, snapper, amberjack, and barracuda. The poisoning brings about symptoms such as nausea, diarrhea, headache, face pain, and nerve problems. These fish are thought to ingest the toxin as a result of eating marine plants that contain it.

Finally, paralytic shellfish poisoning can occur after eating mollusks (clams, mussels, oysters, and scallops) contaminated with marine algae that produce a neurotoxin. The mollusks themselves don't become ill, but people eating them do, experiencing such symptoms as nausea, vomiting, cramps, and muscle weakness. In each of these cases, the toxin is not destroyed by heat. Fish can also harbor viruses, including hepatitis viruses, worms, and other parasites. This is why it is especially important to buy seafood from reputable vendors and to handle it with care.

Numerous herbs have been implicated in liver failure and other health problems. Here are just a few:[12]

chaparral
Jin Bu Huan
ma huang
germander
comfrey
mistletoe
skullcap
margosa oil
maté tea
Gordolobo yerba tea
pennyroyal (squawmint) oil

If you have a question about ciguatera fish poisoning, call the University of Miami Ciguatera Hot Line: 305-361-4619.

If you have a question about seafood safety, call the FDA's Seafood Hotline: 1-800-332-4010.

Safe Food Storage and Preparation

Commercially prepared, canned, or packaged food is usually free of harmful microbial agents when it leaves its manufacturer. When a batch of food *is* contaminated, batch numbering ensures that it can be recalled quickly and the public can be forewarned. When it comes to tampering, the chances are slim that this would occur in a grocery store food. To protect against this unlikely event, however, carefully inspect the seals and wrappers of packages. Jars should be firmly sealed (many have safety buttons—areas of the lid designed to pop up once opened). Packages should be free of holes or tears. A broken seal or mangled package is not providing protection against microorganisms or other contaminants. Likewise, canned goods should be free of dents and cracks or bulges, which can indicate contamination with *Clostridium botulinum*.

As Table 11–4 shows, most cases of food poisoning occur in the home or the restaurant and are caused by improper storage or handling. Those that arise from kitchen mistakes can be avoided by doing three simple things: keep cold food cold; keep your hands, the utensils, and the kitchen clean; and keep hot food hot. Most bacteria flourish in warm environments, whereas heat kills them and chilly temperatures halt their growth. That's why you can keep bacteria in check by paying attention to proper storage and cooking temperatures.

The first step, keeping cold food cold, starts when you leave the grocery store. If you are running errands in a car, shop last so that the groceries do not stay in the car too long, especially in hot weather. Immediately upon arrival at home, pack foods into a refrigerator set at 40 degrees Fahrenheit or a freezer kept at 0 degrees Fahrenheit, and be sure not to leave them in the refrigerator or freezer too long (see Table 11–5).

Place packages of raw meat, poultry, or fish on a plate before refrigerating or store in plastic refrigerator storage containers to prevent bacteria-containing juices from dripping onto other foods. Thaw frozen food in the refrigerator or microwave oven—not on the kitchen counter. Since bacteria can multiply at room temperature, they can thrive in the relatively warm, exterior of a food before the interior has thawed.

Along with keeping foods properly chilled, keeping the kitchen clean prevents contamination of otherwise wholesome foods. Before you handle food, wash your hands in warm, soapy water. In addition, be sure to wash your hands after touching meat, poultry, or fish to prevent the spread of any bacteria that your hands have picked up. Likewise, keep countertops and all kitchen equipment clean with soap and warm water. Because bacteria love to nestle down in the fibers of kitchen cloths, sponges, and wooden cutting boards, take particular care to keep such items clean. Sterilize wet sponges and cloths in the microwave oven—after using, heat them on "high" until they are steamy hot. Or launder them with bleach or sponge bleach solution over a cutting board to sanitize the two items at once. In addition, wash wooden and plastic cutting boards in the dishwasher if possible; the hot temperatures in the dishwasher are especially effective at killing bacteria.

Keeping hot food hot requires cooking food thoroughly to ensure that the heat destroys any bacteria present. See Figure 11–1 on page 426 for proper cooking temperatures. After cooking, foods must be kept hot until serving to prevent bacterial growth. Never leave perishable food at room

| TABLE 11–4 |
| **MAJOR FACTORS THAT CONTRIBUTE TO FOOD POISONING** |

1. Improper cooling
2. Lapse of 12 hours or more between preparation and eating
3. Infected person touching food
4. Mixing contaminated food or ingredient into dish that received no further cooking
5. Inadequate cooking, canning, or heat processing
6. Failure to hold hot food at high temperature
7. Inadequate reheating of food
8. Obtaining food from unsafe source
9. Cross-contamination
10. Improper cleaning of equipment or utensils

SOURCE: Adapted from R. B. Gravani and D. L. Scott, *Today's Food Safety Issues* (Ithaca, NY: Cornell University Institute of Food Science, 1995), p. 7, presented at workshop of the National Foundation for Integrated Pest Management Education and the International Food Information Council, 1995.

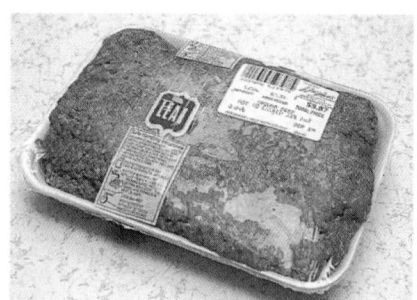

Never thaw food on a kitchen counter. Bacteria can flourish at room temperature.

TABLE 11–5
THE BIG CHILL: STORING FOODS SAFELY

These recommended time limits for refrigeration will help keep foods from spoiling or harboring high levels of bacteria. Foods stored in the freezer can last indefinitely. However, since the food's quality will suffer over time, the limits given here help to ensure that the food will maintain top quality in the freezer.

PRODUCT	REFRIGERATOR (40° F)	FREEZER (0° F)	PRODUCT	REFRIGERATOR (40°F)	FREEZER (40°F)
EGGS			**BACON & SAUSAGE**		
Fresh, in shell	3 weeks	Don't freeze	Bacon	7 days	1 month
Raw yolks, whites	2–4 days	1 year	Sausage, raw from pork,		
Hardcooked	1 week	Don't freeze well	beef, turkey	1–2 days	1–2 months
			Smoked breakfast links, patties	7 days	1–2 months
Liquid pasteurized eggs or			Hard sausage—pepperoni,		
egg substitutes, opened	3 days	Don't freeze	jerky sticks	2–3 weeks	1–2 months
Unopened	10 days	1 year	**HAM, CORNED BEEF**		
MAYONNAISE, COMMERCIAL			Corned beef, in pouch with		Drained,
Refrigerate after opening	2 months	Don't freeze	pickling juices	5–7 days	wrapped 1 month
TV DINNERS, FROZEN CASSEROLES			Ham, canned		
Keep frozen until ready to serve		3–4 months	Label says keep refrigerated	6–9 months	Don't freeze
			Ham, fully cooked—whole	7 days	1–2 months
DELI & VACUUM-PACKED PRODUCTS			Ham, fully cooked—half	3–5 days	1–2 months
Store-prepared (or homemade) egg, chicken, tuna, ham, macaroni salads	3–5 days		Ham, fully cooked—slices	3–4 days	1–2 months
			FRESH MEAT		
Pre-stuffed pork & lamb chops, chicken breasts stuffed with dressing	1 day	These products don't freeze well.	Steaks, beef	3–5 days	6–12 months
			Chops, pork	3–5 days	4–6 months
			Chops, lamb	3–5 days	6–9 months
Store-cooked convenience meals	1–2 days		Roasts, beef	3–5 days	6–12 months
			Roasts, lamb	3–5 days	6–9 months
Commercial brand vacuum-packed dinners with USDA seal	2 weeks, unopened		Roasts, pork & veal	3–5 days	4–6 months
			Variety meats—tongue, brain, kidneys, liver, heart, chitterlings	1–2 days	3–4 months
SOUPS & STEWS			**MEAT LEFTOVERS**		
Vegetable or meat-added	3–4 days	2–3 months	Cooked meat and meat dishes	3–4 days	2–3 months
HAMBURGER, GROUND & STEW MEATS			Gravy and meat broth	1–2 days	2–3 months
Hamburger & stew meats	1–2 days	3–4 months	**FRESH POULTRY**		
Ground turkey, veal, pork, lamb, & mixtures of them	1–2 days	3–4 months	Chicken or turkey, whole	1–2 days	1 year
			Chicken or turkey pieces	1–2 days	9 months
			Giblets	1–2 days	3–4 months
HOT DOGS & LUNCH MEATS			**POULTRY LEFTOVERS**		
Hot dogs, opened package	1 week	In freezer wrap, 1–2 months	Fried chicken	3–4 days	4 months
Unopened package	2 weeks		Cooked poultry dishes	3–4 days	4–6 months
			Pieces, plain	3–4 days	4 months
Lunch meats, opened	3–5 days		Pieces covered with broth, gravy	1–2 days	6 months
Unopened	2 weeks		Chicken nuggets, patties	1–2 days	1–3 months

SOURCE: Adapted from U.S. Department of Agriculture, Food Safety and Inspection Service, *A Quick Consumer Guide to Safe Food Handling* (Washington, D.C.: U.S. Government Printing Office), Home and Garden Bulletin No. 248.

temperature for more than two hours. Before refrigerating large quantities of hot foods, such as a pot of chili or a large casserole, divide it up and place it in shallow containers to allow easy cooling. Otherwise the inside of the pot may stay warm for a dangerously long time, even in the refrigerator.

Meat, poultry, and fish require special handling because they often harbor high levels of bacteria. In addition, they provide a moist, nutritious environment—just right for microbial growth. Wash areas that come into contact with such foods after handling to prevent **cross-contamination.** For instance, after marinating raw meat in a dish, don't put the meat back in the same dish after cooking it, and don't use the marinade unless it has been cooked thoroughly. Wash the dish in hot, soapy water before reusing it, or the bacteria inevitably left in the dish from the raw meat can contaminate and grow in the cooked product or other food—a classic example of cross-contamination. Similarly, wash a cutting board (and your hands) after, say, skinning chicken on it. If you don't, and you chop raw vegetables for a salad on the contaminated board, the vegetables could pick up the bacteria the poultry left behind; since the salad won't be heated, the bacteria won't be killed.

Especially susceptible to bacterial contamination is ground meat. Consider that steaks and roasts are not as risky because bacteria usually settle on the outside of the cuts and are easily destroyed when the outside is heated. But when meat is ground, the bacteria are spread throughout, so more thorough cooking is needed to kill the bacteria in the middle of, say, hamburger patties or meat loaf. To decrease your risk of eating contaminated ground beef, order burgers well done and cook them so that the juices run clear and not a trace of pink is left on the inside. For a meat loaf, use a thermometer to test the internal temperature. Be especially careful when cooking ground meat in the microwave oven, because sometimes that appliance cooks foods unevenly if the foods are not handled properly. The Consumer Tips feature offers advice on the safe use of a microwave oven.

CROSS-CONTAMINATION the inadvertent transfer of bacteria from one food to another that occurs, for instance, by chopping vegetables on the same cutting board used to skin poultry.

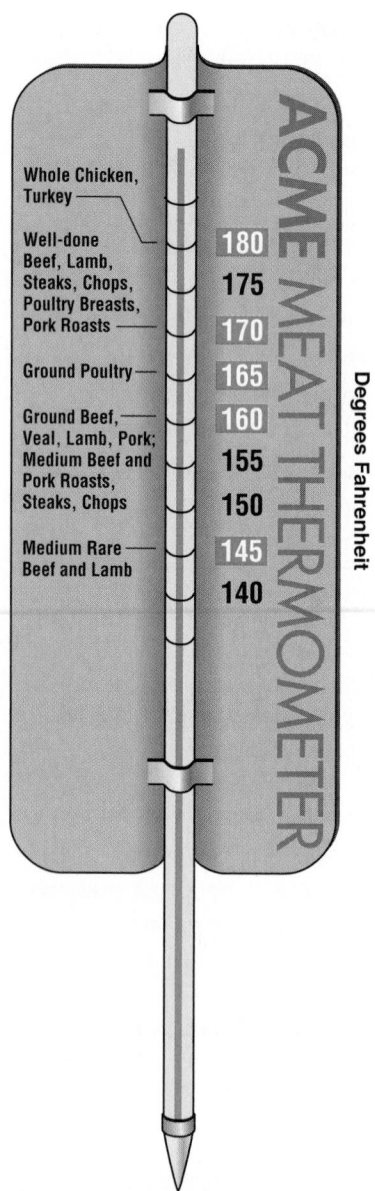

FIGURE 11–1
SAFE INTERNAL TEMPERATURES FOR MEAT AND POULTRY

Never work with raw meat or poultry on the same surface that you use for other foods without thoroughly cleaning the surface after you've finished. Otherwise, bacteria that the meat or poultry left behind can contaminate other foods placed on the cutting board.

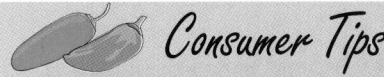 *Consumer Tips*

Microwaving the Safe Way

Some 75 percent of American kitchens have microwave ovens used for thawing, cooking, and reheating foods quickly. Nevertheless, many consumers are not aware of certain safety measures that should be taken when using them to lower the risk of foodborne illness or other health problems. The following tips will help to ensure that you microwave safely.[14]

- Prevent "cold spots" by arranging portions of meat or poultry evenly in a wide, shallow dish. After cooking, check the items' temperature in several places using a probe or meat thermometer. Meat should be at least 160 degrees Fahrenheit; poultry should reach 180 degrees Fahrenheit.

- Cut large pieces of meat or poultry into smaller portions when possible to ensure that all segments are heated thoroughly.

- Cook food that has been thawed in the microwave; don't refreeze it. Unlike defrosting meat or poultry in the refrigerator, thawing in the microwave subjects food to low cooking temperatures in which bacteria can multiply. Refreezing will prevent additional growth, but it won't kill the bacteria that are already present.

- Remember to remove casseroles and other items put in the microwave to thaw. According to the U.S. Department of Agriculture, consumers often forget to

do this. If you accidentally do leave a product in the oven for more than two hours, throw it away.

- Don't partially cook a food ahead of time to speed microwave heating later. Partially cooking food may not generate enough heat to kill any bacteria present; the same goes for microwaving the product later.

- Don't put brown paper bags or recycled paper towels in the microwave. While some recipes suggest microwaving turkeys or ham in those materials to promote tenderness, the paper could start a fire or release dangerous chemicals into the food.

- Cook in dishes that are designed specifically for use in microwave ovens. Margarine tubs or plastic containers made for storing food may melt upon coming into contact with hot foods. In addition, they may leach dangerous chemicals into food during cooking.

- Allow foods to stand for the recommended period of time after cooking to ensure heating through and through. Foods keep cooking even after the microwave is turned off.

- Heat baby bottles on a stove rather than in the microwave. Liquids held in bottles heated in the microwave can be 20 degrees higher than the outside of the bottle. Thus, while the bottle may feel warm to the touch, the formula inside may be hot enough to scald an infant's mouth.

When it comes to picnics, choose foods that last without refrigeration, such as fresh fruits and vegetables, breads and crackers, and canned spreads and cheeses that can be opened and used on the spot. Aged cheeses, such as cheddar and Swiss, do well for an hour or two, but they should be kept in an ice chest for longer periods. Contrary to popular belief, salads made with mayonnaise pose no greater risk than foods prepared with any other type of dressing. Whether a dish contains mayonnaise or not, chill it well before, during, and after the picnic. As for burgers, chicken breasts, and other foods intended for grilling, don't partially cook them ahead of time and then throw them on the fire later. Partial cooking may not kill all the bacteria present, and because half-cooked items may not be heated thoroughly later, chances of bacterial contamination run high. Partial cooking is safe only if you take, say, a burger directly from the microwave oven to place on the grill.[15]

Seafood also should be handled with care, especially fish intended to be eaten raw or only lightly steamed. The foodborne infections that lurk in normal-appearing seafood can be much worse than those of spoilage: worms, parasites, severe viral intestinal disorders, and hepatitis (a prolonged illness of months' or years' duration that greatly increases the risk of liver cancer later). Raw fish dishes such as sushi and sashimi are safe for most healthy people to eat if they are prepared with fresh fish that has been commercially frozen at temperatures lower than most home freezers can attain; freezing kills any parasites that might be present. However, eating raw or undercooked oysters, clams, mussels, and whole scallops is especially risky. Such types of seafood sometimes carry a strain of bacteria called *Vibrios* that can multiply even during refrigeration. While these bacteria are destroyed by thorough cooking, they can thrive in raw shellfish and cause serious illness. In fact, sometimes the bacteria cause a deadly blood poisoning that can kill a person within a day or two.[16] Because of the risk of contamination, the hazards of eating raw or undercooked seafood need to be weighed carefully, especially by vulnerable people, including those with liver disease, diabetes, gastrointestinal disorders, HIV infection, and other diseases that may compromise the body's ability to defend itself against food poisoning. Table 11–6 gives some tips for ensuring a safe catch by carefully buying, storing, and cooking seafood.

In general, remember that fresh food smells fresh. Any food that carries an off odor should not be eaten because the smell is probably the result of bacterial wastes and indicates that the number of bacteria in the food is dangerous. To be sure, not all types of food poisoning are detectable by odor, but if a food smells bad, chances are high that it is spoiled. Refer to Table 11–3 for recommendations for preventing foodborne illness. See also the Kitchen Safety Scorecard to help you rate your kitchen for safety.

Safe Handling Instructions

THIS PRODUCT WAS PREPARED FROM INSPECTED AND PASSED MEAT AND/OR POULTRY. SOME FOOD PRODUCTS MAY CONTAIN BACTERIA THAT CAN CAUSE ILLNESS IF THE PRODUCT IS MISHANDLED OR COOKED IMPROPERLY. FOR YOUR PROTECTION, FOLLOW THESE SAFE HANDLING INSTRUCTIONS.

KEEP REFRIGERATED OR FROZEN. THAW IN REFRIGERATOR OR MICROWAVE.

KEEP RAW MEAT AND POULTRY SEPARATE FROM OTHER FOODS. WASH WORKING SURFACES (INCLUDING CUTTING BOARDS), UTENSILS, AND HANDS AFTER TOUCHING RAW MEAT OR POULTRY.

COOK THOROUGHLY.

KEEP HOT FOODS HOT. REFRIGERATE LEFTOVERS IMMEDIATELY OR DISCARD.

The U.S. Department of Agriculture requires that all fresh meat and poultry products carry this label as a reminder to handle the products carefully.

TABLE 11–6
ENSURING A SAFE CATCH: SEAFOOD SAFETY TIPS

BUYING

- Choose fresh seafood that smells like a "fresh ocean breeze," not unpleasantly "fishy."

- Choose fresh fish steaks and fillets that are moist, with no drying or browning around the edges. The eyes of fresh whole fish should be bright and clear, not cloudy or sunken. Scales should not be "slimy" and should cling tightly to the skin. Gills should be bright pink or red.

- Buy only mollusks in the shell that are alive. When a clam, oyster, mussel, or scallop is alive, its shells will be tightly closed or will close when tapped lightly or iced. To test for freshness, hold the shell between your thumb and forefinger and press as though sliding the two parts of the shell across each other. If the shells move, the shellfish is not fresh.

- Buy seafood only from reputable dealers. You can't know what you're buying from the back of a pickup truck. It may not have undergone FDA or state inspection.

- Cook fish within two days of purchase.

STORING

- Keep fresh fish in the coldest part of your refrigerator—usually under the freezer or in the meat drawer—until ready to cook and serve.

- Store fresh fish in your refrigerator in the same wrapper it had in the store.

- Store live mollusks in your refrigerator in containers covered loosely with a clean, damp cloth. Do not store live shellfish in airtight containers or in water.

- Store canned fish in a clean, covered glass or plastic container in the refrigerator after opening.

- Refrigerate smoked, pickled, vacuum-packed, and modified-atmosphere-packed fish products.

- Keep cooked and raw seafood separate. It's not safe to put cooked seafood back in the original container used for raw seafood or to store raw and cooked seafood together.

COOKING

- For fin fish (baked, broiled, poached, fried, or stewed): allow 10 minutes cooking time for each inch of thickness. Turn the fish over halfway through the cooking time unless it is less than a half inch thick. Add 5 minutes to the total cooking time if the fish is wrapped in foil or cooked in a sauce. Properly cooked fish will flake easily with a fork and should be opaque and firm but not translucent.

- For molluscan shellfish: Boiled—shells will open during boiling. After shells open, boiling should continue 3 to 5 more minutes. Steamed—cook 4 to 9 minutes from the start of steaming.

- Use small pots to boil or steam shellfish. If too many shells are cooking in the same pot, those in the middle might not get thoroughly cooked. Discard any clams, mussels, or oysters that do not open during cooking. Closed shells indicate that they may be undercooked.

- Shucked oysters: Boil or simmer for at least 3 minutes. Fry in oil for at least 10 minutes at 375° F. Bake for at least 10 minutes at 450° F.

SOURCE: Adapted from Department of Health and Human Services, Public Health Service, U.S. Food and Drug Administration, *Getting Hooked on Seafood Safety*, DHHS Publication No. (FDA) 93-2266, May 1993.

KITCHEN SAFETY SCORECARD

 Improper storage of food not only increases the risk of food poisoning but also almost always results in a loss of nutrients and good taste. The following quiz is designed to find out how your kitchen storage savvy rates. To take the quiz, answer whether each statement describes your kitchen, always, sometimes, or never. Then read the comments that follow for additional tips. Score each statement as follows:

Always: 2 points; Sometimes: 1 point; Never: 0 points

1. Highly perishable foods like milk are stored in the refrigerator, not in the refrigerator door.

2. Milk is kept in opaque, closed containers. Orange juice is kept tightly covered.

3. Eggs are stored in their original carton.

4. Fresh produce—especially leafy greens—is in plastic bags or in the vegetable bin.

5. Whole-wheat flour and wheat germ are stored in the refrigerator.

6. Refrigerated leftovers and frozen foods are marked to indicate their contents and the date they were stored.

7. Food is frozen in small containers.

8. Dented cans are checked for seam damage or leaks.

9. Package and can labels are checked for storage directions before being stored.

10. Food is stored in cabinets, not under the sink.

11. Food is stored in cabinets away from the stove.

12. Refrigerator and freezer door seals are periodically cleaned and checked.

Read the following to find out how each of the previous statements relates to kitchen safety:

1. The refrigerator door does not stay as cold as the rest of the refrigerator, so highly perishable foods—especially milk—should not be stored there. Use the door for storing condiments like catsup and mayonnaise.

2. Milk is a good source of riboflavin, but much is lost if milk is exposed to light. Orange juice loses vitamin C upon exposure to air, so use closed containers, or prepare only as much juice as needed.

3. Eggs stay fresh longest when stored large end up in the carton in which they are sold. Use refrigerated eggs within a week for best flavor and cooking quality, although they're safe to eat for three weeks. Eggs that

have cracked shells should be thrown out—they may be contaminated with *Salmonella* bacteria.

4. Most vegetables keep best when stored in the crisper drawer or in plastic bags on the lower shelf of the refrigerator. Either way helps to keep in moisture, which prevents wilting.

5. Most flours and grains can be kept at room temperature but should be tightly covered to prevent insect infestation. Whole grains, however, keep better in the refrigerator. Because of their higher fat content, they are more susceptible to rancidity and insect infestation. Wheat germ should always be refrigerated after opening.

6. Marking the contents of refrigerated and frozen foods eliminates the guessing game. Dating foods is also essential, so foods can be rotated—oldest foods can be used first.

7. The faster foods are cooled, the less time there is for bacteria to grow. Avoid putting hot foods into large containers. The center may be dangerously warm for too long.

8. Buying dented cans is okay, but only if they are free of seam damage and leaks. Check again just before opening. A sticky ring left on the shelf under the can may be an indication of leakage.

9. Some dry packaged foods and canned foods require refrigeration once they are opened; some even before they are opened. Check labels for storage information.

10. Storing food under the sink is potentially dangerous for three reasons. First, cleaning products could leak and soak through cardboard boxes or bags. Second, leaking pipes can rust cans and damage boxes. Finally, openings in the walls for pipes give insects and rodents easy access.

11. Cabinets over the stove get hot. Most foods won't last long under such conditions.

12. Door gaskets should be periodically washed to ensure the cold is sealed in. As a test, close a dollar bill in the door. If the seal is tight, you shouldn't be able to pull it out.

Scoring:
22–24 Excellent food storage savvy.
18–21 Pretty good habits, but try to be more consistent.
13–17 Not so good. Better read the next section carefully.
0–12 Poor storage IQ. Tape a copy of this quiz to the refrigerator as a reminder.

SOURCE: Adapted from S. M. Smith, How to score a kitchen, *Environmental Nutrition* 11 (1988): 1–2. Used with permission.

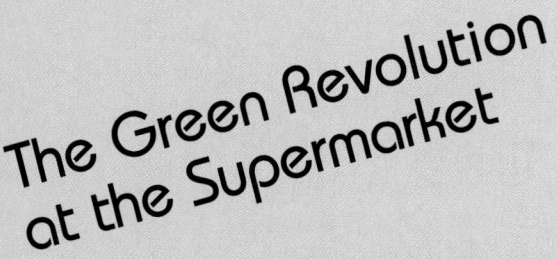

The Green Revolution at the Supermarket

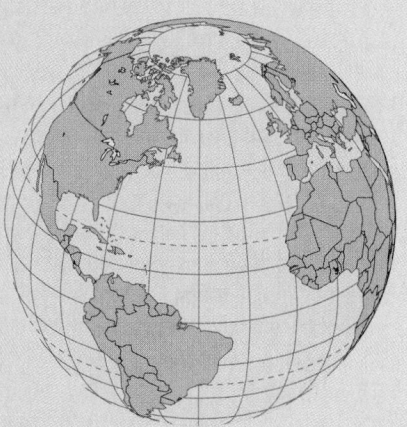

Before her death in 1978, famed anthropologist Margaret Mead wrote: "We are living beyond our means. As a people we have developed a lifestyle that is draining the earth of its priceless and irreplaceable resources without regard for the future of our children and people all around the world."

Mead's was a vision ahead of its time. At the same time that Mead offered her forecast, in fact, one social critic dubbed the era the "Throwaway Age." His description is fitting, given that the United States ranks as the world's top generator of garbage—pitching some 1,400 pounds of waste per person each year, an amount that has been rising since 1960.[17]

Fortunately, news of overflowing landfills, polluted waterways, and environmental disasters such as oil spills has begun to stir a growing environmental consciousness throughout mainstream America. Hundreds of products touted with such claims as "degradable," "environmentally friendly," "recycled," and "safe for the environment" have been introduced into supermarkets since the beginning of this decade, creating a "green revolution" in the grocery store.

On the surface, such efforts on the part of manufacturers are definitely a move in the right direction. Nevertheless, questions have been raised about the reliability of environmental claims used on grocery store items. Since the terms manufacturers use to sell "green" products have not been legally defined, they can sometimes mislead conservation-minded consumers. One manufacturer of garbage bags was sued by a group of state attorneys general for selling an expensive version of bags boasted as being "biodegradable." Although the term suggested that the bags would break down fairly rapidly in garbage heaps, the bags turned out to be photodegradable. In other words, they would degrade when exposed to sunlight but not in the middle of a landfill, making them no better from an environmental standpoint than regular trash bags.[18] The case illustrates why some experts contend that the widely used claims "biodegradable," "photodegradable," and "degradable" are sometimes meaningless in practical terms.

Although virtually everything breaks down eventually upon exposure to air and water, most of our trash ends up buried amid a heap of rubbish in a landfill, where air and moisture can barely penetrate. As a result, even substances that would otherwise degrade rapidly remain intact for years. Consider that archaeologists digging in landfills for the University of Arizona's Garbage Project discovered perfectly legible newspapers, which tend to be highly degradable in theory, dated as far back as 1952.[19]

The claim that a product is made with recycled paper or other materials can also be confusing in some instances. Unless the package spells out what percentage of the item is truly recycled, manufacturers may use as little or as much of the recycled material as they like. A box made with recycled cardboard, for example, can consist of anywhere from one percent to 50 percent to 100 percent recycled material. What's more, much of the "recycled" paper on the market is made of manufacturing waste, such as paper scraps left after envelopes are cut from paper or from punching holes out of notebook paper. Much of this "recycled" paper has always been used. Most "recycled" paper contains only about 10 percent post-consumer waste—that is, paper made from recycled consumer products such as newspaper.[20]

Another point of discrepancy is the oft-used claim that a product is "recyclable." Granted, recycling ranks as an excellent means of helping to preserve our resources. The problem is that many areas of the country lack facilities to recycle certain products, particularly those made of plastic. Hence, experts question whether it's fair to tout them as "recyclable" in the first place.

In addition, products advertised as "safe for the environment," "environmentally friendly," or "eco-safe," without any explanation as to why they are superior, may be nothing more than hype. Those terms, like the others, have not been defined legally.

Finally, "ozone friendly" or "no CFCs" label claims can be misleading. It's true that most aerosol sprays used to contain substances called **chlorofluorocarbons (CFCs),** which appear to play a role in destroying the protective layer of ozone that surrounds the earth and helps filter out cancer-causing rays from the sun. Still, since 1978, CFCs have been virtually eliminated from aerosol sprays sold in the United States. These and other ozone-depleting substances are being phased out gradually. What it all boils down to is that "ozone friendly" or "CFC-free" products are not necessarily any better than similar items on the market.[22]

Beyond the issue of environmental claims is the question of whether recycling, as many consumers believe, is the solution to the garbage problem. It can certainly help, but most experts say the best option is **source reduction**—that is, reducing waste by using fewer materials to begin with, thereby eliminating the use of virgin materials, the need for disposal, and the energy and pollution generated by recycling. Given that about a third of the trash discarded by Americans comes from packaging (much of it for food), practicing source reduction at the supermarket, along with recycling whenever possible, can make a significant impact on the environment. Consider that although some 80 percent of garbage is recyclable, the amount of trash that ends up in landfills increases yearly in the United States—despite stepped-up efforts to encourage source reduction and recycling.[23]

The following tips can help you to practice source reduction and recycling at the supermarket or in the kitchen.

- Buy foods in bulk or in economy-size packages. The more food that fits into a single container, the better.
- Look for products sold in refillable bottles that can be washed and used again or at least be recycled. It takes much less energy to wash out an old bottle than to recycle it or make a new one from scratch. A 12-ounce refillable glass bottle, for example, requires 75 percent less energy per use than a recycled aluminum can or glass bottle and as much as 90 percent less energy than a can or bottle used once and then tossed into the trash.[24]
- Find another use for glass jars or plastic containers. Use empty margarine tubs to store leftovers, for example.

Canada has an eco-labeling program for paper. To qualify, at least half of the materials in the paper must be recycled, and 10 percent of that must be post-consumer recycled materials.[21]

CHLOROFLUOROCARBONS (CFCs) chemicals once used in aerosol sprays and other products and that seem to contribute to the destruction of the earth's ozone layer.

SOURCE REDUCTION (also called precycling) reducing waste by using fewer materials to begin with.

The recycling symbol

- Purchase items made from recycled materials when possible. Check the labels or examine the box. Most cereal boxes that are gray inside are made from 100 percent recycled cardboard.
- Carry your groceries home in a reusable bag, not paper or plastic.
- Store food in reusable containers instead of wrapping it in aluminum foil or plastic wrap.
- Wipe spills with rags that can be washed and reused instead of using paper towels all the time. Then wash and use the rags again.
- Pack your sandwich in a plastic container that can be washed and reused rather than in a plastic bag that will wind up in the garbage.
- Call your local recycling center to find out where you can recycle. Look for it in the Yellow Pages, or call 1-800-CALLEDF, the Environmental Defense Fund, and ask them to help you find your nearest center.
- Remember your power as a consumer. With every purchase, you cast a vote to the manufacturer about your preferences. If no one buys heavily packaged products, companies will stop making them.

Along with conserving material resources, ecology-minded consumers can save energy (and money) by using certain cooking techniques.[25]

- Use the smallest oven possible when you cook. The larger the oven, the more energy needed to heat it.
- Choose the smallest pan needed to cook a food. Smaller pans use less energy.
- Match pan size to the burner size on electric stove tops. Placing a 6-inch pan on an 8-inch burner will waste more than 40 percent of the heat generated by the burner.
- Keep the grease-catching metal pan underneath the burners clean and shiny. Blackened burner pans absorb heat rather than reflect it, thereby reducing the burner's ability to heat efficiently.
- Cover pans with lids whenever possible. Consider that it takes about three times as much energy to cook a pot of spaghetti that's uncovered than one that's covered.
- Turn off electric burners just before heating is completed. The burner will keep putting out heat for a short time after it's shut off.
- Call your gas company if your gas stove's flames are not blue. A yellow flame means the gas might not be burning efficiently.
- Don't preheat your oven. Research indicates that there is little difference in the quality of products cooked in preheated versus non-preheated ovens, making preheating an unnecessary waste of energy.[26]
- Try not to peek into the oven. Each time you open the oven door, heat escapes and considerable energy is wasted. Check on foods by looking through the oven window instead.
- Cook foods in glass or ceramic pans in ovens. That will allow you to turn down the oven temperature about 25 degrees Fahrenheit without prolonging cooking time.
- Keep the inside surfaces of microwave ovens clean to keep the appliance working efficiently.

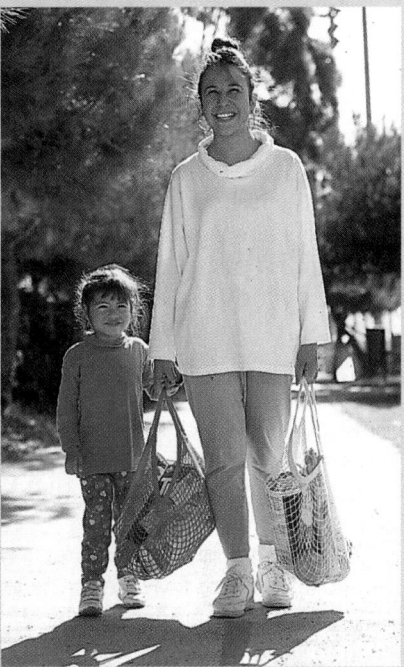

Carry groceries home in reusable bags to conserve resources.

Pesticides and Other Chemical Contaminants

Food producers and food processors exert major efforts to maintain a safe food supply. Some risk of consuming undesirable substances, or **contaminants,** however, is unavoidable. Our industrial society's reliance on chemical processes means that foods may become contaminated by a variety of chemicals introduced into the environment. In addition, agricultural techniques that necessitate the use of pesticides impact the food supply. The following section examines some of the major chemical players in the food supply and looks at some ways that scientists hope to reduce them.

CONTAMINANTS potentially dangerous substances, such as lead, that can accidentally get into foods.

Chemical Agents

Some of the problem industrial chemicals prevalent in the environment and food supply include **organic halogens,** such as polychlorinated biphenyl (PCB) and polybrominated biphenyl (PBB), and **heavy metals,** such as lead and mercury.

Fortunately, episodes of direct, excessive chemical contamination such as chemical spills are few and far between. But when a particular area *does* suddenly become contaminated, the effects can be far-reaching. In 1973, for example, half a ton of PBB was accidentally mixed into some livestock feed that was distributed throughout the state of Michigan. Millions of animals ingested excess PBB, and so did the people who ate the beef that came from the tainted livestock. Dairy farmers recognized the seriousness of the accident when their cows began going dry, aborting their calves, and developing abnormal growths on their hooves. More than 30,000 cattle, sheep, and swine and more than a million chickens died as a result of PBB. Unfortunately, the problem didn't stop with the animals. By 1982, an estimated 97 percent of Michigan's residents had been contaminated with PBB, with side effects that included nervous system aberrations and alterations in the liver and immune systems.[27]

The Michigan incident is just one example of chemical contamination. The number of contaminants we could discuss and the amount of information available about them are far beyond our scope. Still, we illustrate principles that apply to all contaminants by giving details about just a few. A list of several chemical contaminants of particular concern in foods is presented in Table 11–7.

When considering the risks of chemical contamination, remember that even though a substance is toxic, the hazard it poses tends to be small because chemical levels are usually carefully controlled. When a chemical spill or other accident occurs, the risk can suddenly soar. That's why scientists differentiate between **toxicity** (a property of all substances) and **hazard** (the likelihood of a substance's actually causing harm). All substances are potentially toxic, but they are hazardous only if consumed in large enough quantities. In other words, the dose makes the poison. Thus, a chemical that is present in foods in minuscule amounts does not pose a significant hazard until for some reason it becomes concentrated in the food in excess, toxic amounts.

Most experts agree that chemicals in foods pose a small hazard; the chief concern is accidental gross contamination. In some instances, however, chemical contamination can be subtle and insidious. The problem of chronic low-level lead poisoning is a prime example. In the United States, lead poisoning ranks as

ORGANIC HALOGENS compounds that contain one or more of a class of atoms called halogens, including fluorine, chlorine, iodine, or bromine.

HEAVY METALS any of a number of mineral ions, such as mercury and lead, so named because of their relatively high atomic weight. Many heavy metals are poisonous.

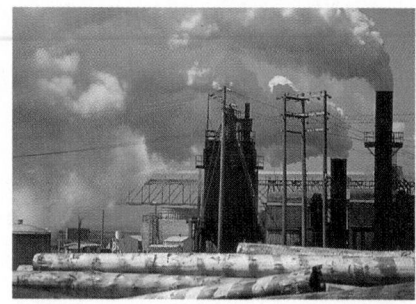

Many of the chemicals that contaminate foods are the waste products of industry.

TOXICITY the ability of a substance to harm living organisms. All substances are toxic if present in high enough concentrations.

HAZARD state of danger; used to refer to any circumstance in which harm is possible.

TABLE 11–7
EXAMPLES OF CONTAMINANTS IN FOODS

NAME AND DESCRIPTION	SOURCES	TOXIC EFFECTS	TYPICAL ROUTE TO FOOD CHAIN
Cadmium (heavy metal)	Used in industrial processes, including electroplating, plastics, batteries, alloys, pigments, smelters, and burning fuels; present in cigarette smoke.	No immediately detectable symptoms; slowly and irreversibly damages kidneys and liver.	Enters air in smokestack emissions, settles on ground and is absorbed into plants, consumed by farm animals, and eaten in meat and produce by people. Sewage sludge and fertilizers leave large amounts in the soil; runoff contaminates shellfish.
Lead (heavy metal)	Lead crystal, improperly manufactured and old ceramic ware, paint, old plumbing, and leaded gasoline.	Displaces calcium, iron, zinc, and other minerals from their sites of action in the nervous system, bone marrow, kidneys, and liver, causing failure to function; harms fetuses, infants, and children, who easily absorb and retain lead; causes breakage of red blood cells (anemia) and interferes with the immune response.	Air pollution, leaded gasoline, water pipes, improperly manufactured and old ceramic ware, and lead crystal.
Mercury (heavy metal)	Widely dispersed in gases from the earth's crust; local high concentrations from industry, electrical equipment, paints, and agriculture.	Poisons the nervous system, especially in fetuses.	Inorganic mercury released into waterways by industry and acid rain is converted to methylmercury by bacteria and ingested by fish (tuna, swordfish, and others).
Polychlorinated biphenyl (PCB) (organic compound)	No natural source; produced for use in electrical equipment.	Causes long-lasting skin eruptions, eye irritation, growth retardation in children of exposed mothers, anorexia, fatigue, and other effects.	Discarded electrical equipment, accidental industrial leakage, or reuse of PCB containers for food.

one of the most common childhood environmental health problems, affecting some three million children under the age of six.[28]

Lead usually does not poison a person all at once; rather, low levels build up gradually in the soft tissues of the kidneys, bone marrow, liver, and brain. Over time, the accumulated lead can cause such health problems as diminished intelligence and impaired development. Pregnant women and young children are particularly vulnerable to the effects of lead because their bodies absorb high levels of calcium to meet their growth needs but the body cannot distinguish between lead and calcium. As a result, they readily absorb lead. If they are calcium or iron deficient, as many women and children are, their bodies take in even more lead.

Historically, lead entered the food and water supply largely through leaded gasoline exhaust, which contaminates rainfall, which in turn pervades crop soil and water supplies. Lead contamination of the water supply has been and continues to be a source of concern (refer to the Spotlight on water in Chapter 7). In addition, lead solder used to seal the seams of cans was long a source of the contaminant. Fortunately, during the past decade, the use of leaded gasoline has been greatly reduced, and lead-soldered cans have been eliminated. Today the levels of lead in foods and beverages are the lowest in history.[29]

Nevertheless, new sources of lead contamination have surfaced during recent years. When it comes to lead exposure via food and beverages, scientists have identified ceramic hollowware, lead crystal ware, and foil capsules on wine bottles as potential sources. Lead can leach from the glaze of ceramic bowls, mugs, and pitchers that have not been properly formulated or fired, especially when the food or beverage inside is hot and acidic, such as coffee, tea, or tomato soup. Wine and other alcoholic beverages also promote the leaching of lead, so experts advise against storing alcohol in pitchers and other containers made with lead crystal. In addition, it's a good idea to wipe with a damp cloth the rims of wine bottles with foil capsules, which have been shown to leach lead.

Many manufacturers have modified or are in the process of modifying their practices to reduce the potential for lead contamination. For help on lowering your own risk, see Table 11–8.

Although chemical contamination is not the greatest hazard posed by the food supply, there are still many unknowns. No one knows what level the contaminants accumulating in the environment may be reaching and threatening the health of the planet and its people. Another unknown factor is the interaction among contaminants; a substance that poses no threat by itself may combine with other chemicals lurking in the environment to form potent carcinogens. Still another unknown is the effect of time. Many potentially hazardous substances have been used for only a short time. What are the effects of prolonged exposure to them?

Despite the uncertainties, keep in mind that more often than not, healthful eating habits and overall good health protect against the toxicity of food contaminants and other environmental pollutants. Eating a wide variety of food ensures an adequate supply of essential nutrients and minimizes exposure to potential environmental contaminants.

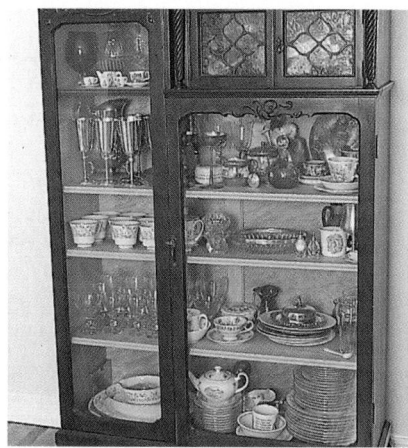

Some antique ceramic and crystal items are best left on the shelf. The older the piece, the higher the chances that it leaches lead.

TABLE 11–8
GETTING THE LEAD OUT

To protect against overexposure to lead, use the following guidelines:

- Do not store fruit juices or other acidic foods in ceramic containers.
- Do not store beverages in lead crystal containers.
- Use antique or collectible housewares for food or beverages only on occasion.
- Do not eat or drink from items that show a dusty or chalky gray residue on the glaze after they are washed.
- Do not feed babies from crystal bottles.
- During pregnancy, avoid frequent use of ceramic mugs for hot beverages such as coffee or tea. In addition, do not use lead crystal ware daily.
- Before pouring from a wine bottle sealed with a foil capsule, wipe the rim of the bottle with a cloth dampened with water or lemon juice.
- Run cold water for several minutes before using it for drinking or cooking.
- If you would like to purchase a home test kit for lead leaching from ceramic ware, contact your local FDA office, listed in the phone directory.
- For a listing of lead-safe ceramic ware, write to the Environmental Defense Fund, P.O. Box 96969, Washington, D.C. 20090-6969.
- For additional questions about lead, call the National Lead Information Center at 1-800-532-3394. Callers may request an information packet in English or Spanish.

SOURCE: Adapted from J.E. Foulke, Lead threat lessens, but mugs pose problem, *FDA Consumer*, April 1993, pp. 19–23.

Pesticide Residues

Pesticides are substances used to prevent, destroy, or repel harmful pests, including insects, spiders, bacteria, weeds, molds and mildews, rodents, and other living things. Unlike many other chemicals present in the food supply, pesticides are intended specifically to poison living things. The trouble with pesticides, of course, is that they can inadvertently harm wildlife, people, and other species.

When farmers first began using pesticides, they chose potent ones—chemicals designed to keep on killing for as long as they remained in the soil. Unfortunately, after years of widespread pesticide use, some unsettling side effects of the chemicals surfaced. They washed from the soil into lakes, rivers, and oceans, contaminating water supplies; they poisoned farm workers, who breathed the chemicals day in and day out; they endangered many species of wildlife, disrupting the animals' abilities to reproduce and wiping out entire populations; and, most disturbing, they would not go away.

For example, in the 1960s, scientists observed that a popular pesticide called DDT had begun accumulating in the body fat of animals. DDT threatened the survival of the American eagle by weakening eggshells to the point of collapse, killing the developing chicks inside. It also appeared in big fish, carnivorous animals, people, and human breast milk. Finally, after years of widespread agricultural use, the United States banned DDT. However, the pesticide still lingers in the environment. Many foreign countries continue to use DDT, including countries from which the United States buys produce. Regrettably, despite the U.S. ban on DDT, U.S. companies are still allowed to sell it (as well as other banned pesticides) to countries where DDT use remains legal. This practice may come back to haunt us, however, when we buy imported produce that has been exposed to DDT. In addition, the DDT situation illustrates the need to consider environmental issues from a global perspective; residues of chemicals banned in one country can travel the entire world not only through the imported and exported foods but also through wind, rain, and waterways.

DDT taught us another lesson about pesticides: A contaminant that builds up in the body carries the greatest potential risk. In the body, a contaminant that is quickly broken down to some harmless compound poses the least risk to health. Likewise, if the body can easily and rapidly excrete a pesticide residue, the body may not be

PESTICIDES chemicals applied intentionally to plants, including foods, to prevent or eliminate pest damage. Pests include all living organisms that destroy or spoil foods: bacteria, molds and fungi, insects, and rats and other rodents, to name a few.

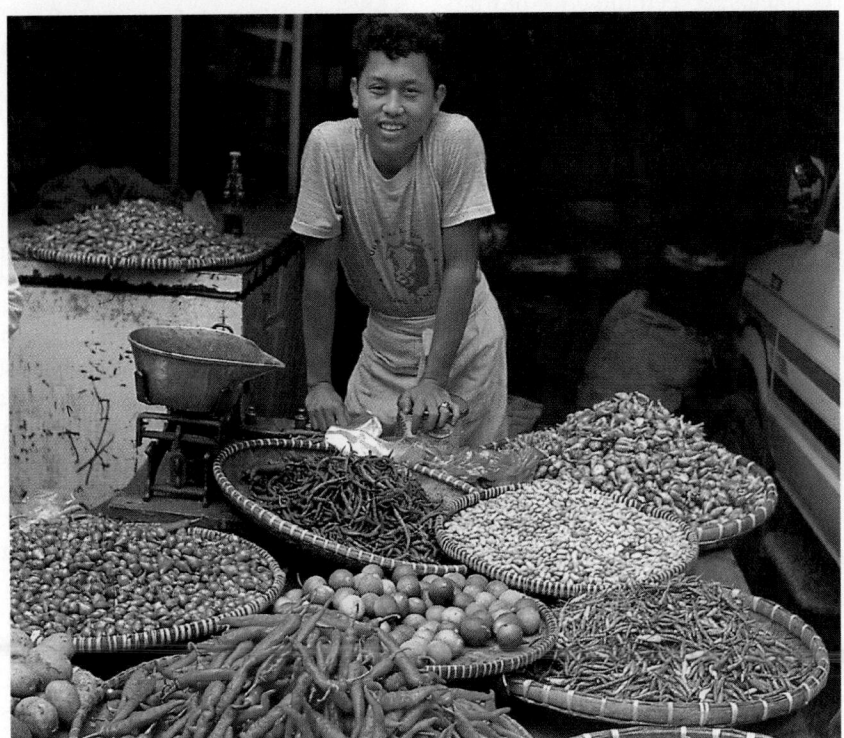

Foods imported from other countries may harbor residues of pesticides that have been banned for use in the United States.

harmed by it. But if the residue enters the body and stays there, all the while interacting with the body's cells and systems, it may wreak havoc. Additional doses piled on top of the first ones compound the damaging effects. Moreover, when a substance resists breakdown either inside the body (by the body's own enzymes) or outside (by microorganisms) and furthermore accumulates from one species to the next, it builds up in the food chain (see Figure 11–2). DDT causes all these problems, which is why it is so deadly.

This is not to say that pesticides have no place in the farming community. Farmers would face daunting obstacles to growing crops without them. Careful use of the chemicals often boosts crop yields, which in turn helps to keep the price of fruits and vegetables down and the availability of a wide variety of produce high. Still, as the DDT experience illustrates, pesticides must be evaluated scrupulously and used judiciously.

The ideal pesticide destroys the target pest and then breaks down quickly to other products that pose minimal hazard to people and other animals. Scientists have made many strides in developing relatively innocuous pesticides over the years, and the search for better, safer pesticides continues. What's more, since the introduction of pesticides decades ago, many national and international agencies have adopted strict **regulations** for pesticide use.

In the United States, the Environmental Protection Agency (EPA) determines whether a particular chemical may be used on U.S. crops. In deciding whether to approve a pesticide, the EPA scrutinizes dozens of studies that assess the substance's possible effects on people, wildlife, fish, or plants as well as its potential to cause such problems as cancer and birth defects. To do so, the EPA examines the estimated amount of a pesticide residue that a person might be exposed to during the course of a 70-year lifetime and the **risk** of harm that amount might pose. If the risk appears unacceptably high, the pesticide will be ruled out. All things considered, the process often requires years of research and costs millions of dollars.[30]

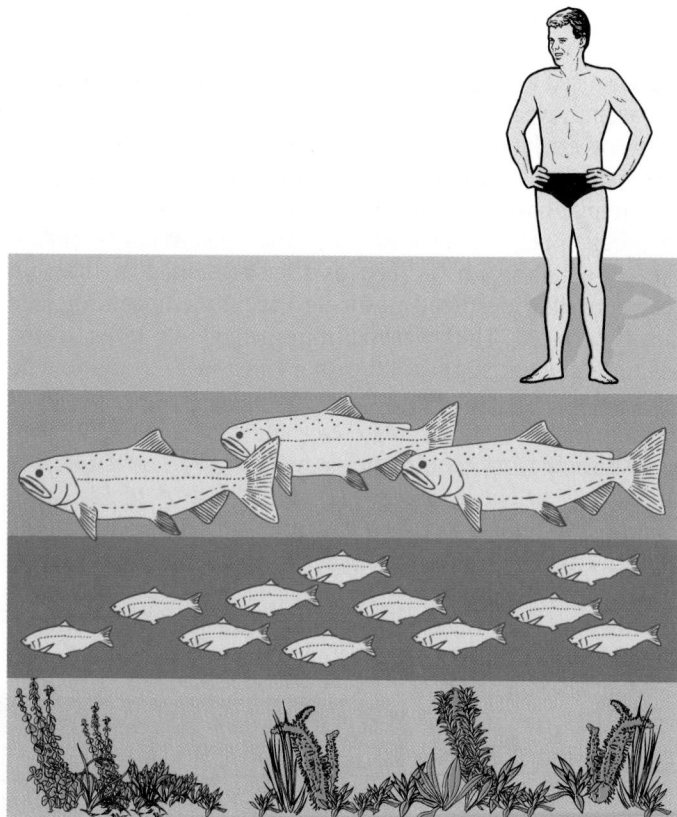

Level 4
A 150-lb. person

Level 3
100-lb. of larger fish

Level 2
A few tons of plant-eating fish

Level 1
Several tons of plants

FIGURE 11–2
HOW A FOOD CHAIN WORKS

A person who eats fish regularly may consume about 100 pounds of it in a year. These fish will, in turn, have eaten a few tons of small plant-eating fish during their lifetime. The little plant eaters will have ingested several tons of plants. If the plants have been contaminated with toxic chemicals, the bodies of the small fish that eat them will contain high concentrations of the chemicals; the larger fish that eat the little fish will harbor even higher amounts of the chemicals; and so on through the food chain. If none of the chemicals are lost along the way, the person at the end of the food chain ultimately eats the same amount of chemical contaminants that was contained in the original *several tons* of plants.

REGULATION a legal mandate that must be obeyed. Failure to follow a regulation brings about serious legal consequences.

RISK the harm a substance may confer. Scientists estimate risk by assessing the amount of a chemical that each person in a population might consume over time (also called *exposure*) and by considering how toxic the substance might be (*toxicity*).

risk = exposure × toxicity
exposure = amount of substance in food × amount of food eaten

Once the EPA approves a pesticide for use, it sets forth safety standards. For those pesticides it allows, it decides which crops may be treated with it and how much may be applied. It also establishes a **tolerance**—that is, the maximum amount of a pesticide residue allowed in or on a food. The EPA also sets forth a **reference dose** for the pesticide. This represents the amount of a chemical that could be consumed daily without posing any health risk. To calculate the reference dose, scientists use animal studies to estimate the maximum amount of the chemical that a person could take in daily without suffering harm. They then take a fraction of this amount, usually 1/100, to ensure an extra **margin of safety.** In other words, the reference dose is 1/100 of the maximum amount of the substance that appears to be safe. Scientists factor in a large margin of safety as a precautionary measure to help ensure that even highly vulnerable people won't be harmed by the substance in question (see Figure 11–3).[31]

After the EPA approves a pesticide for use, the FDA, in its ongoing monitoring program, begins to check for residues of it. Inspectors collect samples from packers, shippers, and other food handlers and then test for pesticide residues. If a food contains residues that exceed the EPA's tolerance limits, the FDA can seize the entire shipment and press criminal charges. In addition, the FDA conducts studies to determine whether pesticide residues from a variety of foods together fall below reference dose levels. Such cross-checks help to ensure that farmers are applying pesticides properly.

While EPA and FDA regulations go a long way in protecting the public from harmful pesticide residues, problems with the monitoring system still exist. As explained earlier, other countries may use pesticides banned in the United States, and imported foods might not be tested for the presence of those pesticides. In addition, consider that in 1993 the National Academy of Sciences issued the results of a large-scale, five-year study on the risk of pesticide residues in the diets of infants and children. Although it concluded that the U.S. food supply is safe for children, it called for changes in the methods used to assess health risks from pesticides to better account for differences between adults and children.[32]

Despite the uncertainties, however, major health organizations, including the American Academy of Pediatrics, the American Cancer Society, and the American Medical Association, agree that the health risks posed by pesticide residues are minimal and that the health risks of *not* eating fruits and vegetables for fear of consuming pesticide residues far outweigh the slight risk linked with those substances. Meanwhile, what can you do to protect yourself against unacceptably high levels of pesticides? The following Nutrition Action feature offers a perspective on that question.

TOLERANCE the maximum amount of a particular substance allowed on food.

REFERENCE DOSE the estimated amount of a chemical that could be consumed daily without causing harmful effects.

MARGIN OF SAFETY from a food safety standpoint, the margin is a zone between the maximum amount of a substance that appears to be safe and the amount allowed in the food supply.

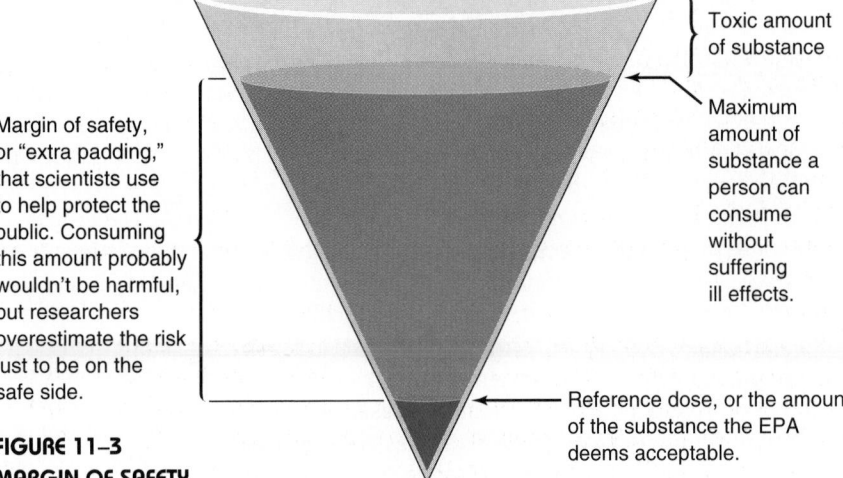

Margin of safety, or "extra padding," that scientists use to help protect the public. Consuming this amount probably wouldn't be harmful, but researchers overestimate the risk just to be on the safe side.

Toxic amount of substance

Maximum amount of substance a person can consume without suffering ill effects.

Reference dose, or the amount of the substance the EPA deems acceptable.

FIGURE 11–3
MARGIN OF SAFETY

Margin of safety, or "extra padding," that scientists use to help protect the public. Consuming this amount probably wouldn't be harmful, but researchers overestimate the risk just to be on the safe side.

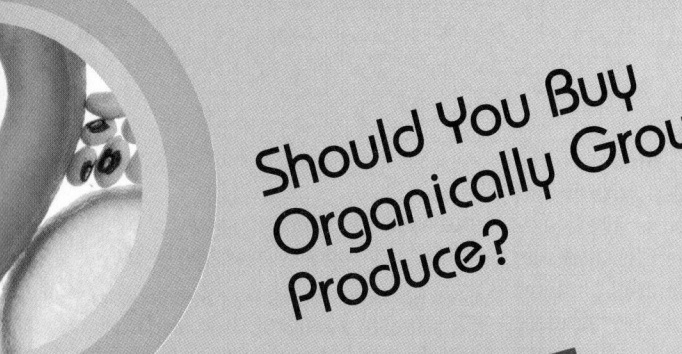

Should You Buy Organically Grown Produce?

It's been more than five years since a consumer group made headlines by contending that Alar, a chemical used to grow apples, posed a serious threat to the health of American children. While the group's exaggerated allegations have long since been put to rest by health experts, the Alar scare and the doubts it raised about the safety of the food supply still linger in the minds of many consumers. So, in the aftermath of the Alar incident, marketers carved out a small but strong niche: "organically grown" and "pesticide-free" produce that commands a premium price. Once sold only in health food stores, "organic" fruits and vegetables can now be found in many mainstream markets.

Consumers who opt for organics often believe that the expensive produce is especially healthful because it has been grown without the use of pesticides and contains no pesticide residues.[33] But organically grown produce is not always what people think it is, for a number of reasons. For one, organic growers often use pesticides naturally found in the environment, such as sulfur, nicotine, and copper, so "organically grown" doesn't always means grown without pesticides.[34]

Second, even though so-called organic foods sometimes are touted as "pesticide-free," they may contain the same levels of pesticide residues or other contaminants as conventional grocery store foods. In some cases, pesticides drift from farm to farm and settle on crops that have not been directly treated with pesticides. In other instances, organic farms may be situated on pesticide-contaminated soil or exposed to tainted water that leaches pesticide residues. In still other cases, farmers use bacteria-laden manure as a fertilizer. If the produce that comes from the crop is not sanitized in some way, it may carry harmful microorganisms. Or a marketer may simply label a product *organic* to boost sales. Unfortunately, that's easy to do, given that the federal government has not, at the time of the publication of this book, set forth federal standards that define the use of the term *organic* on food labels. Granted, a number of states have come up with their own legislation regarding the use of the term *organic.* Nevertheless, many states lack the resources needed to ensure that standards are being met. For instance, few states can afford to pay for regular inspections to assure that organic farmers are following certification protocol.

Similarly, the term *pesticide-free* has never been legally defined and can mislead consumers. While the claim suggests that a product contains no pesticide residue whatsoever, it may simply indicate that no residues were detected in the samples tested. This is a crucial distinction because programs to monitor pesticide residues can vary on a number of counts that influence the ability to detect residues. For instance, the type of test used may not be sensitive

If you grow your own produce, do so with care. Pesticides and disinfectants used on home gardens rank as a major source of chemical residue exposure to consumers. For information on safe use, storage, and disposal of home and garden pesticides, contact your local Cooperative Extension Service or the EPA's Office of Pesticide Programs, Communications Branch, 7506 C, 401 M. Street, Southwest, Washington, DC 20460.

enough to detect residues that a more sophisticated test would be able to spot, or the number of samples of food tested might be low.[35]

What's more, even the very concept of "pesticide-free" produce is misleading because it suggests that produce that's not free of pesticides is harmful. Consider that today scientists can use high-tech laboratory techniques to detect infinitesimal amounts of chemical residues on produce. Table 11–9 gives some comparisons to help put the common measurements for pesticide residues into perspective. As the table suggests, whether a food contains any chemical residues or has been exposed to pesticides at some time in the past is not necessarily the right question to ask about its effect on your health. The real issue is whether the amount of residue that remains in the food at the time you eat it is harmful. If a food has been treated with a pesticide and the chemical has since evaporated, changed into a nontoxic compound, or been diluted below the point at which it can do any harm, the food may not be inferior to an untreated food. In fact, it may be nutritionally superior because it has not been weakened by attacks of pests.

None of this is to say that buying organically grown produce is necessarily a complete waste of money. If you can afford it and you're certain that it comes from a reputable farmer who is following sound organic growing techniques, organically grown food casts a vote in favor of agricultural techniques that promote the well-being of the environment and farming communities over the long run. Reputable organic farmers typically do use fewer pesticides than conventional farmers because they use "eco-friendly" techniques such as crop rotation to help keep pests under control. This helps to protect the soil as well as the groundwater and the farm workers themselves against chemical contamination.

Still, many farmers who aren't meeting "organic" standards per se are using other techniques to keep pesticide use to a minimum. For example, more and more farmers have adopted a system called **integrated pest management**—a technique by which farmers cut back chemical use by combining strategies such as crop rotation, genetic engineering (discussed at the end of the chapter), and biological controls such as the release of a predator insect on a crop to get rid of another pest. What's more, no major health organization advocates eating only organically grown produce. The biggest health hazard, they say, is letting worries about pesticide residues stand in the way of eating a fruit- and vegetable-rich diet. To keep pesticide residues from all types of produce to a minimum, use the produce-handling tips in Table 11–10.

TABLE 11–9
PESTICIDES IN PERSPECTIVE

When you hear about pesticide residues in food, the amounts measured are either parts per million (ppm), parts per billion (ppb), or parts per trillion (ppt). The following comparisons show just how tiny these amounts are.

1 PPM: 1 gram of residue in 1 million grams of food
1 inch in 16 miles
1 minute in 2 years
1 cent in $10,000

1 PPB: 1 gram of residue in 1 billion grams of food
1 inch in 16,000 miles
1 second in 32 years
1 cent in $10 million

1 PPT: 1 gram of residue in 1 trillion grams of food
1 inch in 16 million miles
1 second in 32,000 years
1 square foot on floor tile the size of Indiana

SOURCE: Adapted from International Food Information Council, *Pesticides and Food Safety* (Washington, D.C.: International Food Information Council, 1995), p. 2.

INTEGRATED PEST MANAGEMENT the use of biological controls, crop rotation, genetic engineering, and other tactics to reduce chemical use in the growing of crops.

TABLE 11–10   HANDLING PRODUCE PROPERLY
To keep pesticide residues in fruits and vegetables to a minimum, use the following tips:

- Rinse produce thoroughly with water and scrub with a vegetable brush. When present, most pesticide residues reside on the surface of a product. Consider peeling produce to which wax has been applied; some wax may contain residual from antifungal chemicals.
- Do not use soap to wash produce. Soap was not designed to be used on food and may leave behind undesirable residues of its own.
- Discard the outer leaves of lettuce, cabbage, and other leafy vegetables. Rinse the interior leaves thoroughly to remove dirt and debris.
- Eat a variety of fruits and vegetables. Farmers use different chemicals for different crops, so eating a wide variety of produce helps to cut down on exposure to any particular pesticide residue.

SOURCE: Adapted from C. F. Chaisson and coauthors, *Pesticides in Food: A Guide for Professionals* (Chicago: The American Dietetic Association, 1991), p. 18.

Food Additives

From a safety standpoint, **food additives** rank among the *least* hazardous substances in food, although consumers tend to rank them high on their list of food-related risks. The great majority of food additives enhance the color, flavor, texture, or stability of foods or even improve the nutritional value of certain items, as shown in Table 11–11. Many additives are common substances such as vitamins, herbs, and spices, deliberately added to foods and called direct or **intentional additives.**

On the other hand, **incidental additives,** such as packaging materials or processing chemicals, get into the food by accident during processing. The federal government regulates all types of food additives and requires that food processors perform tests to determine whether additives are present in safe levels.

As Table 11–12 shows, many of the food laws that ensure a safe food supply involve food additives. Manufacturers must go through a lengthy, costly process to get FDA approval for a new food additive. The manufacturer must conduct extensive research to show that the additive in question does what it is supposed to do, that it can be detected and measured in foods to which it has been added, and that it is safe in the amounts in which it will be used.

As with pesticide residues (described earlier), many food additives are allowed only in amounts that ensure a wide margin of safety. Most additives that pose any potential risk are allowed in foods only at levels 1/100 of those at which the risk is still known to be zero. Even nutrient food additives are subject to the margin of

FOOD ADDITIVE any substance added to food, including substances used in the production, processing, treatment, packaging, transportation, or storage of food.

INTENTIONAL FOOD ADDITIVES substances intentionally added to food. Examples include nutrients, colors, spices, and herbs.

INCIDENTAL FOOD ADDITIVES (or indirect additives) substances that accidentally get into food as a result of contact with it during growing, processing, packaging, storing, or some other stage before the food is consumed.

TABLE 11–11
MAJOR USES OF FOOD ADDITIVES

FUNCTION OF ADDITIVE	EXAMPLES	FOODS IN WHICH OFTEN USED
Impart or maintain consistency	Stabilizers, thickeners, anticaking agents, and emulsifiers including alginates, lecithin, mono- and di-glycerides, glycerine, pectin, guar gum.	Baked goods, cake mixes, salad dressings, ice cream, processed cheese, table salt, chocolate.
Improve or maintain nutritional value	Vitamins A and D, thiamin, niacin, folic acid, ascorbic acid (vitamin C), calcium carbonate, zinc oxide, iron.	Flour, bread, biscuits, breakfast cereals, pasta, margarine, milk, iodized salt.
Maintain palatability and wholesomeness	Ascorbic acid, butylated hydroxyanisole (BHA), butylated hydroxytoluene (BHT) benzoates.	Bread, crackers, frozen and dried fruit, margarine, lard, potato chips, cake mixes, meat.
Produce light texture; control acidity or alkalinity	Yeast, sodium bicarbonate, citric acid, lactic acid, phosphoric acid.	Cakes, cookies, quick breads, crackers, butter, soft drinks.
Enhance flavor or impart desired color	Cloves, ginger, fructose, aspartame, MSG, FD&C Red No. 40, caramel, turmeric.	Spice cake, gingerbread, soft drinks, yogurt, soup, candy, cheese, jams, gum.

SOURCE: Adapted from *Food Additives* (Rockville, MD; Washington, D.C.: Food and Drug Administration in cooperation with International Food Information Council, 1992), pp. 7–8.

safety concept. Consider that while iodine has long been added to salt to prevent iodine deficiency, the amounts added have been controlled because excess amounts of the mineral can be deadly.

The GRAS List and the Delaney Clause

Table 11–12 summarizes the impact of many major food laws on the regulation of food additives. Still, attention to two aspects of food law will help you to better understand the issues surrounding them.

Substances Generally Recognized as Safe (GRAS).

For the first half of the twentieth century, scientists evaluated the safety of food additives using a simple approach: An added substance was either "safe" and therefore permitted for use in foods or "poisonous and deleterious" and therefore banned. As the study of toxic agents advanced, scientists realized that eventually they would be able to show that virtually every substance poses a health hazard if the dose is large enough. Consequently, they recognized that simply classifying an additive as "safe" or "poisonous" failed to be an effective means of evaluation.

To get around the problem, Congress set forth the bill that would later become the Food Additives Amendment of 1958. As the members of Congress debated the bill, a question arose as to how to deal with the additives already in use. Congress decided that a "safe"

TABLE 11–12
HISTORY OF FOOD LAW

DATE	LAW	PROVISIONS
1646	Law passed by Massachusetts Bay Colony	Stipulated how much a loaf of bread must weigh to be sold for a penny; example of food regulation prior to the Food and Drugs Act.
1906	Pure Food and Drugs Act	Prohibited interstate shipment of misbranded or adulterated foods and drugs.
1938	Federal Food, Drug, and Cosmetic Act (FFDCA)	Prohibited the addition of poisonous or deleterious substances to foods *except* where such an addition is required in food processing or cannot be avoided by good manufacturing practices; set tolerances for authorized poisonous or deleterious substances added during processing; required labels to identify artificial coloring, artificial flavorings, and other chemical preservatives in food; required labeling of special dietary foods; established standards of purity and quality for foods.
1947	Federal Insecticide, Fungicide, and Rodenticide Act	Allowed the EPA to determine whether a pesticide can be registered or approved for use in the United States.
1954	Pesticide Chemicals Amendment to the FFDCA	Gave the FDA the authority to enforce safety tolerances for registered pesticides in or on agricultural products.
1958	Food Additives Amendment to the FFDCA	Made manufacturers responsible for showing that a new food additive is safe prior to FDA approval; includes Delaney clause, described on page 444.
1960	Color Additives Amendment to the FFDCA	Restricted the addition of color additives to cosmetics, drugs, and foods to those listed by the FDA as safe.
1978	Vitamin and Mineral Amendment to the FFDCA	Gave the FDA more control over product formulation and labeling.
1990	Nutrition Labeling and Education Act	Required manufacturers to include nutrition labeling on a wider range of foods; defined and set standards for use of nutrition and health claims (refer to the Spotlight feature in Chapter 2 for a discussion of food labels).

substance in use prior to 1958 would be deemed a "Substance Generally Recognized as Safe" (a GRAS substance) and be put on the **GRAS list.** Substances not in use before that time would be classified as food additives and subject to regulation under the Food Additives Amendment.

With the establishment of the amendment, the FDA put hundreds of substances on the GRAS list. Everything from vegetable oils, salt, pepper, sugar,

GRAS (GENERALLY RECOGNIZED AS SAFE) LIST a list of ingredients, established by the FDA, that had long been in use and were believed safe. The list is subject to revision as new facts become known.

caffeine, vinegar, and baking powder to meat, poultry, eggs, milk, seafood, cereals, fruit, and vegetables were—and still are—classified as GRAS substances.

The GRAS list came under scrutiny in 1969, however, when safety questions arose about the GRAS substance cyclamate, an artificial sweetener (refer to the Nutrition Action feature in Chapter 3 for more on cyclamate). After reviewing hundreds of studies, the FDA decided to ban cyclamate from use in foods and beverages. As a result of this incident, President Richard Nixon ordered a reevaluation of the safety of all substances on the GRAS list. The FDA conducted a sweeping review and removed about 300 substances from the list. Today, the more than 400 substances classified as GRAS are continually subject to reexamination as new facts and concerns arise.

Delaney Clause.   Another piece of legislature came about during the debate regarding the Food Additives Amendment of 1958. At that time, James J. Delaney (U.S. Representative to New York) sponsored a provision to the bill that forbid the approval of any additive found to cause cancer in animals no matter how small the dose. The rationale for the provision stemmed from the widely held belief that it was possible to completely eliminate cancer-causing agents from the food supply. Congress voted to add the **Delaney clause** into the Food Additives Amendment of 1958, despite considerable debate.

Today, the Delaney clause remains controversial and often puts regulatory agencies in a legal bind because it is virtually impossible to eliminate potential cancer-causing agents from the food supply. Consider that many substances, even those found naturally in a number of foods, can cause cancer when given to animals in large enough amounts. In fact, critics charge that the Delaney clause encourages the use of studies in which animals are fed substances in doses hundreds of thousands of times greater than the dose a person could consume via food. The results of such studies can be meaningless, given that the dose makes the poison, as pointed out earlier in the chapter. In addition, as scientists continue to develop better techniques for detecting chemical residues in foods, the task of completely eliminating minuscule amounts becomes even more complex and unrealistic.

Because of the Delaney clause, the FDA and other regulatory agencies must continually find new ways to interpret the anticancer principle in the regulation of the food supply. The agencies must consider the degree to which people are exposed to the cancer-causing agent and then use animal studies to evaluate the potential risks.

DELANEY CLAUSE a provision in the 1958 Food Additives Amendment that prohibits manufacturers from using any substance that is known to cause cancer in animals or humans at any dose level.

New Technologies on the Horizon

Back in the 1860s, a French scientist named Louis Pasteur came up with a radical, newfangled process by which the disease-producing microorganisms in a food could be destroyed by exposing it to heat. Dubbed pasteurization, after Dr. Pasteur, the process marked a major breakthrough in the science of food safety. At the time, however, Dr. Pasteur's discovery met with widespread fear and opposition. In fact, it wasn't accepted as a vital public health measure until 1909, when the city of Chicago set forth the first U.S. law requiring pasteurization of milk.

Today, of course, few consumers even question the wisdom of drinking pasteurized milk. Still, according to many experts, new technologies such as irradiation have prompted a public outcry similar to the turn-of-the-century resistance to pasteurization.[36] As public health organizations strive to feed a fast-growing world population while ensuring a safe food supply, debate about new ways of doing so is sure to heat up. The following sections explore some of the controversial food technologies under consideration as alternatives to help improve the safety of our food supply and to maintain the nutritional value of the foods available in the marketplace.

Irradiation

Irradiation ranks as one of the foremost technologies earmarked by food safety experts for increased future use in the United States. The process involves exposing food to low doses of radiation, which destroys insects and several types of bacteria, including *Salmonella.* Contrary to popular belief, irradiation does not make a food radioactive. Rather, the radiation rays pass through food, leaving behind no radioactive residues.

Aside from the misunderstanding that irradiation makes food radioactive, many of the criticisms about the process center around substances called **unique radiolytic products**—compounds that are not present in food naturally or after conventional processing. Critics charge that these products may pose health hazards to consumers who eat irradiated food. According to a comprehensive report from the World Health Organization, however, concern about unique radiolytic products is "probably unfounded," because many of the substances found in irradiated foods are similar, if not identical, to compounds found in other foods. Even those that appear to be unique may not have been detected in conventionally processed foods because those items haven't undergone the same kind of extensive testing as have irradiated foods.[37]

Another common concern about irradiation is that it might alter the nutritional value of a food. Again, the World Health Organization, along with numerous other public health agencies, points out that nutrient losses, if any, are insignificant.

To be sure, that's not to say that irradiation poses no risks at all. One of the most troublesome is that the radioactive materials used in the irradiation process may put workers and communities at undue risk. However, as with any technology, the risk of irradiation must be weighed carefully against the benefits and risks of alternative technologies. Consider spices, which typically harbor high levels of pathogens. Often, manufacturers douse them with a toxic, explosive chemical called ethylene oxide to rid them of bacteria. Yet because of its toxic, explosive nature, ethylene oxide puts workers at risk, may pollute the air, and may leave behind residue on the spices. In fact, the gas, which was once used to sterilize medical supplies, has been deemed so dangerous that most manufacturers now use irradiation instead. (Cotton swabs, tampons, teething rings, and a number of other consumer goods are also sterilized via irradiation.)[38] The example of this alternative technology highlights the complexity of the issues surrounding irradiation.

While there are no easy answers about whether this or any other new technology will be best over the long run, it's crucial that both consumers and

IRRADIATION the process of exposing a substance to low doses of radiation to kill insects, bacteria, and other potentially harmful microorganisms.

UNIQUE RADIOLYTIC PRODUCTS substances unique to irradiated food and apparently created during the process of irradiation.

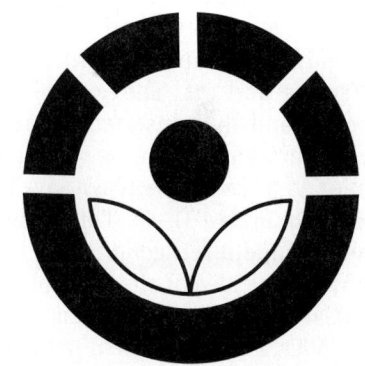

The FDA requires that the labels of all irradiated foods carry this internationally known symbol. The circle in the middle represents an energy source; the five breaks in the outer circle symbolize rays generated by the energy source; and the two petals signify food.

scientists look at all the angles before forming opinions one way or another. The World Health Organization, the Food and Agriculture Organization of the United Nations, the Food and Drug Administration, and numerous other agencies encourage the use of irradiation in the fight against foodborne disease and food loss, and some 35 countries have approved it for use. According to WHO, each year spoilage, insect infestation, and the like lead to losses of as much as 50 percent of the world's food supply, losses that could be eliminated with irradiation. What's more, the process may help prevent deaths resulting from foodborne illness. In the United States, for example, where incidence of *Salmonella* on poultry continues to rise and strains of bacteria such as *E. coli* 0157:H7 keep increasing, irradiation might help to prevent thousands of deaths and illness caused by foodborne disease. Clearly, as the pressures to feed the world safely continue to mount, the public and scientific community will continue to examine the pros and cons of irradiation.

Genetic Engineering

In May 1994, a new breed of tomato made headlines. Called the Flavr Savr, the product garnered national repute as the first food created via **genetic engineering** to hit the market. It wasn't so much the product itself, which is simply a slow-ripening tomato, that caused such a stir, but rather the opening of the regulatory door that can pave the way to a whole new crop of genetically engineered products. What are these high-tech foods, and will we see more of them in the future?

Just as a person's genes determine the person's hair color, eye color, and other characteristics, a plant's genes dictate the plant's structure, resistance to spoilage, and other qualities. With genetic engineering, scientists can alter a plant's genes in an effort to make a particular trait more desirable. To create the Flavr Savr tomato, scientists identified the gene that causes ripe tomatoes to soften and rot. They reversed the gene—or turned it backwards, so to speak—and then inserted the reversed gene back into tomato plants. The backward gene in the new tomatoes suppresses, or "turns off," the rotting gene. As a result, the Flavr Savr tomato stays ripe longer than regular tomatoes (see Figure 11-4). This allows growers more time to ship it to the consumer without refrigeration.[39]

While the idea of altering a plant's genes to create a different version sounds new, scientists have been using a cruder version of the concept for centuries. In the 1500s, farmers crossed, say, a good food crop with another plant resistant to disease to form a hybrid that contained traits of both plants. Many of the fruits and vegetables we enjoy today were produced by this sort of crossbreeding. For example, corn as we know it came from breeding corn with a much harder outer shell on the kernel; kiwi came from a small, hard berry; and nectarines came from modified peaches.[40] What makes genetic engineering different, however, is the speed and precision it affords scientists. Whereas crossbreeding typically takes more than a decade, genetic engineering can yield new products in about five years.

Another distinction is that genetic engineering allows scientists to "mix and match" genes from different species—say, mixing a gene from a fish with the genes of a vegetable. This type of research raises many unanswered ethical

GENETIC ENGINEERING the process of altering the genes of a plant in an effort to create a new plant with different traits. This process of recombining genes is also known as recombinant DNA.

FIGURE 11-4
CREATING THE FLAVR SAVR TOMATO

1. Isolated and cloned the PG (polygalacturonase) gene, which causes ripe tomatoes to soften and rot.

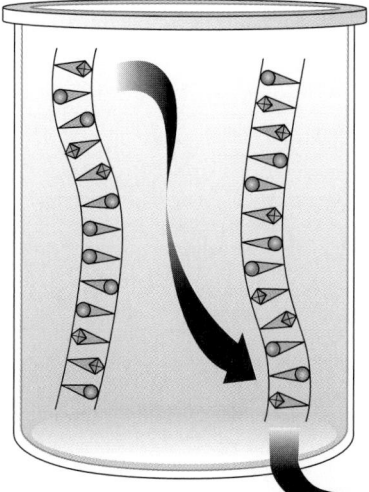

2. Reversed the PG gene sequence so that the gene is backwards (in what scientists call the "antisense" orientation).

9. In the genetically engineered tomato, the natural PG gene's production of the fruit-rotting PG enzyme has been repressed by the reversed gene. This gives the commercial tomato extended shelf life, allowing it to ripen more fully on the vine and still have time to get to market before it spoils.

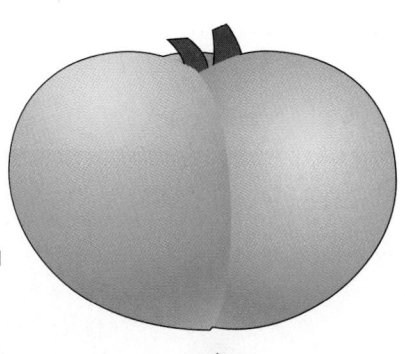

8. Seeds are collected from the genetically engineered greenhouse tomatoes and are planted outdoors for field trials and more seed production.

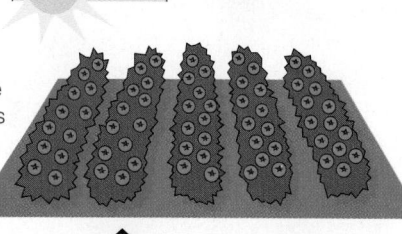

3. Put the reversed PG gene into Agrobacterium, which infects plants and is commonly used by genetic engineers to get modified or foreign genes into target cells.

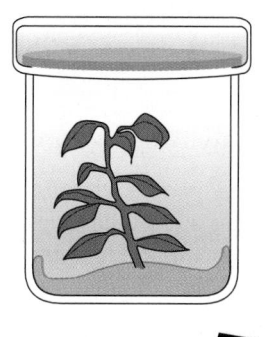

7. Plants sprout roots, are transplanted to soil, and grow to mature tomato plants.

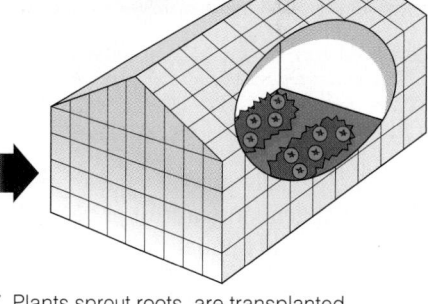

Agrobacterium cell

Altered PG gene is placed in Agrobacterium.

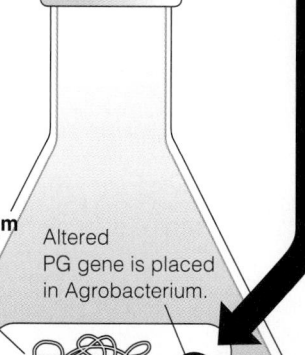

6. Leaf cuttings regenerate tomato plants containing the reversed PG gene.

4. Put Agrobacteria in a petri dish with leaf pieces cut from a tomato plant. The leaves' edges absorb the Agrobacteria and antisense PG gene.

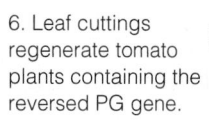

5. Antisense gene becomes part of the genetic material of the tomato plant cells.

Plant cell

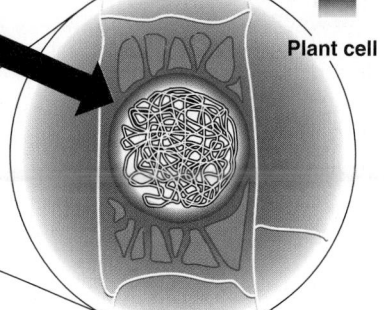

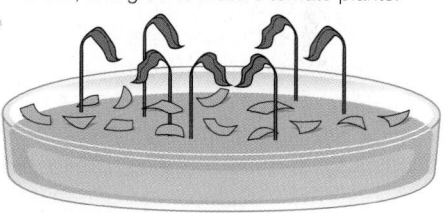

SOURCE: Reprinted with permission from Calgene's recipe for genetically engineered tomatoes, *FDA Consumer,* April 1995, p. 9.

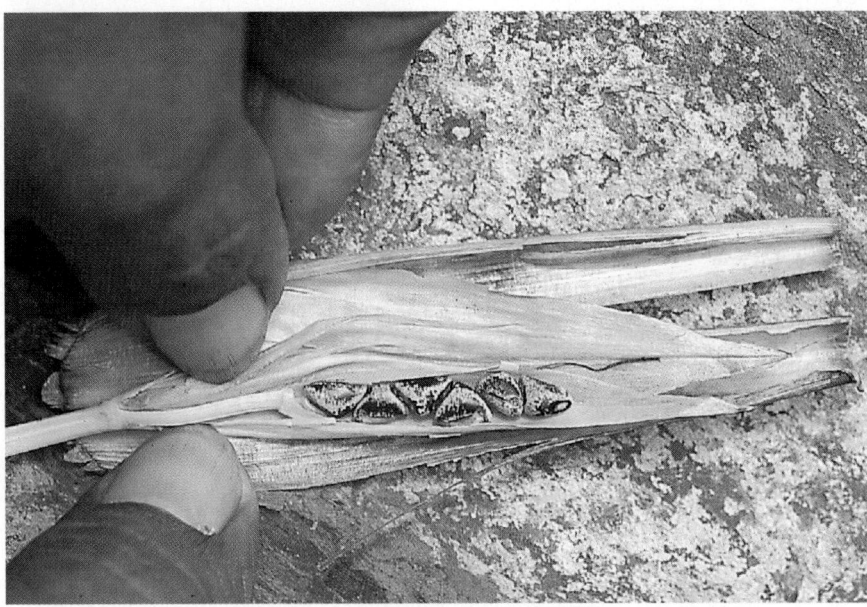

Farmers bred corn as we know it today from this wild corn.

questions, especially among vegetarians and other people who fear that insert-
ing an animal gene into a fruit or vegetable makes a food that is on some level
both vegetable and animal. No such products are expected to enter the marketplace in the near future, but if and when they do, their marketing and labeling
will warrant serious attention.

Another widely debated issue surrounding genetic engineering involves labeling. Many consumer groups have called for across-the-board labels on genetically engineered foods. But according to the FDA, with some exceptions, the
food must carry distinct consequences to consumers who eat it before it must
bear special labeling. When genes from peanuts and
other foods known to be common causes of allergies are
put into a food, the label must indicate that the food contains an allergen unless the manufacturer can prove that
the item's potential to cause allergies has not been transferred via the gene. In
addition, a food that has been genetically engineered to significantly change,
say, its fiber content or nutrient composition must bear a label that states the
nature of the change.[41]

Despite the concerns, many scientists are hopeful that careful use of genetic
engineering will confer long-term benefits. For instance, the development of
insect- and disease-resistant plants may allow farmers to grow crops with fewer
chemicals. The possibilities are enormous, and each new product considered for
entry into the marketplace will require careful scrutiny.

The FDA expects the introduction of 100 to 150 genetically
engineered foods during the next five years.

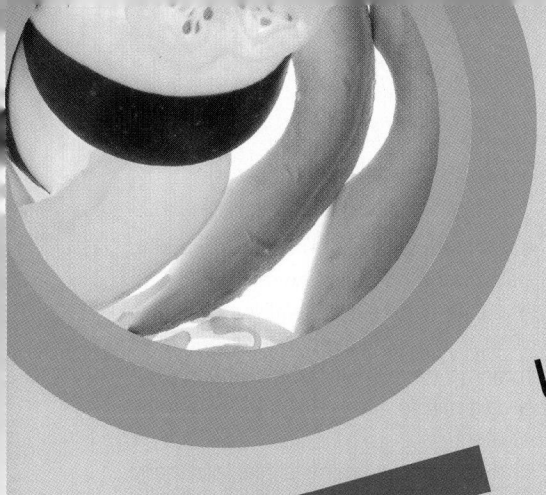

Domestic and World Hunger

This book has focused on the problems of *overnutrition*—obesity, heart disease, cancer, and others—diseases of economically developed nations. People in developing nations as well as people in the less privileged parts of developed nations suffer from problems of **undernutrition,** which is characterized by chronic debilitating hunger and malnutrition. These conditions are most visible in times of **famine,** but they are widespread and persistent even when famine does not occur. They have been with us throughout history, and despite numerous development and assistance programs, they are not disappearing; the number of hungry and malnourished people continues to grow. For these people, hunger is ceaseless, and malnutrition ensues.

Regardless of our race, religion, sex, or nationality, our bodies experience similarly the effects of hunger and its companion **malnutrition**—listlessness, weakness, failure to thrive, stunted growth, mental retardation, muscle wastage, scurvy, pellagra, beriberi, anemia, rickets, osteoporosis, goiter, tooth decay, blindness, and a host of other effects, including death.[42] Apathy and shortened attention span are two of a number of behavioral symptoms often mistaken for laziness, lack of intelligence, or mental illness in undernourished people.

How are hunger and poverty related? The phenomenon of *hunger* is today being discussed in terms of **food security** or **food insecurity.** Food security is defined as access by all people at all times to enough food for an active, healthy life and at a minimum includes the following: 1) the ready availability of nutritionally adequate and safe foods and 2) the ability to acquire personally acceptable foods in a socially acceptable way.[43] Food insecurity was once viewed as a problem of overpopulation and inadequate food production, but now many people recognize it as a problem of **poverty.**[44] Food is *available* but is not *accessible* to the poor, who have neither land nor money. Poverty exists for many reasons, including overpopulation, greed, unemployment, and the lack of productive resources such as land, tools, and credit. If it is at all possible to provide adequate nutrition for all the earth's hungry people, it can be achieved only when the economic, political, and social structures that create a gap between rich and poor—and thereby limit food production, distribution, and consumption—become the targets of change.

Approximately how many people worldwide are affected by food insecurity? The Food and Agriculture Organization (FAO) estimates that of the more than 5 billion people in the world, at least half a billion—one in ten in the human race—suffer from chronic, severe undernutrition, consuming too little food each day to meet even minimum energy requirements.[45] Protein energy malnutrition (PEM) affects more than 780 million persons and contributes to almost 13 million childhood deaths yearly.[46] Worldwide, three micronutrient deficiencies are of particular concern: vitamin A deficiency, the world's most common cause of preventable child blindness and vision impairment; iron deficiency anemia; and

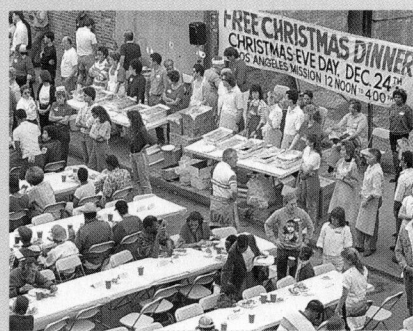

Feeding the hungry—in the United States.

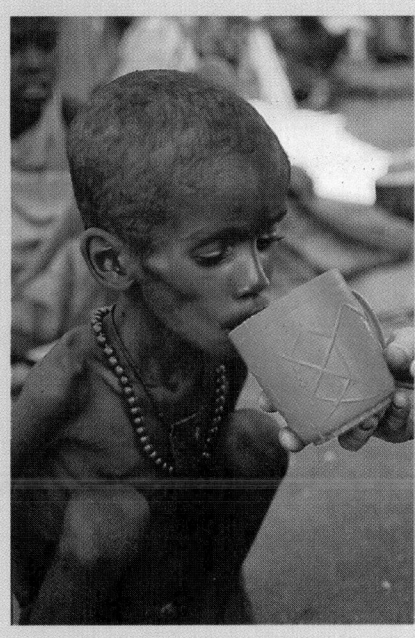

Feeding the hungry—in Somalia.

449

iodine deficiency, causing high levels of goiter and child retardation:[47]

● *Vitamin A deficiency.* Some 13.8 million children below six years of age have **xerophthalmia.** Of these, an estimated 500,000 children become partially or totally blinded, as a result of an insufficiency of vitamin A in the diet. Vitamin A deficiency is also associated with other forms of malnutrition, infection, diarrhea, and a high rate of mortality.

● *Iron deficiency.* Iron deficiency anemia is estimated to affect some 1.5 billion people, or one-fourth of all people living. In infancy and early childhood, iron deficiency is associated with decreased cognitive abilities and resistance to disease.

● *Iodine deficiency.* Iodine deficiency, the major preventable cause of mental retardation worldwide, is a risk factor for both physical and mental retardation in about one billion people. About 200 million people worldwide—especially in mountainous regions—are estimated to have goiter, and over three million suffer overt cretinism.

Worldwide, about 40,000 to 50,000 people die each day as a result of undernutrition. Millions of children die each year from the diseases of poverty: parasitic and infectious diseases such as dysentery, whooping cough, measles, tuberculosis, cholera, and malaria. These diseases interact with poor nutrition to form a vicious cycle in which the outcome for many is death.[48] **UNICEF** estimates that malnutrition and disease claim the lives of 250,000 children *every week.*[49]

When does the risk for undernutrition run high? Undernutrition runs high when nutrient needs are high, as in times of rapid growth. If family food is limited, pregnant and lactating women, infants, and children are the first to show the signs of undernutrition. Effects of food insecurity can be devastating to this group of the population.

During pregnancy, healthy women in developed countries gain an average of about 27 pounds, while low-income women show a weight gain of only 11 to 15 pounds. Babies of these women tend to have low birthweights (less than 5 1/2 pounds). A low-birthweight baby has a greater than normal chance of having physical and mental birth defects, of contracting diseases, and of dying early in life. Low birthweight contributes to more than half of the deaths worldwide of children under five years of age. UNICEF refers to the **under-5 mortality rate** (U5MR) as the single best indicator of children's overall health and well-being.[50] UNICEF argues that the U5MR reflects a country's overall resources directed at children:

> . . . the U5MR reflects the nutritional health and the health knowledge of mothers; the level of immunization and use of **oral rehydration therapy;** the availability of maternal and health services (including prenatal care); income and food availability in the family; the availability of clean water and safe sanitation; and the overall safety of the child's environment.[51]

Until the middle of the twentieth century in most of the developing countries, babies were breastfed for their first year of life, with supplements of other milk and cereal gruel added to their diets after the first several months. Today, the percentage of infants who are exclusively breastfed to the age of four months has dropped to below 10 percent.[52] A number of factors contributed to this unfortunate decline, including the aggressive promotion and sale of infant formula to new mothers; the encouragement by health care practitioners for mothers to bottle feed (with free samples sent home from the hospital after delivery of the newborn); and the global pattern of urbanization and accompanying loss of cultural ties supporting breastfeeding,

combined with more women working outside the home.[53] Overall, WHO estimates that more than a million children's lives could be saved each year if all mothers gave their babies nothing but breast milk for the first four to six months of life.[54]

Breastfeeding permits infants in many developing countries to achieve weight and height gains equal to those of children in developed countries until about six months of age. In fact, replacing breast milk with infant formula in environments and economic circumstances that make it impossible to feed formula safely may lead to infant undernutrition. In the absence of sterilization and refrigeration, formula in bottles is an ideal breeding ground for bacteria. Feeding infants formula made with contaminated water often causes infections leading to diarrhea, dehydration, and inability to absorb nutrients.

Even if infants are protected by breastfeeding at first, they must eventually be weaned. The weaning period is one of the most dangerous periods for children in developing countries. Newly weaned infants often receive nutrient-poor diluted cereals or starchy root crops, and the infants' foods are often prepared with contaminated water, making infection almost inevitable.

What is the status of food insecurity in the United States? Approximately 20 million people in the United States—12 million children and 8 million adults—are suffering from chronic hunger, with the problem getting worse in all regions of the country. A recent analysis of 28 state hunger surveys found consistent results across all surveys and evidence for several broad conclusions:[55]

● Food insufficiency has become a chronic problem in the United States.

● Food insufficiency is not due to food shortages. Hunger results from unequal distribution of economic resources—poverty.

● People who lack access to a variety of resources—not just food—are most at risk of hunger. When income is inadequate to meet the costs of housing, utilities, health care, and other fixed expenses, these items compete with and may take precedence over food.

The United States has become a soup kitchen society to an extent unmatched since the bread lines of the Great Depression. Malnutrition and other health problems associated with chronic hunger—stunted growth, failure to thrive, low-birthweight babies, infant mortality, and anemia—are reported to be either escalating for the first time in many years or slowing in their long-term rates of improvement. In some of these conditions, the United States compares poorly with other industrialized countries.

Who are the hungry in the United States? Through the late 1960s and 1970s, hunger was evident among the chronic poor: migrant workers, Native Americans, southern blacks, unemployed minorities, and some of the elderly as well as the newly unemployed blue-collar workers during the 1970s. Now, hunger is reaching into other segments of the population without regard for age, marital status, previous employment or successes, family ties, or efforts to change the situation. The U.S. farm economy has been burdened by chronic price-depressing surpluses, and available resources are failing to reach many groups. One in 12 goes hungry at least two days a month. The millions who experience hunger today in the United States include the young, the new poor, the elderly, the homeless, low-income women, and ethnic minorities.

What are some of the causes of food insecurity in the United States? The

most compelling single reason is poverty. Poverty and food insecurity are interdependent. Nutrition surveys investigating people's nutritional health in the United States have demonstrated consistently that the lower a family's income, the less adequate the family's nutrition status. Nationally, most studies conducted since 1980 attribute the increases in food insecurity throughout the country to worsening economic conditions among the poor.[56] Major reductions in federal spending for antipoverty programs occurred throughout the 1980s. Severe reductions came in programs directly affecting those deepest in poverty, including Aid to Families with Dependent Children (AFDC), food stamps, low-income housing assistance, and child nutrition. Cuts in college financial aid effectively blocked a pathway out of poverty taken by many in the past.

Although poverty is the major cause of food insecurity in the United States, other problems contribute as well, including alcoholism and chronic substance abuse, mental illness, loneliness, isolation, depression, and despair; the reluctance of people to accept what they perceive as "welfare" or "charity"; delays in receiving public assistance benefits; an increase in the number of single mothers without the means to care for their children; poor management of limited family financial resources; health problems of old age; lack of nutritional adequacy and balance in the food available to hungry people; lack of access to assistance programs; insufficient community food resources for the hungry; and insufficient community transportation systems to deliver food to hungry people who have no transportation.

As a result of the evidence accumulated during the 1960s and 1970s showing that food insecurity was a problem in the United States, the problems of poverty and hunger became national priorities. Old programs were revised and new programs were developed in an attempt to

prevent malnutrition in those people found to be at greatest risk. The Food Stamp Program was expanded to serve more people. School lunch and breakfast programs were enlarged to support children nutritionally while they learned. Feeding programs to reach senior citizens were started. To provide food and nutrition education during the years when nutrition has the most crucial impact on growth, development, and future health, a supplemental food and nutrition program (WIC Program) was established for pregnant and breastfeeding women, infants, and children who were of low income and were nutritionally at risk. The result of these efforts was that food insecurity diminished as a serious problem for this country. Now, however, food insecurity is increasing as a result of rising poverty and cuts in government aid.

What are people doing to help reduce problems of food insecurity? To help remedy the lack of federal solutions, concerned citizens are working through community programs and churches to provide meals to the hungry. **Second Harvest,** the nation's largest supplier of surplus food, distributed over 476.4 million pounds of food (up 18 percent from 1989) to nearly 200 **food banks** and some 50,000 agencies for direct distribution around the nation in 1990.[57] However, even the dramatic increases in the number of food banks, **food pantries, soup kitchens, prepared and perishable food programs,** and other emergency food assistance programs across the nation cannot keep pace with the growth in the number of hungry people seeking food assistance. Each day's worth of meals lasts only for that day, leaving the problem of poverty unsolved, as before. Moreover, one out of every five needy people is not even receiving meals. These people are left to scavenge garbage, to steal food or money to buy food, or to continue to starve.

Exactly how many people in the United States are homeless, and who are the homeless? Estimates of the number of homeless vary and range from 600,000 to 3 million. In addition, nearly 3 million people spend more than 70 percent of their income on rent and are at risk of becoming homeless.[58] The U.S. Conference of Mayors surveyed 28 major cities to assess the status of hunger and homelessness in the urban United States during 1992. Lack of food, inadequate diets, poor nutritional status, and nutrition-related health problems— stunted growth, failure to thrive, low-birth-weight babies, infant mortality, anemia, and compromised immune systems—are common among homeless persons.[59] Increasing numbers of people living with the HIV virus are homeless as a result of the high costs of health care or lack of supportive housing.[60]

The lack of affordable housing leads the list of causes of homelessness identified by the mayors. Without adequate low-income housing, many poor people are forced to choose between shelter and food. Other causes of homelessness include unemployment, underemployment, poverty, inadequate public assistance benefit levels, the high cost of health care, substance abuse and lack of needed services, and mental illness and the lack of needed services. Children accounted for 24 percent of the homeless population in the cities surveyed by the Conference of Mayors.[61]

How are farm families affected by hunger? Changes in the domestic economy are adverse not only on the receiving end but also on the producing end. U.S. farmers today lack significant control over what products they produce, what prices they must pay for supplies, and what prices they receive in return for their commodities. Just before 1980, the USDA urged farmers to increase corn and soybean production for export. To

comply, farmers borrowed heavily to expand their production capabilities. Since that time, the costs to farmers for seed, fertilizer, equipment, and loans have steadily risen while crop prices have declined. Today, thousands of U.S. farmers are hungry, frustrated, and at the point of desperation concerning their debt.[62]

The number of hungry farm families is not known, but agencies that provide aid to the rural poor say the demand for food assistance is increasing. Ironically, farm families do not generally grow fruits, vegetables, and other crops and animals to feed themselves. With modern practices aimed at efficiency, most farmers raise two or three crops—for example, feed, corn, sorghum, and wheat—and buy most of the food they eat themselves from the grocery store. As a result, when crop prices drop, farmers struggle to survive under the sagging prices and realize no significant profits. Eventually, the farmers go out of business entirely from lack of profits, just as would happen in any other type of business in the United States.

How does world hunger differ from hunger in the United States? World hunger is more extreme than domestic hunger. In fact, most people would find it hard to imagine the severity of poverty in the developing world:

> Many hundreds of millions of people in the poorest countries are preoccupied solely with survival and elementary needs. For them, work is frequently not available, or pay is low, and conditions barely tolerable. Homes are constructed of impermanent materials and have neither piped water nor sanitation. Electricity is a luxury. Health services are thinly spread, and in rural areas only rarely within walking distance. Permanent insecurity is the condition of the poor . . . in the wealthy countries, ordinary men and women face genuine economic problems. . . . But they

> rarely face anything resembling the total deprivation found in the poor countries.[63]

World hunger is a problem of supply and demand, of inappropriate technology, of environmental abuse, of demographic distribution, of unequal access to resources, of extremes in dietary patterns, and of unjust economic systems. Oftentimes, people who are poor are powerless to change their situation because they have less access to vital resources such as education, training, food, and health services.

How are international trade and debt connected to hunger? Over the years, developing countries have seen the prices of imported fuels and manufactured items rise much faster than the prices they receive for their export goods (such as bananas, coffee, and various raw materials) on the international market. The combination of high import costs with low export profits often pushes a developing country into accelerating international debt that sometimes leads to bankruptcy.

Debt and trade are closely related to the progress a country can make toward achieving an adequate diet for its people. As import prices increase relative to export prices, more of a country's total money base moves abroad to pay for the imports. With more and more of its money abroad, the country is forced to borrow money, usually at high interest rates, to continue functioning at home. Many of its financial resources must then go to pay the interest on the borrowed money, thus draining the economy further. Creditor nations may not demand much, or any, capital back, but they do require that interest be paid each year, and the interest can consume most of a country's gross national product. Large and growing debts can slow or halt a nation's attempt to deal effectively with its problems of local food insecurity. As more and more of its financial resources are being used to pay off interest on the country's trade debts, less and less money is available to deal with food insecurity at home. Each year, the debt crisis worsens and leads to further problems with hunger.

What about the role of multinational corporations in this issue? Typically, large landowners and **multinational corporations** hire indigenous people for below-subsistence wages to work in the fertile farmlands growing crops to be exported for profit, leaving little fertile land for the local farmers to use to grow food. The local people work hard cultivating cash crops for others, not food crops for themselves. The money they earn is not even enough to buy the products they help to produce. They do not adequately share in the profits realized from the marketing of products grown with their labor. The results: imported foods—bananas, beef, cocoa, coconuts, coffee, pineapples, sugar, tea, winter tomatoes, and others—fill the grocery stores of developed countries, while the poor who labored to grow these foods have less food and fewer resources than when they farmed the land for their own use. Additional cropland is diverted for nonfood, cash crops—tobacco, rubber, cotton, and other agricultural products. These practices have also had an adverse effect on the financial status of many U.S. farmers. The foreign cash crops often undersell the same U.S.-grown produce. The U.S. farmer cannot compete against these lower-priced imported foods and may be forced out of business.

Besides diverting acreage away from the traditional staples of the local diet, some multinational corporations may also contribute to hunger as a result of their marketing techniques. Their advertisements lead many consumers with limited incomes to associate such products as cola beverages, cigarettes, infant formulas, and snack foods with good health and prosperity. Such promotions are tragically inappropriate for these people. A poor family's nutrition status suffers when its tight budget is pinched further by the purchase of such unnecessary goods.

How does overpopulation fit into the picture? The current world population is approximately 5 billion, and for the year 2000, the projected United Nations figure is 6 billion. The earth may not be able to adequately support this many people. The world's present population is certainly of concern, as is the projected increase in that population. As important as the population question is, it is only one cause of the world food problem. Poverty seems to be at the root of both problems—hunger and overpopulation.

Three major factors affect population growth: birthrates, death rates, and standards of living. Low-income countries have high birthrates, high death rates, and low standards of living.

As the world's population continues to grow, it threatens the world's capacity to produce adequate food. The activity of billions of human beings on the earth's limited surface is seriously and adversely affecting our planet: wiping out many of the varieties of plant life, heating up our climate, using up our freshwater supplies, and destroying the protective ozone layer that shields life from the sun's damaging rays—in short, overstraining the earth's ability to support life. Population control is one of the most pressing needs of this time in history.

Is there a better way to distribute world resources? Land reform—giving people a meaningful opportunity to produce food for local consumption for example—can combine with population control to increase everyone's assets. Poor nations must be allowed to increase their agricultural productivity. Much is involved, but to put it simply, poor nations must gain greater access to five things simultaneously: land, capital, water, technology, and knowledge.[64] Equally important, each nation must adopt the political priority of improving the conditions of all its people. International food aid may be required temporarily during the development period, but eventually this aid will become less and less necessary.

Governments can learn from recent history the importance of developing local agricultural technology. A major effort made in the 1960s and 1970s—the green revolution—demonstrated the potential for increased grain production in Asia. It was an effort to bring the agricultural technology of the industrial world to the developing countries, but the high-yielding strains of wheat and rice that were selected required irrigation, chemical fertilizers, and pesticides—all costly and beyond the economic means of too many of the farmers in the developing world.

Instead of transplanting industrial technology into the developing countries, small, efficient farms and local structures for marketing, credit, transportation, food storage, and agricultural education should be developed. International research centers need to examine the conditions of tropical countries and orient their research toward **appropriate technology**—labor-intensive rather than energy-intensive agricultural methods. For example, labor-intensive technology, such as the use of manual grinders for grains, is appropriate in some places because it makes the best use of human, financial, and natural resources. A manual grinder can process 20 pounds of grain per hour, replacing the mortar and pestle, which in the same time can pound a maximum of only 3 pounds.[65] The specific technology that is appropriate for use varies from situation to situation.

MINIGLOSSARY

APPROPRIATE TECHNOLOGY a technology that utilizes locally abundant resources in preference to locally scarce resources. Developing countries usually have a large labor force and little capital; the appropriate technology would therefore be labor intensive.

FAMINE widespread lack of access to food caused by natural disasters, political factors, or war; characterized by a large number of deaths due to starvation and malnutrition.

FOOD BANKS nonprofit community organizations that collect surplus commodities from the government and edible but often unmarketable foods from private industry for use by nonprofit charities, institutions, and feeding programs at nominal cost.

FOOD INSECURITY the inability to acquire or consume an adequate quality or sufficient quantity of food in socially acceptable ways, or the uncertainty that one will be able to do so.

FOOD PANTRIES centers usually attached to existing nonprofit agencies that distribute bags or boxes of groceries to people experiencing food emergencies. Foods distributed by pantries are prepared and consumed elsewhere. Referrals or proof of need is often required. There are roughly two food pantries to every soup kitchen.

FOOD SECURITY access by all people at all times to enough food for an active and healthy life. Food security has two aspects: ensuring that adequate food supplies are available and ensuring that households whose members suffer from undernutrition have the ability to acquire food, either by producing it themselves or by being able to purchase it.

GOBI an acronym formed from the elements of UNICEF's Child Survival campaign—**G**rowth charts, **O**ral rehydration therapy, **B**reast milk, and **I**mmunization.

MALNUTRITION the impairment of health resulting from a relative deficiency or excess of food energy and specific nutrients necessary for health.

MULTINATIONAL CORPORATIONS international companies with direct investments and/or operative facilities in more than one country. U.S. oil and food companies are examples.

ORAL REHYDRATION THERAPY (ORT) the treatment of dehydration (usually due to diarrhea caused by infectious disease) with an oral solution; ORT as developed by UNICEF is intended to enable a mother to mix a simple solution for her child from substances that she has at home.

POVERTY the state of having too little money to meet minimum needs for food, clothing, and shelter. The U.S. Department of Health and Human Services defines the poverty level in the United States as an annual income of $14,350 for a family of four.

PREPARED AND PERISHABLE FOOD PROGRAMS (PPFPs) nonprofit programs that help to feed people in need by linking sources of unused, unserved cooked and fresh food—such as caterers, restaurants, hotel kitchens, and cafeterias—with social service agencies that serve meals to people who would otherwise go hungry. *Foodchain* is the national network of over 125 community-based PPFPs in 41 states and Canada.

SECOND HARVEST a national food banking network to which the majority of food banks belong.

SOUP KITCHEN small feeding operations attached to existing organizations such as churches, civic groups, or nonprofit agencies that serve prepared meals that are consumed on site. Soup kitchens generally do not require clients to prove need or show identification.

UNDER-FIVE MORTALITY RATE (U5MR) the number of children who die before the age of five for every 1,000 live births.

UNDERNUTRITION (also called **HUNGER**) as used in this discussion, a term that describes the domestic and world food problem of a continuous lack of the food energy and nutrients necessary to achieve and maintain health and protection from disease.

UNICEF the United Nations International Children's Emergency Fund, now referred to as the United Nations Children's Fund.

XEROPHTHALMIA (ZEER-AHF-THALL-ME-UH) a severe form of eye disease in which the cornea hardens and may cause blindness. The problem results from vitamin A deficiency.

The cornerstone of true development was best expressed decades ago by Mahatma Gandhi: "Whenever you are in doubt . . . apply the following test. Recall the face of the poorest and the weakest man whom you may have seen, and ask yourself if the step you contemplate is going to be of any use to him. Will he gain anything by it? Will it restore him to a control over his own life and destiny?"[66]

Environmental concerns must be taken more seriously as well. As important as the amount of land available for crop production is the condition of the soil and the availability of water. Soil erosion is now accelerating on every continent at a rate that threatens the world's ability to continue feeding itself.[67] Erosion of soil has always occurred; it is a natural process. But in the past, it has been compensated for by processes that build the soil up, such as the growth of trees.

Where forest has already been converted to farmland and there are no trees, farmers should alternate soil-devouring crops with soil-building crops, a practice known as crop rotation. When farmers must choose whether to make three times as much money planting corn year after year or to rotate crops and possibly go bankrupt, many choose the short-term profits. Ruin may not follow immediately, but it will follow.[68]

Is there hope for a world without hunger for women and children? Women make up 50 percent of the world's population. Any solution to the problems of poverty and hunger is incomplete and even hopeless if it fails to address the role of women in developing countries, for women and their children represent the majority of those living in poverty.

In many countries, over 90 percent of the population live in rural areas. The life of a woman living in rural poverty is oppressive. Typically, these women not only are the primary food producers but also are responsible for child care and food preparation. Often they have to work as harvesters on other people's lands as well. Husbands are frequently required to be absent from their homes, not by choice but because the changing global economy has forced many men to leave home in search of wages.

Women play a vital role in the nutrition of their nation's people. Their nutrition during pregnancy and lactation determines the future health of their children. If women are weakened by malnutrition themselves or are ignorant about how to feed their families, the consequences ripple outward to affect many other individuals. The importance of the role women play in these countries is increasingly appreciated, and many countries now offer development programs with women in mind.

Seven basic strategies are at the heart of women's programs:

- Removing barriers to financial credit.
- Providing access to time-saving technologies.
- Providing appropriate training to promote self-reliance.
- Teaching management and marketing skills.
- Making health and day-care services available.
- Forming women's support groups.[69]
- Providing information and technology to promote planned pregnancies.

The recognition of women's needs by some development organizations is an encouraging trend in the efforts to contend with the world hunger crisis.

There is hopeful news for children in developing countries—the group that is most strongly affected by poverty, malnutrition, and food insecurity and its relationship to the environment.[70] **GOBI,** a child survival plan set forth by UNICEF, has made outstanding progress in cutting the number of hunger-related child deaths. GOBI is an acronym formed from four simple, but profoundly important, elements of UNICEF's Child Survival campaign: **g**rowth charts, **o**ral rehydration therapy (ORT), **b**reast milk, and **i**mmunization.

A mother can learn to weigh her child every month and chart the child's growth on a specially designed paper growth chart. She can learn to detect for herself the early stages of hidden malnutrition that can leave a child irreparably retarded in mind and body. Then at least she can know she needs to take steps to remedy the malnutrition—if she can.

The importance of oral rehydration therapy (ORT) is that most children who die of malnutrition do not starve to death—they die because their health has been compromised by dehydration from infections causing diarrhea. Until recently, there was no easy way of stopping the infection-diarrhea cycle and saving their lives. Now, the spread of ORT is preventing an estimated one million dehydration deaths each year.[71] Oral rehydration therapy is the administration of a simple solution that mothers can make up themselves, using locally available ingredients, which increases a body's ability to absorb fluids 25-fold.[72] International development groups also provide mothers with packets of premeasured salt and sugar to be mixed with water in rural and urban areas. A safe and sanitary supply of drinking water is a prerequisite for the success of the ORT program.

The promotion of breastfeeding among mothers in developing countries has many benefits. Breast milk is hygienic, is readily available, is nutritionally sound, and provides infants with immunologic protection specific for their environment. In the developing world, the advantages of breast-feeding over formula feeding can mean the difference between life and death.

Immunizations (the *I* of GOBI) could prevent most of the 5 million deaths each year from measles, diphtheria, tetanus, whooping cough, poliomyelitis, and tuberculosis. Adequate protein nutrition is necessary, however, for vaccinations to be useful so that the protein in the vaccine itself is not used by the body as a source of protein. The immunization achievements of the 1980s are credited with the prevention of approximately 3 million deaths a year as well as the protection of many millions more from disease, malnutrition, blindness, deafness, and polio.[73]

The first World Summit for Children in history was convened by UNICEF in September of 1990, bringing together representatives of 159 nations for the purpose of making a renewed commitment to ending child deaths and child malnutrition on today's scale by the year 2000.

Significantly, *nutrition* was mentioned for the first time in world history as an internationally recognized human right.[74] An immediate result of this summit has been an increase in the number of governments actively adopting the child survival strategies of UNICEF—universal immunization, oral rehydration therapy, a massive effort to promote breastfeeding as the ideal food for at least the first four to six months of an infant's life, an attack on malnutrition involving nutrition surveillance focusing on growth monitoring and weighing of infants at least once every month for the first 18 months of the child's life, and nutrition and literacy education that will empower women in developing countries and lead to a reduction in nutrition-related diseases among vulnerable children.[75]

What can I do to help alleviate hunger problems? The problems of hunger can appear so great that they sometimes seem approachable only by way of worldwide political decisions. Indeed, the members of the International Conference on Nutrition stressed that worldwide efforts to overcome hunger and malnutrition and to foster self-reliant development must be intensive. To this end, many individuals and groups are working to improve the chances of the future well-being of the world and its people through a number of national and international organizations.*

Solutions to the hunger problem depend on people's willingness to take action and to work together. Regardless of the type and level of involvement a person chooses, each person can make a difference. Individual people can do any of following:

● Assist in government programs as volunteers.

● Help to develop means of informing low-income people of food-related services and programs for which they are eligible.

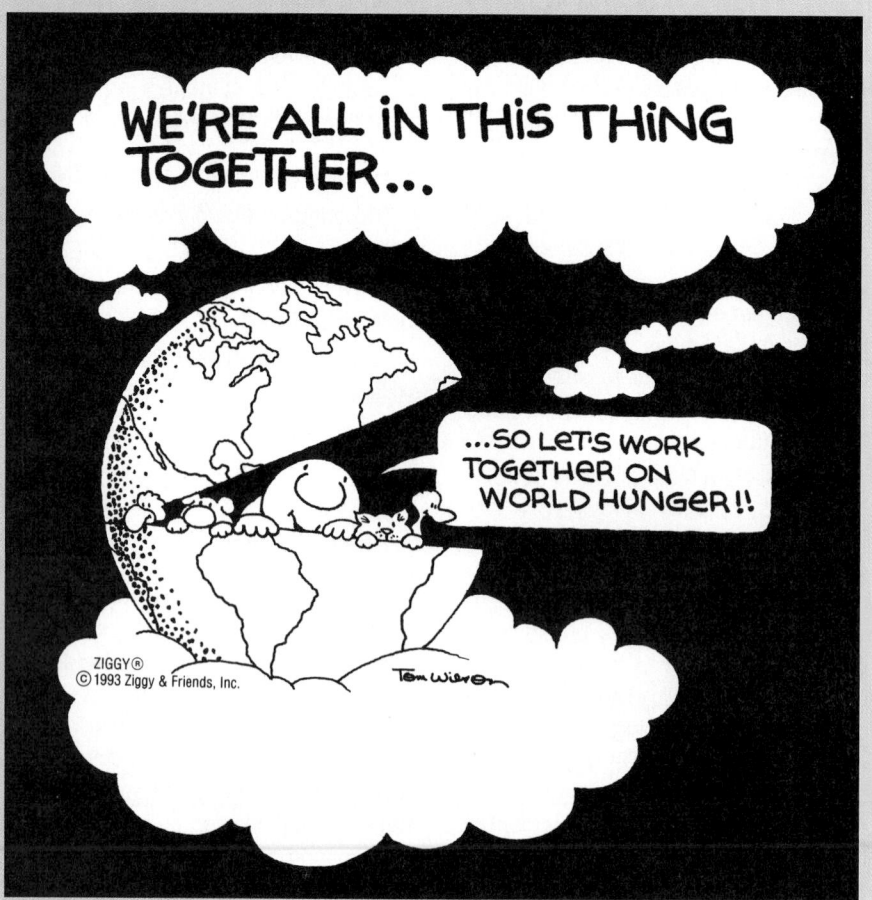

WE'RE ALL IN THIS THING TOGETHER...

...SO LET'S WORK TOGETHER ON WORLD HUNGER!!

ZIGGY®
© 1993 Ziggy & Friends, Inc.

● Help to increase the accessibility of existing programs and services to those who need them.

● Document the needs that exist in their own communities.

● Join with others in the community who have similar interests (support groups that speak for the poor).

● Follow current hunger legislation, call and write legislators about hunger issues, lobby to draw political attention to the need for more job opportunities and a higher minimum wage.

Individuals can also help change the world through the personal choices they make each day.[76] Our choices have an impact on the way the rest of the world's people live and die. Our nation, with 6 percent of the world's population, con-

sumes about 40 percent of the world's food and energy resources. People in affluent nations have the freedom and means to choose their lifestyles. We can find ways to reduce our consumption of the world's nonrenewable resources and use only what is absolutely required.

Choosing a diet at the level of necessity rather than excess would reduce the resource demands made by our industrial agriculture. In fact, those who study the future are convinced that the hope of the world lies in everyone's adopting a simple lifestyle. As one such person put it, "the widespread simplification of life is vital to the well-being of the entire human family."[77] Personal lifestyles do matter, for a society is nothing more than the sum of its individuals. As we go, so goes our world.

---

*Organizations and groups working to end world hunger are listed in Appendix A.

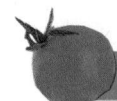

CHECK YOURSELF...

1. Name four of the top ten causes of microbial food contamination.

2. Identify three things you can do to reduce your risk of eating a food contaminated with *E. coli* 0157:H7.

3. Explain cross-contamination.

4. List five ways you can reduce the chances of consuming excess lead.

5. Name three functions of food additives.

6. Describe how overpopulation fits into the world hunger picture.

7. Explain how a food chain works.

8. Identify some of the pros and cons of buying organically grown produce.

9. Describe the Delaney clause and its limitations.

10. List three "eco-friendly" claims that might mislead consumers and explain why they can be confusing.

Answers to selected Check Yourself questions are found in Appendix H.

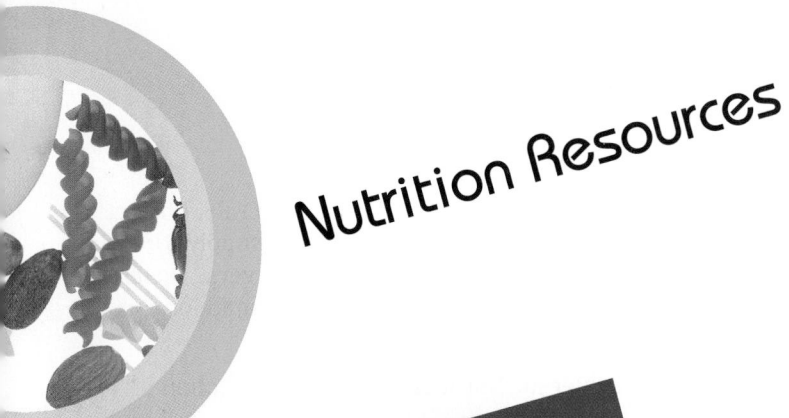

Nutrition Resources

People interested in nutrition often want to know where they can find reliable nutrition information in their own town or county. No matter where you live, there are several sources you can turn to:

- The National Center for Nutrition and Dietetics Consumer Nutrition Hot Line at 1-800-366-1655 is staffed by registered dietitians who will answer food- and nutrition-related questions.

- The Department of Health may have a nutrition expert such as a registered dietitian.

- The local extension agent is often a resource who can provide answers to questions regarding food and nutrition.

- The registered dietitians at your local hospital can serve as sources of reliable nutrition information.

- A nearby college or university may be staffed with knowledgeable professors of nutrition or biochemistry.

Books

Three excellent cookbooks for people wishing to prepare low-fat, heart-healthy meals are the *American Heart Association Cookbook*, 5th ed., New York: Times Books, Random House, 1991; *The Healthy Heart Cookbook*, Birmingham, AL: Oxmoor House, Inc., 1992; *Simply Heartsmart Cooking* by Bonnie Stern, Toronto: Random House of Canada, 1994.

For people with diabetes: *The Joslin Diabetes Gourmet Cookbook* by Bonnie Sanders Polin, PhD, and Frances Towner Giedt, New York: Bantam Books, 1993 and *The American Diabetes Association and The American Dietetic Association Family Cookbook* (Family Cookbook Series v. 1-4), Englewood Cliffs, NJ: Prentice Hall, 1987-1991.

For vegetarian eating: *Laurel's Kitchen Recipes* by Laurel Robertson, Carol Flinders, and Brian Ruppenthal, Berkeley, CA: Ten Speed Press, 1993 and *Moosewood Restaurant Cooks at Home* by The Moosewood Collective, New York: Simon & Schuster/ Fireside, 1994.

For more on sports nutrition: *Eating For Endurance* by Ellen Coleman, Palo Alto, CA: Bull Publishing, 1990 and *Nancy Clark's Sports Nutrition Guidebook* by Nancy Clark, Champaign, IL: Leisure Press, 1990.

For parents: *How to Get Your Kid to Eat . . . But Not Too Much* by Ellyn Satter, Palo Alto, CA: Bull Publishing, 1987.

Journals

Nutrition Today, the publication of the Nutrition Today Society, is an excellent magazine that makes a point of raising controversial issues and providing a forum for conflicting opinions. Six issues per year, from Williams & Wilkins. (See "Addresses" section that follows.)

The *Journal of the American Dietetic Association*, the official publication of the ADA, contains articles of interest to dietitians and nutritionists, news of legislative action on food and nutrition, and a very useful section of abstracts of articles from many other journals of nutrition and related areas. Twelve issues per year, from the American Dietetic Association. (See "Addresses" section that follows.)

Nutrition Reviews, a publication of the International Life Sciences Institute, does much of the work for the library researcher, compiling recent evidence on current topics and presenting extensive bibliographies. Twelve issues per year, from the International Life Sciences Institute. (See "Addresses" section that follows.)

The *Tufts University Diet & Nutrition Letter* is a monthly newsletter that provides up-to-date, easy-to-read, and practical information on nutrition for consumers. (See "Addresses" section that follows.)

Other publications that deserve mention here are *Nutrition and the MD*, the *Journal of Nutrition, Food Technology*, the *American Journal of Clinical Nutrition*, and the *Journal of Nutrition Education. FDA Consumer*, a government publication with many articles of interest to the consumer, is available from the Food and Drug Administration. (See "Addresses" section that follows.) Many of the organizations listed next will provide free publication lists upon request.

Addresses

U.S. Government Agencies

The U.S. Department of Agriculture (USDA) has several divisions. The USDA's Food Safety and Inspection Service (FSIS) inspects and analyzes domestic and imported meat, poultry, and meat and poultry food products; establishes standards and approves recipes and labels of processed meat and poultry products; and monitors the meat and poultry industries for violations of inspection laws. To obtain publications or ask questions, write or call:

FSIS, USDA
Information and Legislative Affairs
Fourteenth and Independence Avenue, SW
2925 South
Washington, D.C. 20250
(202) 690-0351
USDA also maintains a Meat and Poultry Hotline:
1-800-535-4555.

The USDA's Agricultural Research Service (ARS) conducts research to fulfill the diverse needs of agricultural users—from farmers to consumers—in the areas of crop and animal production, protection, processing, and distribution; food safety and quality; and natural resources conservation. Write or call:

ARS, USDA
Information Staff
Room 307, Building 005
BARC—West
Beltsville, MD 20705
(301) 504-6264

The USDA Center for Nutrition Policy and Promotion consists of the Nutrition Education Division from the former Human Nutrition Information Service (HNIS) and the Family Economics Research Group from ARS. Contact the center with questions about the food supply, USDA food plans, dietary analysis of USDA surveys, Dietary Guidelines for Americans, Food Guide Pyramid, or child expenditures.

USDA Center for Nutrition Policy and Promotion
1120 20th St. NW
Suite 200, North Lobby
Washington, D.C. 20036
Nutrition Promotion:
(202) 208-2417
Nutrition Policy:
(202) 208-2331

The USDA's Food and Consumer Service (FCS) administers the Food Stamp Program; the National School Lunch and School Breakfast programs; the Special Supplemental Food Program for Women, Infants, and Children (WIC); and the food distribution, child and adult care food, summer food service, and special milk programs. Write or call:

FCS, USDA
3101 Park Center Drive
Alexandria, VA 22302
(703) 305-2286

The USDA's Agricultural Marketing Service (AMS) operates a variety of marketing programs and services—several of interest to consumers. Its activities include developing grades and standards for the trading of food and other farm products and carrying out grading services on request from packers and processors; inspecting egg products for wholesomeness; administering marketing orders that aid in the marketing of milk, fruits, vegetables, and related specialty crops like nuts; and administering truth-in-seed labeling and other regulatory programs. Write or call:

AMS, USDA
P.O. Box 96456
Washington, D.C. 20090-6456
(202) 720-8998

Other government addresses and telephone numbers follow:

Administration on Aging
330 Independence Avenue, SW
Washington, D.C. 20201
(202) 619-0724

Centers for Disease Control and
   Prevention Information Hotline:
(404) 332-4555

Centers for Disease Control and
   Prevention
Division of Chronic Disease Control and
   Community Intervention
National Center for Chronic Disease
   Prevention and Health Promotion
Community Health Promotion Branch
4770 Buford Highway, NE
Mailstop K-46
Atlanta, GA 30341
(770) 488-5426

Environmental Protection Agency
401 M Street, SW
Washington, D.C. 20460
(202) 260-2090

EPA Safe Drinking Water Hotline:
(800) 426-4791

Federal Trade Commission
Public Reference Branch
Washington, D.C. 20418
(202) 326-2222

Food and Drug Administration
Office of Consumer Affairs
5600 Fishers Lane
HFE 88 Foom 16-59
Rockville, MD 20857
(301) 443-3170

FDA Office of Food Labeling
200 C Street, SW
Washington, D.C. 20204
(202) 205-4561

FDA Seafood Hotline:
(800) FDA-4010

The Food and Nutrition
   Information Center
National Agriculture Library
10301 Baltimore Boulevard,
Room 304
Beltsville, MD 20705-351
(301) 504-5719

National Academy of Sciences/
   National Research Council (NAS/NRC)
2101 Constitution Avenue, NW
Washington, D.C. 20418
(202) 334-2000

National Health Information Center
P.O. Box 1133
Washington, D.C. 20013-1133
(301) 565-4167
(800) 336-4797

Office of Disease Prevention and Health
   Promotion
Public Health Service
U.S. Department of Health and Human
   Services
200 Independence Ave, SW
Room 738G
Washington, D.C. 20201
(202) 205-8611

Consumer and Advocacy Groups

Center on Budget and Policy Priorities
777 N. Capitol Street, NE
Room 705
Washington, D.C. 20002
(202) 408-1080

Center for Science in the Public Interest
1875 Connecticut Avenue, NW
Suite 300
Washington, D.C. 20009
(202) 332-9110

Children's Defense Fund
25 E Street, NW
Washington, D.C. 20001
(202) 628-8787

Children's Foundation
725 Fifteenth Street, NW
Suite 505
Washington, D.C. 20005
(202) 347-3300

Community Nutrition Institute
910 17th Street, NW
Suite 413
Washington, D.C. 20006
(202) 776-0595

Consumer Association of Canada
267 O'Connor St.
Suite 307
Ottawa, Ontario K2P OP7
Canada
(613) 238-2533

The Consumer Information Center
Pueblo, CO 81009
(719) 948-3334

Consumers Union
101 Truman Avenue
Yonkers, N.Y. 10703
(914) 378-2000

Food Research and Action Center
1875 Connecticut Avenue, NW
Suite 540
Washington, D.C. 20009
(202) 986-2200

Interfaith Impact for Justice and Peace
110 Maryland Avenue, NE
Washington, D.C. 20002
(202) 543-2800

National Council of Senior Citizens
1331 F Street, NW
Washington, D.C. 20004
(202) 347-8800

Public Voice for Food and Health Policy
1101 14th Street, NW
Room 710
Washington, D.C. 20005
(202) 371-1840

National Council Against Health
   Fraud, Inc.
P.O. Box 1276
Loma Linda, CA 92354

Nutrition Legislative News
607 4th Street, SW
Washington, D.C. 22024
(202) 488-8879

Urban Institute
2100 M Street, NW, 5th floor
Washington, D.C. 20037
(202) 833-7200

Professional and Service Organizations

AIDS Referral
1620 Eye Street, NW
Washington, D.C. 20006
(202) 293-7330
National AIDS Hotline (CDC):
(800) 342-AIDS (English)
(800) 344-SIDA (Spanish)
(800) 2437-TTY (Deaf)
(900) 820-2437

Alateen
1372 Broadway
New York, NY 10018
(800)356-9996

Alcoholics Anonymous (AA)
World Service
P.O. Box 459
Grand Central Station, NY 10164
(212) 870-3400

Alzheimer's Disease
Information and Referral Service
919 North Michigan Avenue
Chicago, IL 60611
(800) 272-3900

Al-Anon Family Group Headquarters
862 Midtown Station
New York, NY 10018
(212) 302-7240
(800) 356-9996

Alcohol and Drug Abuse
Information Line:
(800) 252-6465

Alliance for Food and Fiber
Food Safety Hotline:
(800) 266-0200

American Academy of Pediatrics
141 Northwest Point Boulevard
Elk Grove Village, IL 60009
(708) 228-5005

American Anorexia/Bulimia
Association, Inc.
293 Central Park West
Suite 1R
New York, NY 10024
(212) 501-8351

American Association of Family and
Consumer Sciences
1555 King Street
Alexandria, VA 22314
(703) 706-4600

American Association of Retired Persons
601 E Street, NW
Washington, D.C. 20049
(202) 434-2277

American Cancer Society
Cancer Information Center
3710 W. Jetton Avenue
Tampa, FL 33629
(800) ACS-2345

American College of Sports Medicine
P.O. Box 1440
Indianapolis, IN 46204
(317) 637-9200

American Council on Science and Health
1995 Broadway, 2nd floor
New York, NY 10023
(212) 362-7044

American Dental Association
211 East Chicago Avenue
Chicago, IL 60611
(312) 440-2500

American Diabetes Association
1660 Duke Street
Alexandria, VA 22314
(703) 549-1500
(800) 232-3472

American Dietetic Association
216 West Jackson Boulevard
Suite 800
Chicago, IL 60606-6995
(312) 899-0040

American Health Foundation
320 E. 43rd Street
New York, NY 10017
(212) 953-1900

American Heart Association
7272 Greenville Avenue
Dallas, TX 75231
(214) 373-6300
(800) 242-8721

American Institute for Cancer Research
1759 R Street, NW
Washington, D.C. 20009
(202) 328-7744
(800) 843-8114

American Institute of Nutrition
9650 Rockville Pike
Bethesda, MD 20814
(301) 530-7050

American Medical Association
515 North State Street
Chicago, IL 60610
(312) 464-5000

American Public Health Association
1015 Fifteenth Street, NW
Washington, D.C. 20005
(202) 789-5600

American Public Welfare Association
(Food Stamp Program Administrators)
810 First Street, NE
Suite 500
Washington, D.C. 20002
(202) 682-0100

American Red Cross
National Headquarters
430 Seventeenth Street, NW
Washington, D.C. 20006
(202) 737-8300

American School Food Service Association
(Child Nutrition Program Personnel)
1600 Duke Street, 7th floor
Alexandria, VA 22314
(703) 739-3900

American SIDS (Sudden Infant Death)
Institute Information Line:
(800) 232-SIDS

American Society for Clinical Nutrition
9650 Rockville Pike
Bethesda, MD 20814
(301) 530-7110

Anorexia Nervosa and Related Eating
Disorders, Inc.
P.O. Box 5102
Eugene, Oregon 97405
(503) 344-1144

Arthritis Foundation
Information Line:
(800) 283-7800

Asthma and Allergy Foundation
of America
Information Line:
(800) 727-8462

Canadian Diabetes Association
15 Toronto Street
Suite 1001
Toronto, Ontario M5C 2E3
Canada
(416) 363-0177

Canadian Dietetic Association
480 University Avenue
Suite 601
Toronto, Ontario M5G 1V2, Canada
(416) 596-0857

Canadian Public Health Association
Publications, Suite 400
1565 Carling Avenue
Ottawa, Ontario K1Z 8R1
Canada

Institute of Food Technologists
221 North LaSalle Street
Chicago, IL 60601
(312) 782-8424

International Life Sciences Institute—
Nutrition Foundation
1126 Sixteenth Street, NW
Suite 111
Washington, D.C. 20036
(202) 659-0074

La Leche League International, Inc.
9616 Minneapolis Avenue
Franklin Park, IL 60131
(800) 525-3243

March of Dimes Birth Defects Foundation
National Headquarters
1275 Mamaroneck Avenue
White Plains, NY 10605
(914) 428-7100

Narcotics Anonymous (NA)
P.O. Box 9999
Van Nuys, CA 91409
(818) 773-9999

National Association for Sickle Cell
Disease Information Line:
(800) 421-8453

National Association of Anorexia Nervosa
and Associated Disorders (ANAD)
P.O. Box 7
Highland Park, IL 60035
(708) 831-3438

National Association of WIC Directors
P.O. Box 53355
Washington, D.C. 20009
(202) 232-5492

National Child Abuse Hotline:
(800) 422-4453

National Council on Alcoholism
2522 St. Paul Street
Baltimore, MD 21218
(800) 527-5344

National Eating Disorder
Information Centre of Canada
200 Elizabeth Street,
College Wing 211
Toronto, Ontario M5G 2C4
Canada
(416) 340-4156

National Osteoporosis Foundation
1150 17th Street, NW
Suite 500
Washington, D.C. 20036
(202) 223-2226

National Pesticide Telecommunications
Network
Agricultural Chemistry Extension
Oregon State University
333 Weniger Hall
Corvallis, OR 97331
NPTN Hotline: (800) 858-PEST

National Safety Council Lead Poisoning
Hotline:
(800) 532-3394

Nutrition Information Service
University of Alabama at Birmingham
Room 447 Webb Building
UAB Station
Birmingham, AL 35294-3360
(800) 231-DIET

Nutrition Screening Initiative
1010 Wisconsin Avenue, NW
Suite 800
Washington, D.C. 20007
(202) 625-1662

Overeaters Anonymous (OA)
6075 Zenith Court, NE
Rio Ranchio, NM 87124
(505) 891-2664

Pennsylvania State Nutrition Center
The Pennsylvania State University
Ruth Building
417 East Calder Way
University Park, PA 16802-5663
(814) 865-6323

PM, Inc.
(Publisher of *Nutrition and the MD*)
Lippincott Raven Publishers
P.O. Box 1610
Hagerstown, MD 21741
(800) 777-2295

Society for Nutrition Education
2001 Killebrew Drive
Suite 340
Minneapolis, MN 55425
(612) 854-0035

Tufts University Diet & Nutrition Letter
Six Beacon Street
Suite 1110
Boston, MA 02108
(800) 274-7581

Weight Watchers
175 Crossways Park W
Woodbury, NY 11797
(800) 651-6000

Williams & Wilkins
(Publisher of *Nutrition Today*)
351 W. Camden Street
Baltimore, MD 21201
(410) 528-4000

Trade Organizations

American Egg Board
1460 Renaissance Drive
Park Ridge, IL 60068
(708) 296-7043

American Meat Institute
1700 North Moore Street
Suite 1600
Arlington, VA 22209
(703) 841-2400

Beech-Nut
Nutrition Corporation
P.O. Box 618
St. Louis, MO 63188
(800) 523-6633

Best Foods
Consumer Service Department
Division of CPC International
International Plaza
P.O. Box 8000
Englewood Cliffs, NJ 07632
(201) 894-4000

Borden Farm Products
Borden Company
Consumer Affairs
180 East Broad Street
Columbus, OH 43215
(614) 225-4000

Campbell Soup Company
Campbell Place
Camden, NJ 08103-1799
(609) 342-4800

General Mills
Nutrition Department
P.O. Box 1113
Minneapolis, MN 55440
(612) 540-2311

Gerber Products Company
445 State Street
Fremont, MI 49413
(616) 928-2000

H. J. Heinz
Consumer Relations
P.O. Box 57
Pittsburgh, PA 15230
(412) 456-5700

Hunt-Wesson Foods
1645 West Valencia Drive
Fullerton, CA 92633
(714) 680-1000

Kellogg Company
Battle Creek, MI 49016-1986
(616) 961-2000

Kraft General Foods Consumer Center
250 North Street
White Plains, NY 10625
(914) 335-2500

Mead Johnson Nutritionals
2400 West Lloyd Expressway
Evansville, IN 47721
(812) 429-5000

Nabisco Consumer Affairs
100 DeForest Avenue
East Hanover, NJ 07936
(800) 932-7800
(800) NABISCO

National Cattlemen's Beef Association
444 North Michigan Avenue
Chicago, IL 60611
(312) 467-5520

National Dairy Council
O'Hare International Center
10255 West Higgins Road
Suite 900
Rosemont, IL 60018-5616
(708) 803-2000

Nestlé Company
Consumer Affairs
800 N. Brand Boulevard
Glendale, N.Y. 91203
(800) 637-8537

NutraSweet Simplesse Company
P.O. Box 830
Deerfield, IL 60015
(800) 321-7254

Oscar Mayer Company
P.O. Box 7188
Madison, WI 53707
(608) 241-3311

Pillsbury Company
200 South Sixth Street
Minneapolis, MN 55402-1464
(612) 330-4966

The Potato Board
7555 E. Hampton Avenue
Suite 412
Denver, CO 80231
(303) 369-7783

Procter and Gamble Company
One Procter and Gamble Plaza
Cincinnati, OH 45202
(513) 983-1100

Rice Council
P.O. Box 740123
Houston, TX 77274
(713) 270-6699

Ross Laboratories
Abbott Laboratory
625 Cleveland Avenue
Columbus, OH 43215
(614) 624-7900
(800) 227-5767

Soy Protein Council
1255 23rd Street, NW
Washington, D.C. 20037
(202) 467-6610

Sunkist Growers
Consumer Service, Division BB
Box 7888
Valley Annex
Van Nuys, CA 91409
(818) 986-4800

United Fresh Fruit and Vegetable
   Association
727 N. Washington Street
Alexandria, VA 22314
(703) 836-3410

Vitamin Nutrition Information
   Service (VNIS)
Hoffman-LaRoche, Inc.
340 Kingsland Street
Nutley, NJ 07110
(201) 235-5000

Organizations Concerned with Hunger and Poverty

Bread for the World Institute
1100 Wayne Avenue
Suite 1000
Silver Spring, MD 20910
(301) 608-2400
For legislative updates:
(301) 588-7439

CARE
Office of Education
151 Ellis Street
Atlanta, GA 30303
(404) 681-2552

Catholic Relief Services
209 West Fayette Street
Baltimore, MD 21201-3443
(410) 625-2220
(800) 235-2772

Center on Hunger, Poverty,
and Nutrition Policy
Tufts University School of Nutrition
11 Curtis Avenue
Medford, MA 02155
(617) 627-3956

Church World Service/CROP
P.O. Box 968
Elkhart, IN 46515
(219) 264-3102
(800) 456-1310

End Hunger Network
365 Sycamore Road
Santa Monica, CA 90402
(310) 454-3716

Food and Agriculture Organization (FAO)
North American Regional Office
1001 22nd Street, NW
Washington, D.C. 20437
(202) 653-2402

Foodchain
970 Jefferson Street
Atlanta, GA 30318
(800) 845-3008

Freedom from Hunger
P.O. Box 2000
1644 DaVinci Court
Davis, CA 95617
(916) 758-6200

The Hunger Project
15 E. 26th Street
Suite 401, 14th floor
New York, NY 10010
(212) 532-4255

Institute for Food and Development Policy
398 60th Street
Oakland, CA 94618
(510) 654-4400

Oxfam America
26 West Street
Boston, MA 02111
(617) 482-1211

Second Harvest
116 Michigan Avenue
Room 4
Chicago, IL 60603
(312) 263-2303

Seeds
P.O. Box 6170
Waco, TX 76706
(817) 755-7745

UNICEF
Information Division
3 UN Plaza
New York, NY 10017
(212) 326-7000

U.S. Agency for International
Development
Office of Nutrition
2201 C Street, NW
Washington, D.C. 20523
(202) 647-4000

U.S. Conference of Mayors
1620 Eye Street, NW,
4th Floor
Washington, D.C. 20006
(202) 293-7330

U.S. National Committee
for World Food Day
1001 22nd Street, NW
Washington, D.C. 20437
(202) 653-2404

World Health Organization
Regional Office
525 23rd Street, NW
Washington, D.C. 20037
(202) 861-3200

World Hunger Education Service
P.O. Box 29056
Washington, D.C. 20017
(202) 298-9503

World Hunger Year
505 8th Avenue
21st floor
New York, NY 10018
(212) 629-8850

World Vision
815-100
P.O. Box 9716
Federal Way, WA 98063
(206) 815-1000

Worldwatch Institute
1776 Massachusetts Avenue, NW
Washington, D.C. 20036
(202) 452-1999

Canadian Government

Federal

Bureau of Nutritional Sciences
Food Directorate
Health Protection Branch
Health Canada
Banting Building
Tunney's Pasture
Ottawa, Ontario K1A OL2
Canada
(613) 957-0911

Nutrition Program Officer
Epidemiology and Community Health,
Indian and Northern Health Services
Health Canada
1911 C, 11th floor
Jeanne Mance Building
Tunney's Pasture
Ottawa, Ontario K1A OL3, Canada
(613) 954-7757

Nutrition Programs Unit
Health Promotion Directorate
Health Canada
Room 456, Jeanne Mance Building
Tunney's Pasture
Ottawa, Ontario K1A 1B4, Canada
(613) 957-8328

Clearinghouses and Information Centers

National Clearinghouse on Bilingual
Education
1118 22nd Street NW
Washington, D.C. 20037
(202) 467-0867

National Clearinghouse for Alcohol and
Drug Information (NCADI)
P.O. Box 2345
Rockville, MD 20847
(301) 468-2600
(800) 729-6686

Cancer Information Service
National Cancer Institute
Information Resources Branch
Bethesda, MD 20892
(800) 4-CANCER
(800) 638-6070 (in Alaska)
(808) 524-1234 (in Oahu, Hawaii)

National Heart, Lung, and Blood
   Institute (NHLBI)
NHLBI Information Center
P.O. Box 30105
Bethesda, MD 20824-0105
(301) 251-1222

National Maternal and Child Health
   Clearinghouse
2070 Chainbridge Road
Suite 450
Vienna, VA 22182
(703) 821-8955

Superintendent of Documents
U.S. Government Printing Office
P.O. Box 371954
Pittsburgh, PA 15250
(202) 512-1800

Selected Sources of Nutrition Information on the Internet

The Internet is a giant collection of worldwide computer networks, consisting of millions of individual computers and users. These users make up small networks, which link together to form regional networks, which then are joined by a "backbone" network to form national and international networks.

Contributors to the Internet include government, academic, commercial, and nonprofit organizations from all over the world. Most users access the Internet by connecting to a "host" computer that belongs to one of these participants. A multitude of commercial vendors also provides access to the Internet. Typically, these vendors offer a variety of Internet services so that subscribers may choose the ones that suit their needs and their equipment:

America Online, Inc.
8619 Westwood Center Dr.
Vienna, VA 22182
(703) 448-8700

CompuServe, Inc.
5000 Arlington Centre Blvd.
Columbus, OH 43220
(614) 457-8650

NewsNet, Inc.
945 Haverford Rd.
Bryn Mawr, PA 19010
(215) 527-8030

Prodigy Services Company
445 Hamilton Ave.
White Plains, NY 10601
(914) 993-8000

Some states provide Internet access for citizens through public libraries and universities. Check with your local library to find out about public service Internet connections in your area.

On the Internet's World Wide Web System, you can find hundreds of sophisticated web sites that have free nutrition resources, research, healthful recipes, government reports, program information, and more. Here is a listing of a selection of nutrition web sites that may help you . . . and they charge nothing for access.*

Get on the web through the "addresses" listed here. Often you can reach sites through different routes, such as gopher and "http." When more than one address is listed, all are useable depending on your access capability. While this list is not comprehensive, it provides a starting point. Moreover, these sites offer "links"—easy access to other related web sites. New nutrition-related home pages open every day and changes are ongoing. Most of the web sites listed here offer consumer-oriented nutrition information as well as resources geared towards professionals.

Government

Department of Agriculture
http://www.usda.gov
http://gopher.nalusda.gov/
Main home page features Guidance of the Administration on the Farm Bill and program descriptions and missions. While many resources are available, often they lead to dead ends, like the "USDA News" service.

- **Food and Nutrition Information Center**
  http://www.nalusda.gov/fnic.html.
  gopher.nalusda.gov
  Features information on food safety and labeling, food guide pyramid and federal regulations.

- **International Food and Nutrition Database**
  Pennsylvania State University
  Gopher to psupen.psu.edu. Search keyword: FNIC
  (Also accessible via: Telnet to psupen.psu.edu. At prompt, type your two-letter state abbreviation.)
  Provides a full-text service.

*The listing of Internet addresses is reprinted from: Community Nutrition Institute, *Nutrition Week,* September 8, 1995.

- **Nutrient Data Bank Bulletin Board**
  Agricultural Research Service
  http://www.inform.umd.edu
  gopher to inform.umd.edu. Select "Educational Resources," "Academic Resources by Topic," "Agriculture and Environment."
  Focuses on the nutrient composition of foods. Also offers FNIC's food composition-related bibliographies.

- **USDA economics and statistics information**
  Cornell University's Mann Library Gateway
  http://usda.mannlib.cornell.edu

- **HACCP Training Program**
  http://www.nalusda.gov/fnic.html
  HACCP (Hazard Analysis Critical Control Points) training programs and resource database.

Food and Drug Administration
http://www/fda/gov
Main site leads to points of interest including: FDA News, Animal Drugs, Biologics and Foods.

- **FDA News**
  http://www/fda/gov/opacom/hpnews.html
  Provides press releases, background reports, new regulations, and FDA Consumer magazine.

- **Center for Food Safety and Applied Nutrition**
  http://vm.cfsan.fda.gov/list.html
  Posts information on biotech, food additives, pesticides, and the "Bad Bug Book" on food safety.

Department of Health and Human Services
http://www.os.dhhs.gov/
As well as program information, the HHS site provides many links to other useful web sites.

National Institute of Health
http://www.nih.gov/icd/
Features health information, scientific resources and grant information as well as a personnel directory of employees.

Environmental Protection Agency
http://www.epa.gov.
User-friendly site has a searchable database and a "people locater" directory.

Government Printing Office
http://www.access.gpo.gov
Location of Government Printing Office's 24 locations and lists of documents for sale. This site will eventually include the Federal Register and the Congressional Record.

FedWorld
http://www.fedworld.gov/
From the National Technical Information Service, FedWorld is designed to be a one-stop shop for locating and obtaining government information. Links to agencies above and more.

Thomas (a congressional resource)
http://thomas.loc.gov/
Full text of bills before Congress and the Congressional Record. Also directs you to "hot legislation" for the week.

Yahoo
http://www/yahoo.com/Government_Agencies/
Executive Branch
Yahoo is a service that organizes information on the web. It can help you find information with its index. The site listed here is an index with links to government agencies, including :USDA information sites, Agricultural Research Service, General Accounting Office. You can also access Yahoo's main site and search the web for nutrition resource links.

General Nutrition Resources

Nutrition Center
University of California at Irvine
http://www-sci.lib.uci.edu/HSG/Nutrition.html
A nutrition resource which includes university resources, information on nutrition education opportunities and programs, and, primarily, links to many nutrition sites on the Internet (including some of the sites listed here). Offers access to on-line journals, consumer-oriented nutrition information, and federal government sites and a database of metabolic pathways and genetic maps.

Arizona Health Sciences Library Nutrition Guide
http://128.196.106.42/nutrition.html
Provides information from the university as well as links to nutrition resources (some are listed here).

International Food Information Council Foundation
http://ificinfo.health.org
Nutrition information for consumers, professionals, and educators in a well-developed site. Presented from perspective of IFIC, supported by the food and beverage industry.

Medweb: Electronic Newsletters and Journals
Emory University's Health Sciences Center Library
http://www.emory.edu/WHSCL/medweb.ejs.html
Has access to hundreds of health and medical periodicals.

Internet Public Library Health and Nutrition Reference
http://ipl.sils.umich.edu/ref/RR/HEA
Provides consumer facts on nutrition and has links to lots of vegetarian recipes. Links to nutrition sites (some of which are listed here).

On-Line Personal Nutrition Profile
Mirical Corporation
http://health.mirical.com/site/form3.html
Plug in your height, weight, gender and a few other stats and get a profile of the optimum food and nutrient intake you should consume based on your attributes.

Vegetarian Pages
http://catless.ncl.ac.uk.vegetarian
Intended to be a worldwide internet guide for vegetarian and vegan-related information.

Vegetarian Resource Group
Baltimore, Maryland
http:www.umanitoba.ca/arrs/VRG/VRG_journals.html
Information and back issues from Baltimore-MD group.

Nutrition Humana WEB
http://www.spin.com.mx/nutrimex/nutrimex.html
Mexican home page for nutrition. (In Spanish)

Dole Five a Day
http://www/dole5aday.com/

Consumer education site from the Dole Food Company. Designed to attract students and teachers to learn about the importance of the federal government's "Five a Day" healthy eating message.

Advocacy/Policy Sites

Handsnet
http://www.igc.apc.org/handsnet/welcome.htmc
Get a feel for Handsnet without subscribing. This web site is updated with key information posted on Handsnet. The full-service, available through paid subscription, links human service advocacy organizations in interactive forums.

"Welfare and Families"
http://epn.org/idea/welfare.html
Hypertext page of Idea Central, a new virtual magazine of the Electronic Policy Network featuring reports and new articles from leading policy and advocacy organizations.

National Center for Children in Poverty
Columbia University School of Public Health
http://cpmcnet.columbia.edu:80/dept/nccp/
Information from the center, including current and back issues of its publication.

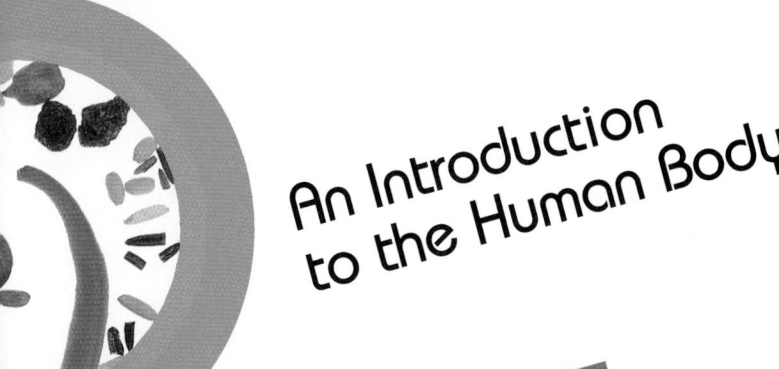

An Introduction to the Human Body

The brief anatomy lesson that follows is a lesson in "anatomy for nutrition's sake" to review the body systems and terminology referred to in this book. To make the body's design understandable, the first few paragraphs are devoted to the life needs of the cells and the evolutionary mechanisms that ensure that they are met.

The Cells

The body is composed of millions of cells, and not one of them knows anything about food. While you get hungry for meat, milk, or bread, each cell of your body sits in its place waiting until the nutrients it needs pass by. Each of the body's **cells** is a self-contained, living entity (Figure B–1), although each depends on the rest of the body to supply its needs. Each cell keeps itself alive just as its single-celled ancestors did, living alone in the ocean 3 billion years ago, by taking up the substances it needs from the surrounding fluid and releasing the wastes it produces into that fluid.

The body cells' most basic need, always, is for energy fuel and the oxygen with which to burn it. Next, they need water, the environment in which they live. Then they need building blocks to maintain themselves—especially the materials they can't make for themselves. These building blocks—the **essential nutrients**—must be supplied preformed from food. These are among the limitations of our heredity from which there is no appeal, and they underlie the first principle of diet planning. Whatever foods we choose, they must provide energy, water, and the essential nutrients. In a sense, the body is only a system organized to provide for these needs of its cells.

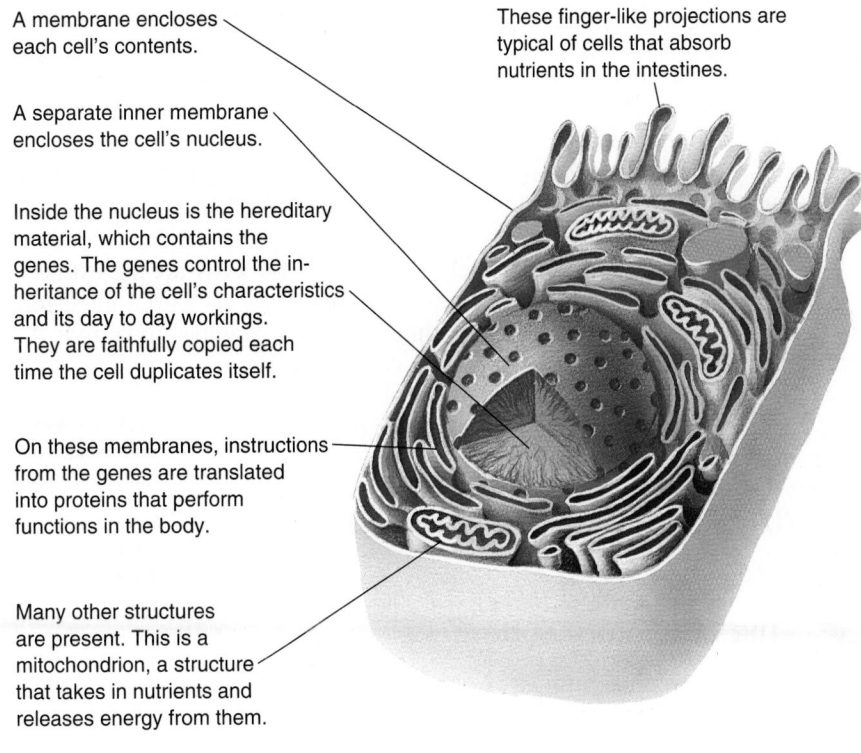

A membrane encloses each cell's contents.

A separate inner membrane encloses the cell's nucleus.

Inside the nucleus is the hereditary material, which contains the genes. The genes control the inheritance of the cell's characteristics and its day to day workings. They are faithfully copied each time the cell duplicates itself.

On these membranes, instructions from the genes are translated into proteins that perform functions in the body.

Many other structures are present. This is a mitochondrion, a structure that takes in nutrients and releases energy from them.

These finger-like projections are typical of cells that absorb nutrients in the intestines.

FIGURE B–1
A TYPICAL CELL (SIMPLIFIED DIAGRAM)

In the human body every cell works in cooperation with every other to support the whole. The cell's **genes** determine the nature of that work. Each gene is a blueprint that directs the making of a piece of protein machinery—most often an **enzyme**—that helps to do the cell's work. Each cell contains a complete set of genes, but different ones are active in different types of cells. For example, in some intestinal cells, the genes for making digestive enzymes are active; in some of the body's fat cells, the genes for making enzymes that make and break down fat are active.

Cells are organized into tissues that perform specialized tasks governed by the genes that are active in them. For example, some cells are joined together to form muscle tissue, which can contract. Tissues also are organized in sets to form whole organs. In the heart organ, for example, muscle tissues, nerve tissues, connective tissues, and other types all work together to pump blood. Some jobs around the body require that several related organs cooperate to perform them. The organs that join together to work on a function are parts of a body system. For example, the heart, lungs, and blood vessels all work to deliver oxygen and nutrients to the body tissues as parts of the cardiovascular system. The next few sections present some body systems with special significance to nutrition.

The Body Fluids

Every cell of the body needs a continuous supply of water, oxygen, energy, and building materials. The body fluids supply these necessities, bathing the outside of all the cells (see Figure B–2). Every cell continuously uses up oxygen (producing carbon dioxide) and nutrients (producing waste products). The body fluids are the transport canals for these materials, carrying oxygen and nutrients to the cells and carbon dioxide and waste away from them. These fluids must circulate to pick up fresh supplies and deliver the wastes to points of disposal.

The fluids that bathe the cells and circulate around the body are the extracellular fluids, the **blood** and **lymph** (Figure B–3). Blood travels within the **arteries, veins,** and **capillaries,** as well as within the heart's chambers (Figure B–4). Lymph is derived from the blood in the capillaries; it squeezes out across their walls and circulates around the cells, permitting exchange of materials. Some of the lymph returns to the blood farther along the capillaries, and the rest travels around the body by way of its own vessels, eventually returning to the bloodstream elsewhere.

The Circulatory System

As the blood, pumped by the heart, travels through the circulatory system, it picks up and delivers materials as needed. Its routing ensures that all cells will be served. Oxygen is picked up and carbon dioxide is released in the **lungs,** and all blood that circulates to the lungs is returned to the heart. From there,

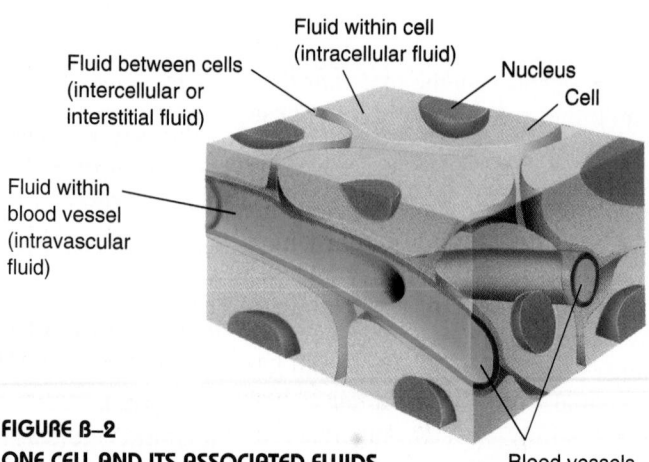

Fluid between cells (intercellular or interstitial fluid)

Fluid within cell (intracellular fluid)

Nucleus

Cell

Fluid within blood vessel (intravascular fluid)

FIGURE B–2
ONE CELL AND ITS ASSOCIATED FLUIDS

Blood vessels

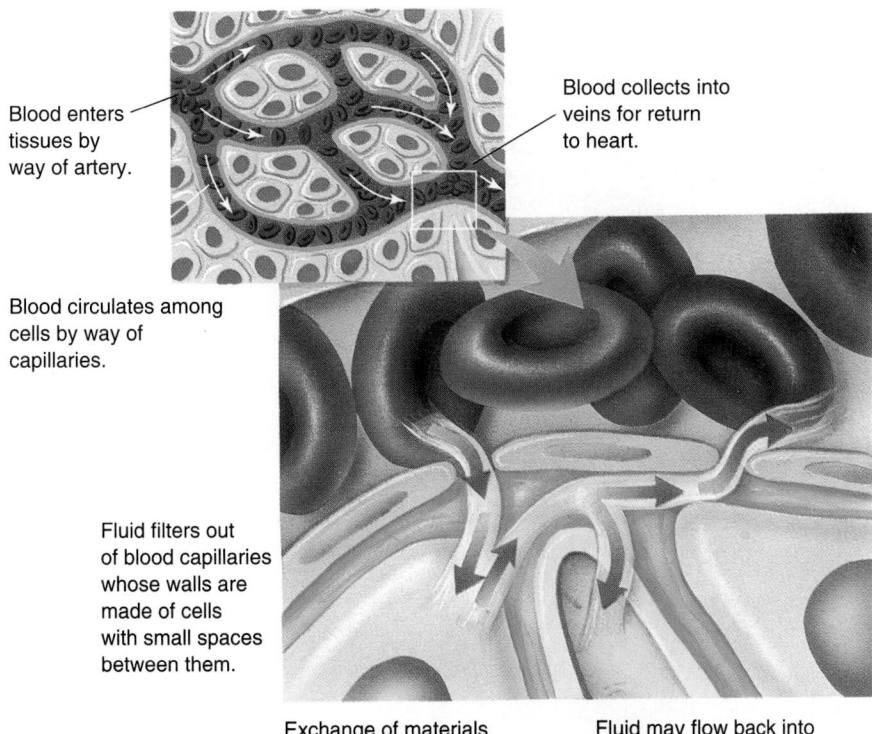

Blood enters tissues by way of artery.

Blood collects into veins for return to heart.

Blood circulates among cells by way of capillaries.

Fluid filters out of blood capillaries whose walls are made of cells with small spaces between them.

Exchange of materials takes place between cell fluid and extracellular fluid.

Fluid may flow back into capillary or into lymph vessel. Lymph enters the bloodstream later through a large lymphatic vessel that empties into a large vein.

FIGURE B–3
HOW THE BODY FLUIDS CIRCULATE AROUND CELLS

The upper left-hand box shows a tiny portion of tissue with blood flowing through its network of capillaries (greatly enlarged). The bottom right-hand box illustrates the movement of the extracellular fluid.

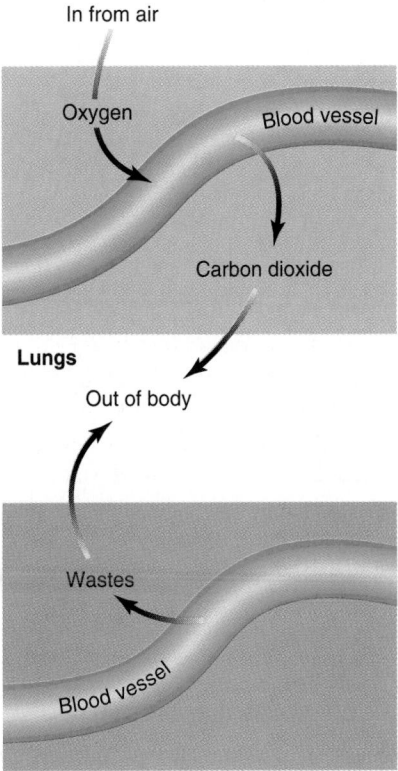

In from air

Oxygen

Blood vessel

Carbon dioxide

Lungs

Out of body

Wastes

Blood vessel

Kidneys

it must go to the other body tissues. Thus all tissues receive freshly oxygenated blood.

As it passes the digestive system, the blood delivers oxygen to the cells there and picks up nutrients from the **intestine** for distribution elsewhere. All blood leaving the digestive system must go next to the **liver,** which has the special task of chemically altering the absorbed materials to make them better suited for use by other tissues. Then, in passing through the **kidneys,** the blood is cleansed of its wastes.

As it flows through the skin, the blood is cooled by radiating heat to the surroundings, helping to maintain the temperature of the body's internal organs. Fluid leaving the blood as lymph may ultimately evaporate from the lungs and skin or be used to make body secretions, such as digestive juices, which will be used within the body for various purposes. On its return to the heart, the blood has delivered most of its oxygen and picked up carbon dioxide from the body cells. Its next stop is the lungs once again, to release its carbon dioxide and

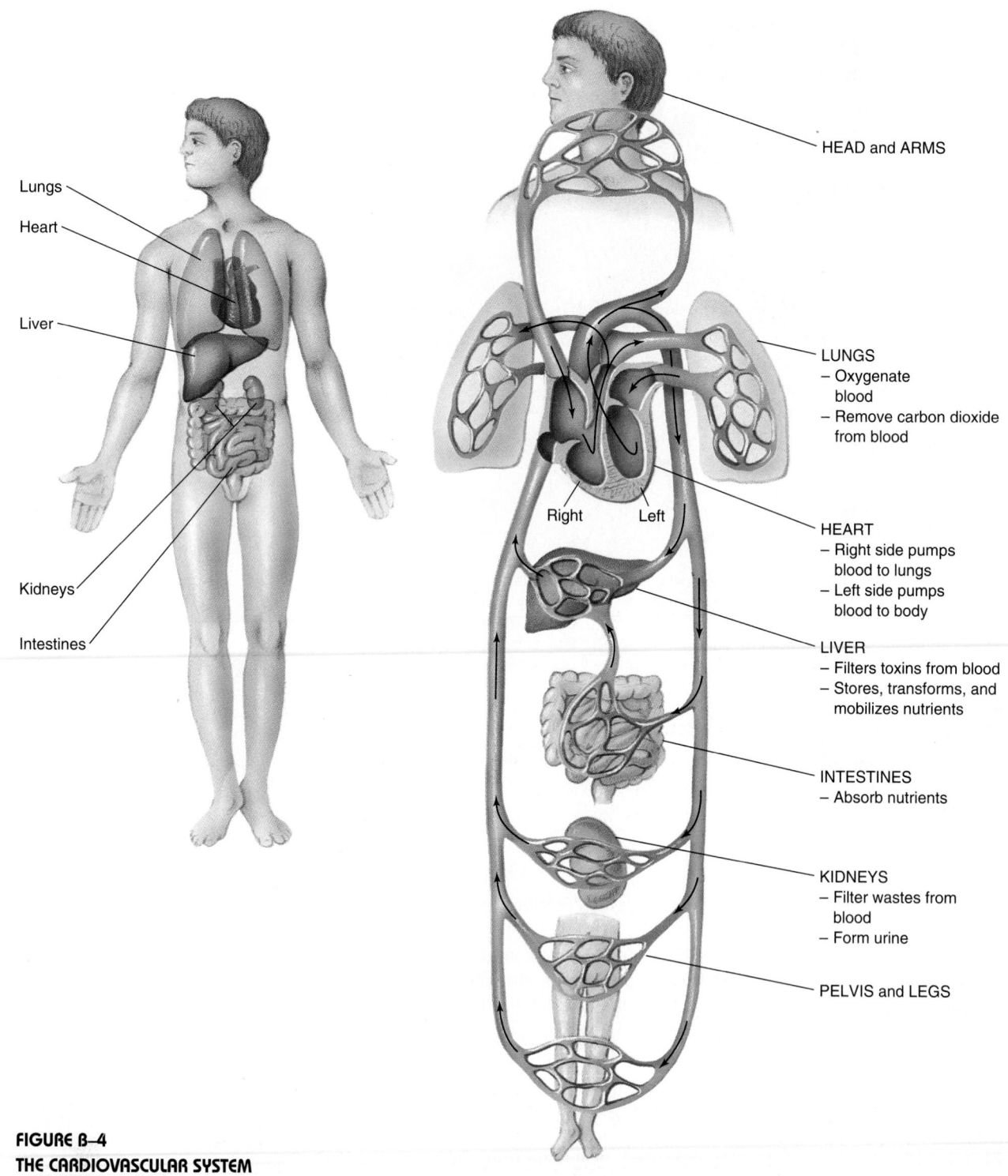

Lungs
Heart
Liver
Kidneys
Intestines

HEAD and ARMS

LUNGS
– Oxygenate
  blood
– Remove carbon dioxide
  from blood

Right   Left

HEART
– Right side pumps
  blood to lungs
– Left side pumps
  blood to body

LIVER
– Filters toxins from blood
– Stores, transforms, and
  mobilizes nutrients

INTESTINES
– Absorb nutrients

KIDNEYS
– Filter wastes from
  blood
– Form urine

PELVIS and LEGS

FIGURE B–4
THE CARDIOVASCULAR SYSTEM

Blood leaves right side of heart, picks up oxygen in lungs, and returns to left side of heart. Blood leaves left side of heart, goes to the head, or to the digestive tract and then to the liver, or to the lower body, and then returns to right side of heart.

cells. Its next stop is the lungs once again, to release its carbon dioxide and replenish its oxygen.

In summary, the routing of the blood is as shown in Figure B–4:

- Heart to body to heart to lungs to heart (repeat).

The portion of the blood that flows by the digestive tract travels from:

- Heart to digestive tract to liver to heart.

The Immune System

Many of the body's cells cooperate to maintain its defenses against infection. The skin presents a physical barrier, and the body's cavities (lungs, digestive tract, and others) are lined with membranes that resist penetration by invading **microbes** or unwanted substances. The body's linings are easily damaged by nutrient deficiencies, and clinicians inspect both the skin and the inside of the mouth to detect signs of malnutrition. (The chapters on protein, vitamins, and minerals present details of the signs of deficiencies.)

When a wound or infection penetrates these first lines of defense (the skin and linings), the lymph and blood present internal defenses: cells and proteins that can inactivate, remove, or destroy microbes and foreign substances. Special cells are able to recognize the chemical structures of some foreign materials and to remember them for a time so that they can quickly mobilize their defenses when they see them again. This ability confers **immunity** against many diseases that you have previously fought and conquered. Some immune cells produce proteins that act as ammunition (**antibodies**) designed to destroy specific targets (**antigens**), and still other cells can gobble up and digest the invaders.

Immune system components reside in tissues all over the body—in the linings of the bones, in the digestive tract, in the blood vessels, in the lymph glands, and in glands of their own. They are in constant flux, being made and dismantled rapidly, and their maintenance requires a continuous supply of nutrients. A deficiency or an overdose of any nutrient is likely to affect the immune system adversely, and a deficiency of nutrients early in an infant's development can weaken that individual's immune defenses against infection for years.

The Hormonal and Nervous Systems

The blood also carries messages, chemical signals from one system of cells to another, that communicate the changing needs of the living system. These chemical messages, or **hormones,** are secreted and released into the blood by the **endocrine** glands. For example, when the **pancreas** (a gland) experiences a too-high concentration of glucose in the blood, it releases **insulin** (a hormone). Insulin stimulates the liver, muscles, and fat cells to remove glucose from the blood and put it away. When the blood glucose level falls too low, the pancreas secretes another hormone, glucagon. The liver responds by releasing glucose into the blood once again.

More about the blood glucose level—Chapter 3.

Glands and hormones abound in the body, each gland a detector system to monitor a condition in the body that needs regulation and each hormone a messenger to stimulate certain tissues to take appropriate action. Examples of the working of these hormones appear throughout this book.

The body's other major communication system is, of course, the nervous system. With the brain and spinal cord as central controllers, the system receives and integrates messages from sensory receptors all over the body—sight, hearing, touch, smell, taste, and others—which all communicate to the brain the state of both the outer and inner worlds, including the availability of food and the need to eat. The system then returns instructions to the muscles and glands, telling them what to do.

The nervous system's part in hunger regulation is coordinated by the brain. The sensations of hunger and appetite are experienced in the **cortex** of the brain, the thinking, outer layer. However, much of the brain's regulatory work goes on in the deep brain centers, without the person's (or the cortex's) awareness. An organ there, the **hypothalamus** (Figure B–5), monitors many body conditions, including the availability of nutrients and water.

The Excretory System

To dispose of waste, the kidneys straddle the circulatory system and filter each pass of the blood (see Figure B–6). Waste materials removed with water are collected as urine in tubes that deliver them to the urinary bladder, which is periodically emptied. Thus the blood is purified continuously throughout the day, and dissolved minerals are excreted as necessary (including sodium, to keep blood pressure from rising too high). As you might expect, the kidneys' work is regulated by hormones secreted by glands responsive to conditions in the blood (such as the sodium concentration).

Temperature Regulation

All the body's cells obtain energy by breaking down the nutrients—carbohydrate, fat, and to some extent protein—and one of the ways this energy is released is as heat. The heat is lost to the air through the skin

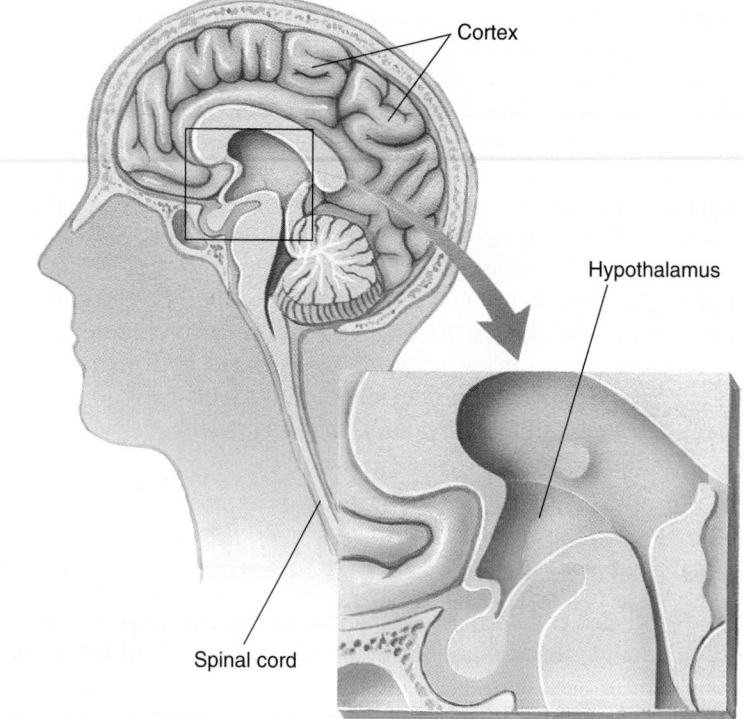

FIGURE B–5

THE BRAIN'S HYPOTHALAMUS AND CORTEX

The hypothalamus monitors the body's conditions and sends signals to the brain's thinking portion, the cortex, which decides on actions.

face. Temperature regulation involves speeding up or slowing down cellular heat production (**metabolism**) and increasing or decreasing heat loss through the skin. Specialized nerve cells in an area of the brain called the hypothalamus serve as a thermostat, measuring the temperature of the blood. These cells signal other cells, near the body surface, to respond appropriately. When the body is too hot, blood vessels immediately under the skin dilate, allowing warm blood to flow near the surface, where its heat can radiate away. The sweat glands also are activated to secrete warm fluid onto the skin surface, where its heat can be lost by evaporation. When the body is cold, these mechanisms shut down and shivering is triggered, generating heat.

By means of these systems of transportation, communication, waste disposal, and heat regulation, the cells of the multicellular human animal cooperate to provide one another with a circulating bath of warm, clean, nutritive fluid whose composition is finely regulated to meet their needs.

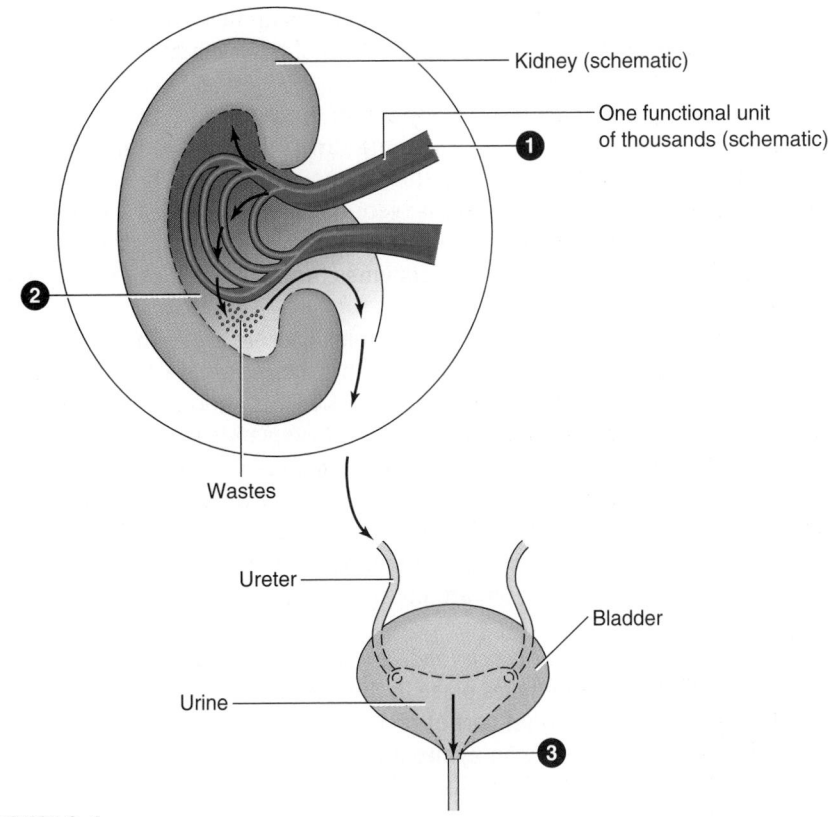

FIGURE B–6
THE EXCRETORY SYSTEM

1. Blood enters kidney by way of arteries and disperses into capillaries.
2. Kidney filters waste from blood and sends it as urine to the bladder.
3. Bladder periodically eliminates urine.

The Digestive System

You may eat meals only two or three times a day, but your body's cells need their nutrients 24 hours a day. Providing the needed nutrients requires the cooperation of millions of specialized cells. When the body's cells are deprived of fuel, certain nerve cells in the brain (the hypothalamus) detect this condition and generate nerve impulses that signal hunger to the conscious part of the brain, the cortex. They also stimulate the stomach to intensify its contractions, creating hunger pangs. Becoming conscious of hunger, then, you eat, delivering a complex mixture of chewed and swallowed food to the intestinal tract.

Many of the cells lining the intestinal tract secrete powerful juices and enzymes to disintegrate nutrients (especially carbohydrate and protein) into their component parts. Two organs outside the digestive tract—the liver with its associated gallbladder and the pancreas—also contribute digestive juices through a common duct into the small intestine. The presence of these digestive juices and enzymes requires that still other cells specialize in protecting the

Digestive tract secretions:

Salivary glands:

Saliva.

Salivary amylase (enzyme that breaks down starch).

Stomach (gastric) glands:

Gastric juice.

Hydrochloric acid (uncoils protein).

Gastric protease (enzyme that breaks down protein).

Mucus (thick coating that protects the stomach wall from these secretions).

digestive system. They secrete a thick, viscous substance known as **mucus,** or the **mucous membrane,** which coats the intestinal tract lining and ensures that it will not itself be digested.

The process of digestion is diagrammed in Figure B–7. The first part, the mouth, is designed for physically breaking down foods. The teeth cut off a bite-size portion and then, aided by the tongue, grind it finely enough to be mixed with saliva and swallowed. The esophagus carries the mixture to the stomach. The stomach is supplied with several sets of muscles to mix and grind it further and secretes acid and enzymes that will begin to break it apart chemically.

During the preparatory stage, as the complex carbohydrate known as starch is released from a food (such as bread), an enzyme present in the saliva starts to break it down chemically to smaller units. But this action is stopped when the carbohydrate units reach the stomach, because glands in the stomach wall exude hydrochloric acid. The salivary enzyme that breaks up starch is digested in the stomach, together with other proteins. Further dismantling of carbohydrate occurs after it leaves the stomach.

Fats and oils, taken as part of such complex foods as meats or nuts or in relatively pure form as butter or oil, are not much affected until after leaving the stomach.

Proteins are eaten as part of such foods as meat, milk, and legumes. Although no chemical action on them takes place in the mouth, chewing and mixing protein with saliva is an important part of preparing it for the chemical action that begins in the stomach. There, enzymes and hydrochloric acid break apart the large, complex protein molecules into smaller pieces known as peptides and finally into dipeptides, tripeptides, and amino acids.

The complicated chemical dismantling that takes place beyond the stomach requires that only small amounts be processed at one time. To accomplish this, the **pylorus,** a circular muscle surrounding the lower end of the stomach, controls the exit of the contents, allowing only a little at a time to be squirted forcefully into the small intestine. Gradually the stomach empties itself by means of these powerful squirts.

The small intestine is "the" organ of digestion and absorption; it finishes the job the mouth and stomach have started. It is actually about 20 feet long, but it is called small because its diameter is small compared with that of the large intestine. Its contents must touch its walls to make contact with the secretions and to be absorbed at the proper places. At the end of the small intestine, a circular muscle (similar in function to the pylorus at the end of the stomach) controls the flow of the contents going into the large intestine (colon).

The small intestine works with the precision of a laboratory chemist. As the thoroughly liquefied and partially digested nutrient mixture arrives there, hormonal messages tell the gallbladder to send its **emulsifier, bile,** in amounts matched to the amount of fat present. Other hormones notify the pancreas to release **bicarbonate** in amounts precisely adjusted to neutralize the stomach acid as well as enzymes of the appropriate kinds and quantities to continue dismantling whatever large molecules remain. Such messages also keep the strong muscles imbedded in the walls of the intestine contracting, in a squeezing activity called **peristalsis,** so that the contents will be pressed along to the next region. Peristalsis is stimulated by the presence of roughage or fiber and is quieted by the presence of fat, which requires a longer time for digestion.

Intestinal cells:

Enzymes (break down carbohydrate and protein).

Mucus (thin coating that protects the intestinal wall).

Liver and gallbladder:

Bile (emulsifier that separates fat into small particles enzymes can attack).

Pancreas:

Bicarbonate (neutralizes acid fluid from stomach so intestinal and pancreatic enzymes can work on its contents).

Enzymes (break down carbohydrate, fat, and protein).

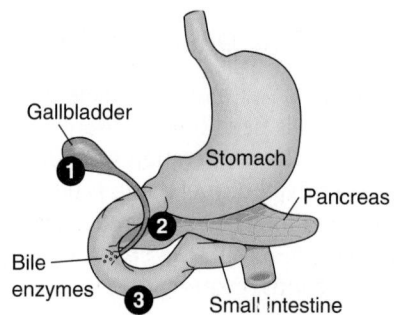

Small intestine—details.

1. The gallbladder sends bile into the small intestine by way of a duct.

2. The pancreas sends enzymes (and bicarbonate).

3. The small intestine also secretes enzymes.

Meanwhile, as the pancreatic and intestinal enzymes act on the bonds that hold the large nutrients together, smaller and smaller units make their appearance in the intestinal fluids. Finally, units that cells can use—glucose, glycerol, fatty acids, and amino acids, among others—are released.

Once the digestive system has broken food down to its nutrient components, it must deliver them to the rest of the body. The cells of the intestinal lining absorb nutrients from the mixture within the intestine and deposit them in the blood and lymph. Every molecule of nutrient must traverse one of these cells if it is to enter the body fluids. The cells are selective: they can recognize the nutrients needed by the body. The cells are also extraordinarily efficient: they absorb enough nutrients to nourish all the body's other cells.

The intestinal tract lining is composed of a single sheet of cells, and the sheet pokes out into millions of finger-shaped projections (**villi**). Each villus has its own capillary network and a lymph vessel so that as nutrients move across the cells, they can immediately mingle into the body fluids. On every villus every cell has a brushlike covering of tiny hairs (**microvilli**) that can trap the nutrient particles. Figure B–8 provides a close look at these details.

The small intestine's lining, villi and all, is wrinkled into thousands of folds, so that its absorbing surface is enormous. If the folds, and the villi that cover them, were spread out flat, the total area would equal a third of a football field in size. The billions of cells of that surface, although they weigh only 4 to 5 pounds, absorb enough nutrients in a few hours a day to nourish the other 150 or so pounds of body tissues.

Nutrients released early in the digestive process, such as simple sugars, and those requiring no special handling, such as the water-soluble vitamins, are absorbed high in the small intestine; nutrients that are released more slowly are absorbed further down. The lymphatic and circulatory systems then take over the job of transporting them to the cell consumers. The lymph at first carries most of the products of fat digestion and the fat-soluble vitamins, later delivering them to the blood. The blood carries the products of carbohydrate and protein digestion, the water-soluble vitamins, and the minerals. By the time the remaining mixture reaches the end of the small intestine, little is left but water, indigestible residue (mostly fiber), and dissolved minerals. The cells lining the colon are specialized for absorbing these minerals and retrieving the water for recycling. The final waste product, the feces, a smooth paste of a consistency suitable for excretion, is stored in the colon until excretion. Such a system can adjust to whatever mixture of foods is presented.

Although a meal may be eaten in half an hour, the nutrients it provides reach the body fluids over a span of about four hours. However, as already mentioned, the cells of the body need their nutrients around the clock. Providing a constant supply requires that there be systems of storage and release to meet the cells' needs between meals.

Storage Systems

Nutrients leave the digestive system by way of both circulatory systems—the blood and the lymph. The blood carries products of carbohydrate and protein digestion and some of the smaller fats; the lymph carries the larger fats in packages called chylomicrons (see Chapter 4).

FIGURE β–7   THE DIGESTIVE SYSTEM

FIBER	CARBOHYDRATE
Mouth The mechanical action of the mouth and teeth crushes and tears fiber in food and mixes it with saliva to moisten it for swallowing.	The salivary glands secrete a watery fluid into the mouth to moisten the food. The salivary enzyme amylase begins digestion: Starch $\xrightarrow{\text{amylase}}$ small polysaccharides, maltose.
Esophagus Fiber is unchanged.	Digestion of starch continues as swallowed food moves down the esophagus.
Stomach Fiber is unchanged.	Stomach acid and enzymes start to digest salivary enzymes, halting starch digestion. To a small extent, stomach acid hydrolyzes maltose and sucrose.
Small intestine Fiber is unchanged.	The pancreas produces enzymes and releases them through the pancreatic duct into the small intestine: Polysaccharides $\xrightarrow{\text{pancreatic amylase}}$ disaccharides. Then enzymes on the surfaces of the small intestinal cells break disaccharides into monosaccharides, and the cells absorb them: Maltose $\xrightarrow{\text{maltase}}$ glucose + glucose. Sucrose $\xrightarrow{\text{sucrase}}$ fructose + glucose. Lactose $\xrightarrow{\text{lactase}}$ galactose + glucose.

Colon (large intestine)
Most fiber passes intact through the digestive tract to the colon. Here, bacterial enzymes digest some fiber:

Some fiber $\xrightarrow{\text{bacterial enzymes}}$ fatty acids, gas.

Fiber holds water; regulates bowel activity; and binds cholesterol and some minerals, carrying them out of the body as it is excreted with feces.

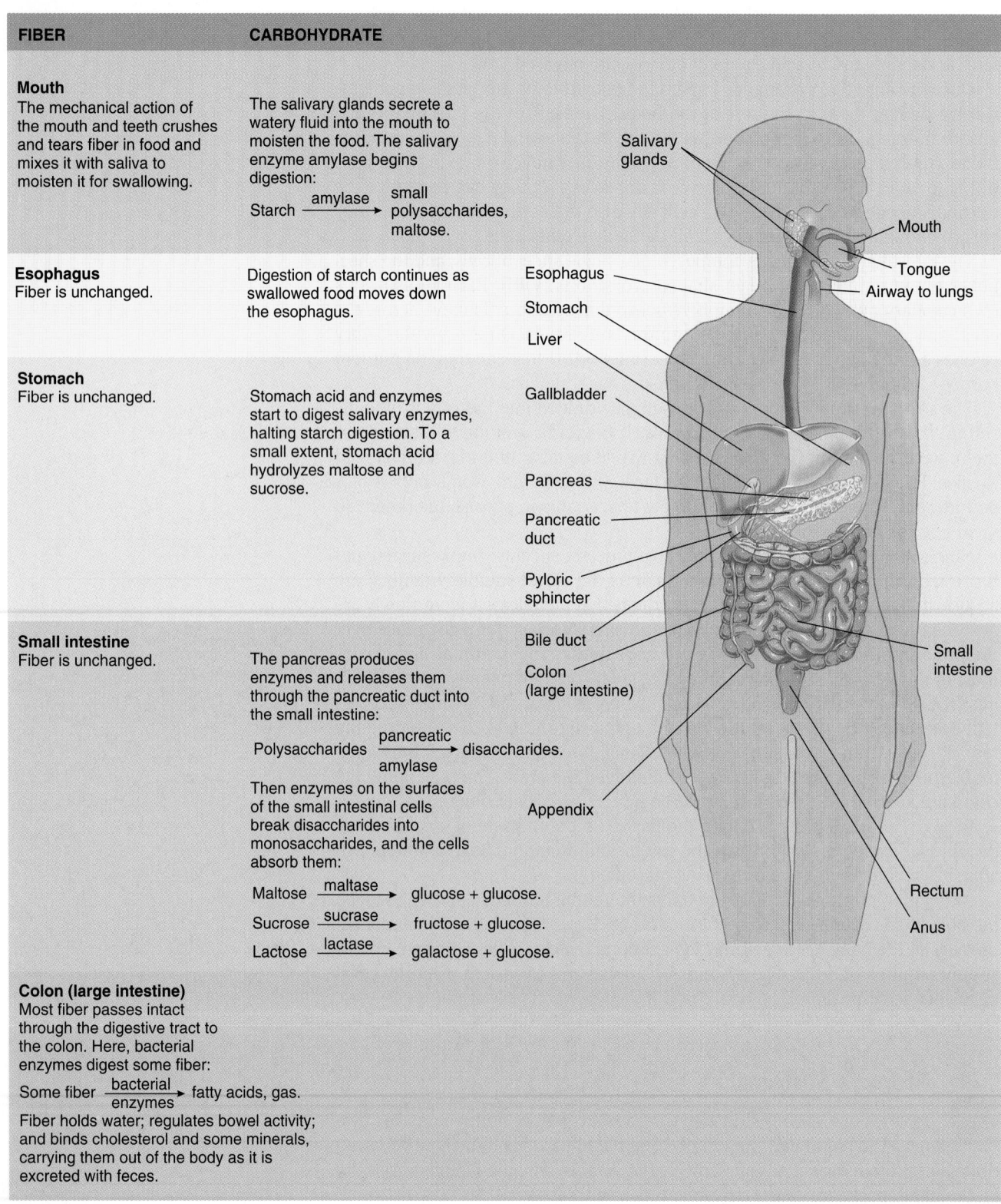

Salivary glands
Mouth
Tongue
Airway to lungs
Esophagus
Stomach
Liver
Gallbladder
Pancreas
Pancreatic duct
Pyloric sphincter
Bile duct
Colon (large intestine)
Appendix
Small intestine
Rectum
Anus

FAT	PROTEIN	VITAMINS	MINERALS AND WATER
Mouth Glands in the base of the tongue secrete a fat-digesting enzyme known as lingual lipase. Some hard fats begin to melt as they reach body temperature.	In the month, chewing crushes and softens protein-rich foods and mixes them with saliva to be swallowed	No action.	The salivary glands add water to disperse and carry food.
Esophagus Fat is unchanged.	No action.	No action.	No action.
Stomach The degree of hydrolysis is slight for most fats but may be appreciable for milk fats. The stomach's churning action mixes fat with water and acid. A gastric enzyme accesses and hydrolyzes a small percentage of fat.	Stomach acid works to uncoil protein strands and activate stomach enzymes. Then the enzymes break the strands into smaller fragments: $$\text{Protein} \xrightarrow[\text{HCl}]{\text{pepsin}} \begin{array}{l}\text{smaller}\\\text{polypeptides}\end{array}$$	Water-soluble vitamins need little action by the digestive organs except absorption in the small intestine. However, vitamin B_{12} requires "intrinsic factor" produced by the stomach in order to be absorbed.	The stomach secretes enough watery fluid to turn a moist, chewed mass of swallowed food into a liquid. Stomach acid acts on iron to make it more absorbable. Vitamin C and a factor in meat also increase iron absorption.
Small intestine The liver secretes bile; the gallbladder stores it and releases it through the common bile duct into the small intestine when fat arrives there. The bile emulsifies the fat, making it ready for enzyme action. The pancreas produces fat-digesting enzymes and releases them through the common bile duct into the small intestine. These enzymes split triglycerides into monoglycerides, free fatty acids, and glycerol, which are absorbed.	In the small intestine, the fragments of protein are split into free amino acids, dipeptides, and tripeptides with the help of enzymes from the pancreas and small intestine. Enzymes on the surface of the small intestinal cells break these peptides into amino acids, and they are absorbed through the cells into the blood. The large intestine carries any undigested protein residue out of the body. Normally, practically all the protein is digested and absorbed.	Bile emulsifies fat-soluble vitamins and aids in their absorption with other fats. Water-soluble vitamins are absorbed.	The small intestine, pancreas, and liver add enough fluid so that approximately 2 gallons are secreted into the intestine in a day. Many minerals are absorbed. Vitamin D aids in the absorption of calcium.
Colon Some fat and cholesterol, trapped in fiber, exit in feces.		Bacteria produce vitamin K, which is absorbed.	More minerals and most of the water are absorbed.

FIGURE B-8   DETAILS OF THE LINING OF THE SMALL INTESTINE

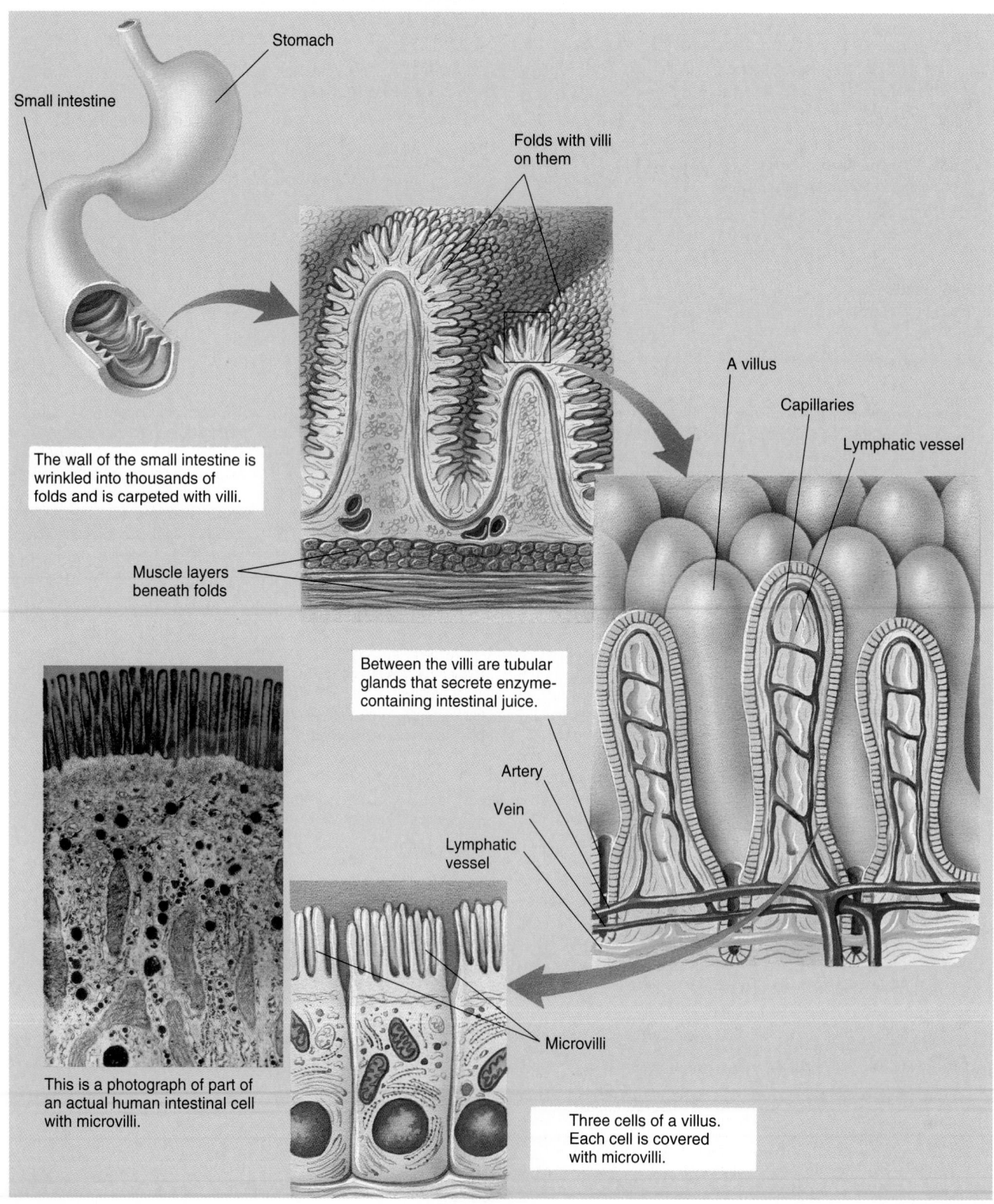

Stomach

Small intestine

Folds with villi on them

The wall of the small intestine is wrinkled into thousands of folds and is carpeted with villi.

Muscle layers beneath folds

A villus

Capillaries

Lymphatic vessel

Between the villi are tubular glands that secrete enzyme-containing intestinal juice.

Artery

Vein

Lymphatic vessel

Microvilli

This is a photograph of part of an actual human intestinal cell with microvilli.

Three cells of a villus. Each cell is covered with microvilli.

All nutrients leaving the digestive system by way of the blood are collected in thousands of capillaries in the membrane that supports the intestine. These converge into veins and then into a single large vein. This vein conveys its contents to the liver and there breaks up once again into a vast network of capillaries that weave among the liver cells, allowing them access to the newly arriving nutrients. The liver cells process these nutrients. They convert the sugars from carbohydrate mostly into the body's sugar, glucose; and if there is a surplus, they store some as glycogen and convert the remainder to fat. They reassemble fatty acids and glycerol from fat into larger fats and package them with protein for transport to other parts of the body. As for the amino acids from protein, the liver cells alter these as needed, making glucose from some if necessary and fat from others if there is an excess, or converting one amino acid into another to use in making proteins.

More about liver glycogen—Chapter 3.
More about lipoproteins—Chapter 4.
More about fasting—Chapter 8.
More about protein deficiency—Chapter 5.

The nutrients leaving the digestive tract by way of the lymph as chylomicrons circulate throughout the body, giving all cells the opportunity to withdraw fats from them. Some also find their way into the blood and circulate through the liver, which removes them, alters their components, and releases new products, including other lipoproteins.

The new products of liver metabolism—glucose, fat packaged with protein (lipoproteins), and amino acids—are released into the bloodstream again and circulated to all other cells of the body. Surplus fat is then removed by cells specialized for its storage; these fat cells are located in deposits all over the body.

The liver's glycogen provides a reserve supply of the body's sugar, glucose, and thus can sustain cell activities if the intervals between meals become so long that glucose absorbed from ingested foods is used up. When the body is depending solely on liver glycogen, however, the supply is used up within three to six hours. Similarly, the fat cells store reserves of fat, the body's other principal energy nutrient. Unlike the liver, however the fat cells have virtually infinite storage capacity and can continue to supply fat for days, weeks, or even months when no food is eaten.

These storage systems for glucose and fat ensure that the cells will not go without energy nutrients even if the body is hungry for food, except under extreme conditions. Body stores also exist for many other nutrients, each with a characteristic capacity. For example, the third energy nutrient, protein, is held in an available pool (the amino acids in the liver and blood) that is rather rapidly depleted during protein deficiency. The liver and fat cells store many vitamins, and the bones provide reserves of calcium, sodium, and other minerals that can be drawn on to keep the blood levels constant and to meet cellular demands.

Metabolism: Breaking Down Nutrients for Energy

The breaking down of body compounds is known as **catabolism.** These reactions usually release energy and are represented, wherever possible, by "down" arrows in chemical diagrams (see Figure B–9). Glycogen can be broken down to glucose, triglycerides to fatty acids and glycerol, and protein to amino acids. When the body needs energy, it breaks any or all of the four basic units—glucose, fatty acids, glycerol, and amino acids—into even smaller units. When the body does not require energy, the end-products of digestion (glucose, amino acids, glycerol, and fatty acids) are used to build body compounds in a process called **anabolism** (see Figure B–9). Anabolic reactions involve the conversion of glucose to glycogen or fat, the conversion of amino acids to body proteins or fat, and the synthesis of body fat from glycerol and fatty acids. Catabolism and anabolism are examples of **energy metabolism.**

Other Systems

In addition to the systems described above, the body has many more: the bones, the muscles, the nerves, the lungs, the reproductive organs, and others. All of these cooperate so that each cell can carry on its own life. Each assures, through hormonal or nerve-mediated messages, that its needs will be met by the others, and each contributes to the welfare of the whole by doing the work it is specialized for.

Of the millions of cells in the body, only a small percentage comprise the cortex of the brain, in which the conscious mind resides. These receive messages from other cells when they require you to "become conscious" of a need for decision and action. In modern life the need may be as complex as, for example, to notice that you feel anxious and to decide to consult an advisor, or it may

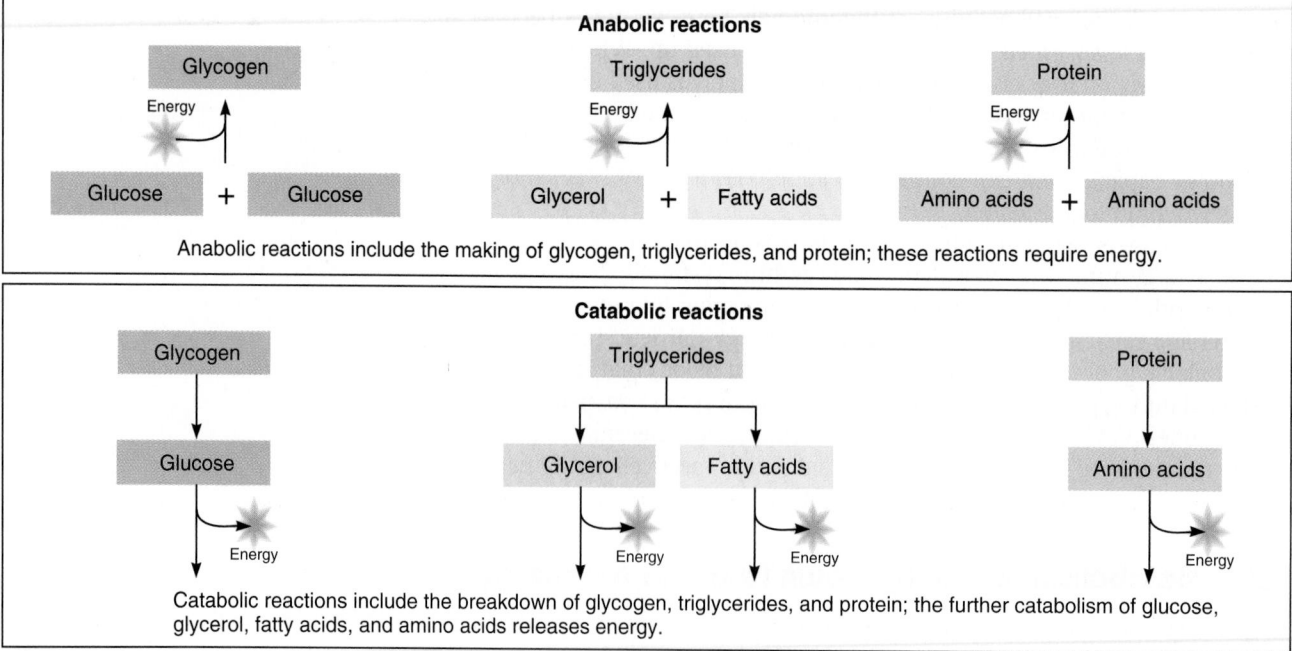

FIGURE B–9
REACTIONS OF ENERGY METABOLISM COMPARED

SOURCE: Reprinted with permission from E. N. Whitney and coauthors, *Nutrition for Health and Health Care* (St. Paul, MN: West Publishing, 1995) p. 120.

be such a "simple" need as "I'm tired, I think I'll go to bed," or "I'm hungry, I guess I'd better eat."

Most of the body's work is done automatically and is finely regulated to achieve a state of well-being. But when your cortex does become involved, you would do well to "listen" to your body and to cultivate an understanding and appreciation of its needs. Then when you make decisions you will act to promote your health.

MINIGLOSSARY

ANABOLISM (ann-ABB-o-lism) reactions in which small molecules are put together to build larger ones. Anabolic reactions consume energy.
   ana = up

ANTIBODIES proteins made by the immune system, expressly designed to combine with and to inactivate specific antigens.

ANTIGENS microbes or substances that are foreign to the body.

ARTERIES blood vessels that carry blood containing fresh oxygen supplies from the heart to the tissues.

BICARBONATE a chemical that neutralizes acid; a secretion of the pancreas.

BILE a compound made from cholesterol by the liver, stored in the gallbladder, and secreted into the small intestine. It emulsifies lipids to ready them for enzymatic digestion.

BLOOD the fluid of the circulatory system—water, red and white blood cells and other formed particles, proteins, nutrients, oxygen, and other constituents.

CAPILLARIES minute, weblike blood vessels that connect arteries to veins and permit transfer of materials between blood and tissues.

CATABOLISM (ca-TAB-o-lism) reactions in which large molecules are broken down to smaller ones. Catabolic reactions usually release energy.
   kata = down

CELLS the smallest units in which independent life can exist. All living things are single cells or organisms made of cells.

CORTEX an outer covering; in the brain, that part in which conscious thought takes place.

EMULSIFIER (ee-MULL-sih-fire) a compound with both water-soluble and fat-soluble portions that can attract lipids into water solution.

ENDOCRINE (EN-doh-crin) a term to describe a gland secreting or a hormone being secreted into the blood.
   endo = into

ENERGY METABOLISM all the reactions by which the body obtains and spends the energy from food or body stores.

ENZYME a protein catalyst. A catalyst is a compound that facilitates (speeds up the rate of) a chemical reaction without itself being altered in the process.

ESSENTIAL NUTRIENTS compounds that can't be synthesized by the body in amounts sufficient to meet physiological needs.

GENE a unit of a cell's inheritance, made of a chemical, DNA, that is copied faithfully so that every time the cell divides, both its offspring get identical copies. Genes direct the cells' machinery to make the proteins that form each cell's structures and to do its work.

HORMONE a chemical messenger, secreted by one organ (a gland) in response to a condition in the body, that acts on another organ or organs to change that condition.

HYPOTHALAMUS (high-poh-THALL-uh-mus) a part of the brain that senses a variety of conditions in the blood, such as temperature, salt content, glucose content, and others, and signals other parts of the brain or body to change those conditions when necessary.

MINIGLOSSARY

IMMUNITY the ability to successfully resist a disease, conferred on the body by way of the immune system's memory of previous exposure to that disease and its ability to mount a specific defense promptly and swiftly.

INSULIN a hormone from the pancreas that helps glucose get into cells.

INTESTINE a long, tubular organ of digestion and the site of nutrient absorption.

KIDNEYS the organs that filter the blood to remove waste material and forward it to the bladder for excretion.

LIVER the large, many-lobed organ that lies under the ribs and filters the blood, removing, processing, and readying for redistribution many of its materials.

LUNGS the organs of gas exchange. Blood circulating through the lungs releases its carbon dioxide and picks up fresh oxygen to carry to the tissues.

LYMPH (LIMF) the fluid outside the circulatory system that bathes the cells, derived from the blood by being pressed through the capillary walls; similar to the blood in composition but without red blood cells.

METABOLISM (meh-TAB-o-lism) total of all chemical reactions that go on in living cells.

MICROBES bacteria, viruses, or other organisms invisible to the naked eye; some cause disease.

MICROVILLI (MY-croh-VILL-ee, MY-croh-VILL-eye) tiny hairlike projections on each cell of the intestinal tract lining that can trap nutrient particles and translocate them into the cells (singular: **microvillus**).

MUCUS (MYOO-cus) a thick, slippery coating of the intestinal tract lining (and other body linings) that protects the cells from exposure to digestive juices. The adjective form is *mucous*, and the coating is often called the mucous membrane.

PANCREAS a gland that secretes the endocrine hormone insulin and also produces the exocrine secretions that aid digestion in the small intestine. (An *exocrine* secretion is one that is expelled through a duct into a body cavity or onto the surface of the skin; *exo* means "out." See also *endocrine*.)

PERISTALSIS (perri-STALL-sis) the wavelike squeezing motions of the stomach and intestines that push their contents along.

PYLORUS (pye-LORE-us) muscle that regulates the opening of the bottom of the stomach.

VEINS blood vessels that carry used blood from the tissues back to the heart.

VILLI (VILL-ee, VILL-eye) poked-out parts of the sheet of cells that line the GI tract; the villi make the surface area much greater than it would otherwise be (singular: **villus**).

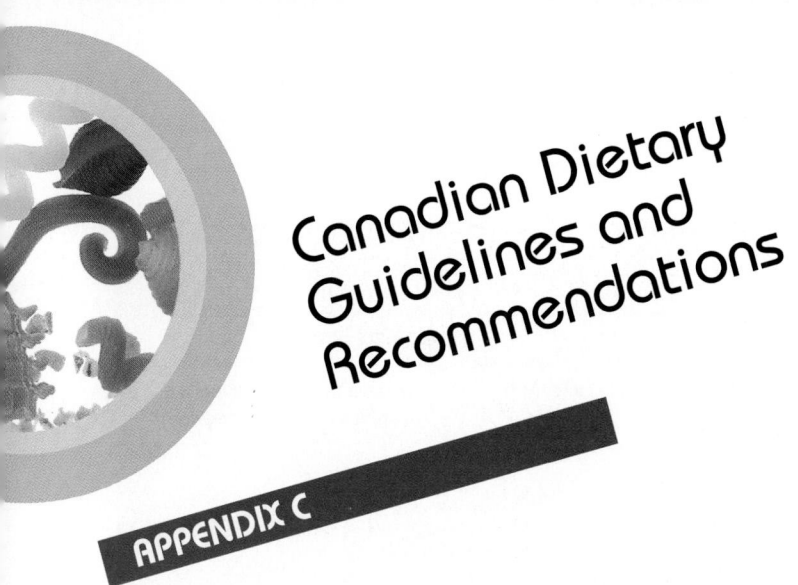

Canadian Dietary Guidelines and Recommendations

Canada's Guidelines For Healthy Eating

Canada's Guidelines for Healthy Eating were developed by the Communications/Implementation Committee as the key nutrition messages to be communicated to healthy Canadians over two years of age. The guidelines encourage people to

- Enjoy a variety of foods.
- Emphasize cereals, breads, other grain products, vegetables, and fruits.
- Choose lower-fat dairy products, leaner meats, and foods prepared with little or no fat.
- Achieve and maintain a healthy body weight by enjoying regular physical activity and healthy eating.
- Limit salt, alcohol, and caffeine.

Canada's Recommended Nutrient Intakes (RNI)

Like the RDA on the inside front cover pages, the Recommended Nutrient Intakes (RNI) for Canadians make recommendations for intakes of vitamins, minerals, protein, and energy. The RNI are presented in Tables C-1 and C-2.

TABLE C-1
RECOMMENDED NUTRIENT INTAKES FOR CANADIANS, 1990

AGE	SEX	WEIGHT (kg)	PROTEIN (g/day)[a]	FAT-SOLUBLE VITAMINS Vitamin A (RE/day)[b]	Vitamin D (μg/day)[c]	Vitamin E (mg/day)[d]
Infants (months)						
0-4	Both	6	12[e]	400	10	3
5-12	Both	9	12	400	10	3
Children and adults (years)						
1	Both	11	13	400	10	3
2-3	Both	14	16	400	5	4
4-6	Both	18	19	500	5	5
7-9	M	25	26	700	2.5	7
	F	25	26	700	2.5	6
10-12	M	34	34	800	2.5	8
	F	36	36	800	5	7
13-15	M	50	49	900	5	9
	F	48	46	800	5	7
16-18	M	62	58	1,000	5	10
	F	53	47	800	2.5	7
19-24	M	71	61	1,000	2.5	10
	F	58	50	800	2.5	7
25-49	M	74	64	1,000	2.5	9
	F	59	51	800	2.5	6
50-74	M	73	63	1,000	5	7
	F	63	54	800	5	6
75+	M	69	59	1,000	5	6
	F	64	55	800	5	5
Pregnancy (additional amount needed)						
1st trimester			5	0	2.5	2
2nd trimester			20	0	2.5	2
3rd trimester			24	0	2.5	2
Lactation (additional amount needed)			22	400	2.5	3

NOTE: Recommended intakes of energy and certain nutrients are not listed in this table because of the nature of the variables upon which they are based. The figures for energy are estimates of average requirements for expected patterns of activity. For nutrients not shown, the following amounts are recommended based on at least 2,000 calories per day and body weights as given: thiamin, 0.4 milligrams per 1,000 calories (0.48 milligrams/5,000 kilojoules); riboflavin, 0.5 milligrams per 1,000 calories (0.6 milligrams/5,000 kilojoules); niacin, 7.2 niacin equivalents per 1,000 calories (8.6 niacin equivalents/5,000 kilojoules); vitamin B_6, 15 micrograms, as pyridoxine, per gram of protein. Recommended intakes during periods of growth are taken as appropriate for individuals representative of the midpoint in each age group. All recommended intakes are designed to cover individual variations in essentially all of a healthy population subsisting upon a variety of common foods available in Canada.

continued

TABLE C-1

continued

| WATER-SOLUBLE VITAMINS | | | MINERALS | | | | | |
Vitamin C (mg/day)[f]	Folate (μg/day)	Vitamin B$_{12}$ (μg/day)	Calcium (mg/day)	Phosphorus (mg/day)	Magnesium (mg/day)	Iron (mg/day)	Iodine (μg/day)	Zinc (mg/day)
20	25	0.3	250	150	20	0.3[g]	30	2[h]
20	40	0.4	400	200	32	7	40	3
20	40	0.5	500	300	40	6	55	4
20	50	0.6	550	350	50	6	65	4
25	70	0.8	600	400	65	8	85	5
25	90	1.0	700	500	100	8	110	7
25	90	1.0	700	500	100	8	95	7
25	120	1.0	900	700	130	8	125	9
25	130	1.0	1,100	800	135	8	110	9
30	175	1.0	1,100	900	185	10	160	12
30	170	1.0	1,000	850	180	13	160	9
40	220	1.0	900	1,000	230	10	160	12
30	190	1.0	700	850	200	12	160	9
40	220	1.0	800	1,000	240	9	160	12
30	180	1.0	700	850	200	13	160	9
40	230	1.0	800	1,000	250	9	160	12
30	185	1.0	700	850	200	13[i]	160	9
40	230	1.0	800	1,000	250	9	160	12
30	195	1.0	800	850	210	8	160	9
40	215	1.0	800	1,000	230	9	160	12
30	200	1.0	800	850	210	8	160	9
0	200	0.2	500	200	15	0	25	6
10	200	0.2	500	200	45	5	25	6
10	200	0.2	500	200	45	10	25	6
25	100	0.2	500	200	65	0	50	6

[a]The primary units are expressed per kilogram of body weight. The figures shown here are examples.

[b]One retinol equivalent (RE) corresponds to the biological activity of 1 microgram of retinol, 6 micrograms of beta-carotene, or 12 micrograms of other carotenes.

[c]Expressed as cholecalciferol or ergocalciferol.

[d]Expressed as 6-a-tocopherol equivalents, relative to which β-and γ-tocopherol and α-tocotrienol have activities of 0.5, 0.1, and 0.3, respectively.

[e]The assumption is made that the protein is from breast milk or is of the same biological value as that of breast milk, and that between 3 and 9 months, adjustment for the quality of the protein is made.

[f]Cigarette smokers should increase intake by 50 percent.

[g]Based on the assumption that breast milk is the source of iron.

[h]Based on the assumption that breast milk is the source of zinc.

[i]After menopause, the recommended intake is 8 milligrams per day.

SOURCE: Health and Welfare Canada, *Nutrition Recommendations: The Report of the Scientific Review Committee* (Ottawa: Canadian Government Publishing Centre, 1990), Table 20, p. 204. Used with permission.

TABLE C–2
AVERAGE ENERGY REQUIREMENTS FOR CANADIANS

Age	Sex	AVERAGE HEIGHT (cm)	AVERAGE WEIGHT (kg)	REQUIREMENTS[a] (cal/kg)[b]	(MJ/kg)[b]	(cal/day)	(MJ/day)	(cal/cm)	(MJ/cm)
Infants (months)									
0-2	Both	55	4.5	120-100	0.50-0.42	500	2.0	9	0.04
3-5	Both	63	7.0	100-95	0.42-0.40	700	2.8	11	0.05
6-8	Both	69	8.5	95-97	0.40-0.41	800	3.4	11.5	0.05
9-11	Both	73	9.5	97-99	0.41	950	3.8	12.5	0.05
Children and adults (years)									
1	Both	82	11	101	0.42	1,100	4.8	13.5	0.06
2-3	Both	95	14	94	0.39	1,300	5.6	13.5	0.06
4-6	Both	107	18	100	0.42	1,800	7.6	17	0.07
7-9	M	126	25	88	0.37	2,200	9.2	17.5	0.07
	F	125	25	76	0.32	1,900	8.0	15	0.06
10-12	M	141	34	73	0.30	2,500	10.4	17.5	0.07
	F	143	36	61	0.25	2,200	9.2	15.5	0.06
13-15	M	159	50	57	0.24	2,800	12.0	17.5	0.07
	F	157	48	46	0.19	2,200	9.2	14	0.06
16-18	M	172	62	51	0.21	3,200	13.2	18.5	0.08
	F	160	53	40	0.17	2,100	8.8	13	0.05
19-24	M	175	71	42	0.18	3,000	12.6		
	F	160	58	36	0.15	2,100	8.8		
25-49	M	172	74	36	0.15	2,700	11.3		
	F	160	59	32	0.13	1,900	8.0		
50-74	M	170	73	31	0.13	2,300	9.7		
	F	158	63	29	0.12	1,800	7.6		
75+	M	168	69	29	0.12	2,000	8.4		
	F	155	64	23	0.10	1,500	6.3		

[a]Requirements can be expected to vary within a range of ±30 percent.

[b]First and last figures are averages at the beginning and end of the three-month period.

SOURCE: Health and Welfare Canada. *Nutrition Recommendations: The Report of the Scientific Review Committee* (Ottawa: Canadian Government Publishing Centre, 1990), Tables 5 and 6, pp. 25, 17. Used with permission.

Canada's Food Guide to Healthy Eating

The 1992 *Canada's Food Guide to Healthy Eating* gives consumers detailed information for selecting foods to meet *Canada's Guidelines for Healthy Eating* (1990). The *Food Guide* was designed to meet the nutritional needs of all Canadians four years of age and older and takes a total diet approach, rather than emphasizing a single food, meal, or day's meals and snacks.

The rainbow side of the Food Guide shows the four food groups with their revised names and pictorial examples of foods in each group. Key statements direct consumers about selecting foods generally from all the groups, and more specifically within each group. The bar side shows the number of servings recommended for each group, using a range of servings instead of a single minimum number. Other notable changes include the number of servings for some food groups and the size of servings for some foods.

Healthy Canada

Health and Welfare Canada | Santé et Bien-étre social Canada

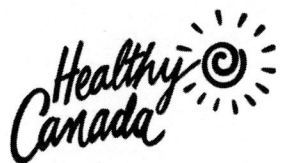

CANADA'S

Food Guide

TO HEALTHY EATING

Enjoy a variety of foods from each group every day.

Choose lower-fat foods more often.

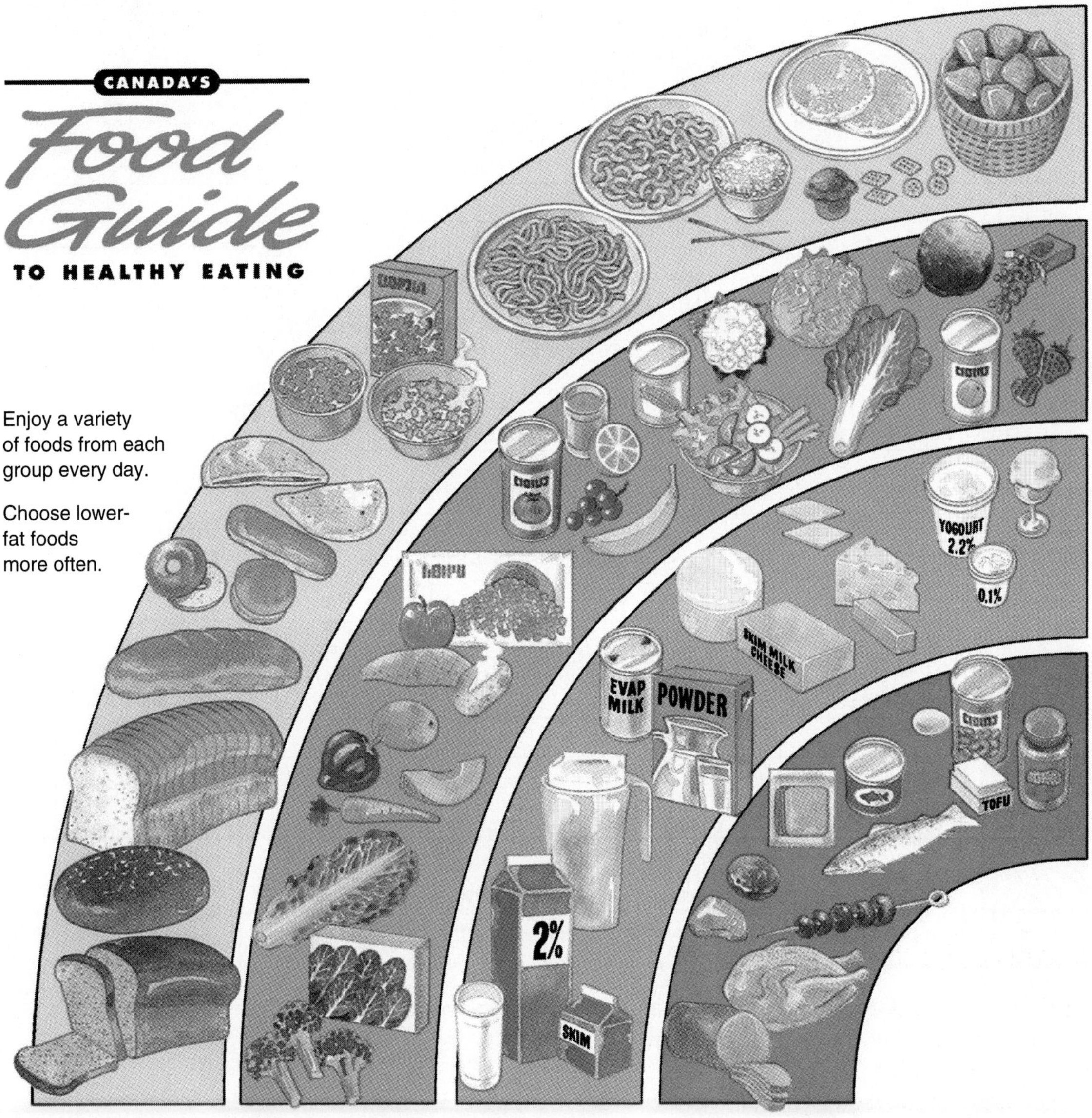

Grain Products
Choose whole grain and enriched products more often.

Vegetables & Fruit
Choose dark green and orange vegetables and orange fruit more often.

Milk Products
Choose lower-fat milk products more often.

Meat & Alternatives
Choose leaner meats, poultry and fish, as well as dried peas, beans and lentils more often.

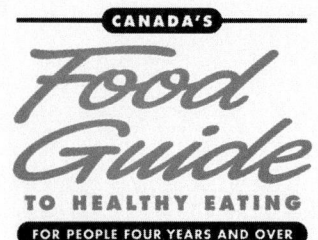

CANADA'S

Food Guide

TO HEALTHY EATING

FOR PEOPLE FOUR YEARS AND OVER

Different People Need Different Amounts of Food

The amount of food you need every day from the 4 food groups and other foods depends on your age, body size, activity level, whether you are male or female and if you are pregnant or breast-feeding. That's why the Food Guide gives a lower and higher number of servings for each food group. For example, young children can choose the lower number of servings, while male teenagers can go to the higher number. Most other people can choose servings somewhere in between.

Grain Products

5–12

SERVINGS PER DAY

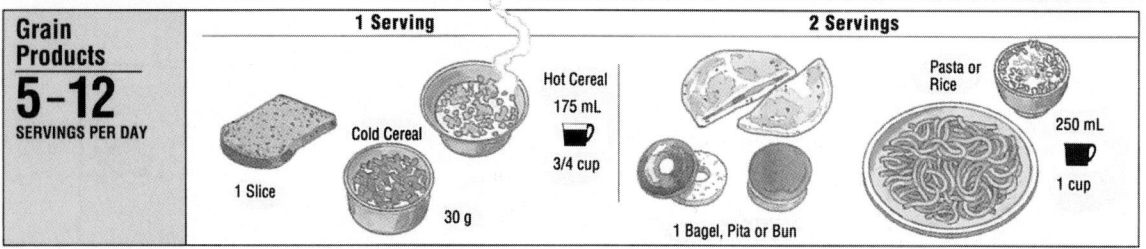

1 Serving

1 Slice · Cold Cereal 30 g · Hot Cereal 175 mL 3/4 cup

2 Servings

1 Bagel, Pita or Bun · Pasta or Rice 250 mL 1 cup

Vegetables & Fruit

5–10

SERVINGS PER DAY

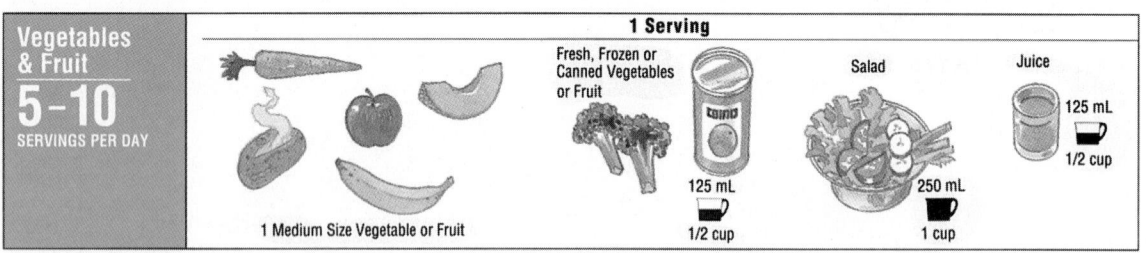

1 Serving

1 Medium Size Vegetable or Fruit · Fresh, Frozen or Canned Vegetables or Fruit 125 mL 1/2 cup · Salad 250 mL 1 cup · Juice 125 mL 1/2 cup

Milk Products

SERVINGS PER DAY

Children 4–9 years: 2–3
Youth 10–16 years: 3–4
Adults: 2–4
Pregnant & Breast-feeding Women: 3–4

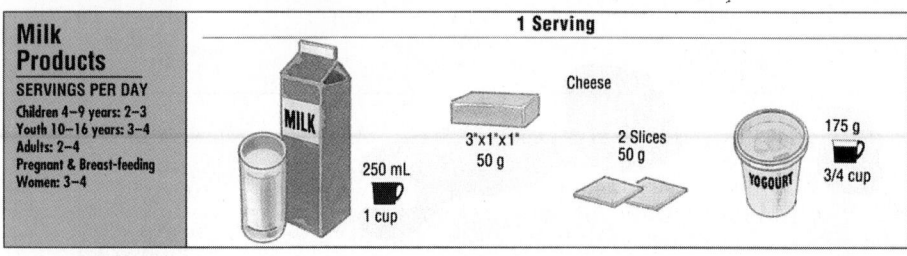

1 Serving

MILK 250 mL 1 cup · Cheese 3"x1"x1" 50 g · 2 Slices 50 g · YOGOURT 175 g 3/4 cup

Other Foods

Taste and enjoyment can also come from other foods and beverages that are not part of the 4 food groups. Some of these foods are higher in fat or Calories, so use these foods in moderation.

Meat & Alternatives

2–3

SERVINGS PER DAY

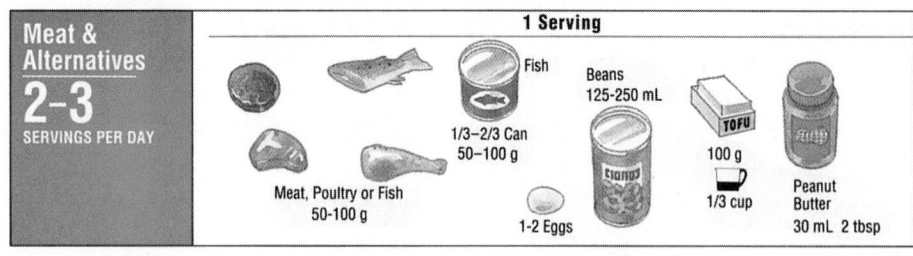

1 Serving

Meat, Poultry or Fish 50-100 g · Fish 1/3–2/3 Can 50–100 g · 1-2 Eggs · Beans 125–250 mL 1/3 cup · TOFU 100 g · Peanut Butter 30 mL 2 tbsp

Enjoy eating well, being active and feeling good about yourself. That's VITALIT

© Minister of Supply and Services Canada 1992   Cat. No. H39-252/1992E   No changes permitted. Reprint permission not required.
ISBN 0-662-19648-1

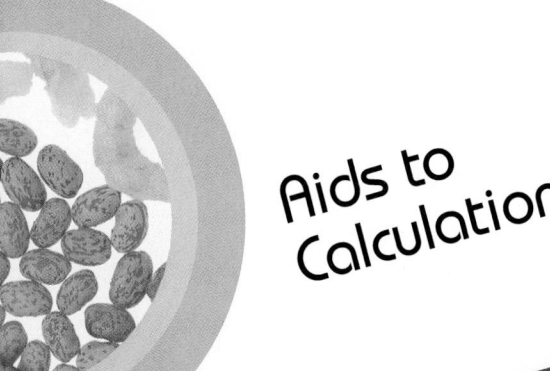

Aids to Calculation

Many mathematical problems have been worked out for you as examples at appropriate places in the text. This appendix aims to help with the use of the metric system and with those problems not fully explained elsewhere.

Conversion Factors*

Conversion factors are useful mathematical tools in everyday calculations, like the ones encountered in the study of nutrition. Skill in the use of conversion factors is especially desirable as the United States and Canada "go metric."

A conversion factor is a fraction in which the numerator (top) and the denominator (bottom) express the same quantity in different units. For example, 2.2 pounds and 1 kilogram are equivalent; they express the same weight. The conversion factor used to change pounds to kilograms or vice versa is:

$$\frac{2.2 \text{ lb}}{1 \text{ kg}} \quad \text{or} \quad \frac{1 \text{ kg}}{2.2 \text{ lb}}$$

Because either of these factors equals 1, a measurement can be multiplied by the factor without changing the value of the measurement. Thus its units can be changed.

The correct factor to use in a problem is the one with the unit you are seeking in the numerator (top) of the fraction. Following are three examples of problems commonly encountered in nutrition study; they illustrate the usefulness of conversion factors.

Example 1

Convert ¼ cup to an approximate number of milliliters for use in a recipe.

1. The conversion factor is:

$$\frac{1 \text{ c}}{250 \text{ ml}} \quad \text{or} \quad \frac{250 \text{ ml}}{1 \text{ c}}$$

2. Multiply 1/4 cup by the factor:

$$¼ \cancel{c} \times \frac{250 \text{ ml}}{1 \cancel{c}} = 62.5 \text{ ml, or about } 60 \text{ ml}$$

*For a listing of specific conversion factors, see inside back cover.

Example 2

Convert the weight of 130 pounds to kilograms.

1. Choose the conversion factor in which the unit you are seeking is on top:

$$\frac{1 \text{ kg}}{2.2 \text{ lb}}$$

2. Multiply 130 pounds by the factor:

$$130 \text{ lb} \times \frac{1 \text{ kg}}{2.2 \text{ lb}} = \frac{130 \text{ kg}}{2.2} = 59 \text{ kg (rounded off to nearest whole number)}.$$

Example 3

How many grams of saturated fat are contained in a 3-ounce hamburger? A 4-ounce hamburger contains 7 grams of saturated fat.

1. You are seeking grams of saturated fat; therefore, the conversion factor is:

$$\frac{7 \text{ g saturated fat}}{4 \text{ oz hamburger}}$$

2. Multiply 3 ounces of hamburger by the conversion factor:

$$3 \text{ oz hamburger} \times \frac{7 \text{ g saturated fat}}{4 \text{ oz hamburger}} = \frac{3 \times 7 \text{ g}}{4} = \frac{21}{4}$$
$$= 5 \text{ g saturated fat (rounded off to nearest whole number)}.$$

Percentages

A percentage is a comparison between a number of items (perhaps your intake of calories) and a standard number (perhaps the number of calories recommended for your age and sex—your energy RDA). The standard number is the number you divide by. The answer you get after the division must be multiplied by 100 to be stated as a percentage (*percent* means "per 100").

Example 4

What percentage of the RDA for calories is your calorie intake?

1. Find your energy RDA (inside front cover). We'll use 2,100 calories to demonstrate.

2. Total your calorie intake for a day—for example, 1,200 calories.

3. Divide your calorie intake by the RDA calories:

1,200 cal (your intake) ÷ 2,100 cal (RDA) = 0.571

4. Multiply your answer by 100 to state it as a percentage:

0.571 × 100 = 57.1 = 57% (rounded off to the nearest whole number).

In some problems in nutrition, the percentage may be more than 100. For example, suppose your daily intake of vitamin A is 3,200 RE and your RDA (male) is 1,000 RE. Your intake as a percentage of the RDA is more than 100 percent (that is, you consume more than 100 percent of your vitamin A RDA). The following calculations show your vitamin A intake as a percentage of the RDA:

$$3,200 \div 1,000 = 3.2$$
$$3.2 \times 100 = 320\% \text{ of RDA.}$$

Sometimes the comparison is between a part of a whole (for example, your calories from protein) and the total amount (your total calories). In this case, the total number is the one you divide by as shown in example 5.

Example 5

What percentages of your total calories for the day come from protein, fat, and carbohydrate?

1. Using Appendix I and your diet record, find the total grams of protein, fat, and carbohydrate you consumed—for example, 60 grams protein, 80 grams fat, and 285 grams carbohydrate.

2. Multiply the number of grams by the number of calories from 1 gram of each energy nutrient (conversion factors):

$$60 \text{ g protein} \times \frac{4 \text{ cal}}{1 \text{ g protein}} = 240 \text{ cal}$$

$$80 \text{ g fat} \times \frac{9 \text{ cal}}{1 \text{ g fat}} = 720 \text{ cal}$$

$$285 \text{ g carbohydrate} \times \frac{4 \text{ cal}}{1 \text{ g carbohydrate}} = 1,140 \text{ cal}$$

$$240 + 720 + 1,140 = 2,100 \text{ cal}$$

3. Find the percentage of total calories from each energy nutrient (see Example 4):

Protein: $240 \div 2,100 = 0.114$
$0.114 \times 100 = 11.4 = 11\%$ of calories.

Fat: $720 \div 2,100 = 0.343$
$0.343 \times 100 = 34.3 = 34\%$ of calories.

Carbohydrate: $1,140 \div 2,100 = 0.543$
$0.543 \times 100 = 54.3 = 54\%$ of calories.

$11\% + 34\% + 54\% = 99\%$ of calories (total).

The percentages total 99 percent rather than 100 percent because a little was lost from each number in rounding off. Either 99 or 101 is a reasonable total in problems like this.

Nutrient Units

To convert IU (International Units) found on supplement labels to the units used in the RDA tables:

Vitamin A

From animal sources:

$3\mu g = 1$ IU

1 RE[a] $= 3.33$ IU

From vegetables and fruits:

$.6 \mu g = 1$ IU

1 RE $= 10$ IU

Vitamin D

$1 \mu g = 40$ IU

Vitamin E

1 mg $= 1$ IU

1α TE[b] $= 1$ IU

Sodium

To convert milligrams of sodium to grams of salt:

mg sodium $\div 400 =$ g of salt

The reverse is also true:

g salt $\times 400 =$ mg sodium

---

[a]Retinol equivalents

[b]Alpha-tocopherol equivalents

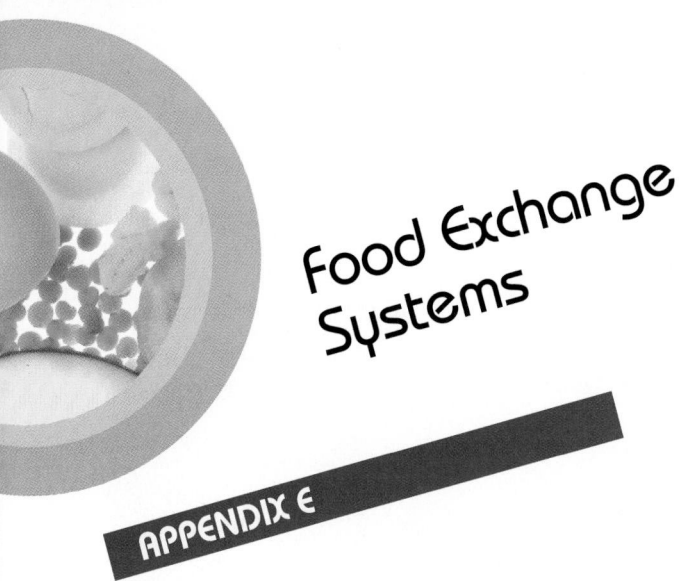

Food Exchange Systems

Chapter 2 introduced dietary guidelines, food group plans, and the exchange system. This appendix provides details of the U.S. and Canadian exchange systems.

The U.S. Exchange System

The U.S. exchange system divides the foods suitable for use in planning a healthy diet into seven lists—the starch, fruit, milk, other carbohydrates, vegetable, meat and meat substitutes, and fat lists.[a] These lists are shown in Tables E-1 through E-7. Following these lists are three other sets of foods: free foods, combination foods, and fast foods (Tables E-8, E-9, and E-10).

---

[a]The U.S. Exchange System presented here is based on material in *Exchange Lists for Meal Planning,* 1995, prepared by committees of the American Diabetes Association and the American Dietetic Association, with permission of both organizations.

TABLE E-1
THE U.S. EXCHANGE SYSTEM: STARCH LIST

15 g carbohydrate, 3 g protein, 0–1 g fat, 80 cal

Cereals, grains, pasta, breads, crackers, snacks, starchy vegetables, and cooked dried beans, peas, and lentils are starches. In general, one starch is:

- ½ cup of cereal, grain, pasta, or starchy vegetable
- 1 ounce of a bread product, such as 1 slice of bread
- ¾ to 1 ounce of most snack foods (some snack foods may also have added fat)

AMOUNT	FOOD
BREAD	
½ (1 oz)	Bagel
2 slices (1½ oz)	Bread, reduced-calorie
1 slice (1 oz)	Bread, white, whole-wheat, pumpernickel, rye
2 (⅔ oz)	Bread sticks, crisp, 4 in. long × ½ in.
½	English muffin
½ (1 oz)	Hot dog or hamburger bun
½	Pita, 6 in. across
1 slice (1 oz)	Raisin bread, unfrosted
1 (1 oz)	Roll, plain, small
1	Tortilla, corn, 6 in. across
1	Tortilla, flour, 7–8 in. across
1	Waffle, 4½ in. square, reduced-fat
CEREALS AND GRAINS	
½ cup	Bran cereals
½ cup	Bulgur
½ cup	Cereals
¾ cup	Cereals, unsweetened, ready-to-eat
3 tbsp	Cornmeal (dry)
⅓ cup	Couscous
3 tbsp	Flour (dry)
¼ cup	Granola, low-fat
¼ cup	Grape-Nuts
½ cup	Grits
½ cup	Kasha
¼ cup	Millet
¼ cup	Muesli
½ cup	Oats
½ cup	Pasta
1½ cups	Puffed cereal
½ cup	Rice milk
⅓ cup	Rice, white or brown
½ cup	Shredded Wheat
½ cup	Sugar-frosted cereal
3 tbsp	Wheat germ

AMOUNT	FOOD
STARCHY VEGETABLES	
⅓ cup	Baked beans
½ cup	Corn
1 (5 oz)	Corn on cob, medium
1 cup	Mixed vegetables with corn, peas, or pasta
½ cup	Peas, green
½ cup	Plantain
1 small (3 oz)	Potato, baked or boiled
½ cup	Potato, mashed
1 cup	Squash, winter (acorn, butternut)
½ cup	Yam, sweet potato, plain
CRACKERS AND SNACKS	
8	Animal crackers
3	Graham crackers, 2½ in. square
¾ oz	Matzoh
4 slices	Melba toast
24	Oyster crackers
3 cups	Popcorn (popped, no fat added or low-fat microwave)
¾ oz	Pretzels
2	Rice cakes, 4 in. across
6	Saltine-type crackers
15–20 (¾ oz)	Snack chips, fat-free (tortilla, potato)
2–5 (¾ oz)	Whole-wheat crackers, no fat added
DRIED BEANS. PEAS, AND LENTILS	
(Count as 1 starch exchange, plus 1 very lean meat exchange)	
½ cup	Beans and peas (garbanzo, pinto, kidney, white, split, black-eyed)
⅔ cup	Lima beans
½ cup	Lentils
3 tbsp	Miso 🥢

🥢 = 400 mg or more of sodium per serving.

TABLE E–1 *continued*
THE U.S. EXCHANGE SYSTEM: STARCH LIST

AMOUNT	FOOD	AMOUNT	FOOD
STARCHY FOODS PREPARED WITH FAT			
(Count as 1 starch exchange, plus 1 fat exchange)			
1	Biscuit, 2½ in. across	2	Pancakes, 4 in. across
½ cup	Chow mein noodles	3 cups	Popcorn, microwave
1 (2 oz)	Corn bread, 2 in. cube	3	Sandwich crackers, cheese or peanut
6	Crackers, round butter type		butter filling
1 cup	Croutons	⅓ cup	Stuffing, bread (prepared)
16–25 (3 oz)	French-fried potatoes	2	Taco shell, 6 in. across
¼ cup	Granola	1	Waffle, 4½ in. square
1 (1½ oz)	Muffin, small	4–6 (1 oz)	Whole-wheat crackers, fat added

TABLE E–2
U.S. EXCHANGE SYSTEM: FRUIT LIST

15 g carbohydrates, 60 cal

Fresh, frozen, canned, and dried fruits and fruit juices are on this list. In general, one fruit exchange is:

- 1 small to medium fresh fruit
- ½ cup of canned or fresh fruit or fruit juice
- ¼ cup of dried fruit

AMOUNT	FOOD	AMOUNT	FOOD
FRUIT		½ fruit (8 oz) or 1 cup cubes	Papaya
		1 (6 oz)	Peach, medium, fresh
1 (4 oz)	Apple, unpeeled, small	½ cup	Peaches, canned
½ cup	Applesauce, unsweetened	½ (4 oz)	Pear, large, fresh
4 rings	Apples, dried	½ cup	Pears, canned
4 whole (5½ oz)	Apricots, fresh	¾ cup	Pineapple, fresh
8 halves	Apricots, dried	½ cup	Pineapple, canned
½ cup	Apricots, canned	2 (5 oz)	Plums, small
1 (4 oz)	Banana, small	½ cup	Plums, canned
¾ cup	Blackberries	3	Prunes, dried
¾ cup	Blueberries	2 tbsp	Raisins
⅓ melon (11 oz) or 1 cup cubes	Cantaloupe, small	1 cup	Raspberries
		1¼ cup whole berries	Strawberries
12 (3 oz)	Cherries, sweet, fresh	2 (8 oz)	Tangerines, small
½ cup	Cherries, sweet, canned	slice (13 ½ oz) or 1¼ cup cubes	Watermelon
3	Dates		
½ large or 2 medium (3½ oz)	Figs, fresh	**FRUIT JUICE**	
1½	Figs, dried	½ cup	Apple juice/cider
½ cup	Fruit cocktail	⅓ cup	Cranberry juice cocktail
½ (11 oz)	Grapefruit, large	1 cup	Cranberry juice cocktail, reduced-calorie
¾ cup	Grapefruit sections, canned		
17 (3 oz)	Grapes, small	⅓ cup	Fruit juice blend, 100% juice
1 slice (10 oz) or 1 cup cubes	Honeydew melon	⅓ cup	Grape juice
1 (3½ oz)	Kiwi	½ cup	Grapefruit juice
¾ cup	Mandarin oranges, canned	½ cup	Orange juice
½ fruit (5½ oz) or ½ cup	Mango, small	½ cup	Pineapple juice
1 (5 oz)	Nectarine, small	⅓ cup	Prune juice
1 (6½ oz)	Orange, small		

TABLE E–3
U.S. EXCHANGE SYSTEM: MILK LIST

Nonfat and very lowfat milk = 12 g carbohydrate, 8 g protein, 0–3 g fat, 90 cal; low-fat milk = 12 g carbohydrate, 8 g protein, 5 g fat, 120 cal; whole milk = 12 g carbohydrate, 8 g protein, 8 g fat, 150 cal.

AMOUNT	FOOD	AMOUNT	FOOD
NONFAT AND VERY LOW-FAT MILK		**LOW-FAT MILK**	
1 c	Nonfat milk	1 c	2% milk
1 c	½% milk	¾ c	Plain low-fat yogurt
1 c	1% milk	1 c	Sweet acidophilus milk
⅓ c	Dry nonfat milk	**WHOLE MILK**	
½ c	Evaporated nonfat milk		
1 c	Nonfat or low-fat buttermilk	1 c	Whole milk
¾ c	Plain nonfat yogurt	½ c	Evaporated whole milk
1 c	Nonfat or low-fat fruit-flavored yogurt sweetened with aspartame or with a nonnutritive sweetener	1 c	Goat's milk
		1 c	Kefir

TABLE E–4
U.S. EXCHANGE SYSTEM: OTHER CARBOHYDRATES LIST

15 grams carbohydrate, or 1 starch, or 1 fruit, or 1 milk.

You can substitute food choices from this list for a starch, fruit, or milk choice on your meal plan. Some choices will also count as one or more fat choices.

AMOUNT	FOOD	EXCHANGES PER SERVING
1/12th cake	Angel food cake, unfrosted	2 carbohydrates
2 in. square	Brownie, small, unfrosted	1 carbohydrate, 1 fat
2 in. square	Cake, unfrosted	1 carbohydrate, 1 fat
2 in. square	Cake, frosted	2 carbohydrates, 1 fat
2 small	Cookie, fat-free	1 carbohydrate
2 small	Cookie or sandwich cookie with creme filling	1 carbohydrate, 1 fat
1 small	Cupcake, frosted	2 carbohydrates, 1 fat
¼ cup	Cranberry sauce, jellied	2 carbohydrates
1 medium (1½ oz)	Doughnut, plain cake	1½ carbohydrates, 2 fats
3¾ in. across (2 oz)	Doughnut, glazed	2 carbohydrates, 2 fats
1 bar (3 oz)	Fruit juice bars, frozen, 100% juice	1 carbohydrate
1 roll (¾ oz)	Fruit snacks, chewy (pureed fruit concentrate)	1 carbohydrate
1 tbsp	Fruit spreads, 100% fruit	1 carbohydrate
½ cup	Gelatin, regular	1 carbohydrate
3	Gingersnaps	1 carbohydrate
1 bar	Granola bar	1 carbohydrate, 1 fat
1 bar	Granola bar, fat-free	2 carbohydrates
⅓ cup	Hummus	1 carbohydrate, 1 fat

continued

TABLE E–4 *continued*
U.S. EXCHANGE SYSTEM: OTHER CARBOHYDRATES LIST

AMOUNT	FOOD	EXCHANGE PER SERVING
½ cup	Ice cream	1 carbohydrate, 2 fats
½ cup	Ice cream, light	1 carbohydrate, 1 fat
½ cup	Ice cream, fat-free, no sugar added	1 carbohydrate
1 tbsp	Jam or jelly, regular	1 carbohydrate
1 cup	Milk, chocolate, whole	2 carbohydrates, 1 fat
⅙ pie	Pie, fruit, 2 crusts	3 carbohydrates, 2 fats
⅛ pie	Pie, pumpkin or custard	1 carbohydrate, 2 fats
12–18 (1 oz)	Potato chips	1 carbohydrate, 2 fats
½ cup	Pudding, regular (made with low-fat milk)	2 carbohydrates
½ cup	Pudding, sugar-free (made with low-fat milk)	1 carbohydrate
¼ cup	Salad dressing, fat-free 🥄	1 carbohydrate
½ cup	Sherbet, sorbet	2 carbohydrates
½ cup	Spaghetti or pasta sauce, canned 🥄	1 carbohydrate, 1 fat
1 (2½ oz)	Sweet roll or Danish	2½ carbohydrates, 2 fats
2 tbsp	Syrup, light	1 carbohydrate
1 tbsp	Syrup, regular	1 carbohydrate
¼ cup	Syrup, regular	4 carbohydrates
6–12 (1 oz)	Tortilla chips	1 carbohydrate, 2 fats
⅓ cup	Yogurt, frozen, low-fat, fat-free	1 carbohydrate, 0–1 fat
½ cup	Yogurt, frozen, fat-free, no sugar added	1 carbohydrate
1 cup	Yogurt, low-fat with fruit	3 carbohydrates, 0–1 fat
5	Vanilla wafers	1 carbohydrate, 1 fat

🥄 = 400 mg or more sodium per exchange.

TABLE E–5
U.S. EXCHANGE SYSTEM: VEGETABLE LIST

5 g carbohydrate, 2 g protein, 25 cal. All portion sizes, except as otherwise noted, are ½ c of any cooked vegetable or vegetable juice, 1 c of any raw vegetable.

Artichoke
Artichoke hearts
Asparagus
Beans (green, wax, Italian)
Bean sprouts
Beets
Broccoli
Brussels sprouts
Cabbage
Carrots
Cauliflower
Celery
Cucumber

Eggplant
Green onions or scallions
Greens (collard, kale, mustard, turnip)
Kohlrabi
Leeks
Mixed vegetables (without corn, peas, or pasta)*
Mushrooms
Okra
Onions
Pea pods
Peppers (all varieties)
Radishes

Salad greens (endive, escarole, lettuce, romaine, spinach)
Sauerkraut 🥄
Spinach
Summer squash
Tomato
Tomatoes, canned
Tomato sauce 🥄

Tomato/vegetable juice 🥄
Turnips
Water chestnuts
Watercress

*Starchy vegetables such as corn, peas, and potatoes are found on the Starch List.
🥄 = 400 mg or more sodium per exchange.

TABLE E–6
U.S. EXCHANGE SYSTEM: MEAT/MEAT SUBSTITUTES

Very-Lean meat = 7 g protein, 0–1 g fat, 35 cal; Lean meat = 7 g protein, 3 g fat, 55 cal; medium-fat meat = 7 g protein, 5 g fat, 75 cal; high-fat meat = 7 g protein, 8 g fat, 100 cal.

Meat and meat substitutes that contain both protein and fat are on this list. In general, one meat exchange is:

- 1 oz meat, fish, poultry, or cheese
- ½ cup dried beans, cooked

Based on the amount of fat they contain, meats are divided into very lean, lean, medium-fat, and high-fat lists.

AMOUNT	FOOD
VERY LEAN MEAT AND SUBSTITUTES LIST	
1 oz	*Poultry:* Chicken or turkey (white meat, no skin), Cornish hen (no skin)
1 oz	*Fish:* Fresh or frozen cod, flounder, haddock, halibut, trout; tuna, fresh or canned in water
1 oz	*Shellfish:* Clams, crab, lobster, scallops, shrimp, imitation shellfish
1 oz	*Game:* Duck or pheasant (no skin), venison, buffalo, ostrich
	Cheese with 1 gram or less fat per ounce:
¼ cup	Nonfat or low-fat cottage cheese
1 oz	Fat-free cheese
1 oz	*Other:* Processed sandwich meats with 1 gram or less fat per ounce, such as deli thin, shaved meats, chipped beef 🖋 , turkey ham
2	Egg whites
¼ cup	Egg substitutes, plain
1 oz	Hot dogs with 1 gram or less fat per ounce 🖋
1 oz	Kidney (high in cholesterol)
1 oz	Sausage with 1 gram or less fat per ounce

Count as one very lean meat and one starch exchange:

AMOUNT	FOOD
½ cup	Dried beans, peas, lentils (cooked)

AMOUNT	FOOD
LEAN MEAT AND SUBSTITUTES LIST	
1 oz	*Beef:* USDA Select or Choice grades of lean beef trimmed of fat, such as round, sirloin, and flank steak; tenderloin; roast (rib, chuck, rump); steak (T-bone, porterhouse, cubed), ground round
1 oz	*Pork:* Lean pork, such as fresh ham; canned, cured, or boiled ham; Canadian bacon 🖋 ; tenderloin, center loin chop

AMOUNT	FOOD
1 oz	*Lamb:* Roast, chop, leg
1 oz	*Veal:* Lean chop, roast
1 oz	*Poultry:* Chicken, turkey (dark meat, no skin), chicken white meat (with skin), domestic duck or goose (well-drained of fat, no skin)
	Fish:
1 oz	Herring (uncreamed or smoked)
6 medium	Oysters
1 oz	Salmon (fresh or canned), catfish
2 medium	Sardines (canned)
1 oz	Tuna (canned in oil, drained)
1 oz	*Game:* Goose (no skin), rabbit
	Cheese:
¼ cup	4.5%-fat cottage cheese
2 tbsp	Grated Parmesan
1 oz	Cheese with 3 grams or less fat per ounce
	Other:
1½ oz	Hot dots with 3 grams or less fat per ounce 🖋
1 oz	Processed sandwich meat with 3 grams or less fat per ounce, such as turkey pastrami or kielbasa
1 oz	Liver, heart (high in cholesterol)

AMOUNT	FOOD
MEDIUM-FAT MEAT AND SUBSTITUTES LIST	
1 oz	*Beef:* Most beef products fall into this category (ground beef, meatloaf, corned beef, short ribs, Prime grades of meat trimmed of fat, such as prime rib)
1 oz	*Pork:* Top loin, chop, Boston butt, cutlet
1 oz	*Lamb:* Rib roast, ground
1 oz	*Veal:* Cutlet (ground or cubed, unbreaded)
1 oz	*Poultry:* Chicken dark meat (with skin), ground turkey or ground chicken, fried chicken (with skin)

🖋 = 400 mg or more sodium per exchange

continued

TABLE E–6 *continued*
U.S. EXCHANGE SYSTEM: MEAT/MEAT SUBSTITUTES

AMOUNT	FOOD	AMOUNT	FOOD
MEDIUM-FAT MEAT AND SUBSTITUTES LIST *(continued)*		**HIGH-FAT MEAT AND SUBSTITUTES LIST**	
1 oz	*Fish:* Any fried fish product	1 oz	*Pork:* Spareribs, ground pork, pork sausage
	Cheese: With 5 grams or less fat per ounce	1 oz	*Cheese:* All regular cheeses, such as
1 oz	Feta		American ✑, cheddar, Monterey Jack,
1 oz	Mozzarella		Swiss
¼ cup	Ricotta	1 oz	*Other:* Processed sandwich meats with
	Other:		8 grams or less fat per ounce, such as
1	Egg (high in cholesterol, limit to 3 per		bologna, pimento loaf, salami
	week)	1 oz	Sausage, such as bratwurst, Italian,
1 oz	Sausage with 5 grams or less fat per		knockwurst, Polish, smoked
	ounce	1 (10/lb)	Hot dog (turkey or chicken) ✑
1 cup	Soy milk	3 slices	Bacon
¼ cup	Tempeh	(20 slices/lb)	
4 oz or	Tofu		
½ cup		**Count as one high-fat meat plus one fat exchange:**	
		1 (10/lb)	Hot dog (beef, pork, or combination) ✑
		2 tbsp	Peanut butter (contains unsaturated fat)

✑ = 400 mg or more sodium per exchange.

TABLE E–7 U.S. EXCHANGE SYSTEM: FAT LIST

5 g fat, 45 cal.

AMOUNT	FOOD	AMOUNT	FOOD
MONOUNSATURATED FATS LIST		1 tbsp	Salad dressing: regular ✑
⅛ (1 oz)	Avocado, medium	2 tbsp	reduced-fat
1 tsp	Oil (canola, olive, peanut)	2 tsp	Miracle Whip Salad Dressing®: regular
8 large	Olives: ripe (black)	1 tbsp	reduced-fat
10 large	green, stuffed ✑	1 tbsp	Seeds: pumpkin, sunflower
	Nuts		
6 nuts	almonds, cashews	**SATURATED FATS LIST***	
6 nuts	mixed (50% peanuts)	1 slice (20 slices/lb)	Bacon, cooked
10 nuts	peanuts	1 tsp	Bacon, grease
4 halves	pecans	1 tsp	Butter: stick
2 tsp	Peanut butter, smooth or crunchy	2 tsp	whipped
1 tbsp	Sesame seeds	1 tbsp	reduced-fat
2 tsp	Tahini paste	2 tbsp (½ oz)	Chitterlings, boiled
		2 tbsp	Coconut, sweetened, shredded
POLYUNSATURATED FATS LIST		2 tbsp	Cream, half and half
1 tsp	Margarine: stick, tub, or squeeze	1 tbsp (½ oz)	Cream cheese: regular
1 tbsp	lower-fat (30% to 50% vegetable oil)	2 tbsp (1 oz)	reduced-fat
1 tsp	Mayonnaise: regular		Fatback or salt pork, see below†
1 tbsp	reduced-fat	1 tsp	Shortening or lard
4 halves	Nuts, walnuts, English	2 tbsp	Sour cream: regular
1 tsp	Oil (corn, safflower, soybean)	3 tbsp	reduced-fat

*Saturated fats can raise blood cholesterol levels.

†Use a piece 1 in. × 1 in. × ¼ in. if you plan to eat the fatback cooked with vegetables. Use a piece 2 in. × 1 in. × ½ in. when eating only the vegetables with the fatback removed.

✑ = 400 mg or more sodium per exchange.

TABLE E–8
U.S. EXCHANGE SYSTEM: FREE FOODS

A free food is any food or drink that contains less then 20 cal/serving. People with diabetes are advised to eat as much as they want of those items that have no serving size specified. They may eat two or three servings per day of those items that have a specific serving size. It is suggested that they spread the servings out through the day. Foods listed without a serving size can be eaten as often as you like.

AMOUNT	FOOD	AMOUNT	FOOD
FAT-FREE OR REDUCED-FAT FOODS			Carbonated or mineral water
1 tbsp	Cream cheese, fat-free	1 tbsp	Cocoa powder, unsweetened
1 tbsp	Creamers, nondairy, liquid		Coffee
2 tsp	Creamers, nondairy, powdered		Club Soda
1 tbsp	Mayonnaise, fat-free		Diet soft drinks, sugar-free
1 tsp	Mayonnaise, reduced-fat		Drink mixes, sugar-free
4 tbsp	Margarine, fat-free		Tea
1 tsp	Margarine, reduced-fat		Tonic water, sugar-free
1 tbsp	Miracle Whip®, nonfat		
1 tsp	Miracle Whip®, reduced-fat	**CONDIMENTS**	
	Nonstick cooking spray	1 tbsp	Catsup
1 tbsp	Salad dressing, fat-free		Horseradish
2 tbsp	Salad dressing, fat-free, Italian		Lemon juice
¼ cup	Salsa		Lime juice
1 tbsp	Sour cream, fat-free, reduced-fat		Mustard
2 tbsp	Whipped topping, regular or light	1½ large	Pickles, dill
			Soy sauce, regular or light
SUGAR-FREE OR LOW-SUGAR FOODS		1 tbsp	Taco sauce
1 candy	Candy, hard, sugar-free		Vinegar
	Gelatin dessert, sugar-free		
	Gelatin, unflavored	**SEASONINGS**	
	Gum, sugar-free		Flavoring extracts
2 tsp	Jam or jelly, low-sugar or light		Garlic
	Sugar substitutes*		Herbs, fresh or dried
2 tbsp	Syrup, sugar-free		Pimento
			Spices
DRINKS			Tabasco® or hot pepper sauce
	Bouillon, broth, consommé		Wine, used in cooking
	Bouillon or broth, low-sodium		Worcestershire sauce

*Sugar substitutes, alternatives, or replacements that are approved by the Food and Drug Administration (FDA) are safe to use. Common brand names include:

Equal® (aspartame)   Sweet-10® (saccharin)
Sprinkle Sweet® (saccharin)   Sugar Twin® (saccharin)
Sweet One® (acesulfame K)   Sweet 'N Low® (saccharin)

= 400 mg or more of sodium per choice.

TABLE E-9
U.S. EXCHANGE SYSTEM: COMBINATION FOODS

Much of the food we eat is mixed together in various combinations. These combination foods do not fit into any one exchange list. It can be quite hard to tell what is in a certain casserole dish or baked food item. This is a list of average values for some typical combination foods. This list will help you fit these foods into your meal plan. Ask your dietitian for information about any other foods you'd like to eat.

AMOUNT	FOOD	EXCHANGES PER SERVING
ENTREES		
1 cup (8 oz)	Tuna noodle casserole, lasagna, spaghetti with meatballs, chili with beans, macaroni and cheese 🥢	2 carbohydrates, 2 medium-fat meats 1 carbohydrate, 2 lean meats 2 carbohydrates, 2 medium-fat meats, 1 fat
2 cups (16 oz)	Chow mein (without noodles or rice)	2 carbohydrates, 2 medium-fat meats, 2 fats
¼ of 10 in. (5 oz)	Pizza, cheese, thin crust 🥢	2 carbohydrates, 1 medium-fat meat, 4 fats
¼ of 10 in. (5 oz)	Pizza, meat topping, thin crust 🥢	
1 (7 oz)	Pot pie 🥢	
FROZEN ENTREES		
1 (11 oz)	Salisbury steak with gravy, mashed potato 🥢	2 carbohydrates, 3 medium-fat meats, 3–4 fats
1 (11 oz)	Turkey with gravy, mashed potato, dressing 🥢	2 carbohydrates, 2 medium-fat meats, 2 fats
1 (8 oz)	Entree with less than 300 calories 🥢	2 carbohydrates, 3 lean meats
SOUPS		
1 cup (8 oz)	Bean 🥢	1 carbohydrate, 1 very lean meat
1 cup (8 oz)	Cream (made with water) 🥢	1 carbohydrate, 1 fat
½ cup (4 oz)	Split pea (made with water) 🥢	1 carbohydrate
1 cup (8 oz)	Tomato (made with water) 🥢	1 carbohydrate
1 cup (8 oz)	Vegetable beef, chicken noodle, or other broth-type 🥢	1 carbohydrate

🥢 = 400 mg or more sodium per exchange.

TABLE E-10
U.S. EXCHANGE SYSTEM: FAST FOODS*

AMOUNT	FOOD	EXCHANGES PER SERVING
2	Burritos with beef 🥢	4 carbohydrates, 2 medium-fat meats, 2 fats
6	Chicken nuggets 🥢	1 carbohydrate, 2 medium-fat meats, 1 fat
1 each	Chicken breast and wing, breaded and fried 🥢	1 carbohydrate, 4 medium-fat meats, 2 fats
1	Fish sandwich/tartar sauce 🥢	3 carbohydrates, 1 medium-fat meat, 3 fats
20–25	French fries, thin	2 carbohydrates, 2 fats
1	Hamburger, regular	2 carbohydrates, 2 medium-fat meats
1	Hamburger, large 🥢	2 carbohydrates, 3 medium-fat meats, 1 fat
1	Hot dog with bun 🥢	1 carbohydrate, 1 high-fat meat, 1 fat
1	Individual pan pizza 🥢	5 carbohydrates, 3 medium-fat meats, 3 fats
1 medium	Soft-serve cone	2 carbohydrates, 1 fat
1 sub (6 in.)	Submarine sandwich 🥢	3 carbohydrates, 1 vegetable, 2 medium-fat meats, 1 fat
1 (6 oz)	Taco, hard shell 🥢	2 carbohydrates, 2 medium-fat meats, 2 fats
1 (3 oz)	Taco, soft shell 🥢	1 carbohydrate, 1 medium-fat meat, 1 fat

*Ask at your fast-food restaurant for nutrition information about your favorite fast foods.

🥢 = 400 mg or more of sodium per serving.

The Canadian Exchange System

The *Good Health Eating Guide* is the Canadian exchange system of meal planning.* It contains several features similar to those of the U.S. exchange system including the following:

- Foods are divided into groups according to carbohydrate, protein, and fat content.
- Foods are interchangeable within a group.
- Most foods are eaten in measured amounts.
- An energy (calorie) value is given for each food group.

Tables E–11 through E-18 present the Canadian exchange system.

TABLE E–11
CANADIAN EXCHANGE SYSTEM: STARCH FOODS GROUP

15 g carbohydrate [starch], 2 g protein, 290 kJ (68 cal).

FOOD	MEASURE	MASS (WEIGHT)	FOOD	MEASURE	MASS (WEIGHT)
BREADS			Rye, coarse or pumpernickel	½ slice	30 g
Bagel	½	30 g	Soda crackers	6	20 g
Bread crumbs	50 mL (¼ cup)	30 g	Tortilla, corn (taco shell)	1	30 g
Bread cubes	250 mL (1 cup)	30 g	Tortilla, flour	1	30 g
Bread sticks	2	20 g	White (French & Italian)	1 slice	25 g
Brewis, cooked	50 mL (¼ cup)	45 g	Whole-wheat, cracked-wheat, rye, white-enriched	1 slice	30 g
Chapati	1	20 g			
Cookies, plain	2	20 g			
English muffin, crumpet	½	30 g	**STARCH VEGETABLES**		
Flour	40 mL (2½ tbsp)	20 g	Beans, peas (dried), cooked	125 mL (½ cup)	80 g
Hamburger bun	½	30 g			
Hot dog bun	½	30 g	Breadfruit	1 slice	75 g
Kaiser roll	½	30 g	Corn, canned whole kernel	125 mL (½ cup)	85 g
Matzo, 15 cm	1	20 g			
Melba toast, rectangular	4	15 g	Corn-on-the-cob	½ medium cob	140 g
Melba toast, rounds	7	15 g	Cornstarch	30 mL (2 tbsp)	15 g
Pita, 20 cm diameter (8" diameter)	¼	30 g	Plantain	⅓ small	50 g
Pita, 15 cm diameter (6" diameter)	½	30 g	Popcorn, air-popped unbuttered	750 mL (3 cups)	20 g
Plain roll	1 small	30 g	Potatoes, whole (with or without skin)	½ medium	95 g
Pretzels	7	20 g			
Raisin bread	1 slice	30 g	Yam, sweet potatoes (with or without skin)	½	75 g
Rice cakes	2	30 g			
Roti	1	20 g			
Rusks	2	20 g			

continued

---

*The tables for the Canadian exchange system are taken from *Good Health Eating Guide* (Toronto: Canadian Diabetes Association, 1994) and are used with the association's permission.

TABLE E–11   *continued*
CANADIAN EXCHANGE SYSTEM: STARCH FOODS GROUP

Each of the following measured foods equals more than 1 Starch choice:

FOOD	MEASURE	FOOD CHOICES	MASS (WEIGHT)
Bran Flakes	150 mL (⅔ cup)	1 Starch + ½ Sugars	24 g
Croissant, small	1 small	1 Starch + 1½ Fats & Oils	35 g
large	½ large	1 Starch + 1½ Fats & Oils	30 g
Corn, canned creamed	12 mL (½ cup)	1 Starch + ½ Fruits & Vegetables	113 g
Potato chips	15 chips	1 Starch + 2 Fats & Oils	30 g
Tortilla chips (nachos)	13 chips	1 Starch + 1½ Fats & Oils	20 g
Corn chips	30 chips	1 Starch + 2 Fats & Oils	30 g
Cheese twists	30 chips	1 Starch + 1½ Fats & Oils	30 g
Cheese puffs	27 chips	1 Starch + 2 Fats & Oils	30 g
Tea Biscuit	1	1 Starch + 2 Fats & Oils	30 g
Pancake, homemade using 50 mL (¼ cup) batter (6" diameter)	1 medium	1½ Starch + 1 Fats & Oils	50 g
Potatoes, French fried (homemade or frozen)	10 regular size	1 Starch & 1 Fats & Oils	35 g
Soup, canned* (prepared with equal volume of water)	250 mL (1 cup)	1 Starch	260 g
Waffle, packaged	1	1 Starch + 1 Fats & Oils	35 g

FOOD	MEASURE	MASS (WEIGHT)	FOOD	MEASURE	MASS (WEIGHT)
CEREALS			**GRAINS**		
Bran flakes, 100% Bran	125 mL (½ cup)	30 g	Barley, cooked	125 mL (½ cup)	120 g
Cooked cereals, cooked	125 mL (½ cup)	125 g	dry	30 mL (2 tbsp)	20 g
dry	30 mL (2 tbsp)	20 g	Bulgar, kasha,		
Cornmeal, cooked	125 mL (½ cup)	125 g	cooked moist	125 mL (½ cup)	70 g
dry	30 mL (2 tbsp)	20 g	cooked crumbly	75 mL (⅓ cup)	40 g
Ready-to-eat	125 mL (½ cup)	20 g	dry	30 mL (2 tbsp)	20 g
unsweetened cereal			Rice, brown & white	125 mL (½ cup)	70 g
Shredded wheat biscuit,	1	20 g	(short & long grain)		
rectangular or round			Rice, wild	75 mL (⅓ cup)	70 g
Shredded wheat,	125 mL (½ cup)	20 g	Tapioca, pearl and	30 mL (2 tbsp)	15 g
bite size			granulated quick		
Wheat germ	75 mL (⅓ cup)	30 g	cooking dry		
Cornflakes	175 mL (⅔ cup)	20 g	Couscous, cooked moist	125 mL (½ cup)	70 g
Rice Krispies	175 mL (⅔ cup)	20 g	dry	30 mL (2 tbsp)	20 g
Cheerios	200 mL (¾ cup)	20 g	Quinoa, cooked moist	125 mL (½ cup)	70 g
Muffets	1 muffet	20 g	dry	30 mL (2 tbsp)	20 g
Puffed rice	300 mL (1¼ cup)	15 g			
Puffed wheat	425 mL (1⅔ cup)	20 g	**PASTA**		
			Macaroni, cooked	125 mL (½ cup)	70 g
			Noodles, cooked	125 mL (½ cup)	80 g
			Spaghetti, cooked	125 mL (½ cup)	70 g

*Soup can vary according to brand and type. Check the label for Food Choice Values and Symbols or the core nutrient listing.

TABLE E–12
CANADIAN EXCHANGE SYSTEM: FRUITS AND VEGETABLES GROUP

10 g carbohydrate, 1 g protein, 190 kJ, (44 cal)

FOOD	MEASURE	MASS (WEIGHT)	FOOD	MEASURE	MASS (WEIGHT)
FRUITS (fresh, frozen, without sugar, canned in water)			canned in water	250 mL (1 cup, includes 30 mL (2 tbsp) liquid	230 g
Apple, raw					
(with or without skin)	½ medium	75 g	Grapefruit, raw with rind	½ small	185 g
sauce unsweetened	125 mL (½ cup)	120 g	raw sectioned	125 mL (½ cup)	100 g
sweetened	*see Combined Food Choices*		canned in water	125 mL (½ cup), includes 30 mL (2 tbsp) liquid)	120 g
Apple butter	20 mL (4 tsp)	20 g			
Apricot, raw	2 medium	115 g	Grapes, raw slip skin	125 mL (½ cup)	75 g
canned in water	4 halves plus 30 mL (2 tbsp) liquid	110 g	raw seedless	125 mL (½ cup)	75 g
Bake-apple	125 mL (½ cup)	120 g	canned in water	75 mL (⅓ cup), includes 30 mL (2 tbsp) liquid	115 g
(cloudberries), raw					
Banana, with peel	½ small	75 g	Honeydew melon,		
peeled	½ small	50 g	raw with rind	½	225 g
Berries			cubed or diced	250 mL (1 cup)	170 g
(blackberries, blueberries, boysenberries, huckleberries, loganberries, raspberries)			Guava, raw	½	50 g
			Kiwi, raw with skin	2	155 g
			Kumquats, raw	3	60 g
			Loquats, raw	8	130 g
raw	125 mL (½ cup)	70 g	Lychee fruit, raw	8	120 g
canned, in water	125 mL (½ cup), includes 30 mL (2 tbsp) liquid	100 g	Mandarin orange,		
			raw with rind	1	135 g
			raw sectioned	125 mL (½ cup)	100 g
Cantaloupe,			canned in water	125 mL (½ cup), includes 30 mL (2 tbsp) liquid	100 g
wedge with rind	¼	240 g			
cubed or diced	250 mL (1 cup)	160 g			
Cherries,			Mango, raw without		
raw with pits	10	75 g	skin and seed		65 g
raw without pits	10	70 g	diced	75 mL (⅓ cup)	65 g
canned in water with pits	75 mL (1/3 cup), includes 30 mL (2 tbsp) liquid	90 g	Nectarine	½ medium	75 g
			Orange, raw with		
canned, in water, without pits	75 mL (1/3 cup), includes 30 mL (2 tbsp) liquid	85 g	rind	1 small	130 g
			raw sectioned	125 mL (½ cup)	95 g
Crabapple, raw	1 small	55 g	Papaya, raw with skin and seeds	¼ medium	150 g
Cranberries, raw	250 mL (1 cup)	100 g	raw without skin and seeds	¼ medium	100 g
Figs, raw	1 medium	50 g			
canned in water	3 medium plus 30 mL (2 tbsp) liquid	100 g	cubed or diced	125 mL (½ cup)	100 g
			Peaches, raw with		
Foxberries, raw	250 mL (1 cup)	100 g	seed and skin	1 large	100 g
Fruit cocktail,	125 mL (½ cup)	120 g	raw sliced or diced	125 mL (½ cup)	100 g
canned in water	includes 30 mL (2 tbsp) liquid		canned in water, halves or slices	125 mL (½ cup) includes 30 mL (2 tbsp) liquid	120 g
Fruit, mixed cut-up	125 mL (½ cup)	120 g			
Gooseberries, raw	250 mL (1 cup)	150 g	Pear, raw with skin and core	½	90 g

continued

CANADIAN EXCHANGE SYSTEM: FRUITS AND VEGETABLES GROUP

FOOD	MEASURE	MASS (WEIGHT)	FOOD	MEASURE	MASS (WEIGHT)
FRUITS (fresh, frozen, without sugar, canned in water)			Dates, without pits	2	15 g
			Peach	½	15 g
raw without skin and core	½	85 g	Pear	½	15 g
halves canned in water	1 half plus 30 mL (2 tbsp liquid)	60 g 90 g	Prunes, raw with pits	2	15 g
			raw without pits	2	10 g
Persimmons,			stewed no liquid	2	20 g
raw native	1	30 g	stewed with liquid	2 plus 15 mL (1 tbsp) liquid	35 g
raw Japanese	¼	50 g	Raisins	30 mL (2 tbsp)	15 g
Pineapple, raw	1 slice	75 g			
raw diced	125 mL (½ cup)	75 g	**JUICES** (no sugar added or unsweetened)		
sliced canned in water	2 slices plus 15 mL (1 tbsp) liquid	100 g	Apricot, grape, guava, mango, prune	50 mL (¼ cup)	55 g
diced canned in water	125 mL (½ cup) includes 30 mL (2 tbsp) liquid	100 g	Apple, carrot, papaya, pear, pineapple, pomegranate	75 mL (⅓ cup)	80 g
sliced canned in juice	1 slice, plus 15 mL (1 tbsp) liquid	55 g	Cranberry (*see Sugars section*)		
			Clamato (*see Sugars section*)		
diced canned in juice	75 mL (⅓ cup) includes 15 mL (1 tbsp) liquid	55 g	Grapefruit, loganberry, orange, raspberry, tangelo, tangerine	125 mL (½ cup)	130 g
Plum, raw	2 small	60 g	Tomato, tomato-based mixed vegetables	250 mL (1 cup)	255 g
Damson	6	65 g			
Japanese	1	70 g	**VEGETABLES** (fresh, frozen or canned)		
canned in water	3 plus 30 mL (2 tbsp) liquid	100 g	Artichokes, French, globe	2 small	50 g
canned in apple juice	2 plus 30 mL (2 tbsp) liquid	70 g	Beets, diced or sliced	125 mL (½ cup)	85 g
Pomegranate, raw	½	140 g	Carrots, diced cooked or uncooked	125 mL (½ cup)	75 g
Strawberries, raw	250 mL (1 cup)	150 g	Chestnuts, fresh	5	20 g
frozen/canned in water	250 mL (1 cup) includes 30 mL (2 tbsp) liquid	240 g	Parsnips, mashed	125 mL (½ cup)	80 g
			Peas, fresh or frozen	125 mL (½ cup)	80 g
			canned	75 mL (⅓ cup)	55 g
Rhubarb	250 mL (1 cup)	150 g	Pumpkin, mashed	125 mL (½ cup)	45 g
Tangelo, raw	1	205 g	Rutabagas, mashed	125 mL (½ cup)	85 g
Tangerine, raw			Sauerkraut	250 mL (1 cup)	235 g
medium-sized	1	115 g	Snowpeas	250 mL (1 cup)	135 g
raw sectioned	125 mL (½ cup)	100 g	Squash, yellow or winter mashed	125 mL (½ cup)	115 g
Watermelon, raw with rind	1 wedge	310 g	Succotash	75 mL (⅓ cup)	55 g
cubed or diced	250 mL (1 cup)	160 g	Tomatoes, canned	250 mL (1 cup)	240 g
			Tomato paste	50 mL (¼ cup)	55 g
DRIED FRUIT			Tomato sauce*	75 mL (⅓ cup)	100 g
			Turnip, mashed	125 mL (½ cup)	115 g
Apple	5 pieces	15 g	Vegetables, mixed	125 mL (½ cup)	90 g
Apricot	4 halves	15 g	Water chestnuts	8 medium	50 g
Banana flakes	30 mL (2 tbsp)	15 g			
Currants	30 mL (2 tbsp)	15 g			

*Tomato sauce varies according to brand name. Check the label or discuss with your dietitian.

TABLE E-13
CANADIAN EXCHANGE SYSTEM: MILK GROUP

TYPE OF MILK	CARBOHYDRATE	PROTEIN	FAT	ENERGY	FOOD	MEASURE	MASS (WEIGHT)
Nonfat	6 g	4 g	0 g	170 kJ (40 cal)	Buttermilk	125 mL (½ c)	125 g
1%	6 g	4 g	1 g	206 kJ (49 cal)	Evaporated milk	50 mL (¼ c)	50 g
					Milk	125 mL (½ c)	125 g
2%	6 g	4 g	2 g	244 kJ (58 cal)	Powdered milk, regular	30 mL (2 tbsp)	15 g
					Instant	50 mL (¼ c)	15 g
Whole	6 g	4 g	4 g	319 kJ (76 cal)	Plain yogurt	125 mL (½ c)	125 g

Each of the following measured foods equals more than 1 Milk choice:

FOOD	FOOD CHOICES	MEASURE	MASS (WEIGHT)
Milkshake	1 Milk + 3 Sugars + ½ Protein	250 mL (1 cup)	300 g
Chocolate Milk 2%	2 Milk 2% + 1 Sugars	250 mL (1 cup)	300 g
Frozen Yogurt	1 Milk + 1 Sugars	125 mL (½ cup)	125 g

TABLE E-14
CANADIAN EXCHANGE SYSTEM: SUGARS

10 g carbohydrate, 167 kJ (40 cal)

FOOD	MEASURE	MASS (WEIGHT)	FOOD	MEASURE	MASS (WEIGHT)
BEVERAGES:			Hard candy mints	2	5 g
Condensed milk	15 ml (1 tbsp)		Honey, molasses corn & cane syrup	10 mL (2 tsp)	15 g
* Flavoured fruit crystals	75 mL (⅓ cup)		Jelly beans	4	10 g
* Iced tea mixes	75 mL (⅓ cup)		Licorice	1 short stick	10 g
Regular soft drinks	125 mL (½ cup)		Marshmallows	2 large	15 g
* Sweet drink mixes	75 mL (⅓ cup)		Popsicle	1 stick (½ popsicle)	
Tonic water	125 mL (½ cup)		Powdered gelatin mix (Jello®) (reconstituted)	50 mL (¼ cup)	
MISCELLANEOUS:			Regular jam, jelly, marmalade	15 mL (1 tbsp)	
Bubble gum (large square)	1 piece	5 g	Sugar, white, brown, icing, maple	10 mL (2 tsp)	10 g
Cranberry cocktail	75 mL (⅓ cup)	80 g	Sweet pickles	2 small	100 g
Cranberry cocktail, light	350 mL (1⅓ cup)	260 g	Sweet relish	30 mL (2 tbsp)	
Cranberry sauce	30 mL (2 tbsp)				

Each of the following measured foods equal more than 1 Sugars choice:

FOOD	CHOICES	MEASURES	MASS (WEIGHT)
Brownie	1 Sugars + 1 Fats & Oils	1	20 g
Clamato juice	1½ Sugars	175 mL (⅔ cup)	
Fruit salad, light syrup	1 Sugars + 1 Fruits & Vegetables	125 mL (½ cup)	130 g
Aero® bar	2½ Sugars + 2½ Fats & Oils	1 bar	43 g
Smarties®	4 ½ Sugars + 2 Fats & Oils	1 box	60 g
Sherbet	3 Sugars + ½ Fats & Oils	125 mL (½ cup)	95 g

*These have been made with water.

TABLE E-15
CANADIAN EXCHANGE SYSTEM: PROTEIN FOODS GROUP

7 g protein, 3 g fat, 230 kJ (55 cal)

FOOD	MEASURE	MASS (WEIGHT)	FOOD	MEASURE	MASS (WEIGHT)
CHEESE:			Shrimp:		
Low fat cheese, about 7% milk fat (M.F.)	1 slice	30 g	fresh	5 large	30 g
Cottage cheese, 2% M.F. or less	50 mL (¼ cup)	55 g	frozen	10 medium	30 g
Ricotta, about 7% M.F.	50 mL (¼ cup)	60 g	canned	18 small	30 g
			dry pack	50 mL (¼ cup)	30 g
FISH:			**MEAT AND POULTRY:**		
Anchovy	*See Extras*		*e.g. beef, chicken, goat, ham, lamb, pork, turkey, veal, wild game:*		
Canned, drained e.g. tuna packed in water, mackerel salmon	50 mL (¼ cup) (⅓ of 6.5 oz can)	30 g	Back, peameal bacon	3 thin slices	30 g
			Chop	½ chop, with bone	40 g
			Minced or ground, lean or extra-lean	30 mL (2 tbsp)	30 g
Cod tongues, cheeks	75 mL (⅓ cup)	50 g	Sliced, lean	1 slice	30 g
Fillet or steak, e.g. Boston blue, cod, flounder, haddock, halibut, mackerel, orange roughy, perch, pickerel, pike, salmon, shad, snapper, sole, swordfish, trout, tuna, whitefish	1 piece	30 g	Steak, lean	1 piece	30 g
			ORGAN MEATS:		
			Heart, liver	1 slice	30 g
			Kidney, sweet breads, chopped	50 mL (¼ cup)	30 g
			Tongue	1 slice	30 g
			Tripe	5 pieces	60 g
Herring	1/3 fish	30 g	**SOYABEAN:**		
Sardines, smelts	2 medium or 3 small	30 g	Bean curd or tofu	½ block	70 g
Squid, octopus	50 mL (¼ cup)	40 g	**EGGS:**		
SHELLFISH:			Egg in shell, raw or cooked	1 medium	50 g
Clams, mussels, oysters, scallops, snails	3 medium	30 g	Egg without shell, cooked or poached in water	1 medium	45 g
Crab, lobster flaked	50 mL (¼ cup)	30 g	Egg, scrambled	50 mL (¼ cup)	55 g

Each of the following measured foods equal more than 1 protein choice:

FOOD	CHOICES	MEASURES	MASS (WEIGHT)
Cheese	1 Protein + 1 Fats & Oils	1 piece	25 g
Cheese, coarsely grated, e.g. cheddar	1 Protein + 1 Fats & Oils	50 mL (¼ cup)	25 g
Cheese, dry, finely grated, e.g. parmesan	1 Protein + 1 Fats & Oils	45 mL	15 g
Cheese, ricotta, high fat	1 Protein + 1 Fats & Oils	50 mL (¼ cup)	55 g
Eel	1 Protein + 1 Fats & Oils	1 slice	50 g
Bologna	1 Protein + 1 Fats & Oils	1 slice	20 g
Canned luncheon meat	1 Protein + 1 Fats & Oils	1 slice	20 g
Corned beef, fresh	1 Protein + 1 Fats & Oils	1 slice	25 g
Corned beef, canned	1 Protein + 1 Fats & Oils	1 slice	25 g
Ground beef, medium fat	1 Protein + 1 Fats & Oils	30 mL (2 tbsp)	25 g
Meat spreads, canned	1 Protein + 1 Fats & Oils	45 mL	35 g
Mutton chop	1 Protein + 1 Fats & Oils	½ chop (with bone)	35 g

continued

TABLE E–15 *continued*
CANADIAN EXCHANGE SYSTEM: PROTEIN FOODS GROUP

FOOD	CHOICES	MEASURES	MASS (WEIGHT)
Pate	*see Fats & Oils group*		
Sausage, pork link	1 Protein + 1 Fats & Oils	1 link	25 g
Sausage, garlic Polish or knockwurst	1 Protein + 1 Fats & Oils	1 slice	50 g
Summer sausage or salami	1 Protein + 1 Fats & Oils	1 slice	40 g
Spareribs or shortribs, with bone	1 Protein + 1 Fats & Oils	1 large	65 g
Stewing beef	1 Protein + 1 Fats & Oils	1 cube	25 g
Weiner, hot dog	1 Protein + 1 Fats & Oils	½ medium	25 g
Blood pudding	1 Protein + 1 Fats & Oils	1 slice	25 g
Peanut butter	1 Protein + 1 Fats & Oils	15 mL (1 tbsp)	15 g

TABLE E–16
CANADIAN EXCHANGE SYSTEM: FATS AND OILS GROUP

5 g fat, 190 kJ (45 cal)

FOOD	MEASURE	MASS (WEIGHT)	FOOD	MEASURE	MASS (WEIGHT)
Avocado	⅛	30 g	in shell	20 nuts	20 g
Bacon, side crisp*	1 slice	5 g	Walnuts	4 halves	10 g
Butter*	5 mL (1 tsp)	5 g	Pumpkin and	20 mL (4 tsp)	10 g
Cheese spread	15 mL (1 tbsp)	15 g	Squash Seeds		
Coconut,			Sesame Seeds	15 mL (1 tbsp)	10 g
fresh*	45 mL (3 tbsp)	15 g	Sunflower Seeds,		
dried*	15 mL (1 tbsp)	10 g	shelled	15 mL (1 tbsp)	10 g
Cream,			in shell	45 mL (3 tbsp)	15 g
half-and-half	30 mL (2 tbsp)	30 g	Oil, cooking and salad	5 mL (1 tsp)	5 g
(cereal) 10%*			Olives,		
light (coffee) 20%*	15 mL (1 tbsp)	15 g	green	10	45 g
whipping 32–37%*	15 mL (1 tbsp)	15 g	black (ripe)	7	57 g
Cream cheese*	15 mL (1 tbsp)	15 g	Pate, liverwurst,	15 mL (1 tbsp)	15 g
Gravy*	30 mL (2 tbsp)	30 g	meat spreads		
Lard*	5 mL (1 tsp)	5 g	Salad dressing:		
Margarine	5 mL (1 tsp)	5 g	blue cheese, French	10 mL (2 tsp)	10 g
Nuts, shelled:			Italian, mayonnaise,		
Almonds	8 nuts	5 g	Thousand Island	5 mL (1 tsp)	5 g
Brazil Nuts	2 nuts	10 g	Salad dressing:		
Cashews	5 nuts	10 g	low-calorie	30 mL (2 tbsp)	30 g
Filberts, Hazelnuts	5 nuts	10 g	Salt pork, raw	5 mL (1 tsp)	5 g
Macadamia	3 nuts	5 g	or cooked*		
Peanuts	10 nuts	10 g	Sesame oil	5 mL (1 tsp)	5 g
Pecans	5 halves	5 g	Sour cream, 12% M.F.	30 mL (2 tbsp)	30 g
Pignolias, Pine nuts	25 mL (5 tsp)	10 g	7% M.F.	60 mL (4 tbsp)	60 g
Pistachios			Shortening*	5 mL (1 tsp)	
shelled	20 nuts	10 g			

*These items contain higher amounts of saturated fat.

TABLE E–17
CANADIAN EXCHANGE SYSTEM: EXTRAS

EXTRA VEGETABLES

Use less than 125 mL (½ cup) for all vegetables listed, larger quantities may need to be counted as Fruits & Vegetables choice.

Artichokes	Cabbage	Kohlrabi	Rhubarb
Asparagus	Cauliflower	Leeks	Sauerkraut
Bamboo shoots	Celery	Lettuce	Shallots
Beans, string, green or	Chard	Mushroom	Spinach
yellow	Cucumber	Okra	Sprouts, alfalfa, radish, etc.
Bean sprouts, mung or soya	Eggplant	Onions, green, mature	Tomato wedges
Bitter melon (balsam pear)	Endive	Parsley	Watercress
Bok choy	Fiddleheads	Peppers, green, red, yellow	Zucchini
Broccoli	Greens, beet, dandelion, etc.	Radish	
Brussels sprouts	Kale	Rapini	

CONDIMENTS

2.5 g carbohydrate, 60 kJ (1 cal), limited to amount indicated

FOOD	MEASURE	FOOD	MEASURE
Anchovies	2 fillets	Dietetic fruit spreads	5 mL (1 tsp)
Barbecue sauce	15 mL (1 tbsp)	Maraschino cherries	1
Bran, natural	30 mL (2 tbsp)	Nondairy coffee whitener	5 mL (1 tsp)
Brewer's yeast	5 mL (1 tsp)	Nuts, chopped pieces	5 mL (1 tsp)
Carob powder	5 mL (1 tsp)	Pickles, unsweetened, dill	2
Catsup	5 mL (1 tsp)	sour mixed	11
Chili sauce	5 mL (1 tsp)	Sugar substitutes, granular	5 mL (1 tsp)
Cocoa powder	5 mL (1 tsp)		(3 to 4 packages)
Cranberry sauce, unsweetened	15 mL (1 tbsp)	Whipped toppings	15 mL (1 tbsp)

May be used without measuring

FREE FOODS

Artificial sweetener, such as	Dulse	Marjoram, cinnamon, etc.	Sugar-free Crystal drink
cyclamate or aspartame	Flavouring and extracts	Mineral water	Tea, clear
Baking powder, soda	Garlic	Mustard	Vinegar
Bouillon or clear broth	Gelatin, unsweetened	Parsley	Water
Bouillon from cube, powder	Ginger root	Pimentos	Worcestershire sauce
or liquid	Herbal teas, unsweetened	Soda water, Club soda	Salt, pepper, thyme
Chow Chow, unsweetened	Horseradish, uncreamed	Soya sauce	
Coffee, clear	Lemon juice/lemon wedge	Sugar-free jelly powder	
Consomme	Lime juice/lime wedge	Sugar-free soft drink	

CANADIAN EXCHANGE SYSTEM: COMBINED FOOD CHOICES

FOOD	CHOICES	MEASURES	MASS (WEIGHT)
Angel food cake	½ Starch + 2½ Sugars	1/12 cake	50 g
Apple crisp (Apples, raisins, oatmeal, flour, brown sugar, butter)	½ Starch + 1½ Fruits & Vegetable + 1 Sugars + 1–2 Fats & Oils	125 mL (½ cup)	
Applesauce, sweetened	1 Fruits & Vegetables + 1 Sugars	125 mL (½ cup)	
Beans and pork in tomato sauce	1 Starch + ½ Fruit & Vegetable + ½ Sugars + 1 Protein	125 mL (½ cup)	135 g
Beef burrito	2 Starch + 3 Protein + 3 Fats & Oils		110 g
Brownie	1 Sugars + 1 Fats & Oils	1 brownie	20 g
Cabbage rolls* (Lean ground pork or lean ground beef, rice, cabbage, sauerkraut)	1 Starch + 2 Protein	3 rolls	310 g
Caesar salad (Romaine lettuce, dressing, sprinkled with croutons and parmesan cheese)	2–4 Fats & Oils	20 mL dressing (4 tsp)	
Cheesecake	½ Starch + 2 Sugars + ½ Protein + 5 Fats & Oils	1 piece	80 g
Chicken fingers (Bread crumbs, chicken breasts, oil)	1 Starch + 2 Protein + 2 Fats & Oils	6 Small	100 g
Chicken and snow pea Oriental (Boneless chicken, snow peas, rice)	2 Starch + ½ Fruits & Vegetables + 3 Protein + 1 Fats & Oil	500 mL (2 cups)	
Chili (Lean ground beef, kidney beans, tomatoes)	1½ Starch + ½ Fruits & Vegetables + 3½ Protein	300 mL (1¼ cup)	325 g
Chips			
Potato chips	1 Starch + 2 Fats & Oils	15 chips	30 g
Corn chips	1 Starch + 2 Fats & Oils	30 chips	30 g
Tortilla chips	1 Starch + 1½ Fats & Oils	13 chips	
Cheese twists	1 Starch + 1½ Fats & Oils	30 chips	30 g
Chocolate bar			
Aero®	2½ Sugars + 2½ Fats & Oils	bar	43 g
Smarties®	4½ Sugars + 2 Fats & Oils	package	60 g
Chocolate cake (without icing) (Flour, sugar, cocoa, oil)	1 Starch + 2 Sugars + 3 Fats & Oils	1/10 of an 8" pan	
Chocolate devil's food cake (without icing)	2 Starch + 2 Sugars + 3 Fats & Oils	1/12 of a 9" pan	
Chocolate milk	2 Milk 2% + 1 Sugars	250 mL (1 cup)	300 g
Clubhouse (tripledecker) sandwich (Cold meat, cheese, tomato, hold the mayo)	3 Starch + 3 Protein + 4 Fats & Oils		
Cookies			
chocolate chip	½ Starch + ½ Sugars + 1½ Fats & Oils	2 cookies	22 g
oatmeal	1 Starch + 1 Sugars + 1 Fats & Oils	2 cookies	40 g

*If eaten with sauce, add ½ Fruits & Vegetables choice.

continued

CANADIAN EXCHANGE SYSTEM: COMBINED FOOD CHOICES

FOOD	CHOICES	MEASURES	MASS (WEIGHT)
Donut (Chocolate glazed, yeast, batter)	1 Starch + 1½ Sugars + 2 Fats & Oils	1 donut	65 g
Egg roll	1 Starch + ½ Protein + 1 Fats & Oils		75 g
Four bean salad (Green beans, wax beans, lima beans, kidney beans, oil & vinegar)	1 Starch + ½ Protein + 1 Fats & Oils	125 mL (½ cup)	
French toast	1 Starch + ½ Protein + 2 Fats & Oils	1 slice	65 g
Fruit in heavy syrup (Fruit, sugar)	1 Fruits & Vegetables + 1 ½ Sugars	125 mL (½ cup)	
Granola bar (Oatmeal, chocolate chips, sugar)	½ Starch + 1 Sugars + 1–2 Fats & Oils		30 g
Granola cereal (Harvest crunch without fruit)	1 Starch + 1 Sugars + 2 Fats & Oils	125 mL (½ cup)	45 g
Hamburger	2 Starch + 3 Protein + 2 Fats & Oils	Junior burger	
Ice cream and cone, plain flavour			
Ice cream	½ Milk + 2–3 Sugars + 1–2 Fats & Oils		100 g
Cone	½ Sugars		4 g
Lasagna (Pasta, meat, cheese, tomato) 13" x 9" Pan;			
regular cheese	1 Starch + 1 Fruits & Vegetables + 3 Protein + 2 Fats & Oils	3" × 4" piece	
low-fat cheese	1 Starch + 1 Fruits & Vegetables + 3 Protein	3" × 4" piece	
Legumes			
Dried beans (kidney, navy, pinto, fava, chick-peas)	2 Starch + 1 Protein	250 mL (1 cup)	180 g
Dried peas	2 Starch + 1 Protein	250 mL (1 cup)	210 g
Lentils	2 Starch + 1 Protein	250 mL (1 cup)	210 g
Macaroni and cheese (Macaroni, cheese, flour, milk, margarine)	2 Starch + 2 Protein + 2 Fats & Oils	250 mL (1 cup)	210 g
Minestrone soup (Lean ground beef, potatoes, carrots, kidney beans, macaroni)	1½ Starch + ½ Fruits & Vegetables + ½ Fats & Oils	250 mL (1 cup)	
Muffin (All bran, flour, raisin, sugar)	1 Starch + ½ Sugars + 1 Fats & Oils	1 small muffin	45 g
Nuts *(dry or roasted without any oil added)*			
Almonds, dried sliced	½ Protein + 2 Fats & Oils	50 mL (¼ cup)	22 g
Brazil nuts, dried unblanched	½ Protein + 2½ Fats & Oils	5 large nuts	23 g
Cashew nuts, dry roasted	½ Starch + ½ Protein + 2 Fats & Oils	50 mL (¼ cup)	28 g
Filbert hazelnut, dry	½ Protein + 3½ Fats & Oils	50 mL (¼ cup)	30 g
Macadamia nuts, dried	½ Protein + 4 Fats & Oils	50 mL (¼ cup)	28 g

continued

FOOD	CHOICES	MEASURES	MASS (WEIGHT)
Nuts *(continued)*			
Peanuts, raw	1 Protein + 2 Fats & Oils	50 mL (¼ cup)	30 g
Pecans, dry roasted	½ Fruits & Vegetables + 3 Fats & Oils	50 mL (¼ cup)	22 g
Pine nuts, pignolia dried	1 Protein + 3 Fats & Oils	50 mL (¼ cup)	34 g
Pistachio nuts, dried	½ Fruits & Vegetables + ½ Protein + 2½ Fats & Oils	50 mL (¼ cup)	27 g
Pumpkin seeds, roasted	2 Protein + 2½ Fats & Oils	50 mL (¼ cup)	47 g
Sesame seeds, whole dried	½ Fruits & Vegetables + ½ Protein + 2½ Fats & Oils	50 mL (¼ cup)	30 g
Sunflower kernel, dried	½ Protein + 1½ Fats & Oils	50 mL (¼ cup)	17 g
Walnuts, dried chopped	½ Protein + 3 Fats & Oils	¼ cup (50 mL)	26 g
Perogies (Potato, cheese, dough)	2 Starch + 1 Protein + 1 Fats & Oils	3 perogies	
Pie, fruit	1 Starch + 1 Fruits & Vegetables + 2 Sugars + 3 Fats & Oils	1 piece	120 g
Pizza, cheese (thin crust) (1/8 of a 12")	1 Starch + 1 Protein + 1 Fats & Oils	1 slice	50 g

Pork stir fry
  (Boneless pork, snow peas,
  peppers, mushrooms)
	½ to 1 Fruits & Vegetables + 3 Protein	200 mL (¾ cup)	

Potato salad
  (Potatoes, onions,
  mayonnaise, celery)
	1 Starch + 1 Fats & Oils	125 mL (½ cup)	130 g

Potatoes, scalloped (Milk, potato, onions)	2 Starch + 1 Milk + 1–2 Fats & Oils	200 mL (¾ cup)	210 g
Pudding, bread or rice (Rice or bread)	1 Starch + 1 Sugar + 1 Fats & Oils	125 mL (½ cup)	
Pudding, vanilla (Milk, sugar)	1 Milk + 2 Sugars	125 mL (½ cup)	
Raisin bran cereal	1 Starch + ½ Fruits & Vegetables + ½ Sugars	175 mL (2/3 cup)	40 g
Rice Krispie squares	½ Starch + 1½ Sugars + ½ Fats & Oils	1 square	30 g

Shepherd's pie
  (Potatoes, lean ground beef,
  frozen mixed vegetables)
	2 Starch + 1 Fruits & Vegetables + 3 Protein	325 mL (1⅓ cup)	

Sherbet, orange	3 Sugars + ½ Fats & Oils	125 mL (½ cup)	

Spaghetti and meat sauce
  (With 175 mL (2/3 cup)
  meat sauce)
	2 Starch + 1 Fruits & Vegetables + 2 Protein + 3 Fats & Oils	250 mL (1 cup)	

Stew
  (Lean stewing beef, carrots,
  peas, potatoes)
	2 Starch + 2 Fruits & Vegetables + 3 Protein + ½ Fats & Oils	200 mL (¾ cup)	

Sundae (Ice cream, chocolate syrup)	4 Sugars + 3 Fats & Oils	125 mL (½ cup)	

Tuna casserole
  (Noodles, tuna, egg, milk,
  cheese, bread crumbs)
	1 Starch + 2 Protein + ½ Fats & Oils	125 mL (½ cup)	

Yogurt, fruit bottom	1 Fruits & Vegetables + 1 Milk + 1 Sugars	125 mL (½ cup)	125 g
(Milk, fruit, sugar)	½ Fruits & Vegetables + 1½ Milk + 1½ Sugars	175 mL (⅔ cup)	175 g
Yogurt, frozen	1 Milk + 1 Sugars	125 mL (½ cup)	125 g

Chapter Notes

CHAPTER 1 NOTES

1. H. A. Guthrie, *Introductory Nutrition* (St. Louis, Mo.: The C. V. Mosby Company, 1983), pp. 2–4.

2. Federal Trade Commission News, General Nutrition Inc. Agrees to Pay $2.4 Million . . . , April 28, 1994.

3. S. H. Short, Health quackery: Our role as professionals, *Journal of the American Dietetic Association* 94 (1994): 607–608; Position of the American Dietetic Association: Identifying food and nutrition misinformation, *Journal of the American Dietetic Association* 88 (1988): 1589–1591.

4. S. H. Short, 1994; R. M. Philen and coauthors, Survey of advertising for nutritional supplements in health and bodybuilding magazines, *Journal of the American Medical Association* 268 (1992): 1008–1011.

5. Top 10 health frauds, *FDA Consumer* (October 1989): 29–31.

6. K. D. Kochanek and coauthors, Advance report of final mortality statistics, 1992, *Monthly Vital Statistics Report* 43 (March 22, 1995): 23.

7. J. M. McGinnis and W. H. Foege, Actual causes of death in the United States, *Journal of the American Medical Association* 270 (1993): 2207–2212.

8. L. Breslow and N. Breslow, Health practices and disability: Some evidence from Alameda County, *Preventive Medicine* 22 (1993): 86–95.

9. U.S. Department of Health and Human Services, Public Health Service, *The Surgeon General's Report on Nutrition and Health: Summary and Recommendations* (Washington, D.C.: U.S. Government Printing Office, 1988), pp. 2–4.

10. Committee on Diet and Health, National Research Council, *Diet and Health: Implications for Reducing Chronic Disease Risk—Executive Summary* (Washington, D.C.: National Academy Press, 1989), pp. 10–15.

11. J. M. McGinnis and W. H. Foege, 1993.

12. U.S. Department of Health and Human Services, Public Health Service, *Healthy People 2000: National Health Promotion and Disease Prevention Objectives* (Washington, D.C.: U.S. Government Printing Office, 1990), pp. 93–94.

13. S. C. Parks and coauthors, President's page: Challenging the future—Changing consumer eating habits create new opportunities in commercial foodservice, *Journal of the American Dietetic Association* 94 (1994): 908.

14. Princeton Survey Research Associates, *Shopping for Health* (Washington, D.C.: Food Marketing Institute, 1992), p. 12.

15. T. A. Pearson and coauthors, Does a cholesterol-lowering diet cost more? American Heart Association 66th Scientific Sessions Abstract, November 1993.

16. Portions of this discussion were adapted from M. A. Boyle and D. H. Morris, *Community Nutrition in Action: An Entrepreneurial Approach* (St. Paul: West Publishing Company, 1994), pp. 240–246.

17. B. W. Hickman and coauthors, Nutrition claims in advertising: A study of four women's magazines, *Journal of Nutrition Education* 25 (1993): 227–235.

18. K. Kotz and M. Story, Food advertisements during children's Saturday morning television programming: Are they consistent with dietary recommendations?, *Journal of the American Dietetic Association* 94 (1994): 1296–1300; G. Pazzaglia Sylvester and coauthors, Children's television and nutrition: Friends or foes?, *Nutrition Today* 30 (1995): 6–15.

19. American Dietetic Association, *Survey of American Dietary Habits* (Chicago: American Dietetic Association, 1993).

20. D. Woznicki and A. G. Case, *Nutrition Accuracy in Popular Magazines* (New York: American Council on Science and Health, Inc., 1994).

21. S. A. Oliveria and coauthors, Parent-child relationships in nutrient intake: The Framingham Children's Study, *American Journal of Clinical Nutrition* 56 (1992): 593–598.

22. J. MacClancy, *Consuming Culture: Why You Eat What You Eat* (New York: Henry Holt and Company, 1992), p. 38.

23. W. H. Glinsmann and G. K. Beauchamp, Babies need sugars in moderation, *Pediatric Basics* 69 (1994): 19–21.

24. U.S. Department of Agriculture, Human Nutrition Information Service, *Shopping for Food and Making Meals in Minutes Using the Dietary Guidelines* (Home and Garden Bulletin No. 232–10), p. 25.

25. Remarks of R. Wyden in *Deception and Fraud in the Diet Industry—Part 1: Hearing Before the House of Representatives, Subcommittee on Regulation, Business Opportunities, and Energy, Committee on Small Business* (Washington, D.C.: U.S. Government Printing Office, March 26, 1990), p. 1.

26. E. Goodman, To swallow or not to swallow: That is the new vitamin question, *Boston Globe,* April 17, 1994, p. A27.

27. E. R. Greenberg and coauthors, A clinical trial of antioxidant vitamins to prevent colorectal adenoma, *New England Journal of Medicine* 331 (1994): 141–147.

28. M. Angell and J. P. Kassirer, Clinical research—What should the public believe?, *New England Journal of Medicine* 331 (1994): 189–190.

29. Ibid.

30. *FDA Consumer,* October 1989.

31. I. Milner, The color of quackery? Fingering the phony nutritionists of the Yellow Pages, *Nutrition Forum* 11 (1994): 19–22.

CHAPTER 2 NOTES

1. A. K. Kant and coauthors, Dietary diversity and subsequent mortality in the First National Health and Nutrition Examination Survey Epidemiologic Follow-up Study, *American Journal of Clinical Nutrition* 57 (1993): 434–440.

2. S. L. Anderson, A look at the Japanese dietary guidelines, *Journal of the American Dietetic Association* 90 (1990): 1527.

3. Personal communication with the Snack Food Association, Alexandria, Virginia, 1994.

4. American Medical Association and American Dietetic Association, *Targets for Adolescent Health: Nutrition and Physical Fitness* (Chicago: American Medical Association, 1991), p. 2.

5. American Heart Association, *Nutritious Nibbles* (Dallas: American Heart Association, 1984), p. 5.

6. U.S. Department of Agriculture, *Making Bag Lunches, Snacks, and Desserts Using the Dietary Guidelines,* USDA HNIS Home and Garden Bulletin No. 232-9 (Washington, D.C.: U.S. Government Printing Office), pp. 2–25.

7. L. S. Sims, A special issue (food labeling reform) deserves a special issue (of *Nutrition Today*)! *Nutrition Today,* September/October 1993, p. 4.

8. Food and Drug Administration, FDA Backgrounder: The New Food Label, April 1994.

9. Food and Drug Administration, Food Safety and Inspection Service, *An Introduction to the New Food Label* (Washington, D.C.: DHHS Publication No. (FDA) 94-2271; USDA-FSIS-41, Ocotober 1993).

10. P. Moriarty, Food labeling and the law, *Food News for Consumers,* Spring–Summer 1993, p. 10.

11. Department of Health and Human Services, Food and Drug Administration, *Federal Register* 58 (June 15, 1993): 33055–33060.

12. S. L. Nightingale, New rule on labeling foods as 'Healthy' issued, *Journal of the American Medical Association* 271 (1994): 1818.

CHAPTER 3 NOTES

1. L. N. Aurisicchio and C. S. Pitchumoni, Lactose intolerance: Recognizing the link between diet and discomfort, *Postgraduate Medicine* 95 (1994):113–116, 119–120.

2. M. Woodward and A. R. Walker, Sugar consumption and dental caries: Evidence from 90 countries, *British Dental Journal* 176 (1994): 297–302.

3. J. H. Shaw, Causes and control of dental caries, *New England Journal of Medicine* 317 (1987): 996–1004.

4. S. Kashket and coauthors, Lack of correlation between food retention on the human dentition and consumer perception of food stickiness, *Journal of Dental Research* 70 (1991): 1314–1319.

5. American Dental Association, *Diet & Dental Health* (Chicago: American Dental Association, 1993), p. 7.

6. M. E. Jensen, Responses of interproximal plaque pH to snack foods and effect of chewing sorbitol-containing gum, *Journal of the American Dental Association* 113 (1986): 262–266.

7. A. S. Papas and coauthors, Dietary models for root caries, *American Journal of Clinical Nutrition* 61 (1995): 417S–422S; American Dental Association, p. 7.

8. American Dental Association, pp. 2–7.

9. C. O. Enwonwu, Interface of malnutrition and periodontal diseases, *American Journal of Clinical Nutrition* 61 (1995): 430S–436S.

10. J. O. Alvarez, Nutrition, tooth development, and dental caries, *American Journal of Clinical Nutrition* 61 (1995): 410S–416S.

11. American Dental Association, p. 2.

12. Personal communication with Marketing Data Enterprises, Inc., Valley Stream, New York, 1994.

13. S. Cohen and coauthors, Saccharin and urothelial proliferation: A threshold phenomenon, *Journal of the American Societies for Experimental Biology* 6 (1992): A-1594.

14. Position of the American Dietetic Association: Appropriate use of nutritive and nonnutritive sweeteners, *Journal of the American Dietetic Association* 87 (1987): 1689–1694.

15. Council on Scientific Affairs, Saccharin: Review of safety issues, *Journal of the American Medical Association* 254 (1985): 2622–2644.

16. S. S. Schiffman and coauthors, Aspartame and susceptibility to headache, *New England Journal of Medicine* 317 (1987): 1181–1185.

17. Council on Scientific Affairs, Aspartame: Review of safety issues, *Journal of the American Medical Association* 254 (1985):400–402; American Council on Science and Health, *Low-Calorie Sweeteners* (New York: American Council on Science and Health, 1993), pp. 7–13; Position of the American Dietetic Association: Use of nutritive and nonnutritive sweeteners, *Journal of the American Dietetic Association* 93 (1993): 817–818.

18. J. E. Blundell and A. J. Hill, Paradoxical effects of an intense sweetener (aspartame) on appetite, *The Lancet* 1 (1986): 1092–1093.

19. B. J. Rolls, Effects of intense sweeteners on hunger, food intake, and body weight: A review, *American Journal of Clinical Nutrition* 53 (1991): 872–878; A. Drewnowski, Comparing the effects of aspartame and sucrose on motivational ratings, taste preferences, and energy intakes in humans, *American Journal of Clinical Nutrition* 59 (1994): 338–345.

20. M. J. Franz and coauthors, Nutrition principles for the management of diabetes and related complications, *Diabetes Care* 17 (1994): 495–496.

21. MRCA Information Services, *Eating in America, Edition II (Eat II),* (Chicago: National Livestock and Meat Board, 1994), pp. 1–35.

22. K. R. Westerterp, Food quotient, respiratory quotient, and energy balance, *American Journal of Clinical Nutrition* 57 (1993): 759S–765S; R. L. Atkinson, Role of diet in obesity treatment, an address presented at the North American Association for the

Study of Obesity and Emory University School of Medicine conference Obesity Update: Pathophysiology, Clinical Consequences, and Therapeutic Options, Atlanta, Georgia, August 1992.

23. E. Giovannucci and coauthors, Relationship of diet to risk of colorectal adenoma in men, *Journal of the National Cancer Institute* 84 (1992): 91–98; J. L. Freudenheim and coauthors, Risks associated with source of fiber and fiber components in cancer of the colon and rectum, *Cancer Research* 50 (1990): 3295–3300.

24. S. R. Glore and coauthors, Soluble fiber and serum lipids: A literature review, *Journal of the American Dietetic Association* 94 (1994): 425–436; M. A. Eastwood, The physiological effects of dietary fiber: An update, *Annual Review of Nutrition,* 12 (1992): 19–35.

25. D. J. Jenkins and coauthors, Effect on blood lipids of very high intakes of fiber in diets low in saturated fat and cholesterol, *New England Journal of Medicine* 329 (1993): 21–26; C. M. Ripsin and coauthors, Oat products and lipid lowering: A meta-analysis, *Journal of the American Medical Association* 267 (1992): 3317–3325.

26. American Dietetic Association, Position of the American Dietetic Association: Health implications of dietary fiber, *Journal of the American Dietetic Association* 93 (1993): 1446–1447.

27. T. M. Wolever and coauthors, The glycemic index: Methodology and clinical implications, *American Journal of Clinical Nutrition* 54 (1991): 846–854.

28. F. Q. Nuttall, Dietary fiber in the management of diabetes, *Diabetes* 42 (1993): 503–508.

29. C. D. Berdanier, Genetic errors that result in diabetes mellitus, *Nutrition Today* 29 (1994): 17–24.

30. Position Statement of the American Diabetes Association, Nutrition Recommendations for people with diabetes mellitus, *Diabetes Care* 17 (1994): 519–522; M. Franz and coauthors, Nutrition principles for the management of diabetes and related complications, *Diabetes Care* 17 (1994): 490–518.

31. A. E. Sloan, The explosion of multi-cultural cuisine, *Food Technology* 48 (1994): 74–75.

32. J. F. Mariani, *Dictionary of American Food and Drink* (New York: Hearst Books, 1994), p. xvi.

33. S. J. Algert and T. H. Ellison, Mexican American food practices, customs, and holidays, *Ethnic and Regional Food Practices, A Series* (Chicago and Alexandria, Va: The American Dietetic Association and American Diabetes Association, 1989), pp. 1–6, 16–23.

34. K. M. Ma, Chinese American food practices, customs, and holidays, *Ethnic and Regional Food Practices, A Series* (Chicago and Alexandria, Va: The American Dietetic Association, 1990), pp. 4–6, 24–27.

35. T. C. Campbell and J. Chen, Diet and chronic degenerative diseases: A summary of results from an ecologic study in rural China, in *Western Diseases* (Totowa, N.J.: Humana Press, 1994), pp. 67–118.

36. Should Americans be eating more Chinese food? *The Tufts University Diet & Nutrition Letter* 8 (1990): 5.

37. M. Nestle, Mediterranean diets: Historical and research overview, *The American Journal of Clinical Nutrition* 61 (1995): 1313S–1320S.

38. Mariani, 1994, p. 295.

39. P. G. Kittler and K. Sucher, *Food and Culture in America* (New York: Van Nostrand Reinhold, 1989), pp. 182–194.

40. Personal communication with the NPD Group's National Eating Trends Service, Park Ridge, Illinois, 1994.

41. C. Higgins and H. S. Warshaw, Jewish food practices, customs, and holidays, *Ethnic and Regional Food Practices, A Series* (Chicago and Alexandria, Va.: The American Dietetic Association and the American Diabetes Association, 1989), pp. 1–3, 7–8, 17–18.

CHAPTER 4 NOTES

1. C. D. Berdanier, ω-3 Fatty acids: A Panacea? *Nutrition Today,* 29 (1994): 28–32.

2. K. K. Carroll, Biological effects of fish oil in relation to chronic diseases, *Lipids* 21 (1986): 731–732.

3. D. Kromhout, E. B. Bosscheiter, and C. D. Coulander, The inverse relation between fish consumption and 20-year mortality from coronary heart disease, *New England Journal of Medicine* 312 (1985): 1205–1209.

4. R. K. Chandra and coauthors, Decreased systemis thromboxane A$_2$ biosynthesis in normal human subjects fed a salmon-rich diet, *American Journal of Clinical Nutrition* 60 (1994): 369–373.

5. R. Vandongen and coauthors, Effects on blood pressure of ω-3 fats in subjects at increased risk of cardiovascular disease, *Hypertension* 22 (1993): 371–379; A. Ascherio and coauthors, Dietary intake of marine n-3 fatty acids, fish intake, and the risk of coronary disease among men, *New England Journal of Medicine* 332 (1995): 977–982.

6. B. E. Phillipson and coauthors, Reduction of plasma lipids, lipoproteins, and apoproteins by dietary fish oil in patients with hypertriglyceridemia, *New England Journal of Medicine* 312 (1985): 1210–1216; A. P. Simopoulos, ω-3 Fatty acids in health and disease and in growth and development, *American Journal of Clinical Nutrition* 54 (1991): 438–463; and W. S. Harris and F. Muzio, Fish oil reduces postprandial triglyceride concentration without accelerating lipid-emulsion removal rates, *American Journal of Clinical Nutrition* 58 (1993): 68–74.

7. W. C. Willett and A. Ascherio, Trans fatty acids: Are the effects only marginal? *American Journal of Public Health* 84 (1994): 722–724.

8. J. T. Judd and coauthors, Dietary *trans* fatty acids: Effects on plasma lipids and lipoproteins of healthy men and women, *American Journal of Clinical Nutrition* 59 (1994): 861–868; R. Troisi and coauthors, Trans fatty acid intake in relation to serum lipid concentrations in adult men, *American Journal of Clinical Nutrition* 56 (1992): 1019–1024; A. H. Lichtenstein and coauthors, Hydrogenation impairs the hypolipidemic effect of corn oil in humans, *Arteriosclerosis and Thrombosis* 13 (1993): 154–161.

9. W. C. Willett and coauthors, Intake of *trans* fatty acids and risk of coronary heart disease among women, *The Lancet* 341 (1993): 581–585.

10. W. C. Willett and A. Ascherio, 1994.

11. Nutrition Committee Advisory, American Heart Association, Trans fatty acids, May 17, 1994; Food and Nutrition Science Alliance, Nutrition groups call condemnation of trans fatty acids extreme, justified, June 20, 1994.

12. Nutrition Committee Advisory, American Heart Association, Trans fatty acids, May 17, 1994.

13. Expert Panel on Detection, Evaluation, and Treatment of High Blood Cholesterol in Adults, Summary of the Second Report of the National Cholesterol Education Program (NCEP) Expert Panel on Detection, Evaluation, and Treatment of High Blood Cholesterol in Adults (Adult Treatment Panel), *Journal of the American Medical Association* 269 (1993): 3014–3023.

14. C. T. Sempos and coauthors, Prevalence of high blood cholesterol among U.S. adults: An update based on guidelines from the second report of the National Cholesterol Education Program Adult Treatment Panel, *Journal of the American Medical Association* 269 (1993): 3009–3014.

15. D. Steinberg and coauthors, Beyond cholesterol: Modification of low-density lipoprotein that increases its atherogenicity, *New England Journal of Medicine* 320 (1989): 915–924.

16. Expert Panel on Detection, Evaluation, and Treatment of High Blood Cholesterol in Adults, Summary of the Second Report of the National Cholesterol Education Program (NCEP) Expert Panel on Detection, Evaluation, and Treatment of High Blood Cholesterol in Adults (Adult Treatment Panel II), *Journal of the American Medical Association* 269 (1993): 3015–3023.

17. G. F. Watts and coauthors, Nutrient intake and progression of coronary artery disease, *American Journal of Cardiology* 73 (1994): 328–332.

18. Adult Treatment Panel II, *Journal of the American Medical Association* 269 (1993): 3015–3023.

19. A. H. Lichtenstein and coauthors, Effects of canola, corn, and olive oils on fasting and postprandial plasma lipoproteins in humans as part of a National Cholesterol Education Program step 2 diet, *Arteriosclerosis and Thrombosis* 13 (1993): 1533–1542; J. M. Hodgson and coauthors, Can linoleic acid contribute to coronary artery disease? *American Journal of Clinical Nutrition* 58 (1993): 228–234; E. S. Sarkkinen and coauthors, Long-term effects of three fat-modified diets in hypercholesterolemic subjects, *Atherosclerosis* 105 (1994): 9–23.

20. C. V. Felton and coauthors, Dietary polyunsaturated fatty acids and composition of human aortic plaques, *The Lancet* 344 (1994): 1195–1196.

21. M. D. Lorgeril and coauthors, Mediterranean alpha-linolenic acid-rich diet in secondary prevention of coronary heart disease, *The Lancet* 343 (1994): 1454–1459.

22. H. Blackburn, Co-investigator, Seven Countries Study, as quoted in D. Schardt, B. Liebman, and S. Schmidt, Going Mediterranean, *Nutrition Action Health Letter* 21 (1994): 1–5.

23. E. B. Rimm and coauthors, Vitamin E consumption and the risk of coronary heart disease in men, *New England Journal of Medicine* 328 (1993): 1450–1456; M. J. Stampfer and coauthors, Vitamin E consumption and the risk of coronary heart disease in women, *New England Journal of Medicine* 328 (1993): 1444–1449; P. Knekt, Antioxidant vitamin intake and coronary mortality in a longitudinal population study, *American Journal of Epidemiology* 139 (1994): 1180–1189.

24. I. Jialal and S. M. Grundy, The effect of dietary supplementation with alpha tocopherol on the oxidative modification of low-density lipoprotein, *Journal of Lipid Research* 6 (1992): 899–906; J. A. Simon, Vitamin C and cardiovascular disease, *Journal of the American College of Nutrition* 11 (1992): 107–125; D. L. Morris, S. B. Kritchevsky, and C. E. Davis, Serum carotenoids and coronary heart disease: The lipid research clinics coronary primary prevention trial and follow-up study, *Journal of the American Medical Association* 272 (1994): 1439–1441.

25. D. Kritchevsky, Antioxidant vitamins in the prevention of cardiovascular disease, *Nutrition Today* 27 (1992): 30–33; D. Steinberg, Antioxidant vitamins and coronary heart disease, *New England Journal of Medicine* 328 (1993): 1487–1489; C. H. Hennekens, J. E. Buring, and R. Peto, Antioxidant vitamins: Benefits not yet proved, *New England Journal of Medicine* 330 (1994): 1080–1081.

26. M. McDowell, Trends in Americans' dietary fat intake, *Journal of the National Cancer Institute* 86 (1994): 889.

27. Personal communication with Consumer Affairs, Entenmann's, Bay Shore, N.Y.

28. Personal communication with Media relations, McDonald's Corporation, Oak Brook, Ill.

29. Personal communication with Consumer Affairs, Kraft, Glenview, Ill.

30. G. E. Ruoff, Reducing fat intake with fat substitutes, *American Family Physician* 43 (April 1991): 1235–1242.

31. *Simplesse All Natural Fat Substitute: A Scientific Overview*, (Deerfield, Ill.: The Simplesse Company, 1991), pp. 3–10.

32. U.S. Department of Health and Human Services, HHS News, FDA Approves Fat Substitute, Olestra, January 24, 1996.

33. The list of food suggestions is from R. M. Mullis and coauthors, Developing nutrient criteria for food-specific dietary guidelines for the general public, *Journal of the American Dietetic Association* 90 (1990): 847–849.

34. The Expert Panel on the Detection, Evaluation, and Treatment of High Blood Cholesterol in Adults: Summary of the Second Report of the National Cholesterol Education Program (Adult Treatment Panel II), *Journal of the American Medical Association* 269 (1993): 3015–3023.

35. D. J. Jenkins and coauthors, Effect on blood lipids of very high intakes of fiber in diets low in saturated fat and cholesterol, *New England Journal of Medicine* 329 (1993): 21–26.

36. D. L. Sprecher and coauthors, Efficacy of psyllium in reducing serum cholesterol levels in hypercholesterolemic patients on high or low-fat diets, *Annals of Internal Medicine* 119 (1993): 545–554.

37. Expert Panel on Detection, Evaluation, and Treatment of High Blood Cholesterol Levels in Adults, *Journal of the American Medical Association* 269 (1993): 3015–3023.

38. R. R. Wing and coauthors, Change in waist-hip ratio with weight loss and its association with change in cardiovascular risk factors, *American Journal of Clinical Nutrition* 55 (1992): 1086–1092.

39. W. S. Harris and F. Muzio, Fish oil reduces postprandial triglyceride concentrations without accelerating lipid-emulsion removal rates, *American Journal of Clinical Nutrition* 58 (1993): 68–74; R. Vandongen, Effects on blood pressure of ω-3 fats in subjects at increased risk of cardiovascular disease, *Hypertension* 22 (1993): 371–379.

40. P. M. Ridker and coauthors, Association of moderate alcohol consumption and plasma concentration of endogenous tissue-type plasminogen activator, *Journal of the American Medical Association* 272 (1994): 929–933.

41. J. M. Gaziano and coauthors, Moderate alcohol intake, increased levels of high-density lipoprotein and its subfractions, and decreased risk of myocardial infarction, *New England Journal of Medicine* 329 (1993): 1829–1834; G. D. Friedman and A. L. Klatsky, Is alcohol good for your heart, *New England Journal of Medicine* 329 (1993): 1882–1883.

42. S. L. Englebardt, Eat, drink, go back to work, *American Health* June 1994, p. 90.

43. T. A. Pearson and P. Terry, What to advise patients about drinking alcohol: The clinician's conundrum, *Journal of the American Medical Association* 272 (1994): 967–968.

44. S. Warshafsky and coauthors, Effect of garlic on total serum cholesterol: A meta-analysis, *Annals of Internal Medicine* 119 (1993): 599–605; T. A. Pearson, The quest for a cholesterol-decreasing diet: Should we subtract, substitute, or supplement? *Annals of Internal Medicine* 119 (1993): 627–628.

45. U.S. Department of Health and Human Services, Report of the Expert Panel on Blood Cholesterol Levels in Children and Adolescents, 1991; S. S. Gidding, The rationale for lowering serum cholesterol levels in American children, *American Journal of Diseases in Children* 147 (1993): 386–392.

CHAPTER 5 NOTES

1. A. A. Albanese and L. A. Orto, The proteins and amino acids, in M. E. Shils, J. A. Olson, and M. Shike, eds., *Modern Nutrition in Health and Disease,* 6th ed. (Philadelphia: Lea and Febiger, 1994), pp. 3-35.

2. W. J. Visek, Arginine needs, physiological state and usual diets: A reevaluation, *Journal of Nutrition* 116 (1986): 36–46.

3. D. W. Wilmore, Glutamine and the gut, Gastroenterology 107 (1994): 1885–1886.

4. Personal communication with Gerald Gleich, M.D., Department of Immunology, Mayo Clinic, Rochester, MN, 1992.

5. Personal communication with EMS Hotline (800-367-2829), 1995.

6. EMS Hotline, 1995; E. A. Belongia and coauthors, An investigation of the cause of eosinophilia-myaligia syndrome associated with tryptophan use, *New England Journal of Medicine* 323 (1990): 357–365.

7. C. Ballentine, The essential guide to amino acids, *FDA Consumer,* September 1985, pp. 23–25.

8. S. A. Anderson and D. J. Raiten, eds., *Safety of Amino Acids Used as Dietary Supplements* (Bethesda, Md.: Life Sciences Research Office, Federation of American Societies for Experimental Biology, 1992), pp. v–x, 193–196, 213–215.

9. C. Ballentine, 1985.

10. P. J. Rasch and coauthors, Protein dietary supplementation and physical performance, *Medicine and Science in Sports* 1 (1969): 195–199.

11. V. Lambert, Using "smart" drugs and drinks may not be smart, *FDA Consumer,* April 1993, pp. 24–26.

12. N. J. Smith and B. Worthington-Roberts, *Food for Sport* (Palo Alto, Calif.: Bull Publishing Company, 1989), p. 21.

13. R. K. Chandra and coauthors, Nutrition and immunity: Lessons from the past and new insights into the future, *American Journal of Clinical Nutrition* 53 (1991): 1087–1101; S. A. Shikora and coauthors, Nutrition and immunology: Clinician's approach, in R. A. Forse, ed., *Diet, Nutrition, and Immunity* (Boca Raton, Fla.: CRC Press, 1994), pp. 9–22.

14. V. R. Young, Soy protein in relation to human protein and amino acid nutrition, *Journal of the American Dietetic Association* 91 (1991): 828–835.

15. B. Torun and F. Chew, Protein-energy malnutrition, in M. E. Shils, J. A. Olson, and M. Shike, eds., *Modern Nutrition in Health and Disease* (Philadelphia: Lea and Febiger, 1994), pp. 950–976.

16. M. Nestle and S. Guttmacher, Hunger in the United States: Rationale, methods, and policy implications of state hunger surveys, *Journal of Nutrition Education* 24 (1992): 18S–22S.

17. M. B. Zemel, Calcium utilization: Effect of varying level and source of dietary protein, *American Journal of Clinical Nutrition* 48 (1988): 880–883.

18. American Dietetic Association, Position of the American Dietetic Association: Vegetarian diets, *Journal of the American Dietetic Association* 93 (1993): 1317–1319.

19. C. Lamberg-Allardt and coauthors, Low serum 25-hydroxyvitamin D concentrations and secondary hyperparathyroidism in middle-aged white strict vegetarians, *American Journal of Clinical Nutrition* 58 (1993): 684–689.

20. D. Ornish and coauthors, Can lifestyle changes reverse coronary heart disease? *The Lancet* 336 (1990): 129–133.

21. S. M. Potter and coauthors, Depression of plasma cholesterol in men by consumption of baked products containing soy protein, *American Journal of Clinical Nutrition* 58 (1993): 501–506; J. T. Dwyer, Nutritional consequences of vegetarianism, *Annual Review of Nutrition* 11 (1991): 61–91.

CHAPTER 6 NOTES

1. J. Jaramillo-Arango, The conquest of nutritional diseases (vitamins), in *The British Contribution to Medicine* (Edinburgh: E. & S. Livingstone, Ltd., 1953), pp. 140–162.

2. R. Hill and coauthors, The discovery of vitamins, in *The Chemistry of Life* (Cambridge: Cambridge University Press, 1970), pp. 156–170.

3. J. M. McKenney and coauthors, A comparison of the efficacy and toxic effects of sustained- vs. immediate-release niacin in hyper-

cholesterolemic patients, *Journal of the American Medical Association* 271 (1994): 672–677; L. Lasagna, Over-the-counter niacin, *Journal of the American Medical Association* 271 (1994): 709–710.

4. A. Bendich, Folic acid and prevention of neural tube birth defects: critical assessment of FDA proposals to increase folic acid intakes, *Journal of Nutrition Education* 26 (1994): 294–299.

5. M. Nestle, Folate fortification and neural tube defects: policy implications, *Journal of Nutrition Education* 26 (1994): 287–293.

6. M. K. Berman and coauthors, Vitamin B_6 in premenstrual syndrome, *Journal of the American Dietetic Association* 90 (1990): 859–860.

7. P. M. Suter and coauthors, Reversal of protein-bound vitamin B_{12} malabsorption with antibiotics in atrophic gastritis, *Gastroenterology* 101 (1991): 1039–1045.

8. J. Selhub and coauthors, Association between plasma homocysteine concentrations and extracranial carotid-artery stenosis, *New England Journal of Medicine* 332 (1995): 286–291; M. J. Stampfer and M. R. Malinow, Can lowering homocysteine levels reduce cardiovascular risk? *New England Journal of Medicine* 332 (1995): 328–329; J. Selhub and coauthors, Vitamin status and intake as primary determinants of homocysteinemia in an elderly population, *Journal of the American Medical Association* 270 (1993): 2693–2698.

9. J. L. Millis and coauthors, Homocysteine metabolism in pregnancies complicated by neural-tube defects, *The Lancet* 345 (1995): 149–151.

10. W. Mertz, A balanced approach to nutrition for health: the need for biologically essential minerals and vitamins, *Journal of the American Dietetic Association* 94 (1994): 1259–1262.

11. L. C. Pauling, *Vitamin C and the Common Cold* (San Francisco: W. H. Freeman, 1970).

12. C. S. Johnston and coauthors, Antihistamine effects and complications of supplemental vitamin C, *Journal of the American Dietetic Association* 92 (1992): 988–989.

13. S. J. VanGarde and M. Woodburn, *Food Preservation and Safety* (Ames, Iowa: Iowa State University Press, 1994), p. 109.

14. J. Bailey, *Keeping Food Fresh* (New York: Harper & Row, 1989), p. 18.

15. VanGarde and Woodburn, p. 110.

16. M. A. McCarthy and R. H. Matthews, *Conserving Nutrients in Foods* Administrative Report No. 384 (Hyattsville, MD: Nutrition Monitoring Division, Human Nutrition Information Service, U.S. Department of Agriculture, 1988), p. 3.

17. VanGarde and Woodburn, pp. 94–98.

18. VanGarde and Woodburn, pp. 123–124.

19. M. F. Hollick and coauthors, The vitamin D content of fortified milk and infant formula, *New England Journal of Medicine* 326 (1992): 1213–1215.

20. National Osteoporosis Foundation, *The Osteoporosis Report* 9 (Winter 1993): 3.

21. Mertz, p. 1260.

22. P. S. Connolly, Treatment of nocturnal leg cramps, *Archives of Internal Medicine* 152 (1992): 1877–1880.

23. A. L. Eldridge and E. T. Sheehan, Food supplement use and related beliefs: Survey of community college students, *Journal of Nutrition Education* 26 (1994): 259–265.

24. J. Hirsh and V. Fuster, Guide to anticoagulant therapy, part 2: oral anticoagulants, *Circulation* 89 (1994): 1473.

25. National Research Council, *Recommended Dietary Allowances, 10th edition* (Washington, D.C.: National Academy Press), 1989, pp. 263–269.

26. *Annual Overview of Nutritional Supplement Industry (1983-1993)* (Washington D.C.: Council for Responsible Nutrition, 1994), p. 10.

27. M. Stampfer and coauthors, Vitamin E consumption and the risk of coronary disease in women, *New England Journal of Medicine* 328 (1993): 1444–1449; E. Rimm and coauthors, Vitamin E consumption and the risk of coronary disease in men, *New England Journal of Medicine* 328 (1993): 1450–1456.

28. D. L. Tribble and coauthors, Reduced plasma ascorbic acid concentrations in nonsmokers regularly exposed to environmental tobacco smoke, *American Journal of Clinical Nutrition* 58 (1993): 886–890.

29. B. Halliwell, Antioxidants: Sense or speculation? *Nutrition Today* 29 (1994): 15–19.

30. The Alpha-Tocopherol, Beta Carotene Cancer Prevention Study Group, The effect of vitamin E and beta carotene on the incidence of lung cancer and other cancers in male smokers, *New England Journal of Medicine* 330 (1994): 1029–1035.

31. C. H. Hennekens and coauthors, Antioxidant vitamins—Benefits not yet proved, *New England Journal of Medicine* 330 (1994): 1080–1081.

CHAPTER 7 NOTES

1. C. M. McCay, Anorganic substances, in *Notes on the History of Nutrition Research,* ed. F. Verzar (Vienna: Hans Huber Publishers, 1973), pp. 156–184.

2. R. P. Heaney, C. M. Weaver, and M. J. Barger-Lux, Food factors influencing calcium availability, in *Nutritional Aspects of Osteoporosis,* eds. P. Burckharat and R. P. Heaney. Proceedings of the 2nd International Symposium on Osteoporosis, Lausanne, Switzerland, May 1994 (New York: Raven Press, 1995).

3. G. D. Miller, J. K. Jarvis, and L. D. McBean, *Handbook of Dairy Foods and Nutrition* (Boca Raton, Fla.: CRC Press, 1994), pp. 28–44.

4. National Digestive Diseases Information Clearinghouse, *Lactose Intolerance,* NIH Publication No. 94-2751, April 1994; L. N. Aurisicchio and C. S. Pitchumoni, Lactose intolerance: Recognizing the link between diet and discomfort, *Postgraduate Medicine* 95 (1994): 113–116, 119–120.

5. Council for Responsible Nutrition, *1993 Overview of the Nutritional Supplement Market* (Washington, D.C.: Council for Responsible Nutrition, 1994).

6. Calcium: How to get enough, *Consumer Reports,* August 1995, pp. 510–513.

7. R. R. Recker, Calcium absorption and achlorhydria, *New England Journal of Medicine* 313 (1985): 70–73.

8. B. P. Bourgoin and coauthors, *American Journal of Public Health* 83:1155 (1993).

9. A. C. Looker, R. R. Briefel, and M. A. McDowell, Calcium intake in the United States, in *Optimal Calcium Intake,* NIH Consensus Development Conference, June 6–8, 1994, p. 19.

10. The opening vignettes are from P. Ola and E. D'Aulaire, The health risk women can no longer ignore, *Reader's Digest,* August 1994, 91–95.

11. National Research Council, *Diet and Health: Implications for Reducing Chronic Risk* (Washington, D.C.: National Academy Press, 1991), p. 121.

12. F. Bronner, Calcium and osteoporosis, *American Journal of Clinical Nutrition* 60 (1994): 831–836.

13. R. L. Smith and coauthors, Prevention of postmenopausal osteoporosis: A comparative study of exercise, calcium supplementation, and hormone replacement therapy, *New England Journal of Medicine* 325 (1991): 1189–1195.

14. W. S. Pollitzer and J. B. Anderson, Ethnic and genetic differences in bone mass: A review with a hereditary versus an environmental perspective, *American Journal of Clinical Nutrition* 50 (1989): 1244–1259.

15. R. P. Heaney, J. Gallagher, and C. Johnson, Calcium nutrition and bone health in the elderly, *American Journal of Clinical Nutrition* 36 (1982): 986–1013.

16. D. V. Porter, Washington Update: NIH Consensus Development Conference Statement: Optimal Calcium Intake, *Nutrition Today* 29 (1994): 37–40; G. D. Miller, Required versus optimal intakes: A look at calcium, *Journal of Nutrition* 124 (1994): 1404S–1430S.

17. U.S. Department of Agriculture, Human Nutrition Information Service, *Food and Nutrient Intakes by Individuals in the United States: 1 Day, 1987–1988,* NFCS Rep. No. 87-1-1, 1993; U.S. Department of Health and Human Services, Public Health Service, National Institutes of Health, *Consensus Development Conference Statement: Optimal Calcium Intake,* June 6–8, 1994.

18. G. Wyshak and R. E. Frisch, Carbonated beverages, dietary calcium, the dietary calcium/phosphorus ratio, and bone fractures in girls and boys, *Journal of Adolescent Health* 15 (1994): 210–215.

19. P. M. Rowe, New U.S. recommendations on calcium intake, *Lancet* 343 (1994): 1559–1560; S. A. Abrams and J. E. Stuff, Calcium metabolism in girls: Current dietary intakes lead to low rates of calcium absorption and retention during puberty, *American Journal of Clinical Nutrition* 60 (1994): 739–743.

20. Top ten advances of 1993, *Harvard Health Letter,* 19(5) (1994): 7.

21. R. L. Prince and coauthors, Prevention of postmenopausal osteoporosis: A comparative study of exercise, calcium supplementation, and hormone-replacement therapy, *New England Journal of Medicine* 325 (1991): 1189–1195.

22. G. Wyshak and R. E. Frisch, *Journal of Adolescent Health* 15 (1994): 210–215.

23. G. G. Krishna and S. C. Kapoor, Potassium depletion exacerbates essential hypertension, *Annals of Internal Medicine* 115 (1991): 77–82.

24. O. Ophir and coauthors, Low blood pressure in vegetarians: The possible role of potassium, *American Journal of Clinical Nutrition* 37 (1983): 755–762.

25. D. Farley, High blood pressure: Controlling the silent killer, *FDA Consumer,* December 1991, pp. 28–33.

26. S. A. Corrigan and coauthors, Weight reduction in the prevention and treatment of hypertension: A review of representative clinical trials, *American Journal of Health Promotion* 5 (1991): 208–214.

27. National High Blood Pressure Education Program Working Group, National High Blood Pressure Education Program Working Group Report on Primary Prevention of Hypertension, *Archives of Internal Medicine* 153 (1993): 186–208.

28. The Joint National Committee on Detection, Evaluation, and Treatment of High Blood Pressure, The Fifth Report of the Joint National Committee on Detection, Evaluation, and Treatment of High Blood Pressure, *Archives of Internal Medicine* 153 (1993): 154–183.

29. Joint National Committee, 1993.

30. National Research Council, *Diet and Health: Implications for Reducing Chronic Disease Risk, Executive Summary* (Washington, D.C.: National Academy Press, 1989), pp. 14–15.

31. B. M. Massie, To combat hypertension, increase activity, *The Physician and Sportsmedicine* 20 (1992): 89–111.

32. R. Stamler and coauthors, Primary prevention of hypertension by nutritional-hygienic means, *Journal of the American Medical Association* 262 (1989): 1801–1807.

33. Joint National Committee, 1993.

34. K. Clark, Calcium and hypertension: Does a relationship exist?, *Nutrition Today* July/August 1989, pp. 21–26; J. A. Cutler, Calcium and blood pressure: An epidemiologic perspective, *American Journal of Hypertension* 3 (1990): 137S–146S, D. A. McCarron and coauthors, Dietary calcium and blood pressure: Modifying factors in specific populations, American Journal of Clinical Nutrition (Supplement) 54 (1991): 215–219.

35. F. C. Luft, Dietary sodium, potassium and chloride intake and arterial hypertension, *Nutrition Today,* May/June 1989, pp. 11–12.

36. Joint National Committee, 1993.

37. M. Moser, *High Blood Pressure & What You Can Do About It* (Elmsford, N.Y.: The Benjamin Company, Inc., 1989), pp. 4–7.

38. N. S. Scrimshaw, Functional consequences of iron deficiency in human populations, *Journal of Nutrition Science and Vitaminology* 30 (1984): 47–63.

39. L. S. Stephenson, Possible new developments in community control of iron-deficiency anemia, *Nutrition Reviews* 53 (1995): 23–30.

40. E. R. Monsen, Iron nutrition and absorption: Dietary factors which impact iron bioavailablity, *Journal of the American Dietetic Association* 88 (1988): 786–790.

41. A. Ascherio and coauthors, Dietary iron intake and risk of coronary disease among men, *Circulation* 89 (1994): 969–974; W. R. Proulx and C. M. Weaver, Ironing out heart disease, *Nutrition Today* 30 (1995): 16–23.

42. J. T. Salonen and coauthors, High stored iron levels are associated with excess risk of myocardial infarction in Eastern Finnish men, *Circulation* 86 (1992): 803–811.

43. A. S. Prasad, Discovery of human zinc deficiency and studies in an experimental human model, *American Journal of Clinical Nutrition* 53 (1991): 403–412.

44. R. J. Cousins and J. M. Hempe, Zinc, in *Present Knowledge in Nutrition*, 6th ed., ed. M. L. Brown (Washington, D.C.: International Life Sciences Institute, Nutrition Foundation, 1990), pp. 251–260.

45. F. Taylor, Iodine—Going from hypo to hyper, *FDA Consumer*, April 1981, pp. 15–18.

46. J. A. Pennington, A review of iodine toxicity reports, *Journal of the American Dietetic Association* 90 (1990): 1571–1581.

47. E. G. Offenbacher and F. X. Pi-Sunyer, Chromium in human nutrition, *Annual Review of Nutrition* 8 (1988): 543–563.

48. F. H. Nielsen, Facts and fallacies about boron, *Nutrition Today*, May/June 1992, pp. 6–12, S. Meacham and coauthors, Effect of boron supplementation on blood and urinary calcium, magnesium, and phosphorus, and urinary boron in athletic and sedentary women, *American Journal of Clinical Nutrition* 61 (1995): 341–345.

49. National Research Council, *Recommended Dietary Allowances—10th Edition* (Washington, D.C.: National Academy Press, 1989), pp. 248–249.

50. U.S. Environmental Protection Agency, Office of Water, *Is Your Drinking Water Safe?* (Washington, D.C.: U.S. Environmental Protection Agency, 1989).

51. U.S. Environmental Protection Agency and Centers for Disease Control and Prevention, Guidance for people with severely weakened immune systems, June 15, 1995.

52. U.S. Environmental Protection Agency Office of Water, *Lead and Your Drinking Water* (Washington, D.C.: U.S. Environmental Protection Agency, 1987).

53. Position of the American Dietetic Association: The impact of fluoride on dental health, *Journal of the American Dietetic Association* 94 (1994): 1428–1431.

54. National Research Council, *Health Effects of Ingested Fluoride* (Washington, D.C.: National Academy Press, 1993), pp. 1–181.

55. Beverage Marketing Corporation, *Bottled Water in the U.S.*, 1994.

56. U.S. General Accounting Office, *Food Safety and Quality: Stronger FDA Standards and Oversight Needed for Bottled Water* (Washington, D.C.: U.S. General Accounting Office, 1991), p. 17.

57. V. Lambert, Bottled water: New trends, new rules, *FDA Consumer*, June 1993, pp. 9–11.

58. J. Stannard and coauthors, Fluoride content of some bottled waters and recommendation for fluoride supplementation, *Journal of Pedodontics* 14 (1990): 103–107.

CHAPTER 8 NOTES

1. Food and Nutrition Board, Institute of Medicine, P. R. Thomas, ed., *Weighing the Options: Criteria for Evaluating Weight-management programs* (Washington, D.C.: National Academy Press, 1995), pp. 1–25.

2. F. X. Pi-Sunyer, Health implications of obesity, *American Journal of Clinical Nutrition* 53 (1991): 1595S–1603S; I-Min Lee and coauthors, Body weight and mortality: A 27-year follow-up of middle-aged men, *Journal of the American Medical Association* 270 (1993): 2823–2828.

3. Federal Trade Commission and Food and Drug Administration, *The Facts About Weight Loss Products and Programs*, DHHS Publication No. (FDA) 92-1189, 1992.

4. S. L. Gortmaker and coauthors, Social and economic consequences of overweight in adolescence and young adulthood, *New England Journal of Medicine* 329 (1993): 1008–1012; J. A. Cassell, Social anthropology and nutrition: A different look at obesity in America, *Journal of the American Dietetic Association* 95 (1995): 424–427.

5. R. Roubenoff, G. E. Dallal, and P. W. Wilson, Predicting body fatness: The body mass index versus estimation by bioelectrical impedance, *American Journal of Public Health* 85 (1995): 726–728.

6. National Research Council, *Diet and Health: Implications for Reducing Chronic Disease Risk* (Washington, D.C.: National Academy Press, 1989), p. 117.

7. Pi-Sunyer, 1991; R. D. Morris and A. A. Rimm, Association of waist to hip ratio and family history with the prevalence of NIDDM among 25,272 adult, white females, *American Journal of Public Health* 81 (1991): 507–509.

8. P. A. Lachance, Human obesity, *Food Technology* 48 (1994): 127–138.

9. J. M. Friedman, Defective gene linked to obesity, *Nature*, December 1, 1994.

10. T. A. Spiegel, E. E. Shrager, and E. Stellar, Responses of lean and obese subjects to preloads, deprivation, and palatability, *Appetite* 13 (1989): 45–69.

11. W. Dietz, Factors associated with childhood obesity, *Nutrition* 7(4) (1991): 290–291.

12. A. J. Stunkard, T. T. Foch, and Z. Hrubec, A twin study of human obesity, *Journal of the American Medical Association* 256 (1986): 51–54; A. J. Stunkard and coauthors, An adoption study of human obesity, *New England Journal of Medicine* 314 (1986): 193–198; A. J. Stunkard and coauthors, The body-mass index of twins who have been reared apart, *New England Journal of Medicine* 322 (1990): 1483–1487.

13. C. Bouchard and L. Perusse, Genetics of obesity, *Annual Review of Nutrition* 13 (1993): 337–354.

14. C. Bouchard and coauthors, The response to long-term overfeeding in identical twins, *New England Journal of Medicine* 322 (1990): 1477–1482.

15. P. Thomas, 1995.

16. K. D. Brownell and T. A. Wadden, Etiology and treatment of obesity: Understanding a serious, prevalent, and refractory disorder, *Journal of Consulting and Clinical Psychology* 60 (1992): 505–517.

17. L. Lissner and coauthors, Dietary fat and the regulation of energy intake in human subjects, *American Journal of Clinical Nutrition* 46 (1987): 886–892; I. Romieu, Energy intake and other determinants of relative weight, *American Journal of Clinical Nutrition* 47 (1988): 406–412.

18. B. J. Rolls and D. J. Shide, The influence of dietary fat on food intake and body weight, *Nutrition Reviews* 50 (1992): 283–290.

19. J. Beedoe and coauthors, A review of low-calorie and very-low-calorie diet plans and possible metabolic consequences, *Topics in Clinical Nutrition* 6(1) (1990): 68–83.

20. National Task Force on the Prevention and Treatment of Obesity, Very low calorie diets, *Journal of the American Medical Association* 270 (1993): 967–974.

21. F. M. Berg, Drug treatment for obesity, *Obesity and Health* 7 (1993): 8–12.

22. G. A. Bray, Drug treatment of obesity, *American Journal of Clinical Nutrition* 55 (1992): 538S–544S.

23. E. Jequier, Thermogenic drugs in obesity treatment, *American Journal of Clinical Nutrition* 55 (1992): 249S–251S.

24. P. R. Thomas, 1995.

25. J. Stevens and coauthors, Effect of psyllium gum and wheat bran on spontaneous energy intake, *American Journal of Clinical Nutrition* 46 (1987): 812–817.

26. F. M. Berg, Chromium picolinate: Scam of the hour, *Obesity and Health* 7 (1993): 54–55.

27. A. M. Macgregor and C. S. Rand, Gastric surgery in morbid obesity: Outcome in patients aged 55 years and older, *Archives of Surgery* 128 (1993): 1153–1157.

28. M. G. Perri, Confronting the maintenance problem in the treatment of obesity, *Journal of Cardiopulmonary Rehabilitation* 13 (1993): 164–166.

29. P. Thomas, 1995.

30. M. Shah and coauthors, Comparison of a low-fat, ad libitum complex carbohydrate diet with a low energy diet in moderately obese women, *American Journal of Clinical Nutrition* 59 (1994): 980–984.

31. C. O'Neil and coauthors, Factors associated with maintenance of weight loss: Prevention of relapse, *Nutrition* 7 (1991): 302–306.

32. K. Brownell, Yo-yo dieting, in *Nutrition 91/92*, ed. C. C. Cook-Fuller with S. Barrett (Guilford, Conn.: The Dushkin Publishing Group, 1991), pp. 132–134.

33. C. E. Ross, Overweight and depression, *Journal of Health and Social Behavior* 35 (1994): 63–78.

34. National Task Force on the Prevention and Treatment of Obesity, Weight cycling, *Journal of the American Medical Association* 275 (1994): 1196–1202.

35. F. X. Pi-Sunyer, The fattening of America, *Journal of the American Medical Association* 272 (1994): 238.

36. J. P. Foreyt and G. K. Goodrick, *Living Without Dieting* (New York: Warner Books, 1992), p. 28.

37. Ibid., 30.

38. K. D. Brownell, *The LEARN Program for Weight Control* (Dallas, Texas: American Health Publishing Company, 1994), pp. 102–103.

39. Foreyt and Goodrick, pp. 43–58.

40. J. O. Prochaska, *Changing for Good* (New York: William Morrow and Company, 1994), p. 47.

41. Ibid., 38–50.

42. R. Lemberg, *Controlling Eating Disorders with Facts, Advice, and Resources* (Oryx Press, 1992).

43. D. Neumark-Sztainer, Excessive weight preoccupation: Normative but not harmless, *Nutrition Today* 30 (1995): 68–74.

44. Ibid., 1995.

45. Task force on DSM-IV, 307.50 Eating Disorders Not Otherwise Specified, *DSM-IV Draft Criteria* (Washington, D.C.: American Psychiatric Association, 1993), p. P:2.

46. R. T. Harris, Anorexia nervosa and bulimia nervosa in female adolescents, *Nutrition Today,* March/April 1991, pp. 30–34.

47. D. Williamson, *Assessment of Eating Disorders: Obesity, Anorexia, and Bulimia Nervosa,* (New York: Pergamon Press, 1990); Practice guidelines for eating disorders, *American Journal of Psychiatry* 150 (1993): 212–218.

48. D. W. Reiff and K. K. L. Reiff, Position of the American Dietetic Association: Nutrition intervention in the treatment of anorexia nervosa, bulimia nervosa, and binge eating, *Journal of the American Dietetic Association* 94 (1994): 902–907.

CHAPTER 9 NOTES

1. S. N. Blair and coauthors, Changes in physical fitness and all-cause mortality: a prospective study of healthy and unhealthy men, *Journal of the American Medical Association* 273 (1995): 1093–1098; K. E. Powell and coauthors, Physical activity and chronic diseases, *American Journal of Clinical Nutrition* 49 (1989): 999–1006.

2. R. Pate and coauthors, Physical activities and public health, *Journal of the American Medical Association* 273 (1995): 402–407.

3. S. N. Blair, Diet and activity: The synergistic merger, *Nutrition Today* 30 (1995): 108–112.

4. The idea of positive addiction and this list of prerequisites for it originate with the psychologist W. Glasser, *Positive Addiction* (New York: Harper and Row, 1976), p. 93.

5. S. N. Blair, 1995.

6. U.S. Centers for Disease Control and Prevention and American College of Sports Medicine, Summary statement: Workshop on physical activity and public health, July 29, 1993.

7. M. A. Fiatarone and coauthors, Exercise training and nutritional supplementation for physical fraility in very elderly people, *New England Journal of Medicine* 330 (1994): 1769–1775.

8. B. Hurley, Aerobic or strength training for coronary risk factor intervention? *Annals of Internal Medicine* 26 (1994): 153–154.

9. F. Katch and W. McArdle, *Introduction to Nutrition, Exercise, and Health* (Philadelphia: Lea and Febiger, 1993) p. 329.

10. American College of Sports Medicine, Position Paper: The Recommended Quantity and Quality of Exercise for Developing and Maintaining Cardiorespiratory and Muscular Fitness in Healthy Adults, *Medicine and Science in Sports and Exercise* 22 (1990): 265.

11. American College of Sports Medicine, *Guidelines for Exercise Testing and Prescription*, 4th ed. (Philadelphia: Lea and Febiger, 1991), Chapter 3.

12. PAR-Q Validation Report. British Columbia Department of Health, June 1975 (modified version). From American College of Sports Medicine, *Guidelines for Exercise Testing and Prescription*, 4th ed. (Philadelphia: Lea and Febiger, 1991), Chapter 3.

13. Katch and McArdle, 1993, p. 174.

14. E. Hultman, R. C. Harris, and L. L. Spriet, Work and exercise, in *Modern Nutrition in Health and Disease*, 8th ed., M. E. Shils, J. A. Olson, and M. Shike, eds. (Philadelphia: Lea and Febiger, 1994), pp. 663–680.

15. E. Hultman, 1994.

16. J. A. Romijn and coauthors, Regulation of endogenous fat and carbohydrate metabolism in relation to exercise intensity and duration, *American Journal of Physiology* 265 (1993): E380–E391.

17. G. A. Brooks and J. Mercier, Balance of carbohydrate and lipid utilization during exercise: The "crossover" concept, *Journal of Applied Physiology* 76 (1994): 2253–2261.

18. S. Blair, *Living with Exercise* (Dallas, Tx: American Health Publishing Company, 1991), p. 85.

19. D. C. Nieman, *Fitness and Sports Medicine: An Introduction* (Palo Alto, Calif.: Bull Publishing Company, 1990), pp. 246–258.

20. Position of the American Dietetic Association and the Canadian Dietetic Association, Nutrition for physical fitness and athletic performance for adults, *Journal of the American Dietetic Association* 93 (1993): 691–695.

21. A. Grandjean, What are the protein requirements for athletes? *Food and Nutrition News* 65 (2), March/April 1993, p. 11; M. E. Houston, Protein and amino acid needs of athletes, *Nutrition Today*, September/October 1992, pp. 36–39.

22. M. L. Stefanick, Exercise and weight control, *Exercise, Sports, and Science Review* 21 (1993): 363–396.

23. C. E. Broeder, The effects of either high-intensity resistance or endurance training on resting metabolic rate, *American Journal of Clinical Nutrition* 55 (1992): 802–810.

24. J. A. Romijn and coauthors, Strenuous endurance training increases lipolysis and triglyceride-fatty acid cycling at rest, *Journal of Applied Physiology* 75 (1993): 108–113; T. J. Horton and C. A. Geissler, Effect of habitual exercise on daily energy expenditure and metabolic rate during standardized activity, *American Journal of Clinical Nutrition* 59 (1994): 13–19.

25. C. E. Broeder, 1992.

26. C. M. Cumming, P. B. Brevard, and J. M. Pearson, Recreational runners' beliefs and practices concerning water intake, *Journal of Nutrition Education* 26 (1994): 195–197.

27. R. J. Maughn, Fluid and electrolyte loss and replacement in exercise, in C. Williams and J. T. Devlin, eds., *Foods, Nutrition and Sports Performance: An International Scientific Consensus.* (London, E & FN Spon, 1992) pp. 19–33.

28. K. B. Wheeler and A. M. Cameron, Plasma volume: The hidden key to performance, *American Fitness Quarterly* (April 1990): 24–26.

29. M. Millard-Stafford, Fluid replacement during exercise in the heat, *Sports Medicine* 13 (1992): 223–233.

30. C. V. Gisolfi and S. M. Duchman, Guidelines for optimal replacement beverages for different athletic events, *Medicine and Science in Sports and Exercise* 24 (1992): 679–687.

31. R. J. Maughn, 1992.

32. Wheeler and Cameron, 1990.

33. Wheeler and Cameron, 1990.

34. Katch and McArdle, 1993.

35. M. Meydani and coauthors, Protective effect of vitamin E on exercise-induced oxidative damage in young and older adults, *American Journal of Physiology* 264 (1993).

36. L. Bucci, *Nutrients as Ergogenic Aids for Sports and Exercise* (Boca Raton, Fla.: CRC Press, 1993), pp. 1–161; M. Kaminski and R. Boal, An effect of ascorbic acid on delayed-onset muscle soreness, *Pain* 50 (1992): 317.

37. L. M. Weight, P. Jacobs, and T. D. Noakes, Dietary iron deficiency and sports anemia, *British Journal of Nutrition* 68 (1992): 253–260.

38. Nutrition and physical performance, in Nieman, 1990, pp. 221–268.

39. Hultman and coauthors, 1994.

40. P. M. Rowe, New U.S. recommendations on calcium intake, *The Lancet* 343 (1994): 1559–1560.

41. T. Lloyd and coauthors, Interrelationships of diet, athletic activity, menstrual status, and bone density in collegiate women, *American Journal of Clinical Nutrition* 46 (1987): 681–684.

42. K. Beals and M. M. Manore, The prevalence and consequence of subclinical eating disorders in female athletes, *International Journal of Sports Nutrition* 4 (1994): 175–195.

43. U.S. Department of Health and Human Services, Public Health Service, National Institutes of Health, *Consensus Development Conference Statement: Optimal Calcium Intake*, June 6–8, 1994.

44. T. H. Murray, The ethics of drugs and sports, in *Drugs and Performance in Sports*, R. H. Strauss, ed. (Philadelphia: W. B. Saunders Company, 1987), pp. 11–21.

45. V. S. Cowart, Dietary supplements: Alternatives to anabolic steroids? *The Physician and Sportsmedicine* 20 (1992): 189–198.

46. Position of the American Dietetic Association and Canadian Dietetic Association: Nutrition for physical fitness and athletic performance for adults, *Journal of the American Dietetic Association* 93 (1993): 691–696; L. Bucci, *Nutrients as Ergogenic Aids for Sports and Exercise* (Boca Raton, Fla.: CRC Press, 1993), pp. 1–161.

47. D. C. Nieman, *Fitness and Sports Medicine: An Introduction* (Palo Alto, Calif.: Bull Publishing Company, 1990), pp. 243–256.

48. G. Mirkin, Can bee pollen benefit health? *Journal of the American Medical Association* 262 (1989): 1854.

49. A. Z. Belko, Vitamins and Exercise—An Update, *Medicine and Science in Sports and Exercise* 19 (1987): S191–S196; E. J. Vander Beek, Vitamins and endurance training: Food for running or faddish claims? *Sports Medicine* 2 (1985): 175–197; Nutrition and physical performance, in Nieman, 1990, pp. 221–268.

50. Food and Drug Administration, *Anabolic Steroids: Losing at Winning*, DHHS Publication No. (FDA) 88-3171; K. L. Ropp, No-win situation for athletes, *FDA Consumer*, December 1992, pp. 8–12; National Academy of Sports Medicine Policy Statement and Position Paper: Anabolic androgenic steroids, growth hormones, stimulants, ergogenics, and drug use in sports, in *Death in the Locker Room II: Drugs and Sports*, B. Goldman and R. Klatz (Chicago: Elite Sports Medicine Publications, 1992), pp. 328–373.

51. C. E. Yesalis and coauthors, Anabolic steroid use in the United States, *Journal of the American Medical Association* 270 (1993): 1217–1221.

52. American College of Sports Medicine, 1990.

53. Nieman, 1990.

54. W. S. Holt, Jr., Nutrition and athletes, *American Family Physician* 47 (1993): 1757–1764.

55. A. N. Bosch, S. C. Dennis, and T. D. Noakes, Influence of carbohydrate loading on fuel substrate turnover and oxidation during prolonged exercise, *Journal of Applied Physiology* 74 (1993): 1921–1927.

56. W. M. Sherman and D. A. Wright, Preevent nutrition for prolonged exercise, in *The Theory and Practice of Athletic Nutrition: Bridging the Gap. Report of the Ross Synposium*, A. S. Grandjean and J. Storlie, eds. (Columbus, Ohio: Ross Laboratories, 1989), pp. 30–46.

57. A. R. Coggan and S. C. Swanson, Nutritional manipulations before and during endurance exercise, *Medicine and Science in Sports and Exercise* 24 (1992): S331–S335.

58. Secretary of Health and Human Services, *Eighth Special Report to the U.S. Congress on Alcohol and Health* (Rockville, Md.: U.S. Department of Health and Human Services, 1993), pp. 1–15.

59. L. T. Medanik and W. B. Clark, The demographic distribution of U.S. drinking patterns in 1990: Description and trends from 1984, *American Journal of Public Health* 84 (1994): 1218–1222.

60. L. Guohua, G. S. Smith, and S. P. Baker, Drinking behavior in relation to cause of death among U.S. adults, *American Journal of Public Health* 84 (1994): 1402–1406.

61. Alcohol-related traffic fatalities, *FDA Consumer*, March 1993, p. 26; L. Archer, B. F. Grant, and D. A. Dawson, What if Americans drank less? The potential effect on the prevalence of alcohol abuse and dependence, *American Journal of Public Health* 85 (1995): 61–66.

62. Committee on Diet and Health, *Diet and Health* (Washington, D.C.: National Academy Press, 1989), pp. 16, 431–464.

63. Eighth Special Report to the U.S. Congress on Alcohol and Health, 1993.

64. R. A. Dietrich, Genetics of alcoholism: How do we find the answers and what do we do then? *Alcohol and Alcoholism* 25 (1990): 571–572.

65. P. Avogaro, Alcohol—A risk or protective factor in aging, in *Sedentary Life and Nutrition*, F. Fabris, L. Pernigotti, and E. Farrario, eds. (New York: Raven Press, Ltd., 1990), pp. 163–172.

66. R. Doll and coauthors, Mortality in relation to consumption of alcohol: 13 years' observations on male British doctors, *British Medical Journal* 309 (1994): 911–918; P. M. Ridker and coauthors, Association of moderate alcohol consumption and plasma concentration of endogenous tissue-type plasminogen activator, *Journal of the American Medical Association* 272 (1994): 929–933.

67. T. A. Pearson and P. Terry, What to advise patients about drinking alcohol: The clinician's conundrum, *Journal of the American Medical Association* 272 (1994): 967–968.

68. Summary of the Report of a Working Group of the Royal Colleges of Physicians, Psychiatrists, and General Practitioners, Alcohol and the heart in perspective: Sensible limits reaffirmed, *Journal of the Royal College of Physicians of London* 29 (1995): 266–271.

69. J. M. Gaziano and coauthors, Moderate alcohol intake, increased levels of high-density lipoprotein and its subfractions, and decreased risk of myocardial infarction, *New England Journal of Medicine* 329 (1993): 1829–1834; and G. D. Friedman and A. L. Klatsky, Is alcohol good for your heart, *New England Journal of Medicine* 329 (1993): 1882–1883.

70. S. E. Hankinson and W. C. Willett, Alcohol and breast cancer: Is there a conclusion? *Nutrition* 11 (1995): 320–321.

71. M. Frezza and co-authors, High blood alcohol levels in women—The role of decreased gastric alcohol dehydrogenase activity and first-pass metabolism, *New England Journal of Medicine* 322 (1990): 95–99.

72. L. Marsano, Alcohol and malnutrition, *Alcohol, Health, and Research World* 17 (1993): 284–291; M.C. Mitchell, Alcohol, in *Present Knowledge in Nutrition*, 6th ed., ed. M. L. Brown (Washington, D.C.: International Life Sciences Institute, 1990), pp. 457–462.

73. B. J. Sonko and coauthors, Effect of alcohol on postmeal fat storage, *American Journal of Clinical Nutrition* 59 (1994): 619–625.

74. J. J. B. Anderson and B. R. Switzer, Effects of alcohol on nutritional status: Part I—Minerals, *Internal Medicine* 8 (1987): 69, 73–75, 79, 81–82, 85.

75. The questions are taken from the *CAGE* questionnaire to screen for alcohol abuse, in M. Carethers, Health promotion in the elderly, *American Family Physician* 45 (1992): 2253.

CHAPTER 10 NOTES

1. L. Breslow and N. Breslow, Health practices and disability: Some evidence from Alameda County, *Preventive Medicine* 22 (1993): 86–95.

2. N. M. Lien, K. K. Meyer, and M. Winick, Early malnutrition and "late" adoption: A study of the effects of the development of

Korean orphans adopted into American families, *American Journal of Clinical Nutrition* 30 (1977): 1734–1739.

3. Food and Nutrition Board, Subcommittee on the Tenth Edition of the RDAs, *Recommended Dietary Allowances,* 10th ed. (Washington, D.C.: National Academy Press, 1989).

4. Institute of Medicine, National Academy of Sciences, Food and Nutrition Board, *Nutrition During Pregnancy* (Washington, D.C.: National Academy Press, 1990), p. 17.

5. Ibid., 1990.

6. Nutrition during pregnancy and lactation, *Dairy Council Digest* 62 (1991): 13–18.

7. Folate supplements prevent recurrence of neural tube defects, *Nutrition Reviews* 50 (1992): 22–26.

8. M. M. Werler, M. B. Shapiro, and A. A. Mitchell, Periconceptual folic acid exposure and risks of occurent neural tube defects, *Journal of the American Medical Association* 269 (1993): 1257–1261; D. T. Burk and P. E. Mirkes, Summary of the 1993 Teratology Society Public Affairs Committee Symposium: Folic acid prevention of neural tube defects: Public policy issues, *Teratology* 49 (1994): 239–241.

9. Institute of Medicine, 1990.

10. B. Worthington-Roberts and R. M. Pitkin, Women's nutrition for optimal reproductive health, in *Call to Action: Better Nutrition for Mothers, Children, and Families,* ed. C. Sharbaugh (Washington, D.C.: National Center for Education in Maternal and Child Health, 1991), p. 124.

11. Institute of Medicine, 1990; C. W. Suitor and J. D. Gardner, *Journal of the American Dietetic Association* 90 (1990): 268.

12. M. Bonati, S. Nannini, and A. Addis, Vitamin A supplementation during pregnancy in developed countries, *Lancet* 345 (1995): 736–737; *New England Journal of Medicine,* November 23, 1995.

13. Institute of Medicine, 1990.

14. U.S. Department of Health and Human Services, Public Health Service, *Healthy People 2000: National Health Promotion and Disease Prevention Objectives* (Washington, D.C.: U.S. Government Printing Office, 1990).

15. C. M. Olson, Promoting positive nutritional practices during pregnancy and lactation, *American Journal of Clinical Nutrition* 59 (1994): 525S–531S.

16. Institute of Medicine, 1990.

17. S. Rodwell Williams and B. Worthington-Roberts, *Nutrition Throughout the Lifecycle* (St. Louis: Mosby Year Book, 1992), pp. 127–128.

18. Ibid., 127.

19. A. Nehlig and G. Debry, Potential teratogenic and neurodevelopmental consequences of coffee and caffeine exposure: A review of human and animal data, *Neurotoxicology and Teratology* 16 (1994): 531–543.

20. Food and Nutrition Board, *Nutrition During Pregnancy* (Washington, D.C.: National Academy Press, 1990), pp. 397–399.

21. X. Ou Shu and coauthors, Maternal smoking, alcohol drinking, caffeine consumption, and fetal growth: Results from a prospective study, *Epidemiology* 6 (1995): 115–120.

22. U.S. Department of Health and Human Services, *Healthy People 2000,* 1990.

23. M. G. Bulterys, S. Greenland, and J. F. Kraus, Chronic fetal hypoxia and sudden infant death syndrome: Interaction between maternal smoking and low hematocrit during pregnancy, *Pediatrics* 86 (1990): 535–540; E. A. Mitchell and coauthors, Smoking and sudden infant death syndrome, *Pediatrics* 91 (1993): 893–896.

24. B. Worthington-Roberts and R. M. Pitkin, Women's nutrition for optimal reproductive health, pp. 113–136.

25. Ibid., 129.

26. L. Eldridge and coauthors, Frequent alcohol consumption among women of childbearing age— Behavioral risk factor surveillance system, *Morbidity and Mortality Weekly Report* 43 (1994): 328–329, 335.

27. N. I. Hahn and M. Erick, Battling morning (noon and night) sickness: New approaches for treating an age-old problem, *Journal of the American Dietetic Association* 94 (1994): 147–148.

28. J. C. King and J. Weininger, Pregnancy and lactation, in *Present Knowledge in Nutrition,* 6th ed., ed., M. L. Brown (Washington, D.C.: Nutrition Foundation, 1990), pp. 314–319.

29. J. M. Belizan and coauthors, Calcium supplementation to prevent hypertensive disorders of pregnancy, *New England Journal of Medicine* 325 (1991): 1399–1405; C. Guillermo and coauthors, Calcium supplementation during pregnancy: A systematic review of randomized controlled trials, *British Journal of Obstetrics and Gynecology* 101 (1994): 753–758; K. Cong and coauthors, Calcium supplementation during pregnancy for reducing pregnancy induced hypertension, *Chinese Medical Journal* 108 (1995): 57–59.

30. U.S. Department of Health and Human Services, Public Health Service, *Surgeon General's Report on Nutrition and Health* (Washington, D.C.: U.S. Government Printing Office, DHHS Pub. No. 88-50210, 1988), pp. 345–380.

31. D. R. Hollingsworth, *Pregnancy, Diabetes, and Birth,* 2nd ed. (Baltimore: Williams and Wilkins, 1992).

32. Position of the American Dietetic Association: Nutrition care for pregnant adolescents, *Journal of the American Dietetic Association* 94 (1994): 449–450.

33. M. Story and I. Alton, Nutrition issues, and adolescent pregnancy, *Nutrition Today* 30 (1995): 142–151.

34. E. Whitney and S. Rolfes, *Understanding Nutrition* (St. Paul: West Publishing, 1993), p. 491.

35. M. L. Hediger and coauthors, Rate and amount of weight gain during adolescent pregnancy: Associations with maternal weight-for-height and birth weight, *American Journal of Clinical Nutrition* 52 (1990): 793–799.

36. Position of the American Dietetic Association: Nutrition care for pregnant adolescents, 1994.

37. R. Tannahil, *Food in History* (New York: Crown Publishers, 1988), p. 275.

38. R. Urgert and coauthors, Effects of cafestol and kahweol from coffee grounds on serum lipids and serum liver enzymes in humans, *American Journal of Clinical Nutrition* 61 (1995): 149–154.

39. A. Leviton and E. N. Allred, Correlates of decaffeinated coffee choice, *Epidemiology* 5 (1994): 537–540.

40. E. C. Strain and coauthors, Caffeine dependence syndrome, *Journal of the American Medical Association* 272 (1994): 1043–1048.

41. S. G. Oei and coauthors, Fetal arrhythmia caused by excessive intake of caffeine by pregnant women, *British Medical Journal* 298 (1989): 1075–1076.

42. C. Infante-Rivard and coauthors, Fetal loss associated with caffeine intake before and during pregnancy, *Journal of the American Medical Association* 270 (1993): 2940–2943; B. Eskenazi, Caffeine during pregnancy: Grounds for concern? *Journal of the American Medical Association* 270 (1993): 2973–2974.

43. N. L. Benowitz and coauthors, Persistent increase in caffeine concentrations in people who stop smoking, *British Medical Journal* 298 (1989): 1075–1076.

44. Institute of Medicine, National Academy of Sciences, Food and Nutrition Board, *Nutrition During Lactation* (Washington, D.C.: National Academy Press, 1991), pp. 1–19.

45. R. D. Williams, Breastfeeding best bet for babies, *FDA Consumer* 29 (1995): 19–23.

46. Ibid., 1991.

47. U.S. Department of Health and Human Services, *Healthy People 2000*, pp. 379–380.

48. American Academy of Pediatrics, Committee on Nutrition, The use of whole cow's milk in infancy, *Pediatrics* 89 (1992): 1105.

49. E. E. Ziegler, S. J. Fomon, and S. E. Nelson, *Journal of Pediatrics* 116 (1990): 11.

50. M. Irigoyen and coauthors, *Pediatrics* 88 (1991): 320.

51. The discussion of food allergies is adapted from infant nutrition in the 1990s, *Dairy Council Digest* 63 (1992): 31–36.

52. Food and Nutrition Board, National Research Council, *Recommended Dietary Allowances*, 10th ed. (Washington, D.C.: National Academy Press, 1989), pp. 24–38.

53. L. L. Birch and coauthors, The variability of young children's energy intake, *New England Journal of Medicine* 324 (1991): 232–235; M. Sigman-Grant, Feeding Preschoolers: Balancing nutritional and developmental needs, *Nutrition Today* 27 (1992): 13–17.

54. E. Satter, *How to Get Your Kids to Eat . . . But Not Too Much* (Palo Alto, Calif.: Bull Publishing Company, 1987), pp. 13–28.

55. Community Nutrition Institute, USDA finalizes school food dietary guidelines, *Nutrition Week* 25 (1995): 3.

56. R. Yip and coauthors, Pediatric nutrition surveillance system—United States, 1980–1991, *Morbidity and Mortality Weekly Report*, November 27, 1992, pp. 1–24.

57. P. C. DuRousseau and coauthors, Children in foster care: Are they at nutritional risk? *Journal of the American Dietetic Association* 91 (1991): 83–85; M. L. Taylor and S. A. Koblinsky, Dietary intake and growth status of young homeless children, *Journal of the American Dietetic Association* 93 (1993): 464–466.

58. ADA Reports, Position of the American Dietetic Association: Domestic hunger and inadequate access to food, *Journal of the American Dietetic Association* 90 (1990): 1437–1441.

59. J. Dwyer and J. Arent, Child nutrition, in *Call to Action: Better Nutrition for Mothers, Children, and Families,* ed. C. O. Sharbaugh (Washington, D.C., National Center for Education in Maternal and Child Health, 1991), pp. 151–168.

60. L. Mellin, Combating Childhood Obesity, *Journal of the American Dietetic Association* 93 (1993): 265–267.

61. M. Knip and O. Nuutinen, Long-term effects of weight reduction on serum lipids and plasma insulin in obese children, *American Journal of Clinical Nutrition* 57 (1993): 490–493; W. H. Dietz, Prevention of childhood obesity, *Pediatric Clinics of North America* 33 (1986): 823–833.

62. R. A. Behrens and M. E. Longe, *Hospital-Based Health Promotion Programs for Children and Youth* (USA: American Hospital Publishing, Inc., 1987), pp. 9–21.

63. G. P. Sylvester and coauthors, Children's television and nutrition: Friend or foes? *Nutrition Today* 30 (1995): 6–10; K. Kotz and coauthors, Food advertisements during children's Saturday morning television programming, *Journal of the American Dietetic Association* 94 (1994): 1296–1299.

64. A. Leung and coauthors, Children and television, *American Family Physician* 50 (1994): 909–913.

65. Yip and coauthors, Pediatric Nutrition Surveillance System.

66. National Cholesterol Education Program, *Report of the Expert Panel on Blood Cholesterol Levels in Children and Adolescents* (Washington, D.C.: U.S. Department of Health and Human Services, Public Health Service, National Institutes of Health, NIH Publication No. 91-2732, 1991), pp. 1–22; F. E. Thompson and B. A. Dennison, Dietary sources of fats and cholesterol in U.S. children aged 2 through 5 years, *American Journal of Public Health* 84 (1994): 799–806.

67. U.S. Department of Health and Human Services, Report of the Expert Panel on Blood Cholesterol Levels in Children and Adolescents, 1991; S. S. Gidding, The rationale for lowering serum cholesterol levels in American children, *American Journal of Diseases in Children* 147 (1993): 386–392.

68. C. N. Bianculli, Physical growth and development in adolescents, in *Health of Adolescents and Youths in the Americas* (Washington, D.C.: Pan American Health Organization, Scientific Publication No. 489, 1985), pp. 45–50.

69. F. P. Heald, Nutrition in adolescence, in *Health of Adolescents and Youths in the Americas*, pp. 51–61.

70. M. Story and coauthors, Adolescent nutrition: Trends and critical issues for the 1990s, in *Call to Action: Better Nutrition for Mothers, Children, and Families* ed. C. O. Sharbaugh (Washington, D.C.: National Center for Education in Maternal and Child Health, 1991), pp. 169–189.

71. L. E. Underwood, Normal adolescent growth and development, *Nutrition Today* 26 (1991): 11–16; G. B. Forbes, Body composition of adolescent girls, *Nutrition Today* 26 (1991): 17–20.

72. D. J. Sherman, The neglected health care needs of street youth, *Public Health Reports* 107 (1992): 433–440.

73. M. Story and coauthors, Adolescent nutrition, 1991.

74. G. Kolata, Obese children: A growing problem, *Science* 232 (1986): 20–21.

75. U.S. Department of Health and Human Services, Public Health Service, *Surgeon General's Report,* pp. 539–593.

76. L. Brabin and B. J. Brabin, The cost of successful adolescent growth and development in girls in relation to iron and vitamin A status, *American Journal of Clinical Nutrition* 55 (1992): 955–958.

77. L. Hallberg and L. Rossander-Hulten, Iron requirements in menstruating women, *American Journal of Clinical Nutrition* 54 (1991): 1047–1058.

78. V. Matkovic, Diet, genetics, and peak bone mass of adolescent girls, *Nutrition Today* 26 (1991): 21–24.

79. Ibid.

80. National Cholesterol Education Program, *Report of the Expert Panel on Blood Cholesterol Levels in Children,* 1991.

81. U.S. Department of Health and Human Services, Public Health Service, *Surgeon General's Report on Nutrition and Health* (Washington, D.C.: U.S. Government Printing Office, DHHS Pub. No. 88-50210, 1988), pp. 345–380.

82. U.S. Department of Health and Human Services, *Healthy People 2000,* pp. 571–578.

83. R. A. Thompson and R. T. Sherman, *Helping Athletes with Eating Disorders* (Champaign, Ill.: Human Kinetics Publishers, 1993).

84. National Center for Health Statistics, *Health United States, 1988* (Washington, D.C.: U.S. Department of Health and Human Services, December 1988).

85. A. E. Harper, Nutrition, aging, and longevity, *American Journal of Clinical Nutrition* (supplement) 36 (October 1982): 737–749.

86. The discussion of demographic trends is adapted from B. Senauer, E. Asp, and J. Kinsey, *Food Trends and the Changing Consumer* (St. Paul: Eagan Press, 1991), pp. 199–213.

87. Ibid., 199.

88. U.S. Department of Health and Human Services, *Healthy People 2000,* pp. 579–592.

89. J. M. McGinnis and M. Nestle, The Surgeon General's report on nutrition and health: Policy implications and implementation strategies, *American Journal of Clinical Nutrition* 49 (1989): 23–28.

90. Institute of Medicine, *The Second Fifty Years, Promoting Health and Preventing Disability* (Washington, D.C.: National Academy Press, 1992), pp. 1–21.

91. Institute of Medicine, *Extending Life, Enhancing Life: A National Research Agenda on Aging* (Washington, D.C.: National Academy Press, 1991) pp. 1–39.

92. J. E. Kerstetter, B. A. Holthausen, and P. A. Fitz, Malnutrition in the institutionalized older adult, *Journal of the American Dietetic Association* 92 (1992): 1109–1116.

93. J. T. Dwyer, J. J. Gallo, and W. Reichel, Assessing nutritional status in elderly patients, *American Family Physician* 47 (1993): 613–620.

94. R. Chernoff, Thirst and fluid requirements, *Nutrition Reviews* 52 (1994): S3–S5.

95. J. B. Blumberg, Changing nutrient requirements in older adults, *Nutrition Today,* September/October 1992, pp. 15–20.

96. J. Blumberg, Nutrient requirements of the healthy elderly—Should there be specific RDAs? *Nutrition Reviews* 52 (1994): S15–S18.

97. U.S. Department of Health and Human Services, *The Surgeon General's Report on Nutrition and Health* (Washington, D.C.: DHHS, 1988), pp. 595–617.

98. H. Payette and K. Gray-Donald, Do vitamin and mineral supplements improve the dietary intake of elderly Canadians? *Canadian Journal of Public Health* 82 (1993): 58–60.

99. Nutrition of the elderly, *Dairy Council Digest* 48 (1977): 1–2.

100. E. L. Smith, P. E. Smith, and C. Gilligan, Diet, exercise, and chronic disease patterns in older adults, *Nutrition Reviews* 46 (1988): 52–61.

101. Institute of Medicine, *Extending Life,* pp. 1–39.

102. Institute of Medicine, *The Second Fifty Years,* pp. 168–169.

103. Kerstetter, Holthausen, and Fitz, Malnutrition, p. 1113.

104. F. G. Abdellah and S. R. Moore, eds., *Surgeon General's Workshop on Health Promotion and Aging: Proceedings* (Washington, D.C.: Office of the Surgeon General, 1988), pp. G1–G19.

105. M. T. Fanelli and M. Kaufman, Nutrition and older adults, in *Aging and Public Health,* ed. H. T. Philips and S. H. Gaylord (New York: Springer Publishing, 1985), pp. 70–100.

106. Community Nutrition Institute, *Nutrition Week,* April 30, 1993, p. 3.

107. *Nutrition Screening Initiative Survey* (Washington, D.C.: Peter D. Hart Research Associates, February 1990; President's page: The Nutrition Screening Initiative—An emerging force in public policy, *Journal of the American Dietetic Association* 93 (1993): 822.

108. Kerstetter, Holthausen, and Fitz, Malnutrition, p. 1114.

109. M. A. Hess, President's page: ADA as an advocate for older Americans, *Journal of the American Dietetic Association* 91 (1991): 847–849.

110. J. V. White and coauthors, Nutrition Screening Initiative: Development and implementation of the public awareness checklist and screening tools, *Journal of the American Dietetic Association* 92 (1992): 163–167.

111. J. Weinberg, Psychologic implications of the nutritional needs of the elderly, *Journal of the American Dietetic Association* 60 (1972): 293–296.

112. D. M. Czajka-Narins and coauthors, Nutritional and biochemical effects of nutrition programs in the elderly, *Clinics in Geriatric Medicine* 3 (1987): 275–288; Nestle and Gilbride, Nutrition policies for health promotion, pp. 314–317.

113. D. L. Edwards and coauthors, Home-delivered meals benefit the diabetic elderly, *Journal of the American Dietetic Association* 93 (1993): 585–587.

114. Institute of Medicine, *The Second Fifty Years,* p. 182.

115. *Meals-on-Wheels America: More Meals for the Homebound Through Public/Private Partnerships—A Technical Assistant Guide* (New York: New York City Department for the Aging, 1989).

116. The list of advantages is adapted from D. A. Roe, *Geriatric Nutrition,* 3rd ed. (Englewood Cliffs, N.J.: Prentice-Hall, 1992), pp. 1–9.

117. J. Austoker, Diet and cancer: Cancer prevention in primary care, *British Medical Journal* 308 (1994): 1610–1614.

118. E. Giovannucci and W. C. Willett, Dietary factors and risk of colon cancer, *Annals of Medicine* 26 (1994): 443–452.

119. E. Giovannucci and coauthors, Intake of fat, meat, and fiber in relation to risk of colon cancer in men, *Cancer Research* 54 (1994): 2390–2397.

120. W. C. Willett and coauthors, Relation of meat, fat, and fiber intake to the risk of colon cancer in a prospective study among women, *New England Journal of Medicine* 323 (1990): 1664–1672.

121. J. Dwyer, Dietary fiber and colorectal cancer risk, *Nutrition Reviews* 51 (1993): 147–148.

122. M. Ferraroni and coauthors, Selected micronutrient intake and the risk of colorectal cancer, *British Journal of Cancer* 70 (1994): 1150–1155.

123. K. K. Carroll, Dietary fats and cancer, *American Journal of Clinical Nutrition* 53 (1991): 1064S–1067S; C. W. Welsch, Dietary fat, calories, and mammary gland tumorigenesis, In *Advances in Experimental Medicine and Biology* (New York: Plenum Press, 1992), pp. 203–221.

124. R. L. Prentice and coauthors, Dietary fat and breast cancer: A quantitative assessment of the epidemiological literature and a discussion of methodological issues, *Cancer Research* 49 (1989): 3147–3156; P. Toniolo and coauthors, Consumption of meat, animal products, protein, and fat and risk of breast cancer: A prospective cohort study in New York, *Epidemiology* 5 (1994): 391–397.

125. K. Katsouyanni and coauthors, The association of fat and other macronutrients with breast cancer: A case-controlled study from Greece, *British Journal of Cancer* 70 (1994): 537–541.

126. Xiu-Ying Qi and coauthors, The association between breast cancer and diet and other factors, *Asia Pacific Journal of Public Health* 7 (1994): 98–104.

127. L. N. Kolonel, Dietary fat and breast cancer: The evidence in perspective, *Nutrition* 10 (1994): 578–579.

128. G. Block, Vitamin C and cancer prevention: The epidemiologic evidence, *American Journal of Clinical Nutrition* 53 (1991): 270S–282S.

129. P. Knekt and coauthors, Vitamin E and cancer prevention, *American Journal of Clinical Nutrition* 53 (1991): 283S–286S.

130. C. F. Garland and coauthors, Can colon cancer incidence and death rates be reduced with calcium and vitamin D? *American Journal of Clinical Nutrition* 54 (1991): 193S–201S; M. Wargovich and coauthors, Modulating effects of calcium in animal models of colon carcinogenesis and short-term studies in subjects at increased risk for colon cancer, *American Journal of Clinical Nutrition* 54 (1991): 202S–205S.

131. M. A. Rogers and coauthors, Consumption of nitrate, nitrite, and nitrosodimethylamine and the risk of upper aerodigestive tract cancer, *Cancer Epidemiology, Biomarkers, and Prevention* 4 (1995): 29–36; L. E. Hansson and coauthors, Nutrients and gastric cancer risk. A population-based case-control study in Sweden, *International Journal of Cancer* 57 (1994): 638–644.

132. S. E. Hankinson and W. C. Willett, Alcohol and breast cancer: Is there a conclusion? *Nutrition* 11 (1995): 320–321; F. Houn, The association between alcohol and breast cancer: Popular press coverage of research, *American Journal of Public Health* 85 (1995): 1082–1086.

133. G. Howe and coauthors, The association between alcohol and breast cancer risk: Evidence from the combined analysis of six dietary case-control studies, *International Journal of Cancer* 47 (1991): 707–710; L. Holmberg and coauthors, Diet and breast cancer risk: Results from a population-based, case-control study in Sweden, *Archives of Internal Medicine* 154 (1994): 1805–1811; J. L. Freudenheim and coauthors, Lifetime alcohol consumption and risk of breast cancer, *Nutrition and Cancer* 23 (1995): 1–11.

134. R. Sankaranarayanan and coauthors, A case-control study of diet and lung cancer in Kerala, South India, *International Journal of Cancer* 58 (1994): 644–649.

135. A. Bloch and C. A. Thompson, Position of the American Dietetic Association: Phytochemicals and functional foods, *Journal of the American Dietetic Association* 95 (1995): 493–496.

136. J. Childers and coauthors, Chemoprevention of cervical cancer with folic acid: A Phase III Southwest Oncology Group Intergroup Study, *Cancer Epidemiology, Biomarkers, and Prevention* 4 (1995): 155–159.

137. American Cancer Society, Dietary Guidelines, 1992.

138. T. Byers, Dietary trends in the United States: Relevance to cancer prevention, *Cancer* 72 (1993): 1015–1018.

139. J. Dwyer, Diet and nutritional strategies for cancer risk reduction: Focus on the 21st century, *Cancer* 72 (1993): 1024–31.

140. J. M. Coon, Natural food toxicants: A perspective, in *Nutrition Reviews' Present Knowledge in Nutrition,* 4th ed. (Washington, D.C.: Nutrition Foundation, 1976), pp. 528–546.

CHAPTER 11 NOTES

1. Council for Agricultural Science and Technology, *Foodborne Pathogens: Risks and Consequences,* Task Force Report No. 122, 1994, pp. 1–87; T. Roberts and L. Unnevehr, New approaches to regulating food, *Food Review* 17 (1994): 2.

2. D. O. Cliver, *Eating Safely* (New York: American Council on Science and Health, 1993), p. 19.

3. P. Kurtzweil, HACCP patrolling for food hazards, *FDA Consumer,* January–February 1995, p. 9.

4. Get rid of the garlic, FDA says, *FDA Consumer,* June 1989, p. 2.

5. B. P. Bell and coauthors, A multistate outbreak of *Escherichia coli* 0157:H7-associated bloody diarrhea and hemolytic uremic syndrome from hamburgers: The Washington experience, *Journal of the American Medical Association* 272 (1994): 1349–1353.

6. U.S. Department of Agriculture Food Safety and Inspection Service, *E. coli* 0157:H7 at a glance, *Food News for Consumers* 10 (1993), p. 5.

7. R. E. Besser and coauthors, An outbreak of diarrhea and hemolytic uremic syndrome from *Escherichia coli* 0157:H7 in fresh-pressed apple cider, *Journal of the American Medical Association* 269 (1993): 2217–2219.

8. S. C. Witt, *Biotechnology, Microbes and the Environment* (San Francisco: Center for Science Information, 1990), pp. 182–183.

9. E. Hilton and coauthors, Ingestion of yogurt containing *lactobacillus acidophilus* as prophylaxis for candidal vaginitis, *Annals of Internal Medicine* 116 (1992): 353–357.

10. R. S. Horowitz and coauthors, Jin Bu Huan toxicity in children—Colorado 1993, *Morbidity and Mortality Weekly Report* 42 (1993): 633–635.

11. U.S. Department of Health and Human Services, Public Health Service, FDA warns consumers against Nature's Nutrition Formula One, statement issued February 28, 1995.

12. R. S. Koff, Herbal hepatotoxicity: Revisiting a dangerous alternative, *Journal of the American Medical Association* 273 (1995): 502.

13. N. D. Vietmeyer, The preposterous puffer, *National Geographic* 166 (1984): 260–270.

14. U.S. Department of Agriculture News Division, News Feature, *Quick, Safe Microwave Technique*, April 17, 1989; U.S. Department of Agriculture—FSIS, *Food News for Consumers*, Hotline calling, but the recipe says . . ., Winter 1989.

15. U.S. Department of Agriculture Office of Public Affairs, News Division, "Grill" the USDA Hotline experts about safe summer cooking, Release No. 0483.94, 1994.

16. Department of Health and Human Services, Public Health Service, U.S. Food and Drug Administration, *Getting Hooked on Seafood Safety*, DHHS Publication No. (FDA) 93-2266, May 1993.

17. J. E. Young, Reducing waste, Saving materials, in *State of the World 1991,* Worldwatch Institute (New York: W.W. Norton, 1991), pp. 42–49.

18. Personal communication with Cheryl Sutton, Assistant Communications Director for Attorney General Hubert H. Humphrey III, St. Paul, Minnesota.

19. W. Rathje and C. Murphy, *Rubbish! The Archaeology of Garbage* (New York: HarperCollins Publishers, 1992), p. 113.

20. M. Ryan, Paper recycling on a roll, in *Vital Signs 1994,* Worldwatch Institute (New York: W.W. Norton, 1994), p. 121.

21. Ibid.

22. Environmental Protection Agency, *Green Advertising Claims*, EPA 530-F-92-024, October 1992.

23. G. C. Saign, *Green Essentials* (San Francisco: Mercury House, 1994), pp. 356–357.

24. J. E. Young, 1991.

25. A. Wilson, *Consumer Guide to Home Energy Savings* (Washington, D.C.: The American Council for an Energy-Efficient Economy, 1990), pp. 183–187.

26. D. Odland and C. Davis, Products cooked in preheated versus non-preheated ovens, *Journal of the American Dietetic Association* 81 (1982): 135–145.

27. 97% of Michigan population contaminated by 1973 spills, *Tallahassee Democrat,* April 16, 1982.

28. U.S. Public Health Service, Screening for lead exposure in children, *American Family Physician* 51 (1995): 139–143.

29. J. E. Foulke, Lead threat lessens, but mugs pose problem, *FDA Consumer,* April 1993, pp. 19–23.

30. International Food Information Council, *Pesticides and Food Safety* (Washington, D.C.: International Food Information Council Foundation, 1995), p. 2.

31. Ibid., 2–4; C. F. Chaisson and coauthors, *Pesticides in Food: A Guide for Professionals* (Chicago: The American Dietetic Association, 1991), pp. 4–8.

32. National Academy of Sciences, National Research Council, *Pesticides in the Diets of Infants and Children* (Washington, D.C.: National Academy Press, 1993).

33. Council for Agricultural Science and Technology (CAST), *Public Perceptions of Agrichemicals* (Ames, Iowa: CAST Task Force Report No. 123, 1995), pp. 17–21.

34. C. F. Chaisson and coauthors, *Pesticides in Food: A Guide for Professionals* (Chicago: The American Dietetic Association, 1991), p. 16.

35. Ibid., 17.

36. World Health Organization, *Safety and Nutritional Adequacy of Irradiated Food* (Geneva, Switzerland: World Health Organization, 1994), pp. 4–5.

37. Ibid., 39–45.

38. C. Lochhead, The high-tech food process foes find hard to swallow, *Food Technology,* August 1989, pp. 56–60.

39. J. Henkel, Genetic engineering: Fast forwarding to the future, *FDA Consumer,* April 1995, pp. 6–11.

40. H. I. Miller, Foods of the future: The new biotechnology and FDA regulation, *Journal of the American Medical Association* 269 (1993): 910–912.

41. Henkel, 1995.

42. G. G. Graham, Starvation in the modern world, *New England Journal of Medicine* 328 (1993): 1058–1061.

43. C. C. Campbell, Food insecurity: A nutritional outcome or a predictor variable?, *Journal of Nutrition* 121 (1991): 408–415.

44. The description of food insecurity in the miniglossary is from World Bank, *The Challenge of Hunger in Africa: A Call to Action* (Washington, D.C.: World Bank, 1988), p. 1.

45. World food supplies and prevalence of chronic undernutrition in developing regions as assessed in 1992 (Rome: FAO Statistical Analysis Service, 1992).

46. Nutrition: The global challenge, International Conference of Nutrition, Rome, December 1992, FAO/WHO.

47. B. A. Carlson and T. M. Wardlaw, A global, regional, and country assessment of child malnutrition, *UNICEF Staff Working papers,* no. 7 (New York: UNICEF, 1990), pp. 1–30.

48. D. R. Gwatkin, How many die? A set of demographic estimates of the annual number of infant and child deaths in the world, *American Journal of Public Health* 70 (1980): 1286–1289.

49. This estimate is from UNICEF, *The State of the World's Children 1993* (London: Oxford University Press, 1993), p. 57.

50. Y. W. Bradshaw and coauthors, Borrowing against the future: children and third world indebtedness, *Social Forces* 71 (1993): 629–656.

51. UNICEF, *The State of the World's Children* (London: Oxford University Press, 1989), p. 82.

52. UNICEF, 1993, p. 44.

53. L. Robertson, Breastfeeding practices in maternity wards in Swaziland, *Journal of Nutrition Education* 23 (1991): 284–287.

54. UNICEF, *The State of the World's Children* (London: Oxford University Press, 1992).

55. M. Nestle and S. Guttmacher, Hunger in the United States: Rationale, methods, and policy implications of state hunger surveys, *Journal of Nutrition Education* 24 (1992): 208–228.

56. K. Radimer and coauthors, Understanding hunger and developing indicators to assess it in women and children, *Journal of Nutrition Education* 24 (1992): 365–455.

57. Bread for the World Institute, *Hunger 1992: Second Annual Report of the State of World Hunger* (Washington, D.C.: Bread for the World Institute, 1991), p. 15.

58. Bread for The World Institute, *Hunger 1993: Uprooted People* (Washington, D.C.: Bread for the World Institute, 1992), p. 107.

59. J. L. Wiecha, J. T. Dwyer, and M. Dunn-Strohecker, Nutrition and health services needs among the homeless, *Public Health Reports* 106(4) (1991): 364–374.

60. The discussion about homelessness and the steps to end homelessness is adapted from Bread for the World Institute, 1993, pp. 108–109.

61. The U.S. Conference of Mayors, 1992.

62. Select Committee on Hunger, *Farm Crisis: Growing Poverty and Hunger Among America's Food Producers* (Washington, D.C.: U.S. Government Printing Office, 1987), p. 163.

63. Independent Commission on International Issues, *North-South: A Program for Survival* (Cambridge, Mass.: MIT Press, 1980), pp. 49–50.

64. E. O'Kelly, Appropriate technology for women, *Development Forum*, June 1984, p. 2.

65. National Agricultural Lands Study, *Soil Degradation: Effects on Agricultural Productivity*, Interim Report No. 4 (Washington, D.C.: U.S. Department of Agriculture, November 1980), as cited by L. R. Brown, World population growth, soil erosion, and food security, *Science* 214 (1981): 995–1002.

66. A. Durning, Life on the Brink, *World Watch Papers* 3(1990): 29.

67. B. Stutz, The landscape of hunger, *Audubon*, March-April 1993, pp. 54–57; Newsbreaks: Effects of environmental degradation on nutrition, *Nutrition Today*, March/April 1992, p. 4.

68. T. Peterson, Hunger and the environment, *Seeds*, October 1987, pp. 6–13.

69. Oxfam America, *Facts for Action: Women Creating a New World*, no. 3 (Boston: Oxfam America, 1991), pp. 2–3.

70. S. Lewis, Food security, environment, poverty, and the world's children, *Journal of Nutrition Education* 24 (1992): 35–55.

71. UNICEF, *The State of the World's Children 1993* (London: Oxford University Press, 1993), p. 1.

72. Oral rehydration therapy, *World Health* (Geneva: World Health Organization), June 1985.

73. UNICEF, 1993, p. 1.

74. S. Lewis, 1992.

75. S. Lewis, 1992, p. 55.

76. The case for optimism, in E. Cornish, *The Study of the Future: An Introduction to the Art and Science of Understanding and Shaping Tomorrow's World* (Washington, D.C.: World Future Society, 1977), pp. 34–37.

77. D. Elgin, *Voluntary Simplicity: Toward a Way of Life That Is Outwardly Simple, Inwardly Rich* (New York: William Morrow, 1981), p. 25.

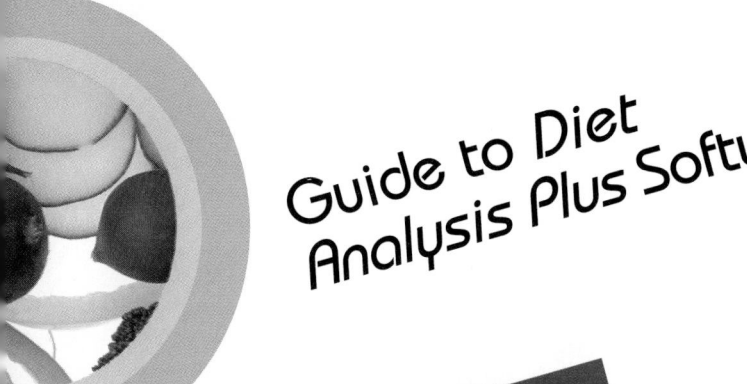

Guide to Diet Analysis Plus Software

Use the West *Diet Analysis Plus* software to analyze your dietary intake and compare it to the recommended intake of nutrients for your personal profile. You will enter personal data (age, weight, height, gender, activity level) and three days of food intake. The West *Diet Analysis Plus* program will calculate the nutrients in the foods you eat (each day separately and the average) and compare the values to the current recommended standards. It will also provide lists of foods that contribute various nutrients to your diet.

Instructions for Recording Dietary Intake

Please adhere to the following instructions when recording your dietary intake for analysis using the West *Diet Analysis Plus* program. As is the case with computer programs, the more accurate the input, the more reliable the output.

1. Record all of the foods, snacks, and beverages you consume for three days. Use the *Food Record—Input Form* in this appendix to record your food intake. (Feel free to make copies of the form.) Since most people eat differently on weekdays than on weekends, you should include two weekdays and one weekend day. (The West *Diet Analysis Plus* allows you to analyze up to five days of intakes.)

2. Carry a copy of your *Food Record—Input Form* with you. Write down each food, snack, and beverage you consume. Fully describe the foods and indicate the amounts or ingredients (see the accompanying example). Be specific when recording amounts and method of preparation (for example, boiled, baked, fried). You can also enter names by food codes. (See Step 5.)

Sample Food Intake Record

Amount	Description of Food or Ingredient
1	Egg McMuffin
1 c	Orange juice, from frozen concentrate
2 c	Coffee with
2 Tbsp	Half and half
4 oz	Turkey breast
2 slices	Wheat bread
1 tsp	Mustard
1 tsp	Mayonnaise, low-calorie
1 c	Frozen low-fat vanilla yogurt
3 c	Popcorn, air-popped

3. Weigh, measure, or count food items carefully. Use household measures. Refer to food labels if you are uncertain about amounts.

4. Do not enter vitamin and mineral supplements. They should be considered separately from your food intake.

5. *Option—Enter foods by code number rather than by name.* Before going to the computer, you may choose to find the description of the foods that you have eaten in the Food Composition Table in Appendix I in this text. The far left-hand column of the table provides a computer code number for each food. You can enter that code number on your form (see the next example) and use the codes to enter foods into the program.

Example of a Food Record Using Food Codes

Code	Amount	Description
1241	1	Egg McMuffin
273	1 c	Orange juice, from frozen concentrate
20	2 c	Coffee with
70	2 Tbsp	Half and half
653	4 oz	Turkey breast
357	2 slices	Wheat bread
979	1 tsp	Mustard
1493	1 tsp	Mayonnaise, low-calorie
1584	1 c	Frozen low-fat vanilla yogurt
540	3 c	Popcorn, air popped

The manual packaged with *Diet Analysis Plus* provides you with system requirements; detailed instructions for loading, starting up, and running the program; and information about additional features including ways to enter personalized exercises and adjust calorie/nutrient levels for weight gain/loss. The following instructions will help you complete a basic diet analysis.

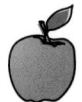

West *Diet Analysis Plus* Software Instructions for DOS Version (IBM-PC and Compatibles)*

1. Start the West *Diet Analysis Plus* program, and the Main Menu window will be displayed. Select "Create new personal record and daily intake data" by using the arrow keys to highlight this choice and press Enter (or type C, the highlighted letter).

2. Enter Student Information in the window that appears—your name, student ID number, instructor, class days and time, and date. This information will be on all your printed reports. Press Enter after each entry. When finished, press ESC, and you will continue to a new screen.

3. You will now be at the Personal Information/Recommended Daily Nutrients screen. Enter your name, age, weight, height, gender, and activity level. Press Enter after each entry; when you have completed your entries, the recommended daily nutrients will be on-screen. Press ESC to continue to the next screen.

4. You will now be at the Options List window. Select Day 1 by typing 1, or highlight "View/Edit Daily Intake—Day 1" and press Enter. Type in the food name—for example, milk, and press Enter. A window will display a list of milk items or items that match your entry. Alternatively, you may type in the computer code number for the food from the table in Appendix I.

   Then type in the amount and measure. For example, for 1 cup, type 1, press Enter, type c, and press Enter. Use this process to enter all of your foods.

   Continue entering all your foods for Day 1. When all entries for Day 1 are completed, press ESC. You will be asked if you want to see the analysis. If you press N for No, you will return to the Options List where you can select Day 2.

   Note: If you press Y for Yes first, the analysis of Day 1 will appear on-screen. Use the arrow keys to highlight calories or any other nutrient, then press Enter. A new bar-graph analysis will show which foods contributed to that nutrient. Try it! When you have finished, press ESC to continue.

5. You will now be at the Options List window. Select Day 2 by typing 2, or highlight "View/Edit Daily Intake—Day 2" and press Enter. Enter foods as described in Step 4 and press ESC when entries for Day 2 are completed.

6. You will be back at the Options List window. Select Day 3 by typing 3, or highlight "View/Edit Daily Intake—Day 3" and press Enter. Enter foods as described in Step 4 and press ESC when food entries are completed.

---

*A Windows version of *Diet Analysis Plus* is also now available. For further instructions on how to use that version, you may refer to the *User's Guide* packaged with the software. Go to the next section on the following page for Macintosh instructions.

7. You will again be back at the Options List window. Highlight "Print Various Reports" and press Enter. Another window will open for you to select the reports you want. If you select "Print all," it will print all reports for which there is saved information.

Or you can print each report separately. To print the recommended nutrients, select RDA or RNI (Canadian version). To print your average daily food intake, select Average. When you select Analysis or Spreadsheet reports, another window will open where you can select each day you want to print.

Helpful Hints (DOS)

- *Out of time? Can't finish?* Press ESC to exit (press several times, if necessary). You will be asked if you want to save. Press Y to save your record. When you return, you will be able to look up your record, finish your entries, and print your reports. See (2) under the next item.
- *Want to change a mistaken entry or make additions?*
  1. *When the program is still on:* Press ESC until you have the Options List window again. Select the day you want and press Enter. Move the highlight to the entry to change and overwrite with the correct information. Press ESC when done.
  2. *Retrieve your record and make changes:* Start the program and from the main menu, highlight "Retrieve stored personal record." Press Enter and follow on-screen instructions.
- *Do you want more detail such as which foods contributed which nutrients?*
  1. The Spreadsheet report prints all nutrients for all foods.
  2. You can also see individual nutrient data on-screen. With the Bar-Graph Analysis on-screen, move the highlight to the nutrient you are interested in and press Enter. A new bar graph will display the food sources for that nutrient.
- *Where do I enter 24 hours of exercises or make weight gain/loss adjustments?* At the Personal Information screen. See Step 3 and move your cursor to the activity level. When it is highlighted, choose the "personalized" activity and follow on-screen instructions.

West *Diet Analysis Plus* Software Instructions for Macintosh Version

1. Start the West *Diet Analysis Plus* program and the Main Menu Bar will be displayed. Select File-New, and a personal profile entry screen will appear.
2. Enter your personal information: name, age, weight, height (feet and inches), gender, activity level, student ID number (if applicable), and any class information. Press Enter after each entry or click on the next field. When you are finished, click on OK. This information will be on all your printed reports.
3. The Profile & Exercises screen will appear with the recommended nutrients. The Foodlist:Day 1 screen will also appear behind the profile screen. Click

on the Foodlist:Day 1 screen to bring it to the front (to make it active). You are now ready to enter your foodlist.

4. At the Foodlist screen, type in the food name—for example, type milk and press return. A window will display a list of milk items or items that match your entry. (Or you may type in the computer code number from the table in Appendix I.) Double click on the highlighted item to select it or click the OK button.

   Then, type in the number of servings in the highlighted servings box. The standard serving size for your food selection will be displayed in parentheses on-screen for your reference. To enter 1 serving, type 1 and press Enter. To enter a half-serving, type .5 and press Enter. When done, press Enter again (or click on ADD) to add the item to your foodlist. Use this process to enter all of your foods.

   When all entries for Day 1 are completed, click on Foodlist—Analyze Day 1 at the Main Menu Bar. An analysis will appear on screen showing the percentage of the recommended nutrients for that foodlist. For quick reference, you can see the percentage on a pie chart in the lower left-hand section of the window.

5. To enter foodlists for days 2-3, click on the arrow in the Current Day box of the Foodlist screen and then move to the day you want. Enter foods as described in Step 4 for up to three days.

6. Once you have entered foods for more than one day, you can average two or more foodlists to see how you're doing overall. To average your foodlists, click on Foodlists—Average All Days. The Analysis-Foodlist Average screen will show your average daily intake.

7. You can save your personal profile, foodlists, and analyses by selecting File-Save from the Main Menu Bar. You can also print any of the reports by clicking on File-Print.

8. Once you have saved your record and closed the windows, or quit the program, you can retrieve them by selecting File-Open. Highlight the record you want and press Enter (or click on Open). Any reports you may have saved are now retrievable as well.

Helpful Hints (Mac)

- *Out of time? Can't finish?* Select File-Save from the Main Menu Bar. Everything you have entered on-screen will be saved in one record, until you reopen your record later.

- *Need to retrieve your record and make additions or changes?* Select File-Open from the Main Menu Bar. Select the record you want by highlighting it and pressing Enter (or click on Open).

- *Want to learn which foods contributed to the nutrient totals or find other special reports?* With your foodlist on-screen:

  - Click on Foodlist—Single Nutrient to see the contribution from a single nutrient.

  - Click on Foodlist—Spreadsheet to see all nutrients for all foods.

  - Click on Foodlist—High/Low Search to search for foods high or low in a specific nutrient.

- *Want to correct your personal profile?* Select Profile—Edit Personal Information from the Main Menu Bar.

- *Want to make weight gain/loss and exercise adjustments?* Select Exercise—Exercise and Diet Weight Gain/Loss from the Main Menu Bar to adjust your recommended nutrients for exercise. Enter an exercise—for example, running. A window will open showing the exercises that match your entry (just as with the food entry). Double click on an item to select it, or highlight it and then click on OK. Enter the amount of time spent, in minutes, doing the exercise. Press Enter or click on ADD to add the exercise to your list.

To adjust your dietary needs to gain or lose weight, use the Weight Gain/Loss option. Click on the up arrow to "gain" and then down arrow to "lose." Your daily caloric needs will be adjusted accordingly. Click OK when you are finished.

Food Record—Input Form

TITLE OF ANALYSIS: _____ **DATE:** _____

Name _____

Age _____

Gender [ ] Male   [ ] Female-Pregnant
       [ ] Female   [ ] Female-Nursing

Weight _____   Height _____

Activity Level # _____
    Enter number from choices on right.

1. *Sedentary:* Very inactive, sometimes under someone else's care.
2. *Lightly Active:* Most office workers & professionals. Equals 8 hours sleep, 16 hours of sitting/standing of which 3 hours is light and 1 hour is moderate activity.
3. *Moderately Active:* Most persons in light industry, building trades; many farm workers, child care providers, active students, mechanics, commerical fishermen.
4. *Very Active:* Full-time athletes, mine or steel workers, unskilled laborers, some agricultural workers, army recruits and soldiers in active service.
5. *Exceptionally Active:* Lumberjacks, construction workers, heavy manual laborers.

Code	Amount	Description of Food or Ingredient	Code	Amount	Description of Food or Ingredient

Form 101 ESHA Research, Nutrition & Fitness Software P.O. Box 13028 Salem, OR 97309. 1-800-659-ESHA

TITLE OF ANALYSIS: _____

DATE: _____

TITLE OF ANALYSIS: _____

DATE: _____

Code	Amount	Description of Food or Ingredient	Code	Amount	Description of Food or Ingredient

Form 101 ESHA Research, Nutrition & Fitness Software P.O. Box 13028 Salem, OR 97309.   1-800-659-ESHA

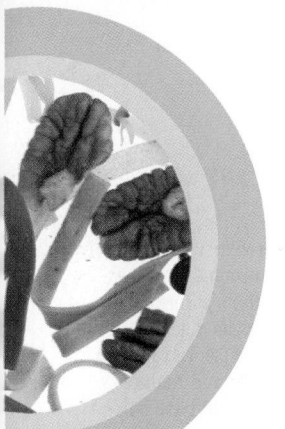

Answers to Selected Check Yourself Questions*

Chapter 1

1. Overnutrition contributes to heart disease, cancer, and stroke. It also contributes to a number of other conditions including diabetes and hypertension. **2.** As defined in the chapter, a *nutritionist* is someone who claims to be capable of advising people about their diets; some nutritionists are registered dietitians, whereas others are self-described experts whose training is questionable. In contrast, a *registered dietitian* is a nutrition professional who has graduated from a college program in dietetics approved by the American Dietetic Association, has completed an internship program or the equivalent, has passed a national registration examination, and maintains competencies in the field through regular continuing education. **3.** Four of the many factors that influence our eating habits are personal preference, cultural traditions, economic considerations, and advertising (other factors include availability, social and psychological factors, and personal beliefs). **4.** Health fraud or quackery is conscious deceit practiced for profit (for example, the promotion of an unproven product or therapy). **6.** Three red flags that can help you spot a quack are 1) promoter claims that the medical establishment (or government) is against him or her and won't accept the new "alternative" treatment, 2) the promoter uses testimonials and anecdotes from satisfied customers to support claims, and 3) the promoter uses a computer-scored questionnaire for diagnosing "nutrient deficiencies." Other red flags: The promoter claims that the product will make weight loss easy; the promoter promises that the product is made with a "secret formula," available only through this one company; or the treatment is only available through the back pages of magazines, over the phone, or by mail-order ads in the form of news stories or infomercials. **7.** Many of our eating habits arise from the traditions, belief systems, technologies, values, and norms of the culture in which we live. **8.** Three factors other than diet that influence longevity include avoiding excess alcohol, not smoking, and maintaining desirable weight. Other factors include exercising regularly and sleeping seven to eight hours a night. **9.** The Food and Drug Administration holds the authority to prosecute companies that display false nutrition information on product labels or enclosures, and the Federal Trade Commission can prosecute manufacturers who make fraudulent or misleading statements in their advertisements. **10.** Two government reports that recognize the role of nutrition in health are *The Surgeon General's Report on Nutrition and Health* and *Diet and Health.*

Chapter 2

1. Characteristics of a healthful diet can include any of the following: nutrient adequacy, balance, calorie control, moderation, and variety.

2. Nutrient density refers to foods that are rich in nutrients (protein, vitamins, minerals) but relatively low in calories and fat. **3.** The Food Guide Pyramid recommends 6 to 11 servings from the *Bread, Cereal, Rice and Pasta Group*, 3 to 5 servings from the *Vegetable Group*, 2 to 4 servings from the *Fruit Group*, 2 to 3 servings from the *Milk, Yogurt, and Cheese Group*, and 2 to 3 servings from the *Meat, Poultry, Fish, Dry Beans, Eggs, and Nuts Group*. **4.** Nutrients that must appear on virtually all food labels include fat (total fat, saturated fat, cholesterol), carbohydrate (total carbohydrate, simple sugars, dietary fiber), sodium, protein, vitamins A and C, calcium, and iron. **5.** The % Daily Value on food labels can be used to check how the foods you eat fit into a healthful diet in terms of their fats, carbohydrates, fiber, and sodium. For example, if a label shows that a serving of a food contains 3 grams of fat (and a Daily Value for fat of 5 percent), this means that the food supplies 5 percent of the total fat that a person eating a 2,000 calorie diet should consume. **6.** The seven Dietary Guidelines are 1) Balance the food you eat with physical activity; maintain or improve your weight; 2) Eat a variety of foods; 3) Choose a diet low in fat, saturated fat, and cholesterol; 4) Choose a diet with plenty of grain products, vegetables, and fruit; 5) Choose a diet moderate in sugars; 6) Choose a diet moderate in salt and sodium; and 7) If you drink alcoholic beverages, do so in moderation. **7.** You can use the RDA to get a feel for the adequacy of your own diet. However, the RDA should not be used as nutritional "goals" to be met daily, since you cannot know your exact nutrient requirements and the RDA include a large margin of safety. **9.** Items in the ingredients list are listed in descending order by weight. **10.** The three calorie-yielding nutrients are carbohydrate, fat, and protein.

Chapter 3

1. The simple carbohydrates include glucose, fructose, galactose, maltose, sucrose, and lactose. These sugars are found as naturally occurring sugars in fresh fruits and vegetables (glucose and fructose), in milk and milk products (lactose), and in concentrated form in honey, corn syrup, table sugar, cakes, cookies, candy, soda pop, and other foods with added sugars. **2.** Complex carbohydrates include starch and fiber. Starch is found mostly as grains—as in wheat, rice, and corn products; fiber is found in plant foods such as whole grains, fruits, legumes, and vegetables. **3.** The primary role of carbohydrates in the body is to provide energy, and for certain cells (brain and nervous system) carbohydrates are the preferred energy source. Carbohydrate-rich foods are usually less expensive than protein as an energy source, and unlike fat—the other energy nutrient—carbohydrates are not associated with chronic diseases such as heart disease and cancer. **4.** The *Dietary Guidelines for Americans* recommend that we 1) choose a diet with

---

*Answers to all Check Yourself questions can be found within the chapters. Although most Check Yourself questions are answered in this appendix, we have left questions that require essay-style answers, or that have multiple answers, for you to complete.

plenty of grain products, vegetables, and fruits and 2) choose a diet moderate in sugars. **5.** Sugar-containing foods can be incorporated into a carefully designed eating plan for the person with diabetes, since blood glucose levels are affected by a number of dietary factors, including the total amounts of carbohydrate (complex and simple), fiber, and fat consumed in a meal. **6.** Enrichment of refined grain products makes them comparable to whole-grain products with respect to four nutrients (thiamin, riboflavin, niacin, and iron). However, since enrichment does not add back other important nutrients (for example, magnesium, vitamin B_6, zinc, and chromium) to refined products, whole-grain products are preferred choices over enriched products. **7.** Some of the health effects of fiber include 1) fiber serves as an aid to weight control by providing satiety; high-fiber foods are typically lower in calories than high-fat, low-fiber foods; 2) fiber provides bulk in the large intestine and promotes regularity; 3) fiber speeds transit time through the colon and may protect against colon cancer; 4) fiber may stabilize blood sugar levels by delaying glucose absorption; and 5) certain fibers may lower blood cholesterol. **10.** The body maintains normal blood glucose concentrations by releasing the hormone insulin from the pancreas in response to high blood glucose concentrations. Insulin stimulates body cells to absorb the excess glucose. The body responds to low blood concentrations of glucose by releasing the hormone glucagon from the pancreas. Glucagon stimulates the liver to release its stored glucose into the blood.

Chapter 4

1. Fat in the diet provides calories, satiety, fat-soluble vitamins, aroma, and flavor. **2.** Fat in the body serves as a concentrated energy reserve, nourishes the skin and hair, provides the major components of cell membranes, insulates the body from extremes of body temperature, and cushions the vital organs to protect them from shock. **3.** Examples of food sources of highly saturated fats are beef tallow, butter, coconut and palm oil, and lard. Examples of highly monounsaturated fats include avocados, canola and olive oils, and peanuts. Examples of highly polyunsaturated fats include corn and safflower oils, fish, almonds, and walnuts. Examples of cholesterol-containing foods include animal-derived products such as liver, meat, egg yolks, and whole milk products. **4.** Hydrogenation adds hydrogen to unsaturated fat to make it more solid and more resistant to chemical damage. **5.** *Chylomicrons* serve as a means of transporting newly digested fat from the intestine through the lymph and blood to body cells; *very-low-density lipoproteins (VLDL)* carry fats packaged or made by the liver to various tissues in the body; *low-density lipoproteins (LDL)* carry cholesterol (much of it synthesized in the liver) to body cells; *high-density lipoproteins (HDL)* carry cholesterol in the blood back to the liver for recycling or disposal. **6.** A high LDL level or a low HDL level are associated with increased risk of heart disease; a high HDL level is associated with a decreased risk of heart disease. **8.** The current recommendations for fat in the diet are 1) eat no more than 30 percent of calories as fat; 2) eat no more than 10 percent of calories as saturated fat; 3) eat no more than 10 percent of calories as polyunsaturated fat; 4) eat 10 percent to 15 percent of calories as monounsaturated fat; and 5) limit daily cholesterol intake to no more than 300 milligrams. **9.** The leading risk factors for heart disease include high blood cholesterol (especially high LDL), cigarette smoking, high blood pressure, and obesity. **10.** People can raise their HDL levels by losing weight if they are overweight and by following a regular exercise routine.

Chapter 5

1. Nitrogen is the element that appears exclusively in protein. **2.** Protein synthesis will be halted if an essential amino acid is missing from the diet. **3.** The quality of a dietary protein depends on both its assortment of essential amino acids relative to human needs and on its digestibility. **4.** We are advised to consume about 12 percent of our calories from protein. **5.** The proteins in the body are used for growth and maintenance, enzyme action, hormones, antibodies, fluid and acid-base balance, transportation, body structures, and energy. **6.** Some of the risks associated with using amino acid supplements include irritability, insomnia, gastrointestinal illness, amino acid imbalances, and impaired growth. **7.** Complementary proteins are two or more food proteins whose amino acid assortments complement each other in such a way that the essential amino acids limited in or missing from each other are supplied by the others. **9.** Yes, a vegetarian diet can meet protein needs when varied plant-based protein sources are included in the diet on a daily basis. **10.** Without careful planning the vegan diet may be limited in iron, vitamin D, calcium, riboflavin, vitamin B_{12}, and high-quality protein.

Chapter 6

2. Beta-carotene, a precursor of vitamin A, is an orange pigment found in plants that is converted into active vitamin A inside the body; preformed vitamin A is vitamin A already in its active form. **3.** People following very-low-calorie diets, strict vegetarians, women who are pregnant or breastfeeding, among others, may need a multivitamin/mineral supplement. **5.** People need not obtain all their vitamin D from food because the body can synthesize it with the help of sunlight. **6.** Retinal, one of the active forms of vitamin A, is synthesized from dietary vitamin A and functions as a portion of the visual pigments in the eyes. These pigments serve to transform light into nerve impulses that are interpreted by the brain as visual images. **7.** Women of childbearing age are advised to consume generous amounts of folate (in the form of folic acid) before and during the first few weeks of pregnancy to reduce the risk of producing a baby with neural tube defects. **8.** Phytochemicals are chemicals found in plants that are not nutrients but that appear to help fight diseases such as cancer. **10.** Look for a supplement that meets high standards (USP standards) for manufacturing. Consider cost; a thirty-day supply of a multivitamin/mineral supplement should cost no more than about $10. Look for a bottle or package with an expiration date. Also, choose a supplement that contains both vitamins and minerals in amounts no more than 100 to 150 percent of the RDA for each. Consider child-proof bottles if there are children in the home.

Chapter 7

1. Major minerals are essential mineral nutrients found in the body in amounts greater than 5 grams; trace minerals are essential mineral nutrients found in the human body in amounts less than 5 grams. **2.** Chloride, the major negatively charged ion of the fluids outside the cells, helps maintain acid-base balance in the blood and is part of hydrochloric acid in the stomach. As the body's chief positively charged ion inside the cells, potassium plays a major role in maintaining water balance and cell integrity, and it is critical to maintaining the heartbeat. Magnesium is a part of the body's protein-making machinery, is necessary for the release of energy, and it helps to relax muscles after contraction. Sulfur helps strands of protein to assume and hold a particular shape, thus enabling them to perform their specific roles. **3.** Phosphorus is the mineral least likely to be deficient in the diet. **4.** Processing affects the sodium-potassium ratio in foods; the more processed a food is, the more sodium and the less potassium it contains. **7.** The bone minerals are calcium, phosphorus, magnesium, and fluoride. **8.** Iodine functions as part of the thyroid hormones, which regulate body temperature, metabolic rate, reproduction, and growth. Iodine deficiency can cause goiter (enlargement of the thyroid gland) and cretinism (severe mental and physical retardation of an infant exposed to a deficiency during pregnancy). **9.** Vitamin C and the MFP factor enhance absorption of iron from a meal. Phytic acid, tannic acid, and fiber can interfere with or inhibit the absorption of iron. **10.** Iron deficiency results in anemia, diagnosed by a low blood hemoglobin level. Meats, fish, and poultry contain heme iron, which is readily absorbed by the body. **11.** Deficiency symptoms of zinc in children include growth retardation, delayed sexual development, poor appetite, and decreased taste sensitivity; zinc deficiency in adults results in poor taste perception and impaired wound healing. **12.** Water in the body serves many functions including transporting nutrients to cells, acting as a shock absorber in joints and around the spinal cord, and helping to maintain body temperature.

Chapter 8

1. A primary factor influencing basal metabolic rate is body composition. The more lean tissue in a body, the higher the metabolic rate. **2.** The two major components of energy expenditure are energy for basal metabolism and energy for physical activity. **3.** The fatfold test gives a fair approximation of total body fat. **4.** Risk factors associated with obesity include arthritis, certain types of cancer, heart disease, decreased longevity, diabetes, gallbladder and liver disease, hypertension, respiratory problems, and varicose veins. **5.** It is likely that the most important single contributor to the obesity problem in this country is underactivity. **6.** A successful weight-loss program includes healthful eating habits, exercise, behavior modification, and a weight-maintenance component. **7.** A weekly weight loss of one to two pounds (or less) is recommended. **9.** Exercise increases one's calorie expenditure, alters body composition in a desirable direction, and offers the psychological benefits of looking and feeling healthy. **10.** Central obesity refers to excess fat on the abdomen and around the trunk and is associated with a greater risk for developing diabetes, hypertension, and heart disease. **11.** The measure of a successful weight-loss program is keeping off the lost weight. **12.** A person with anorexia nervosa has an intense fear of gaining weight, a refusal to maintain body weight at or above a minimal normal weight for age and height, a disturbance in self perception of weight status, and amenorrhea. The person with bulimia nervosa experiences repeated episodes of uncontrolled binge eating followed by recurrent compensatory behaviors such as self-induced vomiting, misuse of laxatives and diuretics, or excessive exercise.

Chapter 9

1. The four components of fitness are strength, flexibility, muscle endurance, and cardiovascular endurance. Cardiovascular endurance has top priority. **3.** Aerobic exercise (running, swimming, rollerblading) requires oxygen and uses fat as the main source of energy. Anaerobic exercise (sprinting) burns stored glycogen as fuel without relying on a source of oxygen. **4.** Target heart rate is the heartbeat rate that will achieve a cardiovascular conditioning effect for a given person—fast enough to push the heart but not so fast as to strain it. To determine your target heart rate, subtract your age from 220 and then multiply this number by 60 percent and 85 percent to find lower and upper limits. **5.** The recommended prescription for cardiovascular fitness is that you exercise within your target heart rate range at least three times per week for 20 to 60 minutes. **6.** The training effect is the effect of regular exercise on the cardiovascular system—including improvements in heart, lung, and muscle function and increased blood volume. **7.** Anabolic steroids are synthetic male hormones that appear to help build muscle. There are numerous side effects including acne, liver abnormalities, temporary infertility, roid rages, dizziness, hypertension, heart disease, stroke, and stunted growth. **8.** The American Dietetic Association recommends that athletes consume 1 to 1.5 grams of protein per kilogram of healthy body weight. **9.** Water is always an adequate fluid-replacement beverage; properly balanced sports drinks may also be considered by the endurance athlete. **10.** The diet that best supports athletic performance is similar to the diet recommended for good health. The eating plan should consist mostly of whole, minimally processed foods low in fat, and high in complex carbohydrates, vitamins, and minerals.

Chapter 10

1. During pregnancy, a woman has increased needs for nearly all nutrients; a 30 milligram supplement of iron is recommended. Other supplements sometimes recommended are folate, vitamin D, vitamin B_{12}, calcium, or a balanced multivitamin/mineral supplement. **2.** The recommended weight gain for pregnancy is 25 to 35 pounds for women entering pregnancy at a healthful weight, 28 to 40 pounds for women who are underweight, and 16 to 25 pounds for obese women. This weight includes the weight of the infant, placenta, blood and fluid volume, breasts, uterus, and supporting muscles, amniotic fluid, and maternal fat stores. **3.** Birthweight is the most potent indicator of the infant's future health status. **5.** Three advantages of breastfeeding are immunological protection, the receipt of *Lactobacillus bifidus* (favors growth of friendly intestinal bacteria), and protection from allergy development. **7.** Much of an infant's body water is found between cells and in the vascular spaces and is easier to lose. **8.** Adequate intakes of calcium are needed during preadolescence in preparation for the significant skeletal growth to occur during adolescence. **10.** Marked changes in physical development (menstruation) take place in females between the ages of 10 and 18 years and in boys (increased muscle development) between the ages of 12 and 20 years. **11.** Three nutrition-related problems common among teenagers are undernutrition, low calcium intakes, and eating disorders. **12.** Physiological changes associated with aging include sensory impairments, altered endocrine, gastrointestinal, and cardiovascular functions, oral problems, and changes in the skeletal system. **13.** Calorie needs decline with age; nutrient requirements generally remain the same as one ages, but some evidence suggests an increased need for certain vitamins. **15.** Nutrients thought to be protective of cancer formation include beta-carotene, fiber, vitamin C, vitamin E, selenium, and calcium. High fat intakes are associated with increased risk of cancer formation.

Chapter 11

2. To reduce your risk of eating a food contaminated with *E. coli*, be sure to cook all meat and poultry to 160 degrees Fahrenheit, avoid cross-contamination, and do not drink raw milk. **3.** Cross contamination refers to the accidental transfer of bacteria from one food to another that occurs, for example, by chopping vegetables on the same cutting board used to skin poultry. **4.** To reduce your chances of consuming excess lead, do not store foods or beverages in lead crystal containers; run cold water for several minutes before using it for drinking or cooking; don't store fruit juices or other acidic foods in ceramic containers; use antique or collectible housewares for food or beverages only occasionally; and do not eat or drink from items that show a dusty or chalky gray residue on the glaze after they are washed. **5.** Food addi-

tives function to enhance flavor, impart color, and improve nutritional value of foods (other functions include improving texture or stability of foods). **7.** If the food eaten by one species has been contaminated by chemicals, it will accumulate in the food chain from one species to the next. **9.** The Delaney Clause prohibits manufacturers from using any substance that is known to cause cancer in animals or humans at any dose level. The Delaney Clause is limited because it is virtually impossible to eliminate potential cancer-causing agents from the food supply, and it overlooks the principle that it is the dose that matters in cancer formation.

TABLE OF FOOD COMPOSITION

This edition of the table of food composition contains more complete values for several nutrients than any comparable table.[1] These include dietary fiber; saturated, monounsaturated, and polyunsaturated fat; vitamin B_6; folate; magnesium; and zinc. The table includes a wide variety of foods from all food groups and is updated yearly to reflect current food patterns. For example, this edition includes many new nonfat items; several new ethnic items such as basmati rice, calamata olives, and gai choy chinese mustard; and a new selection of baby foods.

Sources of Data To achieve a complete and reliable listing of nutrients for all the foods, over 1000 sources of information are researched. Government sources are the primary base for all the data: the USDA *Handbook* series and its current supplemental data, as well as current data on baked goods, snacks, and sweets. In addition, provisional USDA information—both published and unpublished—is included. The data are refined through information obtained in many conversations with professional staff members at the USDA Human Nutrition Information Service in Hyattsville, Maryland.

Even with all the government sources available, however, some nutrient values are still missing; and as the USDA updates various data, it sometimes reports conflicting values for the same items. To fill in the missing values and resolve discrepancies, other reliable sources of information are used. These sources include refereed journal articles, food composition tables from Canada and England, information from other nutrient data banks and publications, unpublished scientific data, and manufacturers' data.

Accuracy of Estimates The energy and nutrients in recipes and combination foods vary widely, depending on the ingredients. The amounts of various fatty acids and cholesterol are influenced by the type of fat used (the specific type of oil, vegetable shortening, butter, margarine, etc.).

Estimates of nutrient amounts for foods and nutrients include all possible adjustments in the interest of accuracy. When multiple values are reported for a nutrient, the numbers are averaged and weighted with consideration of the original number of samples in the separate sources. Whenever water percentages are available, estimates of nutrient amounts are adjusted for water content. When no water is given, water percentage is assumed to be that shown in the table. Whenever a reported weight appeared inconsistent (cooked eggplant and collards, for example), many kitchen tests were made, and the average weight of the typical product was given as tested.

When estimates of nutrient amounts in cooked foods are derived from reported amounts in raw foods, published retention factors are applied. Some reported data for combination foods are modified in this table to include newer data available for major ingredients. For example, since the "pies" were analyzed and reported, newer data on fruits have been published. Bakery items reflect the most current data with the new enrichment levels for certain nutrients.

Considerable effort has been made to report the most accurate data available and to eliminate missing values. The table is updated annually, and the authors welcome any suggestions or comments for future editions.

Average Values It is important to know that many different nutrient values can be reported for foods, even by reliable sources. Many factors influence the amounts of nutrients in foods, including the mineral content of the soil, the method of processing, genetics, the diet of the animal or the fertilizer of the plant, the season of the year, methods of analysis, the difference in moisture content of the samples analyzed, the length and method of storage, and methods of cooking the food.

Although each nutrient from USDA government data is presented as a single number in some USDA publications, each number is actually an average of a range of data. The more detailed reports (Handbook 8 series) indicate the number of samples and the standard deviation of the data. One can also find different reported values for foods, as older USDA data are replaced with newer data in more recent publications. Therefore, nutrient data should be viewed and used only as a guide, a close approximation of nutrient content.

Dietary Fiber Dietary fiber deserves a special word. Estimates of dietary fiber are included for all the foods in this table. This information comes primarily from extensive published and unpublished data from the USDA Human Nutrition Information Service in Hyattsville, Maryland; *Composition of Foods by Southgate* (England); and many journal articles.

It is important to recognize that data for dietary fiber are still undergoing review in the scientific community. No doubt, these estimates will change as analytical techniques are refined and interpretations clarified.

Vitamin A Vitamin A is reported in retinol equivalents. The amount of this vitamin can vary by the season of the year and the maturity of the plant. Reported values in both dairy products and plants are higher in summer and early fall than in winter. The values reported here represent year-round averages. The organ meats of all animal products (liver especially) contain large amounts of vitamin A, which vary widely, depending on the background of the animal. The vitamin is also present in very small amounts in regular meat and is often reported as a trace.

Newer reported vitamin A values for some plant foods have increased significantly due to additional information and sometimes to improved plant genetics. Recent vitamin A values for canned pumpkin, for example, are 3.5 times greater than the previously reported values.

Fats Total fats, as well as the breakdown of total fats to saturated, monounsaturated, and polyunsaturated fats, are listed in the table. The fatty acids seldom add up to the total. This discrepancy is due to rounding and to the existence of small amounts of other fatty acid components that are not included in the three basic categories, including *trans*-fatty acids and glycerol.

Niacin Niacin values are for preformed niacin and do not include additional niacin that may form in the body from the conversion of tryptophan.

Using the Table The items in this table have been organized into several categories, which are listed at the head of each right-hand page. As the key shows, each group has been color-coded to make it easier to find individual items.

In an effort to conserve space, the following abbreviations have been used in the food descriptions and nutrient breakdowns:

diam = diameter
ea = each
enr = enriched
f/ = from
g = grams
liq = liquid
pce = piece
pkg = package
w/ = with
w/o = without
t = trace
0 = zero (no nutrient value)
— = information not available

TABLE I-1
FOOD COMPOSITION

Computer Code Number	Food Description	Measure	Wt (g)	H2O (%)	Ener (cal)	Prot (g)	Carb (g)	Dietary Fiber (g)	Fat (g)	Fat Breakdown (g)		
										Sat	Mono	Poly
BEVERAGES												
	Alcoholic:											
	Beer:											
1	Regular (12 fl oz)	1½ c	356	92	146	1	13	3	0	0	0	0
2	Light (12 fl oz)	1½ c	354	95	99[1]	1	5	1	0	0	0	0
1506	Nonalcoholic (12 fl oz)	1 ea	360	98	32	1	5	0	0	0	0	0
	Gin, rum, vodka, whiskey:											
3	80 proof	1½ fl oz	42	67	97	0	0	0	0	0	0	0
4	86 proof	1½ fl oz	42	64	105	0	<1	0	0	0	0	0
5	90 proof	1½ fl oz	42	62	110	0	0	0	0	0	0	0
	Liqueur:											
1359	Coffee liqueur, 53 proof	1½ fl oz	52	31	175	<1	24	0	<1	.1	t	.1
1360	Coffee & cream liqueur, 34 proof	1½ fl oz	47	46	154	1	10	0	7	4.5	2.1	.3
1361	Crème de menthe, 72 proof	1½ fl oz	50	28	186	0	21	0	<1	t	t	.1
	Wine:											
6	Dessert (4 fl oz)	½ c	118	72	181[2]	<1	14	0	0	0	0	0
7	Red	3½ fl oz	103	88	74	<1	2	0	0	0	0	0
8	Rosé	3½ fl oz	103	89	73	<1	1	0	0	0	0	0
9	White medium	3½ fl oz	103	90	70	<1	1	0	0	0	0	0
1592	Nonalcoholic	1 c	232	98	14	1	3	0	0	0	0	0
1593	Nonalcoholic light	1 c	251	98	15	1	3	0	0	0	0	0
1409	Wine cooler, bottle (12 fl oz)	1½ c	340	90	169	<1	20	<1	<1	0	0	t
1595	Wine cooler, cup	1 c	227	90	113	<1	13	<1	<1	0	0	t
	Carbonated:[3]											
10	Club soda (12 fl oz)	1½ c	355	100	0	0	0	0	0	0	0	0
11	Cola beverage (12 fl oz)	1½ c	370	89	152	0	38	0	<1	.02	.03	.1
12	Diet cola w/aspartame (12 fl oz)	1½ c	355	100	4	<1	<1	0	0	0	0	0
13	Diet cola w/saccharin (12 fl oz)	1½ c	355	100	0	0	<1	0	0	0	0	0
14	Ginger ale (12 fl oz)	1½ c	366	91	124	0	32	0	0	0	0	0
15	Grape soda (12 fl oz)	1½ c	372	89	160	0	42	0	0	0	0	0
16	Lemon-lime (12 fl oz)	1½ c	368	90	147	0	38	0	0	0	0	0
17	Orange (12 fl oz)	1½ c	372	88	179	0	46	0	0	0	0	0
18	Pepper-type soda (12 fl oz)	1½ c	368	89	151	0	38	0	<1	.3	0	0
19	Root beer (12 fl oz)	1½ c	370	89	152	0	39	0	0	0	0	0
20	Coffee,[3] brewed	1 c	240	99	5[4]	<1	1	0	<1	0	0	0
21	Coffee,[3] prepared from instant	1 c	240	99	5[4]	<1	1	0	<1	0	0	0
	Fruit drinks, noncarbonated:[5]											
22	Fruit punch drink, canned	½ c	126	88	59	0	15	0	<1	0	0	0
1358	Gatorade	1 c	240	94	60	0	15	0	0	0	0	0
23	Grape drink, canned	½ c	125	87	63	<1	16	<1	0	0	0	0
1304	Kool-Aid, with sugar	1 c	240	90	89	0	23	0	<1	0	0	0
1356	Kool-Aid, with NutraSweet	1 c	240	95	43	0	11	0	0	0	0	0

[1]Calories can vary from 78 to 131 for 12 fl. oz.

[2]Values are for sweet dessert wine. Dry dessert wines contain 149 cal and 5 g of carbohydrate.

[3]Mineral content varies depending on water source.

[4]Calorie values from USDA vary from 1 to 5 cal per cup.

[5]Usually less than 10% fruit juice.

(Computer code number is for West Diet Analysis program)

I-4

Chol (mg)	Calc (mg)	Iron (mg)	Magn (mg)	Phos (mg)	Pota (mg)	Sodi (mg)	Zinc (mg)	VT-A (RE)	Thia (mg)	Ribo (mg)	Niac (mg)	V-B6 (mg)	Fola (µg)	VT-C (mg)
0	18	.11	21	43	89	18	.07	0	.04	.11	1.60	.18	21	0
0	18	.14	18	42	64	11	.11	0	.04	.11	1.38	.11	15	0
0	25	.04	32	112	90	18	.04	0	.02	.09	1.63	.18	22	0
0	0	.02	0	2	1	<1	.02	0	<.01	0	0	0	0	0
0	0	.02	0	2	1	<1	.02	0	<.01	0	0	0	0	0
0	0	.02	0	2	1	<1	.02	0	<.01	0	0	0	0	0
0	1	.03	2	3	16	4	.02	0	0	.01	.07	0	0	0
7	8	.06	1	24	15	43	.08	20	0	.03	.04	.01	0	0
0	0	.04	0	0	0	2	.02	0	0	0	0	0	0	0
0	9	.28	11	11	108	11	.08	0	.02	.02	.25	0	<1	0
0	8	.44	13	14	116	5	.09	0	.01	.03	.08	.03	2	0
0	8	.39	10	15	102	5	.06	0	0	.02	.07	.02	1	0
0	9	.33	10	14	83	5	.07	0	0	.01	.07	.01	<1	0
0	21	.93	23	35	204	16	.19	0	0	.02	.23	.05	2	0
0	23	1	25	38	221	18	.2	0	0	.03	.25	.05	3	0
0	19	.92	18	22	152	29	.2	1	.02	.02	.16	.04	4	6
0	13	.61	12	15	101	19	.13	<1	.01	.02	.10	.03	3	4
0	18	.04	4	0	7	75	.36	0	0	0	0	0	0	0
0	11	.11	4	44	4	15	.04	0	0	0	0	0	0	0
0	14	.11	4	32	0	21[6]	.28	0	.02	.08	0	0	0	0
0	14	.14	4	39	7	57	.18	0	0	0	0	0	0	0
0	11	.66	4	0	4	26	.18	0	0	0	0	0	0	0
0	11	.3	4	0	4	56	.26	0	0	0	0	0	0	0
0	7	.26	4	0	4	40	.18	0	0	0	.06	0	0	0
0	19	.22	4	4	7	45	.37	0	0	0	0	0	0	0
0	11	.15	0	40	4	37	.15	0	0	0	0	0	0	0
0	19	.19	4	0	4	48	.26	0	0	0	0	0	0	0
0	5	.12	12	2	130	5	.05	0	0	0	.53	0	<1	0
0	7	.12	10	7	86	7	.07	0	0	<.01	.68	0	0	0
0	10	.26	3	1	32	28	.15	2	.03	.03	.03	0	2	37
0	0	.12	2	22	26	96	.05	0	.01	0	0	0	0	0
0	4	.13	5	5	44	1	.04	0	.01	.01	.13	.03	1	20
0	38	.12	2	48	2	34	.07	0	0	<.01	<.01	0	<1	28
0	17	.65	5	5	50	50	.26	2	.02	.05	.05	0	5	77

[6]Value for product sweetened with aspartame only; sodium is 32 mg if a blend of aspartame and sodium saccharin is used.

(For purposes of calculations, use "0" for t, <1, <.1, <.01, etc.)

TABLE I–1
FOOD COMPOSITION

Computer Code Number	Food Description	Measure	Wt (g)	H$_2$O (%)	Ener (cal)	Prot (g)	Carb (g)	Dietary Fiber (g)	Fat (g)	Fat Breakdown (g)		
										Sat	Mono	Poly
	BEVERAGES—Cont.											
	Fruit drinks, noncarbonated—Cont.											
26	Lemonade, frozen concentrate (6-oz can)	¾ c	219	52	396	1	103	1	< 1	.1	t	.1
27	Lemonade, from concentrate	1 c	248	89	99	< 1	26	< 1	< 1	t	t	t
28	Limeade, frozen concentrate (6-oz can)	¾ c	218	50	408	< 1	107	1	< 1	t	t	.1
29	Limeade, from concentrate	1 c	247	89	101	0	27	< 1	< 1	0	0	t
24	Pineapple grapefruit, canned	1 c	250	88	118	< 1	29	< 1	< 1	t	t	.1
25	Pineapple orange, canned	1 c	250	87	125	3	30	< 1	0	0	0	0
	Fruit and vegetable juices: see Fruit and Vegetable sections											
	Slim Fast:[1]											
1612	Chocolate malt with nonfat milk	1 c	273	82	190	14	32	2	1	.3	.1	t
1613	Strawberry with nonfat milk	1 c	273	82	190	14	32	2	1	.3	.1	t
1611	Vanilla with nonfat milk	1 c	273	82	190	14	32	2	1	.3	.1	t
	Ultra Slim Fast:[1]											
1616	Chocolate with nonfat milk	1 c	278	81	200	14	36	5	1	.3	.1	t
1614	French vanilla with nonfat milk	1 c	278	81	190	14	36	4	1	.3	.1	t
1615	Strawberry Supreme with nonfat milk	1 c	278	81	190	14	36	4	1	.3	.1	t
1357	Water, bottled: Perrier (6½ fl oz)	1 ea	192	100	0	0	0	0	0	0	0	0
1594	Water, bottled: Tonic water	1½ c	366	91	124	0	32	0	0	0	0	0
	Tea:[2]											
30	Brewed, regular	1 c	240	100	2	0	1	0	< 1	0	0	t
1662	Brewed, herbal	¾ c	178	100	2	0	< 1	0	t	0	0	t
32	From instant, sweetened	1 c	262	91	89	< 1	22	0	< 1	t	0	t
31	From instant, unsweetened	1 c	237	100	2	0	< 1	0	0	0	0	0
	DAIRY											
	Butter: see Fats and Oils, #158,159,160											
	Cheese, natural:											
33	Blue	1 oz	28	42	100	6	1	0	8	5.3	2.2	.2
34	Brick	1 oz	28	41	105	7	1	0	8	5.3	2.4	.2
35	Brie	1 oz	28	48	95	6	< 1	0	8	4.9	2.3	.2
36	Camembert	1 oz	28	52	85	6	< 1	0	7	4.3	2	.2
37	Cheddar:	1 oz	28	37	114	7	< 1	0	9	6	2.7	.3
38	1" cube	1 ea	17	37	69	4	< 1	0	6	3.6	1.6	.2
39	Shredded	1 c	113	37	455	28	1	0	37	23.8	10.6	1.1
1406	Low fat, low sodium	1 oz	28	65	49	7	1	0	2	1.3	0.6	0.1
	Cottage:											
984	Low sodium, low fat	1 c	225	84	162	28	6	0	2	1.4	.6	.07
40	Creamed, large curd	1 c	225	79	232	28	6	0	10	6.4	2.9	.3
41	Creamed, small curd	1 c	210	79	216	26	6	0	9	6	2.7	.3
42	With fruit	1 c	226	72	280	22	30	0	8	4.9	2.2	.2
43	Low fat 2%	1 c	226	79	203	31	8	0	4	2.8	1.2	.1
44	Low fat 1%	1 c	226	82	164	28	6	0	2	1.5	.7	.1
46	Cream	1 oz	28	54	99	2	1	0	10	6.2	2.8	.4
983	Cream, low fat	1 oz	28	64	65	3	2	0	5	3.1	1.4	0.2
47	Edam	1 oz	28	42	101	7	< 1	0	8	5	2.3	.2
48	Feta	1 oz	28	55	75	4	1	0	6	4.2	1.3	.2

[1]See Chapter 9 for healthy weight loss strategies. The formulas for these products change periodically; these data reflect nutrient values as of our publication date.

[2]Mineral content varies depending on water source.

(Computer code number is for West Diet Analysis program)

Chol (mg)	Calc (mg)	Iron (mg)	Magn (mg)	Phos (mg)	Pota (mg)	Sodi (mg)	Zinc (mg)	VT-A (RE)	Thia (mg)	Ribo (mg)	Niac (mg)	V-B6 (mg)	Fola (μg)	VT-C (mg)
0	15	1.58	11	20	146	9	.18	21	.06	.21	.16	.05	22	39[3]
0	7	.4	5	5	37	7	.1	5	.01	.05	.04	.01	5	10[3]
0	11	.22	9	13	128	0	.09	0	.02	.02	.22	0	9	26
0	7	.07	2	2	32	5	.05	0	0	0	.05	0	2	7
0	18	.78	15	15	152	35	.15	9	.08	.04	.67	.1	26	115
0	13	.68	15	10	115	7	.15	133	.08	.05	.52	.12	27	56
4	450	6.3	140	400	690	230	5.25	350	.53	.59	7	.7	120	21
4	450	6.3	140	400	720	220	5.25	350	.53	.59	7	.7	120	21
4	450	6.31	140	401	721	220	5.24	350	.53	.59	7	.7	120	21
<1	450	6.3	140	400	800	230	5.25	350	.52	.59	7	.7	120	21
<1	450	6.3	140	400	730	250	5.25	350	.52	.59	7	.7	120	21
<1	450	6.3	140	400	710	250	5.25	350	.52	.59	7	.7	120	21
0	27	0	0	0	0	2	0	0	0	0	0	0	0	0
0	4	.04	0	0	0	15	.37	0	0	0	0	0	0	0
0	0	.05	7	2	89	7	.05	0	0	.03	0	0	12	0
0	4	.14	2	0	16	2	.07	0	.02	.01	0	0	1	0
0	5	.05	5	3	50	8	.08	0	0	.05	.09	.01	10	0
0	5	.05	5	2	47	7	.07	0	0	<.01	.09	0	1	0
21	150	.09	6	110	73	395	.75	65	.01	.11	.29	.05	10	0
27	191	.12	7	128	39	159	.74	86	0	.1	.03	.02	6	0
28	52	.14	6	53	43	178	.67	52	.02	.15	.11	.07	18	0
20	110	.09	6	98	53	239	.67	71	.01	.14	.18	.06	18	0
30	204	.19	8	145	28	176	.88	86	.01	.11	.02	.02	5	0
18	123	.12	5	87	17	106	.53	51	0	.06	.01	.01	3	0
119	815	.77	31	579	111	702	3.53	342	.03	.43	.09	.08	21	0
6	199	.2	8	137	32	6	.88	18	.01	.01	.03	.02	5	0
9	137	.32	11	302	193	29	.86	25	.05	.36	.3	.15	27	0
33	135	.32	12	297	190	911	.83	108	.05	.37	.28	.15	27	0
31	126	.29	11	277	177	851	.78	101	.04	.34	.26	.14	26	0
25	108	.25	9	237	151	915	.65	81	.04	.29	.23	.12	22	0
19	155	.36	14	341	217	918	.95	45	.05	.42	.33	.17	30	0
10	138	.32	12	303	193	918	.86	25	.05	.37	.29	.15	28	0
31	23	.34	2	29	34	84	.15	124	0	.06	.03	.01	4	0
16	32	.48	2	41	47	84	.22	63	.01	.08	.04	.02	5	0
25	207	.12	8	152	53	274	1.07	72	.01	.11	.02	.02	5	0
25	140	.18	5	96	18	316	.82	36	.04	.24	.28	.12	9	0

a[3]Vitamin C can range from 5 to 72 mg in a small can of frozen concentrate, and from 1 to 18 mg in 1 c of prepared lemonade.

(For purposes of calculations, use "0" for t, <1, <.1, <.01, etc.)

TABLE I–1
FOOD COMPOSITION

Computer Code Number	Food Description	Measure	Wt (g)	H$_2$O (%)	Ener (cal)	Prot (g)	Carb (g)	Dietary Fiber (g)	Fat (g)	Fat Breakdown (g) Sat	Mono	Poly
	DAIRY—Cont.											
	Cheese—Cont.											
49	Gouda	1 oz	28	42	101	7	1	0	8	5	2.2	.2
50	Gruyère	1 oz	28	33	117	8	<1	0	9	5.4	2.8	.5
51	Gorgonzola	1 oz	28	39	111	7	0	0	9	5.5	2.4	.5
52	Liederkranz	1 oz	28	53	87	5	<1	0	8	5.3	2.2	.2
1676	Limburger	1 oz	28	48	93	6	<1	0	8	4.7	2.4	.1
53	Monterey Jack	1 oz	28	41	106	7	<1	0	9	5.4	2.5	.3
54	Mozzarella, whole milk	1 oz	28	54	80	5	1	0	6	3.7	1.9	.2
55	Mozzarella, part-skim milk, low moisture	1 oz	28	49	79	8	1	0	5	3.1	1.4	.1
56	Muenster	1 oz	28	42	104	7	<1	0	9	5.4	2.5	.2
1399	Nonfat (Kraft Singles)	1 oz	28	60	45	6	4	0	0	0	0	0
	Parmesan, grated:											
57	Cup, not pressed down	1 c	100	18	456	42	4	0	30	19	8.7	.7
58	Tablespoon	1 tbs	5	18	23	2	<1	0	2	1	.4	t
59	Ounce	1 oz	28	18	129	12	1	0	9	5.4	2.5	.2
60	Provolone	1 oz	28	41	100	7	1	0	8	4.8	2.1	.2
61	Ricotta, whole milk	1 c	246	72	428	28	8	0	32	20.4	8.9	1
62	Ricotta, part-skim milk	1 c	246	74	339	28	13	0	19	12.1	5.7	.6
63	Romano	1 oz	28	31	109	9	1	0	8	4.8	2.2	.2
64	Swiss	1 oz	28	37	106	8	1	0	8	5	2.1	.3
976	Swiss, low fat	1 oz	28	60	51	8	1	0	1	.9	.4	<.1
	Pasteurized processed cheese products:											
65	American	1 oz	28	39	106	6	<1	0	9	5.6	2.5	.3
66	Swiss	1 oz	28	42	94	7	1	0	7	4.6	2	.2
67	American cheese food, jar	1 oz	28	43	93	6	2	0	7	4.4	2	.2
68	American cheese spread	1 oz	28	48	82	5	2	0	6	3.8	1.8	.2
982	Velveeta cheese spread, low fat, low sodium	1 oz	28	63	51	7	1	0	2	1.3	0.6	0.1
69	Cream, sweet:	1 c	242	81	315	7	10	0	28	17.3	8	1
	Half & half (cream & milk):											
70	Tablespoon	1 tbs	15	81	19	<1	1	0	2	1.1	.5	.1
71	Light, coffee or table:	1 c	240	74	468	6	9	0	46	28.8	13.4	1.7
72	Tablespoon	1 tbs	15	74	29	<1	1	0	3	1.8	.8	.1
73	Light whipping cream, liquid:[1]	1 c	239	64	698	5	7	0	74	46.1	21.7	2.1
74	Tablespoon	1 tbs	15	64	44	<1	<1	0	5	2.9	1.4	.1
75	Heavy whipping cream, liquid:[1]	1 c	238	58	821	5	7	0	88	54.7	25.5	3.3
76	Tablespoon	1 tbs	15	58	52	<1	<1	0	6	3.4	1.6	.2
77	Whipped cream, pressurized:	1 c	60	61	154	2	8	0	13	8.3	3.8	.5
78	Tablespoon	1 tbs	4	61	10	<1	<1	0	1	.6	.3	t
79	Cream, sour, cultured:	1 c	230	71	492	7	10	0	48	29.9	13.9	1.8
80	Tablespoon	1 tbs	14	71	30	<1	1	0	3	1.8	.8	.1
	Cream products—imitation and part dairy:											
81	Coffee whitener, frozen or liquid	1 tbs	15	77	20	<1	2	0	2	1.4	t	0
82	Coffee whitener, powdered	1 tsp	2	2	11	<1	1	0	1	.6	t	t
83	Dessert topping, frozen, nondairy:	1 c	75	50	239	1	17	0	19	16.4	1.2	.4
84	Tablespoon	1 tbs	5	50	16	<1	1	0	1	1.1	.1	t
85	Dessert topping, mix with whole milk:	1 c	80	67	151	3	13	0	10	8.6	.7	.2
86	Tablespoon	1 tbs	5	67	9	<1	1	0	1	.5	t	t

[1]For whipped cream, (non-pressurized), double the liquid cream volume of codes 73, 74 or 75, 76. One tablespoon liquid cream becomes 2 tablespoons when "whipped."

(Computer code number is for West Diet Analysis program)

Chol (mg)	Calc (mg)	Iron (mg)	Magn (mg)	Phos (mg)	Pota (mg)	Sodi (mg)	Zinc (mg)	VT-A (RE)	Thia (mg)	Ribo (mg)	Niac (mg)	V-B6 (mg)	Fola (μg)	VT-C (mg)
32	198	.07	8	155	34	232	1.11	49	.01	.09	.02	.02	6	0
31	286	.05	10	171	23	95	1.11	85	.02	.08	.03	.02	3	0
25	149	.12	8	121	26	512	.57	103	.01	.09	.2	.04	9	0
21	110	.12	7	100	68	389	.7	91	.01	.18	.1	.04	34	0
26	141	.04	6	111	36	227	.6	90	.02	.14	.04	.02	16	0
25	211	.2	8	126	23	152	.85	72	0	.11	.03	.02	5	0
22	146	.05	5	105	19	105	.63	68	0	.07	.02	.02	2	0
15	207	.07	7	148	27	149	.89	54	.01	.1	.03	.02	3	0
27	203	.12	8	132	38	178	.8	90	0	.09	.03	.02	3	0
5	224	0	–	165	81	438	–	128	–	.10	–	–	–	0
79	1375	.95	51	807	107	1861	3.19	173	.04	.39	.31	.1	8	0
4	69	.05	3	40	5	93	.16	9	0	.02	.02	.01	< 1	0
22	390	.27	14	229	30	528	.9	49	.01	.11	.09	.03	2	0
20	214	.15	8	140	39	247	.92	75	0	.09	.04	.02	3	0
124	509	.93	28	389	258	206	2.88	330	.03	.48	.26	.11	30	0
76	669	1.08	36	450	308	308	3.3	278	.05	.45	.19	.05	32	0
29	300	.22	12	215	24	340	.73	40	.01	.1	.02	.02	2	0
26	272	.05	10	171	31	74	1.11	72	.01	.1	.03	.02	2	0
10	272	.05	10	72	31	74	1.11	18	.01	.1	.03	.02	2	0
27	174	.11	6	211	46	405	.85	82	.01	.1	.02	.02	2	0
24	219	.17	8	216	61	388	1.03	65	0	.08	.01	.01	2	0
18	163	.24	9	130	79	336	.85	62	.01	.13	.04	.04	2	0
16	159	.09	8	202	69	380	.73	54	.01	.12	.04	.03	2	0
10	194	.12	7	234	51	2	.94	18	.01	.11	.02	.02	3	0
89	254	.17	25	230	315	98	1.23	259	.08	.36	.19	.09	6	2
6	16	.01	2	14	19	6	.08	16	.01	.02	.01	.01	< 1	< 1
158	230	.1	21	191	293	95	.65	437	.08	.35	.14	.08	6	2
10	14	.01	1	12	18	6	.04	27	.01	.02	.01	0	< 1	< 1
265	165	.07	17	146	231	82	.6	705	.06	.3	.1	.07	9	1
17	10	0	1	9	14	5	.04	44	.01	.02	.01	0	1	< 1
326	153	.07	17	148	179	89	.55	1001	.05	.26	.09	.06	9	1
21	10	0	1	9	11	6	.03	63	0	.02	.01	0	1	< 1
46	61	.03	6	54	88	78	.22	124	.02	.04	.04	.02	2	0
3	4	0	< 1	4	6	5	.01	8	0	0	0	0	< 1	0
102	267	.14	26	195	331	122	.62	449	.08	.34	.15	.04	25	2
6	16	.01	2	12	20	7	.04	27	0	.02	.01	0	2	< 1
0	1	< .01	< 1	10	29	12	0	1	0	0	0	0	0	0
0	< 1	.02	< 1	8	16	4	.01	< 1	0	0	0	0	0	0
0	5	.09	1	6	14	19	.02	64[2]	0	0	0	0	0	0
0	< 1	.01	< 1	< 1	1	1	0	4[2]	0	0	0	0	0	0
8	72	.03	8	69	120	53	.22	39[2]	.02	.09	.05	.02	3	1
< 1	5	0	< 1	4	8	3	.01	2[2]	0	.01	0	0	< 1	< 1

[2]Vitamin A value is from beta-carotene used for coloring.

(For purposes of calculations, use "0" for t, < 1, < .1, < .01, etc.)

TABLE I–1
FOOD COMPOSITION

Computer Code Number	Food Description	Measure	Wt (g)	H₂O (%)	Ener (cal)	Prot (g)	Carb (g)	Dietary Fiber (g)	Fat (g)	Fat Breakdown (g) Sat	Mono	Poly
DAIRY—Cont.												
88	Dessert topping, pressurized:	1 c	70	60	185	1	11	0	16	13.2	1.3	.2
87	Tablespoon	1 tbs	4	60	11	<1	1	0	1	.8	.1	t
91	Sour cream, imitation:	1 c	230	71	478	6	15	<1	45	40.9	1.3	.1
92	Tablespoon	1 tbs	14	71	29	<1	1	0	3	2.5	.1	t
89	Sour dressing, part dairy:	1 c	235	75	418	8	11	0	39	31.3	4.6	1.1
90	Tablespoon	1 tbs	15	75	27	<1	1	0	2	2	.3	.1
	Milk, fluid:											
93	Whole milk	1 c	244	88	150	8	11	0	8	5.1	2.3	.3
94	2% low-fat milk	1 c	244	89	121	8	12	0	5	2.9	1.3	.2
95	2% milk solids added[1]	1 c	245	89	124	9	12	0	5	2.9	1.4	.2
96	1% low-fat milk	1 c	244	90	102	8	12	–	3	1.6	.8	.1
97	1% milk solids added[1]	1 c	245	90	104	9	12	0	2	1.5	.7	.1
98	Nonfat milk, vitamin A added	1 c	245	91	86	8	12	0	<1	.3	.1	t
99	Nonfat milk solids added[1]	1 c	245	90	90	9	12	0	1	.4	.2	t
100	Buttermilk, nonfat	1 c	245	90	99	8	12	0	2	1.3	.6	.1
	Milk, canned:											
101	Sweetened condensed	1 c	306	27	982	24	166	0	27	16.8	7.4	1
102	Evaporated, whole	1 c	252	74	338	17	25	0	19	11.6	5.9	.6
103	Evaporated, nonfat	1 c	255	79	199	19	29	0	1	.3	.2	t
	Milk, dried:											
104	Buttermilk, sweet	1 c	120	3	464	41	59	0	7	4.3	2	.3
105	Instant, nonfat, envelope[2]	1 ea	91	4	325	32	47	0	1	.4	.2	t
106	Instant nonfat, cup	1 c	68	4	243	24	35	0	<1	.3	.1	t
107	Goat milk	1 c	244	87	167	9	11	0	10	6.5	2.7	.4
108	Kefir, 2% milkfat[3]	1 c	233	82	122	9	9	0	5	2.9	1.2	.1
	Milk beverages and powdered mixes:											
	Chocolate:											
109	Whole	1 c	250	82	208	8	26	3	9	5.2	2.5	.3
110	2% fat	1 c	250	83	178	8	26	3	5	3.1	1.5	.2
111	1% fat	1 c	250	85	157	8	26	3	3	1.5	.7	.1
	Chocolate-flavored beverages:											
112	Powder containing nonfat dry milk:	1 oz	28	2	102	3	22	<1	1	.7	.4	t
113	Prepared with water	¾ c	206	86	103	4	22	<1	1	.7	.4	t
114	Powder without nonfat dry milk:	¾ oz	22	1	77	1	20	1	1	.4	.2	t
115	Prepared with whole milk	1 c	266	81	226	9	31	<1	9	5.5	2.6	.3
116	Eggnog, commercial	1 c	254	74	343	10	34	0	19	11.3	5.7	.9
974	Eggnog, low fat	1 c	254	85	189	12	17	0	8	3.8	2.7	0.7
1027	Instant Breakfast, envelope, powder only:	1 ea	37	7	131	7	24	<1	1	.3	.1	t
1028	Prepared with whole milk	1 c	281	77	280	15	36	<1	9	5.4	2.5	.3
1029	Prepared with 2% milk	1 c	281	78	252	15	36	<1	5	3.3	1.5	.2
1283	Prepared with 1% milk	1 c	281	79	233	16	36	<1	3	2	.9	t
1284	Prepared with nonfat milk	1 c	281	80	215	16	36	<1	1	.6	.3	t
117	Malted milk, chocolate, powder:[4]	¾ oz	21	1	79	1	18	<1	1	.5	.2	.1
118	Prepared with whole milk	1 c	265	81	228	9	30	1	9	5.5	2.6	.4
1661	Ovaltine with whole milk	1 c	265	81	225	9	29	1	9	5.5	2.6	.4
119	Malted milk, regular, powder:[4]	¾ oz	21	2	87	2	16	<1	2	.9	.4	.3
120	Prepared with whole milk	1 c	265	81	236	10	27	<1	10	5.9	2.8	.6

[1] Milk solids added, label claims less than 10 g protein per cup.

[2] Yields 1 qt fluid milk when reconstituted according to package directions.

[3] Most values provided by product labeling.

[4] The latest USDA data from *Handbook 8–14* on beverages updates previous USDA data.

(Computer code number is for West Diet Analysis program)

Chol (mg)	Calc (mg)	Iron (mg)	Magn (mg)	Phos (mg)	Pota (mg)	Sodi (mg)	Zinc (mg)	VT-A (RE)	Thia (mg)	Ribo (mg)	Niac (mg)	V-B6 (mg)	Fola (µg)	VT-C (mg)
0	4	.01	1	13	13	43	.01	33[2]	.0	0	0	0	0	0
0	<1	0	<1	1	1	2	0	2[2]	0	0	0	0	0	0
0	6	.9	15	102	370	235	2.74	0	0	0	0	0	0	0
0	<1	.05	1	6	23	14	.16	0	0	0	0	0	0	0
13	266	.07	23	204	381	113	.87	5[5]	.09	.38	.17	.04	28	2
1	17	0	1	13	24	7	.06	<1[5]	.01	.02	.01	0	2	<1
33	290	.12	33	228	371	120	.93	76	.09	.39	.2	.1	12	2
18	298	.12	33	232	376	122	.95	139	.09	.4	.21	.1	12	2
18	311	.12	35	244	397	128	.98	140	.1	.42	.22	.11	13	2
10	300	.12	34	235	381	123	.95	144	.09	.41	.21	.1	12	2
10	311	.12	35	244	397	128	.98	145	.1	.42	.22	.11	13	2
4	301	.1	28	247	407	126	.98	149	.09	.34	.22	.1	13	2
5	316	.12	35	255	419	129	1	149	.1	.43	.22	.11	13	2
9	284	.12	27	219	370	257	1.03	20	.08	.38	.14	.08	12	2
104	869	.58	79	774	1135	389	2.88	248	.27	1.27	.64	.16	34	8
74	658	.48	61	512	764	267	1.94	136	.12	.8	.49	.13	20	5
9	740	.74	69	497	847	293	2.29	298	.11	.79	.44	.14	22	3
83	1421	.36	132	1120	1910	620	4.84	65	.47	1.9	1.05	.41	57	7
17	1119	.28	106	896	1552	500	4.01	646[6]	.38	1.58	.81	.31	45	5
12	836	.21	80	670	1159	373	3	483[6]	.28	1.18	.61	.23	34	4
28	327	.12	34	271	498	122	.73	137	.12	.34	.68	.11	1	3
10	350	.5	28	319	205	50	.9	155	.45	.44	.3	.09	23	<1
30	280	.6	33	253	418	149	1.03	73	.09	.41	.31	.1	12	2
17	285	.6	33	255	423	151	1.03	143	.09	.41	.32	.1	12	2
7	288	.6	33	258	425	152	1.03	148	.09	.42	.32	.1	12	2
1	92	.34	24	89	202	143	.41	1	.03	.16	.17	.03	0	1
2	97	.35	25	89	202	148	.45	1	.03	.17	.18	.04	3	1
0	8	.69	22	28	129	46	.34	<1	.01	.03	.11	<.01	1	<1
32	301	.8	53	255	497	164	1.28	77	.1	.43	.32	.1	12	2
149	330	.51	47	277	419	138	1.17	203	.09	.48	.27	.13	2	4
194	269	.71	32	269	367	155	1.26	197	.11	.55	.21	.15	30	2
4	105	4.74	84	158	350	142	3.16	554	.31	.07	5.25	.42	105	28
38	396	4.86	117	356	721	262	4.09	630	.41	.47	5.46	.52	118	31
23	403	4.87	118	390	726	264	4.12	693	.41	.48	5.46	.53	118	31
14	406	4.87	118	393	731	266	4.12	698	.41	.48	5.45	.52	118	31
9	406	4.84	112	404	755	268	4.14	703	.4	.42	5.47	.52	118	31
1	13	.48	15	37	129	53	.17	4	.04	.04	.42	.03	4	<1
34	305	.61	48	265	498	172	1.09	80	.13	.44	.62	.13	16	3
34	385	4	53	313	620	244	1.17	901	.74	1.26	10.9	1.02	32	34
4	63	.15	20	75	159	104	.21	18	.11	.19	1.1	.09	10	1
37	355	.26	53	302	530	223	1.14	95	.2	.59	1.31	.19	22	3

[5] Vitamin A value is from beta-carotene used for coloring.

[6] With added vitamin A.

(For purposes of calculations, use "0" for t, <1, <.1, <.01, etc.)

TABLE I–1
FOOD COMPOSITION

Computer Code Number	Food Description	Measure	Wt (g)	H₂O (%)	Ener (cal)	Prot (g)	Carb (g)	Dietary Fiber (g)	Fat (g)	Fat Breakdown (g)		
										Sat	Mono	Poly
DAIRY—Cont.												
121	Milk shakes, chocolate (10 fl oz)	1¼ c	283	72	359	10	58	< 1	10	6.5	3	.4
122	Milk shakes, vanilla (10 fl oz)	1¼ c	283	75	314	10	51	< 1	8	5.3	2.4	.3
	Milk desserts:											
134	Custard, baked	1 c	265	79	278	13	28	0	12	6.2	4	1
1548	Low-fat frozen dessert bars	1 ea	81	72	90	2	18	0	1	.2	.1	.4
	Ice cream, vanilla (about 10% fat):											
123	Hardened: ½ gallon	1 ea	1064	61	2138	37	251	1	117	72.4	33.8	4.4
124	Cup	1 c	133	61	267	5	31	< 1	15	9	4.2	.6
125	Fluid ounces	3 oz	50	61	101	2	12	< 1	6	3.4	1.6	.2
126	Soft serve	1 c	173	60	372	7	38	< 1	22	12.9	6	.8
	Ice cream, rich vanilla (16% fat):											
127	Hardened: ½ gallon	1 ea	1188	60	2554	49	264	1	154	88.9	41.5	5.5
128	Cup	1 c	148	57	357	5	33	< 1	24	14.8	6.9	.9
1724	Ben & Jerry's	½ c	106	64	230	4	21	0	17	10	–	–
	Ice milk, vanilla (about 4% fat):											
129	Hardened: ½ gallon	1 ea	1048	68	1456	40	238	1	45	27.7	12.9	1.7
130	Cup	1 c	131	68	182	5	30	< 1	6	3.5	1.6	.2
131	Soft serve (about 3% fat)	1 c	175	70	221	9	38	< 1	5	2.8	1.3	.2
	Pudding, canned (5-oz can = .55 cup):											
135	Chocolate	1 ea	142	69	189	4	32	1	6	1	2.4	2
136	Tapioca	1 ea	142	74	169	3	27	< 1	5	.9	2.2	1.9
137	Vanilla	1 ea	142	71	185	3	31	< 1	5	.8	2.2	1.9
	Puddings, dry mix with whole milk:											
138	Chocolate, instant	1 c	260	75	289	8	49	3	8	4.8	2.4	.5
139	Chocolate, regular, cooked	½ c	130	74	144	4	23	1	4	2.7	1.3	.2
140	Rice, cooked	½ c	132	72	161	4	27	1	4	2.3	1.1	.2
141	Tapioca, cooked	½ c	130	74	148	4	25	< 1	4	2.3	1.1	.1
142	Vanilla, instant	½ c	130	74	148	4	26	< 1	4	2.3	1.1	.2
143	Vanilla, regular, cooked	½ c	130	75	144	4	24	< 1	4	2.4	1.1	.2
132	Sherbet (2% fat): ½ gallon	1 ea	1542	66	2127	17	469	0	31	17.9	8.3	1.2
133	Cup	1 c	193	66	266	2	59	0	4	2.2	1	.2
144	Soy milk	1 c	240	93	79	7	4	3	5	.5	.8	2
1584	Yogurt, frozen, low-fat[1]	½ c	87	65	138	3	21	0	5	3	1.4	.2
1512	Scoop	1 ea	79	74	78	4	16	0	< 1	.1	t	0
	Yogurt, low-fat:											
1172	Fruit added with low-calorie sweetener	1 c	241	86	122	11	19	1	< 1	.2	.1	t
145	Fruit added[2]	1 c	227	75	232	10	43	< 1	2	1.6	.7	.1
146	Plain	1 c	227	85	144	12	16	0	4	2.3	1	.1
147	Vanilla or coffee flavor	1 c	227	79	194	11	31	0	3	1.8	.8	.1
148	Yogurt, made with nonfat milk	1 c	227	85	127	13	17	0	< 1	.3	.1	t
149	Yogurt, made with whole milk	1 c	227	88	139	8	11	0	7	4.8	2	.2
EGGS[3]												
	Raw, large:											
150	Whole, without shell	1 ea	50	75	74	6	1	0	5	1.5	1.9	.7
151	White	1 ea	33	88	17	4	< 1	0	0	0	0	0
152	Yolk	1 ea	17	49	59	3	< 1	0	5	1.6	1.9	.7

[1]Data is from 1992 USDA data on snacks and sweets.

[3]This data is newest revised information from the USDA with 24% less cholesterol.

[2]Carbohydrate and calories vary widely—consult label if more precise values are needed.

(Computer code number is for West Diet Analysis program)

Chol (mg)	Calc (mg)	Iron (mg)	Magn (mg)	Phos (mg)	Pota (mg)	Sodi (mg)	Zinc (mg)	VT-A (RE)	Thia (mg)	Ribo (mg)	Niac (mg)	V-B6 (mg)	Fola (µg)	VT-C (mg)
37	320	.88	48	289	566	275	1.16	65	.16	.69	.46	.14	10	1
31	345	.25	34	289	492	232	1.02	91	.13	.52	.52	.15	9	2
231	297	.79	37	299	405	204	1.4	159	.09	.6	.22	.13	27	1
1	82	.07	10	65	111	47	.26	38	.03	.11	.06	.03	3	1
468	1362	.96	149	1117	2117	851	7.34	1245	.44	2.55	1.23	.51	53	6
59	170	.12	19	140	265	106	.92	156	.05	.32	.15	.06	7	1
22	64	.04	7	53	100	40	.34	59	.02	.12	.06	.02	3	<1
157	227	.36	21	201	306	106	.9	266	.08	.31	.16	.08	16	1
1081	1556	2.49	143	1378	2102	725	6.18	1829	.58	2.16	1.13	.57	107	10
90	173	.07	16	141	235	83	.59	272	.06	.24	.12	.06	7	1
95	150	.36	–	–	–	55	–	225	–	–	–	–	–	0
147	1456	1.05	157	1142	2211	891	4.61	493	.61	2.78	.94	.68	63	8
18	182	.13	20	143	276	111	.58	62	.08	.35	.12	.08	8	1
21	275	.1	25	212	387	123	.93	51	.09	.35	.21	.08	11	2
4	128	.72	30	114	256	183	.6	16	.04	.22	.49	.04	4	3
1	119	.33	11	112	148	168	.38	0	.03	.14	.44	.14	6	1
10	125	.18	11	97	160	192	.35	9	.03	.2	.36	.02	0	0
29	265	.75	47	621	432	738	1.09	55	.09	.37	.25	.1	10	2
16	144	.47	20	121	212	134	.58	34	.04	.23	.13	.05	5	1
15	133	.5	17	114	165	140	.6	26	.1	.18	.6	.04	5	1
16	135	.08	16	107	172	157	.44	35	.04	.18	.09	.05	5	1
14	131	.09	16	256	166	372	.43	33	.04	.18	.1	.05	5	1
16	139	.06	17	107	177	208	.45	35	.04	.18	.1	.04	5	1
77	833	2.16	123	617	1480	709	7.4	216	.39	1.05	1.48	.52	62	66
10	104	.27	15	77	185	89	.93	27	.05	.13	.18	.07	8	8
0	10	1.39	46	117	338	29	.55	7	.39	.17	.35	.1	4	0
2	124	.26	12	112	184	76	.36	50	.03	.19	.25	.07	5	1
1	137	.07	13	108	175	53	.67	1	.03	.16	.09	.04	8	1
3	369	.61	41	291	550	139	1.83	6	.1	.45	.5	.11	32	26
10	345	.16	33	270	440	133	1.68	25	.08	.4	.22	.09	21	2
14	415	.18	40	327	529	159	2.02	36	.1	.49	.26	.11	25	2
11	388	.16	37	306	497	149	1.88	30	.09	.46	.24	.1	24	2
4	452	.2	43	356	579	174	2.2	5	.11	.53	.28	.12	28	2
29	275	.11	26	215	350	105	1.34	68	.07	.32	.17	.07	17	1
213	25	.72	5	89	61	63	.55	96	.03	.25	.04	.07	24	0
0	2	.01	4	4	47	54	0	0	<.01	.15	.03	0	1	0
218	23	.59	2	83	16	7	.52	99	.03	.11	0	.06	25	0

(For purposes of calculations, use "0" for t, <1, <.1, <.01, etc.)

TABLE I–1
FOOD COMPOSITION

Computer Code Number	Food Description	Measure	Wt (g)	H₂O (%)	Ener (cal)	Prot (g)	Carb (g)	Dietary Fiber (g)	Fat (g)	Fat Breakdown (g)		
										Sat	Mono	Poly
	EGGS—Cont.											
	Cooked:											
153	Fried in margarine	1 ea	46	69	92	6	1	0	7	1.9	2.8	1.3
154	Hard-cooked, shell removed	1 ea	50	75	78	6	1	0	5	1.6	2	.7
155	Hard-cooked, chopped	1 c	136	75	211	17	2	0	14	4.5	5.6	1.9
156	Poached, no added salt	1 ea	50	75	75	6	1	0	5	1.6	1.9	.7
157	Scrambled with milk & margarine	1 ea	61	73	101	7	1	0	7	2.2	2.9	1.3
1681	Egg substitute, liquid	½ c	126	83	106	15	1	0	4	.8	1.1	2
1254	Egg Beaters, Fleischmann's	.25 c	61	–	30	6	1	0	0	0	0	0
1256	Eggs, scrambled, f/frozen	0.33 c	50	70	92	6	2	0	6	1.1	1.4	3.6
1262	Eggs, Second Nature, prepared	0.33 c	69	81	66	9	1	0	3	.5	.7	1.3
	FATS and OILS											
158	Butter: Stick	½ c	113	16	810	1	< 1	0	92	57.1	27.6	3.4
159	Tablespoon	1 tbs	14	16	100	< 1	< 1	0	11	7.1	3.4	.4
160	Pat (about 1 tsp)[1]	1 ea	5	16	36	< 1	< 1	0	4	2.5	1.2	.2
1682	Whipped	1 tsp	3	16	22	< 1	< 1	0	3	1.5	.7	.1
	Fats, cooking:											
1363	Bacon fat	1 tbs	14	0	125	0	0	0	14	6.4	5.9	1.1
1362	Beef fat/tallow	1 c	205	0	1849	0	0	0	205	103	85.7	8.2
1364	Chicken fat	1 c	205	< 1	1845	0	0	0	205	61.1	91.6	42.8
161	Vegetable shortening:	1 c	205	0	1812	0	0	0	205	51.5	91.2	53.5
162	Tablespoon	1 tbs	13	0	115	0	0	0	13	3.3	5.8	3.4
163	Lard:	1 c	205	0	1849	0	0	0	205	80.4	92.5	23
164	Tablespoon	1 tbs	13	0	117	0	0	0	13	5.1	5.9	1.5
	Margarine:											
165	Imitation (about 40% fat), soft:	1 c	227	58	783	1	1	0	88	14.5	33	37
166	Tablespoon	1 tbs	14	58	48	< 1	< 1	0	5	.9	2	2.3
167	Regular, hard (about 80% fat):	½ c	113	16	812	1	1	0	91	14.8	42	29.6
168	Tablespoon	1 tbs	14	16	101	< 1	< 1	0	11	1.8	5	3.6
169	Pat	1 ea	5	16	36	< 1	< 1	0	4	.8	1.8	1.3
170	Regular, soft (about 80% fat):	1 c	227	16	1625	2	1	0	183	30.7	83	61
171	Tablespoon	1 tbs	14	16	100	< 1	< 1	0	11	1.9	5.1	3.8
	Saffola:											
2056	Unsalted	1 tbs	14	20	101	0	0	0	11	1.9	4.8	4.7
2057	Reduced fat	1 tbs	14	5.27	71	0	0	0	9	1.3	2.7	4.5
172	Spread (about 60% fat), hard:	½ c	113	37	610	1	0	0	69	15.9	29.4	20.5
173	Tablespoon	1 tbs	14	37	76	< 1	0	0	9	2	3.6	2.5
174	Pat[1]	1 ea	5	37	27	< 1	0	0	3	.7	1.2	1
175	Spread (about 60% fat), soft:	1 c	227	37	1226	1	0	0	138	29.1	71.5	31.3
176	Tablespoon	1 tbs	14	37	76	< 1	0	0	9	1.8	4.4	1.9
2160	Touch of Butter (47% fat)	1 tbs	14	36	77	< 1	0	0	9	2	4.4	1.9
	Oils:											
1585	Canola:	1 c	218	0	1927	0	0	0	218	15.5	128	64.5
1586	Tablespoon	1 tbs	14	0	124	0	0	0	14	1	8.2	4.1
177	Corn:	1 c	218	0	1927	0	0	0	218	29.4	52.8	127
178	Tablespoon	1 tbs	14	0	124	0	0	0	14	1.8	3.4	8.2

[1]Pat is 1" square, ⅓" thick; about 1 tsp; 90 per lb.

(Computer code number is for West Diet Analysis program)

Chol (mg)	Calc (mg)	Iron (mg)	Magn (mg)	Phos (mg)	Pota (mg)	Sodi (mg)	Zinc (mg)	VT-A (RE)	Thia (mg)	Ribo (mg)	Niac (mg)	V-B6 (mg)	Fola (µg)	VT-C (mg)
211	25	.72	5	89	61	162	.55	114	.03	.24	.04	.07	17	0
212	25	.59	5	86	63	62	.53	84	.03	.26	.03	.06	22	0
577	68	1.62	14	234	171	169	1.44	228	.09	.7	.09	.17	60	0
212	25	.72	5	89	60	61	.56	95	.02	.22	.03	.06	18	0
215	43	.73	7	104	84	171	.62	119	.03	.27	.05	.07	18	< 1
1	67	2.65	11	152	416	223	1.65	272	.14	.38	.14	< .01	19	0
0	40	1.08	–	–	85	100	–	–	–	–	–	–	–	–
1	42	1.14	9	41	122	114	.56	77	.06	.21	.08	.07	7	< 1
1	42	1.65	7	95	260	139	1.02	170	.07	.22	.08	0	9	0
247	27	.18	2	26	29	935[2]	.06	852[3]	.01	.04	.05	< .01	3	0
31	3	.02	< 1	3	4	117[2]	.01	107[3]	< .01	< .01	.01	0	< 1	0
11	1	.01	< 1	1	1	41[2]	< .01	38[3]	0	< .01	< .01	0	< 1	0
7	1	0	< 1	1	1	26[2]	< .01	24[3]	0	< .01	< .01	0	< 1	0
14	< 1	0	< 1	0	< 1	76	< .01	0	0	0	0	0	0	0
223	0	0	0	0	< 1	< 1	0	0	0	0	0	0	0	0
174	0	0	0	0	0	0	0	351	0	0	0	0	0	0
0	0	0	0	0	0	0	0	0	0	0	0	0	0	0
0	0	0	0	0	0	0	0	0	0	0	0	0	0	0
195	< 1	0	< 1	0	< 1	< 1	.23	0	0	0	0	0	0	0
12	< 1	0	< 1	0	< 1	< 1	.01	0	0	0	0	0	0	0
0	40	0	4	31	57	800[4]	0	2254[5]	.01	.05	.03	.01	2	< 1
0	2	0	< 1	2	4	49[4]	0	139[5]	< .01	< .01	< .01	< .01	< 1	< 1
0	34	0	3	26	48	1065[4]	.23	1122[5]	.01	.04	.03	.01	1	< 1
0	4	0	< 1	3	6	132[4]	.03	139[5]	< .01	< .01	< .01	< .01	< 1	< 1
0	2	0	< 1	1	2	47[4]	.01	50[5]	< .01	< .01	< .01	0	< 1	< 1
0	60	0	5	46	86	1678[4]	0	2254[5]	.02	.07	.04	.02	2	< 1
0	4	0	< 1	3	5	103[4]	0	139[5]	< .01	< .01	< .01	< .01	< 1	< 1
52	0	0	–	–	–	0	–	–	–	–	–	–	–	0
–	0	0	–	–	–	116	–	52	–	–	–	–	–	0
0	24	0	2	18	34	1122[4]	.17	1122[5]	.01	.03	.02	.01	1	< 1
0	3	0	< 1	2	4	139[4]	0	139[5]	< .01	< .01	< .01	< .01	< 1	< 1
0	1	0	< 1	1	1	50[4]	0	50[5]	0	< .01	< .01	0	< 1	< 1
0	47	0	4	37	68	2256[4]	0	2254[5]	.02	.06	.04	.01	2	< 1
0	3	0	< 1	2	4	139[4]	0	139[5]	< .01	< .01	< .01	< .01	< 1	< 1
1	3	< .01	< 1	2	4	140	0	152	< .01	< .01	< .01	< .01	< 1	< .1
0	0	0	0	0	0	0	0	0	0	0	0	0	0	0
0	0	0	0	0	0	0	0	0	0	0	0	0	0	0
0	0	0	0	0	0	0	0	0	0	0	0	0	0	0
0	0	0	0	0	0	0	0	0	0	0	0	0	0	0

[2] For salted butter, unsalted butter contains 12 mg sodium per stick or ½ c, 1.5 mg/tbs, or .5 mg/pat.

[3] Values for vitamin A are a year-round average.

[4] For salted margarine.

[5] Based on average vitamin A content of fortified margarine. Federal specifications require a minimum of 15,000 IU/lb.

(For purposes of calculations, use "0" for t, < 1, < .1, < .01, etc.)

TABLE I-1
FOOD COMPOSITION

Computer Code Number	Food Description	Measure	Wt (g)	H₂O (%)	Ener (cal)	Prot (g)	Carb (g)	Dietary Fiber (g)	Fat (g)	Fat Breakdown (g)		
										Sat	Mono	Poly
	FATS and OILS—Cont.											
	Oils—Cont.											
179	Olive:	1 c	216	0	1909	0	0	0	216	29.2	159	18.4
180	Tablespoon	1 tbs	14	0	124	0	0	0	14	1.9	10.3	1.2
1683	Olive, extra virgin	1 tbs	14	< 1	126	0	0	0	14	1.96	10.8	1.3
181	Peanut:	1 c	216	0	1909	0	0	0	216	35.6	113	56.8
182	Tablespoon	1 tbs	14	0	124	0	0	0	14	2.4	7.3	3.7
183	Safflower:	1 c	218	0	1927	0	0	0	218	19.8	26.4	162
184	Tablespoon	1 tbs	14	0	124	0	0	0	14	1.3	1.7	10.4
185	Soybean:	1 c	218	0	1927	0	0	0	218	31.4	50.8	126
186	Tablespoon	1 tbs	14	0	124	0	0	0	14	2	3.3	8.1
187	Soybean/cottonseed:	1 c	218	0	1927	0	0	0	218	40	64.3	105
188	Tablespoon	1 tbs	14	0	124	0	0	0	14	2.5	4.1	6.7
189	Sunflower:	1 c	218	0	1927	0	0	0	218	25	45	144
190	Tablespoon	1 tbs	14	0	124	0	0	0	14	1.5	2.9	9.2
	Salad dressings/sandwich spreads:											
191	Blue cheese, regular	1 tbs	15	32	76	1	1	< 1	8	1.5	1.9	4.4
1040	Low calorie	1 tbs	15	80	15	1	< 1	< 1	1	.2	.5	.4
1684	Caesar's	1 tbs	12	36	55	1	< 1	< 1	5	.9	3.5	.5
192	French, regular	1 tbs	16	38	69	< 1	3	< 1	9	1.5	1.2	3.4
193	Low calorie	1 tbs	16	69	21	< 1	3	< 1	1	.1	.2	.5
194	Italian, regular	1 tbs	15	38	70	< 1	1	< 1	9	1	1.6	4.1
195	Low calorie	1 tbs	15	82	16	< 1	1	< 1	1	.2	.3	.9
	Kraft, Deliciously Right											
2150	1000 Island	2 tbs	32	–	70	0	8	0	4	1	–	–
2153	Bacon & Tomato	2 tbs	31	–	60	1	3	0	5	1	–	–
2154	Cucumber Ranch	2 tbs	31	–	60	0	2	0	5	1	–	–
2151	French	2 tbs	32	–	50	0	6	0	3	.5	–	–
2152	Ranch	2 tbs	31	–	100	0	5	0	9	1.5	–	–
199	Mayo type, regular	1 tbs	15	40	58	< 1	3	0	5	.7	1.4	2.7
1030	Low calorie	1 tbs	15	54	39	< 1	1	0	3	.4	.8	1.4
196	Mayonnaise:											
196	Regular (soybean)	1 tbs	14	15	100	< 1	< 1	0	11	1.6	3.1	5.7
197	Imitation, low calorie	1 tbs	15	63	35	< 1	2	0	3	.5	.7	1.6
1488	Regular, low calorie, low sodium	1 tbs	14	63	32	< 1	2	0	3	.5	.6	1.4
1493	Regular, low calorie	1 tbs	16	63	37	< 1	3	0	3	.5	.7	1.6
2058	Saffola Light	1 tbs	15	–	44	0	1	0	4	.5	1	2.9
198	Ranch, regular	½ c	119	35	436	4	6	0	45	6.7	19.4	17
1042	Low calorie	1 tbs	15	70	32	0	1	0	3	.5	–	1
1685	Russian	1 tbs	15	35	74	< 1	2	0	8	1.1	1.8	4.5
1502	Salad dressing, low calorie, oil free	1 tbs	15	88	4	< 1	1	< 1	< 1	0	0	0
	Salad dressing, no cholesterol											
1605	(Miracle Whip)	1 tbs	15	57	48	0	2	0	4	1.1	1.1	2.1
203	Salad dressing, from recipe, cooked[1]	1 tbs	16	69	25	1	2	< 1	2	.5	.6	.3
200	Tartar sauce, regular	1 tbs	14	34	74	< 1	1	< 1	8	1.5	2.6	4.1
1503	Low calorie	1 tbs	14	63	31	< 1	2	< 1	2	.4	.6	1.3
201	Thousand island, regular	1 tbs	16	46	60	< 1	2	< 1	6	1	1.3	3.2
202	Low calorie	1 tbs	15	69	24	< 1	2	< 1	2	.2	.4	.9
204	Vinegar & oil	1 tbs	16	47	72	0	< 1	0	8	1.5	2.4	3.9

[1]Fatty acid values apply to product made with regular margarine.

(Computer code number is for West Diet Analysis program)

Chol (mg)	Calc (mg)	Iron (mg)	Magn (mg)	Phos (mg)	Pota (mg)	Sodi (mg)	Zinc (mg)	VT-A (RE)	Thia (mg)	Ribo (mg)	Niac (mg)	V-B6 (mg)	Fola (µg)	VT-C (mg)
0	<1	.82	<1	3	0	<1	.13	0	0	0	0	0	0	0
0	<1	.05	<1	<1	0	<1	.01	0	0	0	0	0	0	0
0	–	–	–	–	–	–	–	0	0	0	0	0	0	0
0	<1	.06	<1	0	<1	<1	.02	0	0	0	0	0	0	0
0	<1	0	<1	0	0	<1	0	0	0	0	0	0	0	0
0	0	0	0	0	0	0	0	0	0	0	0	0	0	0
0	0	0	0	0	0	0	0	0	0	0	0	0	0	0
0	<1	.04	<1	1	0	0	0	0	0	0	0	0	0	0
0	<1	<.01	<1	<1	0	0	0	0	0	0	0	0	0	0
0	0	0	0	0	0	0	0	0	0	0	0	0	0	0
0	0	0	0	0	0	0	0	0	0	0	0	0	0	0
0	0	0	0	0	0	0	0	0	0	0	0	0	0	0
3	12	.03	0	11	6	164	0	10	<.01	.02	.02	.01	1	<1
<1	13	.08	1	12	1	180	.04	<1	<.01	.02	.01	<.01	<1	<1
12	22	.19	3	19	20	202	.12	6	<.01	.02	.49	.01	2	1
9	2	.06	0	2	13	219	.01	3	<.01	<.01	<.01	<.01	1	0
1	2	.06	0	2	13	126	.03	0	0	0	0	0	0	0
0	2	.03	<1	1	2	118	.02	4	<.01	<.01	0	<.01	1	0
1	<1	.03	0	1	2	118	.02	0	0	0	0	0	0	0
5	0	0	–	–	55	320	–	0	–	–	–	–	–	0
3	0	0	–	–	40	300	–	0	–	–	–	–	–	0
0	0	0	–	–	20	450	–	0	–	–	–	–	–	0
0	0	0	–	–	15	260	–	100	–	–	–	–	–	0
0	0	0	–	–	0	320	–	0	–	–	–	–	–	0
4	2	.03	<1	4	1	107	.03	13	<.01	<.01	<.01	<.01	1	0
4	2	.03	<1	4	1	107	.03	10	<.01	<.01	0	0	1	0
8	3	.07	<1	4	5	80	.02	12	0	0	<.01	.08	1	0
4	<1	0	<1	<1	2	75	.02	0	0	0	0	0	0	0
3	0	0	0	0	1	15	.02	1	0	<.01	0	0	<1	0
4	<1	0	<1	<1	2	80	02	0	0	0	0	0	0	0
–	0	0	–	–	–	103	–	0	–	–	–	–	–	0
47	119	.31	12	100	158	522	.44	86	.04	.17	.08	.05	6	1
5	11	0	–	–	5	150	–	0	–	–	–	–	–	0
3	3	.1	.23	6	24	130	.06	31	.01	.01	.1	<.01	1.59	1
0	1	.04	2	1	7	256	<.01	<1	0	0	<.01	<.01	<1	<1
0	0	<.01	0	0	0	102	0	2	0	0	0	0	0	0
9	13	.08	0	14	19	117	0	20	.01	.02	.04	0	0	<1
7	3	.13	<1	4	11	99	.02	9	<.01	<.01	0	.01	1	<1
3	2	.09	<1	1	5	83	.02	2	<.01	<.01	.01	<.01	<1	<1
4	2	.09	<1	3	18	112	.02	15	<.01	<.01	<.01	<.01	1	0
2	2	.09	<1	3	17	150	.02	14	<.01	<.01	<.01	<.01	1	0
0	0	0	0	0	1	<1	0	0	0	0	0	0	0	0

(2)Sodium bisulfite used to preserve color; unsulfured product would contain lower levels of sodium.

(For purposes of calculations, use "0" for t, <1, <.1, <.01, etc.)

TABLE I–1
FOOD COMPOSITION

Computer Code Number	Food Description	Measure	Wt (g)	H$_2$O (%)	Ener (cal)	Prot (g)	Carb (g)	Dietary Fiber (g)	Fat (g)	Fat Breakdown (g) Sat	Mono	Poly
	FATS and OILS—Cont.											
	Salad dressings/sandwich spreads—Cont.											
	Wishbone											
2179	Fat Free French	1 tbs	16	–	6	0	1	–	0	0	–	.1
2180	Lite Creamy Italian	1 tbs	15	–	26	< 1	2	–	2	.4	–	.7
2166	Lite Italian	1 tbs	16	77	6	0	1	7	–	0	–	.1
2167	Lite Ranch	1 tbs	15	–	42	< 1	3	0	4	.7	–	2.3
	FRUITS and FRUIT JUICES											
	Apples:											
	Fresh, raw, with peel:											
205	2 ¾" diam (about 3 per lb w/cores)	1 ea	138	84	81	< 1	21	3	< 1	.1	t	.1
206	3 ¾" diam (about 2 per lb w/cores)	1 ea	212	84	125	< 1	32	4	1	.1	t	.2
207	Raw, peeled slices	1 c	110	85	63	< 1	16	2	< 1	.1	t	.1
208	Dried, sulfured	10 ea	64	32	155	1	42	6	< 1	t	t	.1
209	Apple juice, bottled or canned	1 c	248	88	116	< 1	29	< 1	< 1	< 1	t	< .1
210	Applesauce, sweetened	1 c	255	80	193	< 1	51	3	< 1	.1	t	.1
211	Applesauce, unsweetened	1 c	244	88	104	< 1	28	3	< 1	< 1	t	t
	Apricots:											
212	Raw, w/o pits (about 12 per lb w/ pits)	3 ea	106	86	51	1	12	2	< 1	t	.2	.1
	Canned (fruit and liquid):											
213	Heavy syrup	1 c	258	78	214	1	55	3	< 1	t	.1	t
214	Halves	3 ea	85	78	70	< 1	18	1	< 1	t	t	t
215	Juice pack	1 c	248	87	119	2	30	3	< 1	t	t	t
216	Halves	3 ea	84	87	40	1	10	1	< 1	t	t	t
217	Dried, halves	10 ea	35	31	83	1	22	3	< 1	t	.1	t
218	Dried, cooked, unsweetened, w/liquid	1 c	250	76	212	3	55	9	< 1	t	.2	.1
219	Apricot nectar, canned	1 c	251	85	140	1	36	2	< 1	t	.1	t
	Avocados, raw, edible part only:											
220	California (2 lb with refuse)	1 ea	173	73	306	4	12	6	30	4.5	19.4	3.5
221	Florida (1 lb with refuse)	1 ea	304	80	340	5	27	8	27	5.3	14.8	4.5
222	Mashed, fresh, average	1 c	230	74	370	5	17	9	35	5.6	22.1	4.5
	Bananas, raw, without peel:											
223	Whole, 8¾" long (175 g w/peel)	1 ea	114	74	104	1	27	2	1	.2	t	.1
224	Slices	1 c	150	74	137	2	35	3	1	.3	.1	.1
1285	Bananas, dehydrated slices	1 oz	28	3	98	1	25	2	1	.2	t	.1
225	Blackberries, raw	1 c	144	86	75	1	18	6	1	.3	.1	.1
	Blueberries:											
226	Fresh	1 c	145	85	81	1	20	4	1	t	.2	.3
227	Frozen, sweetened	10 oz	284	77	230	1	62	6	< 1	.1	.1	.2
228	Frozen, thawed	1 c	230	77	186	1	50	5	< 1	.1	.1	.2
	Cherries:											
229	Sour, red pitted, canned water pack	1 c	244	90	88	2	22	2	< 1	.1	.1	.1
230	Sweet, red pitted, raw	10 ea	68	81	49	1	11	< 1	1	.1	.2	.2
231	Cranberry juice cocktail[1]	1 c	253	85	144	0[2]	36	< 1	< 1	.1	t	.1
1411	Cranberry juice, low calorie	¾ c	178	95	34	0	8	1	0	0	0	0
232	Cranberry-apple juice	1 c	253	83	169	< 1	43	< 1	< 1[3]	t	t	.1

[1]Data here are from the newest USDA *Handbook 8–14* on beverages. These data are somewhat different from that presented in *Handbook 8–9* on fruits and fruit juices.

[2]The newest USDA *Handbook 8–14* data on beverages indicates "0" for protein.

[3]The newest USDA *Handbook 8–14* data on beverages indicates "0" for fat.

(Computer code number is for West Diet Analysis program)

Chol (mg)	Calc (mg)	Iron (mg)	Magn (mg)	Phos (mg)	Pota (mg)	Sodi (mg)	Zinc (mg)	VT-A (RE)	Thia (mg)	Ribo (mg)	Niac (mg)	V-B6 (mg)	Fola (µg)	VT-C (mg)
0	–	–	–	–	–	249	–	–	–	–	–	–	–	–
<1	0	0	–	–	–	148	–	–	0	0	0	–	–	0
0	1	0	–	–	–	249	–	–	0	0	0	–	–	–
5	0	0	0	0	0	148	0	–	0	0	0	–	–	0
0	10	.25	7	10	159	0	.05	7	.02	.02	.11	.07	4	8
0	15	.38	11	15	244	0	.08	11	.04	.03	.16	.1	6	12
0	4	.08	3	8	124	0	.04	5	.02	.01	.1	.05	<1	4
0	9	.9	10	24	288	56[2]	.13	6	0	.1	.59	.08	0	2
0	17	.92	7	17	295	7	.07	<1	.05	.04	.25	.07	<1	2
0	10	.89	8	18	155	8	.1	3	.03	.07	.48	.07	2	4[4]
0	7	.29	7	17	183	5	.07	7	.03	.06	.46	.06	1	3[4]
0	15	.57	8	20	313	1	.28	277	.03	.04	.64	.06	9	11
0	23	.77	18	31	361	10	.28	317	.05	.06	.97	.14	4	8
0	8	.25	6	10	119	3	.09	105	.02	.02	.32	.05	1	3
0	30	.74	25	50	409	10	.27	419	.04	.05	.85	.13	4	12
0	10	.25	8	17	139	3	.09	142	.01	.02	.29	.04	1	4
0	16	1.65	16	41	482	4	.26	253	<.01	.05	1.05	.05	4	1
0	40	4.18	42	102	1222	8	.66	590	.01	.07	2.36	.28	0	4
0	18	.95	13	23	286	8	.23	331	.02	.03	.65	.05	3	2[5]
0	19	2.04	71	73	1096	21	.73	106	.19	.21	3.32	.48	113	14
0	33	1.61	103	118	1483	15	1.28	185	.33	.37	5.84	.85	162	24
0	25	2.37	90	94	1377	23	.97	140	.25	.28	4.42	.64	142	18
0	7	.35	33	23	451	1	.18	9	.05	.11	.62	.66	22	10
0	9	.46	43	30	594	2	.24	12	.07	.15	.81	.87	29	14
0	6	.33	31	21	417	1	.17	9	.05	.07	.79	.15	11	2
0	46	.82	29	30	282	0	.39	24	.04	.06	.58	.08	49	30
0	9	.25	7	14	129	9	.16	15	.07	.07	.52	.05	9	19
0	17	1.11	6	20	170	3	.17	13	.06	.15	.72	.17	19	3
0	14	.9	5	16	138	2	.14	10	.05	.12	.58	.14	15	2
0	27	3.37	15	24	239	17	.17	183	.04	.1	.43	.11	19	5
0	10	.26	7	13	152	0	.04	14	.03	.04	.27	.02	3	5
0	8	.38	5	5	45	5	.18	1	.02	.02	.09	.05	1	90[6]
0	16	.07	4	2	39	5	.04	1	.02	.02	.06	.03	<1	57
0	18	.15	5	8	68	5	.1	1	.01	.05	.15	.05	1	81[6]

[4]Value based on products without added vitamin C. Bottled apple juice with added vitamin C usually contains 41.6 mg/100 g, or 103 mg per cup. Check label for specific vitamin C values.

[5]Without added vitamin C. Products with added vitamin C contain 136 mg per cup. Check label.

[6]Nutrient added.

(For purposes of calculations, use "0" for t, <1, <.1, <.01, etc.)

TABLE I-1
FOOD COMPOSITION

Computer Code Number	Food Description	Measure	Wt (g)	H₂O (%)	Ener (cal)	Prot (g)	Carb (g)	Dietary Fiber (g)	Fat (g)	Fat Breakdown (g)		
										Sat	Mono	Poly
	FRUITS and FRUIT JUICES—Cont.											
233	Cranberry sauce, canned, strained	1 c	277	61	418	1	107	3	<1	t	.1	.2
234	Dates, whole, without pits	10 ea	83	22	228	2	61	6	<1	.2	.1	t
235	Dates, chopped	1 c	178	22	490	4	130	13	1	.3	.2	t
236	Figs, dried	10 ea	187	28	477	6	122	17	2	.4	.5	1
	Fruit cocktail, canned, fruit and liq:											
237	Heavy syrup pack	1 c	255	80	186	1	48	3	<1	t	t	.1
238	Juice pack	1 c	248	87	114	1	29	3	<1	t	t	t
	Grapefruit:											
	Raw 3¾" diam (half w/rind = 241 g)											
239	Pink/red, half fruit, edible part	1 ea	123	91	37	1	9	2	<1	t	t	t
240	White, half fruit, edible part	1 ea	118	90	39	1	10	2	<1	t	t	t
241	Canned sections with light syrup	1 c	254	84	152	1	39	1	<1	t	t	.1
	Grapefruit juice:											
242	Fresh, raw	1 c	247	90	96	1	23	<1	<1	t	t	.1
243	Canned, unsweetened	1 c	247	90	94	1	22	<1	<1	t	t	.1
244	Sweetened	1 c	250	87	115	1	28	<1	<1	t	t	.1
	Frozen concentrate, unsweetened:											
245	Undiluted, 6-fl-oz can	¾ c	207	62	302	4	71	1	1	.1	.1	.2
246	Diluted with 3 cans water	1 c	247	89	101	1	24	<1	<1	.1	t	.1
	Grapes, raw European (adherent skin):											
247	Thompson seedless	10 ea	50	81	35	<1	9	<1	<1	.1	t	.1
248	Tokay/Emperor, seeded types	10 ea	57	81	40	<1	10	<1	<1	.1	t	.1
	Grape juice:											
249	Bottled or canned	1 c	253	84	154	1	38	2	<1	.1	t	.1
	Frozen concentrate, sweetened:											
250	Undiluted, 6-fl-oz can	¾ c	216	54	387	1	96	<1	1	.2	t	.2
251	Diluted with 3 cans water	1 c	250	87	127	<1	32	<1	<1	.1	t	.1
1410	Low calorie	1 c	250	84	153	1	37	<1	<1	.1	t	.1
252	Kiwi fruit, raw, peeled (88 g with peel)	1 ea	76	83	46	1	11	1	<1	t	.1	.1
253	Lemons, raw, without peel and seeds (about 4 per lb whole)	1 ea	58	89	17	1	5	2	<1	t	t	.1
	Lemon juice:											
254	Fresh:	1 c	244	91	61	1	21	1	<1	.1	t	.2
255	Tablespoon	1 tbs	15	91	4	<1	1	<1	<1	t	t	t
256	Canned or bottled, unsweetened:	1 c	244	93	51	1	16	1	1	.1	t	.2
257	Tablespoon	1 tbs	15	93	3	<1	1	<1	<1	t	t	t
258	Frozen, single strength, unsweetened:	1 c	244	92	54	1	16	1	1	.1	t	.2
259	Tablespoon	1 tbs	15	92	3	<1	1	<1	<1	t	t	t
	Lime juice:											
260	Fresh:	1 c	246	90	66	1	22	1	<1	t	t	.1
261	Tablespoon	1 tbs	15	90	4	<1	1	<1	<1	t	t	t
262	Canned or bottled, unsweetened	1 c	246	93	52	1	16	1	1	.1	.1	.2
263	Mangoes, raw, edible part (300 g w/skin & seeds)	1 ea	207	82	134	1	35	6	1	.1	.2	.1

(Computer code number is for West Diet Analysis program)

Chol (mg)	Calc (mg)	Iron (mg)	Magn (mg)	Phos (mg)	Pota (mg)	Sodi (mg)	Zinc (mg)	VT-A (RE)	Thia (mg)	Ribo (mg)	Niac (mg)	V-B6 (mg)	Fola (μg)	VT-C (mg)
0	11	.61	8	17	72	80	.14	6	.04	.06	.28	.04	2	6
0	27	.95	29	33	541	2	.24	4	.07	.08	1.83	.16	10	0
0	57	2.05	62	71	1160	5	.52	9	.16	.18	3.92	.34	22	0
0	269	4.19	110	127	1331	21	.95	24	.13	.16	1.3	.42	14	2
0	15	.74	13	28	224	15	.2	51	.05	.05	.95	.13	7	5
0	20	.52	17	35	235	10	.22	77	.03	.04	1	.13	6	7
0	13	.15	10	11	159	0	.09	32[1]	.04	.02	.23	.05	15	47
0	14	.07	11	9	175	0	.08	1	.04	.02	.32	.05	12	39
0	36	1.02	25	25	328	5	.2	2	.1	.05	.62	.05	22	54
0	22	.49	30	37	400	2	.12	2[2]	.1	.05	.49	.11	25	94
0	17	.49	25	27	378	2	.22	2	.1	.05	.57	.05	26	72
0	20	.9	25	27	405	5	.15	2	.1	.06	.8	.05	26	67
0	56	1.01	79	101	1001	6	.37	6	.3	.16	1.6	.32	26	248
0	20	.35	27	35	336	2	.12	2	.1	.05	.54	.11	9	83
0	6	.13	3	7	92	1	.03	3	.05	.03	.15	.05	2	5
0	6	.15	3	7	105	1	.03	4	.05	.03	.17	.06	2	6
0	23	.61	25	28	334	8	.13	3	.07	.09	.66	.16	7	<1
0	28	.78	32	32	159	15	.28	6	.11	.2	.93	.32	9	179[3]
0	10	.25	10	10	52	5	.1	2	.04	.06	.31	.1	3	60[3]
0	22	.6	25	27	330	8	.12	2	.06	.09	.65	.16	6	<1
0	20	.31	23	30	252	4	.08[4]	13	.01	.04	.38	.04	17	74
0	15	.35	5	9	80	1	.03	2	.02	.01	.06	.05	6	31
0	17	.07	15	15	303	2	.12	5	.07	.02	.24	.12	31	112
0	1	0	1	1	19	<1	.01	<1	0	0	.01	.01	2	7
0	27	.32	19	22	249	51	.15	4	.1	.02	.48	.1	25	60
0	2	.02	1	1	15	3	.01	<1	.01	0	.03	.01	2	4
0	19	.29	19	19	217	2	.12	3	.14	.03	.33	.15	23	77
0	1	.02	1	1	13	<1	.01	<1	.01	0	.02	.01	1	5
0	22	.07	15	17	268	2	.15	2	.05	.02	.25	.11	20	72
0	1	0	1	1	16	<1	.01	<1	0	0	.01	.01	1	4
0	29	.57	17	25	184	39[5]	.15	4	.08	.01	.4	.07	19	16
0	21	.27	19	23	323	4	.08	805	.12	.12	1.21	.28	39	57

[1]Vitamin A in Texas red grapefruit would be 74 RE.

[2]This is vitamin A for white grapefruit juice; pink or red grapefruit juice = 109 RE per cup.

[3]With added vitamin C (ascorbic acid).

[4]Data are estimated from other fruit data.

[5]Sodium benzoate and sodium bisulfite added as preservatives.

(For purposes of calculations, use "0" for t, < 1, < .1, < .01, etc.)

Table I-1
Food Composition

Computer Code Number	Food Description	Measure	Wt (g)	H₂O (%)	Ener (cal)	Prot (g)	Carb (g)	Dietary Fiber (g)	Fat (g)	Fat Breakdown (g)		
										Sat	Mono	Poly
	FRUITS and FRUIT JUICES—Cont.											
	Melons, raw, without rind and contents:											
264	Cantaloupe, 5" diam (2 ⅓ lb whole with refuse), orange flesh	½ ea	267	90	93	2	22	2	1	.1	.1	.2
265	Honeydew, 6½" diam (5¼ lb whole with refuse), slice = ¹⁄₁₀ melon	1 pce	129	90	45	1	12	1	<1	t	t	t
266	Nectarines, raw, w/o pits, 2½" diam	1 ea	136	86	67	1	16	2	1	.1	.2	.3
	Oranges, raw:											
267	Whole w/o peel and seeds, 2 ⅝" diam (180 g with peel and seeds)	1 ea	131	87	62	1	15	3	<1	t	t	t
268	Sections, without membranes	1 c	180	87	85	2	21	4	<1	t	t	t
	Orange juice:											
269	Fresh, all varieties	1 c	248	88	112	2	26	<1	<1	.1	.1	.1
270	Canned, unsweetened	1 c	249	89	105	1	24	<1	<1	t	.1	.1
271	Chilled	1 c	249	88	110	2	25	<1	1	.1	.1	.2
	Frozen concentrate:											
272	Undiluted (6-oz can)	¾ c	213	58	339	5	81	2	<1	.1	.1	.1
273	Diluted w/3 parts water by volume	1 c	249	88	112	2	27	<1	<1	t	t	t
1345	Orange juice, from dry crystals	1 c	248	88	114	0	29	0	<1	t	t	t
274	Orange and grapefruit juice, canned	1 c	247	89	106	1	25	<1	<1	t	t	t
	Papayas, raw:											
275	½" slices	1 c	140	89	54	1	14	3	<1	.1	.1	t
276	Whole, 3½" diam by 5⅛" w/o seeds and skin (1 lb w/refuse)	1 ea	304	89	118	2	30	5	<1	.1	.1	.1
1031	Papaya nectar, canned	1 c	250	85	142	<1	36	2	<1	.1	.1	.1
	Peaches:											
277	Raw, whole, 2½" diam, peeled, pitted (about 4 per lb whole)	1 ea	87	88	37	1	10	2	<1	t	t	t
278	Raw, sliced	1 c	170	88	73	1	19	3	<1	t	.1	.1
	Canned, fruit and liquid:											
279	Heavy syrup pack:	1 c	256	79	189	1	51	3	<1	t	.1	.1
280	Half	1 ea	81	79	60	<1	16	1	<1	t	t	t
281	Juice pack:	1 c	248	88	109	2	29	4	<1	t	t	t
282	Half	1 ea	77	88	34	<1	9	1	<1	t	t	t
283	Dried, uncooked	10 ea	130	32	311	5	80	12	1	.1	.4	.5
284	Dried, cooked, fruit and liquid	1 c	258	78	198	3	51	7	1	.1	.2	.3
	Frozen, slice, sweetened:											
285	10-oz package	1 ea	284	75	266	2	68	4	<1	t	.1	.2
286	Cup, thawed measure	1 c	250	75	235	2	60	4	<1	t	.1	.2
1032	Peach nectar, canned	1 c	249	86	134	1	35	1	<1	t	t	t
	Pears:											
	Fresh, with skin, cored:											
287	Bartlett, 2½" diam (about 2½ per lb)	1 ea	166	84	98	1	25	4[1]	1	t	.1	.2
288	Bosc, 2 1/5" diam (about 3 per lb)	1 ea	141	84	83	1	21	3[1]	1	t	.1	.1
289	D'Anjou, 3" diam (about 2 per lb)	1 ea	200	84	118	1	30	5[1]	1	t	.2	.2
	Canned, fruit and liquid:											
290	Heavy syrup pack:	1 c	255	80	188	1	49	5[1]	<1	t	.1	.1
291	Half	1 ea	79	80	58	<1	15	2[1]	<1	t	t	t
292	Juice pack:	1 c	248	86	124	1	32	5[1]	<1	t	t	t
293	Half	1 ea	77	86	38	<1	10	2[1]	<1	t	t	t

[1]Dietary fiber data vary 2.4 to 3.4 g/100 g for fresh pears; 1.6 to 2.6 g/100 g for canned pears.

(Computer code number is for West Diet Analysis program)

Chol (mg)	Calc (mg)	Iron (mg)	Magn (mg)	Phos (mg)	Pota (mg)	Sodi (mg)	Zinc (mg)	VT-A (RE)	Thia (mg)	Ribo (mg)	Niac (mg)	V-B6 (mg)	Fola (µg)	VT-C (mg)
0	29	.56	29	45	825	24	.43	860	.1	.06	1.53	.31	45	113
0	8	.09	9	13	350	13	.11	5	.1	.02	.77	.08	39	32
0	7	.2	11	22	288	0	.12	101	.02	.06	1.35	.03	5	7
0	52	.13	13	18	237	0	.09	27	.11	.05	.37	.08	40	70
0	72	.18	18	25	326	0	.13	38	.16	.07	.51	.11	54	96
0	27	.5	27	42	496	2	.12	50	.22	.07	.99	.1	75	124
0	20	1.1	27	35	436	5	.17	45	.15	.07	.78	.22	45	86
0	25	.42	27	27	473	3	.1	20[2]	.19	.28	.05	.7	45[2]	82[2]
0	68	.75	72	121	1435	6	.38	59	.6	.14	1.53	.33	330	294
0	22	.25	25	40	473	3	.12	20	.2	.04	.5	.11	109	97
0	62	.2	2	37	50	12	.1	551	0	.04	0	0	142	121
0	20	1.14	25	35	390	7	.17	30	.14	.07	.83	.06	35	72
0	34	.14	14	7	360	4	.1	39	.04	.04	.47	.03	53	86
0	73	.3	30	15	781	9	.21	85	.08	.1	1.03	.06	115	187
0	25	.85	7	0	77	13	.37	27	.01	.01	.37	.02	5	8
0	4	.1	6	10	171	0	.12	47	.01	.04	.86	.02	3	6
0	8	.19	12	20	335	0	.24	92	.03	.07	1.68	.03	6	11
0	8	.69	13	28	235	15	.23	84	.03	.06	1.57	.05	8	7
0	2	.22	4	9	74	5	.07	27	.01	.02	.5	.01	3	2
0	15	.67	17	42	317	10	.27	94	.02	.04	1.44	.05	8	9
0	5	.21	5	13	99	3	.08	29	.01	.01	.45	.01	3	3
0	36	5.28	55	153	1293	9	.74	281	< .01	.28	5.69	.09	< 1	6
0	23	3.38	33	98	826	5	.46	52	.01	.05	3.92	.1	< 1	10
0	9	1.05	14	31	369	17	.14	81	.04	.1	1.85	.05	9	267[3]
0	8	.92	12	27	325	15	.12	71	.03	.09	1.63	.04	8	236[3]
0	12	.47	10	15	100	17	.2	64	.01	.03	.72	.02	3	13
0	18	.41	10	18	208	0	.2	3	.03	.07	.17	.03	12	7
0	16	.35	8	16	176	0	.17	3	.03	.06	.14	.02	10	6
0	22	.5	12	22	250	0	.24	4	.04	.08	.2	.04	15	8
0	13	.56	10	18	165	13	.2	1	.03	.06	.62	.04	3	3
0	4	.17	3	6	51	4	.06	< 1	.01	.02	.19	.01	1	1
0	22	.72	17	30	238	10	.22	2	.03	.03	.5	.03	3	4
0	7	.22	5	9	74	3	.07	1	.01	.01	.15	.01	1	1

[2]Values for juice from California oranges indicate the following values for 1 c: 36 RE of vitamin A, 72 µg of folate, and 106 mg of vitamin C.

[3]With added vitamin C (ascorbic acid).

(For purposes of calculations, use "0" for t, < 1, < .1, < .01, etc.)

TABLE I–1
FOOD COMPOSITION

Computer Code Number	Food Description	Measure	Wt (g)	H$_2$O (%)	Ener (cal)	Prot (g)	Carb (g)	Dietary Fiber (g)	Fat (g)	Fat Breakdown (g)		
										Sat	Mono	Poly
	FRUITS and FRUIT JUICES—Cont.											
294	Dried halves	10 ea	175	27	459	3	121	13	1	.1	.2	.3
1033	Pear nectar, canned	1 c	250	84	150	< 1	39	2	< 1	t	t	t
	Pineapple:											
295	Fresh chunks, diced	1 c	155	87	76	1	19	2	1	t	.1	.2
	Canned, fruit and liquid:											
	Heavy syrup pack:											
296	Crushed, chunks, tidbits	⅓ c	84	79	65	< 1	17	1	< 1	t	t	t
297	Slices	1 ea	58	79	45	< 1	12	< 1	< 1	t	t	t
	Pineapple, canned—Cont.											
298	Juice pack, crushed, chunks, tidbits	1 c	250	84	150	1	39	2	< 1	t	t	.1
299	Juice pack, slices	1 ea	58	84	35	< 1	9	< 1	< 1	t	t	t
300	Pineapple juice, canned, unsweetened	1 c	250	86	140	1	35	< 1	< 1	t	t	.1
	Plantains, without peel:											
301	Raw slices (whole = 179 g w/o peel)	1 c	148	65	181	2	47	3[1]	1	.3	.1	.1
302	Cooked, boiled, sliced	1 c	154	67	179	1	48	4	< 1	.1	t	.1
	Plums:											
303	Fresh, medium, 2⅛" diam	1 ea	66	85	36	1	9	1	< 1	t	.3	.1
304	Fresh, small, 1½" diam	1 ea	28	85	15	< 1	4	< 1	< 1	t	.1	t
	Canned, purple, with liquid:											
305	Heavy syrup pack:	1 c	258	76	229	1	60	3	< 1	t	.2	.1
306	Plums	3 ea	110	76	98	< 1	26	1	< 1	t	.1	t
307	Juice pack:	1 c	252	84	146	1	38	3	< 1	t	t	t
308	Plums	3 ea	95	84	55	< 1	14	1	< 1	t	t	t
1698	Pomegranate, fresh	1 ea	154	81	105	1	27	5	< 1	–	–	–
	Prunes, dried, pitted:											
309	Uncooked (10 = 97 g w/pits, 84 g w/o pits)	10 ea	84	32	200	2	53	8[2]	< 1	t	.3	.1
310	Cooked, unsweetened, fruit & liq (250 g w/pits)	1c	212	70	227	3	60	14	< 1	t	.3	.1
311	Prune juice, bottled or canned	1c	256	81	182	2	45	3	1	t	.5	t
	Raisins, seedless:											
312	Cup, not pressed down	1 c	145	15	435	5	115	5	1	.2	t	.2
313	One packet, ½ oz	½ oz	14	15	42	< 1	11	1	< 1	t	t	t
	Raspberries:											
314	Fresh	1 c	123	87	60	1	14	5	1	t	.1	.4
315	Frozen, sweetened:	10 oz	284	73	293	2	74	13	< 1	t	t	.3
316	Cup, thawed measure	1 c	250	73	258	2	66	11	< 1	t	t	.2
317	Rhubarb, cooked, added sugar	1 c	240	68	278	1	75	5	< 1	t	t	.1
	Strawberries:											
318	Fresh, whole, capped	1 c	149	92	45	1	10	2	1	t	.1	.3
	Frozen, sliced, sweetened:											
319	10-oz container	10 oz	284	73	272	2	74	5	< 1	t	.1	.2
320	Cup, thawed measure	1 c	255	73	244	1	66	5	< 1	t	t	.2
	Tangerines, without peel and seeds:											
321	Fresh (2⅜" whole) 116 g w/refuse	1 ea	84	88	37	1	9	1	< 1	t	t	t
322	Canned, light syrup, fruit and liquid	1 c	252	83	153	1	41	2	< 1	t	t	t
323	Tangerine juice, canned, sweetened	1 c	249	87	124	1	30	< 1	< 1	t	t	.1

[1] Dietary fiber value partially derived from data for bananas.

[2] Dietary fiber data can vary between 6 and 13 g for 10 prunes.

(Computer code number is for West Diet Analysis program)

Chol (mg)	Calc (mg)	Iron (mg)	Magn (mg)	Phos (mg)	Pota (mg)	Sodi (mg)	Zinc (mg)	VT-A (RE)	Thia (mg)	Ribo (mg)	Niac (mg)	V-B6 (mg)	Fola (µg)	VT-C (mg)
0	59	3.68	58	103	933	10	.68	1	.01	.25	2.4	.13	0	12
0	12	.65	7	7	32	10	.17	<1	<.01	.03	.32	.03	3	3
0	11	.57	22	11	175	2	.12	4	.14	.06	.65	.13	16	24
0	12	.32	13	6	87	1	.1	1	.08	.02	.24	.06	4	6
0	8	.22	9	4	60	1	.07	1	.05	.01	.17	.04	3	4
0	35	.7	35	15	305	3	.25	10	.24	.05	.71	.18	12	24
0	8	.16	8	3	71	1	.06	2	.05	.01	.16	.04	3	6
0	42	.65	32	20	335	3	.27	1	.14	.05	.64	.24	58	27[3]
0	4	.89	55	50	739	6	.21	167[4]	.08	.08	1.02	.44	33	27
0	3	.89	49	43	716	8	.2	140	.07	.08	1.16	.37	40	17
0	3	.07	5	7	113	0	.07	21	.03	.06	.33	.05	1	6
0	1	.03	2	3	48	0	.03	9	.01	.03	.14	.02	1	3
0	23	2.17	13	33	234	49	.18	67	.04	.1	.75	.07	6	1
0	10	.92	5	14	100	21	.08	29	.02	.04	.32	.03	3	<1
0	25	.86	20	38	388	3	.28	255	.06	.15	1.19	.07	7	7
0	10	.32	8	14	146	1	.1	96	.02	.06	.45	.03	2	3
0	5	.46	5	12	399	5	–	0	.05	.05	.46	.16	–	9
0	43	2.08	38	66	625	3	.44	167	.07	.14	1.65	.22	3	3
0	49	2.35	42	74	708	4	.51	65	.05	.21	1.53	.46	<1	6
0	31	3	36	64	707	10	.54	1	.04	.18	2	.56	1	11
0	71	3.02	48	141	1088	17	.39	1	.23	.13	1.19	.36	5	5
0	7	.29	5	14	105	2	.04	<1	.02	.01	.11	.03	<1	<1
0	27	.7	22	15	186	0	.57	16	.04	.11	1.11	.07	32	31
0	43	1.85	37	48	324	3	.51	17	.05	.13	.65	.1	74	47
0	37	1.63	32	42	285	3	.45	15	.05	.11	.57	.08	65	41
0	348	.5	29	19	230	2	.19	17	.04	.05	.48	.05	13	8
0	21	.57	15	28	247	1	.19	4	.03	.1	.34	.09	26	84
0	31	1.68	20	37	278	9	.17	7	.04	.14	1.14	.08	42	117
0	28	1.51	18	33	250	8	.15	6	.04	.13	1.02	.08	38	105
0	12	.08	10	8	131	1	.2	77	.09	.02	.13	.06	17	26
0	18	.93	20	25	196	15	.6	212	.13	.11	1.12	.11	12	50
0	45	.5	20	35	443	3	.07	105	.15	.05	.25	.08	11	55

[3]If vitamin C is added, it contains 96 mg per cup.

[4]Vitamin A values range from 1.5 RE for white-fleshed varieties to 178 RE for yellow-fleshed varieties.

(For purposes of calculations, use "0" for t, <1, <.1, <.01, etc.)

TABLE I–1
FOOD COMPOSITION

Computer Code Number	Food Description	Measure	Wt (g)	H₂O (%)	Ener (cal)	Prot (g)	Carb (g)	Dietary Fiber (g)	Fat (g)	Fat Breakdown (g)		
										Sat	Mono	Poly
	FRUITS and FRUIT JUICES—Cont.											
	Watermelon, raw, without rind & seeds:											
324	Piece, 1" by 10" diam (2 lb w/refuse or 926 g)	1 pce	482	91	154	3	35	1	2	.6	.4	1.1
325	Diced	1 c	160	91	51	1	11	1	1	.2	.1	.4
	BAKED GOODS: BREADS, CAKES, COOKIES, CRACKERS, PIES											
326	Bagels, plain, enriched, 3½" diam	1 ea	68	33	187	7	36	2	1	.1	.1	.5
1663	Bagel, oat bran	1 ea	68	33	173	7	36	8	1	.1	.2	.3
	Biscuits:											
327	From home recipe	1 ea	28	29	100	2	13	<1	5	1.2	2	1.2
328	From mix	1 ea	28	29	94	2	14	1	3	.8	1.2	1.2
329	From refrigerated dough	1 ea	20	27	75	1	9	<1	4	2	1	.1
330	Bread crumbs, dry, grated (see #364, 365 for soft crumbs)	1 c	100	6	395	12	72	4	5	1.3	2.1	2
	Breads:											
331	Boston brown, canned, 3¼" slice	1 pce	45	47	88	2	19	2	1	.1	.1	.3
332	Cracked wheat (¼ cracked-wheat & ¾ enr wheat flour): 1-lb loaf	1 ea	454	36	1180	39	225	27	18	4.2	8.6	3.1
333	Slice (18 per loaf)	1 pce	25	36	65	2	12	2	1	.2	.5	.2
334	Slice, toasted	1 pce	21	30	59	2	11	1	1	.2	.4	.2
335	French/Vienna, enriched: 1-lb loaf	1 ea	454	34	1243	40	236	13	14	2.9	5.5	3.1
337	Slice, 4¾ x 4 x ½"	1 pce	25	34	68	2	13	1	1	.2	.3	.2
336	French, slice, 5 x 2½"	1 pce	35	34	96	3	18	1	1	.2	.4	.2
	French toast: see Mixed Dishes, and Fast Foods, #691											
2083	Honey Wheatberry	1 pce	38	2	100	3	18	2	2	0	.5	0
338	Italian, enriched: 1-lb loaf	1 ea	454	36	1230	40	227	14	16	3.9	3.7	6.3
339	Slice, 4½ x 3¼ x ¾"	1 pce	30	36	81	3	15	1	1	.3	.2	.4
340	Mixed grain, enriched: 1-lb loaf	1 ea	454	38	1135	45	211	32	17	3.7	6.9	4.2
341	Slice (18 per loaf)	1 pce	25	38	62	3	12	2	1	.2	.4	.2
342	Slice, toasted	1 pce	23	32	63	3	12	2	1	.2	.4	.2
343	Oatmeal, enriched: 1-lb loaf	1 ea	454	37	1221	38	220	18	20	3.2	7.2	7.7
344	Slice (18 per loaf)	1 pce	25	37	67	2	12	1	1	.2	.4	.4
345	Slice, toasted	1 pce	23	31	67	2	12	1	1	.2	.4	.4
346	Pita pocket bread, enr, 6½" round	1 ea	60	32	165	5	33	1	1	.1	.1	.3
347	Pumpernickel (⅔ rye & ⅓ enr wheat flour): 1-lb loaf	1 ea	454	38	1135	39	216	33	14	2	4.2	5.6
348	Slice, 5 x 4 x ⅜"	1 pce	32	38	80	3	15	2	1	.1	.3	.4
349	Slice, toasted	1 pce	29	32	80	3	15	2	1	.1	.3	.4
350	Raisin, enriched: 1-lb loaf	1 ea	454	34	1243	36	237	20	20	4.9	10.4	3.1
351	Slice (18 per loaf)	1 pce	25	34	68	2	13	1	1	.3	.6	.2
352	Slice, toasted	1 pce	21	28	62	2	12	1	1	.2	.5	.2
353	Rye, light (⅓ rye & ⅔ enr wheat flour): 1-lb loaf	1 ea	454	37	1177	39	219	28	15	2.8	6	3.6
354	Slice, 4¾ x 3¾ x ⁷⁄₁₆"	1 pce	25	37	65	2	12	2	1	.2	.3	.2
355	Slice, toasted	1 pce	22	31	62	2	12	2	1	.2	.3	.2

[1]A blend of white and whole-wheat flour—no official ratio specified.

(Computer code number is for West Diet Analysis program)

Chol (mg)	Calc (mg)	Iron (mg)	Magn (mg)	Phos (mg)	Pota (mg)	Sodi (mg)	Zinc (mg)	VT-A (RE)	Thia (mg)	Ribo (mg)	Niac (mg)	V-B6 (mg)	Fola (µg)	VT-C (mg)
0	39	.82	53	43	559	10	.34	178	.39	.1	.96	.69	11	46
0	13	.27	18	14	186	3	.11	59	.13	.03	.32	.23	4	15
0	50	2.43	20	65	69	363	.6	0	.37	.21	3.1	.03	15	0
0	8	2.1	39	112	139	345	1.42	< 1	.23	.23	2.01	.14	31	< 1
1	67	.81	5	46	34	163	.15	6	.1	.09	.84	.01	3	< 1
1	52	.58	7	131	53	267	.17	7	.1	.1	.86	.02	2	< 1
1	24	.44	2	70	23	158	.08	7	.07	.05	.44	.01	2	0
0	227	6.13	46	147	221	862	1.23	.1	.76	.43	6.85	.1	25	0
< 1	31	.95	28	50	143	284	.22	5	.01	.05	.5	.04	3	0
0	195	12.8	236	695	804	2452	5.68	0	1.63	1.09	16.7	1.38	177	0
0	11	.7	13	38	44	135	.31	0	.09	.06	.92	.08	10	0
0	10	.64	12	35	40	123	.29	0	.07	.05	.75	.06	6	0
0	341	11.5	123	477	513	2764	3.95	0	2.36	1.49	21.6	.19	141	0
0	19	.63	7	26	28	152	.22	0	.13	.08	1.19	.01	8	0
0	26	.89	9	37	40	213	.3	0	.18	.11	1.66	.01	11	0
0	20	.72	–	–	–	200	–	0	.12	.07	.8	–	–	0
0	354	13.4	123	468	499	2648	3.9	0	2.15	1.33	19.9	.22	136	0
0	23	.88	8	31	33	175	.26	0	.14	.09	1.31	.01	9	0
0	413	15.8	241	799	926	2216	5.81	0	1.85	1.55	19.8	1.51	218	1
0	23	.87	13	44	51	122	.32	0	.1	.09	1.09	.08	12	< 1
0	23	.87	13	44	51	122	.32	0	.08	.08	.98	.07	9	< 1
0	300	12.3	168	572	645	2724	4.68	9	1.81	1.09	14.3	.31	123	2
0	16	.68	9	32	36	150	.26	< 1	.1	.06	.78	.02	7	< 1
0	17	.68	9	32	35	150	.26	< 1	.08	.05	.71	.01	5	< 1
0	52	1.58	16	58	72	322	.5	0	.36	.2	2.78	.02	14	0
0	309	13.1	245	808	944	3050	6.76	0	1.48	1.38	14	.57	155	0
0	22	.92	17	57	67	215	.48	0	.1	.1	.99	.04	11	0
0	22	.92	17	57	66	214	.47	0	.08	.09	.89	.04	8	0
0	300	13.2	118	495	1030	1770	3.27	.9	1.54	1.81	15.8	.31	154	2
0	17	.73	7	27	57	97	.18	.05	.08	.1	.87	.02	9	< 1
0	15	.66	6	25	52	89	.16	.42	.06	.08	.71	.01	5	< 1
0	331	12.9	182	568	754	2996	5.22	0	1.97	1.52	17.3	.34	232	0
0	18	.71	10	31	42	165	.29	0	.11	.08	.95	.02	13	0
0	18	.68	9	30	40	160	.28	0	.08	.07	.83	.02	9	< 1

(For purposes of calculations, use "0" for t, < 1, < .1, < .01, etc.)

TABLE I–1
FOOD COMPOSITION

Computer Code Number	Food Description	Measure	Wt (g)	H₂O (%)	Ener (cal)	Prot (g)	Carb (g)	Dietary Fiber (g)	Fat (g)	Fat Breakdown (g) Sat	Mono	Poly
	BAKED GOODS: BREADS, CAKES, COOKIES, CRACKERS, PIES—Cont.											
356	Wheat (enr wheat & whole-wheat flour):[1] 1-lb loaf	1 ea	454	37	1180	41	213	25	19	3.9	7.3	4.5
357	Slice (18 per loaf)	1 pce	25	37	64	2	12	1	1	.2	.4	.2
358	Slice, toasted	1 pce	23	32	65	2	12	1	1	.2	.4	.2
359	White, enriched: 1-lb loaf	1 ea	454	37	1213	38	225	12	16	3.7	7.3	3.4
360	Slice (18 per loaf)	1 pce	25	37	67	2	12	1	1	.2	.4	.2
361	Slice, toasted	1 pce	22	30	64	2	12	1	1	.2	.4	.2
362	Slice (22 per loaf)	1 pce	20	37	53	2	10	1	1	.2	.3	.2
363	Slice, toasted	1 pce	17	30	50	2	9	< 1	1	.2	.3	.1
364	White bread cubes, soft	1 c	30	36	81	3	15	1	1	.2	.5	.2
365	White bread crumbs, soft	1 c	45	36	120	4	23	1	1	.3	.6	.4
366	Whole-wheat: 1-lb loaf	1 ea	454	38	1116	44	209	28	19	4.2	7.6	4.5
367	Slice (16 per loaf)	1 pce	28	38	69	3	13	2	1	.3	.5	.3
368	Slice, toasted	1 pce	25	30	69	3	13	2	1	.3	.5	.3
	Bread stuffing, prepared from mix:											
369	Dry type	1 c	140	65	249	4	30	4	12	2.4	5.3	3.6
370	Moist type, with egg and margarine	1 c	203	65	341	8	45	4	15	3	6.5	4.3
	Cakes, prepared from mixes:[1] Angel food:											
371	Whole cake, 9¾" diam tube	1 ea	635	33	1641	38	367	10	5	.8	.5	2.3
372	Piece, 1/12 of cake	1 pce	53	33	137	3	31	1	< 1	.1	t	.2
373	Boston cream pie, 1/8 of cake	1 pce	120	45	302	3	52	2	10	3	5.3	1.2
	Coffee cake:											
374	Whole cake, 7¾ x 5⅛ x 1¼"	1 ea	430	31	1368	24	227	7	41	8	16.6	13.6
375	Piece, 1/6 of cake	1 pce	72	31	229	4	38	1	7	1.3	2.8	2.3
	Devil's food, chocolate frosting:											
376	Whole cake, 2 layer, 8 or 9" diam	1 ea	1107	23	4059	45	605	31	182	51.4	99.6	21.1
377	Piece, 1/16 of cake	1 pce	69	23	253	3	38	2	11	3.2	6.2	1.3
378	Cupcake, 2½" diam	1 ea	42	23	154	2	23	1	7	1.9	3.8	.8
	Gingerbread:											
379	Whole cake, 8" square	1 ea	570	33	1764	23	289	18	58	14.8	21.9	7.6
380	Piece, 1/9 of cake	1 pce	63	33	195	3	32	2	6	1.6	3.5	.8
	Yellow, chocolate frosting, 2 layer:											
381	Whole cake, 8 or 9" diam	1 ea	1108	22	4207	42	613	20	193	52.4	107	23.2
382	Piece, 1/16 of cake	1 pce	69	22	262	3	38	1	12	3.3	6.7	1.4
	Cakes from recipes w/enr flour: Carrot cake, cream cheese frosting:[2]											
383	Whole, 9 x 13" cake	1 ea	1536	21	6693	71	725	20	406	75.1	100	208
384	Piece, 1/16 of cake, 2¼ x 3¼" slice	1 pce	112	23	488	5	53	1	30	5.5	7.3	15.2
	Fruitcake, dark:											
385	Whole cake, 7½" diam tube, 2¼" high	1 ea	1361	25	4409	39	838	48	124	15.2	56.8	44.1
386	Piece, 1/32 of cake, ⅔" arc	1 pce	43	25	139	1	26	2	4	.5	1.8	1.4
	Sheet, plain, no frosting:[3]											
387	Whole cake, 9" square	1 ea	777	23	2773	42	444	6	96	25	41.3	24.5
388	Piece, 1/9 of cake	1 pce	86	23	307	5	48	< 1	11	3.3	5	2.8

[1]Excepting angel food cake, cakes were made from mixes containing vegetable shortening, and frostings were made with margarine. All mixes use enriched flour.

[2]Made with vegetable oil.

[3]Cake made with vegetable shortening.

[4]Made with margarine.

(Computer code number is for West Diet Analysis program)

Chol (mg)	Calc (mg)	Iron (mg)	Magn (mg)	Phos (mg)	Pota (mg)	Sodi (mg)	Zinc (mg)	VT-A (RE)	Thia (mg)	Ribo (mg)	Niac (mg)	V-B6 (mg)	Fola (µg)	VT-C (mg)
0	476	15	209	681	913	2414	4.77	0	2	1.28	18.7	.49	185	0
0	26	.83	12	38	50	133	.26	0	.11	.08	1.13	.03	11	0
0	26	.83	12	38	50	132	.26	0	.08	.06	.93	.02	7	0
5	490	12.9	109	427	541	2452	2.81	0	2.13	1.5	17	.29	154	0
<1	27	.71	6	24	30	135	.15	0	.12	.09	.99	.01	9	0
<1	26	.73	6	23	29	130	.15	0	.09	.08	.86	.01	6	0
<1	22	.57	5	19	24	108	.12	0	.09	.07	.75	.01	7	0
<1	20	.57	4	18	22	101	.12	0	.07	.06	.67	.01	4	0
<1	25	.84	6	28	32	151	.19	0	.14	.1	1.19	.02	10	0
<1	38	1.3	9	44	48	227	.28	0	.18	.11	1.5	.15	16	0
0	327	15	390	1039	1144	2382	8.85	0	1.59	.93	17.4	.81	227	0
0	20	.94	24	64	72	147	.55	0	.1	.06	1.09	.05	14	0
0	20	.93	24	65	71	148	.55	0	.08	.05	.97	.05	10	0
0	45	1.54	17	59	104	760	.39	113	.19	.15	2.07	.06	24	0
0	130	3.35	30	99	266	936	.65	140	.34	.29	3.23	.11	35	3
0	889	3.3	76	1473	591	4756	.44	0	.65	3.12	5.61	.2	19	0
0	74	.28	6	123	49	397	.04	0	.05	.26	.47	.02	2	0
44	28	.46	7	59	47	173	.19	28	.49	.32	.23	.03	10	<1
211	585	6.19	77	925	482	1810	1.94	172	.72	.75	6.54	.21	52	1
35	98	1.04	13	155	81	303	.32	29	.12	.13	1.09	.04	9	<1
509	476	24.5	376	1350	2214	3690	7.64	310	.3	1.47	6.39	.41	89	1
32	30	1.52	23	84	138	230	.48	19	.02	.09	.4	.03	6	<1
19	18	.93	14	51	84	140	.29	12	.01	.06	.24	.02	3	<1
200	393	18.9	91	958	1375	2615	2.34	91	1.08	1.06	8.89	.22	57	1
22	43	2.09	10	106	152	289	.26	10	.12	.12	.98	.02	6	<1
609	410	23.2	332	1783	1975	3742	6.87	299	1.33	1.74	13.9	.32	89	1
38	25	1.44	21	111	123	233	.43	19	.08	.11	.86	.02	6	<1
829	384	19.4	276	1090	1714	3	7.53	5897	2.09	2.4	15.5	1.17	184	17
60	28	1.41	20	79	125	276	.55	480	.15	.17	1.13	.08	13	1
68	449	28.3	218	708	2082	3674	3.67	475	.68	1.35	10.8	.63	41	5
2	14	.89	7	22	66	116	.12	15	.02	.04	.34	.02	1	<1
505	497	11.7	108	793	613	2331	2.75	130	1.24	1.4	10.1	.26	54	2
56	55	1.3	12	88	68	258	.3	14	.14	.15	1.12	.03	6	<1

(For purposes of calculations, use "0" for t, <1, <.1, <.01, etc.)

TABLE I–1
FOOD COMPOSITION

Computer Code Number	Food Description	Measure	Wt (g)	H_2O (%)	Ener (cal)	Prot (g)	Carb (g)	Dietary Fiber (g)	Fat (g)	Fat Breakdown (g) Sat	Mono	Poly
	BAKED GOODS: BREADS, CAKES, COOKIES, CRACKERS, PIES—Cont.											
	Sheet, plain, uncooked white frosting:[4]											
389	Whole cake, 9" square	1 ea	1096	22	4085	38	644	10	159	26.1	67	56.1
390	Piece, ⅑ of cake	1 pce	121	22	451	4	71	1	18	2.9	7.4	6.2
	Pound cake:											
391	Loaf, 8½ x 3½ x 3¼"	1 ea	478	25	1863	26	234	4	95	53	26.7	5.21
392	Piece, 1/17 of loaf, ½" slice	1 pce	28	25	109	2	14	<1	6	3	1.5	.31
	Cakes, commercial:											
	Cheesecake:											
401	Whole cake, 9" diam	1 ea	1110	46	3559	61	283	23	250	128	86	15.3
402	Piece, 1/12 of cake	1 pce	92	46	295	5	23	2	21	10.6	7.1	1.3
	Pound cake:											
393	Loaf, 8½ x 3½ x 3"	1 ea	500	25	1948	27	244	3	99	55.5	27.9	5.4
394	Slice, 1/17 of loaf, 2" slice	1 pce	29	25	113	2	14	<1	6	3.2	1.6	.3
	Snack: 2 small cakes per package											
395	Chocolate w/creme filling (Ding Dong)	1 ea	28	20	105	1	17	<1	4	.9	1.5	1.2
396	Sponge w/creme filling (Twinkie)	1 ea	42	20	153	1	27	<1	5	1.1	1.9	1.5
1677	Sponge cake, 1/12 of 12" cake	1 pce	65	30	188	4	40	<1	2	.5	.6	.3
1678	Strawberry shortcake, fresh	1 ea	254	74	327	5	40	4	17	10.1	4.9	1
	White, white frosting, 2 layer:											
397	Whole cake, 8 or 9" diam	1 ea	1140	20	4271	38	718	11	154	45.7	68.1	39.8
398	Piece, 1/16 of cake	1 pce	71	20	266	2	45	1	10	2.8	4.2	2.5
	Yellow, chocolate frosting, 2 layer:											
399	Whole cake, 8 or 9" diam	1 ea	1108	22	4207	42	614	20	193	52.4	107	23.2
400	Piece, 1/16 of cake	1 pce	69	22	262	3	38	1	12	3.3	6.7	1.4
1332	Bagel chips	5 pce	70	4	298	6	52	6	7	1.2	1.9	3.3
2225	Bagel chips, Onion Garlic, Toasted	0.5 oz	14	–	70	2	9	–	2	0	2	0
1035	Cheese puffs/Cheetos	1 oz	28	1	155	2	15	<1	10	1.9	5.8	1.3
	Cookies made with enriched flour:											
	Brownies with nuts:											
403	Commercial w/frosting, 1½ x 1¾ x ⅞"	1 ea	25	14	101	1	16	1	4	1.1	2.1	.6
404	Home recipe, 1¾ x 1¾ x ⅞"[1]	1 ea	20	13	93	1	10	<1	6	1.5	2.2	1.9
1902	Fat Free, Entenmann's	1 pce	40	24	110	2	27	1	0	0	0	0
	Chocolate chip:											
405	Commercial, 2¼" diam	4 ea	42	12	192	1	25	1	10	3.1	5.5	1.1
406	Home recipe, 2¼" diam	4 ea	40	6	195	2	23	1	11	3.2	4.2	3.4
407	From refrigerated dough, 2¼" diam	4 ea	48	13	213	2	29	1	10	3.3	4.8	1
408	Fig bars	4 ea	56	16	195	2	40	3	4	.7	2.2	.7
2052	Fruit Bar, No Fat	1 ea	28	–	90	2	21	0	0	0	0	0
2162	Fudge, Fat Free, Snackwell	16 g	16	14	53	1	12	<1	<1	.1	.1	<.1
2002	Granola Cookie, Fat Free	3 ea	28	17	85	2	19	2	0	0	0	0
409	Oatmeal raisin, 2⅝" diam	4 ea	52	6	226	3	36	2	8	1.7	3.6	2.6
410	Peanut butter, home recipe, 2⅝" diam[2]	4 ea	48	6	228	4	28	1	11	2.1	5.2	3.5
411	Sandwich-type, all	4 ea	40	2	189	2	28	1	8	1.7	4.7	1.1
412	Shortbread, commercial, small	4 ea	32	4	161	2	21	1	8	2	4.3	1
413	Shortbread, home recipe, large[3]	2 ea	28	3	153	2	16	1	9	5.8	2.7	.4

(1)Made with vegetable oil.
(2)Made with vegetable shortening.
(3)Made with margarine.

(Computer code number is for West Diet Analysis program)

Chol (mg)	Calc (mg)	Iron (mg)	Magn (mg)	Phos (mg)	Pota (mg)	Sodi (mg)	Zinc (mg)	VT-A (RE)	Thia (mg)	Ribo (mg)	Niac (mg)	V-B6 (mg)	Fola (μg)	VT-C (mg)
614	680	11.8	66	1567	581	3770	2.74	208	1.1	.77	5.48	.38	99	2
68	75	1.31	7	173	64	416	.3	23	.12	.08	.6	.04	11	<1
0	85	1.71	–	–	324	1502	–	745	0	.51	6.26	.07	53	0
0	5	.1	–	–	19	88	–	44	0	.03	.4	<.01	3	0
611	566	6.99	122	1032	999	2297	5.66	1787	.31	2.14	2.16	.58	167	7
51	47	.58	10	86	83	190	.47	148	.03	.18	.18	.05	14	1
1105	175	6.95	55	685	595	1983	2.3	779	.68	1.15	6.55	.17	55	1
64	10	.4	3	40	34	115	.13	45	.04	.07	.38	.01	3	<1
5	21	.94	12	26	35	119	.16	1	.06	.08	.69	.01	2	<1
7	19	.55	3	32	38	153	.13	2	.06	.06	.51	.01	2	<1
66	46	1.77	7	89	64	158	.33	30	.16	.18	1.25	.03	8	0
53	209	2.33	29	289	359	510	.57	172	.29	.33	2.26	.13	40	95
91	547	9.12	60	742	661	2665	1.77	369	1.14	1.48	10.3	.16	64	1
6	34	.57	4	46	41	166	.11	23	.07	.09	.64	.01	4	<1
609	410	23.2	332	1783	1975	3742	6.87	299	1.33	1.74	13.9	.32	89	1
38	25	1.44	21	111	123	233	.43	19	.08	.11	.86	.02	6	<1
0	9	1.38	41	145	137	418	.88	0	.1	.12	1.57	.1	58	0
0	–	–	–	–	–	80	–	–	.09	.03	1.20	–	–	–
1	16	.67	5	31	47	294	.11	10	.07	.1	.92	.04	34	<1
4	7	.56	8	25	37	78	.18	5	.06	.05	.43	.01	3	<1
15	11	.37	11	26	35	69	.19	40	.03	.04	.2	.02	3	<1
0	0	1.08	–	–	90	140	–	0	–	–	–	–	–	0
0	6	1.02	15	21	39	137	.19	21	.05	.08	.68	.07	2	0
13	16	.99	22	40	90	144	.37	66	.07	.07	.54	.03	5	<1
11	12	1.08	11	33	86	100	.24	8	.09	.09	.95	.02	4	0
0	36	1.63	15	35	116	196	.22	2	.09	.12	1.05	.04	6	<1
0	0	.36	–	–	–	95	–	0	–	–	–	–	–	0
0	3	.29	5	11	26	71	.08	–	.02	.02	.26	0	–	0
0	–	.72	–	–	85	80	–	–	.09	.03	.40	–	–	4
17	52	1.38	22	84	124	280	.45	85	.13	.09	.65	.04	6	<1
15	19	1.08	19	56	111	249	.39	75	.11	.1	1.68	.04	9	<1
0	10	1.56	18	39	70	242	.32	.04	.03	.07	.83	.01	2	0
6	11	.88	5	35	32	146	.17	4	.11	.1	1.07	.01	3	0
25	5	.75	4	20	20	132	.12	85	.1	.07	.83	.01	3	0

(For purposes of calculations, use "0" for t, < 1, < .1, < .01, etc.)

TABLE I–1
FOOD COMPOSITION

Computer Code Number	Food Description	Measure	Wt (g)	H₂O (%)	Ener (cal)	Prot (g)	Carb (g)	Dietary Fiber (g)	Fat (g)	Fat Breakdown (g)		
										Sat	Mono	Poly
	BAKED GOODS: BREADS, CAKES, COOKIES, CRACKERS, PIES—Cont.											
414	Sugar, from refrigerated dough, 2" diam	4 ea	48	5	232	2	31	< 1	11	2.8	6.2	1.4
1874	Vanilla Sandwich, Snackwell's	26 g	26	3	109	1	21	1	2	.5	.8	.2
415	Vanilla wafers	10 ea	40	5	176	2	29	8	6	1.4	2.4	1.5
416	Corn chips	1 oz	28	1	151	2	16	1	9	1.3	2.7	4.7
	Crackers:[1]											
1034	Armenian cracker bread	4 pce	28	4	110	3	23	1	.3	< .1	< .1	< .1
417	Cheese	10 ea	10	3	50	1	6	< 1	3	.9	.9	.5
418	Cheese with peanut butter	4 ea	30	4	145	4	17	< 1	7	1.5	3.6	1.3
	Fat Free:											
2161	Cracked Pepper, Snackwell	15 g	15	2	60	2	13	< 1	< 1	.1	.1	.2
2159	Wheat, Snackwell	7 ea	15	1	60	2	12	1	< 1	.1	.1	.1
2075	Whole Wheat, Herb seasoned	.5 oz	14	.709	45	2	9	2	0	0	0	0
2077	Whole Wheat, Onion	.5 oz	14	.709	45	2	9	2	0	0	0	0
419	Graham	2 ea	14	4	59	1	11	< 1	1	.4	.7	.2
420	Melba toast, plain	1 pce	5	5	19	1	4	< 1	< 1	< .1	< .1	< .1
1514	Rice cakes, unsalted	2 ea	18	6	69	1	14	< 1	1	.2	.2	.2
421	Rye wafer, whole grain	2 ea	14	5	47	1	11	2	< 1	< .1	< .1	< .1
422	Saltine®[2]	4 ea	12	4	52	1	9	< 1	1	.3	.8	.2
1971	Saltine®, Unsalted Tops	2 ea	6	–	25	1	4	0	1	0	0	0
423	Snack-type, round like Ritz	3 ea	9	3	45	1	5	< 1	2	.4	1	.8
424	Wheat, thin	4 ea	8	3	38	1	5	1	2	.7	.8	.2
425	Whole-wheat wafers	2 ea	8	3	35	1	5	1	1	.2	.8	.2
426	Croissants, 4½ x 4 x 1¾"	1 ea	57	23	231	5	26	1	12	6.7	3.2	.7
1699	Croutons, seasoned	½ c	15	4	70	2	10	< 1	3	.8	1.4	.4
	Danish pastry:											
427	Packaged ring, plain, 12 oz	1 ea	340	21	1349	19	181	1	65	13.5	40.8	6.4
428	Round piece, plain, 4¼" diam, 1" high	1 ea	57	21	226	3	30	< 1	11	2.3	6.8	1.1
429	Ounce, plain	1 oz	28	21	111	2	15	< 1	5	1.1	3.4	.5
430	Round piece with fruit	1 ea	65	29	231	3	31	–	11	2.3	7	1.1
	Desserts, 3 x 3" piece:											
1348	Apple crisp	1 pce	78	61	127	1	25	–	3	.6	1.2	.8
1353	Apple cobbler	1 pce	104	57	199	2	35	1	6	1.3	2.7	1.9
1349	Cherry crisp	1 pce	138	75	158	2	27	1	5	1	2.4	1.7
1352	Cherry cobbler	1 pce	129	66	198	2	34	1	6	1.3	2.7	1.9
1350	Peach crisp	1 pce	139	73	166	1	30	1	5	1	2.3	1.6
1351	Peach cobbler	1 pce	130	65	204	2	36	1	6	1.3	2.7	1.9
	Doughnuts:											
431	Cake type, plain, 3¼" diam	1 ea	50	21	211	3	25	1	11	1.9	4.8	4.1
432	Yeast-leavened, glazed, 3¾" diam	1 ea	60	25	242	4	27	1	14	3.5	7.7	1.7
	English muffins:											
433	Plain, enriched	1 ea	57	42	134	4	26	2	1	.1	.2	.5
434	Toasted	1 ea	50	37	128	4	25	2	1	.1	.2	5
1504	Whole wheat	1 ea	50	46	102	4	20	5	1	.2	.3	.4
2010	Fruit & Fitness bar, fat free	1 ea	38	20	110	2	27	1	0	0	0	0
1414	Granola bar, soft	1 ea	42	6	188	3	29	2	7	3.1	1.6	2.3
1415	Granola bar, hard	1 ea	28	4	132	3	18	2	6	.7	1.2	3.4

[1]Crackers made with enriched white (wheat) flour except for rye wafers and whole-wheat wafers.   [2]Made with lard.

(Computer code number is for West Diet Analysis program)

Chol (mg)	Calc (mg)	Iron (mg)	Magn (mg)	Phos (mg)	Pota (mg)	Sodi (mg)	Zinc (mg)	VT-A (RE)	Thia (mg)	Ribo (mg)	Niac (mg)	V-B6 (mg)	Fola (µg)	VT-C (mg)
15	43	.89	4	90	78	225	.13	5	.09	.06	1.16	.01	3	0
<1	17	.61	5	36	28	95	.16	–	.05	.07	.69	.01	–	0
23	19	.96	6	42	39	125	.14	7	.11	.13	1.24	.03	4	0
0	36	.37	21	52	40	179	.36	3	.01	.04	.33	.07[3]	6[4]	<1
0	5	1.4	7	32	32	140	.2	0	.19	.13	1.6	.01	5	0
1	15	.48	4	22	14	99	.11	9	.06	.04	.47	.05	3	0
2	24	.88	17	97	73	298	.33	3	.12	.1	1.96	.45	8	0
<1	26	.73	4	51	19	148	.14	–	.05	.06	.78	.01	–	<1
<1	28	.58	7	61	43	169	.21	–	.04	.07	.73	.02	–	0
0	.36	–	–	–	70	80	–	–	.06	–	.4	–	–	–
0	.36	–	–	–	70	80	–	–	.06	–	.4	–	–	–
0	3	.52	4	15	19	85	.11	0	.03	.04	.58	.01	2	0
0	5	.19	3	10	10	41	.1	0	.02	.01	.21	<.01	1	0
0	2	.37	25	63	52	5	.54	1	0	.03	1.4	.02	4	0
0	6	.83	17	47	69	111	.39	<1	.06	.04	.22	.04	6	<1
0	14	.65	3	13	15	156	.09	0	.07	.05	.63	<.01	4	0
0	–	.36	–	–	5	50	–	–	–	–	–	–	–	–
0	11	.32	2	21	12	76	.06	0	.03	.03	.36	<.01	1	0
2	3	.25	6[5]	15	17	69	.24[5]	0	.04	.03	.4	.01	1	0
0	4	.25	8[5]	24	24	53	.17	0	.02	.01	.36	.01	2	0
43	21	1.16	9	60	67	424	.43	78	.22	.14	1.25	.03	16	<1
<1	14	.42	6	21	27	186	.14	1	.08	.06	.7	.01	6	0
105	143	6.94	54	286	371	1261	1.87	20	.99	.75	8.5	.2	54	10
18	24	1.16	9	48	62	211	.31	3	.16	.12	1.43	.03	9	2
9	12	.58	4	24	31	105	.16	2	.08	.06	.71	.02	5	1
13	15	.97	10	47	76	230	.33	17	.2	.14	1.24	.04	10	1
0	22	.58	5	19	76	142	.12	24	.07	.06	.6	.03	4	2
1	31	.78	6	44	87	304	.16	76	.1	.09	.74	.04	3	<1
0	29	2.15	12	23	164	73	.15	145	.07	.08	.59	.06	10	3
1	37	1.81	10	48	114	311	.2	135	.1	.11	.85	.05	9	2
0	23	.95	13	31	198	69	.2	104	.05	.05	1.03	.03	6	5
1	33	.91	10	54	140	308	.23	105	.09	.09	1.18	.03	6	3
18	22	.98	10	135	63	273	.27	9	.11	.12	.92	.03	4	<1
4	26	1.23	13	56	65	205	.46	6	.22	.13	1.71	.03	13	0
0	99	1.43	12	76	75	264	.4	0	.25	.16	2.21	.02	21	<1
0	94	1.37	11	72	71	252	.38	0	.19	.14	1.9	.02	14	<1
0	133	1.23	35	141	105	319	.8	0	.15	.07	1.71	.08	24	0
0	–	1.08	–	–	120	35	–	–	.12	.07	.8	–	–	6
<1	45	1.09	31	98	136	118	.64	0	.12	.07	.22	.04	10	0
0	17	.84	27	79	95	83	.58	4	.07	.03	.45	.02	7	<1

[3]Vitamin B$_6$ values vary between brands. Check the label.

[4]Values from 1992 USDA data for snacks and sweets.

[5]Values derived from whole-wheat recipes and retention values.

(For purposes of calculations, use "0" for t, <1, <.1, <.01, etc.)

Table I–1
Food Composition

Computer Code Number	Food Description	Measure	Wt (g)	H₂O (%)	Ener (cal)	Prot (g)	Carb (g)	Dietary Fiber (g)	Fat (g)	Fat Breakdown (g) Sat	Mono	Poly
	BAKED GOODS: BREADS, CAKES, COOKIES, CRACKERS, PIES—Cont.											
	Granola bar, Fat free:											
1985	Blueberry	1 ea	43	7	140	3	33	3	0	0	0	0
2012	Chocolate	1 ea	43	7	140	3	33	3	0	0	0	0
1983	Date Almond	1 ea	43	7	140	3	33	3	0	0	0	0
1984	Raisin	1 ea	43	7	140	3	33	3	0	0	0	0
2011	Strawberry	1 ea	43	7	140	3	33	3	0	0	0	0
	Muffins, 2½" diam, 1½" high:											
	From home recipe											
435	Blueberry[1]	1 ea	45	39	131	3	18	7	5	1.1	1.2	2.4
436	Bran, wheat[2]	1 ea	45	35	130	3	19	3	6	1.2	1.4	2.8
437	Cornmeal	1 ea	45	32	144	3	20	2	6	1.2	1.4	2.8
	From commercial mix:											
438	Blueberry	1 ea	45	36	135	2	22	1	4	.7	1.6	1.4
439	Bran, wheat	1 ea	45	35	124	3	21	4	4	1.1	2.1	.6
440	Cornmeal	1 ea	45	30	144	3	22	2	5	1.3	2.4	.6
	Nabisco Newtons, Fat free:											
1864	Cranberry	1 ea	23	–	68	1	16	–	0	0	0	0
1867	Fig	1 ea	23	–	68	1	16	–	0	0	0	0
1865	Raspberry	1 ea	23	–	68	1	16	–	0	0	0	0
1868	Strawberry	1 ea	23	–	68	1	16	–	0	0	0	0
	Pancakes, 4" diam:											
441	Buckwheat, from mix w/ egg and milk	1 ea	27	54	56	2	8	1	2	.5	.5	.8
442	Plain, from home recipe	1 ea	27	53	61	2	8	< 1	3	.6	.7	1.2
443	Plain, from mix; egg, milk, oil added	1 ea	27	53	52	1	10	< 1	1	.1	.2	.2
1468	Pan Dulce, Sweet roll w/topping	1 ea	79	21	291	5	48	1	9	2	3.9	2.7
	Piecrust, with enriched flour, vegetable shortening, baked:											
444	Home recipe, 9" shell	1 ea	180	10	949	11	85	3	62	15.5	27.4	16.4
	From mix:											
445	For 2-crust pie	1 ea	320	10	1686	20	152	6	111	27.6	48.6	29.2
446	1 pie shell	1 ea	180	11	902	12	91	3	55	13.9	31.1	6.9
	Pies, 9" diam; crust made with vegetable shortening, enriched flour:											
447	Apple:[3] Whole pie	1 ea	945	52	2239	18	321	16	104	19.9	56.1	19.8
448	Piece, ⅙ of pie	1 pce	158	52	374	3	54	3	17	3.3	9.4	3.3
449	Banana cream: Whole pie	1 ea	1188	48	3195	52	391	–	162	44.7	68	39.2
450	Piece, ⅙ of pie	1 pce	198	48	533	9	65	–	27	7.4	11.3	6.5
451	Blueberry:[3] Whole pie	1 ea	945	51	2315	25	317	13	112	27.6	48.4	29.1
452	Piece, ⅙ of pie	1 pce	158	51	387	4	53	2	19	4.6	8.1	4.9
453	Cherry:[3] Whole pie	1 ea	945	46	2551	26	364	14	115	28.3	50.2	30.7
454	Piece, ⅙ of pie	1 pce	158	46	427	4	61	2	19	4.7	8.4	5.1
455	Chocolate cream:[4] Whole pie	1 ea	1194	46	3367	57	372	6	192	62	78	40
456	Piece, ⅙ of pie	1 pce	199	46	561	10	62	1	32	10	13	6.7
457	Custard:[3] Whole pie	1 ea	910	61	1911	50	189	11	106	25.3	52.4	17.5
458	Piece, ⅙ of pie	1 pce	152	61	319	8	32	2	18	4.2	8.8	2.9
459	Lemon meringue:[3] Whole pie	1 ea	840	42	2251	13	396	10	73	13.1	30.5	24.3
460	Piece, ⅙ of pie	1 pce	140	42	375	2	66	2	12	2.2	5.1	4

[1] Made with vegetable shortening.

[2] Made with vegetable oil

[3] Values from latest USDA data for Baked Goods.

[4] Values based on recipe: pie crust, cooked chocolate pudding, whipped cream topping.

(Computer code number is for West Diet Analysis program)

Chol (mg)	Calc (mg)	Iron (mg)	Magn (mg)	Phos (mg)	Pota (mg)	Sodi (mg)	Zinc (mg)	VT-A (RE)	Thia (mg)	Ribo (mg)	Niac (mg)	V-B6 (mg)	Fola (µg)	VT-C (mg)
0	20	3.6	–	–	120	10	–	–	.03	.07	.4	–	–	–
0	20	3.6	–	–	120	10	–	–	.03	.07	.4	–	–	–
0	20	3.6	–	–	120	10	–	–	.03	.07	.4	–	–	–
0	20	3.6	–	–	120	10	–	–	.03	.07	.4	–	–	–
0	20	3.6	–	–	120	10	–	–	.03	.07	.4	–	–	–
18	85	1.03	7	65	55	198	.24	13	.12	.13	.99	.02	5	1
16	84	1.89	35	128	143	265	1.24	108	.15	.2	1.81	.14	23	4
20	116	1.18	10	79	65	263	.27	18	.14	.14	1.07	.04	8	< 1
21	11	.51	5	85	35	197	.17	10	.07	.14	1.01	.03	5	< 1
31	14	1.14	26	150	66	210	.52	14	.09	.11	1.29	.08	7	0
28	34	.88	9	173	59	358	.29	20	.11	.12	.94	.05	5	< 1
–	–	–	–	–	–	76	–	–	–	–	–	–	–	–
–	–	–	–	–	–	76	–	–	–	–	–	–	–	–
–	–	–	–	–	–	76	–	–	–	–	–	–	–	–
–	–	–	–	–	–	76	–	–	–	–	–	–	–	–
18	69	.51	15	110	63	144	.32	18	.05	.07	.36	.04	5	< 1
16	59	.49	4	43	36	119	.15	15	.05	.08	.42	.01	3	< 1
3	34	.42	5	90	47	170	.1	2	.06	.06	.46	.03	2	< 1
26	13	1.82	10	56	57	140	.35	88	.23	.21	1.98	.04	22	< 1
0	18	5.22	25	121	121	976	.79	0	.7	.5	5.96	.04	20	0
0	32	9.28	45	214	214	1734	1.41	0	1.25	.89	10.6	.08	35	0
0	108	3.89	27	151	112	1312	.7	0	.54	.33	4.27	.1	22	0
0	104	4.25	66	227	614	2513	1.51	284	.26	.25	2.49	.36	38	30
0	17	.71	11	38	103	420	.25	47	.04	.04	.42	.06	6	5
606	891	12.5	190	1092	1960	2851	5.7	832	1.65	2.46	12.5	1.58	131	19
101	149	2.08	32	182	327	475	.95	139	.27	.41	2.08	.26	22	3
0	66	11.7	76	284	473	1748	1.89	38	1.45	1.25	11.2	.32	47	7
0	11	1.96	13	47	79	292	.32	6	.24	.21	1.88	.05	8	1
0	94	17.6	85	284	728	1804	1.89	454	1.4	1.18	12.1	.32	66	9
0	16	2.94	14	47	122	302	.32	76	.23	.2	2.02	.05	11	2
632	967	15.3	311	1313	1755	2924	7.6	872	1.6	2.4	12	.56	119	6
105	161	2.04	52	219	292	487	1.3	145	.27	.4	2	.09	20	1
300	728	5.28	100	1019	965	2184	4.73	456	.35	1.89	2.66	.44	182	3
50	122	.88	17	170	161	365	.79	76	.06	.32	.44	.07	30	< 1
378	470	5.12	126	882	748	1226	4.12	437	.52	1.76	5.45	.25	67	27
63	78	.85	21	147	125	204	.69	73	.09	.29	.91	.04	11	4

(For purposes of calculations, use "0" for t, < 1, < .1, < .01, etc.)

I–35

TABLE I–1
FOOD COMPOSITION

Computer Code Number	Food Description	Measure	Wt (g)	H₂O (%)	Ener (cal)	Prot (g)	Carb (g)	Dietary Fiber (g)	Fat (g)	Fat Breakdown (g)		
										Sat	Mono	Poly
	BAKED GOODS: BREADS, CAKES, COOKIES, CRACKERS, PIES—Cont.											
461	Peach: Whole pie	1 ea	945	45	2603	22	377	13	108	26.4	49	31.8
462	Piece, ⅙ of pie	1 pce	158	45	435	4	63	2	18	4.4	8.2	5.3
463	Pecan:[1] Whole pie	1 ea	825	19	3300	33	472	29	153	31	88	24.5
464	Piece, ⅙ of pie	1 pce	138	19	552	6	79	5	25	5.2	14.9	4.1
465	Pumpkin:[1] Whole pie	1 ea	1240	58	2604	48	339	33	118	25	62.1	19.8
466	Piece, ⅙ of pie	1 pce	206	58	433	8	56	6	20	4.2	10.3	3.3
467	Pies, fried, commercial: Apple	1 ea	85	40	266	2	33	2	14	6.5	5.8	1.2
468	Pies, fried, commercial: Cherry	1 ea	85	40	269	3	36	2	14	2	6	4.6
	Pretzels, made with enriched flour:											
469	Thin sticks, 2¼" long	10 ea	3	3	11	<1	2	<1	<1	t	t	t
470	Dutch twists, 2¾ x 2⅝"	1 ea	16	3	61	1	13	<1	1	.1	.2	.2
471	Thin twists, 3¼ x 2¼ x ¼"	10 ea	60	3	229	5	47	2	2	.4	.8	.7
	Rolls & buns, enriched, commercial:											
472	Cloverleaf rolls, 2½" diam, 2" high	1 ea	28	32	85	2	14	1	2	.5	1.1	.3
473	Hot dog buns	1 ea	40	34	114	3	20	1	2	.5	1	.4
474	Hamburger buns	1 ea	45	34	129	4	23	1	2	.5	1.1	.4
475	Hard roll, white, 3¾" diam, 2" high	1 ea	50	31	147	5	26	1	2	.3	.6	.9
476	Submarine rolls/hoagies, 11½ x 3 x 2½"	1 ea	135	31	392	12	75	4	4	.9	1.3	1.4
	Rolls & buns, enriched, home recipe:											
477	Dinner rolls 2½" diam, 2" high	1 ea	35	29	112	3	19	1	3	.7	1.1	.7
478	Toaster pastries, fortified (Poptarts)	1 ea	54	12	212	3	38	1	6	.8	2.2	2.1
2132	Toaster Strudel pastry—Cream Cheese	1 ea	53	32	184	3	28	<1	9	2.8	–	–
2134	Toaster Strudel pastry—French Toast	1 ea	53	31	177	3	27	1	7	2.8	–	–
	Tortilla chips:											
1271	Plain	1 oz	28	7	140	2	18	2	6	2	4.4	1
1036	Nacho flavor	1 oz	28	2	139	2	18	1	7	1.4	4.3	1
1037	Taco flavor	1 oz	28	2	134	2	18	2	7	1.3	4	1
	Tortillas:											
479	Corn, enriched, 6" diam	1 ea	30	44	67	2	14	2	1	.1	.2	.3
480	Flour, 8" diam	1 ea	35	27	115	3	20	1	2	.4	1	1
1301	Flour, 10" diam	1 ea	57	27	185	5	32	1	4	.6	1.6	1.6
481	Taco shells	1 ea	14	4	66	1	9	1	3	.4	1.5	.6
	Waffles, 7" diam:											
482	From home recipe	1 ea	75	42	218	6	25	1	11	2.1	2.6	5.1
483	From mix, egg/milk added	1 ea	75	42	218	5	26	1	10	1.7	2.7	5.2
1510	Whole grain, prepared from frozen	1 ea	39	44	106	4	12	1	5	1.6	1.9	1
	GRAIN PRODUCTS: CEREAL, FLOUR, GRAIN, PASTA and NOODLES, POPCORN											
484	Barley, pearled, dry, uncooked	1 c	200	10	704	20	155	27	2	.5	.3	1.1
485	Barley, pearled, cooked	1 c	157	69	193	4	44	8	1	.1	.1	.3
	Breakfast bars, fat free:											
2009	Apple	1 ea	38	21	110	2	24	3	0	0	0	0
2005	Chocolate	1 ea	38	21	110	2	24	3	0	0	0	0
2003	Strawberry	1 ea	38	21	110	2	24	3	0	0	0	0

[1] Values from latest USDA data for Baked Goods.

(Computer code number is for West Diet Analysis program)

Chol (mg)	Calc (mg)	Iron (mg)	Magn (mg)	Phos (mg)	Pota (mg)	Sodi (mg)	Zinc (mg)	VT-A (RE)	Thia (mg)	Ribo (mg)	Niac (mg)	V-B6 (mg)	Fola (µg)	VT-C (mg)
17	79	3	68	256	1132	2660	1.59	187	.28	.5	1	.42	49	11
3	13	.57	11	43	789	445	.27	31	.05	.09	.2	.07	8	2
264	140	8.66	149	635	611	3498	4.7	388	.75	1.01	2.05	.17	49	9
44	23	1.45	25	106	102	585	.79	65	.13	.17	.34	.03	8	2
248	744	9.8	186	880	1909	3496	5.58	5951[2]	.68	1.9	2.32	.71	186	19
41	124	1.63	31	146	317	581	.93	989[2]	.11	.31	.38	.12	31	3
13	13	.88	8	37	51	325	.17	8	.1	.08	.98	.03	4	2
13	19	.88	9	37	55	318	.17	15	.1	.08	.98	.03	3	1
0	1	.13	1	3	4	51	.03	0	.01	.02	.16	<.01	2	0
0	6	.69	6	18	23	274	.14	0	.07	.1	.84	.02	13	0
0	22	2.59	21	68	88	1029	.51	0	.28	.37	3.15	.07	50	0
<1	34	.89	6	33	38	148	.22	0	.14	.09	1.14	.01	8	<1
0	56	1.27	8	35	56	224	.25	0	.19	.12	1.57	.02	11	0
0	63	1.43	9	40	63	252	.28	0	.22	.14	1.77	.02	12	0
0	47	1.65	14	50	54	272	.47	0	.24	.17	2.12	.03	8	0
0	122	3.78	27	115	122	783	.85	0	.54	.33	4.47	.05	41	0
13	21	1.04	7	44	53	145	.24	28	.14	.14	1.21	.02	15	<1
0	14	1.89	10	60	60	226	.36	57[3]	.16	.2	2.13	.21	43	<1
12	12	.95	–	–	–	–	–	17	–	–	–	–	–	0
6	6	.84	–	–	–	191	–	2	–	–	–	–	–	0
0	0	0	25	58	65	135	.43	0	.02	.05	.36	.08	3	0
1	42	.4	23	69	61	198	.34	12	.04	.05	.4	.08	4	1
1	44	.57	25	68	61	221	.36	25	.07	.06	.57	.08	6	<1
0	52	.42	19	94	46	48	.28	8	.03	.02	.45	.07	5	0
0	44	1.17	9	44	46	169	.25	0	.19	.1	1.26	.02	4	0
0	71	1.88	15	70	74	272	.4	0	.3	.17	2.03	.03	7	0
0	22	.35	15	35	25	51	.18	5	.04	.02	.23	.04	1	0
52	191	1.74	14	143	119	383	.51	49	.2	.26	1.55	.04	11	<1
52	91	1.23	14	143	119	383	.5	49	.15	.3	1.55	.04	11	<1
39	84	.7	15	83	91	150	.41	25	.08	.12	.75	.05	7	<1
0	58	5	158	442	560	18	4.26	4	.38	.23	9.22	.52	46	0
0	17	2.09	34	85	146	5	1.29	2	.13	.1	3.23	.18	25	0
0	20	.72	–	–	160	65	–	–	.09	.03	.4	–	–	2
0	20	.72	–	–	160	65	–	–	.09	.03	.4	–	–	2
0	20	.72	–	–	160	65	–	–	.09	.03	.4	–	–	2

[2]Latest USDA values of vitamin A for canned pumpkin are almost 3.5 times greater than previously published values. Canned pumpkin is usually a blend of pumpkin and winter squash.

[3]Vitamin A values from label declarations vary.

(For purposes of calculations, use "0" for t, <1, <.1, <.01, etc.)

Table I–1
Food Composition

Computer Code Number	Food Description	Measure	Wt (g)	H$_2$O (%)	Ener (cal)	Prot (g)	Carb (g)	Dietary Fiber (g)	Fat (g)	Fat Breakdown (g)		
										Sat	Mono	Poly
	GRAIN PRODUCTS: CEREAL, FLOUR, GRAIN, PASTA and NOODLES, POPCORN—Cont.											
	Breakfast cereals, hot, cooked:											
	Corn grits (hominy) enriched:											
486	Regular and quick, prepared, yellow	1 c	242	85	145	3	31	5	<1	.1	.1	.2
487	Instant, prepared from packet, white	1 ea	137	85	82	2	18	<1	<1	t	t	<.1
	Cream of wheat:											
488	Regular, quick, instant	1 c	244	87	131	4	27	1	<1	.1	.1	.2
489	Mix and eat, plain, packet	1 ea	142	82	102	3	21	<1	<1	t	t	.1
1664	Farina cereal, cooked	½ c	117	87	58	2	12	2	<1	t	t	t
490	Malt-O-Meal	1 c	240	88	122	4	26	1	<1	t	t	.1
494	Maypo	1 c	242	83	172	6	32	6	2	.4	.8	.1
	Oatmeal or rolled oats:											
491	Regular, quick, instant, nonfort	1 c	234	85	145	6	25	4	2	.4	.7	.9
	Instant, fortified:											
492	Plain, from packet	¾ c	177	85	104	4	18	3	2	.3	.6	.7
493	Flavored, from packet	¾ c	164	76	167	4	33	2	2	.3	.6	.7
	Breakfast cereals, ready to eat:											
495	All-Bran	⅓ c	28	3	70	4	21	10	1	.1	.1	.3
1306	Alpha Bits	1 c	28	1	109	2	24	1	1	.1	.2	.3
1307	Apple Jacks	1 c	28	2	109	2	25	1	<1	t	t	t
1308	Bran Buds	1 c	84	3	217	12	64	31	2	.4	.3	1.1
1305	Bran Chex	1 c	49	2	156	5	39	8	1	.2	.2	.8
1309	Honey BucWheat Crisp	¾ c	28	5	109	3	23	2	1	.2	.2	.4
1310	C. W. Post, plain	1 c	97	2	432	9	70	7	15	11.3	1.7	1.4
1311	C. W. Post, with raisins	1 c	103	4	446	9	74	14	15	11	1.7	1.4
496	Cap'n Crunch	1 c	37	2	156	2	30	1	3	2.2	.4	.5
1312	Cap'n Crunchberries	1 c	38	3	160	2	31	1	3	2.1	.4	.5
1313	Cap'n Crunch, peanut butter	1 c	38	2	167	3	29	<1	5	2.1	1.5	1.1
497	Cheerios	1 c	23	5	90	3	16	2	1	.3	.5	.6
1314	Cocoa Krispies	1 c	36	2	139	2	32	<1	1	.1	.1	.2
1316	Cocoa Pebbles	1 c	31	2	127	1	27	<1	2	t	t	t
1315	Corn Bran	1 c	36	2	125	2	30	7	1	.2	.3	.7
1317	Corn Chex	1 c	28	2	110	2	25	<1	1	.1	.2	.6
498	Corn Flakes, Kellogg's	1¼ c	28	3	109	2	24	1	<1	t	t	t
499	Corn Flakes, Post Toasties	1¼ c	28	3	108	2	24	1	<1	t	t	t
1340	Corn Pops	1 c	28	3	107	1	25	<1	<1	t	t	.1
1318	Cracklin' Oat Bran	1 c	60	4	229	6	41	10	9	2.1	2.3	3.5
1038	Crispy Wheat `N Raisins	1 c	43	7	150	3	35	3	1	.1	.1	.4
1319	Fortified Oat Flakes	1 c	48	3	177	9	35	1	1	.1	.3	.3
500	40% Bran Flakes, Kellogg's	1 c	39	3	127	5	31	6	1	.1	.1	.4
501	40% Bran Flakes, Post	1 c	47	3	152	5	37	9	1	.2	.2	.3
502	Froot Loops	1 c	28	3	111	2	25	1	1	.2	.1	.1
518	Frosted Flakes	1 c	35	3	133	2	32	1	<1	t	t	t
1320	Frosted Mini-Wheats	4 ea	31	5	111	3	26	2	<1	.1	t	.2
1321	Frosted Rice Krispies	1 c	28	3	108	1	26	<1	<1	t	t	t
1324	Fruit & Fibre w/dates	½ c	28	9	95	2	21	4	1	.2	.6	.5
1325	Fruitful Bran	¾ c	34	1	144	3	37	6	<1	.1	.1	.2

(Computer code number is for West Diet Analysis program)

Chol (mg)	Calc (mg)	Iron (mg)	Magn (mg)	Phos (mg)	Pota (mg)	Sodi (mg)	Zinc (mg)	VT-A (RE)	Thia (mg)	Ribo (mg)	Niac (mg)	V-B6 (mg)	Fola (μg)	VT-C (mg)
0	0	1.55[1]	10	29	53	0[2]	.17	14[3]	.24[1]	.14[1]	1.96[1]	.06	2	0
0	7	1.01[1]	5	16	29	343	.08	0	.18[1]	.08[1]	1.3[1]	.03	1	0
0	51[1]	10.5[1]	12	102[4]	46	141[4]	.34	0	.24[1]	0[1]	1.46[1]	.03	10	0
0	20[1]	8.09[1]	7	20[1]	38	241	.24	376[1]	.43[1]	.28[1]	4.97[1]	.57	101	0
0	2	.58	2	14	15	0[5]	.08	0	.09	.06	.64	.01	2	0
0	5	9.6[1]	5	24[1]	31	2[5]	.17	0	.48[1]	.24[1]	5.76[1]	.02	5	0
0	126	8.47	51	249	213	9.7	1.5	709	.73	.73	9.44	.97	10	29
0	19	1.59	56	177	131	2[5]	1.15	4	.26	.05	.3	.05	9	0
0	162[1]	6.3[1]	42	132	99	283[1]	.87	453[1]	.53[1]	.28[1]	5.47[1]	.74	150	0
0	172[1]	7[1]	38	138	156	235[1]	1	458[1]	.53[1]	.38[1]	5.9[1]	.76	156	0
0	23	4.52[1]	105	261	345	315	3.75	371[1]	.37[1]	.43[1]	5[1]	.51	100	15[1]
0	8	2.7	17	51	108	177	1.51	371	.37	.43	5	.51	100	0
0	3	4.52	6	30	23	124	3.75	370	.37	.43	5	.51	100	15
0	56	13.4	267	729	1403	515	11.1	1111	1.09	1.26	14.8	1.51	296	44
0	29	7.79	125	326	393	454	2.14	11	.64	.26	8.62	.88	172	26
0	40	8.12	32	80	106	266	.51	673	.68	.77	9	1.4	9	27
<1	47	15.4	67	224	197	166	1.64	1283	1.26	1.46	17.1	1.75	342	0
<1	50	16.4	74	231	260	160	1.64	1362	1.34	1.55	18.1	1.85	363	0
0	6	9.81[1]	15	47	48	278	4	5[1]	.66[1]	.71[1]	8.62[1]	1	238	0
<1	12	9.8	15	51	54	265	3.88	5	.65	.74	8.92	1.02	140	0
0	8	10	20	53	62	291	4.15	6	.66	.77	9.73	1.14	265	0
0	39	3.66[1]	32	109	82	249	.64	304[1]	.3[1]	.34[1]	4.05[1]	.41	5	12[1]
<1	6	2.27	12	47	53	275	1.91	476	.47	.54	6.34	.65	127	19
0	5	1.97	13	24	52	148	1.66	411	.41	.47	5.52	.56	109	0
0	41	12.2	18	52	70	310	4	8	.37	.7	10.9	.86	232	0
0	3	1.8	4	11	23	268	.1	14	.37	.07	5	.51	100	15
0	1	1.8[1]	3	18	26	286	.08	370[1]	.36[1]	.42[1]	4.93[1]	.5	99	15[1]
0	1	.74[1]	4	12	32	293	.08	370[1]	.36[1]	.42[1]	4.93[1]	.5	99	0
0	1	1.8	2	28	17	103	1.51	370	.37	.43	5	.51	100	15
0	40	3.78	116	241	355	487	3.18	794	.78	.9	10.6	1.08	212	32
0	71	6.84	34	117	173	204	.51	569	.56	.64	7.57	.77	15	0
0	68	13.7	58	176	343	429	1.5	635	.62	.72	8.45	.86	169	0
0	19	24.8[1]	71	191	247	302	5.15	516[1]	.51[1]	.58[1]	6.86[1]	.7	137	0
0	21	7.47[1]	101	296	250	430	2.49	622[1]	.61[1]	.7[1]	8.27[1]	.85	165	0
0	3	4.52[1]	7	24	26	144	3.75	370[1]	.37[1]	.43[1]	5[1]	.51	100	15[1]
0	1	2.21[1]	3	26	22	283	.05	463[1]	.45[1]	.52[1]	6.16[1]	.63	123	19[1]
0	10	1.95	25	81	105	9	1.64	410	.4	.46	5.46	.56	109	16
0	1	1.79	5	27	21	237	.31	370	.37	.43	5	.51	100	15
0	15	5	40	108	167	132	1.51	356	.37	.43	5	.5	100	0
0	23	5	67	152	276	264	1.3	270	.46	.43	6	.5	100	<1

[1]Nutrient added (values sometimes based on label declaration).

[2]Cooked without salt. If salt is added according to label recommendation, sodium content is **540 mg**.

[3]Value for yellow corn grits; cooked white corn grits contain 0 RE of vitamin A.

[4]Values for quick cereal.

[5]Cooked without salt. If added according to label recommendations, sodium content is 390 mg for Cream of Wheat; 324 mg for Malt-O-Meal; 374 mg for oatmeal; 385 mg for Farina.

(For purposes of calculations, use "0" for t, <1, <.1, <.01, etc.)

Table I–1
Food Composition

Computer Code Number	Food Description	Measure	Wt (g)	H$_2$O (%)	Ener (cal)	Prot (g)	Carb (g)	Dietary Fiber (g)	Fat (g)	Fat Breakdown (g)		
										Sat	Mono	Poly
	GRAIN PRODUCTS: CEREAL, FLOUR, GRAIN, PASTA and NOODLES, POPCORN—Cont.											
	Breakfast cereals, ready to eat—Cont.											
1322	Fruity Pebbles	1 c	32	3	131	1	28	1	2	.4	.3	.4
503	Golden Grahams	1 c	39	2	150	2	33	1	1	1	.1	.2
504	Granola, homemade	½ c	61	3	297	8	34	6	17	2.9	4.7	8.6
1670	Granola, low fat, commercial	½ c	47	3	179	4	36	3	3	0	–	–
505	Grape Nuts	½ c	57	3	203	7	47	6	<1	t	t	.2
1326	Grape Nuts Flakes	1 c	32	3	116	3	26	3	<1	.1	t	.1
1665	Heartland Natural with raisins	1 c	101	5	430	10	70	6	14	–	–	–
1327	Honey & Nut Corn Flakes	1 c	38	4	151	2	31	1	2	.3	.7	1
506	Honey Nut Cheerios	1 c	33	3	126	4	27	1	1	.1	.3	.3
1328	HoneyBran	1 c	35	2	119	3	29	4	1	.1	.1	.4
1329	HoneyComb	1 c	22	1	86	1	20	<1	<1	.1	.1	.2
1330	King Vitaman	1 c	19	2	77	1	16	1	1	.7	.1	.2
1039	Kix	1 c	19	3	74	2	16	<1	<1	.1	.1	.2
1331	Life	1 c	43	5	158	8	31	3	1	.1	.2	.4
507	Lucky Charms	1 c	32	3	125	3	26	1	1	.2	.4	.5
1323	Mueslix Five Grain	1 c	82	5	279	7	63	7	3	.5	1	1.2
1416	Granola, low-fat	⅓ c	31	3	119	3	25	2	2	0	–	–
	Health Valley Granola, fat-free:											
2081	Date & Almond	1 oz	28	7	90	2	21	3	0	0	0	0
2080	Raisin Cinnamon	1 oz	28	7	90	2	21	3	0	0	0	0
2082	Tropical Fruit	1 oz	28	7	90	21	2	3	0	0	0	0
508	Nature Valley Granola	1 c	113	4	502	12	75	6	20	13	2.9	2.8
1666	Nutri Grain Almond Raisin	⅔ c	40	9	140	3	31	3	2	0	–	–
1333	Nutri-Grain—corn	1 c	42	3	160	3	35	3	1	.1	.2	.6
1335	Nutri-Grain—wheat	1 c	44	3	158	4	37	3	<1	.1	.1	.3
1336	100% Bran	1 c	66	3	177	8	48	20	3	.6	.6	1.9
509	100% Natural cereal, plain	½ c	57	2	267	7	36	5	12	8.2	2.3	1.1
1337	100% Natural with apples & cinnamon	1 c	104	2	478	11	70	7	20	15.4	1.8	1.3
1338	100% Natural with raisins & dates	1 c	110	3	496	11	72	7	20	13.6	3.7	1.7
510	Product 19	1 c	33	3	125	3	27	1	<1	t	t	.1
1339	Quisp	1 c	30	2	124	2	25	<1	2	1.5	.3	.3
511	Raisin Bran, Kellogg's	1 c	49	8	152	5	37	5	1	.2	.1	.4
512	Raisin Bran, Post	1 c	56	9	171	5	42	8	1	.2	.2	.4
1667	Raisin Squares	½ c	28	8	90	2	23	2	0	0	0	0
1041	Rice Chex	¾ c	19	3	75	1	17	<1	1	.2	.2	.3
513	Rice Krispies, Kellogg's	1 c	29	3	114	2	25	<1	<1	t	t	.1
514	Rice, puffed	1 c	14	3	56	1	13	<1	<1	t	t	t
515	Shredded Wheat	1 c	43	5	155	5	34	4	1	.2	.2	.5
516	Special K	1 c	21	2	83	4	16	1	<1	t	t	t
517	Super Golden Crisp	1 c	33	1	123	2	30	1	<1	t	t	.1
519	Honey Smacks	1 c	38	3	142	3	33	<1	1	.1	.1	.3
1341	Tasteeos	1 c	24	2	94	3	19	3	1	.2	.2	.3
1342	Team	1 c	42	4	164	3	36	<1	1	.2	.2	.3
520	Total, wheat, with added calcium	1 c	33	4	116	3	26	4	1	.1	.1	.3
521	Trix	1 c	28	2	109	2	25	<1	<1	.2	.1	.1
1344	Wheat Chex	1 c	46	2	168	5	38	4	1	.2	.2	.6

(Computer code number is for West Diet Analysis program)

Chol (mg)	Calc (mg)	Iron (mg)	Magn (mg)	Phos (mg)	Pota (mg)	Sodi (mg)	Zinc (mg)	VT-A (RE)	Thia (mg)	Ribo (mg)	Niac (mg)	V-B6 (mg)	Fola (µg)	VT-C (mg)
0	4	2.04	9	19	25	178	1.73	424	.42	.49	5.6	.58	114	0
< 1	24	6.21[1]	16	56	86	386	.34	517[1]	.51[1]	.59[1]	6.87[1]	.7	6	21[1]
0	38	2.42	71	247	306	6	2.23	2	.37	.15	1.07	.21	49	1
0	19	7	38	108	136	47	5.66	329	.55	.64	7.55	.76	146	–
0	5	2.47[1]	38	143	190	396	1.25	755[1]	.74[1]	.85[1]	9.98[1]	1.03	201	0
0	13	9.28	36	95	113	181	.65	423	.42	.49	5.71	.58	114	0
0	61	3.7	130	346	382	207	2.61	6	.29	.13	1.43	.18	41	1
0	5	2.39	8	17	48	302	.14	503	.49	.57	6.67	.68	133	20
0	23	5.3[1]	39	122	116	299	.87	437[1]	.43[1]	.5[1]	5.87[1]	.6	22	18[1]
0	16	5.57	46	131	150	202	.9	463	.45	.52	6.16	.63	23	19
0	4	2.09	7	22	70	123	1.17	291	.29	.33	3.87	.4	78	0
0	2	11.4	6	24	23	145	.15	644	.83	.95	11.6	1.06	259	30
0	24	5.44	8	26	30	194	.16	252	.25	.28	3.35	.34	67	10
0	150	11.3	14	232	192	224	1.42	9	.93	.97	11.3	.08	36	0
0	36	5.09[1]	27	89	66	227	.56	424[1]	.42[1]	.48[1]	5.63[1]	.58	6	17[1]
0	38	8.94	82	215	369	107	7.46	747	.75	.84	9.84	.99	197	1
0	–	1.8	24	80	95	60	3.74	150	.37	.42	4.99	.5	100	–
0	–	.36	–	–	85	35	–	–	.06	–	.4	–	–	–
0	–	.36	–	–	85	35	–	–	.06	–	.4	–	–	–
0	–	.36	–	–	85	35	–	–	.06	–	.4	–	–	–
0	71	3.77	115	353	388	232	2.19	7	.4	.19	.82	.09	85	0
0	16	.8	11	77	130	220	3.75	–	.38	.43	5	.5	100	–
0	1	.89	27	120	98	276	5.54	556	.55	.63	7.39	.76	148	22
0	12	1.24	34	164	119	299	5.81	583	.57	.66	7.74	.79	155	23
0	46	8.12	312	801	824	457	5.74	0	1.58	1.78	20.9	2.11	47	63
< 1	99	1.68	68	209	281	24	1.28	3	.17	.31	1.3	.1	17	0
1	157	2.9	72	351	515	52	2	6	.33	.57	1.88	.11	17	1
1	159	3.12	124	347	537	47	2.11	6	.31	.65	2.09	.16	45	0
0	4	21[1]	12	46	51	378	.49	1746[1]	1.75[1]	1.98[1]	23.3[1]	2.34	465	70[1]
0	9	6.33	12	25	45	240	.18	5	.54	.76	5.79	.91	8	0
0	17	22.2[1]	63	182	254	271	5	498[1]	.49[1]	.59[1]	6.66[1]	.69	132	0
0	26	8.9[1]	95	234	344	365	2.97	741[1]	.73[1]	.84[1]	9.86[1]	1.01	197	0
0	10	8.1	26	84	110	0	1.5	0	.38	.43	5	.5	100	–
0	3	1.2	5	19	22	158	.26	1	.25	.01	3.34	.34	67	10
0	5	1.83[1]	12	32	28	213	.49	0[1]	.12[1]	.03[1]	.2[1]	.05	3	15[1]
0	1	.15[1]	4	14	16	< 1	.14	0	.01[1]	.01[1]	.42[1]	.01	3	0
0	16	1.8	57	152	156	4	1.41	0	.11	.12	2.24	.11	21	0
< 1	6	3.39[1]	12	41	37	196	2.82	275[1]	.28[1]	.32[1]	3.75[1]	.38	75	11[1]
0	7	2.08[1]	20	60	123	29	1.75	437[1]	.43[1]	.49[1]	5.81[1]	.59	116	0
0	4	2.39[1]	18	41	56	100	.38	503[1]	.49[1]	.57[1]	6.67[1]	.68	133	20[1]
0	11	3.82	26	96	71	182	.69	318	.31	.36	4.22	.43	9	13
0	6	2.57	19	65	71	259	.58	556	.55	.63	7.39	.76	7	22
0	282	21[1]	37	136	123	326	.78	1746[1]	1.75[1]	1.98[1]	23.3[1]	2.34	465	70[1]
0	6	4.52[1]	6	19	27	179	.13	371[1]	.37[1]	.43[1]	5[1]	.51	3	15[1]
0	18	7.31	58	181	173	308	1.23	0	.6	.17	8.1	.83	162	24

[1]Nutrient added (values sometimes based on label declaration).

(For purposes of calculations, use "0" for t, < 1, < .1, < .01, etc.)

Table I–1
Food Composition

Computer Code Number	Food Description	Measure	Wt (g)	H₂O (%)	Ener (cal)	Prot (g)	Carb (g)	Dietary Fiber (g)	Fat (g)	Fat Breakdown (g)		
										Sat	Mono	Poly
	GRAIN PRODUCTS: CEREAL, FLOUR, GRAIN, PASTA and NOODLES, POPCORN—Cont.											
1043	Wheat cereal, puffed, fortified	1 c	12	3	44	2	10	1	< 1	t	t	.1
522	Wheaties	1 c	29	5	101	3	23	3	< 1	.1	t	.2
	Buckwheat flour:											
523	Dark	1 c	98	11	328	12	69	8	3	.7	.9	.9
524	Light	1 c	98	12	340	6	78	6	1	.2	.4	.4
525	Buckwheat, whole grain, dry	1 c	175	10	600	23	125	18	6	1.3	1.8	1.8
526	Bulgar, dry, uncooked	1 c	140	9	479	17	106	26	2	.3	.2	.8
527	Bulgar, cooked	1 c	182	78	151	6	34	8	< 1	< .1	< .1	.2
	Cereal bar, Snackwell											
2165	Apple-Cinnamon	37 g	37	16	119	1	29	1	0	0.1	< .1	.1
2164	Blueberry	37 g	37	16	121	1	29	1	0	0.1	< .1	.1
2163	Strawberry	37 g	37	16	120	1	29	1	0	< .1	< .1	.1
	Cornmeal:											
528	Whole-ground, unbolted, dry	1 c	122	10	442	10	94	9	4	.6	1.2	2
529	Bolted, nearly whole, dry	1 c	122	10	441	10	94	12	4	.6	1.2	2
530	Degermed, enriched, dry	1 c	138	12	505	12	107	10	2	.3	.6	1
531	Degermed, enriched, cooked	1 c	240	78	209	5	44	4	1	.1	.2	.4
	Macaroni, cooked:											
532	Enriched	1 c	140	66	197	7	40	2	1	.1	.1	.4
533	Whole wheat	1 c	140	67	174	7	37	5	1	.1	.1	.3
534	Vegetable, enriched	1 c	134	68	172	6	36	6	< 1	t	t	.1
535	Millet, cooked	½ c	120	71	143	4	28	2	1	.2	.2	.6
	Noodles (see also Pasta and Spaghetti)											
1507	Cellophane noodles	1 c	190	79	160	< 1	39	< 1	< 1	t	t	t
1995	Cellophane noodles, dry	½ c	70	13	246	< 1	60	< 1	< 1	< .1	< .1	< .1
537	Chow mein, dry	1 c	45	1	237	4	26	2	14	2	3.5	7.8
536	Egg noodles, cooked, enriched	1 c	160	69	213	8	40	2	2	.5	.7	.7
538	Spinach noodles, dry	3½ oz	100	8	372	13	75	11	2	.2	.2	.6
1343	Oat bran, dry	¼ c	23	7	57	4	16	4	2	.3	.6	.7
	Pasta, cooked (see also #953–956):											
1418	Fresh	2 oz	57	69	74	3	14	1	1	.1	.1	.2
1417	Linguini	1 c	140	66	197	7	40	2	1	.1	.1	.4
1598	Rotini	1 c	140	66	197	7	40	2	1	.1	.1	.4
	Popcorn:											
539	Air popped, plain	1 c	8	4	31	1	6	1	< 1	< .1	.1	.2
1042	Microwaved, low fat, low sodium	1 c	6	3	24	1	4	1	1	.1	.2	.3
540	Popped in vegetable oil/salted	1 c	11	2	55	1	6	1	3	.5	.9	1.5
541	Sugar-syrup coated	1 c	35	2	151	1	28	2	4	1.3	1	1.6
	Rice:											
542	Brown rice, cooked	1 c	195	73	216	5	45	4	2	.4	.6	.6
2215	Mexican rice	½ c	113	–	410	8	90	3	15	2	.1	.1
2216	Spanish rice	½ c	123	85	65	2	14	1	1	–	–	–
	White, enriched, all types:											
543	Regular/long grain, dry	1 c	185	11	675	13	148	2	1	.3	.4	.3
544	Regular/long grain, cooked	1 c	205	68	267	6	58	1	< 1	.2	.2	.2
545	Instant, prepared without salt	1 c	165	76	161	3	35	1	< 1	.1	.1	.1

(Computer code number is for West Diet Analysis program)

Chol (mg)	Calc (mg)	Iron (mg)	Magn (mg)	Phos (mg)	Pota (mg)	Sodi (mg)	Zinc (mg)	VT-A (RE)	Thia (mg)	Ribo (mg)	Niac (mg)	V-B6 (mg)	Fola (µg)	VT-C (mg)
0	3	.57	17	43	42	<1	.28	0	.02	.03	1.3	.02	4	0
0	44	4.61[1]	32	100	108	276	.65	384[1]	.38[1]	.43[1]	5.1[1]	.52	102	15[1]
0	40	3.98	246	330	565	11	3.06	0	.41	.19	6.03	.57	53	0
0	11	1	47	86	314	1	2.56	0	.09	.05	.47	.09	100	0
0	32	3.85	405	606	805	2	4.2	0	.18	.74	12.3	.37	52	0
0	49	3.44	230	420	574	24	2.7	0	.32	.16	7.15	.48	38	0
0	18	1.75	58	73	123	9	1.04	0	.1	.05	1.82	.15	33	0
<1	17	5	6	37	68	103	3.88	–	.39	.44	5.2	.52	–	<1
<1	14	4.83	5	35	44	107	3.85	–	.39	.44	5.2	.52	–	<1
<1	14	4.82	6	35	47	102	3.83	–	.39	.44	5.2	.52	–	2
0	7	4.21	155	294	350	43	2.22	57	.47	.24	4.43	.37	31	0
0	7	4.21	154	294	350	43	2.22	57	.37	.1	2.3	.37	31	0
0	7	5.7	55	115	224	4	.99	57	.99	.56	6.96	.35	66	0
0	3	2.35	22	48	91	1	.41	23	.3	.21	2.42	.12	22	0
0	10	1.96	25	76	43	1	.74	0	.29	.14	2.34	.05	10	0
0	21	1.48	42	124	62	4	1.13	0	.15	.06	.99	.11	7	0
0	15	.66	26	67	41	8	.59	7	.15	.08	1.43	.03	8	0
0	4	.76	53	120	74	2	1.09	0	.13	.1	1.6	.13	23	0
0	14	1	3	15	5	9	.23	0	.07	0	.09	.02	1	0
0	18	1.53	2	22	7	7	.29	0	.11	.0	.14	.04	1	0
0	18	1.53	2	22	7	7	.29	0	.11	0	.14	.04	1	0
53	19	2.54	30	110	45	11	.99	10	.3	.13	2.38	.06	11	0
0	58	2.13	174	332	376	36	2.76	46	.37	.2	4.55	.32	48	0
0	13	1.27	55	169	130	1	.73	0	.27	.05	.22	.04	12	0
19	3	.65	10	36	14	3	.32	3	.12	.09	.56	.02	4	0
0	10	1.96	25	76	43	1	.74	0	.29	.14	2.34	.05	10	0
0	10	1.96	25	76	43	1	.74	0	.29	.14	2.34	.05	10	0
0	1	.21	11	24	24	<1	.27	2	.02	.02	.15	.02	2	0
0	1	.13	9	15	14	28	.22	1	.02	.01	.12	.01	1	0
0	1	.31	12	27	25	97	.29	2	.01	.01	.17	.02	2	<1
2	15	.61	12	29	38	72	.2	4	.02	.02	.77	.01	1	0
0	19	.82	84	162	84	10	1.23	0	.19	.05	2.98	.28	8	0
0	150	4.5	–	–	–	1350	–	–	–	–	–	–	–	48
0	–	.36	–	–	–	670	–	–	–	–	–	–	–	–
0	52	8	46	213	213	9	2.02	0	1.07	.09	7.75	.3	15	0
0	20	2.48	25	88	72	2	1	0	.33	.03	3.03	.19	6	0
0	13	1.04	8	23	7	5[2]	.4	0	.12	.08	1.45	.02	7	0

[1]Nutrient added (values sometimes based on label declaration).

[2]If prepared with salt according to label recommendation, sodium would be 608 mg.

(Computer code number is for West Diet Analysis program)

Table I–1
Food Composition

Computer Code Number	Food Description	Measure	Wt (g)	H₂O (%)	Ener (cal)	Prot (g)	Carb (g)	Dietary Fiber (g)	Fat (g)	Fat Breakdown (g) Sat	Mono	Poly
	GRAIN PRODUCTS: CEREAL, FLOUR, GRAIN, PASTA and NOODLES, POPCORN—Cont.											
	Parboiled/converted rice:											
546	Raw, dry	1 c	185	10	686	13	151	3	1	.3	.3	.3
547	Cooked	1 c	175	73	200	4	43	1	<1	.1	.1	.1
1486	Sticky rice (glutinous), cooked	1 c	241	76	234	5	51	2	<1	.1	.2	.2
548	Wild rice, cooked	1 c	164	73	166	7	35	2	1	.1	.1	.4
1700	Rice and pasta (Rice-a-Roni), cooked	½ c	109	71	133	3	23	4	3	.6	1.2	1
549	Rye flour, medium	1 c	102	10	361	10	79	15	2	.2	.2	.8
1044	Soy flour, low-fat	1 c	88	2	324	45	30	1	6	.9	1.3	3.3
	Spaghetti pasta:											
550	Without salt, enriched	1 c	140	66	197	7	40	2	1	.1	.1	.4
551	With salt, enriched	1 c	140	66	197	7	40	2	1	.1	.1	.4
552	Whole-wheat spaghetti, cooked	1 c	140	67	174	7	37	6	1	.1	.1	.3
1302	Tapioca, pearl, dry	1 c	152	11	518	<1	134	2	<1	.01	.01	.01
553	Wheat bran, crude	½ c	30	10	65	5	19	13	1	.2	.2	.7
554	Wheat germ, raw	1 c	100	11	360	23	52	15	10	1.7	1.4	6
555	Wheat germ, toasted	1 c	113	5	432	33	56	16	12	2.1	1.7	7.5
1669	Wheat germ, with brown sugar & honey	½ c	57	5	215	12	35	3	5	.8	.7	2.8
556	Rolled wheat, cooked	1 c	240	83	149	5	33	4	1	.2	.2	.4
557	Whole-grain wheat, cooked	⅓ c	50	86	28	1	7	1	<1	t	t	.1
	Wheat flour (unbleached):											
	All-purpose white, enriched:											
558	Sifted	1 c	115	11	419	12	88	3	1	.2	.1	.5
559	Unsifted	1 c	125	11	455	13	95	3	1	.2	.1	.5
560	Cake or pastry, enriched, sifted	1 c	96	12	348	8	75	2	1	.1	.1	.4
561	Self-rising, enriched, unsifted	1 c	125	11	443	12	93	3	1	.2	.1	.5
562	Whole wheat, from hard wheats	1 c	120	10	406	16	87	15	2	.4	.3	.9
	MEATS: FISH and SHELLFISH											
1045	Bass, baked or broiled	4 oz	113	68	166	27	0	0	5	1.1	2.1	1.5
1046	Bluefish, baked or broiled	4 oz	113	62	180	29	0	0	6	1.3	2.6	1.5
1047	Bluefish, fried in bread crumbs	4 oz	113	61	232	26	5	<1	11	2.4	4.9	2.8
1686	Catfish, breaded/flour fried	4 oz	113	48	325	21	14	1	20	5	9	5
	Clams:											
563	Raw meat only	4 oz	113	81	84	14	3	0	1	.1	.1	.3
564	Canned, drained	4 oz	113	72	168	29	6	0	2	.2	.2	.6
1290	Steamed, meat only	20 ea	90	71	133	23	5	0	2	.2	.2	.5
	Cod:											
565	Baked with butter	4 oz	113	75	150	26	0	0	4	.4	.3	.6
566	Batter fried	4 oz	113	76	196	20	8	<1	9	2.2	3.6	2.6
567	Poached, no added fat	4 oz	113	77	116	25	0	0	1	.2	.1	.3
	Crab, meat only:											
1048	Blue crab, cooked	4 oz	113	77	115	23	0	0	2	.3	.3	.8
1049	Dungeness crab, cooked	4 oz	113	73	124	25	1	0	1	.2	.2	.5
568	Blue crab, canned	4 oz	113	76	112	23	0	0	1	.3	.2	.5
1587	Crab, imitation, from surimi	4 oz	113	74	115	14	12	0	1	.3	.2	.8
569	Fish sticks, breaded pollock	2 ea	57	46	155	9	14	<1	7	1.8	2.9	1.8
	Flounder/sole, baked w/lemon juice:											
570	With butter	4 oz	113	73	160	21	<1	0	8	4.3	2	.7
571	With margarine	4 oz	113	73	160	21	<1	0	8	1.6	3.1	2.5

(Computer code number is for West Diet Analysis program)

Chol (mg)	Calc (mg)	Iron (mg)	Magn (mg)	Phos (mg)	Pota (mg)	Sodi (mg)	Zinc (mg)	VT-A (RE)	Thia (mg)	Ribo (mg)	Niac (mg)	V-B6 (mg)	Fola (μg)	VT-C (mg)
0	111	6.6	57	252	222	9	1.78	0	1.1	.13	6.72	.65	31	0
0	33	1.98	21	73	65	5	.54	0	.44	.03	2.45	.03	7	0
0	5	.34	12	19	24	12	.99	0	.05	.03	.7	.06	2	0
0	5	.98	52	134	166	5	2.2	0	.08	.14	2.12	.22	43	0
1	9	1.02	13	40	46	619	.31	0	.13	.08	1.94	.11	8	< 1
0	24	2.16	76	211	347	3	2.03	0	.29	.12	1.76	.27	19	0
0	165	5.27	201	521	2260	16	1.04	4	.33	.25	1.9	.46	360	0
0	10	1.96	25	76	43	1	.74	0	.29	.14	2.34	.05	10	0
0	10	1.96	25	76	43	140	.74	0	.29	.14	2.34	.05	10	0
0	21	1.48	42	125	62	4	1.13	0	.15	.06	.99	.11	7	0
0	30	2.4	2	11	17	2	.18	0	.01	0	0	.01	6	0
0	22	3.18	183	304	355	1	2.18	0	.16	.17	4.08	.39	24	0
0	39	6.26	239	842	892	12	12.3	0	1.88	.5	6.81	1.3	281	0
0	51	10.3	362	1294	1070	5	18.8	0	1.89	.93	6.32	1.11	398	7
0	19	3.86	136	490	405	2	7.06	0	.71	.35	2.37	.42	150	7
0	17	1.49	53	166	170	0	1.15	0	.17	.12	2.14	.17	26	0
0	3	.29	12	26	33	< 1	.24	0	.04	.01	.5	.03	4	0
0	17	5.34	25	124	122	2	.8	0	.9	.57	6.79	.05	30	0
0	19	5.8	27	135	133	2	.87	0	.98	.62	7.38	.05	32	0
0	13	7	15	82	101	2	.6	15	.36	.4	6.5	.03	18	0
0	423	5.84	24	743	155	1586	.77	0	.84	.52	7.29	.06	52	0
0	41	4.66	166	415	486	6	3.52	0	.54	.26	7.64	.41	53	0
98	116	2.17	43	290	517	102	.94	40	.1	.1	1.72	.16	19	2
86	10	.7	48	328	539	87	1.19	155	.08	.11	8.22	.53	2	0
68	9	.6	42	323	468	76	1.02	136	.07	.09	6.24	.41	2	< 1
92	40	1.44	34	270	576	597	1.03	32	.4	.22	3.2	.22	19	< 1
38	52	15.9	10	191	355	63	1.54	102	.09	.24	2	.07	18	15
76	104	31.6	20	383	707	127	3.1	194	.17	.48	3.81	.12	33	25
60	83	25.2	16	304	565	101	2.46	154	.13	.38	3.02	.1	26	20
68	23	.56	48	159	278	254	.66	34	.1	.09	2.85	.32	11	< 1
64	43	.9	36	230	443	124	.61	17	.12	.12	2.54	.23	10	1
61	23	.54	41	259	496	69	.64	14	.09	.08	2.48	.28	8	1
113	118	1.03	37	234	367	316	4.79	2	.11	.06	3.74	.2	57	4
86	67	.49	66	198	461	427	6.21	35	.06	.23	4.11	.2	48	4
100	114	.95	44	295	423	378	4.56	2	.09	.09	1.55	.17	48	3
23	15	.44	49	320	102	951	.37	23	.04	.03	.2	.03	2	0
64	11	.42	14	103	148	331	.38	18	.07	.1	1.21	.03	10	0
91	21	.37	67	249	363	193	.71	72	.09	.13	2.47	.27	13	1
73	21	.37	67	249	364	201	.71	92	.09	.13	2.47	.27	13	1

(For purposes of calculations, use "0" for t, < 1, < .1, < .01, etc.)

Table I–1
Food Composition

Computer Code Number	Food Description	Measure	Wt (g)	H₂O (%)	Ener (cal)	Prot (g)	Carb (g)	Dietary Fiber (g)	Fat (g)	Fat Breakdown (g)		
										Sat	Mono	Poly
	MEATS: FISH and SHELLFISH—Cont.											
572	Without added fat	4 oz	113	73	133	27	0	0	2	.4	.3	.5
1599	Grouper, baked or broiled	4 oz	113	73	133	28	0	0	1	.3	.3	.5
573	Haddoc, breaded, fried[1]	4 oz	113	55	264	22	14	1	13	3.2	5.4	3.3
1050	Haddock, smoked	4 oz	113	72	131	29	0	0	1	.2	.2	.4
	Halibut:											
1600	Baked or broiled	4 oz	113	72	158	30	0	0	3	.5	1.1	1.1
574	Baked with butter & lemon juice	4 oz	113	69	186	29	0	0	7	2.7	2.1	1.1
1051	Smoked	1 oz	28	49	63	6	0	0	4	.7	1.3	1.9
1054	Raw	4 oz	113	78	124	24	0	0	3	.4	.7	.9
575	Herring, pickled	3 oz	85	55	223	12	8	0	15	2	10.1	1.4
1052	Lobster meat, cooked w/moist heat	1 c	145	76	142	30	2	0	1	.2	.2	.1
1687	Ocean perch, baked/broiled	4 oz	113	73	137	27	0	0	2	.4	.9	.6
576	Ocean perch, breaded/fried	4 oz	113	59	249	22	9	1	13	3.2	5.7	3.4
1056	Octopus, raw	4 oz	113	80	93	17	3	0	1	.3	.2	.3
	Oysters:											
577	Raw, Eastern	1 c	248	85	169	18	10	0	6	1.9	.8	2.4
578	Raw, Pacific	1 c	248	82	201	23	12	0	6	1.3	.9	2.2
	Cooked:											
579	Eastern, breaded, fried, medium	6 ea	88	65	173	8	10	< 1	11	2.8	4.1	2.9
580	Western, simmered	4 oz	113	64	184	21	11	0	5	1.2	.8	2
581	Pollock, baked or broiled	4 oz	113	74	128	27	0	0	1	.3	.2	.6
1055	Pollock, moist heat, poached	4 oz	113	74	128	27	0	0	1	.3	.2	.6
	Salmon:											
582	Canned pink, solids and liquid	4 oz	113	69	157	22	0	0	7	1.7	2.1	2.3
583	Broiled or baked	4 oz	113	62	244	31	0	0	13	2.2	6	2.7
584	Smoked	4 oz	113	72	132	21	0	0	5	1	2.3	1.1
585	Atlantic sardines, canned, drained, 2 = 24 g	4 oz	113	60	235	28	0	0	13	1.7	4.4	5.8
586	Scallops, breaded, cooked from frozen	6 ea	93	58	199	17	9	< 1	10	2.5	4.2	2.7
1588	Scallops, imitation, from surimi	4 oz	113	74	112	14	12	0	< 1	.1	.1	.2
1688	Scallops, steamed/boiled	½ c	60	81	64	10	1	0	2	.3	.7	.6
	Shrimp:											
587	Cooked, boiled, 2 large = 14 g	6 ea	86	77	85	18	0	0	1	.2	.2	.4
588	Canned, drained	½ c	64	73	77	15	1	0	1	.2	.2	.5
589	Fried, 2 large = 15 g[1]	12 ea	90	53	218	19	10	< 1	11	1.9	3.6	4.6
1057	Raw, large, about 7 g each	14 ea	100	76	106	20	1	0	2	.3	.3	.7
1589	Shrimp, imitation, from surimi	4 oz	113	75	114	14	10	0	2	.3	.2	.9
1053	Snapper, baked or broiled	4 oz	113	70	145	30	0	0	2	.4	.4	.7
1060	Squid, fried in flour[2]	4 oz	113	65	198	20	9	< 1	8	2.1	3.1	2.4
1590	Surimi[3]	4 oz	113	76	112	17	8	0	1	.2	.2	.5
1058	Swordfish, raw	4 oz	113	76	137	22	0	0	5	1.2	1.8	1
1059	Swordfish, baked or broiled	4 oz	113	69	176	29	0	0	6	1.6	2.2	1.3
590	Trout, baked or broiled	4 oz	113	71	170	26	0	0	7	1.8	2	2.1
	Tuna, light, canned, drained solids:											
591	Oil pack	3 oz	85	60	168	25	0	0	7	1.3	2.5	2.4
592	Water pack	3 oz	85	74	98	22	0	0	1	.2	.1	.3
1061	Bluefin tuna, fresh	4 oz	113	68	163	26	0	0	6	1.4	1.8	1.9

[1]Dipped in egg, bread crumbs, and flour; fried in vegetable shortening.

[2]Recipe is 94.6% squid, 4.9% flour, and 0.6% salt.

[3]Surimi is processed from Walleye (Alaska) pollock. Also see Imitation crab, shrimp, scallops.

(Computer code number is for West Diet Analysis program)

Chol (mg)	Calc (mg)	Iron (mg)	Magn (mg)	Phos (mg)	Pota (mg)	Sodi (mg)	Zinc (mg)	VT-A (RE)	Thia (mg)	Ribo (mg)	Niac (mg)	V-B6 (mg)	Fola (μg)	VT-C (mg)
77	20	.39	66	327	390	119	.72	13	.09	.13	2.47	.27	10	2
53	24	1.29	42	162	537	60	.58	57	.09	.01	.43	.4	12	0
96	63	1.93	46	228	346	524	.59	33	.08	.14	4.51	.28	19	<1
87	56	1.59	61	285	469	862	.57	25	.05	.06	5.75	.45	17	0
47	68	1.21	121	323	652	78	.6	61	.08	.1	8.07	.45	16	0
54	66	1.17	116	308	636	112	.57	93	.08	.1	7.69	.43	16	5
28	14	.24	23	63	128	136	.12	13	.01	.02	1.64	.09	1	<1
36	53	.95	94	252	510	61	.48	53	.07	.08	6.62	.39	14	0
11	65	1.04	7	76	59	740	.45	219	.03	.12	2.81	.14	2	0
104	88	.57	51	268	510	551	4.23	38	.01	.1	1.55	.11	16	0
61	155	1	44	314	395	109	.7	16	.15	.15	2.77	.31	12	1
71	136	1.58	38	263	324	432	.67	23	.14	.18	2.69	.24	15	1
54	60	6.01	34	211	395	261	1.91	51	.03	.04	2.38	.41	18	6
131	112	16.5	117	335	387	523	225	74	.25	.24	3.42	.15	25	9
124	20	12.6	55	402	417	263	41.2	201	.17	.58	4.98	.12	25	20
71	55	6.12	51	139	214	366	76.7	79	.13	.18	1.45	.06	12	3
113	18	10.4	50	276	342	240	37.6	169	.14	.5	4.11	.1	17	15
108	7	.32	83	544	437	132	.68	26	.08	.09	1.87	.08	4	0
108	7	.32	83	544	437	132	.68	26	.08	.09	1.87	.08	4	0
62	242[4]	.95	38	373	368	626	1.04	19	.03	.21	7.42	.34	17	0
99	8	.62	35	312	425	75	.58	71	.24	.19	7.56	.25	6	0
26	12	.96	20	185	197	885	.35	29	.03	.11	5.35	.31	2	0
160	433[4]	3.31	44	553	450	572	1.5	76	.09	.26	5.95	.19	13	0
57	39	.76	55	219	309	431	.99	20	.04	.1	1.4	.13	17	2
25	9	.35	49	320	117	899	.37	23	.01	.02	.35	.03	2	0
19	15	.15	33	95	168	246	.55	31	.01	.04	.6	.08	7	1
167	33	2.65	29	117	156	192	1.34	57	.03	.03	2.22	.11	3	2
110	38	1.75	26	148	135	108	.8	11	.02	.02	1.76	.07	1	1
159	60	1.13	36	196	202	309	1.24	50	.12	.12	2.76	.09	7	1
152	52	2.41	37	205	185	148	1.11	54	.03	.03	2.55	.1	3	2
41	21	.68	49	320	101	797	.37	23	.03	.04	.19	.03	2	0
53	45	.27	42	228	590	65	.5	40	.06	<.01	.39	.52	7	2
295	44	1.15	43	285	316	347	1.97	12	.06	.52	2.95	.07	6	5
34	10	.29	49	319	127	162	.37	22	.02	.02	.25	.03	2	0
44	5	.92	31	297	326	102	1.3	41	.04	.11	11	.37	2	1
57	7	1.18	38	381	417	130	1.67	46	.05	.13	13.3	.43	3	1
78	97	.43	35	304	507	63	.58	17	.17	.11	6.54	.39	22	2
15	11	1.18	26	264	175	301	.77	20	.03	.1	10.5	.09	5	0
25	9	1.3	23	139	201	287	.65	14	.03	.06	11.3	.3	3	0
43	9	1.16	57	288	286	44	.68	740	.27	.28	9.81	.52	2	0

[4] If bones are discarded, calcium value is greatly reduced.

(For purposes of calculations, use "0" for t, <1, <.1, <.01, etc.)

Table I–1
Food Composition

Computer Code Number	Food Description	Measure	Wt (g)	H₂O (%)	Ener (cal)	Prot (g)	Carb (g)	Dietary Fiber (g)	Fat (g)	Fat Breakdown (g) Sat	Mono	Poly
	MEATS: BEEF, LAMB, PORK, and others											
	BEEF, cooked:[1]											
	Braised, simmered, pot roasted:											
	Relatively fat, choice chuck blade:											
593	Lean and fat, piece 2½ x 2½ x ¾"4 oz	4 oz	113	47	393	30	0	0	29	11.6	12.6	1.1
594	Lean only	4 oz	113	55	297	35	0	0	16	6.3	7	.5
	Relatively lean, like choice round:											
595	Lean and fat, pce 4⅛ x 2½ x ¾"	4 oz	113	52	311	32	0	0	19	7.2	8.3	.7
596	Lean only	4 oz	113	57	249	36	0	0	11	3.6	4.7	.4
	Ground beef, broiled, patty 3 x ⅝":											
597	Extra lean, about 16% fat	4 oz	113	54	299	32	0	0	18	7	7.8	.7
598	Lean, 21% fat	4 oz	113	53	316	32	0	0	20	7.9	8.7	.7
	Roasts, oven cooked, no added liquid:											
	Relatively fat, prime rib:											
601	Lean and fat, pce 4⅛ x 2¼ x ½"	4 oz	113	46	425	25	0	0	35	14.3	15.2	1.3
602	Lean only	4 oz	113	58	274	31	0	0	16	6.6	6.8	.5
	Relatively lean, choice round:											
603	Lean and fat, pce 2½ x 2½ x ¾"	4 oz	113	59	273	30	0	0	16	6.2	6.9	.6
604	Lean only	4 oz	113	65	198	33	0	0	6	2.3	2.7	.2
1701	Steak, rib, broiled, lean	4 oz	113	58	250	32	0	0	13	5	5	.4
	Steak, broiled, relatively lean, choice sirloin:											
605	Lean and fat, pce 2½ x 2½ x ¾"	4 oz	113	52	320	31	0	0	21	8.7	9.3	.8
606	Lean only	4 oz	113	62	228	34	0	0	9	3.5	3.9	.4
	Steak, broiled, relatively fat, choice T-bone:											
1063	Lean and fat	4 oz	113	53	337	28	0	0	24	9.7	10.1	.9
1064	Lean only	4 oz	113	60	242	32	0	0	12	4.7	4.7	.4
	Variety meats:											
1086	Brains, panfried	4 oz	113	71	221	15	0	0	18	4.2	4.5	2.6
599	Heart, simmered	4 oz	113	64	197	33	<1	0	6	1.9	1.4	1.5
600	Liver, fried	4 oz	113	56	245	30	9	0	9	3	1.8	1.9
1062	Tongue, cooked	4 oz	113	56	320	25	<1	0	23	10.3	11	.9
607	Beef, canned, corned	4 oz	113	58	282	31	0	0	17	7	6.8	.7
608	Beef, dried, cured	1 oz	28	57	46	8	<1	0	1	.5	.5	.1
	LAMB, domestic, cooked:											
	Chop, arm, braised (5.6 oz raw w/bone):											
609	Lean and fat	1 ea	70	44	242	21	0	0	17	6.9	7.1	1.2
610	Lean only	1 ea	55	49	153	20	0	0	8	2.8	3.4	.5
	Chop, loin, broiled (4.2 oz. raw w/bone):											
611	Lean and fat	1 ea	64	52	202	16	0	0	15	6.3	6.2	1.1
612	Lean only	1 ea	46	61	99	14	0	0	4	1.6	2	.3
1067	Cutlet, avg of lean cuts, cooked	4 oz	113	54	330	28	0	0	23	9.9	9.9	1.7
	Leg, roasted, 3 oz = 4⅛ x 2¼ x ½":											
613	Lean and fat	4 oz	113	57	292	29	0	0	19	7.8	7.9	1.3
614	Lean only	4 oz	113	64	216	32	0	0	9	3.1	3.8	.6
615	Rib, roasted, lean and fat	4 oz	113	48	406	24	0	0	34	14.5	14.2	2.5
616	Rib, roasted, lean only	4 oz	113	60	262	30	0	0	15	5.4	6.6	1
1065	Shoulder, roasted, lean and fat	4 oz	113	56	312	25	0	0	23	9.6	9.2	1.8

[1]Outer layer of fat removed to about ½" of the lean. Deposits of fat within the cut remain.

(Computer code number is for West Diet Analysis program)

I–48

Chol (mg)	Calc (mg)	Iron (mg)	Magn (mg)	Phos (mg)	Pota (mg)	Sodi (mg)	Zinc (mg)	VT-A (RE)	Thia (mg)	Ribo (mg)	Niac (mg)	V-B6 (mg)	Fola (µg)	VT-C (mg)
112	11	3.46	22	244	274	67	7.61	0	.08	.27	3.55	.32	10	0
120	15	4.17	26	265	297	81	11.7	0	.09	.32	3.03	.33	7	0
109	7	3.54	25	278	319	57	5.57	0	.08	.27	4.23	.37	11	0
109	6	3.92	28	308	348	58	6.21	0	.08	.29	4.63	.41	12	0
112	10	3.14	28	214	418	93	7.29	0	.08	.36	6.63	.36	12	0
114	14	2.78	27	205	396	101	7.03	0	.07	.27	6.77	.34	12	0
96	12	2.62	22	195	334	71	5.94	0	.08	.19	3.81	.26	8	0
90	11	2.96	28	242	422	81	7.87	0	.09	.24	4.67	.34	9	0
81	7	2.09	27	234	405	67	4.89	0	.09	.18	3.93	.4	7	0
78	6	2.21	31	256	447	70	5.38	0	.1	.19	4.25	.43	8	0
90	15	3	31	235	445	78	8	0	.11	.25	5.92	.45	9	0
102	12	3.4	32	247	407	70	6.5	0	.13	.3	4.38	.45	10	0
101	12	3.81	36	277	456	75	7.39	0	.15	.33	4.85	.51	11	0
94	9	3.01	28	208	401	69	5.31	0	.11	.25	4.63	.39	8	0
91	8	3.4	33	235	460	74	6.12	0	.13	.28	5.26	.44	9	0
2253	10	2.52	17	436	400	178	1.53	0	.15	.29	4.29	.44	7	4
219	7	8.52	28	282	264	71	3.55	0	.16	1.75	4.62	.24	2	2
545	12	7.12	26	522	411	120	6.18	12123[2]	.24	4.69	16.4	1.63	249	26
121	8	3.84	19	160	204	68	5.44	0	.03	.4	2.44	.18	6	1
97	14	2.36	16	126	153	1136	4.04	0	.02	.17	2.77	.15	10	2
12	2	1.28	9	49	126	972	1.49	0	.02	.06	1.55	.1	3	4
84	18	1.68	18	144	214	50	4.26	0	.05	.18	4.67	.08	13	0
67	14	1.49	16	127	186	42	4.01	0	.04	.15	3.48	.07	12	0
64	13	1.16	15	125	209	49	2.23	0	.06	.16	4.54	.08	12	0
44	9	.92	13	104	173	39	1.9	0	.05	.13	3.15	.07	11	0
110	12	2.27	25	206	340	77	4.68	0	.13	.32	7.51	.16	19	0
105	12	2.25	27	217	355	75	4.99	0	.11	.31	7.47	.17	23	0
101	9	2.4	29	234	383	77	5.6	0	.13	.33	7.19	.19	26	0
110	25	1.81	23	188	307	83	3.96	0	.1	.24	7.65	.13	17	0
100	24	2.01	26	221	356	92	5.07	0	.1	.26	6.99	.17	25	0
104	23	2.22	26	209	285	75	5.94	0	.1	.27	6.97	.15	24	0

[2] Value varies widely.

(For purposes of calculations, use "0" for t, < 1, < .1, < .01, etc.)

Table I–1
Food Composition

Computer Code Number	Food Description	Measure	Wt (g)	H$_2$O (%)	Ener (cal)	Prot (g)	Carb (g)	Dietary Fiber (g)	Fat (g)	Fat Breakdown (g)		
										Sat	Mono	Poly
MEATS: BEEF, LAMB, PORK, and others—Cont.												
1066	Shoulder, roasted, lean only	4 oz	113	63	231	28	0	0	12	4.6	4.9	1.1
	Variety meats:											
1069	Brains, panfried	4 oz	113	76	164	14	0	0	12	2.9	2.1	1.2
1068	Heart, braised	4 oz	113	64	209	28	2	0	9	3.6	2.5	.9
1070	Sweetbreads, cooked	4 oz	113	60	264	26	0	0	17	7.8	6.2	.8
1071	Tongue, cooked	4 oz	113	58	311	24	0	0	23	8.9	11.3	1.4
	PORK, cured, cooked (see also #669–672):											
617	Bacon, medium slices	3 pce	19	13	109	6	< 1	0	9	3.3	4.5	1.1
1087	Breakfast strips, cooked	2 pce	23	27	106	7	< 1	0	8	2.9	3.7	1.3
618	Canadian-style bacon	2 pce	47	62	87	11	1	0	4	1.3	1.9	.4
	Ham, roasted:											
619	Lean and fat, 2 pces 4⅛ x 2¼ x ¼"	4 oz	113	65	275	24	0	0	19	6.8	8.9	2.1
620	Lean only	4 oz	113	68	177	24	0	0	6	2	3	.7
621	Ham, canned, roasted, 8% fat	4 oz	113	69	189	24	1	0	10	3.2	4.6	1
	PORK, fresh, cooked:											
	Chops, loin (cut 3 per lb with bone):											
1291	Braised, lean and fat	1 ea	71	44	170	19	0	0	10	3.6	4.3	1
1292	Braised, lean only	1 ea	55	51	112	16	0	0	5	1.9	2.3	1
622	Broiled, lean and fat	1 ea	87	50	211	24	0	0	12	4.6	5.4	1
623	Broiled, lean only	1 ea	72	57	151	21	0	0	7	2.6	3.4	1
624	Panfried, lean and fat	1 ea	89	45	247	27	0	0	15	5.4	6.3	1.7
625	Panfried, lean only	1 ea	67	53	161	17	0	0	10	3.5	4	1.7
626	Leg, roasted, lean and fat	4 oz	113	53	308	30	0	0	20	7	9	2
627	Leg, roasted, lean only	4 oz	113	59	233	35	0	0	9	3	4	1
628	Rib, roasted, lean and fat	4 oz	113	51	288	31	0	0	17	6.7	7.9	1
629	Rib, roasted, lean only	4 oz	113	57	252	32	0	0	13	4.9	5.9	.96
630	Shoulder, braised, lean and fat	4 oz	113	47	391	32	0	0	26	9.6	11.8	2.6
631	Shoulder, braised, lean only	4 oz	113	54	281	37	0	0	14	4.8	6.5	1.3
1088	Spareribs, cooked, yield from 1 lb raw with bone	4 oz	113	40	450	33	0	0	34	12.5	15	3
1095	Rabbit, roasted (1 cup meat = 140 g)	4 oz	113	61	223	33	0	0	9	2.7	2.5	1.8
	VEAL, cooked:											
632	Cutlet, braised or broiled, 4⅛ x 2¼ x ½"	4 oz	113	52	322	34	0	0	19	7.6	7.6	1.3
633	Rib roasted, lean, 2 pieces 4⅛ x 2¼ x ¼"	4 oz	113	60	257	27	0	0	16	6.1	6.2	1.1
634	Liver, panfried	4 oz	113	67	187	24	3	0	8	2.9	1.7	1.2
1096	Venison (deer meat), roasted	4 oz	113	65	179	34	0	0	4	1.4	1	.7
MEATS: POULTRY and POULTRY PRODUCTS												
	CHICKEN, cooked:											
	Fried, batter dipped:[1]											
635	Breast (5.6 oz with bones)	1 ea	140	52	364	35	13	< 1	18	4.9	7.6	4.3
636	Drumstick (3.4 oz with bones)	1 ea	72	53	192	16	6	< 1	11	3	4.6	2.7
637	Thigh	1 ea	86	51	238	19	8	< 1	14	3.8	5.8	3.3
638	Wing	1 ea	49	46	158	10	5	< 1	11	2.9	4.4	2.5
	Fried, flour coated:[1]											
639	Breast (4.2 oz with bones)	1 ea	98	57	217	31	2	< 1	9	2.4	3.4	1.9

[1]Fried in vegetable shortening.

(Computer code number is for West Diet Analysis program)

Chol (mg)	Calc (mg)	Iron (mg)	Magn (mg)	Phos (mg)	Pota (mg)	Sodi (mg)	Zinc (mg)	VT-A (RE)	Thia (mg)	Ribo (mg)	Niac (mg)	V-B6 (mg)	Fola (μg)	VT-C (mg)
99	21	2.42	28	227	301	77	6.48	0	.1	.29	6.53	.17	28	0
2309	14	1.91	16	381	232	152	1.54	0	.12	.27	2.8	.12	6	14
281	16	6.26	27	288	213	71	4.17	0	.19	1.35	4.94	.34	2	8
452	14	2.4	21	489	328	59	3.04	0	.02	.24	2.9	.06	15	23
213	11	2.99	18	151	179	76	3.39	0	.09	.48	4.18	.19	3	8
16	2	.31	5	64	92	303	.62	0	.13	.05	1.39	.05	1	6[2]
24	3	.45	6	61	107	483	.83	0	.17	.08	1.72	.08	1	10
27	5	.38	10	139	183	726	.8	0	.39	.09	3.25	.21	2	10[2]
70	8	1	21	242	323	1341	2.6	0	.68	.25	5.04	.43	3	0
62	8	1	25	257	357	1500	2.9	0	.77	.29	5.67	.53	5	0
46	8	1	23	250	397	1207	2.6	0	1.09	.28	5.68	.45	6	26[2]
57	15	.77	13	129	266	34	1.7	2	.43	.18	3	.26	2	<1
43	15	.77	13	129	266	34	1.7	1	.38	.2	3	.25	2	<1
70	17	.76	24	214	368	54	2	3	.76	.28	4.37	.35	4	<1
57	12	.66	21	182	315	46	1.8	1	.66	.22	3.99	.34	4	<1
82	24	.81	26	231	378	71	2	3	.91	.27	5	.35	5	<1
55	15	.7	17	148	245	52	2.6	1	.49	.25	3.03	.27	3	<1
106	16	1.15	25	297	398	68	3.36	3	.72	.35	5.16	.45	11	<1
108	8	1.29	33	322	442	73	3.41	3	.91	.4	5.56	.38	3	<1
82	32	1.01	24	261	476	52	2.34	2	.82	.34	7	.34	3	<1
80	29	1.13	25	268	494	53	2.4	2	.86	.35	7	.39	3	<1
123	20	1.83	21	240	417	99	4.7	3	.61	.35	6	.4	5	<1
129	9	2.22	25	255	458	115	5.64	2	.68	.41	6.74	.46	6	<1
137	53	2.1	27	295	362	105	5.22	3	.46	.43	6.2	.4	5	0
93	21	2.57	24	297	433	53	2.59	0	.1	.24	9.56	.53	12	0
134	32	1.24	27	249	316	91	4.13	0	.04	.34	10.3	.29	16	0
125	12	1.1	25	222	333	104	4.64	0	.06	.31	7.92	.28	15	0
635	8	2.97	22	360	232	60	10.8	9095[3]	.15	2.2	9.62	.56	858	35
127	8	5.07	27	256	379	61	3.12	0	.2	.68	7.61	.43[4]	5[4]	0
119	28	1.75	34	259	281	385	1.33	28	.16	.2	14.7	.6	8	0
62	12	.97	14	105	133	193	1.68	19	.08	.15	3.67	.19	6	0
80	15	1.25	18	133	165	247	1.75	25	.1	.19	4.91	.22	8	0
39	10	.63	8	59	68	156	.68	17	.05	.07	2.58	.15	3	0
87	16	1.17	29	228	253	74	1.08	15	.08	.13	13.5	.57	4	0

[2]Values based on products containing added ascorbic acid or sodium ascorbate. If none added, ascorbic acid content would be negligible.

[3]Value varies widely.

[4]Values estimated from other game meat.

(For purposes of calculations, use "0" for t, <1, <.1, <.01, etc.)

Table I–1
Food Composition

Computer Code Number	Food Description	Measure	Wt (g)	H₂O (%)	Ener (cal)	Prot (g)	Carb (g)	Dietary Fiber (g)	Fat (g)	Fat Breakdown (g)		
										Sat	Mono	Poly
MEATS:	POULTRY and POULTRY PRODUCTS—Cont.											
	CHICKEN—Cont.											
1212	Breast, without skin	1 ea	86	60	160	29	< 1	.02	4	1.1	1.5	.9
640	Drumstick (2.6 oz with bones)	1 ea	49	57	120	13	1	< 1	7	1.8	2.7	1.6
641	Thigh	1 ea	62	54	162	17	2	< 1	9	2.5	3.6	2.1
1099	Thigh, without skin	1 ea	52	59	113	15	1	< 1	5	1.4	2	1.3
642	Wing	1 ea	32	49	102	8	1	< 1	7	1.9	2.8	1.6
	Roasted:											
643	All types of meat	1 c	140	64	266	40	0	0	10	2.9	3.7	2.4
644	Dark meat	1 c	140	63	287	38	0	0	14	3.7	5	3.2
645	Light meat	1 c	140	65	242	43	0	0	6	1.8	2.2	1.4
646	Breast, without skin	1 ea	86	65	141	27	0	0	3	.9	1.1	.7
647	Drumstick	1 ea	44	67	95	12	0	0	5	1.4	2	1
1703	Leg, without skin	1 ea	95	65	163	26	0	0	5	1.4	2	1
648	Thigh	1 ea	62	59	153	15	0	0	10	2.7	3.8	2.1
1100	Thigh, without skin	1 ea	52	63	108	13	0	0	6	1.6	2.2	1.3
649	Stewed, all types:	1 c	140	67	248	38	0	0	9	2.6	3.3	2.2
656	Canned, boneless chicken	4 oz	113	69	187	25	0	0	9	2.5	3.6	2
1102	Gizzards, simmered	3 ea	66	67	101	18	1	0	2	.7	.6	.7
1101	Hearts, simmered	8 ea	25	65	45	6	< 1	0	2	.6	.5	.6
650	Liver, simmered: Ounce	3 oz	85	68	133	21	1	0	5	1.6	1.1	.8
1098	Liver, simmered: Piece = 20 g	6 ea	120	68	187	29	1	0	7	2.2	1.6	1.1
	DUCK, roasted:											
1293	Meat with skin, about 2.7 cups	½ ea	382	52	1287	73	0	0	108	36.9	49.3	13.9
651	Meat only, about 1.5 cups	½ ea	221	64	444	52	0	0	25	9.2	8.2	3.2
	GOOSE, domesticated, roasted:											
1294	Meat only, 4.2 cups	½ ea	591	57	1406	171	0	0	75	26.9	25.6	9.1
1295	Meat with skin, about 5.5 cups	½ ea	774	52	2360	194	0	0	169	53.2	78.9	19.5
	TURKEY:											
	Roasted, meat only:											
652	Dark meat	4 oz	113	63	250	31	0	0	13	4	4	3.5
653	Light meat	4 oz	113	66	223	32	0	0	9	2.7	3.8	2.3
	Roasted, meat only—Cont.											
654	All types, chopped or diced	1 c	140	65	238	41	0	0	7	2.3	1.5	2
655	All types, sliced	4 oz	113	65	193	33	0	0	6	1.9	1.2	1.6
1103	Ground, cooked	4 oz	113	59	266	31	0	0	15	3.8	5.5	3.7
1104	Breast, barbecued	2 oz	57	69	72	11	2	0	2	.6	.6	.4
1105	Breast, hickory smoked	2 oz	57	72	62	13	0	0	1	.3	.3	.2
1106	Gizzard, cooked	2 ea	134	65	218	39	1	0	5	1.5	1	1.5
1107	Heart, cooked	4 ea	64	64	113	17	1	0	4	1.1	.8	1.1
1108	Liver, cooked	1 ea	75	66	126	18	3	0	4	1.4	1.1	.8
	POULTRY FOOD PRODUCTS (see also items in Sausages and Lunchmeats section):											
658	Chicken roll, light meat	2 pce	57	69	91	11	1	0	4	1.1	1.7	.9
1567	Chicken patty, breaded, cooked	1 ea	75	49	213	12	11	< 1	13	4	6	1.7
659	Turkey and gravy, frozen package	3 oz	85	85	57	5	4	< 1	2	.7	.8	.4
	Turkey breast, Louis Rich											
1943	Hickory Smoked	1 pce	80	–	80	16	2	0	1	0	–	–

(Computer code number is for West Diet Analysis program)

Chol (mg)	Calc (mg)	Iron (mg)	Magn (mg)	Phos (mg)	Pota (mg)	Sodi (mg)	Zinc (mg)	VT-A (RE)	Thia (mg)	Ribo (mg)	Niac (mg)	V-B6 (mg)	Fola (µg)	VT-C (mg)
78	14	.98	27	211	237	68	.93	6	.07	.11	12.7	.55	3	0
44	6	.66	11	86	112	44	1.42	12	.04	.11	2.96	.17	4	0
60	9	.92	16	115	146	55	1.56	18	.06	.15	4.31	.2	5	0
53	7	.76	14	103	134	49	1.45	11	.05	.13	3.7	.2	5	0
26	5	.4	6	48	57	25	.56	12	.02	.04	2.14	.13	1	0
124	21	1.69	35	273	340	120	2.94	22	.1	.25	12.8	.66	8	0
130	21	1.86	32	251	336	130	3.92	31	.1	.32	9.17	.5	11	0
119	21	1.48	38	302	346	107	1.72	13	.09	.16	17.4	.84	6	0
73	13	.89	25	196	220	64	.86	5	.06	.1	11.8	.52	3	0
41	5	.57	10	77	101	40	1.4	8	.03	.1	2.67	.15	4	0
88	11	1.26	23	174	234	90	3.03	18	.07	.22	5.8	.35	9	0
58	7	.83	14	107	137	52	1.46	30	.04	.13	3.95	.19	4	0
49	6	.68	12	95	123	46	1.34	10	.04	.12	3.39	.18	4	0
116	20	1.64	29	210	252	98	2.79	21	.07	.23	8.55	.36	8	0
70	16	1.79	14	126	155	570	1.6	39	.02	.15	7.18	.4	5	2
128	7	2.74	13	102	118	44	2.89	37	.02	.16	2.63	.08	35	1
61	5	2.22	5	49	33	12	1.8	2	.01	.18	.69	.08	20	< 1
536	12	7.23	18	264	119	42	3.68	4177	.13	1.49	3.78	.5	655	13
757	17	10.2	25	373	168	61	5.21	5894	.18	2.1	5.34	.7	924	19
320	42	10.3	61	596	779	225	7.11	241	.66	1.03	18.4	.69	23	0
196	26	5.97	44	449	557	143	5.75	51	.57	1.04	11.3	.55	22	0
567	83	17	147	1826	2293	449	18.7	71	.54	2.3	24.1	2.78	71	0
704	100	21.9	170	2089	2546	541	20.3	163	.6	2.5	32.3	2.86	15	0
101	37	2.64	27	221	310	86	4.7	0	.07	.28	3.99	.36	10	0
86	24	1.53	29	235	322	71	2.31	0	.07	.15	7.11	.53	7	0
106	35	2.49	36	298	417	98	4.34	0	.09	.25	7.62	.64	10	0
86	28	2.02	29	242	338	79	3.52	0	.07	.21	6.17	.52	8	0
116	28	2.2	27	222	306	121	3.25	0	.06	.19	5.47	.44	8	0
22	10	.4	12	184	166	609	.5	0	.02	.06	5.45	.22	2	< 1
23	4	.23	11	130	158	816	.64	0	.02	.06	4.72	.2	2	0
310	20	7.28	25	172	281	72	5.57	75	.04	.44	4.11	.16	69	2
145	8	4.4	14	131	117	35	3.37	5	.04	.56	2.08	.2	50	1
469	8	5.85	11	204	145	48	2.32	2805	.04	1.07	4.46	.39	500	1
28	24	.55	11	89	129	332	.41	14	.04	.07	3.02	.12	1	0
45	7	.86	18	195	208	352	.61	21	.11	.1	5.18	.26	8	< 1
15	12	.79	7	69	52	471	.59	11	.02	.11	1.53	.08	3	0
35	0	.72	–	–	–	1060	–	0	–	–	–	–	–	0

(1)If sodium ascorbate is added, product contains 11 mg ascorbic acid.

(For purposes of calculations, use "0" for t, < 1, < .1, < .01, etc.)

Table I–1
Food Composition

Computer Code Number	Food Description	Measure	Wt (g)	H₂O (%)	Ener (cal)	Prot (g)	Carb (g)	Dietary Fiber (g)	Fat (g)	Fat Breakdown (g)		
										Sat	Mono	Poly
MEATS:	POULTRY and POULTRY PRODUCTS TURKEY—Cont.											
1947	Honey roasted	1 pce	80	–	80	16	3	0	1	.5	–	–
1945	Oven roasted	1 pce	80	–	70	16	–	0	1	0	–	–
660	Turkey loaf, breast meat	4 oz	113	72	125	25	0	0	2	.5	.5	.3
661	Turkey patty, breaded, fried	2 oz	57	50	160	8	9	<1	10	2.7	4.2	2.7
662	Turkey, frozen, roasted, seasoned	4 oz	113	68	175	24	3	0	7	2.2	1.4	1.9
1704	Turkey roll, light meat	1 pce	28	72	42	5	<1	0	2	.6	.7	.5
MEATS:	SAUSAGES and LUNCHMEATS (see also Poultry Food Products)											
1072	Beerwurst/beer salami, beef	1 oz	28	53	93	4	<1	0	8	3.7	4	.3
1074	Beerwurst/beer salami, pork	1 oz	28	61	67	4	1	0	5	1.8	2.5	.7
1075	Berliner sausage	1 oz	28	61	65	4	1	0	5	1.7	2.3	.4
	Bologna:											
1297	Beef	1 pce	23	55	72	3	<1	0	7	2.8	3.2	.3
663	Beef & pork	1 pce	28	54	88	3	1	0	8	3	3.8	.7
2155	Healthy Favorites	2 ea	46	–	45	7	2	0	1	0	–	–
1298	Pork	1 pce	23	61	57	4	<1	0	5	1.6	2.2	.5
664	Turkey	1 pce	28	65	56	4	<1	0	4	1.4	1.4	1.2
	Bologna, Oscar Mayer											
2115	Beef, light	1 pce	28	–	60	3	2	0	4	1.5	–	–
2114	Regular, light	1 pce	28	–	60	3	2	0	4	1.5	–	–
665	Braunschweiger sausage	2 pce	57	48	205	8	2	0	18	6.2	8.5	2.1
1073	Bratwurst, link	1 ea	70	51	226	10	2	0	19	6.9	9.3	2
666	Brown & serve sausage links, cooked	2 ea	26	45	102	4	1	0	10	3.4	4.4	1
1089	Cheesefurter/cheese smokie	2 ea	86	52	280	12	1	0	25	9	11.8	2.6
2157	Chicken breast, Healthy Favorites	4 pce	52	–	40	9	1	0	0	0	0	0
1556	Chorizo, pork & beef	3 oz	85	32	387	20	2	0	33	12.2	15.6	2.9
1950	Coldcuts, Louis Rich, Deli Thin	1 pce	13	–	10	2	1	0	0	0	0	0
1090	Corned beef loaf, jellied	1 pce	28	69	43	6	0	0	2	.7	.8	.1
	Frankfurters (see also #657):											
1077	Beef, large link, 8/package	1 ea	57	55	180	7	1	0	16	6.9	7.7	.8
1078	Beef and pork, large link, 8/package	1 ea	57	54	182	6	1	0	17	6.2	7.8	1.6
667	Beef and pork, small link, 10/pkg	1 ea	45	54	144	5	1	0	13	4.9	6.2	1.2
657	Chicken frankfurter, 10/package	1 ea	45	57	115	6	3	0	9	2.5	3.8	1.8
668	Turkey frankfurter, 10/package	1 ea	45	63	101	6	1	0	8	2.7	2.5	2.2
1968	Turkey/Chicken frank 8/pkg	1 ea	43	–	80	6	1	0	6	2	–	–
	Ham:											
669	Ham lunchmeat, canned, 3 x 2 x ½"	1 pce	21	52	70	3	<1	0	6	2.3	3	.7
670	Chopped ham, packaged	2 pce	42	64	76	7	1.3	0	4.5	1.4	2.1	.5
671	Ham lunchmeat, regular	2 pce	57	65	103	10	2	0	6	1.9	2.8	.7
672	Ham lunchmeat, extra lean	2 pce	57	71	74	11	1	0	3	.9	1.3	.3
2156	Honey ham, Healthy Favorites	4 pce	52	–	50	9	2	0	2	.5	–	–
2113	Oscar Mayer Lower Sodium Ham	1 pce	21	–	23	3	1	0	1	0.3	–	–
673	Turkey ham lunchmeat	2 pce	57	71	73	11	<1	0	3	1	.7	.9
1091	Kielbasa sausage	1 pce	26	54	81	3	1	0	7	2.6	3.4	.8
1092	Knockwurst sausage, link	1 ea	68	55	209	8	1	0	19	6.9	8.7	2
1093	Mortadella lunchmeat	2 pce	30	52	93	5	1	0	8	2.9	3.4	.9
1097	Olive loaf lunchmeat	2 pce	57	58	134	7	5	<1	9	3.3	4.5	1.1
1970	Turkey Bologna, Louis Rich	1 pce	28	–	50	3	1	0	4	1	–	–

(Computer code number is for West Diet Analysis program)

Chol (mg)	Calc (mg)	Iron (mg)	Magn (mg)	Phos (mg)	Pota (mg)	Sodi (mg)	Zinc (mg)	VT-A (RE)	Thia (mg)	Ribo (mg)	Niac (mg)	V-B6 (mg)	Fola (μg)	VT-C (mg)
35	0	.72	–	–	–	940	–	0	–	–	–	–	–	0
35	0	–	–	–	–	910	–	0	–	–	–	–	–	0
46	8	.45	23	260	315	1617	1.28	0	.04	.12	9.45	.41	5	0[1]
35	8	1.25	9	153	156	456	.82	6	.06	.11	1.3	.11	5	0
60	6	1.86	25	277	338	768	2.88	0	.05	.19	7.11	.31	6	0
12	11	.37	4	52	71	137	.45	0	.03	.06	1.98	.09	1	0
17	3	.43	3	27	49	288	.69	0	.02	.03	.96	.05	1	4
17	2	.22	4	29	72	347	.49	0	.16	.05	.92	.1	1	8
13	3	.33	4	37	80	363	.7	0	.11	.06	.88	.06	1	2
13	3	.38	3	20	36	226	.5	0	.01	.02	.55	.03	1	5
15	3	.43	3	26	51	288	.55	0	.05	.04	.73	.05	1	6[2]
15	–	.36	–	–	–	510	–	–	–	–	–	–	–	–
14	3	.18	3	32	65	272	.47	0	.12	.04	.9	.06	1	8
28	24	.43	4	37	56	246	.49	0	.02	.05	1	.06	2	0
10	–	–	–	–	–	310	–	–	–	–	–	–	–	–
15	–	–	–	–	–	310	–	–	–	–	–	–	–	–
89	5	5.34	6	96	113	652	1.6	2405	.14	.87	4.77	.19	25	6[2]
44	34	.72	11	94	196	778	1.47	0	.17	.16	2.31	.09	4	20
16	2	.62	4	42	70	248	.3	0	.21	.09	.96	.06	1	0
58	50	.93	11	153	177	930	1.94	33	.21	.14	2.5	.11	3	17
25	–	.72	–	–	–	620	–	–	–	–	–	–	–	–
75	7	1.35	15	128	338	1049	2.9	0	.54	.25	4.36	.45	2	0
4	0	.18	–	–	–	153	–	0	–	–	–	–	–	0
13	3	.58	3	20	29	267	1.16	0	0	.03	.5	.03	2	2
35	11	.81	2	50	95	585	1.24	0	.03	.06	1.38	.07	2	14
28	6	.66	6	49	95	638	1.05	0	.11	.07	1.5	.07	2	15
22	5	.52	4	39	75	504	.83	0	.09	.05	1.18	.06	2	12[2]
45	43	.9	6	48	38	616	.47	17	.03	.05	1.39	.14	2	0
39	48	.83	6	60	81	641	1.4	0	.02	.08	1.86	.1	4	0
40	60	1.08	–	–	–	480	–	0	–	–	–	–	–	0
13	1	.15	2	17	45	270	.31	0	.08	.04	.65	.04	1	<1
21	3	.35	7	65	134	576	.9	0	.36	.09	2.2	.15	1	12[2]
32	4	.56	11	140	188	746	1.21	0	.49	.14	2.98	.19	2	16[2]
27	4	.43	10	124	198	810	1.09	0	.53	.13	2.74	.26	2	15[2]
25	–	.72	–	–	–	630	–	–	–	–	–	–	–	–
10	–	.24	–	–	–	173	–	–	–	–	–	–	–	–
32	6	1.57	9	108	185	567	1.68	0	.03	.14	2.01	.14	3	0
17	11	.38	4	38	70	279	.52	0	.06	.06	.75	.05	1	5
39	7	.62	7	67	135	687	1.13	0	.23	.09	1.86	.12	1	18
17	5	.42	3	29	49	374	.63	0	.04	.05	.8	.04	1	8
22	62	.31	11	72	169	846	.79	11	.17	.15	1.05	.13	1	5
20	20	.36	–	–	–	250	–	0	–	–	–	–	–	0

[2]Values based on products containing added ascorbic acid or sodium ascorbate. If none added, ascorbic acid content would be negligible.

(For purposes of calculations, use "0" for t, < 1, < .1, < .01, etc.)

Table I–1
Food Composition

Computer Code Number	Food Description	Measure	Wt (g)	H₂O (%)	Ener (cal)	Prot (g)	Carb (g)	Dietary Fiber (g)	Fat (g)	Fat Breakdown (g)		
										Sat	Mono	Poly
	MEATS: SAUSAGES and LUNCHMEATS (see also Poultry Food Products)—Cont.											
1952	Turkey breast, fat free	1 pce	28	–	25	4	1	0	0	0	0	0
1080	Turkey pastrami	2 pce	57	71	80	10	1	0	4	1	1.2	.9
1969	Turkey salami	1 pce	28	–	45	5	0	0	3	1	–	–
1081	Pepperoni sausage	2 pce	11	27	54	2	<1	0	5	1.8	2.3	.5
1094	Pickle & pimento loaf	2 pce	57	57	149	7	3	<1	12	4.5	5.5	1.5
1082	Polish sausage	1 oz	28	53	92	4	<1	0	8	2.9	3.9	.9
674	Pork sausage, cooked,[1] link, small	2 ea	26	45	96	5	<1	0	8	2.8	3.6	1
1079	Pork sausage, cooked, patty	4 oz	113	45	418	22	1	0	35	12.2	15.8	4.3
675	Salami, pork and beef	2 pce	57	60	143	8	1	0	11	4.6	5.2	1.1
676	Salami, turkey	2 pce	57	66	111	9	<1	0	8	2.3	2.6	2
677	Beef & pork, dry	3 pce	30	35	125	7	1	0	10	3.7	5.1	1
	Sandwich spreads:											
1300	Ham salad spread	1 c	240	63	518	21	26	0	37	12.2	17.3	6.5
678	Pork and beef	2 tbs	30	60	70	2	4	<1	5	1.8	2.3	.8
1296	Chicken/turkey	2 tbs	26	66	52	3	2	0	4	.9	.8	1.6
1084	Smoked link sausage, beef and pork	1 ea	68	52	228	9	1	0	21	7.2	9.7	2.2
1083	Smoked link sausage, pork	1 ea	68	39	265	15	1	0	22	7.7	9.9	2.6
1085	Summer sausage	2 pce	46	51	154	7	<1	0	14	5.5	6	.6
1076	Turkey breakfast sausage	1 pce	28	60	65	6	0	0	5	1.6	1.8	1.2
679	Vienna sausage, canned	2 ea	32	60	89	3	1	0	8	3	4	.5
	MIXED DISHES and FAST FOODS											
	MIXED DISHES:											
1445	Almond chicken	1 c	242	77	275	20	18	4	14	2	5.3	5.8
1454	Bean cake	1 ea	32	23	130	2	16	1	7	1	2.9	2.6
680	Beef stew w/ vegetables, homemade	1 c	245	82	218	16	15	2	10	4.9	4.5	.5
1109	Beef stew w/ vegetables, canned	1 c	245	82	194	14	17	2	8	2.4	3.1	.3
1116	Beef, macaroni, tomato sauce casserole	1 c	226	73	284	21	25	3	11	4.2	4.7	.6
1452	Beef fajita	1 ea	189	63	347	15	39	3	15	4.3	6.4	1
1265	Beef flauta	1 ea	113	49	360	17	13	2	27	4.9	11.6	9.1
681	Beef pot pie, homemade[2]	1 pce	210	55	517	21	39	3	31	8.4	14.9	7.4
1898	Broccoli, batter fried	1 c	85	74	123	3	9	2	9	1.3	2.2	4.9
1462	Buffalo wings/spicy chicken wings	2 ea	32	53	98	8	<1	<1	7	1.8	2.8	1.6
1675	Carrot raisin salad	½ c	88	58	202	1	21	3	14	2.1	3.9	7.1
682	Chicken à la king, homemade	1 c	245	68	468	27	12	1	34	12.7	14.3	6.2
683	Chicken & noodles, homemade	1 c	240	71	367	22	26	2	18	5.9	7.1	3.5
684	Chicken chow mein, canned	1 c	250	89	95	6	18	2	1	0	.1	.8
685	Chicken chow mein, homemade	1 c	250	78	255	31	10	1	10	2.4	4.3	3.1
1451	Chicken fajitas	1 ea	189	61	344	17	43	4	11	2	5	1
1264	Chicken flauta	1 ea	113	53	343	14	13	2	27	4.3	11.1	9.6
686	Chicken pot pie, homemade (⅓)	1 pce	232	57	545	23	42	3	33	10.9	15.5	6.6
1672	Chili con carne	½ c	127	77	128	12	11	2	4	1.7	1.7	.3
1112	Chicken salad with celery	2 c	78	53	268	11	1	<1	25	4	7.2	12.1
1382	Chicken teriyaki-breast	1 pce	128	67	176	26	7	<1	4	.9	1.0	0.9
687	Chili with beans, canned	1 c	255	76	286	15	30	11	14	6	5.9	.9
1479	Chinese pastry	1 oz	28	46	67	1	13	<1	1	.2	.4	.8
688	Chop suey with beef & pork	1 c	250	63	483	26	35	4	25	5.7	9.8	3.9

[1]Cooked weight is half the weight of raw sausage.

[2]Crust made with vegetable shortening and enriched flour.

(Computer code number is for West Diet Analysis program)

Chol (mg)	Calc (mg)	Iron (mg)	Magn (mg)	Phos (mg)	Pota (mg)	Sodi (mg)	Zinc (mg)	VT-A (RE)	Thia (mg)	Ribo (mg)	Niac (mg)	V-B6 (mg)	Fola (µg)	VT-C (mg)
10	0	0	–	–	–	310	–	0	–	–	–	–	–	0
31	5	.95	8	114	148	595	1.23	0	.03	.14	2.01	.15	3	0
20	0	0	–	–	–	290	–	0	–	–	–	–	–	0
9	1	.15	2	13	38	224	.27	0	.03	.03	.54	.03	<1	0
21	54	.58	10	80	194	792	.8	4	.17	.14	1.17	.11	3	8
20	3	.41	4	39	67	245	.55	0	.14	.04	.97	.05	1	<1
22	8	.32	4	48	94	336	.65	0	.19	.07	1.18	.09	1	<1
94	36	1.42	19	209	409	1462	2.84	0	.84	.29	5.13	.37	2	2
37	7	1.51	9	65	112	607	1.21	0	.14	.21	2.01	.12	1	7[8]
47	11	.92	9	60	139	572	1.03	0	.04	.1	2.01	.14	2	0
24	2	.45	5	43	113	558	.97	0	.18	.09	1.46	.15	1	8[8]
89	19	1.42	24	288	360	2188	2.64	0	1.04	.29	5.04	.36	2	14
11	4	.24	2	18	33	304	.31	3	.05	.04	.52	.04	1	0
8	3	.16	3	9	48	98	.27	11	.01	.02	.43	.03	1	<1
48	7	.99	8	73	128	642	1.43	0	.18	.12	2.19	.12	1	13
46	20	.79	13	110	228	1020	1.92	0	.48	.17	3.08	.24	3	1
33	6	1.17	6	51	125	571	1.18	0	.07	.15	1.98	.12	1	9
23	5	.52	6	52	76	188	.97	0	.03	.08	1.42	.08	1	0
17	3	.28	2	16	32	304	.51	0	.03	.03	.51	.04	1	0
35	81	2.12	59	238	550	615	1.56	75	.08	.19	8.59	.4	31	10
0	3	.65	6	21	56	55	.15	0	.06	.04	.49	.02	9	0
64	29	2.94	40	184	613	292	5.29	568	.15	.17	4.66	.28	37	17
34	29	2.21	39	110	426	1006	4.24	262	.07	.12	2.45	.2	31	7
57	28	3.11	42	161	559	841	4.3	93	.23	.25	5.22	.33	22	13
22	64	3	32	170	362	721	2	44	.3	.26	4	.27	21	24
45	50	2.15	29	199	292	187	4.18	15	.07	.15	2.13	.25	10	14
44	29	3.78	6	149	334	596	3.17	519	.29	.29	4.83	.24	29	6
16	67	.94	20	71	242	62	.38	102	.08	.13	.75	.11	43	53
26	5	.4	6	47	59	61	.56	17	.01	.04	2.06	.13	1	<1
10	26	.74	14	46	317	117	.18	1462	.08	.05	.63	.22	9	5
186	127	2.45	20	358	404	760	1.8	272	.1	.42	5.39	.23	11	12
96	26	2.16	26	247	149	600	1.53	10	.05	.17	4.32	.19	10	0
8	45	1.25	14	85	418	725	1.3	28	.05	.1	1	.09	12	12
78	57	2.5	28	293	473	718	2.12	50	.07	.22	4.25	.41	19	10
35	71	3	43	174	451	372	1.5	47	.41	.34	5.6	.03	35	19
37	52	.97	28	146	243	189	1.18	21	.05	.1	3.21	.22	8	14
72	70	3.02	25	232	343	594	2	735	.32	.32	4.87	.46	29	5
67	34	2.62	23	99	347	506	1.8	84	.06	.57	1.25	.17	15	<1
47	16	.62	11	80	138	201	.8	31	.03	.07	3.27	.34	8	1
80	27	1.75	36	199	309	1866	1.94	16	.08	.2	8.69	.46	13	3
43	120	8.75	115	393	931	1331	5.1	87	.12	.27	.91	.34	58	4
0	7	.55	6	16	28	3	.2	<1	.04	<.01	.35	.02	1	0
52	44	4.45	61	284	586	930	3.9	152	.42	.42	6.4	.47	50	23

[8]Values based on products containing added ascorbic acid or sodium ascorbate. If none added, ascorbic acid content would be negligible.

(For purposes of calculations, use "0" for t, <1, <.1, <.01, etc.)

Table I–1
Food Composition

Computer Code Number	Food Description	Measure	Wt (g)	H₂O (%)	Ener (cal)	Prot (g)	Carb (g)	Dietary Fiber (g)	Fat (g)	Fat Breakdown (g)		
										Sat	Mono	Poly
	MIXED DISHES and FAST FOOD—Cont.											
	MIXED DISHES—Cont.											
690	Coleslaw[1]	1 c	120	74	178	2	15	2	13	2	2.9	7.7
689	Corn pudding[2]	1 c	250	76	273	11	32	4	13	6.3	4.3	1.7
1110	Corned beef hash, canned	1 c	220	67	398	19	24	1	25	11.9	10.9	.9
1255	Deviled egg (½ egg 1 filling)	1 ea	31	69	63	4	< 1	0	5	1.2	1.7	1.5
	Egg foo yung patty:											
1467	Meatless	1 ea	86	94	26	3	< 1	0	1	.4	.5	.2
1458	With beef	1 ea	86	74	129	9	3	< 1	9	2.2	3.2	2.4
1465	With chicken	1 ea	86	74	130	9	4	< 1	9	2.1	3.1	2.5
1602	Egg roll, meatless	1 ea	64	70	101	3	10	1	6	1.2	2.5	1.6
1550	Egg roll, with meat	1 ea	64	66	114	5	9	1	6	1.6	2.9	1.6
1113	Egg salad	1 c	183	57	586	17	3	0	56	10.6	17.5	24.2
691	French toast w/wheat bread, homemade[3]	1 pce	65	54	151	5	16	< 1	7	2	3	1.7
1355	Green pepper, stuffed	1 ea	172	74	236	11	20	2	12	5.3	5.3	.6
1487	Hot & sour soup (Chinese)	1 c	244	88	133	12	5	< 1	6	2	2.9	1.2
1997	Hummous/Hummus	¼ c	62	64	105	3	12	2	5	0.8	2.2	2.0
	Lasagna:											
1346	With meat, homemade	1 pce	245	66	382	22	39	3	15	7.7	5	.8
1111	Without meat, homemade	1 pce	218	68	298	15	39	3	9	5.4	2.4	.6
1117	Frozen entree	1 pce	205	74	235	15	25	3	9	4	3.3	.5
1606	Lo mein, meatless	1 c	200	83	123	6	23	3	1	.3	.3	.4
1607	Lo mein, with meat	1 c	200	71	284	16	27	3	13	2.9	4.2	4.7
692	Macaroni & cheese, canned[4]	1 c	240	80	228	9	26	1	10	4.2	3.1	1.4
693	Macaroni & cheese, homemade[5]	1 c	200	58	430	17	40	1	22	8.9	8.8	3.6
1115	Macaroni salad, no cheese	1 c	141	60	363	3	21	3	30	4.4	8.5	15.5
1120	Meat loaf, beef	1 pce	87	62	185	14	5	< 1	11	4	4.8	.6
1119	Meat loaf, beef and pork (⅓)	1 pce	87	57	221	17	4	< 1	15	5.4	6.4	1.2
1303	Moussaka (lamb & eggplant)	1 c	250	83	209	18	14	3	9	2.7	3.7	1.5
1899	Mushrooms, batter fried	5 ea	70	66	148	2	8	1	12	2.1	3.0	6.4
715	Potato salad with mayonnaise and eggs[6]	½ c	125	76	179	3	14	2	10	1.8	3.1	4.7
1674	Pizza, combination, 1/12 of 12" round	1 pce	53	48	123	9	14	–	4	1	1.7	.6
1673	Pizza, pepperoni, 1/12 of 12" round	1 pce	47	46	121	7	13	–	5	1.5	2.1	.8
694	Quiche Lorraine, ⅛ of 8" quiche[7]	1 pce	176	54	508	20	20	1	39	18	13.8	4.9
1449	Ramen noodles, cooked	1 c	227	83	156	5	29	3	2	.4	.4	.4
1671	Ravioli, meat	½ c	125	68	194	11	18	1	9	3	3.6	1
1597	Fried rice (meatless)	1 c	166	68	264	5	34	1	11	1.7	2.9	6.2
2142	Roast beef hash	½ c	95	68	158	11	10	1	8	2.5	2.9	1.7
	Spaghetti (enriched) in tomato sauce:											
	With cheese:											
695	Canned	1 c	250	80	190	5	38	2	1	0	.4	.5
696	Homemade	1 c	250	77	260	9	37	2	9	2	5.4	1.2

[1]Recipe: 41% cabbage; 12% celery; 12% table cream; 12% sugar; 7% green pepper; 6% lemon juice; 4% onion; 3% pimento; 3% vinegar; 2% each for salt, dry mustard, and white pepper.
[2]Recipe: 55% yellow corn, 23% whole milk, 14% egg, 4% sugar, 3% salt, and 1% pepper.
[3]Recipe: 35% whole milk, 32% white bread, 29% egg, and cooked in 4% margarine.
[4]Made with corn oil.
[5]Made with margarine.
[6]Recipe: 62% potatoes; 12% egg; 8% mayonnaise; 7% celery; 6% sweet pickle relish; 2% onion; 1% each for green pepper, pimento, salt, and dry mustard.
[7]Crust made with vegetable shortening and enriched flour.

(Computer code number is for West Diet Analysis program)

Chol (mg)	Calc (mg)	Iron (mg)	Magn (mg)	Phos (mg)	Pota (mg)	Sodi (mg)	Zinc (mg)	VT-A (RE)	Thia (mg)	Ribo (mg)	Niac (mg)	V-B6 (mg)	Fola (μg)	VT-C (mg)
6[9]	41	.88	11	43	215	324	.24	60	.05	.04	.1	.13	47	10
250	100	1.4	37	143	403	138	1.25	90	1.03	.32	2.47	.29	63	7
73	29	4.4	36	147	440	1188	3.3	0	.02	.2	4.62	.43	20	0
121	15	.35	3	49	37	94	.3	49	.02	.14	.02	.05	13	0
37	7	.26	2	38	77	257	.17	14	.01	.07	1.07	.02	5	0
180	26	1.1	11	112	143	185	1.16	92	.05	.24	.73	.16	22	3
182	28	.85	12	102	143	188	.81	95	.05	.24	.95	.13	22	3
30	12	.74	9	39	97	307	.25	15	.07	.1	.75	.05	13	3
38	12	.77	10	58	124	305	.5	14	.13	.12	1.31	.09	8	2
574	74	1.8	13	236	180	666	1.44	262	.08	.66	.08	.47	61	0
76	64	1.09	11	76	86	311	.44	81	.13	.21	1.06	.05	15	< 1
38	17	1.88	20	89	230	203	2.2	44	.14	.09	2.91	.31	17	55
22	29	1.87	27	160	351	1562	1.15	2	.19	.22	4.56	.15	12	1
0	31	.97	18	69	107	150	.68	2	.06	.03	.25	.24	37	5
56	258	3.43	50	289	461	745	3.19	158	.21	.33	4	.21	19	16
31	252	2.5	44	239	375	714	1.7	156	.2	.28	2.49	.17	17	15
33	158	2.17	39	185	453	496	2.19	149	.16	.24	3.06	.19	17	25
22	48	2.18	30	115	396	624	.91	163	.18	.23	2.48	.18	41	13
61	25	2.2	34	177	260	276	1.85	38	.42	.27	3.4	.26	39	9
24	199	.96	31	182	139	730	1.2	73	.12	.24	.96	.02	8	< 1
42	362	1.8	37	322	240	1086	1.2	234	.2	.4	1.8	.05	10	1
22	27	.67	16	51	137	289	.38	39	.08	.05	.75	.26	16	3
72	35	1.61	18	129	236	329	2.92	14	.07	.22	3.36	.11	10	1
91	35	1.55	16	129	236	389	3.12	23	.2	.22	3.18	.19	11	1
101	104	2.2	38	204	578	400	2.84	105	.21	.31	4.01	.26	45	6
14	54	.77	8	103	180	121	.42	10	.07	.22	1.65	.05	8	1
85	24	.81	19	65	318	661	.39	41	.1	.07	1.11	.18	8	13
14	68	1.03	12	88	119	255	.75	68	.14	.12	1.31	.06	18	1
10	43	.63	6	50	102	178	.35	36	.09	.16	2.04	.04	35	1
205	201	1.9	27	271	271	549	1.48	243	.22	.45	4.71	.1	17	3
38	20	1.78	24	82	51	1349	.61	204	.22	.09	1.42	.07	8	< 1
84	33	1.99	20	109	259	619	1.67	94	.13	.20	2.85	.15	13	11
42	30	1.84	24	94	134	286	.84	62	.21	.11	2.25	.1	22	4
29	10	1.24	18	103	294	427	2.53	< 1	.08	.1	1.89	.25	8	4
8	40	2.75	21	87	303	955	1.12	120	.35	.27	4.5	.13	6	10
8	80	2.25	26	135	408	955	1.3	140	.25	.17	2.25	.2	8	12

[9]From dairy cream in recipe.

(For purposes of calculations, use "0" for t, < 1, < .1, < .01, etc.)

Table I–1
Food Composition

Computer Code Number	Food Description	Measure	Wt (g)	H₂O (%)	Ener (cal)	Prot (g)	Carb (g)	Dietary Fiber (g)	Fat (g)	Fat Breakdown (g)		
										Sat	Mono	Poly
	MIXED DISHES and FAST FOODS—Cont.											
	MIXED DISHES—Cont.											
	With meatballs:											
697	Canned	1 c	250	78	258	12	28	6	10	2.1	3.9	3.9
698	Homemade	1 c	248	70	332	19	39	8	12	3.3	6.3	2.2
716	Spinach soufflé[1]	1 c	136	74	219	11	3	4	18	7.1	6.8	3.1
1553	Sweet & sour pork	1 c	226	76	231	14	25	1	8	2.8	3.8	2.9
1263	Sweet & sour chicken breast	1 ea	131	79	117	8	15	1	3	0.6	0.8	1.5
1515	Three bean salad	1 ea	340	82	316	9	30	7	19	2.8	4.3	11.1
717	Tuna salad[2]	1 c	205	63	383	33	19	1	19	3.2	5.9	8.4
1121	Tuna noodle casserole, homemade	1 c	202	75	238	17	25	2	7	1.9	1.5	3.2
1270	Waldorf salad	1 c	142	59	411	3	13	2	41	5.4	10.9	22.2
	FAST FOODS and SANDWICHES (see end of this appendix for additional Fast Foods):											
699	Burrito,[3] beef & bean	1 ea	175	52	385	17	50	4	14	6.3	5.3	.9
700	Burrito, bean	1 ea	174	53	358	11	57	7	11	5.5	3.8	1
2106	Burrito, chicken con queso	1 ea	306	77	280	12	53	5	6	1.5	–	–
701	Cheeseburger with bun, regular	1 ea	112	55	261	13	20	–	14	6.7	5.2	1.1
702	Cheeseburger with bun, 4-oz patty	1 ea	194	51	487	25	41	–	25	10.2	9.1	3.1
703	Chicken patty sandwich	1 ea	157	47	444	21	33	1	25	7.4	9	7.2
704	Corndog	1 ea	111	47	292	11	35	–	12	3.3	5.8	2.2
1922	Corndog, chicken	1 ea	113	59	272	13	26	–	13	–	–	–
705	Enchilada	1 ea	230	63	451	14	40	–	27	15	8.9	1.1
706	English muffin with egg, cheese, bacon	1 ea	138	49	362	19	30	1	19	8.6	6.4	1.9
	Fish sandwich:											
707	Regular, with cheese	1 ea	140	45	400	16	36	< 1	22	6.2	6.8	7.2
708	Large, no cheese	1 ea	170	47	464	18	44	< 1	24	5.6	8.3	8.9
709	Hamburger with bun, regular	1 ea	98	45	252	12	30	1	9	3.2	3.4	1.6
710	Hamburger with bun, 4-oz patty	1 ea	174	51	466	26	31	–	26	9.7	11.4	2.2
711	Hot dog/frankfurter with bun	1 ea	85	54	210	9	16	–	13	4.4	5.9	1.5
	Lunchables											
2129	Bologna & American cheese	1 ea	128	–	450	18	19	0	34	15	–	–
2130	Ham & swiss cheese	1 ea	128	–	320	22	19	0	17	8	–	–
2117	Honey ham & Amer. w/choc pudding	1 ea	176	–	390	18	34	1	20	9	–	–
2118	Honey turkey & cheddar w/Jello	1 ea	163	–	320	17	27	1	16	9	–	–
2131	Pepperoni & American cheese	1 ea	128	–	480	20	19	0	36	17	–	–
2125	Salami & American cheese	1 ea	128	–	430	18	18	0	32	15	–	–
2127	Turkey & cheddar	1 ea	128	–	360	20	20	1	22	11	–	–
712	Pizza, cheese, ⅛ of 15" round[4]	1 pce	120	49	268	15	39	2	6	2.9	1.9	.9
	SANDWICHES:											
	Avocado, cheese, tomato, & lettuce:											
1276	On white bread, firm	1 ea	205	57	489	15	40	4	32	9	12.7	8
1278	On part whole wheat	1 ea	195	58	454	14	33	5	31	9	12.6	8
1277	On whole wheat	1 ea	209	57	481	16	39	7	32	9	12.9	8

[1] Recipe: 29% whole milk, 26% spinach, 13% egg white, 13% cheddar cheese, 7% egg yolk, 7% butter, 4% flour, 1% salt and pepper.

[2] Made with drained chunk light tuna, celery, onion, pickle relish, and mayonnaise-type salad dressing.

[3] Made with a 10½"-diameter flour tortilla.

[4] Crust made with vegetable shortening and enriched flour.

(Computer code number is for West Diet Analysis program)

Chol (mg)	Calc (mg)	Iron (mg)	Magn (mg)	Phos (mg)	Pota (mg)	Sodi (mg)	Zinc (mg)	VT-A (RE)	Thia (mg)	Ribo (mg)	Niac (mg)	V-B6 (mg)	Fola (μg)	VT-C (mg)
22	52	3.25	20	113	245	1220	2.39	100	.15	.17	2.25	.12	5	5
74	124	3.72	40	236	665	1009	2.45	159	.25	.3	3.97	.2	10	22
184	230	1.35	38	231	201	763	1.29	676	.09	.3	.48	.12	62	3
38	28	1.49	34	148	390	1220	1.7	27	.55	.22	3.62	.35	11	23
23	16	.8	21	75	187	732	.66	20	.06	.08	3.06	.18	6	12
0	80	3.21	57	147	508	1164	1.22	52	.16	.21	.91	.1	120	10
27	35	2.05	39	365	365	824	1.15	55	.06	.14	13.7	.17	15	5
41	34	2.3	31	156	182	775	1.21	13	.18	.15	7.81	.2	10	1
22	42	.85	36	78	268	250	.59	41	.09	.05	.35	.37	27	6
37	80	3.71	63	107	497	1011	2.91	49	.4	.63	4.1	.28	56	1
3	90	3.62	70	78	524	790	1.22	26	.5	.49	3.25	.24	94	2
10	40	.72	–	–	–	600	–	40	–	–	–	–	–	15
38	132	1.93	19	157	167	710	1.9	51	.23	.17	4.64	.11	16	2
70	200	4	35	283	392	1228	4.07	76	.41	.33	9.41	.21	27	2
52	52	4.03	30	201	305	826	1.62	27	.28	.2	5.87	.17	25	8
50	64	3.92	11	105	167	617	.83	23	.18	.44	2.64	.06	38	0
65	–	–	–	–	–	670	–	–	–	–	–	–	–	–
62	458	1.86	71	189	338	1106	3.54	262	.11	.6	2.69	.55	48	1
221	196	3.11	32	302	201	741	1.71	149	.45	.5	3.71	.15	41	1
52	141	2.67	28	238	270	718	.9	74	.35	.32	3.23	.08	24	2
60	90	2.81	36	228	366	661	1.07	32	.36	.24	3.66	.12	48	3
39	47	2.25	21	101	197	516	1.88	12	.23	.29	4.3	.12	16	2
84	75	4.49	37	230	426	600	4.7	3	.28	.33	5.45	.3	37	1
38	20	2.01	11	84	124	581	1.72	0	.2	.24	3.16	.04	26	< 1
85	300	2.70	–	–	–	1620	–	60	–	–	–	–	–	0
60	300	1.80	–	–	–	1770	–	80	–	–	–	–	–	–
55	250	2.7	–	–	–	1540	–	–	–	–	–	–	–	–
50	20	6	–	–	–	1360	–	–	–	–	–	–	–	–
95	250	2.70	–	–	–	1840	–	–	–	–	–	–	–	–
80	250	2.70	–	–	–	1740	–	60	–	–	–	–	–	–
70	300	1.80	–	–	–	1650	–	60	–	–	–	–	–	–
18	222	1.1	30	215	209	640	1.56	140	.35	.31	4.73	.08	112	2
35	282	2.98	52	232	554	552	1.67	146	.36	.38	3.59	.3	77	11
32	277	3.01	64	248	584	525	1.85	136	.33	.37	3.73	.36	76	11
33	269	3.45	97	323	648	594	2.63	137	.34	.36	4.18	.41	88	11

(For purposes of calculations, use "0" for t, < 1, < .1, < .01, etc.)

Table I–1
Food Composition

Computer Code Number	Food Description	Measure	Wt (g)	H₂O (%)	Ener (cal)	Prot (g)	Carb (g)	Dietary Fiber (g)	Fat (g)	Fat Breakdown (g)		
										Sat	Mono	Poly
	FAST FOODS and SANDWICHES (see end of this appendix for additional Fast Foods)—Cont.											
	SANDWICHES—Cont.											
	Bacon, lettuce & tomato:											
1137	On white bread, soft	1 ea	135	46	401	12	34	2	24	6	9	8
1139	On part whole wheat	1 ea	136	47	398	13	32	3	25	6	9.5	8
1138	On whole wheat	1 ea	149	47	421	14	37	6	26	6	9.6	8
	Cheese, grilled:											
1140	On white bread, soft	1 ea	117	37	393	17	29	1	23	12.2	7.6	2.1
1142	On part whole wheat	1 ea	117	37	389	18	27	2	24	12.3	7.7	2.2
1141	On whole wheat	1 ea	131	38	416	19	33	5	24	12.5	8	2.4
1596	Chicken fillet	1 ea	182	47	515	24	39	1	29	8.5	10.4	8.4
	Chicken salad:											
1143	On white bread, soft	1 ea	105	39	371	10	28	1	24	4	7.3	12
1145	On part whole wheat	1 ea	105	40	366	10	27	2	25	4	7	12
1144	On whole wheat	1 ea	118	40	389	12	32	5	25	4	7.6	12
1146	Corned beef & swiss on rye	1 ea	147	45	457	28	25	3	28	9.8	9	6.4
	Egg salad:											
1147	On white bread, soft	1 ea	111	42	380	9	29	1	26	4.5	8	11.8
1149	On part whole wheat	1 ea	111	42	375	9	27	2	26	4.5	8	11.8
1148	On whole wheat	1 ea	125	42	403	11	33	5	27	4.7	8	12
	Ham:											
1279	On rye bread	1 ea	116	56	241	16	20	3	10	2.2	3.8	3.6
1151	On white bread, soft	1 ea	122	55	260	17	23	1	11	2.3	4.1	3.6
1153	On part whole wheat	1 ea	122	55	257	17	22	2	11	2.3	4.1	3.7
1152	On whole wheat	1 ea	136	54	284	19	27	4	12	2.5	4.4	3.9
	Ham & cheese:											
1280	On white bread, soft	1 ea	151	49	388	21	29	1	20	7.8	6.8	4.6
1282	On part whole wheat	1 ea	151	50	384	22	27	3	21	7.8	6.9	4.7
1281	On whole wheat	1 ea	165	49	411	24	33	5	22	8	7.1	4.9
1150	Ham & swiss on rye	1 ea	145	50	368	23	25	3	19	7.2	6.2	4.6
	Ham salad:											
1154	On white bread, soft	1 ea	125	46	365	10	34	1	21	5	8	7.5
1156	On part whole wheat	1 ea	125	46	360	10	33	2	22	5	8	7.5
1155	On whole wheat	1 ea	139	46	387	12	38	5	22	5	8	7.8
1157	Patty melt: Ground beef & cheese on rye	1 ea	177	42	600	36	24	3	40	13.8	14.5	7.9
	Peanut butter & jelly:											
1158	On white bread, soft	1 ea	100	27	345	10	47	3	14	2.7	6.6	3.9
1160	On part whole wheat	1 ea	100	27	341	11	46	4	14	2.8	6.6	4
1159	On whole wheat	1 ea	114	28	368	13	51	7	15	2.9	6.9	4.2
1161	Reuben, grilled: Corned beef, swiss cheese, sauerkraut on rye	1 ea	233	51	639	29	40	5	40	13.7	12.8	9.7
	Roast beef:											
713	On a bun	1 ea	150	49	374	23	36	–	15	3.9	7.3	1.8
1162	On white bread, soft	1 ea	122	46	315	23	27	1	13	2.7	4.3	4.9
1164	On part whole wheat	1 ea	122	47	311	23	25	2	13	2.8	4.3	5
1163	On whole wheat	1 ea	136	46	339	25	30	4	14	3	4.6	5.3
	Tuna salad:											
1165	On white bread, soft	1 ea	116	45	331	13	32	2	17	3	5	8
1167	On part whole wheat	1 ea	116	46	326	13	30	3	17	3	5	8

(Computer code number is for West Diet Analysis program)

Chol (mg)	Calc (mg)	Iron (mg)	Magn (mg)	Phos (mg)	Pota (mg)	Sodi (mg)	Zinc (mg)	VT-A (RE)	Thia (mg)	Ribo (mg)	Niac (mg)	V-B6 (mg)	Fola (µg)	VT-C (mg)
28	60	2.33	22	144	252	731	1.16	35	.4	.23	3.8	.19	31	13
27	73	2.6	38	177	313	753	1.43	35	.4	.25	4.3	.23	35	14
26	62	3.18	75	257	378	818	2.29	35	.4	.23	4.6	.29	47	13
55	393	1.79	26	473	152	1129	2.03	209	.28	.39	2.27	.08	24	< 1
53	405	2.08	38	502	206	1143	2.27	209	.25	.36	2.35	.09	27	< 1
53	398	2.53	73	581	269	1219	3.05	211	.26	.34	2.72	.16	39	< 1
60	60	4.68	35	233	353	957	1.87	31	.33	.24	6.81	.2	29	9
32	56	1.98	17	95	129	447	.73	26	.23	.17	3.36	.25	24	< 1
31	67	2.13	30	124	181	461	.98	26	.24	.18	3.78	.29	27	< 1
31	58	2.58	63	196	240	526	1.72	26	.25	.17	4.17	.34	39	< 1
79	307	2.75	39	290	193	1064	3.69	80	.23	.35	3.26	.19	32	1
147	65	2.21	15	112	106	507	.69	73	.24	.29	1.82	.2	34	0
146	77	2.36	29	141	161	521	.93	73	.26	.32	2.25	.24	38	0
147	69	2.81	61	215	217	592	1.68	74	.27	.31	2.61	.3	49	0
35	38	1.72	29	197	303	1289	1.76	6	.78	.28	4.66	.38	23	17
36	47	1.86	24	193	287	1263	1.59	6	.8	.25	4.67	.36	19	17
35	56	2.09	34	216	329	1274	1.79	6	.8	.27	5.03	.39	21	17
36	50	2.5	62	283	389	1364	2.45	6	.83	.27	5.45	.46	31	18
59	224	2.2	29	381	304	1564	2.26	87	.78	.35	4.47	.34	24	14
57	236	2.49	43	412	356	1578	2.5	87	.75	.37	4.92	.38	27	14
57	228	2.93	77	488	419	1655	3.27	88	.76	.36	5.29	.45	39	14
56	309	1.99	41	353	313	1289	2.74	77	.73	.38	4.52	.37	29	14
31	53	1.93	17	125	148	872	.98	11	.47	.26	3	.18	20	3
29	64	2.2	31	154	200	886	1.22	11	.48	.23	3.45	.2	24	3
28	57	2.65	64	228	262	961	1.98	11	.49	.21	3.82	.29	36	3
116	219	3.76	43	407	369	895	6.79	137	.28	.47	6.39	.35	39	< 1
2	61	2.23	51	132	256	290	1.02	< 1	.3	.17	5.17	.13	43	< 1
0	73	2.52	65	162	309	305	1.26	< 1	.27	.19	5.63	.17	47	< 1
0	64	2.97	99	238	374	375	2.04	< 1	.28	.18	6.03	.24	59	< 1
114	411	3.68	47	413	318	1685	5.44	130	.25	.41	4	.3	39	15
55	58	4.56	33	258	341	855	3.66	22	.4	.33	6.33	.28	43	2
34	47	3.21	23	157	335	1243	2.95	9	.26	.28	5	.32	23	10
34	56	3.33	33	182	377	1254	3.14	9	.24	.25	5.36	.33	26	10
34	50	3.77	61	247	438	1343	3.85	9	.25	.25	5.78	.4	36	10
16	56	2	21	143	149	543	.62	24	.23	.17	5	.13	23	1
14	67	2.35	34	172	200	557	.86	24	.25	.19	5	.17	27	1

(For purposes of calculations, use "0" for t, < 1, < .1, < .01, etc.)

Table I–1
Food Composition

Computer Code Number	Food Description	Measure	Wt (g)	H₂O (%)	Ener (cal)	Prot (g)	Carb (g)	Dietary Fiber (g)	Fat (g)	Fat Breakdown (g)		
										Sat	Mono	Poly
	FAST FOODS and SANDWICHES (see end of this appendix for additional Fast Foods)—Cont.											
1166	On whole wheat	1 ea	130	45	353	15	36	5	18	3	5	8
	Turkey:											
1168	On white bread, soft	1 ea	122	54	270	19	22	1	11	2	3.5	5
1170	On part whole wheat	1 ea	122	54	267	19	21	2	11	2	3.5	5
1169	On whole wheat	1 ea	136	53	294	21	26	4	12	2.2	3.8	5.3
	Turkey ham:											
1272	On rye bread	1 ea	116	57	239	16	19	3	10	2.2	3.1	4.3
1273	On white bread, soft	1 ea	122	55	259	17	23	1	11	2.3	3.3	4.4
1275	On part whole wheat	1 ea	122	56	255	17	22	2	11	2.4	3.3	4.4
1274	On whole wheat	1 ea	136	55	282	19	27	4	12	2.6	3.6	4.7
714	Taco	1 ea	78	58	168	9	12	–	9	5.2	3	.4
	Tostada:											
1114	With refried beans	1 ea	157	66	243	10	29	8	11	5.9	3.3	.8
1118	With beans & beef	1 ea	192	70	284	14	25	3	14	9.8	3	.5
1354	With beans & chicken	1 ea	157	67	253	19	19	3	11	4.5	4.4	1.6
	Vegetarian foods:											
1511	Baked beans, canned	½ c	127	73	118	6	26	6	1	.1	t	.2
1175	Breakfast links	1 ea	34	50	87	6	3	1	6	1	2	3.2
1171	Nuteena	1 pce	67	58	160	8	5	2	12	1.7	4.6	3.7
1173	Redi-burger	1 pce	68	57	130	14	5	1	6	.7	1.3	3.3
1174	Vege-burger	½ c	108	73	110	22	4	1	1	.1	.1	.4
	Vegetarian Foods, Worthington											
1854	Burger, no salt added	½ c	113	–	150	22	7	–	4	–	–	–
1846	Chik slices, canned	2 pce	60	–	90	4	2	–	8	–	–	–
1833	Chili, canned	½ c	106	–	144	8	11	–	8	–	–	–
1835	Choplets	2 pce	92	–	100	18	4	–	2	–	–	–
1831	Country stew	9.5 oz	269	–	219	1	23	–	10	–	–	–
1836	Non-meat balls	3 ea	54	–	100	6	5	–	6	–	–	–
1838	Numete, slices	1 pce	68	–	150	7	7	–	11	–	–	–
1839	Prime steaks, canned	1 pce	92	–	160	10	7	–	10	–	–	–
1840	Protose, slices	1 pce	76	–	180	17	9	–	8	–	–	–
1842	Saucettes, canned links	2 pce	67	–	150	10	3	–	11	–	–	–
1844	Savory slices	2 pce	56	–	100	8	4	–	6	–	–	–
1849	Skallops, no salt added	½ c	85	–	80	13	4	–	1	–	–	–
1847	Turkee slices	2 pce	63	–	130	9	3	–	9	–	–	–
	NUTS, SEEDS, and PRODUCTS											
	Almonds:											
1365	Dry roasted, salted	1 c	138	3	810	22	33	14	71	6.7	46.2	14.9
718	Slivered, packed, unsalted	1 c	135	4	795	27	27	13[1]	70	6.7	45.8	14.9
719	Whole, dried, unsalted:	1 c	142	4	836	28	29	13[1]	74	7	48.1	15.6
720	Ounce	1 oz	28	4	165	6	6	3[1]	15	1.4	9.6	3.1
721	Almond butter	1 tbs	16	1	101	2	3	1	9	.9	6.1	2
722	Brazil nuts, dry (about 7)	1 oz	28	3	184	4	4	2	19	4.6	6.5	6.8
	Cashew nuts, salted:											
723	Dry roasted:	1 c	137	2	786	21	45	4	64	12.5	37.4	10.7
724	Ounce	1 oz	28	2	161	4	9	1	13	2.6	7.7	2.2

[1]Values reported for dietary fiber in almonds vary from 7.0 to 14.3 g/100 g.

(Computer code number is for West Diet Analysis program)

Chol (mg)	Calc (mg)	Iron (mg)	Magn (mg)	Phos (mg)	Pota (mg)	Sodi (mg)	Zinc (mg)	VT-A (RE)	Thia (mg)	Ribo (mg)	Niac (mg)	V-B6 (mg)	Fola (µg)	VT-C (mg)
14	59	2.79	67	246	262	629	1.66	24	.26	.18	6	.22	39	1
34	44	1.57	24	198	236	1238	1.05	9	.2	.18	7	.33	19	0
34	53	1.8	34	223	279	1249	1.24	9	.21	.19	7.39	.35	22	0
35	47	2.19	62	289	336	1339	1.89	9	.22	.19	7.88	.41	32	0
41	40	3.03	28	178	287	1004	2.43	6	.2	.29	3.81	.23	24	0
43	49	3.29	23	172	271	976	2.27	6	.21	.27	3.81	.23	20	0
41	58	3.42	33	197	313	987	2.46	6	.22	.29	4.17	.25	23	0
43	52	3.86	61	263	371	1069	3.15	6	.23	.28	4.57	.31	33	0
26	101	1.1	32	93	216	366	1.79	67	.07	.2	1.47	.11	11	1
33	229	2.06	64	127	440	592	2.07	93	.11	.36	1.44	.17	82	1
63	161	2.09	58	148	419	743	2.71	148	.08	.42	2.44	.21	83	3
53	171	1.81	49	240	367	435	2.29	87	.11	.2	4.49	.32	54	3
0	63	.37	41	132	376	504	1.78	22	.19	.08	.54	.17	30	4
0	21	1.27	12	77	79	302	.5	22	.8	.14	3.8	.2	9	0
0	21	1.2	40	111	200	120	.87	10	.47	.58	.14	.45	60	<1
0	19	1.4	13	56	120	370	1.2	10	.6	.4	6.7	.8	17	<1
0	32	2.7	24	105	110	190	1.1	10	.53	.68	5	.56	27	<1
–	–	1.80	–	–	40	170	–	–	.30	.10	8	.50	–	–
–	–	.72	–	–	20	330	–	–	.03	.03	.80	.12	–	–
–	–	.82	–	–	136	417	–	–	.11	.05	3.79	.15	–	–
–	–	.36	–	–	10	440	–	–	–	–	–	–	–	–
–	40	2.69	–	–	299	758	–	–	.38	.34	7.98	.30	–	–
–	20	.72	–	–	30	210	–	–	.90	.03	.20	–	–	–
–	20	–	–	–	150	410	–	–	.09	–	6	.04	–	–
–	–	1.08	–	–	35	410	–	–	.15	.17	3	.12	–	–
–	20	1.80	–	–	120	470	–	–	.23	.17	8	.30	–	–
–	–	–	–	–	15	430	–	–	.03	.03	.14	.12	–	–
–	–	.36	–	–	35	340	–	–	.03	.07	.20	.08	–	–
–	–	.72	–	–	5	80	–	–	–	–	–	–	–	–
–	–	.72	–	–	25	430	–	–	.90	.07	3	.16	–	–
0	389	5.24	420	756	1062	1076	6.76	0	.18	.83	3.89	.1	88	1
0	359	4.94	400	702	988	15	3.94	0	.28	1.05	4.54	.15	79	1
0	378	5.2	420	738	1039	16[3]	4.15	0	.3	1.11	4.77	.16	83	1
0	75	1.04	84	147	205	3[3]	.83	0	.06	.22	.95	.03	17	<1
0	43	.59	48	84	121	2[4]	.49	0	.02	.1	.46	.01	10	<1
0	50	.96	64	168	170	1	1.3	0	.28	.03	.46	.07	1	<1
0	62	8.22	356	671	774	877[5]	7.67	0	.27	.27	1.92	.35	95	0
0	13	1.7	74	137	158	179[5]	1.59	0	.06	.06	.4	.07	19	0

[3] Salted almonds contain 1108 mg sodium per cup, 221 mg per ounce.

[4] Salted almond butter contains 72 mg sodium per tablespoon.

[5] Dry-roasted cashews without salt contain 21 mg sodium per cup, or 4 mg per ounce.

(For purposes of calculations, use "0" for t, <1, <.1, <.01, etc.)

Table I–1
Food Composition

Computer Code Number	Food Description	Measure	Wt (g)	H₂O (%)	Ener (cal)	Prot (g)	Carb (g)	Dietary Fiber (g)	Fat (g)	Fat Breakdown (g)		
										Sat	Mono	Poly
	NUTS, SEEDS, and PRODUCTS—Cont.											
725	Oil roasted:	1 c	130	4	748	21	37	4	63	12.4	36.9	10.6
726	Ounce	1 oz	28	4	161	5	8	1	14	2.7	8	2.3
1366	Cashew nuts, unsalted, dry roasted	1 c	137	2	786	21	45	4	64	12.5	37.4	10.7
1367	Cashew nuts, unsalted, oil roasted	1 c	130	4	748	21	37	4	63	12.4	36.9	10.6
727	Cashew butter, unsalted	1 tbs	16	3	94	3	4	1	8	1.6	4.7	1.3
728	Chestnuts, European, roasted (1 cup = approx 17 kernels)	1 c	143	40	350	5	76	9	3	.6	1.1	1.2
	Coconut, raw:											
729	Piece 2 x 2 x ½"	1 pce	45	47	159	2	7	4	15	13.4	.6	.2
730	Shredded/grated, unpacked[1]	½ c	40	47	142	1	6	4	13	11.9	.6	.2
	Coconut, dried, shredded/grated:											
731	Unsweetened	1 c	78	3	514	5	19	13	50	44.6	2.1	.6
732	Sweetened	1 c	93	13	465	3	44	4	33	29.3	1.4	.4
733	Filberts/hazelnuts, chopped:	1 c	115	5	726	15	18	9	72	5.3	56.4	6.9
734	Ounce	1 oz	28	5	177	4	4	2	18	1.3	13.9	1.7
735	Macadamias, oil roasted, salted:	1 c	134	2	962	10	17	12	102	15.3	80.9	1.8
736	Ounce	1 oz	28	2	201	2	4	3	21	3.2	16.9	.4
1368	Macadamias, oil roasted, unsalted	1 c	134	2	962	10	17	12	102	15.3	80.9	1.8
	Mixed nuts:											
737	Dry roasted, salted	1 c	137	2	814	24	35	12	71	9.4	43	14.7
738	Oil roasted, salted	1 c	142	2	876	24	30	13	80	12.4	45	18.9
1369	Oil roasted, unsalted	1 c	142	2	876	24	30	13	80	12.4	45	18.9
	Peanuts:											
739	Oil roasted, salted:	1 c	144	2	837	38	27	10	71	9.8	35.3	22.5
740	Ounce	1 oz	28	2	163	7	5	2	14	1.9	6.9	4.4
1370	Oil roasted, unsalted	1 c	144	2	837	38	27	9	71	9.8	35.3	22.5
741	Dried, unsalted:	1 c	146	2	854	35	31	10	73	10.1	36.1	22.9
742	Ounce	1 oz	28	2	166	7	6	2	14	2	7	4.4
743	Peanut butter:	½ c	129	1	759	32	27	8	64	12.3	30.4	18.6
1371	Tablespoon	2 tbs	32	1	188	8	7	2	16	3.1	7.6	4.6
744	Pecan halves, dried, unsalted:	1 c	108	5	720	8	20	5[2]	73	5.8	45.5	18.1
745	Ounce	1 oz	28	5	187	2	5	1[2]	19	1.5	11.8	4.8
1372	Pecan halves, dry roasted, salted	¼ c	28	1	185	2	6	1	18	1.5	11.4	4.5
746	Pine nuts/piñons, dried	1 oz	28	6	159	3	5	3	17	2.7	6.5	7.3
747	Pistachios, dried, shelled	1 oz	28	4	162	6	7	3	14	1.7	9.3	2.1
1373	Pistachios, dry roasted, salted, shelled	1 c	128	2	776	19	35	14	68	8.6	45.6	10.2
748	Pumpkin kernels, dried, unsalted	1 oz	28	7	151	7	5	4	13	2.5	4	5.9
1374	Pumpkin kernels, roasted, salted	1 c	227	7	1184	75	30	15	96	18.1	29.7	43.6
749	Sesame seeds, hulled, dried	¼ c	38	5	223	10	4	3	21	2.9	7.9	9.1
	Sunflower seed kernels:											
750	Dry	¼ c	36	5	205	8	7	2	18	1.9	3.4	11.8
751	Oil roasted	¼ c	34	3	209	7	5	2	19	2	3.7	12.9
752	Tahini (sesame butter)	1 tbs	15	3	91	3	3	1	8	1.2	3.2	3.7
1334	Trail Mix w/chocolate chips	1 c	146	7	707	21	66	–	47	8.9	19.8	16.5
753	Black walnuts, chopped:	1 c	125	4	758	30	15	6	71	4.5	15.9	46.9

[1] ½ cup packed = 65 g.

[2] Dietary fiber data calculated/derived from data on other nuts.

(Computer code number is for West Diet Analysis program)

Chol (mg)	Calc (mg)	Iron (mg)	Magn (mg)	Phos (mg)	Pota (mg)	Sodi (mg)	Zinc (mg)	VT-A (RE)	Thia (mg)	Ribo (mg)	Niac (mg)	V-B6 (mg)	Fola (µg)	VT-C (mg)
0	53	5.33	332	553	689	813[3]	6.18	0	.55	.23	2.34	.32	88	0
0	11	1.16	72	120	148	175[3]	1.35	0	.12	.05	.51	.07	19	0
0	62	8.22	356	671	774	22	7.67	0	.27	.27	1.92	.35	95	0
0	53	5.33	332	553	689	22	6.18	0	.55	.23	2.34	.32	88	0
0	7	.8	41	73	87	2[4]	.83	0	.05	.03	.26	.04	11	0
0	41	1.3	47	153	847	3	.81	3	.35	.25	1.92	.71	100	37
0	6	1.09	14	51	160	9	.49	0	.03	.01	.24	.02	12	1
0	6	.97	13	45	142	8	.44	0	.03	.01	.22	.02	11	1
0	20	2.59	70	160	423	29	1.57	0	.05	.08	.47	.23	7	1
0	14	1.79	46	99	313	243	1.69	0	.03	.02	.44	.25	8	1
0	216	3.76	327	358	511	3	2.76	8	.57	.13	1.31	.7	83	1
0	53	.93	80	88	126	1	.68	2	.14	.03	.32	.17	20	< 1
0	60	2.41	157	268	440	348[5]	1.47	1	.28	.15	2.71	.26	21	0
0	13	.5	32	56	92	73[5]	.31	< 1	.06	.03	.57	.05	4	0
0	60	2.41	155	268	440	9	1.47	1	.28	.15	2.71	.26	21	0
0	96	5.07	308	596	817	917[6]	5.21	1	.27	.27	6.44	.41	69	1
0	153	4.56	334	659	825	926[6]	7.21	3	.71	.31	7.19	.34	118	1
0	153	4.56	334	659	825	16	7.21	3	.71	.31	7.19	.34	118	1
0	126	2.64	266	744	982	624[7]	9.55	0	.36	.16	20.4	.37	181	0
0	25	.52	52	147	193	123[7]	1.88	0	.07	.03	4.03	.07	36	0
0	126	2.64	266	744	982	9	9.55	0	.36	.16	20.4	.37	181	0
0	79	3.3	256	523	961	9	4.83	0	.64	.14	19.7	.37	212	0
0	15	.64	49	101	187	2	.94	0	.12	.03	3.83	.07	41	0
0	44	2.15	203	417	930	617[8]	3.24	0	.18	.13	16.9	.48	101	0
0	11	.54	50	104	232	153[8]	.81	0	.04	.03	4.22	.12	25	0
0	39	2.3	138	314	423	1[9]	5.91	14	.92	.14	.96	.2	42	2
0	10	.6	36	82	111	< 1[9]	1.55	4	.24	.04	.25	.05	11	1
0	10	.62	38	86	105	218	1.61	4	.09	.03	.26	.05	11	1
0	2	.87	66	10	176	20	1.22	1	.35	.06	1.24	.03	16	1
0	38	1.92	45	142	306	2[10]	.38	7	.23	.05	.31	.07	16	2
0	90	4.06	166	609	1241	998	1.74	31	.54	.31	1.8	.33	76	9
0	12	4.24	152	332	226	5[11]	2.12	11	.06	.09	.49	.06	16	1
0	98	33.8	1212	2658	1829	1305	16.9	86	.48	.72	3.95	.2	130	4
0	50	2.96	132	295	155	15	3.91	3	.27	.03	1.78	.05	36	0
0	42	2.44	127	253	248	1[12]	1.82	2	.82	.09	1.62	.28	82	1
0	19	2.28	43	387	164	1[12]	1.77	2	.11	.09	1.4	.27	80	< 1
0	21	.95	53	118	69	< 1	1.58	1	.24	.02	.85	.02	15	0
5.84	159	4.96	253	565	946	177	4.28	6	.6	.33	6.44	.38	95	2
0	73	3.85	253	580	655	1	4.58	37	.27	.14	.26	.69	82	4

[3]Oil-roasted cashews without salt contain 22 mg sodium per cup, or 5 mg per ounce.
[4]Salted cashew butter contains 98 mg sodium per tablespoon.
[5]Macadamia nuts without salt contain 9 mg sodium per cup, or 2 mg per ounce.
[6]Mixed nuts without salt contain about 15 mg sodium per cup.
[7]Peanuts without salt contain 22 mg sodium per cup, or 4 mg per ounce.
[8]Peanut butter without added salt contains 3 mg sodium per tablespoon.
[9]Salted pecans contain 816 mg sodium per cup, or 214 mg per ounce.
[10]Salted pistachios contain approx 221 mg sodium per ounce.
[11]Salted pumpkin/squash kernels contain approximately 163 mg sodium per ounce.
[12]Unsalted sunflower seeds contain 1 mg sodium per ¼ cup.

(For purposes of calculations, use "0" for t, < 1, < .1, < .01, etc.)

Table I–1
Food Composition

Computer Code Number	Food Description	Measure	Wt (g)	H₂O (%)	Ener (cal)	Prot (g)	Carb (g)	Dietary Fiber (g)	Fat (g)	Fat Breakdown (g)		
										Sat	Mono	Poly
	NUTS, SEEDS, and PRODUCTS—Cont.											
754	Ounce	1 oz	28	4	170	7	3	1	16	1	3.6	10.6
755	English walnuts, chopped:	1 c	120	4	770	17	22	5	74	6.7	17	47
756	Ounce	1 oz	28	4	180	4	5	1	17	1.6	4	11.1
	SWEETENERS and SWEETS (see also Dairy [milk desserts] and Baked Goods)											
757	Apple butter	2 tbs	35	52	64	< 1	17	< 1	< 1	t	t	.1
1124	Butterscotch topping	2 tbs	41	32	103	1	27	< 1	< 1	t	t	0
1125	Caramel topping	2 tbs	41	32	103	1	27	< 1	< 1	t	t	0
	Cake frosting, creamy vanilla:											
1127	Canned	2 tbs	31	13	131	< 1	22	0	5	1.5	2.7	.7
1123	From mix	2 tbs	31	12	132	< 1	22	0	5	1	2.1	1.8
	Cake frosting, lite:											
2061	Milk chocolate	1 tbs	29	18	105	0	21	1	2	.7	–	–
2062	Vanilla	1 tbs	29	15	110	0	22	< 1	2	.6	–	–
	Candy:											
1128	Almond Joy candy bar	1 oz	28	8	130	1	16	2	8	4.7	1.5	.7
2069	Butterscotch morsels	¼ c	43	1	243	0	29	0	12	12.3	–	–
758	Caramel, plain or chocolate	1 oz	28	8	107	1	22	< 1	2	1.9	.2	.1
1961	Chewing gum, sugarless	1 pce	3	–	5	0	2	–	0	–	0	0
	Chocolate (see also #784, 785, 971):											
	Milk chocolate:											
759	Plain	1 oz	28	1	143	2	17	1	9	5.2	2.8	.3
760	With almonds	1 oz	28	2	147	3	15	2	10	4.8	3.8	.6
761	With peanuts	1 oz	28	5	155	5	11	2	12	3.4	5.1	2.6
762	With rice cereal	1 oz	28	2	139	2	18	1	7	4.5	2.4	.2
763	Semisweet chocolate chips	1 c	170	1	811	7	108	10	50	29.8	16.9	1.6
764	Sweet dark chocolate (candy bar)	1 oz	28	1	133	1	17	2	8	5.9	3.3	.3
1133	SKOR English toffee candy bar	1 ea	32	4	169	1	18	< 1	11	7	2.5	2
765	Fondant candy, uncoated (mints, candy corn, other)	1 oz	28	7	100	0	26	0	< 1	.1	0	–
1697	Fruit Roll-up (small)	1 ea	14	21	41	< 1	11	< 1	< 1	t	t	.1
766	Fudge, chocolate	1 oz	28	10	107	< 1	22	< 1	2	1.5	.7	.1
767	Gumdrops	1 oz	28	1	108	0	28	0	< 1	0	t	.1
768	Hard candy, all flavors	1 oz	28	1	104	0	28	0	0	0	0	0
769	Jellybeans	1 oz	28	6	104	0	26	0	< 1	0	t	.1
1134	M&M's plain chocolate candy	1 pkg	48	1	228	3	33	1	11	5	3	.3
1135	M&M's peanut chocolate candy	1 pkg	47	2	234	5	28	2	13	5	5.1	2
1130	Mars almond bar	1 ea	50	5	234	4	31	1	11	4.8	4.4	.8
1129	Milky Way candy bar	1 ea	60	2	251	3	43	1	9	4.7	3.3	.3
1708	Milk chocolate-coated peanuts	½ c	85	2	441	11	42	4	29	12.4	11	3.7
1709	Peanut brittle, recipe	½ c	74	2	335	6	51	1	14	3.7	6.2	3.5
1132	Reese's peanut butter cup	2 ea	45	8	218	5	21	2	14	10.4	.9	.9
1131	Snickers candy bar (2.2oz)	1 ea	61	6	278	6	37	2	14	7.3	4.1	.5
1482	Fruit juice bar (2.5 fl oz)	1 ea	77	78	63	1	16	–	< 1	–	–	–
771	Gelatin dessert/Jello, prepared	½ c	120	85	71	1	17	0	0	0	0	0
1702	SugarFree	½ c	113	98	8	1	1	0	0	0	0	0
772	Honey:	1 c	339	17	1030	1	279	0	0	0	0	0
773	Tablespoon	1 tbs	21	17	64	< 1	17	< 1	0	0	0	0

(Computer code number is for West Diet Analysis program)

Chol (mg)	Calc (mg)	Iron (mg)	Magn (mg)	Phos (mg)	Pota (mg)	Sodi (mg)	Zinc (mg)	VT-A (RE)	Thia (mg)	Ribo (mg)	Niac (mg)	V-B6 (mg)	Fola (µg)	VT-C (mg)
0	16	.87	57	132	149	<1	.97	9	.06	.03	.2	.16	18	1
0	113	2.93	203	380	602	12	3.28	15	.46	.18	1.25	.67	79	4
0	27	.69	48	90	142	3	.77	4	.11	.04	.29	.16	18	1
0	2	.05	1	2	32	0	.02	0	0	<.01	.03	.01	0	1
<1	22	.07	3	19	34	143	.08	11	0	.04	.02	.01	1	<1
<1	22	.07	3	19	34	143	.08	11	0	.04	.02	.01	1	<1
0	1	.03	<1	12	11	28	0	70	0	<.01	<.01	0	0	0
0	3	.07	1	8	7	69	.03	33	.01	.01	.11	<.01	0	0
0	3	.43	–	–	–	72	–	0	–	–	–	–	–	0
0	1	.03	–	–	–	53	–	0	–	–	–	–	–	0
1	22	.34	19	40	105	38	.23	3	.01	.04	.13	.02	2	<1
0	0	0	–	–	79	45	–	0	.03	.04	.03	–	–	0
2	39	.04	5	32	61	69	.12	2	<.01	.05	.07	.01	1	<1
–	–	–	–	–	0	0	–	–	–	–	–	–	–	–
6	54	.39	17	61	109	23	.39	14	.02	.08	.09	.01	2	<1
5	63	.46	25	75	124	21	.38	4	.02	.12	.21	.01	3	<1
3	33	.53	35	83	150	11	.69	6	.08	.05	2.14	.04	23	0
5	48	.21	14	55	97	41	.32	3	.02	.08	.13	.02	3	<1
0	54	5.32	196	224	621	19	2.75	3	.09	.15	.73	.08	5	0
0	5	.59	33	45	96	3	.42	1	.01	.07	.19	.01	1	0
19	36	.13	11	48	76	74	.24	22	.01	.11	.03	.01	2	<1
0	1	.02	<1	1	4	11	.01	0	<.01	<.01	<.01	<.01	0	0
0	6	.55	13	6	12	2	.01	<1	<.01	.01	.2	.03	0	<1
4	12	.14	7	16	29	18	.11	13	<.01	.02	.03	<.01	1	<1
0	1	.11	<1	<1	1	12	0	0	0	<.01	<.01	0	0	0
0	1	.08	1	1	1	11	<.01	0	<.01	<.01	<.01	<.01	0	0
0	1	.31	1	1	10	7	.01	0	0	0	0	0	0	0
0	81	.73	32	94	188	49	.61	12	.03	.12	.26	.03	4	0
0	63	.7	39	130	184	44	.72	5	.03	.1	1.51	.08	26	0
4	84	.55	36	114	163	85	.55	22	.02	.16	.47	.03	7	1
12	78	.46	20	98	145	144	.43	28	.02	.13	.21	.03	5	1
8	88	1.12	77	180	427	35	1.61	0	.1	.15	3.61	.18	7	0
10	22	1.02	37	82	153	334	.71	35	.14	.04	2.57	.08	52	0
7	35	.49	38	108	180	131	.63	9	.02	.09	1.79	.04	13	0
7	70	.48	37	129	200	164	.7	19	.03	.11	1.83	.11	24	<1
0	4	.15	3	5	41	3	.04	2	.01	.01	.12	.02	5	7
0	2	.04	1	26	1	50	.04	0	0	<.01	<.01	<.01	0	0
0	2	.01	1	31	0	54	.03	0	0	<.01	<.01	<.01	0	0
0	20	1.42	7	14	176	14	.75	0	0	.13	.41	.08	7	8
0	1	.09	<1	1	11	1	.05	0	0	.01	.03	.01	<1	<1

(For purposes of calculations, use "0" for t, <1, <.1, <.01, etc.)

Table I–1
Food Composition

Computer Code Number	Food Description	Measure	Wt (g)	H$_2$O (%)	Ener (cal)	Prot (g)	Carb (g)	Dietary Fiber (g)	Fat (g)	Fat Breakdown (g)		
										Sat	Mono	Poly
	SWEETENERS and SWEETS (see also Dairy [milk desserts] and Baked Goods)—Cont.											
774	Jams or preserves:	1 tbs	20	35	48	< 1	13	< 1	< 1	0	t	0
775	Packet	1 ea	14	34	34	< 1	9	< 1	< 1	t	t	0
776	Jellies:	1 tbs	18	28	49	< 1	13	< 1	< 1	t	t	t
777	Packet	1 ea	14	28	38	< 1	10	< 1	< 1	t	t	t
1136	Marmalade	2 tbs	40	33	98	< 1	26	< 1	0	0	0	0
770	Marshmallows	4 ea	28	16	90	1	23	< 1	< 1	0	0	0
1126	Marshmallow creme topping	3 tbs	50	18	155	1	40	0	< 1	0	0	0
778	Popsicle/ice pops	1 ea	95	80	68	0	18	0	0	0	0	0
	Sugars:											
779	Brown sugar	1 c	220	2	827	0	214	0	0	0	0	0
780	White sugar, granulated:	1 c	200	< 1	774	0	200	0	0	0	0	0
781	Tablespoon	1 tbs	12	< 1	46	0	12	0	0	0	0	0
782	Packet	1 ea	6	< 1	23	0	6	0	0	0	0	0
783	White sugar, powdered, sifted	1 c	100	< 1	389	0	100	0	< 1	0	0	0
	Sweeteners:											
1711	Equal, packet	1 ea	1	5	4	1	0	0	0	0	0	0
1712	Sweet 'N Low, packet	1 ea	1	< 1	4	0	1	0	0	0	0	0
	Syrups:											
	Chocolate:											
785	Hot fudge type	2 tbs	38	22	131	2	22	< 1	5	2.2	1.4	1.2
784	Thin type	2 tbs	38	37	83	1	22	1	< 1	.2	.1	< .1
786	Molasses, blackstrap[1]	2 tbs	40	29	94	0	24	0	0	0	0	0
1710	Light cane	1 tbs	21	26	56	0	14	0	< 1	0	0	0
787	Pancake table syrup (corn and maple)	¼ c	79	24	227	0	60	0	0	0	0	0
	VEGETABLES and LEGUMES											
788	Alfalfa sprouts	1 c	33	91	10	1	1	1	< 1	t	t	.1
1815	Amaranth leaves, raw, chopped	1 c	28	93	7	1	1	< 1	< 1	< .1	< .1	< .1
1816	Amaranth leaves, raw, each	1 ea	14	93	4	0	1	< 1	< 1	< .1	< .1	< .1
1817	Amaranth leaves, cooked	1 c	132	92	28	3	5	2	< 1	.1	.1	.1
1987	Argula, raw, chopped	5 ea	10	92	3	0	0	–	0	–	–	–
789	Artichokes, cooked globe (300 g w/refuse)	1 ea	120	84	60	4	13	6	< 1	t	t	.1
1177	Artichoke hearts, cooked from frozen	9 oz	240	86	108	7	22	13	1	.3	t	.5
1176	Artichoke hearts, marinated	6 oz	170	59	168	4	13	8	14	2	3	7.7
2021	Artichoke hearts in water	.6 c	101	86	44	2	10	6	0	< .1	< .1	.1
	Asparagus, green, cooked:											
	From fresh:											
790	Cuts and tips	½ c	90	92	22	2	4	2	< 1	.1	t	.1
791	Spears, ½" diam at base	6 ea	90	92	22	2	4	2	< 1	.1	t	.1
	From frozen:											
792	Cuts and tips	½ c	90	91	25	3	4	2	< 1	.1	t	.2
793	Spears, ½" diam at base	6 ea	90	91	25	3	4	2	< 1	.1	t	.2
794	Canned, spears, ½" diam at base	6 ea	120	94	23	3	3	2	1	.2	t	.3
795	Bamboo shoots, canned, drained slices	1 c	131	94	25	2	4	3	1	.1	t	.2
1795	Bamboo shoots, raw	1 c	151	91	41	4	8	3	< 1	.1	0	.2
1798	Bamboo shoots, cooked	1 c	120	96	14	2	2	1	0	.1	< .1	.1

[1]Light molasses would contain about 66 mg calcium, 2.1 mg iron, 18 mg magnesium, and 366 mg potassium for 2 tbsp.

(Computer code number is for West Diet Analysis program)

Chol (mg)	Calc (mg)	Iron (mg)	Magn (mg)	Phos (mg)	Pota (mg)	Sodi (mg)	Zinc (mg)	VT-A (RE)	Thia (mg)	Ribo (mg)	Niac (mg)	V-B6 (mg)	Fola (µg)	VT-C (mg)
0	4	.2	1	2	15	8	.01	<1	0	<.01	.01	<.01	7	2
0	3	.07	1	2	11	6	.01	<1	0	<.01	.01	<.01	5	1
0	1	.04	1	1	12	6	.01	<1	<.01	<.01	.01	<.01	<1	<1
0	1	.03	1	1	9	5	.01	<1	<.01	<.01	.01	<.01	<1	<1
0	15	.06	1	2	15	22	.02	2	<.01	<.01	.02	.01	14	2
0	1	.06	1	2	1	13	.01	<1	<.01	<.01	.02	<.01	<1	0
0	2	.11	1	4	3	23	.02	<1	<.01	<.01	.04	0	1	0
0	0	0	1	0	4	11	.02	0	0	0	0	0	0	0
0	187	4.2	64	48	761	86	.4	0	.02	.01	.18	.06	2	0
0	2	.13	0	4	4	2	.07	0	0	.04	0	0	0	0
0	<1	.01	0	<1	<1	<1	<.01	0	0	<.01	0	0	0	0
0	<1	<.01	0	<1	<1	<1	<.01	0	0	<.01	0	0	0	0
0	1	.06	1	2	2	1	.03	0	0	0	0	0	0	0
0	<1	.02	–	0	<1	<1	–	0	0	0	0	–	–	0
0	<1	–	<1	–	1	1	–	–	–	–	–	–	–	–
5	38	.46	18	65	82	49	.3	8	.01	.08	.08	.01	2	<1
0	5	.81	25	49	85	36	.28	1	<.01	.02	.12	<.01	2	<1
0	344[2]	7[1]	86[1]	16	997[1]	22	.4	0	.01	.02	.43	.28	<1	0
0	43	.99	51	7	307	8	.06	0	.01	<.01	.2	.14	0	0
0	1	.07	2	7	2	66	.03	0	.01	.01	.02	0	0	0
0	11	.32	9	23	26	2	.3	5	.03	.04	.16	.01	12	3
0	61	.66	16	14	174	6	.26	83	.01	.04	.19	.05	24	12
0	30	.32	8	7	86	3	.13	41	0	.02	.09	.03	12	6
0	276	2.98	73	95	846	28	1.16	366	.03	.18	.74	.23	75	54
0	16	.15	5	5	37	3	.05	24	0	.01	.03	.01	10	2
0	54	1.55	72	103	425	114	.59	21	.08	.08	1.2	.13	61	12
0	50	1.34	74	146	634	127	.86	39	.15	.38	2.2	.21	286	12
0	39	1.62	48	102	439	899	.54	28	.06	.17	1.38	.15	149	52
0	40	1.36	40	60	265	66	.3	15	.06	.05	.59	.09	45	7
0	18	.66	9	49	144	10	.38	49	.11	.11	.97	.11	131	10
0	18	.66	9	49	144	10	.38	49	.11	.11	.97	.11	131	10
0	21	.58	12	49	196	4	.5	74	.06	.09	.94	.02	122	22
0	21	.58	12	49	196	4	.5	74	.06	.09	.94	.02	122	22
0	19	2.2	12	52	206	468[2]	.48	64	.07	.12	1.14	.13	115	22
0	10	.42	5	33	105	9	.85	1	.03	.03	.18	.18	4	1
0	20	.76	5	89	805	6	1.68	3	.23	.11	.91	.36	11	6
0	14	.29	4	24	640	5	.56	0	.02	.06	.36	.12	3	0

[2]Low sodium pack contains 3 mg sodium.

(For purposes of calculations, use "0" for t, <1, <.1, <.01, etc.)

Table I–1
Food Composition

Computer Code Number	Food Description	Measure	Wt (g)	H$_2$O (%)	Ener (cal)	Prot (g)	Carb (g)	Dietary Fiber (g)	Fat (g)	Fat Breakdown (g)		
										Sat	Mono	Poly
	VEGETABLES AND LEGUMES—Cont.											
	Beans (see also alphabetical listing in this section):											
796	Black beans, cooked	½ c	86	66	114	8	20	7	<1	.1	t	.2
	Canned beans (white/navy):											
803	With pork and tomato sauce	½ c	126	73	123	7	24	6	1	.5	.6	.2
804	With sweet sauce	1 c	253	71	281	13	53	11	4	1.4	1.6	.5
805	With frankfurters	1 c	257	69	365	17	40	18	17	6	7.3	2.2
	Lima beans:											
797	Thick seeded (Fordhooks), cooked from frozen	½ c	85	74	85	5	16	6	<1	.1	t	.1
798	Thin seeded (Baby), cooked from frozen	½ c	90	72	95	6	18	6	<1	.1	t	.1
799	Cooked from dry, drained	½ c	94	70	108	7	20	7	<1	.1	t	.2
1998	Red Mexican, cooked f/dry	1 c	224	70	252	15	47	18	1	.2	.2	.3
	Snap bean/green string beans cuts and french style:											
800	Cooked from fresh	½ c	62	89	22	1	5	2	<1	t	t	.1
801	Cooked from frozen	½ c	67	92	17	1	4	2	<1	t	t	.1
802	Canned, drained	½ c	67	93	13	1	3	1	<1	t	t	t
1713	Snap bean, yellow, cooked f/fresh	½ c	63	89	22	1	5	1	<1	t	t	.1
	Bean sprouts (mung):											
806	Raw	1 c	104	90	31	3	6	2	<1	.1	t	.1
807	Cooked, stir-fried	1 c	124	84	62	5	13	4	<1	.1	.1	.1
808	Cooked, boiled, drained	1 c	124	93	26	3	5	1	<1	t	t	t
1788	Canned, drained	1 c	125	96	15	2	3	1	0	<.1	<.1	<.1
	Beets, cooked from fresh:											
809	Sliced or diced	½ c	85	87	37	1	8	1	<1	t	t	.1
810	Whole beets, 2" diam	2 ea	100	87	44	2	10	2	<1	t	t	.1
	Beets, canned:											
811	Sliced or diced	½ c	85	91	26	1	6	2	<1	t	t	t
812	Pickled slices	½ c	114	82	74	1	19	2	<1	t	t	t
813	Beet greens, cooked, drained	½ c	72	89	19	2	4	2	<1	t	t	.1
	Broccoli, raw:											
817	Chopped	1 c	88	91	25	3	5	3	<1	.1	t	.2
818	Spears	1 ea	151	91	42	4	8	5	1	.1	t	.3
	Broccoli, cooked from fresh:											
819	Spears	1 ea	180	91	50	5	9	5	1	.1	t	.3
820	Chopped	1 c	156	91	44	5	8	5	1	.1	t	.3
	Broccoli, cooked from frozen:											
821	Spear, small piece	3 ea	90	91	25	3	5	2	<1	t	t	.1
822	Chopped	1 c	184	91	51	6	10	5	<1	t	t	.1
1603	Broccoflower, steamed	3½ oz	100	90	32	3	6	3	<1	t	t	.1
823	Brussels sprouts, cooked from fresh	½ c	78	87	30	2	7	4	<1	.1	t	.2
824	Brussels sprouts, cooked from frozen	½ c	77	87	33	3	6	3	<1	.1	t	.2
	Cabbage, common varieties:											
825	Raw, shredded or chopped	1 c	70	92	17	1	4	1	<1	t	t	.1

(Computer code number is for West Diet Analysis program)

Chol (mg)	Calc (mg)	Iron (mg)	Magn (mg)	Phos (mg)	Pota (mg)	Sodi (mg)	Zinc (mg)	VT-A (RE)	Thia (mg)	Ribo (mg)	Niac (mg)	V-B6 (mg)	Fola (μg)	VT-C (mg)
0	23	1.81	60	120	305	1	.97	1	.21	.05	.43	.06	128	0
9	71	4.15	44	148	378	554	7.4	16	.07	.06	.63	.09	28	4
18	154	4.23	86	266	673	850	3.82	29	.12	.15	.89	.22	95	8
15	123	4.47	72	267	604	1105	4.83	40	.15	.14	2.32	.12	77	6
0	19	1.16	29	54	347	45	.37	16	.06	.05	.91	.1	18	11
0	25	1.76	50	101	370	26	.5	15	.06	.05	.69	.1	14	5
0	16	2.26	40	104	478	2	.89	0	.15	.05	.4	.15	78	0
0	84	3.72	96	279	738	481	1.74	1	.27	.13	.75	.23	188	4
0	29	.79	16	24	185	2	.22	41[1]	.05	.06	.38	.03	21	6
0	30	.55	14	16	75	9	.42	35[2]	.03	.05	.28	.04	5	5
0	17	.6	9	13	73	168[3]	.19	23[4]	.01	.04	.13	.02	21	3
0	29	.8	16	25	188	2	.23	5	.05	.06	.39	.04	21	6
0	14	.95	22	56	154	6	.43	2	.09	.13	.78	.09	63	14
0	16	2.36	41	98	272	11	1.12	4	.17	.22	1.49	.16	86	20
0	15	.81	17	35	125	12	.58	2	.06	.13	1.01	.07	36	14
0	18	.54	11	40	34	175	.35	3	.04	.09	.28	.04	12	<1
0	14	.67	20	32	259	65	.3	3	.02	.03	.28	.06	68	3
0	16	.79	23	38	305	77	.35	4	.03	.04	.33	.07	80	4
0	13	1.55	14	14	125	232[5]	.18	1	.01	.03	.13	.05	26	3
0	13	.47	17	19	168	301	.3	1	.01	.05	.29	.06	30	3
0	82	1.37	49	29	654	174	.36	367	.08	.21	.36	.09	10	18
0	42	.77	22	58	286	24	.35	136[6]	.06	.1	.56	.14	62	82
0	72	1.33	38	100	491	41	.6	233[6]	.1	.18	.96	.24	107	141
0	83	1.51	43	106	526	47	.68	250[6]	.1	.2	1.03	.26	90	134
0	72	1.31	37	92	456	41	.59	217[6]	.09	.18	.89	.22	78	116
0	46	.55	18	49	162	22	.27	170[6]	.05	.07	.41	.12	27	36
0	94	1.12	37	101	331	44	.55	348[6]	.1	.15	.84	.24	103	74
0	32	.7	20	64	322	23	.5	67	.07	.09	.76	.18	48	63
0	28	.94	16	44	247	16	.26	56	.08	.06	.47	.14	47	48
0	19	.57	19	42	252	18	.28	46	.08	.09	.42	.22	78	35
0	33	.41	10	16	172	13	.13	9	.03	.03	.21	.07	30	22

[1] Data is for green varieties; yellow beans contain 10 RE per cup.

[2] Data is for green varieties; yellow beans contain 15 RE per cup.

[3] Low sodium pack contains 3 mg sodium per cup.

[4] For green varieties; yellow beans contain 14 RE per cup.

[5] Low sodium pack contains 39 mg sodium.

[6] Vitamin A for whole plant: leaves are 1600 RE/100 g raw; flower clusters are 300/100 g raw; stalks are 40 RE/100 g raw.

(For purposes of calculations, use "0" for t, < 1, < .1, < .01, etc.)

Table I–1
Food Composition

Computer Code Number	Food Description	Measure	Wt (g)	H₂O (%)	Ener (cal)	Prot (g)	Carb (g)	Dietary Fiber (g)	Fat (g)	Fat Breakdown (g)		
										Sat	Mono	Poly
	VEGETABLES AND LEGUMES—Cont.											
826	Cooked, drained	1 c	150	94	33	2	7	4	1	.1	t	.3
	Cabbage, Chinese:											
1178	Bok choy, raw, shredded	1 c	70	95	9	1	2	1	<1	t	t	.1
827	Bok choy, cooked, drained	1 c	170	96	20	3	3	3	<1	t	t	.1
828	Pe tsai, raw, chopped	1 c	76	94	12	1	2	1	<1	t	t	.1
1796	Pe Tsai, cooked	1 c	119	95	17	2	3	2	0	<.1	<.1	.1
1937	Cabbage, Kim Chee style	1 c	150	92	31	2	6	2	0	<.1	<.1	.2
	Cabbage, red, coarsely chopped:											
829	Raw	1 c	70	92	19	1	4	2	<1	t	t	.1
830	Cooked, drained	½ c	75	94	16	1	3	2	<1	t	t	.1
831	Cabbage, savoy, coarsely chopped, raw	1 c	70	91	19	1	4	2	<1	t	t	t
1785	Cabbage, savoy, cooked	1 c	145	92	35	3	8	4	0	<.1	<.1	.1
1896	Capers	5 g	5	86	0	0	0	0	0	–	–	–
	Carrots, raw:											
832	Whole, 7 ½ x 1 ⅛"	1 ea	72	88	31	1	7	2	<1	t	t	.1
833	Grated	½ c	55	88	24	1	6	2	<1	t	t	t
	Carrots, cooked, sliced, drained:											
834	From fresh	½ c	78	87	35	1	8	2	<1	t	t	.1
835	From frozen	½ c	73	90	26	1	6	3	<1	t	t	t
836	Carrots, canned, sliced, drained	½ c	73	93	17	<1	4	2	<1	t	t	.1
837	Carrot juice, canned	½ c	123	89	49	1	11	2	<1	t	t	.1
	Cauliflower, flowerets:											
838	Raw	½ c	50	92	12	1	3	1	<1	t	t	.1
839	Cooked from fresh, drained	½ c	62	93	14	1	3	1	<1	.1	t	.1
840	Cooked, from frozen, drained	½ c	90	94	17	1	3	2	<1	t	t	.1
	Celery, pascal type, raw:											
841	Large outer stalk, 8 x 1½" (root end)	1 ea	40	95	6	<1	1	1	<1	t	t	t
842	Diced	1 c	120	95	19	1	4	2	<1	t	t	.1
1789	Celery/Celeric root, cooked	3.5 oz	99	93	25	1	6	4	<1	<.1	<.1	.1
1179	Chard, swiss, raw, chopped	1 c	36	93	7	1	1	1	<1	t	t	t
1180	Chard, swiss, cooked	1 c	175	93	35	3	7	4	<1	t	t	.1
1855	Chayote fruit, raw	1 ea	203	93	49	2	11	6	1	–	–	–
1856	Chayote fruit, cooked	1 c	160	93	38	1	8	1	1	–	–	–
	Chickpeas (see Garbanzo Beans #854)											
	Collards, cooked, drained:											
843	From fresh	½ c	64	95	17	1	4	2	<1	t	t	.1
844	From frozen	½ c	85	88	31	3	6	3	<1	.1	t	.1
	Corn, cooked, drained:											
845	From fresh, on cob, 5" long	1 ea	77	70	83	3	19	2	1	.2	.3	.5
846	From frozen, on cob, 3½" long	1 ea	63	73	59	2	14	2	<1	.1	.1	.2
847	Kernels, cooked from frozen	½ c	82	76	66	2	17	2	<1	t	t	t
	Corn, canned:											
848	Cream style	½ c	128	79	92	2	23	2	1	.1	.2	.3
849	Whole kernel, vacuum pack	½ c	105	77	83	3	20	6	1	.1	.2	.3
	Cowpeas (see Black-eyed peas #814–816)											
850	Cucumber slices with peel	7 pce	28	96	4	<1	1	<1	<1	t	t	t
1948	Cucumber, Kim Chee style	1 c	150	91	32	2	7	2	<1	.1	0	.1

(Computer code number is for West Diet Analysis program)

Chol (mg)	Calc (mg)	Iron (mg)	Magn (mg)	Phos (mg)	Pota (mg)	Sodi (mg)	Zinc (mg)	VT-A (RE)	Thia (mg)	Ribo (mg)	Niac (mg)	V-B6 (mg)	Fola (µg)	VT-C (mg)
0	46	.25	12	22	146	12	.13	19	.09	.08	.42	.17	30	30
0	73	.56	13	26	176	45	.13	210	.03	.05	.35	.14	46	31
0	158	1.77	19	49	631	58	.29	437	.05	.11	.73	.28	69	44
0	58	.24	10	22	180	7	.17	91	.03	.04	.3	.18	60	20
0	38	.36	12	46	268	11	.21	115	.05	.05	.6	.21	64	19
0	145	1.28	28	59	375	995	.35	426	.07	.1	.75	.34	88	80
0	36	.34	11	29	144	8	.15	3	.03	.02	.21	.15	14	40
0	28	.26	8	22	105	6	.11	2	.03	.01	.15	.1	9	26
0	24	.28	20	29	161	20	.19	70	.05	.02	.21	.13	56	22
0	44	.55	35	48	267	35	.33	129	.07	.03	.03	.22	67	25
0	2	.05	–	–	–	105	–	1	–	–	–	–	–	0
0	19	.36	11	32	232	25	.14	2024	.07	.04	.67	.11	10	7
0	15	.27	8	24	177	19	.11	1546	.05	.03	.51	.08	8	5
0	24	.48	10	23	177	51	.23	1913	.03	.04	.39	.19	11	2
0	20	.34	7	19	115	43	.17	1291	.02	.03	.32	.09	8	2
0	18	.47	6	17	130	175[1]	.19	1004	.01	.02	.4	.08	7	2
0	29	.57	17	52	359	36	.22	3166	.11	.07	.47	.27	5	10
0	11	.22	7	22	152	15	.14	1	.03	.03	.26	.11	28	23
0	10	.2	6	20	88	9	.11	1	.03	.03	.25	.11	27	27
0	15	.37	8	22	125	16	.12	2	.03	.05	.28	.08	37	28
0	16	.16	4	10	115	35	.05	5	.02	.02	.13	.03	11	3
0	48	.48	13	30	344	104	.16	16	.06	.05	.39	.1	34	8
0	26	.43	12	65	172	61	.2	0	.03	.04	.42	.1	3	4
0	18	.65	29	17	136	77	.13	119	.01	.03	.14	.04	5	11
0	101	3.96	150	58	961	313	.58	550	.06	.15	.63	.15	15	31
0	39	.81	28	53	305	8	.71	11	.06	.08	1.02	.27	56	22
0	21	.35	19	46	277	2	.5	8	.04	.06	.67	.19	29	13
0	15	.1	4	5	83	10	.07	175	.01	.03	.19	.03	4	8
0	179	.95	25	23	213	42	.23	508	.04	.1	.54	.1	64	22
0	2	.47	25	79	193	13	.37	17[2]	.17	.06	1.24	.05	36	5
0	2	.38	18	47	158	3	.4	13[2]	.11	.04	.96	.14	19	3
0	2	.25	15	38	113	4	.29	20[2]	.06	.06	1.05	.08	19	2
0	4	.49	22	65	172	364[3]	.68	12[2]	.03	.07	1.23	.08	57	6
0	5	.44	24	67	195	286[4]	.48	25[2]	.04	.08	1.23	.06	51	9
0	4	.07	3	6	41	1	.06	6	.01	.01	.06	.01	4	2
0	14	7.23	12	20	176	1532	.77	50	.05	.05	.69	.17	35	5

[1]Low sodium pack contains 31 mg sodium.

[2]For yellow varieties; white varieties contain only a trace of vitamin A.

[3]Low sodium pack contains 4 mg sodium per ½ cup.

[4]Low sodium pack contains 6 mg sodium per cup.

(For purposes of calculations, use "0" for t, < 1, < .1, < .01, etc.)

Table I–1
Food Composition

Computer Code Number	Food Description	Measure	Wt (g)	H$_2$O (%)	Ener (cal)	Prot (g)	Carb (g)	Dietary Fiber (g)	Fat (g)	Fat Breakdown (g)		
										Sat	Mono	Poly
	VEGETABLES AND LEGUMES—Cont.											
	Dandelion greens:											
851	Raw	1 c	55	86	25	1	5	2	<1	.1	t	.2
852	Chopped, cooked, drained	1 c	105	90	35	2	7	3	1	.1	.1	.4
853	Eggplant, cooked	1 c	160	92	45	1	11	4	<1	.1	t	.2
1714	Endive, fresh, chopped	¼ c	13	94	2	<1	<1	<1	<1	t	t	t
856	Escarole/curly endive, chopped	1 c	50	94	8	1	2	1	<1	t	t	t
854	Garbanzo beans (chickpeas), cooked	1 c	164	60	269	15	45	8	4	.4	1	1.9
1939	Grape leaves, raw	10 g	10	79	7	0	1	–	0	–	–	–
855	Great northern beans, cooked	1 c	177	69	209	15	37	10	1	.3	t	.3
857	Jerusalem artichoke, raw slices	1 c	150	78	114	3	26	2	<1	0	t	t
1016	Jicama	1 c	120	90	46	1	11	6	0	<.1	0	.1
	Kale, cooked, drained:											
858	From fresh	½ c	65	91	21	1	4	1	<1	t	t	.1
859	From frozen	½ c	65	90	19	2	3	1	<1	t	t	.2
860	Kidney beans, canned	1 c	256	77	217	13	40	16	1	.1	.1	.5
1181	Kohlrabi, raw slices	1 c	140	91	38	2	9	5	<1	t	t	.1
861	Kohlrabi, cooked	1 c	165	90	48	3	11	3	<1	t	t	.1
1183	Leeks, raw, chopped	1 c	104	83	63	2	15	3	<1	t	t	.2
1182	Leeks, cooked, chopped	½ c	52	91	16	<1	4	2	<1	t	t	.1
862	Lentils, cooked from dry	½ c	99	70	115	9	20	5	<1	.1	.1	.2
1288	Lentils, sprouted, stir-fried	4 oz	113	69	115	10	24	4	1	.1	.1	.2
1289	Lentils, sprouted, raw	1 c	77	67	82	7	17	3	<1	t	.1	.2
	Lettuce:											
	Butterhead/Boston types:											
863	Head, 5" diameter	¼ ea	41	96	5	1	1	1	<1	t	t	.1
864	Leaves, inner or outer	4 ea	30	96	4	<1	1	<1	<1	t	t	t
	Iceberg/crisphead:											
865	Head, 6" diameter	¼ ea	135	96	17	1	3	1	<1	t	t	.1
866	Wedge, ¼ head	1 ea	135	96	18	1	3	1	<1	t	t	.1
867	Chopped or shredded	1 c	56	96	7	1	1	1	<1	t	t	.1
868	Looseleaf, chopped	½ c	28	94	5	<1	1	<1	<1	t	t	t
869	Romaine, chopped	½ c	28	95	4	<1	1	<1	<1	t	t	t
870	Romaine, inner leaf	3 ea	30	95	5	<1	1	<1	<1	t	t	t
1930	Luffa, cooked	1 c	178	89	57	3	13	6	0	.1	<.1	.1
	Mushrooms:											
871	Raw, sliced	½ c	35	92	9	1	2	<1	<1	t	t	.1
872	Cooked from fresh, pieces	½ c	78	91	21	2	4	2	<1	t	t	.1
1962	Stir fried, shitake	1 c	145	84	80	2	21	3	<1	.1	.1	<.1
873	Canned, drained	½ c	78	91	19	1	4	2	<1	t	t	.1
1951	Mushroom caps, pickled	8 ea	47	92	11	1	2	1	<1	<.1	0	.1
	Mustard greens:											
874	Cooked from fresh	½ c	70	95	11	2	1	1	<1	t	.1	t
875	Cooked from frozen	½ c	75	94	14	2	2	2	<1	t	.1	t
876	Navy beans, cooked from dry	1 c	182	63	258	16	48	16	1	.3	.1	.4
	Okra, cooked:											
877	From fresh pods	8 ea	85	90	27	2	6	2	<1	t	t	t
878	From frozen slices	½ c	92	91	34	2	8	3	<1	.1	t	.1
1236	Batter fried from fresh	1 c	92	69	175	3	12	2	13	2.1	3.4	7.1
1930	Chinese, (Luffa), cooked	1 c	178	89	57	3	13	6	0	.1	<.1	.1

(Computer code number is for West Diet Analysis program)

Chol (mg)	Calc (mg)	Iron (mg)	Magn (mg)	Phos (mg)	Pota (mg)	Sodi (mg)	Zinc (mg)	VT-A (RE)	Thia (mg)	Ribo (mg)	Niac (mg)	V-B6 (mg)	Fola (µg)	VT-C (mg)
0	102	1.71	20	36	218	42	.23	770	.1	.14	.44	.14	15	19
0	147	1.89	25	44	243	46	.29	1229	.14	.18	.54	.17	13	19
0	10	.56	21	35	397	5	.24	10	.12	.03	.96	.14	23	2
0	7	.10	2	4	41	3	.1	27	.01	.01	.05	< .01	18	1
0	26	.41	8	14	157	11	.39	103	.04	.04	.2	.01	71	3
0	80	4.74	79	276	477	11	2.51	4	.19	.1	.86	.23	282	2
0	72	.69	–	4	26	2	–	86	.02	.01	.12	–	–	3
0	120	3.77	88	292	692	4	1.56	< 1	.28	.1	1.21	.21	181	2
0	21	5.1	25	117	644	6	.18	3	.3	.09	1.95	.12	20	6
0	14	.72	14	22	180	5	.19	2	.02	.03	.24	.05	14	24
0	47	.58	12	18	148	15	.16	481	.03	.05	.32	.09	9	27
0	90	.61	12	18	209	10	.12	413	.03	.07	.44	.06	9	16
0	61	3.23	72	240	658	873	1.41	< 1	.27	.22	1.17	.06	129	3
0	34	.56	27	64	490	28	.04	5	.07	.03	.56	.21	22	87
0	41	.66	31	74	561	35	.51	6	.07	.03	.64	.25	20	89
0	61	2.18	29	36	187	21	.12	10	.06	.03	.42	.24	67	12
0	16	.57	7	9	45	5	.03	2	.01	.01	.1	.06	13	2
0	19	3.3	36	178	365	2	1.26	1	.17	.07	1.05	.18	178	1
0	16	3.52	40	174	322	11	1.81	5	.25	.1	1.36	.19	76	14
0	19	2.47	28	133	247	8	1.16	3	.18	.1	.87	.15	77	13
0	13	.12	5	9	104	2	.07	40	.02	.02	.12	.02	30	3
0	10	.09	4	7	76	2	.05	29	.02	.02	.09	.01	22	2
0	25	.67	12	27	213	12	.3	45	.06	.04	.25	.05	76	5
0	25	.67	12	27	213	12	.3	45	.06	.04	.25	.05	76	5
0	11	.28	5	11	88	5	.12	18	.03	.02	.1	.02	31	2
0	19	.39	3	7	74	3	.08	53	.01	.02	.11	.01	14	5
0	10	.31	2	13	81	2	.07	73	.03	.03	.14	.01	38	7
0	11	.33	2	14	87	2	.07	78	.03	.03	.15	.01	41	7
0	112	.8	101	99	570	420	.97	103	.23	.1	1.54	.33	81	29
0	2	.43	3	36	129	1	.26	0	.04	.16	1.44	.03	7	1
0	5	1.36	9	68	277	2	.68	0	.06	.23	3.48	.07	14	3
0	4	.64	20	42	170	6	1.94	0	.05	.25	2.18	.23	30	.44
0	9	.62	12	51	101	331	.56	0	.07	.02	1.24	.05	10	0
0	2	.5	5	38	139	95	.28	0	.03	.16	1.42	.03	6	1
0	51	.49	11	29	141	11	.08	212	.03	.04	.3	.07	51	18
0	76	.84	10	18	104	19	.15	335	.03	.04	.19	.08	52	10
0	127	4.51	107	286	670	2	1.93	< 1	.37	.11	.97	.3	255	2
0	54	.38	48	48	273	4	.47	49	.11	.05	.74	.16	39	14
0	88	.62	47	42	215	3	.57	47	.09	.11	.72	.04	133	11
15	104	.77	37	106	214	137	.5	43	.13	.1	.75	.13	37	10
0	112	.8	101	99	570	420	.97	103	.23	.1	1.54	.33	81	29

(For purposes of calculations, use "0" for t, < 1, < .1, < .01, etc.)

Table I–1
Food Composition

Computer Code Number	Food Description	Measure	Wt (g)	H$_2$O (%)	Ener (cal)	Prot (g)	Carb (g)	Dietary Fiber (g)	Fat (g)	Fat Breakdown (g) Sat	Mono	Poly
	VEGETABLES AND LEGUMES—Cont.											
	Onions:											
879	Raw, chopped	1 c	160	90	61	2	14	3	<1	t	t	.1
880	Raw, sliced	1 c	115	90	44	1	10	2	<1	t	t	.1
881	Cooked, drained, chopped	½ c	105	88	46	1	11	1	<1	t	t	.1
882	Dehydrated flakes	¼ c	14	4	45	1	12	1	<1	t	t	t
1934	Onions, pearl, cooked	1 c	185	87	81	3	19	3	<1	.1	.1	.1
	Spring/green onions, chopped:											
883	Bulb and top	½ c	50	90	16	1	4	1	<1	t	t	t
1185	Green tops only	1 c	100	92	34	2	6	3	<1	.1	.1	.2
1184	White part only	½ c	50	92	25	1	5	1	<1	t	t	t
884	Onion rings, breaded, heated f/frozen	2 ea	20	28	81	1	8	<1	5	1.7	2.2	1
1917	Palm Hearts, cooked slices	1 c	146	70	150	4	39	2	<1	.1	.1	<.1
	Parsley:											
885	Raw, chopped	½ c	30	88	11	1	2	1	<1	t	.1	t
886	Raw, sprigs	5 ea	5	88	2	<1	<1	<1	<1	t	t	t
887	Freeze dried	¼ c	1	2	3	<1	<1	<1	<1	t	t	t
888	Parsnips, sliced, cooked	½ c	78	78	63	1	15	3	<1	t	.1	t
	Peas:											
	Black-eyed, cooked:											
814	From dry, drained	½ c	85	70	99	7	18	6	<1	.1	t	.2
815	From fresh, drained	½ c	82	76	80	3	17	4	<1	.1	t	.1
816	From frozen, drained	½ c	85	66	112	7	20	7	1	.2	.1	.2
889	Edible pod peas, cooked	1 c	160	89	67	5	11	4	<1	.1	t	.2
890	Green, canned, drained	½ c	85	82	59	4	11	3	<1	.1	t	.1
891	Green, cooked from frozen	½ c	80	80	62	4	11	4	<1	t	t	.1
1786	Snow peas, raw, cup	1 c	145	89	61	4	11	4	0	.1	<.1	.1
1787	Snow peas, raw each	10 ea	29	89	12	1	2	1	0	<.1	<.1	<.1
892	Split, green, cooked from dry	½ c	98	70	116	8	21	3	<1	.1	.1	.2
1187	Peas & carrots, cooked from frozen	½ c	80	86	38	2	8	3	<1	.1	t	.2
1186	Peas & carrots, canned w/liquid	½ c	128	88	49	3	11	4	<1	.1	t	.2
	Peppers, hot:											
893	Hot green chili, canned	½ c	68	93	17	1	4	1	<1	t	t	t
894	Hot green chili, raw	1 ea	45	88	18	1	4	1	<1	t	t	.1
1715	Hot red chili, raw, diced	1 tbs	9	88	4	<1	1	<1	<1	t	t	t
1988	Jalapeno, raw	2 oz	57	90	25	–	–	–	–	–	–	–
895	Jalapeno, chopped, canned	½ c	68	89	16	1	3	2	<1	t	t	.2
1918	Wheels in brine (Ortega)	2 tbs	29	–	10	0	2	–	0	0	0	0
	Peppers, sweet, green:											
896	Whole pod (90 g with refuse), raw	1 ea	74	92	20	1	5	1	<1	t	t	.1
897	Cooked, chopped (1 pod cooked = 73 g)	½ c	68	92	19	1	5	1	<1	t	t	.1
	Peppers, sweet, red:											
1286	Raw, chopped	1 c	100	92	27	1	6	2	<1	t	t	.1
1807	Raw, each	1 ea	74	92	20	1	5	1	<1	<.1	<.1	.1
1287	Cooked, chopped	½ c	68	92	19	1	5	1	<1	t	t	.1
	Peppers, sweet, yellow:											
1872	Raw, large	1 ea	186	92	50	2	12	4	<1	.1	.1	2.1
1873	Strips (pieces)	10 pce	52	92	14	1	3	1	<1	0	<.1	.6
898	Pinto beans, cooked from dry	½ c	85	64	116	7	22	7	<1	t	.1	.2

(Computer code number is for West Diet Analysis program)

Chol (mg)	Calc (mg)	Iron (mg)	Magn (mg)	Phos (mg)	Pota (mg)	Sodi (mg)	Zinc (mg)	VT-A (RE)	Thia (mg)	Ribo (mg)	Niac (mg)	V-B6 (mg)	Fola (µg)	VT-C (mg)
0	32	.35	16	53	251	5	.3	0	.07	.03	.24	.19	30	10
0	23	.25	12	38	181	3	.22	0	.05	.02	.17	.13	22	7
0	23	.25	12	37	174	3	.22	0	.04	.02	.17	.13	16	5
0	36	.22	13	42	227	3	.26	0	.07	.01	.14	.22	23	10
0	41	.44	20	64	305	433	.39	0	.08	.04	.30	.24	28	10
0	36	.74	10	19	138	8	.19	19	.03	.04	.26	.03	32	9
0	56	2.2	21	39	260	7	.22	40	.07	.1	.6	0	80	51
0	20	.44	8	20	115	3	.12	< 1	.03	.02	.17	.05	18	13
0	6	.34	4	16	26	75	.08	5	.06	.03	.72	.01	3	< 1
0	26	2.47	15	204	2637	20	5.45	10	.07	.25	1.25	1.06	30	10
0	41	1.86	15	17	166	17	.32	156	.03	.03	.39	.03	46	40
0	6	.31	3	3	27	3	.04	26	< .01	< .01	.02	< .01	8	7
0	2	.54	4	5	63	4	.06	63	.01	.03	.15	.02	21	1
0	29	.45	23	53	286	8	.2	0	.06	.04	.56	.07	45	10[1]
0	20	2.15	45	133	238	3	1.1	1	.17	.05	.42	.09	177	< 1
0	106	.92	43	42	343	3	.85	65	.08	.12	1.16	.05	104	2
0	20	1.8	43	104	319	4	1.21	6	.22	.05	.62	.08	120	2
0	67	3.15	42	88	384	6	.59	21	.2	.12	.86	.23	47	77
0	17	.81	14	57	147	186[2]	.6	65	.1	.07	.62	.05	38	8
0	19	1.26	23	72	134	70	.75	54	.23	.08	1.18	.09	47	8
0	62	3.02	35	77	290	6	.39	21	.22	.12	.87	.23	60	87
0	12	.6	7	15	58	1	.08	4	.04	.02	.17	.05	12	17
0	14	1.26	35	97	355	2	.98	1	.19	.05	.87	.05	64	< 1
0	18	.75	13	39	126	54	.36	621	.18	.05	.92	.07	21	6
0	29	.96	18	59	128	332	.74	739	.09	.07	.74	.11	23	8
0	5	.34	10	12	127	797	.12	41[3]	.01	.03	.54	.1	7	46
0	8	.54	11	21	153	3	.13	35[3]	.04	.04	.43	.13	11	109
0	2	.11	2	4	32	1	.03	101	.01	.01	.09	.03	2	22
–	–	–	–	–	3	3	–	38	–	–	–	–	–	66
0	18	1.9	8	12	92	995	.13	116	.02	.03	.34	.14	9	9
0	–	–	–	–	55	390	–	–	–	–	–	–	–	21
0	7	.34	7	14	131	1	.09	47	.05	.02	.38	.18	16	66
0	6	.31	7	12	113	1	.08	40	.04	.02	.32	.16	11	51
0	9	.46	10	19	177	2	.12	570	.07	.03	.51	.25	22	190
0	7	.34	7	14	131	1	.09	422	.05	.02	.38	.18	16	141
0	6	.31	7	12	112	1	.08	256	.04	.02	.32	.16	11	116
0	20	.86	22	45	394	4	.32	44	.05	.05	1.66	.31	48	342
0	6	.24	6	12	110	1	.09	12	.01	.01	.46	.09	14	96
0	41	2.23	47	137	398	2	.92	< 1	.16	.08	.34	.13	147	2

[1] Value for Vitamin C is highest right after harvest and drops after that.

[2] Low sodium pack contains 1.7 mg sodium.

[3] Data is for green chili peppers; red varieties contain 809 RE vitamin A per ¼ cup; 484 RE per whole pepper.

(For purposes of calculations, use "0" for t, < 1, < .1, < .01, etc.)

Table I–1
Food Composition

Computer Code Number	Food Description	Measure	Wt (g)	H₂O (%)	Ener (cal)	Prot (g)	Carb (g)	Dietary Fiber (g)	Fat (g)	Fat Breakdown (g)		
										Sat	Mono	Poly
	VEGETABLES AND LEGUMES—Cont.											
1191	Poi, two finger	¼ c	60	72	67	< 1	16	< 1	< 1	t	t	t
	Potatoes:[1]											
	Baked in oven, 4¾" x 2⅓" diam:											
899	With skin	1 ea	202	71	220	5	51	5	< 1	.1	1	.1
900	Flesh only	1 ea	156	75	145	3	34	2	< 1	t	t	.1
901	Skin only	1 ea	58	47	115	2	27	2	< 1	t	t	t
	Baked in microwave, 4¾" x 2⅓" diam:											
902	With skin	1 ea	202	72	212	5	49	5	< 1	.1	t	.1
903	Flesh only	1 ea	156	74	156	3	36	2	< 1	t	t	.1
904	Skin only	1 ea	58	64	77	3	17	2	< 1	t	t	t
	Boiled, about 2½" diam:											
905	Peeled after boiling	1 ea	136	77	118	3	27	2	< 1	t	t	.1
906	Peeled before boiling	1 ea	135	78	116	2	27	2	< 1	t	t	.1
	French fried, strips 2–3½" long:											
907	Oven heated	10 pce	50	35	163	2	19	1	9	3.8	4.2	.9
908	Fried in vegetable oil	10 ea	50	40	155	2	19	2	8	2.5	4	1.2
1188	Fried in veg and animal oil	10 ea	50	38	158	2	20	2	8	3.4	4	.5
909	Hashed browns from frozen	1 c	156	56	340	5	44	3	18	7	8	2.1
	Mashed:											
910	Home recipe with whole milk[2]	½ c	105	79	81	2	18	2	1	.3	.2	.1
911	Home recipe with milk and marg	½ c	105	76	111	2	18	2	4	1.1	1.9	1.3
912	Prepared from flakes; water, milk, margarine, salt added	½ c	110	76	124	2	17	1	6	1.6	2.5	1.7
	Potato products, prepared:											
	Au gratin:											
913	From dry mix	½ c	122	79	114	3	16	2	5	3.2	1.4	.2
914	From home recipe[3]	½ c	122	74	162	6	14	2	9	4.3	3.2	1.3
	Scalloped:											
915	From dry mix	½ c	122	79	114	3	16	1	5	3.2	1.5	.2
916	From home recipe[4]	½ c	122	81	105	4	13	1	5	1.7	1.6	.9
	Potato salad (see Mixed Dishes #715)											
1192	Potato puffs, cooked from frozen	½ c	62	61	107	1	16	1	6	1.1	1.9	0
917	Potato chips	14 ea	28	2	150	2	15	1	10	3.1	2.8	3.5
918	Pumpkin, cooked from fresh, mashed	1 c	245	94	49	2	12	2	< 1	.1	t	t
919	Pumpkin, canned	½ c	123	90	42	1	10	3	< 1	.2	.1	t
1891	Radicchio, raw, shredded	0.5 c	20	93	5	0	1	–	< 1	–	–	–
1894	Radicchio leaf, raw	10 ea	80	93	18	1	4	–	< 1	–	–	–
920	Red radishes	10 ea	45	95	8	< 1	2	< 1	< 1	t	t	t
1793	Daikon radishes (Chinese) raw	0.5 c	44	95	8	< 1	2	1	< .1	< .1	< .1	< .1
921	Refried beans, canned	½ c	126	72	135	8	23	7	1	.5	.6	.2
1375	Rutabaga, cooked cubes	½ c	85	89	33	1	7	2	< 1	t	t	.1
922	Sauerkraut, canned with liquid	½ c	118	93	22	1	5	3	< 1	t	t	.1
923	Seaweed, kelp, raw	1 oz	28	82	12	< 1	3	< 1	< 1	.1	t	t
924	Seaweed, spirulina, dried	1 oz	28	5	31	16	7	1	2	.8	.2	.6
1866	Shallots, raw, chopped	1 tbs	10	80	7	0	2	0	< 1	0	0	0

[1] Vitamin C varies with length of storage. After 3 months of storage approximately two-thirds of the ascorbic acid remains; after 6 to 7 months, about one-third remains.

[2] Recipe: 84% potatoes, 15% whole milk, 1% salt.

[3] Recipe: 55% potatoes, 30% whole milk, 9% cheddar cheese, 3% butter, 2% flour, 1% salt.

[4] Recipe: 59% potatoes, 36% whole milk, 2% butter, 2% flour, 1% salt.

(Computer code number is for West Diet Analysis program)

Chol (mg)	Calc (mg)	Iron (mg)	Magn (mg)	Phos (mg)	Pota (mg)	Sodi (mg)	Zinc (mg)	VT-A (RE)	Thia (mg)	Ribo (mg)	Niac (mg)	V-B6 (mg)	Fola (μg)	VT-C (mg)
0	10	.53	14	23	110	7	.13	1	.08	.02	.66	.16	13	2
0	20	2.75	55	115	844	16	.65	0	.22	.07	3.31	.7	22	26[1]
0	8	.55	39	78	610	8	.45	0	.16	.03	2.18	.47	14	20[1]
0	20	4.08	25	59	332	12	.28	0	.07	.06	1.78	.36	13	8[1]
0	22	2.5	55	212	903	16	.73	0	.24	.06	3.45	.69	24	30[1]
0	8	.64	39	170	641	11	.51	0	.2	.04	2.54	.5	19	24[1]
0	27	3.45	21	48	377	9	.3	0	.04	.04	1.29	.28	10	9[1]
0	7	.42	30	60	515	5	.41	0	.14	.03	1.96	.41	14	18[1]
0	11	.42	27	54	443	7	.36	0	.13	.03	1.77	.36	12	10[1]
0	6	.83	11	48	270	306	.2	0	.04	.02	1.33	.11	11	3
0	8	.68	17	67	356	82	.26	1	.07	.02	1.14	.12	17	3
6	10	.38	17	47	366	108	.19	0	.09	.01	1.63	.12	15	5
0	23	2.36	26	112	680	53	.5	0	.17	.03	3.78	.2	10	10
2	27	.28	19	50	314	318	.3	6	.09	.04	1.18	.24	9	7[1]
2[5]	27	.27	19	48	303	310	.28	57	.09	.04	1.13	.23	8	6[1]
4[5]	54	.24	20	62	256	365	.2	59	.12	.05	.73	.01	8	11
6	102	.39	18	116	268	536	.29	38	.02	.1	1.15	.05	8	4
18[6]	146	.78	24	138	483	528	.84	47	.08	.14	1.22	.21	10	12
13	44	.47	17	68	249	416	.31	54	.02	.07	1.26	.05	12	4
7[7]	70	.7	23	77	463	410	.49	38	.08	.11	1.29	.22	11	13
0	19	0	12	30	162	251	.19	1	.12	.01	1.05	.14	10	1
0	7	.46	19	46	357	166[8]	.31	0	.05	.06	1.07	.19	13	9
0	37	1.4	22	74	564	2	.56	2651	.08	.19	1.01	.11	21	12
0	32	1.71	28	43	253	6	.21	2712	.03	.07	.45	.07	15	5
0	4	.11	3	8	60	4	.12	1	0	.01	.05	.01	12	2
0	15	.45	10	32	242	18	.50	2	.01	.02	.20	.05	48	6
0	9	.13	4	8	104	11	.13	<1	<.01	.02	.13	.03	12	10
0	12	.18	7	10	100	9	.07	0	.01	.01	.09	.02	12	10
0	58	2.24	49	106	495	534	1.73	<1	.06	.07	.61	.13	105	8
0	41	.45	20	48	277	17	.3	48	.07	.03	.61	.09	13	16
0	35	1.73	15	24	201	780	.22	2	.02	.03	.17	.15	28	17
0	48	.81	34	12	25	66	.35	3	.01	.04	.13	<.01	50	<1
0	34	8.08	55	33	382	293	.57	16	.67	1.04	3.63	.1	26	3
0	4	.12	2	6	33	1	.04	0	.01	0	.02	.03	3	1

(5)Data is for margarine; if butter is used, cholesterol = 25 mg for 29 total mg.

(6)Data is for butter; if margarine is used, cholesterol = 37 mg.

(7)Data is for butter; if margarine is used cholesterol = 15 mg.

(8)If no salt added, sodium = 2 mg.

(For purposes of calculations, use "0" for t, <1, <.1, <.01, etc.)

Table I–1
Food Composition

Computer Code Number	Food Description	Measure	Wt (g)	H₂O (%)	Ener (cal)	Prot (g)	Carb (g)	Dietary Fiber (g)	Fat (g)	Fat Breakdown (g)		
										Sat	Mono	Poly
	VEGETABLES AND LEGUMES—Cont.											
1557	Snow peas, stir-fried	1 c	165	89	69	5	12	4	<1	.1	t	.1
925	Soybeans, cooked from dry	½ c	86	63	149	14	9	5	8	1.1	1.7	4.4
1996	Soybeans, dry roasted	½ c	86	–	387	34	28	7	19	2.7	4.1	10.5
	Soybean products:											
926	Miso	½ c	138	42	284	16	39	7	8	1.2	1.8	4.7
927	Tofu (soybean curd, regular)	½ c	124	85	94	10	2	1	6	.9	1.3	3.3
	Spinach:											
928	Raw, chopped	1 c	56	92	12	2	2	2	<1	t	t	.1
929	Cooked, from fresh, drained	½ c	90	91	21	3	3	2	<1	t	t	.1
930	Cooked from frozen (leaf)	½ c	95	90	27	3	5	2	<1	t	t	.1
931	Canned, drained solids	½ c	107	92	25	3	4	3	1	.1	t	.2
	Spinach soufflé (see Mixed Dishes)											
	Squash, summer varieties, cooked:											
932	Varieties averaged	½ c	90	94	18	1	4	1	<1	.1	t	.1
933	Crookneck	½ c	90	94	18	1	4	1	<1	.1	t	.1
934	Zucchini	½ c	90	95	14	1	4	1	<1	t	t	t
	Squash, winter varieties, cooked:											
	Average of all varieties, baked:											
935	Mashed	1 c	245	89	96	2	21	7	2	.3	.1	.7
936	Cubes	1 c	205	89	80	2	18	6	1	.3	.1	.5
937	Acorn, baked, mashed	½ c	122	83	68	1	18	5	<1	t	t	.1
1218	Acorn, boiled, mashed	½ c	122	90	41	1	11	3	<1	t	t	t
	Butternut:											
938	Baked cubes	1 c	205	88	82	2	22	6	<1	t	t	.1
1219	Baked, mashed	½ c	122	88	49	1	13	3	<1	t	t	t
1193	Cooked from frozen	½ c	120	88	47	1	12	3	<1	t	t	t
1194	Hubbard, baked, mashed	½ c	120	85	60	3	13	3	1	.2	.1	.3
1195	Hubbard, boiled, mashed	½ c	118	91	35	2	8	3	<1	.1	t	.2
1196	Spaghetti, baked or boiled	½ c	77	92	22	1	5	1	<1	t	t	.1
1189	Succotash, cooked from frozen	½ c	85	74	79	4	17	5	1	.1	.1	.4
	Sweet potatoes:											
939	Baked in skin, peeled, 5 x 2" diam	1 ea	114	67	140	3	28	4	<1	t	t	.1
940	Boiled without skin, 5 x 2" diam	1 ea	151	73	159	3	37	3	<1	.1	t	.2
941	Candied, 2½ x 2"	1 pce	105	67	143	1	29	2	3	1.4	.7	.2
	Canned:											
942	Solid pack	½ c	128	74	129	3	30	2	<1	.1	t	.1
943	Vacuum pack, mashed	½ c	127	76	116	2	27	4	<1	.1	t	.1
944	Vacuum pack, 3¾ x 1"	2 pce	80	76	73	1	17	2	<1	t	t	.1
1940	Taro shoots, cooked	1 c	140	95	20	1	4	–	0	<.1	<.1	<.1
	Tomatillos:											
1877	Raw, each	1 ea	34	92	11	0	2	1	<1	–	–	–
1875	Raw, chopped	0.5 c	66	92	21	1	4	1	1	–	–	–
	Tomatoes:											
945	Raw, whole, 2⅗" diam	1 ea	123	94	26	1	6	1	<1	.1	.1	.2
946	Raw, chopped	1 c	180	94	38	2	8	2	1	.1	.1	.2

(Computer code number is for West Diet Analysis program)

PAGE KEY: I–4 = BEV   I–6 = DAIRY   I–12 = EGGS   I–14 = FAT/OIL   I–18 = FRUIT   I–26 = BAKERY   I–36 = GRAIN   I–44 = FISH   I–48 = MEATS   I–50 = POULTRY   I–54 = SAUSAGE   I–56 = MIXED/FAST   I–64 = NUTS/SEEDS   I–68 = SWEETS   I–70 = VEG/LEG   I–84 = MISC   I–88 = SOUPS/SAUCES   I–90 = FAST   I–106 = FRZN ENTREE   I–112 = BABY FOODS

Chol (mg)	Calc (mg)	Iron (mg)	Magn (mg)	Phos (mg)	Pota (mg)	Sodi (mg)	Zinc (mg)	VT-A (RE)	Thia (mg)	Ribo (mg)	Niac (mg)	V-B6 (mg)	Fola (μg)	VT-C (mg)
0	71	3.43	40	87	330	7	.45	21	.22	.12	.94	.25	55	84
0	88	4.42	74	211	443	1	.99	1	.13	.24	.34	.2	46	1
0	232	3.41	196	558	1173	2	4.11	2	.37	.65	.91	.19	176	4
0	92	3.76	58	211	226	5033	4.57	12	.13	.34	1.19	.3	46	0
0	130	6.65	126	120	150	9	.99	11	.1	.06	.24	.06	19	< 1
0	55	1.52	44	27	312	44	.3	376	.04	.11	.4	.11	109	16
0	122	3.21	78	50	419	63	.68	737	.09	.21	.44	.22	131	9
0	139	1.44	65	46	283	82	.66	739	.06	.16	.4	.14	103	12
0	136	2.46	81	47	370	29[1]	.49	939	.02	.15	.41	.11	105	15
0	24	.32	22	35	173	1	.35	26[2]	.04	.04	.46	.06	18	5
0	24	.32	22	35	173	1	.35	26[2]	.04	.04	.46	.08	18	5
0	12	.31	20	36	228	3	.16	22[2]	.04	.04	.38	.07	15	4
0	34	.81	20	49	1070	2	.64	871	.21	.06	1.72	.18	69	24
0	29	.68	16	41	896	2	.53	729	.17	.05	1.44	.15	57	20
0	54	1.14	52	55	535	5	.21	52	.2	.02	1.08	.24	23	13
0	32	.68	32	33	322	4	.13	31	.12	.01	.65	.14	14	8
0	84	1.23	59	55	582	8	.27	1435	.15	.03	1.99	.25	39	31
0	50	.73	35	33	348	5	.16	854	.09	.02	1.19	.15	23	18
0	23	.69	11	17	160	2	.14	401	.06	.05	.56	.08	20	4
0	20	.56	26	28	430	10	.18	725	.09	.06	.67	.21	19	11
0	12	.33	15	16	253	6	.12	473	.05	.03	.39	.12	11	8
0	16	.26	8	11	91	14	.15	8	.03	.02	.63	.08	6	3
0	13	.75	20	60	225	38	.38	20	.06	.06	1.11	.08	28	5
0	32	2	28	74	396	11	.33	1928	.08	.14	.69	.27	26	25
0	32	.85	15	41	276	20	.41	2575	.08	.21	.97	.37	17	26
8[3]	27	1.19	12	27	198	73	.16	440	.02	.04	.41	.04	12	7
0	38	1.7	31	67	268	96	.27	1937	.03	.11	1.22	.3	14	7
0	28	1.13	28	62	398	67	.23	1013	.05	.07	.94	.24	21	34
0	18	.71	18	39	250	42	.14	638	.03	.05	.59	.15	13	21
0	20	.57	11	36	482	3	.76	7	.05	.07	1.13	.16	4	26
0	2	.21	7	13	91	< 1	.07	4	.01	.01	.63	.02	2	4
0	5	.41	13	26	177	1	.15	8	.03	.02	1.22	.04	5	8
0	6	.55	13	29	273	11	.11	76	.07	.06	.77	.1	18	23[4]
0	9	.81	20	43	400	16	.16	112	.11	.09	1.13	.14	27	34[4]

[1] Dietary pack contains 58 mg sodium.

[2] Applies to squash including skin; flesh has no appreciable vitamin A value.

[3] For recipe using butter.

[4] Year-round average. From June through October, ascorbic acid is approximately 32 mg and 47 mg, respectively, for one tomato and 1 c chopped tomato. From November through May, market samples average around 12 and 18 mg, respectively.

(For purposes of calculations, use "0" for t, < 1, < .1, < .01, etc.)

Table I–1
Food Composition

Computer Code Number	Food Description	Measure	Wt (g)	H₂O (%)	Ener (cal)	Prot (g)	Carb (g)	Dietary Fiber (g)	Fat (g)	Fat Breakdown (g) Sat	Mono	Poly
	VEGETABLES AND LEGUMES—Cont.											
	Tomatoes—Cont.:											
947	Cooked from raw	1 c	240	92	65	3	14	2	1	.1	.2	.4
948	Canned, solids and liquid	1 c	240	94	48	2	10	2	1	.1	.1	.2
	Tomatoes, sundried:											
1879	Cup measure	1 c	54	15	139	8	30	7	2	.2	.3	.6
1881	Pieces	10 pce	20	15	52	3	11	2	1	.1	.1	.2
1885	Oil pack, drained	33 ea	100	54	213	5	23	7	14	1.9	8.7	2.1
2020	Tomato, Roma, fresh	1 ea	123	94	26	1	6	1	< 1	.1	.1	.2
949	Tomato juice, canned	1 c	244	94	41	2	10	1	< 1	t	t	.1
	Tomato products, canned:											
950	Paste	1 c	262	80	220	10	49	11	2	.3	.4	.9
951	Puree	1 c	250	87	102	4	25	6	< 1	t	t	.1
952	Sauce	1 c	245	89	73	3	18	3	< 1	.1	.1	.2
953	Turnips, cubes, cooked from fresh	½ c	78	94	14	1	4	2	< 1	t	t	t
	Turnip greens, cooked:											
954	From fresh, leaves and stems	1 c	144	93	29	2	6	4	< 1	.1	t	.1
955	From frozen, chopped	1 c	164	90	49	6	8	7	1	.2	.1	.3
956	Vegetable juice cocktail, canned	½ c	121	93	23	1	6	1	< 1	t	t	t
	Vegetables, mixed:											
957	Canned, drained	½ c	81	87	38	2	8	3	< 1	t	t	.1
958	Frozen, cooked, drained	½ c	91	83	53	3	12	5	< 1	t	t	.1
1888	Water chestnuts, Chinese, raw	½ c	62	74	66	1	15	2	0	< .1	< .1	< .1
959	Water chestnuts, canned, slices	½ c	70	86	35	1	9	2	< 1	t	t	t
960	Water chestnuts, canned, whole	4 ea	28	86	14	< 1	3	1	< 1	t	t	t
1190	Watercress, fresh, chopped	½ c	17	95	2	< 1	< 1	< 1	< 1	t	t	t
	MISCELLANEOUS											
	Baking powders for home use:											
	Sodium aluminum sulfate:											
962	With monocalcium phosphate monohydrate	1 tsp	3	2	4	< 1	1	0	0	0	0	0
963	With monocalcium phosphate monohydrate, calcium sulfate	1 tsp	3	5	2	0	1	0	0	0	0	0
964	Straight phosphate	1 tsp	4	4	2	< 1	1	0	0	0	0	0
965	Low sodium	1 tsp	4	6	4	< 1	2	0	< 1	0	0	0
1204	Baking soda	1 tsp	3	< 1	0	0	0	0	0	0	0	0
966	Basil, dried	1 tbs	4	6	10	1	2	1	< 1	–	–	–
2068	Cajun Seasoning	1 tsp	3	.5	6	< 1	1	< 1	< 1	–	–	–
961	Carob flour	1 c	103	4	394	5	92	41	1	.1	.2	.2
967	Catsup:	¼ c	61	67	64	1	17	1	< 1	t	t	.1
968	Tablespoon	1 tbs	15	67	16	< 1	4	< 1	< 1	t	t	t
1200	Cayenne/red pepper	1 tbs	5	8	16	1	3	1	1	.2	.1	.4
969	Celery seed	1 tsp	2	6	8	< 1	1	< 1	1	t	.3	.1
1203	Chili powder:	1 tbs	8	8	25	1	4	3	1	.3	.3	.6
970	Teaspoon	1 tsp	3	8	8	< 1	2	1	< 1	.1	.1	.2
	Chocolate:											
971	Baking, unsweetened, square	1 oz	28	1	146	3	8	4	15	9.2	5.2	.5

(Computer code number is for West Diet Analysis program)

Chol (mg)	Calc (mg)	Iron (mg)	Magn (mg)	Phos (mg)	Pota (mg)	Sodi (mg)	Zinc (mg)	VT-A (RE)	Thia (mg)	Ribo (mg)	Niac (mg)	V-B6 (mg)	Fola (µg)	VT-C (mg)
0	14	1.34	34	74	670	26	.26	178	.17	.14	1.8	.23	31	55
0	62[1]	1.46	29	46	530	391[2]	.38	144	.11	.07	1.76	.22	19	36
0	59	4.91	105	192	1851	1131	1.08	47	.29	.26	4.89	.18	37	21
0	22	1.82	39	71	685	419	.40	17	.11	.10	1.81	.07	14	8
0	47	2.68	81	139	1565	266	.78	129	.19	.38	3.63	.32	23	102
0	6	.55	14	30	273	11	.11	77	.07	.06	.77	.10	18	23
0	22	1.42	27	46	537	881[3]	.34	137	.11	.08	1.64	.27	49	45
0	92	7.83	133	206	2441	2070[4]	2.1	647	.41	.5	8.44	1	59	110
0	37	2.33	60	100	1050	998[5]	.55	340	.18	.13	4.3	.38	27	88
0	34	1.89	47	78	909	1482[6]	.61	240	.16	.14	2.82	.38	23	32
0	17	.17	6	15	105	39	.16	0	.02	.02	.23	.05	7	9
0	197	1.15	32	42	292	42	.2	792	.06	.1	.59	.26	170	39
0	248	3.18	43	56	366	25	.67	1308	.09	.12	.77	.11	65	36
0	13	.51	13	21	234	442	.24	142	.05	.03	.88	.17	25	33
0	22	.86	13	34	237	121	.33	944	.04	.04	.47	.06	19	4
0	23	.74	20	46	154	32	.45	389	.06	.11	.77	.07	17	3
0	7	.04	14	39	362	9	.31	0	.09	.12	.62	.20	10	2
0	3	.61	3	13	83	6	.27	<1	.01	.02	.25	.11	4	1
0	1	.25	1	5	33	2	.11	<1	<.01	.01	.1	.04	2	<1
0	20	.03	4	10	56	7	.02	80	.01	.02	.03	.02	2	7
0	58	0	<1	87	4	328	0	0	0	0	0	0	0	0
0	176	.32	1	63	1	318	<.01	0	0	0	0	0	0	0
0	295	.43	1	377	<1	316	<.01	0	0	0	0	0	0	0
0	173	.35	1	295	434	4	.03	0	0	0	0	0	0	0
0	0	0	0	0	0	821	0	0	0	0	0	0	0	0
0	85	1.68	19	22	154	2	.26	38	.01	.01	.31	–	–	2
–	–	–	–	–	30	474	–	–	–	–	–	–	–	–
0	358	3.04	56	81	852	36	.95	1	.05	.47	1.96	.38	30	<1
0	12	.43	13	24	295	723	.14	62	.05	.04	.84	.11	9	9
0	3	.1	3	6	72	178	.03	15	.01	.01	.21	.03	2	2
0	8	.41	8	15	106	2	.13	209	.02	.05	.44	–	–	4
0	35	.9	9	11	28	3	.14	<1	.01	.01	.1	–	–	<1
0	22	1.12	14	24	149	81	.21	279	.03	.06	.61	–	4	5
0	7	.43	5	8	50	30	.07	105	.01	.02	.2	–	2	2
0	21	1.79	88	117	233	4	1.14	3	.02	.05	.31	.03	2	0

(1)Calcium is added as a firming agent.

(2)Dietary pack contains 31 mg sodium.

(3)If no salt is added, sodium content is 24 mg.

(4)If salt is added, sodium content is 2070 mg.

(5)If salt is added, sodium content is 998 mg.

(6)With salt added.

(For purposes of calculations, use "0" for t, <1, <.1, <.01, etc.)

Table I–1
Food Composition

Computer Code Number	Food Description	Measure	Wt (g)	H₂O (%)	Ener (cal)	Prot (g)	Carb (g)	Dietary Fiber (g)	Fat (g)	Fat Breakdown (g)		
										Sat	Mono	Poly
	MISCELLANEOUS—Cont.											
	For other chocolate items, see Sweeteners & Sweets											
972	Cilantro/coriander, fresh	1 tbs	1	93	< 1	< 1	< 1	< 1	< 1	t	t	t
1197	Cornstarch	1 tbs	8	8	30	< 1	7	< 1	< 1	t	t	t
973	Cinnamon	1 tsp	2	10	5	< 1	2	1	< 1	t	t	t
974	Curry powder	1 tsp	2	10	7	< 1	1	1	< 1	t	.2	t
1202	Dill weed, dried	1 tbs	3	7	8	1	2	1	< 1	–	–	–
1705	Dip, french onion	1 tbs	14	70	31	< 1	< 1	< 1	3	1.9	.9	.1
975	Garlic cloves	1 ea	3	59	4	< 1	1	< 1	< 1	t	0	t
976	Garlic powder	1 tsp	3	6	10	1	2	< 1	< 1	t	t	t
977	Gelatin, dry, unsweetened: Envelope	1 ea	7	13	23	6	0	0	< 1	t	t	t
978	Ginger root, slices, raw	2 pce	4	81	3	< 1	1	< 1	< 1	t	t	t
1198	Horseradish, prepared	1 tbs	15	87	6	< 1	1	< 1	< 1	t	t	t
1199	Hummous/hummus	1 c	246	65	421	12	50	10	21	3	9	8
1909	Mustard, country dijon	1 tsp	5	–	5	0	0	0	0	0	0	0
979	Mustard, prepared (1 packet = 1 tsp)	1 tsp	5	80	4	< 1	< 1	< 1	< 1	t	.2	t
	Miso (see #926 under Vegetables and Legumes, Soybean products)											
2067	No msg seasoning blend	1 tsp	5	.5	3	< 1	1	< 1	< 1	–	–	–
980	Olives, green	5 ea	19	78	22	< 1	< 1	< 1	2	.3	1.9	.2
981	Olives, ripe, pitted	5 ea	22	80	25	< 1	1	1	2	.3	1.8	.2
982	Onion powder	1 tsp	2	5	7	< 1	2	< 1	< 1	t	t	t
983	Oregano, ground	1 tsp	1	7	3	< 1	1	< 1	< 1	t	t	.1
2066	Oriental seasoning blend	1 tsp	3	.5	10	< 1	2	< 1	< 1	–	–	–
984	Paprika	1 tsp	2	10	6	< 1	1	< 1	< 1	t	t	.2
985	Black pepper	1 tsp	2	11	5	< 1	1	1	< 1	t	t	t
	Pickles:											
986	Dill, medium, 3¾ x 1¼" diam	1 ea	65	92	12	< 1	3	1	< 1	t	t	.1
987	Fresh pack, slices, 1½" diam x ¼"	2 pce	15	92	3	< 1	3	< 1	< 1	t	t	t
988	Sweet, medium	1 ea	35	65	41	< 1	11	< 1	< 1	t	t	t
989	Pickle relish, sweet	2 tbs	30	63	41	< 1	10	1	< 1	.1	t	.1
	Popcorn (see Grain Products #539–541)											
1201	Sage, ground	1 tsp	1	8	3	< 1	1	< 1	< 1	.1	t	t
1347	Salsa, from recipe	1 tbs	14	93	3	< 1	1	< 1	< 1	t	t	t
2118	Salsa, pico de Gallo-med	2 tbs	30	92	5	0	2	.5	0	0	0	0
990	Salt	1 tsp	5	< 1	0	0	0	0	0	0	0	0
	Salt substitutes:											
1205	Morton, salt substitute	1 tsp	2	2	< 1	0	< 1	0	0	0	0	0
1207	Morton, Light Salt	1 tsp	6	0	0	0	0	0	0	0	0	0
1206	Norcliff Thayer, No Salt, packet	1 ea	1	0	0	0	0	0	0	0	0	0
	Sports/Fitness bar:											
2043	Forza energy bar	1 ea	70	18	231	11	45	4	1	–	–	–
2042	Power bar	1 ea	65	21	225	10	40	3	1	–	–	–
2041	Tiger sports bar	1 ea	65	17	230	11	40	4	2	–	–	–
991	Vinegar, cider	½ c	120	94	17	0	7	0	0	0	0	0
	Vinegar, Fleischmann's											
2172	Balsamic	1 tbs	15	64	21	0	5	0	0	0	0	0
2176	Malt	1 tbs	15	90	5	0	< 1	0	0	0	0	0
2182	Tarragon	1 tbs	15	95	3	0	< 1	0	0	0	0	0
2181	White wine	1 tbs	15	89	5	0	< 1	0	0	0	0	0

(Computer code number is for West Diet Analysis program)

Chol (mg)	Calc (mg)	Iron (mg)	Magn (mg)	Phos (mg)	Pota (mg)	Sodi (mg)	Zinc (mg)	VT-A (RE)	Thia (mg)	Ribo (mg)	Niac (mg)	V-B6 (mg)	Fola (μg)	VT-C (mg)
0	1	.02	<1	<1	5	<1	<.01	3	<.01	<.01	.01	<.01	<1	<1
0	<1	.04	<1	1	<1	1	<.01	0	0	0	0	0	0	0
0	25	.76	1	1	10	1	.04	1	<.01	<.01	.03	.02	–	1
0	10	.59	5	7	31	1	.08	2	<.01	.01	.07	–	–	<1
0	54	1.46	14	17	99	6	.1	0	.01	.01	.09	.04	–	–
6	17	.01	2	13	22	27	.04	28	.01	.02	.02	<.01	2	<1
0	5	.05	1	5	12	1	.03	0	.01	<.01	.02	.04	<1	1
0	2	.08	2	13	33	1	.07	0	.01	<.01	.02	.61	2	<1
0	4	.08	2	3	1	14	.01	0	<.01	.02	.01	<.01	2	0
0	1	.02	2	1	17	1	.01	0	<.01	<.01	.03	.01	<1	<1
0	9	.13	4	5	44	14	.18	0	0	0	0	.01	2	0
0	123	4	71	276	428	600	2.7	6	.23	.13	1	.98	146	19
0	–	–	–	–	10	120	–	–	–	–	–	–	–	–
0	4	.1	2	4	6	63	.03	0	0	0	0	<.01	0	0
–	–	–	–	–	13	1390	–	–	–	–	–	–	–	–
0	12	.31	4	3	10	456	.01	6	0	0	0	<.01	<1	0
0	19	.74	1	1	2	192	.05	9	<.01	0	.01	<.01	0	<1
0	8	.06	2	7	19	1	.05	0	.01	<.01	.01	.03	3	<1
0	16	.44	3	2	17	<1	.04	7	<.01	<.01	.06	–	–	1
–	–	–	–	–	12	107	–	–	–	–	–	–	–	–
0	4	.5	4	7	47	1	.08	121	.01	.04	.32	–	–	1
0	9	.58	4	3	25	1	.03	<1	<.01	<.01	.02	0	–	0
0	6	.34	7	14	75	833	.09	21	.01	.02	.04	.01	1	1
0	5	.08	2	3	17	192	.02	5	<.01	<.01	.01	<.01	<1	<1
0	1	.21	1	4	11	328	.03	4	<.01	.01	.06	.01	<1	<1
0	6	.24	1	4	60	214	.02	3	0	.01	0	<.01	0	2
0	17	.28	4	1	11	<1	.05	6	.01	<.01	.06	–	–	<1
0	1	.06	1	3	23	55	.02	21	.01	<.01	.06	.01	2	5
0	–	–	–	–	–	260	–	–	–	–	–	–	–	–
0	1	.01	<1	0	<1	1938	0	0	0	0	0	0	0	0
0	11	–	<1	10	1006	<1	–	0	–	–	–	–	–	–
0	3	0	4	0	1500	1099	0	0	0	0	0	0	0	0
0	–	–	–	–	385	0	–	0	0	0	0	0	0	0
0	300	6.3	160	350	220	65	5.25	–	1.5	1.7	20	2	400	60
–	300	5.4	140	350	120	20	5.25	–	1.5	1.7	20	2	400	60
–	350	4.5	140	400	280	100	–	50	1.5	1.7	20	2	400	60
0	7	.7	26	11	120	1	0	0	0	0	0	0	0	0
–	2	.07	–	3	11	3	–	–	.07	.07	.07	–	–	<1
–	2	.07	–	2	14	5	–	–	.07	.07	.07	–	–	2
–	<1	.07	–	<1	2	1	–	–	.07	.07	.07	–	–	<1
–	1	.07	–	15	12	1	–	–	.07	.07	.07	–	–	<1

(For purposes of calculations, use "0" for t, <1, <.1, <.01, etc.)

Table I–1
Food Composition

Computer Code Number	Food Description	Measure	Wt (g)	H₂O (%)	Ener (cal)	Prot (g)	Carb (g)	Dietary Fiber (g)	Fat (g)	Fat Breakdown (g)		
										Sat	Mono	Poly
	MISCELLANEOUS—Cont.											
	Yeast:											
992	Baker's, dry, active, package	1 ea	7	8	21	3	3	2	< 1	t	.2	t
993	Brewer's, dry	1 tbs	8	5	23	3	3	3	< 1	t	t	0
	SOUPS, SAUCES, AND GRAVIES											
	SOUPS, canned, condensed:											
	Unprepared, condensed:											
1210	Cream of celery	1 c	251	85	181	3	18	2	11	2.8	2.6	5
1215	Cream of chicken	1 c	251	82	233	7	19	1	15	4.2	6.5	3
1216	Cream of mushroom	1 c	251	81	259	4	19	1	19	5.1	3.6	8.9
1220	Onion	1 c	246	86	113	8	16	2	4	.5	1.5	1.3
	Prepared w/equal volume whole milk:											
994	Clam chowder, New England	1 c	248	85	164	9	17	1	7	2.9	2.3	1.1
1209	Cream of celery	1 c	248	87	164	6	15	1	10	3.9	2.5	2.6
995	Cream of chicken	1 c	248	85	191	7	15	< 1	11	4.6	4.5	1.6
996	Cream of mushroom	1 c	248	85	203	6	15	1	14	5.1	3	4.6
1214	Cream of potato	1 c	248	87	149	6	17	1	6	3.8	1.7	.6
1213	Oyster stew	1 c	245	89	135	6	10	0	8	5	2.1	.3
997	Tomato	1 c	248	85	161	6	22	1	6	2.9	1.6	1.1
	Prepared with equal volume of water:											
998	Bean with bacon	1 c	253	84	172	8	23	9	6	1.5	2.2	1.8
999	Beef broth/bouillon/consommé	1 c	240	98	17	3	< 1	0	1	.3	.2	t
1000	Beef noodle	1 c	244	92	83	5	9	1	3	1.1	1.2	.5
1001	Chicken noodle	1 c	241	92	75	4	9	1	2	.7	1.1	.6
1002	Chicken rice	1 c	241	94	60	4	7	1	2	.5	.9	.4
1208	Chili beef	1 c	250	85	170	7	21	9	7	3.3	2.8	.3
1003	Clam chowder, Manhatten	1 c	244	92	78	2	12	1	2	.4	.4	1.3
1004	Cream of chicken	1 c	244	91	117	3	9	< 1	7	2.1	3.3	1.5
1005	Cream of mushroom	1 c	244	90	129	2	9	< 1	9	2.4	1.7	4.2
1006	Minestrone	1 c	241	91	82	4	11	1	3	.6	.7	1.1
1211	Onion	1 c	241	93	58	4	8	1	2	.3	.8	.7
1007	Split pea & ham	1 c	253	82	190	10	28	5	4	1.8	1.8	.6
1008	Tomato	1 c	244	90	85	2	17	< 1	2	.4	.4	1
1009	Vegetable beef	1 c	244	92	78	6	10	< 1	2	.9	.8	.1
1010	Vegetarian vegetable	1 c	241	92	72	2	12	< 1	2	.3	.8	.7
1707	Ready to serve											
	Chunky chicken soup	½ c	126	84	89	6	9	< 1	3	1	1.5	.7
	SOUPS, dehydrated:											
	Unprepared, dry products:											
1011	Beef bouillon, packet	1 ea	6	3	14	1	1	< 1	1	.3	.2	t
1012	Onion soup, packet	1 ea	34	4	100	4	18	4	2	.5	1.2	.2
	Prepared with water:											
1299	Beef broth/bouillon	1 c	244	97	20	1	2	0	1	.3	.3	t
1376	Chicken broth	1 c	244	97	22	1	1	0	1	.3	.4	.4
1013	Chicken noodle	1 c	251	94	53	3	8	< 1	1	.3	.5	.4
1122	Cream of chicken	1 c	261	91	107	2	13	1	5	3.4	1.2	.4
1014	Onion	1 c	246	96	27	1	5	< 1	1	.1	.3	.1
1217	Split pea	1 c	255	87	125	7	21	3	1	.4	.7	.3
1015	Tomato vegetable	1 c	252	93	55	2	10	1	1	.4	.3	.1

(Computer code number is for West Diet Analysis program)

Chol (mg)	Calc (mg)	Iron (mg)	Magn (mg)	Phos (mg)	Pota (mg)	Sodi (mg)	Zinc (mg)	VT-A (RE)	Thia (mg)	Ribo (mg)	Niac (mg)	V-B6 (mg)	Fola (μg)	VT-C (mg)
0	4	1.16	7	90	140	4	.45	< 1	.16	.38	2.79	.11	164	< 1
0	17[1]	1.38	18	140	151	10	.63	0	1.25	.34	3.03	.4	313	0
28	80	1.26	13	75	245	1900	.3	60	.06	.1	.66	.02	5	1
20	68	1.2	5	75	175	1972	1.26	113	.06	.12	1.64	.03	3	< 1
3	65	1.05	10	85	168	2033	1.19	0	.06	.17	1.62	.02	8	2
0	54	1.35	5	22	137	2115	1.23	0	.07	.05	1.21	.1	30	2
22	186	1.49	22	156	300	992	.8	40	.07	.24	1.03	.13	10	3
32	186	.69	22	151	310	1009	.2	67	.07	.25	.44	.06	8	1
27	181	.67	17	151	273	1047	.67	94	.07	.26	.92	.07	8	1
20	179	.59	20	156	270	1076	.64	37	.08	.28	.91	.06	10	2
22	166	.55	17	161	322	1061	.67	67	.08	.24	.64	.09	9	1
32	166	1.05	20	162	235	1041	10.3	44	.07	.23	.34	.06	10	4
17	159	1.81	22	149	449	932	.29	109	.13	.25	1.52	.16	21	68
3	81	2.05	46	132	402	951	1.03	89	.09	.03	.57	.04	32	2
0	14	.41	5	31	130	782	0	0	< .01	.05	1.87	.02	5	0
5	15	1.1	5	46	100	952	1.54	63	.07	.06	1.07	.04	4	< 1
7	17	.77	5	36	55	1106	.39	71	.05	.06	1.39	.03	2	< 1
7	17	.75	0	22	101	815	.26	66	.02	.02	1.13	.02	1	< 1
13	43	2.13	30	148	525	1035	1.4	151	.06	.07	1.07	.16	18	4
2	27	1.63	12	41	187	578	.98	96	.03	.04	.82	.1	10	4
10	34	.61	2	37	88	986	.63	56	.03	.06	.82	.02	2	< 1
2	46	.51	5	49	100	1032	.59	0	.05	.09	.72	.01	5	1
2	34	.92	7	55	313	911	.73	234	.05	.04	.94	.1	16	1
0	27	.67	2	12	67	1053	.61	0	.03	.02	.6	.05	15	1
8	23	2.28	48	213	400	1006	1.32	45	.15	.08	1.47	.07	3	2
0	12	1.76	7	34	264	871	.24	69	.09	.05	1.42	.11	15	66
5	17	1.12	5	41	173	956	1.54	189	.04	.05	1.03	.08	10	2
0	22	1.08	7	34	210	822	.46	301	.05	.05	.92	.05	11	1
15	13	.87	4	57	88	446	.5	65	.04	.09	2.21	.03	2	1
1	4	.06	3	19	27	1019	0	< 1	< .01	.01	.27	.01	2	0
2	48	.51	22	110	226	3044	.2	1	.1	.21	1.73	.03	6	1
0	10	.02	7	24	37	1362	.07	1	< .01	.02	.36	0	0	0
0	15	.07	5	12	24	1484	.01	12	.01	.03	.19	0	2	0
3	32	.5	7	32	31	1278	.2	6	.07	.06	.88	.01	2	< 1
3	76	.26	5	97	214	1185	1.57	123	.1	.2	2.61	.05	5	1
0	12	.15	5	29	64	849	.06	< 1	.03	.06	.48	0	1	< 1
3	20	.94	43	124	224	1148	.56	5	.21	.14	1.26	.05	40	0
0	8	.63	20	31	104	1142	.17	19	.06	.04	.79	.05	10	7

(For purposes of calculations, use "0" for t, < 1, < .1, < .01, etc.)

Table I–1
Food Composition

Computer Code Number	Food Description	Measure	Wt (g)	H₂O (%)	Ener (cal)	Prot (g)	Carb (g)	Dietary Fiber (g)	Fat (g)	Fat Breakdown (g)		
										Sat	Mono	Poly
	SAUCES											
	From dry mixes, prepared with milk:											
1016	Cheese sauce	1 c	279	77	307	16	23	1	17	9.3	5.3	1.6
1017	Hollandaise	1 c	259	84	240	5	14	< 1	20	11.6	5.9	.9
1018	White sauce	1 c	264	82	240	10	21	< 1	13	6.4	4.7	1.7
	From home recipe:											
1019	White sauce, medium[1]	1 c	250	77	355	9	20	< 1	27	7.8	9.1	8.8
1206	Lofat cheese sauce	¼ c	61	73	85	6	4	0	5	2.1	1.9	.9
	Ready to serve:											
2202	Alfredo sauce	¼ c	69	–	170	5	16	0	10	6	–	–
1020	Barbeque sauce	1 tbs	16	81	10	< 1	1	< 1	< 1	t	.1	.1
1706	Chili sauce, tomato base	1 tbs	17	68	18	< 1	4	< 1	< 1	t	t	t
2126	Creole sauce	¼ c	62	–	25	1	4	1	1	0	–	–
2124	Hoison sauce	2 tbs	34	48	70	1	14	0	2	0	–	–
2199	Pesto sauce	2 tbs	29	21	155	5	2	< 1	14	3.6	9.1	1.1
1021	Soy sauce	1 tbs	18	71	10	< 1	2	0	< 1	t	t	t
2123	Szechuan sauce	2 tbs	31	82	23	1	4	< 1	1	.1	.2	.2
1380	Teriyaki sauce	1 tbs	18	68	15	< 1	3	0	0	0	0	0
	Spaghetti sauce, canned:											
1377	Plain	1 c	249	75	271	5	40	8	12	1.7	6.1	3.3
1378	With meat	1 c	257	74	309	9	39	8	15	2.8	7.2	3.3
1379	With mushrooms	½ c	123	75	108	2	13	1	3	.4	1.5	.8
	GRAVIES											
	Canned:											
1022	Beef	1 c	233	88	123	9	11	1	6	2.7	2	.2
1023	Chicken	1 c	238	85	188	5	13	< 1	14	3.4	6.1	3.5
1024	Mushroom	1 c	238	89	119	3	13	< 1	6	1	2.8	2.4
1025	From dry mix, brown	1 c	258	92	75	2	13	< 1	2	.8	.7	.1
1026	From dry mix, chicken	1 c	260	91	83	3	14	< 1	2	.5	.9	.4
	FAST FOOD RESTAURANTS											
	ARBY'S											
1402	Bac'n cheddar deluxe	1 ea	226	59	501	21	38	< 1	31	8.5	12.4	11.2
	Roast beef sandwiches:											
1403	Regular	1 ea	147	47	363	21	34	1	17	6.6	7.6	2.4
1404	Junior	1 ea	86	48	275	11	22	< 1	10	3.9	5	1.7
1405	Super	1 ea	234	58	509	22	50	1	26	7	11	5.4
1407	Beef 'n cheddar	1 ea	197	34	516	25	44	1	27	7.6	12.1	7.1
1408	Chicken breast sandwich	1 ea	184	52	401	20	47	1	20	3	8.8	10.3
1412	Ham'n cheese sandwich	1 ea	156	54	328	23	32	< 1	13	4.7	5.4	2.7
1726	Italian sub sandwich	1 ea	297	–	671	34	47	–	39	12.8	15.7	8.5
1413	Turkey sandwich, deluxe	1 ea	197	61	263	20	33	< 1	6	1.6	2.3	7.8
1680	Turkey sub sandwich	1 ea	277	62	486	33	47	–	19	5.3	6	7
	Milk shakes:											
1419	Chocolate	1 ea	340	74	451	10	77	< 1	12	2.8	7	1.7
1420	Jamocha	1 ea	326	75	368	9	59	0	11	2.5	6.4	1.6
1421	Vanilla	1 ea	312	75	330	11	46	0	12	3.9	5.3	2.3
1728	Salad, roast chicken	1 ea	400	89	204	24	12	–	7`	3.3	.9	.9
1729	Sports drink, Upper Ten, svg	1 ea	358	88	169	0	42	–	0	0	0	0

Source: Arby's Inc. for the basic nutrients. Values for some nutrients from known values of major ingredients.

[1]Made with enriched flour, margarine, and whole milk.

(Computer code number is for West Diet Analysis program)

Chol (mg)	Calc (mg)	Iron (mg)	Magn (mg)	Phos (mg)	Pota (mg)	Sodi (mg)	Zinc (mg)	VT-A (RE)	Thia (mg)	Ribo (mg)	Niac (mg)	V-B6 (mg)	Fola (µg)	VT-C (mg)
53	569	.28	47	438	552	1565	.97	117	.15	.56	.32	.14	13	2
52	124	.9	8	127	124	1564	.7	220	.04	.18	.06	.5	22	<1
34	425	.26	264	256	444	797	.55	92	.08	.45	.53	.07	16	3
29	261	.73	32	217	344	369	.94	310	.19	.42	.98	.1	14	2
11	165	.25	10	181	99	387	.73	58	.03	.14	.16	.03	4	0
30	150	0	–	100	80	600	–	80	0	.1	0	–	–	0
0	3	.12	1	3	27	128	.03	14	<.01	<.01	.06	.01	1	1
0	3	.14	2	9	63	227	.05	24	.02	.01	.27	.02	1	3
0	20	0	–	–	–	340	–	40	–	–	–	–	–	0
0	0	0	–	–	–	500	–	0	–	–	–	–	–	0
9	209	1.22	17	104	103	211	.52	43	.01	.05	.22	.04	8	3
0	3	.36	6	20	32	1029	.07	0	.01	.02	.6	.03	3	3
0	6	.28	6	6	54	255	.06	27	.01	.01	.28	.02	1	2
0	4	.31	11	28	41	690	.02	0	.01	.01	.23	.02	4	0
0	70	1.62	60	90	956	1235	.52	306	.14	.15	3.76	.88	54	28
16	69	2	61	117	978	1213	1.41	299	.14	.17	4.64	.9	54	27
0	15	1	15	30	333	494	.34	242	.08	.08	.93	.16	13	9
7	14	1.63	5	70	188	1304	2.33	0	.07	.08	1.54	.02	5	0
5	48	1.12	5	69	259	1373	1.9	264	.04	.1	1.05	.02	5	0
0	17	1.57	5	36	252	1356	1.67	0	.08	.15	1.6	.05	29	0
3	67	.23	10	44	57	1075	.31	0	.04	.08	.81	0	0	0
3	39	.26	10	47	62	1133	.32	0	.05	.15	.78	.03	3	3
37	108	4.5	–	–	422	1672	3	39	.34	.45	9.4	–	–	11
41	57	4.6	15	114	400	888	3.56	1	.28	.46	10.4	.2	13	1
21	39	2.6	8	58	194	502	1.5	–	.17	.25	6.4	.1	7	–
40	83	6	23	175	491	1082	3.45	28	.36	.5	11.4	.3	19	8
53	152	6.2	24	260	326	1184	3.05	–	.43	.64	10	–	19	1
41	54	2.6	27	162	298	919	.14	–	.2	.51	8	.34	16	5
51	157	2.7	29	374	353	1292	.83	37	.77	.34	7	.31	24	22
69	410	4.32	–	–	565	2062	–	100	.92	.49	8.2	–	–	11
33	131	2.7	30	253	357	1275	1.5	40	.08	.43	15.6	.52	20	12
51	400	4.68	–	–	500	2033	–	–	13.2	.54	18.8	–	–	–
36	250	2.7	48	350	410	341	1.5	40	.06	.85	.8	.14	14	5
35	250	2.7	36	350	525	262	1.5	60	.06	.77	5	.14	14	2
32	300	2.7	36	350	686	281	1.5	100	.23	.85	4	.14	37	2
43	170	1.98	–	–	877	508	–	485	.33	.54	5.6	–	–	51
0	–	–	–	–	0	40	–	–	–	–	–	–	–	–

(For purposes of calculations, use "0" for t, <1, <.1, <.01, etc.)

Table I-1
Food Composition

Computer Code Number	Food Description	Measure	Wt (g)	H₂O (%)	Ener (cal)	Prot (g)	Carb (g)	Dietary Fiber (g)	Fat (g)	Fat Breakdown (g)		
										Sat	Mono	Poly
	BURGER KING											
	Croissant sandwiches:											
1422	Egg, bacon, & cheese	1 ea	119	50	353	15	18	<1	24	8.1	12.1	3
1423	Egg, sausage, & cheese	1 ea	163	47	543	21	22	1	42	14	20.5	5.1
1424	Egg, ham, & cheese	1 ea	145	57	352	18	19	<1	22	7	11.1	2
	Whopper sandwiches:											
1425	Whopper	1 ea	265	58	618	27	44	3	38	10.8	10.8	12.8
1426	Whopper with cheese	1 ea	289	57	708	32	44	3	45	15.7	12.8	12.8
1427	Double beef	1 ea	351	57	860	46	45	3	56	19	19	13
1428	Double beef & cheese	1 ea	374	57	947	52	45	3	63	23.9	21.9	14
1429	Hamburger deluxe	1 ea	136	53	339	15	28	<1	19	5.9	5.9	6.9
1430	Cheeseburger deluxe	1 ea	158	52	408	19	30	<1	24	8.4	7.3	7.3
1431	Hamburger	1 ea	109	47	275	15	30	1	11	4	5	1
1432	Cheeseburger	1 ea	120	49	313	18	29	1	15	6.3	6.3	1
1433	Double cheeseburger with bacon	1 ea	159	49	460	32	20	1	28	13	12.9	2
1434	Chicken sandwich	1 ea	230	45	703	26	54	2	43	8	11	20.1
1629	BK broiler chicken sandwich	1 ea	248	59	540	30	41	2	29	6	–	–
1739	Chicken caesar pita sandwich	1 ea	237	59	520	27	44	4	26	6	–	–
1435	Chicken tenders	1 ea	95	50	270	17	15	2	13	3.2	5.3	3.2
1436	Ham & cheese sandwich	1 ea	230	59	471	24	44	<1	23	10	8	4
1437	Ocean catch fish fillet	1 ea	189	47	534	19	44	1	36	6	5.8	12.7
1740	Monterey roast beef sandwhich	1 ea	238	57	540	30	40	3	30	9	–	–
1439	French fries (salted)	1 ea	74	38	255	3	27	2	13	3	6	1
1630	French toast sticks-svg	1 ea	141	33	500	4	60	1	27	–	–	–
1440	Onion rings	1 ea	79	51	198	3	26	3	9	1.3	5.1	2.6
1441	Milk shakes, chocolate	1 ea	273	75	298	9	52	3	7	3.9	3.9	0
1442	Milk shakes, vanilla	1 ea	273	75	298	9	51	1	7	3.9	2.9	0
1443	Fried apple pie	1 ea	125	47	343	3	43	2	17	3.3	8.9	1

Source: Burger King Corporation.

Computer Code Number	Food Description	Measure	Wt (g)	H₂O (%)	Ener (cal)	Prot (g)	Carb (g)	Dietary Fiber (g)	Fat (g)	Fat Breakdown (g)		
	DAIRY QUEEN											
	Ice cream cones:											
1446	Small vanilla	1 ea	85	64	140	4	22	0	4	3	1	–
1447	Regular vanilla	1 ea	142	65	230	6	36	0	7	5	1	1
1448	Large vanilla	1 ea	213	66	340	9	53	0	10	7	1	1
1450	Chocolate dipped	1 ea	156	60	330	6	40	<1	16	8	4	3
1453	Chocolate sundae	1 ea	177	62	300	6	54	<1	7	5	1	1
1455	Banana split	1 ea	383	68	529	9	97	2	11	8.3	3.1	.4
1456	Peanut Buster Parfait	1 ea	305	53	710	16	94	1	32	10	10	9
1457	Hot Fudge Brownie Delight	1 ea	266	53	619	10	89	1	25	12.2	10.5	1.7
1459	Buster bar	1 ea	149	45	450	11	40	<1	29	9	10	8
1645	Breeze, strawberry, regular	1 ea	354	70	420	12	90	–	1	–	–	–
1460	Dilly bar	1 ea	85	55	210	3	21	<1	13	6	3	3
1461	DQ ice cream sandwich	1 ea	60	48	138	3	24	<1	4	2	1	1
1463	Milk shakes, regular	1 ea	418	71	548	13	93	<1	15	8.4	2.1	2.1
1464	Milk shakes, large	1 ea	489	72	636	14	107	<1	17	10.6	2.1	2.1
1466	Malted milkshake	1 ea	418	68	610	13	106	<1	14	8	2	2
1468	Float	1 ea	397	76	410	5	82	0	7	5	1	1
1469	Freeze	1 ea	397	72	500	9	89	0	12	7.5	3.4	.4
1640	Sundae, waffle cone, strawberry	1 ea	173	–	173	8	56	–	12	5	3	3

(Computer code number is for West Diet Analysis program)

Chol (mg)	Calc (mg)	Iron (mg)	Magn (mg)	Phos (mg)	Pota (mg)	Sodi (mg)	Zinc (mg)	VT-A (RE)	Thia (mg)	Ribo (mg)	Niac (mg)	V-B6 (mg)	Fola (μg)	VT-C (mg)
227	151	1.8	–	–	–	797	–	81	.32	.3	2.02	.11	–	2
261	154	2.97	–	–	–	1025	–	82	.37	.33	4.1	.12	–	<1
232	151	1.8	–	–	–	1400	–	81	.49	.32	3.02	.22	–	10
88	59	4.4	–	–	–	834	–	98	.32	.4	6.87	.34	–	9
113	246	4.4	–	–	–	1248	–	147	.33	.47	6.88	.32	–	9
169	80	7.3	–	–	–	920	–	100	.34	.56	10	–	–	9
193	249	7.28	–	–	–	1336	–	150	.35	.63	9.97	–	–	9
42	39	2.76	–	–	–	489	–	30	.23	.25	3.94	.14	–	6
59	110	2.93	–	–	–	682	–	89	.24	.3	4.19	–	–	6
32	42	1.9	–	–	–	529	–	21	.23	.25	4.23	–	–	3
47	104	1.88	–	–	–	741	–	63	.23	.29	4.17	–	–	3
104	144	3.24	–	–	–	863	–	58	.22	.3	4.32	–	–	1
60	100	3.62	–	–	–	1406	–	13	.45	.31	10	–	–	1
80	40	5.4	–	–	–	480	–	40	–	–	–	–	–	6
55	250	2.7	–	–	490	1050	–	80	–	–	–	–	–	2
38	19	.78	–	–	–	571	–	5	.08	.08	7.56	–	–	<1
70	195	3.2	–	–	–	1534	–	85	.87	.42	6	–	–	7
45	44	2.67	–	–	–	808	–	15	.21	.2	2.96	–	–	1
75	300	3.6	–	–	500	1270	–	80	–	–	–	–	–	5
0	6	.69	–	–	–	153	–	0	.06	.2	5	–	–	2
0	60	2.7	–	–	–	490	–	–	–	–	–	–	–	–
0	79	.51	–	–	–	516	–	0	.04	.03	.46	–	–	<1
19	192	1.73	–	–	–	221	–	58	.12	.53	.12	–	–	0
19	288	–	–	–	–	221	–	58	.11	.55	.12	–	–	3
0	17	1.6	–	–	–	254	–	4	.27	.18	.6	–	–	7
15	100	.4	–	100	150	60	–	20	.03	.17	.06	–	–	<1
20	150	.7	–	150	260	95	–	40	.06	.26	.11	.09	–	0
30	200	1.4	–	200	380	140	–	60	.12	.34	.17	–	–	0
20	300	.7	–	150	290	100	–	40	.06	.26	.11	.09	–	0
20	150	1.1	–	150	290	140	–	40	.06	.26	.3	.14	–	0
31	311	3.74	–	42	893	259	–	156	.16	.27	.41	.21	–	16
30	350	3.6	–	450	660	410	–	60	.15	.51	3	.22	–	2
30	262	4.71	–	523	445	297	–	70	.1	.6	.26	.16	–	1
15	300	1.1	–	250	400	220	–	20	.12	.17	3	.08	–	1
–	500	1.8	–	350	490	170	–	–	.12	.68	–	–	–	24
10	250	.72	–	80	170	50	–	20	.03	.14	–	.06	–	1
5	59	.71	–	59	103	133	–	15	.03	.26	.39	.05	–	<1
47	421	1.52	–	369	600	242	–	84	.24	.63	.84	.2	–	0
53	477	1.53	–	477	700	276	–	212	.16	.72	.85	–	–	0
45	400	1.44	–	350	570	230	–	80	.12	.66	.8	.19	–	0
20	200	1.1	–	200	–	85	–	40	.06	.26	.05	.09	–	<1
30	300	1.8	–	350	–	180	–	98	.15	.51	–	.15	–	2
20	150	1.44	–	200	330	220	–	40	.09	.26	–	–	–	6

(For purposes of calculations, use "0" for t, <1, <.1, <.01, etc.)

Table I-1
Food Composition

Computer Code Number	Food Description	Measure	Wt (g)	H₂O (%)	Ener (cal)	Prot (g)	Carb (g)	Dietary Fiber (g)	Fat (g)	Fat Breakdown (g)		
										Sat	Mono	Poly
	DAIRY QUEEN—Cont.											
	Mr. Misty:											
1470	Regular	1 ea	330	81	250	0	63	0	0	0	0	0
1471	Kiss	1 ea	89	81	70	0	17	0	0	0	0	0
1472	Freeze	1 ea	411	72	500	9	91	0	12	7.4	3.4	.4
1473	Float	1 ea	411	78	390	5	74	0	7	4.3	2	.3
	Yogurt											
1641	Yogurt cone	1 ea	142	67	180	6	38	–	1	–	–	–
1643	Yogurt sundae-strawberry	1 ea	170	70	200	6	43	–	1	–	–	–
	Sandwiches:											
1474	Chicken	1 ea	202	56	455	25	39	< 1	21	4.2	7.4	8.5
1647	Grilled chicken fillet	1 ea	184	63	300	25	33	–	8	2	2	3
1475	Fish fillet	1 ea	177	58	385	17	41	< 1	17	3.1	5.2	8.3
1476	Fish fillet with cheese	1 ea	191	56	436	20	42	< 1	22	6.2	7.3	8.3
1477	Hamburger, single	1 ea	148	55	323	18	30	< 1	17	6.2	6.2	1
1478	Hamburger, double	1 ea	210	57	488	33	31	< 1	26	12.7	11.7	2.1
1480	Cheeseburger, single	1 ea	162	55	379	21	31	< 1	19	9.3	7.3	1
1481	Cheeseburger, double	1 ea	239	54	603	39	33	< 1	36	19	13.7	2.1
	Hot dog:											
1483	Regular	1 ea	100	51	283	9	23	< 1	16	6.1	7.1	2
1484	With cheese	1 ea	114	49	333	12	24	< 1	21	9.1	8.1	2
1485	With chili	1 ea	128	53	323	11	26	2	19	7.1	8.1	2
1489	French fries, small	1 ea	71	38	210	3	29	1	10	2	5	3
1490	French fries, large	1 ea	113	50	344	4	46	2	16	3.5	7.1	5.3
1491	Onion rings	1 ea	85	46	240	4	29	< 1	12	3	5	4

Source: International Dairy Queen.

	HARDEE'S											
1734	Frisco burger hamburger	1 ea	242	–	760	36	43	–	50	18	–	–
1735	Frisco grilled chicken sandwich	1 ea	244	–	620	35	44	–	34	10	–	–
1736	Frisco grilled chicken salad	1 ea	278	–	120	18	2	–	4	1	–	–
1737	Peach shake	1 ea	345	–	390	10	77	–	4	3	–	–
	JACK IN THE BOX											
	Breakfast items:											
1492	Breakfast Jack sandwich	1 ea	126	50	312	19	31	–	13	5.2	5	2.5
1494	Sausage crescent	1 ea	156	39	580	22	28	–	43	15.5	21.5	5.7
1495	Supreme crescent	1 ea	146	39	506	22	32	–	31	13.2	18.9	7.8
1496	Pancake platter	1 ea	231	45	610	15	87	–	22	8.6	7.6	3.5
1497	Scrambled egg platter	1 ea	249	52	655	21	58	–	37	10.2	19.4	5.1
	Sandwiches:											
1654	Bacon bacon cheeseburger	1 ea	242	49	710	35	41	0	45	15	15.7	8.7
1498	Hamburger	1 ea	98	39	283	13	31	0	11	4.1	4.9	2
1499	Cheeseburger	1 ea	113	39	339	16	33	0	14	6	6	2.3
1500	Jumbo Jack burger	1 ea	205	55	501	23	37	0	31	9	11.6	7.4
1501	Jumbo Jack burger with cheese	1 ea	246	55	620	29	42	0	37	12	15.2	9.1
1655	Chicken sandwich	1 ea	160	52	400	20	38	0	18	4	–	–
1505	Chicken supreme	1 ea	228	55	577	23	45	0	34	10	13.8	10.6

(Computer code number is for West Diet Analysis program)

Chol (mg)	Calc (mg)	Iron (mg)	Magn (mg)	Phos (mg)	Pota (mg)	Sodi (mg)	Zinc (mg)	VT-A (RE)	Thia (mg)	Ribo (mg)	Niac (mg)	V-B6 (mg)	Fola (μg)	VT-C (mg)
0	0	0	–	–	–	10	–	0	0	0	–	0	–	2
0	0	0	–	–	–	10	–	0	0	0	–	0	–	0
30	300	1.4	–	200	–	140	–	98	.12	.51	–	.18	–	2
20	200	.7	–	200	–	95	–	49	.06	.26	–	.09	–	1
–	200	.72	–	150	190	80	–	–	.06	.26	–	–	–	–
–	250	.72	–	150	240	80	–	–	.06	.34	–	–	–	12
58	42	1.9	–	370	370	804	–	21	.4	.36	12	–	–	3
50	60	3.6	–	350	330	800	–	20	.3	1.02	12	–	–	2
47	42	1.9	–	156	292	656	–	16	.3	.24	3	–	–	–
62	104	1.9	–	260	301	882	–	83	.3	.27	5	–	–	–
47	104	3.75	–	156	271	605	–	21	.31	.27	4	–	–	1
101	42	5.7	–	265	440	668	–	21	.3	.46	7	–	–	1
62	156	3.74	–	260	280	831	–	83	.31	.35	4	–	–	1
127	212	5.7	–	423	465	1132	–	159	.3	.54	7.4	–	–	1
25	40	1.41	–	61	172	707	–	0	.23	.14	2	–	–	<1
35	101	1.41	–	151	182	928	–	89	.23	.17	2	–	–	<1
30	40	1.45	–	60	262	726	–	60	.23	.14	3	–	–	<1
0	10	.72	–	100	430	115	–	0	.09	.02	2	–	–	5
0	13	1.27	–	132	689	177	–	0	.13	.03	2.65	–	–	8
0	20	.72	–	60	90	135	–	15	.09	.05	.4	–	–	2
70	–	–	–	–	–	1280	–	–	–	–	–	–	–	–
95	–	–	–	–	–	1730	–	–	–	–	–	–	–	–
60	–	–	–	–	–	520	–	–	–	–	–	–	–	–
25	–	–	–	–	–	290	–	–	–	–	–	–	–	–
193	208	2.8	–	–	229	927	–	83	.47	.41	3	–	–	9
185	150	2.7	–	–	260	1010	–	100	.6	.51	4.6	–	–	0
200	143	3.4	–	–	258	887	–	143	.65	.54	4.2	–	–	11
100	100	1.8	–	–	310	890	–	80	.03	.85	7	–	–	6
444	175	5.73	–	–	526	1239	–	175	–	.77	5.85	–	–	11
110	250	5.4	–	–	540	1240	–	80	.24	.48	8.8	.39	–	9
26	101	1.8	–	–	–	556	–	–	.15	.26	2	–	–	–
41	205	2.72	–	–	–	753	–	40	.23	.23	3.03	–	–	–
67	80	2.86	–	–	–	677	–	–	.33	.27	1.66	–	–	–
104	203	3.86	–	–	–	1108	–	–	.37	.45	1.63	–	–	–
45	150	1.8	–	–	180	1290	–	40	–	–	–	–	–	0
79	186	2.7	–	–	–	1368	–	74	.36	.3	10.2	–	–	6

(For purposes of calculations, use "0" for t, <1, <.1, <.01, etc.)

Table I–1
Food Composition

Computer Code Number	Food Description	Measure	Wt (g)	H₂O (%)	Ener (cal)	Prot (g)	Carb (g)	Dietary Fiber (g)	Fat (g)	Fat Breakdown (g) Sat	Mono	Poly
	JACK IN THE BOX—Cont.											
1656	Chicken sandwich, Sourdough ranch	1 ea	225	73	205	14	41	7	0	0	0	0
1583	Double cheeseburger	1 ea	149	41	441	24	34	0	27	11.8	11.6	3.1
1651	Grilled Sourdough burger	1 ea	223	48	670	32	39	0	43	16	17.8	7.9
1508	Tacos, regular	1 ea	81	58	191	7	16	2	11	4.2	–	–
1509	Tacos, super	1 ea	135	59	300	13	24	3	17	6.4	–	–
1513	Taco salad	1 ea	402	76	503	34	28	–	31	13.4	11.9	1.6
	Teriyaki bowl:											
1668	Chicken	1 ea	440	62	580	28	115	6	2	–	–	–
1679	Beef	1 ea	440	62	640	28	124	7	3	1	–	–
1516	French fries	1 ea	109	37	351	5	45	5	17	4	11	.6
1517	Hash browns	1 ea	62	51	174	1	15	1	12	2.8	7.4	.3
1518	Onion rings	1 ea	108	34	398	5	40	0	24	6.3	15.9	.9
	Milk shakes:											
1519	Chocolate	1 ea	322	72	390	9	74	0	6	3.5	2.1	–
1520	Strawberry	1 ea	328	67	363	10	66	0	8	4.3	2	–
1521	Vanilla	1 ea	317	73	365	9	65	0	7	4.2	1.8	–
1522	Apple turnover	1 ea	119	34	379	3	52	0	21	4.3	11.5	1.8

Source: Jack in the Box Restaurant, Inc.

Computer Code Number	Food Description	Measure	Wt (g)	H₂O (%)	Ener (cal)	Prot (g)	Carb (g)	Dietary Fiber (g)	Fat (g)	Fat Breakdown (g) Sat	Mono	Poly
	KENTUCKY FRIED CHICKEN											
	Rotisserie Gold:											
1472	Dark Qtr–no skin	1 ea	117	60	217	27	0	–	12	3.5	–	–
1473	Dark Qtr–w/skin	1 ea	146	54	333	30	1	–	24	6.6	–	–
1513	White Qtr with wing w/skin	1 ea	176	59	335	40	1	–	19	5.4	–	–
1525	White Qtr with wing–no skin	1 ea	117	20	199	37	0	–	6	1.7	–	–
	Original recipe:											
1253	Center breast	1 ea	95	52	240	23	8	<1	13	3.5	7.2	1.8
1251	Side breast	1 ea	69	47	204	14	7	<1	12	3.5	7.3	1.7
1250	Drumstick	1 ea	47	51	125	11	2	<1	7	1.8	3.4	1.1
1252	Thigh	1 ea	88	49	266	17	7	<1	19	4.9	8.7	2.6
1249	Wing	1 ea	42	41	136	9	4	<1	9	2.3	4.6	1.4
	Dinners:											
1254	2-pce dinner, white	1 ea	322	59	702	32	56	2	39	9.5	18.4	7.9
1255	2-pce dinner, dark	1 ea	346	71	721	33	57	1	40	10.1	17.9	8.5
1256	2-pce dinner, combo	1 ea	341	47	741	32	58	1	42	10.7	19.3	8.8
	Hot & Spicy											
1451	Chicken Center breast	1 ea	125	48	360	28	13	–	22	5	–	–
1452	Chicken Side breast	1 ea	120	43	400	22	16	–	28	6	–	–
1430	Chicken Thigh	1 ea	119	47	370	24	10	–	27	6	–	–
1471	Chicken Whole Wing	1 ea	61	38	220	14	5	–	16	4	–	–
	Extra crispy recipe:											
1261	Center breast	1 ea	104	48	291	25	9	<1	17	4	9.5	1.9
1259	Side breast	1 ea	84	40	290	17	11	<1	20	4.2	9.3	1.7
1258	Drumstick	1 ea	58	48	170	11	5	<1	11	3	6.8	1.5
1260	Thigh	1 ea	107	43	373	18	13	<1	29	7.6	15.7	4
1257	Wing	1 ea	53	32	216	10	8	<1	15	4	9.6	2
	Dinners:											
1262	2-pce dinner, white	1 ea	348	57	829	34	62	1	49	11.8	25.6	8.6
1263	2-pce dinner, dark	1 ea	375	59	878	36	62	1	54	13.3	26.9	9.9

(Computer code number is for West Diet Analysis program)

Chol (mg)	Calc (mg)	Iron (mg)	Magn (mg)	Phos (mg)	Pota (mg)	Sodi (mg)	Zinc (mg)	VT-A (RE)	Thia (mg)	Ribo (mg)	Niac (mg)	V-B6 (mg)	Fola (µg)	VT-C (mg)
0	0	4.91	–	–	–	136	–	341	–	–	–	–	–	82
72	245	2.7	–	–	–	842	–	98	.15	.34	6	–	–	–
110	200	4.5	–	–	510	1140	–	150	.65	.48	8	.33	–	6
21	104	1.1	35	152	249	426	1.2	0	.07	.17	1	.13	–	0
37	161	1.6	45	212	316	771	1.8	0	.12	.08	1.4	.18	–	3
92	410	3.8	–	–	–	1600	–	270	.29	.53	5.8	–	–	9
30	100	1.8	–	–	380	1220	–	1100	–	–	–	–	–	9
25	150	4.5	–	–	430	930	–	1000	–	–	–	–	–	6
0	0	1.3	–	–	–	194	–	–	.18	.03	3.8	–	–	29
0	0	.39	–	–	–	339	–	0	.05	–	1.09	–	–	7
0	31	2.31	–	–	–	473	–	–	.3	.18	2.73	–	–	3
25	300	.72	–	–	680	210	–	–	.15	.6	.4	–	–	0
33	330	.36	–	–	605	198	–	–	.15	.43	.4	–	–	0
31	313	–	–	–	594	188	–	–	.15	.34	.4	–	–	0
0	0	2.12	–	–	87	498	–	–	.24	.14	2.12	–	–	10
128	10	.18	–	–	–	772	–	15	–	–	–	–	–	1
163	10	.18	–	–	–	980	–	15	–	–	–	–	–	1
157	10	.18	–	–	–	1104	–	15	–	–	–	–	–	1
97	10	.18	–	–	–	667	–	15	–	–	–	–	–	1
85	28	.83	–	–	–	562	–	14	.07	.14	9.5	–	–	–
65	57	.92	–	–	–	502	–	12	.05	.1	5.29	–	–	–
62	17	.91	–	–	–	222	–	12	.04	.1	2.64	–	–	–
104	37	1.1	–	–	–	547	–	29	.07	.25	4.65	–	–	–
47	24	.92	–	–	–	304	–	12	.02	.06	2.83	–	–	–
119	215	3.71	–	–	–	1854	–	76	.22	.38	11.8	.5	–	36
164	197	3.84	–	–	–	1738	–	76	.25	.57	10.6	.46	–	37
160	217	3.88	–	–	–	1801	–	57	.24	.53	10.9	.47	–	38
80	20	.72	–	–	–	750	–	15	–	–	–	–	–	6
80	40	1.08	–	–	–	850	–	15	–	–	–	–	–	6
100	20	1.08	–	–	–	670	–	15	–	–	–	–	–	6
65	20	.72	–	–	–	440	–	65	30	–	–	–	–	–
66	29	.62	–	–	–	652	–	13	.08	.1	11.5	–	–	–
54	14	.61	–	–	–	514	–	11	.07	.08	6.49	–	–	–
58	12	.59	–	–	–	277	–	27	.05	.1	3.11	–	–	–
88	48	1.08	–	–	–	510	–	29	.09	.19	6.38	–	–	–
58	18	.05	–	–	–	287	–	27	–	.03	.05	2.69	–	–
125	161	2.51	–	–	–	1915	–	76	.31	.34	12.8	.56	–	36
176	180	3.48	–	–	–	1869	–	77	.32	.5	12	.53	–	36

(For purposes of calculations, use "0" for t, < 1, < .1, < .01, etc.)

Table I–1
Food Composition

Computer Code Number	Food Description	Measure	Wt (g)	H₂O (%)	Ener (cal)	Prot (g)	Carb (g)	Dietary Fiber (g)	Fat (g)	Fat Breakdown (g)		
										Sat	Mono	Poly
	KENTUCKY FRIED CHICKEN—Cont.											
1264	2-pce dinner, combo	1 ea	371	57	919	35	65	1	58	14.1	29.4	10.6
1265	Mashed potatoes	⅓ c	80	81	60	2	12	1	1	.2	.4	t
1526	Breadstick	1 ea	33	10	110	3	17	0	3	0	–	–
1268	Corn-on-the-cob	1 ea	143	70	210	5	32	8	11	.5	1	1.5
1527	Cornbread	1 pce	56	26	228	3	25	1	13	2	–	–
1269	Coleslaw	⅓ c	79	75	100	1	12	< 1	5	.9	1.5	3
1429	Chicken Hot Wings	1 ea	119	38	415	24	16	–	29	–	–	–
1381	Kentucky nuggets	6 ea	96	41	287	16	15	< 1	18	4	8.7	2.2
	Kentucky nugget sauce:											
1382	Barbeque	2 tsp	30	68	37	< 1	8	–	1	.1	–	.3
1383	Sweet & sour	2 tbs	30	48	61	< 1	14	–	1	.1	–	.3
1384	Honey	2 tbs	30	8	104	0	26	–	–	–	–	–
1385	Mustard	2 tbs	30	69	38	1	6	–	1	.1	–	1.2
1386	Kentucky fries	1 ea	119	42	352	5	40	5	18	5	12.5	1.1
1534	Macaroni & Cheese	1 ea	114	71	162	7	15	0	8	3	–	–
1387	Mashed potatoes & gravy	⅓ c	86	80	74	1	11	< 1	4	.4	.4	.2
1388	Buttermilk biscuit	1 ea	75	28	270	6	32	< 1	15	3.7	6.7	2.5
1530	Pasta Salad	1 ea	108	78	135	2	14	1	8	1	–	–
1389	Potato salad	⅓ c	90	74	130	2	13	1	8	1.4	2.8	3.5
1383	Potato Wedges	1 ea	92	55	192	3	25	3	9	3	–	–
1390	Baked beans	⅓ c	89	70	107	4	19	3	2	.4	.5	.2
1391	Chicken Little sandwich	1 ea	57	32	205	7	17	1	12	2.4	–	4.1
1535	Red Beans & Rice	1 ea	111	76	113	4	18	3	3	1	–	–
1529	Vegetable Medley Salad	1 ea	114	77	126	1	21	3	4	1	–	–

Source: Kentucky Fried Chicken Corporation.

	LONG JOHN SILVER'S											
	Fish, batter fried:											
1523	Fish & Fryes (fries), 3 piece	1 ea	350	54	893	28	84	–	46	10	26	9
1524	Fish & Fryes, 2 piece	1 ea	260	54	608	27	52	–	37	8	23	5
1525	Fish dinner, 3 piece	1 ea	540	60	1180	47	93	–	70	–	–	–
	Fish, breaded & fried:											
1526	Fish dinner, 3 piece	1 ea	450	60	940	35	84	–	52	–	–	–
1527	Fish dinner, 2 piece	1 ea	400	60	818	26	76	–	46	–	–	–
	Chicken:											
1528	Chicken Plank dinner, 3 piece	1 ea	370	56	825	30	94	–	41	9	23	9
1529	Chicken Plank dinner, 4 piece	1 ea	440	60	1037	41	82	–	59	–	–	–
1530	Chicken Nugget dinner, 6 piece	1 ea	300	60	699	23	54	–	45	–	–	–
1531	Clam chowder	1 ea	185	86	131	10	9	1	6	2	2	2
1532	Clam dinner	1 ea	460	47	1262	31	145	–	66	14	40	13
1533	Fish & chicken dinner	1 ea	460	52	1014	38	109	–	52	11	31	10
1534	Oyster dinner	1 ea	360	60	789	17	78	–	45	–	–	–
1535	Scallop dinner	1 ea	320	60	747	17	66	–	45	–	–	–
1536	Seafood platter	1 ea	410	60	976	29	85	–	58	–	–	–
1537	Shrimp dinner, batter fried	1 ea	300	54	761	16	80	–	43	9	25	8
1538	Fish sandwich platter	1 ea	400	59	835	30	84	–	42	–	–	–
	Salads:											
1539	Ocean chef salad	1 ea	320	89	150	16	18	3	1	6	6	3
1540	Seafood salad	1 ea	480	89	656	26	21	3	54	9	14	30

(Computer code number is for West Diet Analysis program)

Chol (mg)	Calc (mg)	Iron (mg)	Magn (mg)	Phos (mg)	Pota (mg)	Sodi (mg)	Zinc (mg)	VT-A (RE)	Thia (mg)	Ribo (mg)	Niac (mg)	V-B6 (mg)	Fola (µg)	VT-C (mg)
172	183	2.96	–	–	–	1949	–	76	.31	.45	11.7	.49	–	36
<1	21	.28	14	41	218	228	.16	5	.01	.04	.96	.11	7	4
0	30	.18	–	–	–	15	–	0	–	–	–	–	–	0
688	0	.34	–	–	72	–	–	19	.14	.11	1.8	–	–	2
42	60	.72	–	–	–	194	–	10	–	–	–	–	–	–
4	26	.32	–	–	–	155	–	28	.03	.03	.17	–	–	24
132	35	2.86	–	–	–	1084	–	13	–	–	–	–	–	5
67	2	.1	–	–	–	874	–	15	.02	.02	1	.05	–	<1
–	6	.21	–	–	–	477	–	39	–	.01	.2	–	–	–
–	5	.21	–	–	–	157	–	60	–	.02	.04	–	–	–
–	1	.21	–	–	–	–	–	0	–	.01	.08	–	–	–
–	11	.32	–	–	–	367	–	1	–	.01	.17	–	–	–
7	17	1.5	–	–	–	826	–	0	.23	.08	3.09	–	–	0
16	120	.72	–	–	–	531	–	–	–	–	–	–	–	0
<1	14	.3	–	–	–	278	–	11	–	.03	.86	–	–	–
3	49	2.2	–	–	–	652	–	32	.28	.22	3	–	–	–
1	20	1.08	–	–	–	663	–	110	–	–	–	–	–	7
8	7	1.6	11	23	184	305	.29	58	.05	.02	.4	.14	5	–
3	–	–	–	–	–	428	–	–	–	–	–	–	–	–
2	32	1.2	23	73	185	433	1.29	40	.05	.04	.4	.07	26	2
21	27	2.05	–	–	–	401	–	6	.19	.14	2.65	–	–	–
4	10	.71	–	–	–	312	–	–	–	–	–	–	–	–
0	20	.36	–	–	–	240	–	375	–	–	–	–	–	5
64	182	4	–	–	1021	1395	2.7	36	.41	.39	7.3	–	–	14
60	40	2	–	–	897	1474	1.2	–	.38	.34	8	–	–	9
119	–	–	–	–	–	2797	–	–	–	–	–	–	–	–
101	–	–	–	–	–	1900	–	–	–	–	–	–	–	–
76	–	–	–	–	–	1526	–	–	–	–	–	–	–	–
51	185	4	–	–	1085	1855	2.78	37	.49	.47	14.8	–	–	8
25	–	–	–	–	–	2433	–	–	–	–	–	–	–	–
25	–	–	–	–	–	853	–	–	–	–	–	–	–	–
19	187	1.68	–	–	355	551	1.56	140	.1	.24	1.87	–	–	–
96	255	5.73	–	–	1160	2332	3.8	51	.96	.55	15	–	–	15
80	213	4.8	–	–	1366	2231	3	43	.64	.64	15	–	–	10
55	–	–	–	–	–	763	–	–	–	–	–	–	–	–
37	–	–	–	–	–	1579	–	–	–	–	–	–	–	–
95	–	–	–	–	–	2161	–	–	–	–	–	–	–	–
91	181	3.26	–	–	761	1477	2.7	36	.41	.4	8	–	–	8
75	–	–	–	–	–	1402	–	–	–	–	–	–	–	–
55	137	5	–	–	130	998	.4	684	1.6	.2	4	–	–	29
95	259	8	–	–	224	1692	1.5	345	.26	.45	5	–	–	36

(For purposes of calculations, use "0" for t, <1, <.1, <.01, etc.)

Table I–1
Food Composition

Computer Code Number	Food Description	Measure	Wt (g)	H₂O (%)	Ener (cal)	Prot (g)	Carb (g)	Dietary Fiber (g)	Fat (g)	Fat Breakdown (g)		
										Sat	Mono	Poly
	LONG JOHN SILVER'S—Cont.											
1541	Coleslaw	1 ea	98	70	140	1	20	1	6	1	1.5	3.5
1542	Fryes (fries) serving	1 ea	85	43	250	3	28	1	15	2.5	7.4	5
1543	Hush puppies	1 ea	47	38	137	4	20	<1	4	1.8	2.6	1.4

Source: Long John Silver's, Lexington, KY.

Computer Code Number	Food Description	Measure	Wt (g)	H₂O (%)	Ener (cal)	Prot (g)	Carb (g)	Dietary Fiber (g)	Fat (g)	Sat	Mono	Poly
	McDONALD'S											
	Sandwiches:											
1221	Big Mac	1 ea	215	53	508	25	46	3	26	9	7.4	4.1
1444	McChicken	1 ea	187	52	486	17	41	2	28	5	8.4	10
1591	McLean Deluxe	1 ea	206	64	332	23	36	2	11	4	3.5	1
	Sandwiches—Cont.											
1438	McLean Deluxe with Cheese	1 ea	219	63	382	25	37	2	15	7	4	1.3
1222	Quarter-Pounder	1 ea	166	52	403	22	34	2	20	8	7	1
1223	Quarter-Pounder with Cheese	1 ea	194	50	507	27	34	2	28	12	1	2
1224	Filet-O-Fish	1 ea	142	49	357	13	40	2	16	3.6	4	5
1225	Hamburger	1 ea	102	49	251	12	33	2	8	3	2.7	9
1226	Cheeseburger	1 ea	116	55	302	14	34	2	12	5	3.6	1
1227	French fries, small serving	1 ea	68	40	207	3	26	2	10	1.7	3.1	2.5
1228	Chicken McNuggets	6 ea	112	51	1224	19	16	0	18	3.8	5.7	3.7
	Sauces (packet):											
1229	Hot mustard	1 ea	30	60	63	5	8	<1	4	.47	1.1	2
1230	Barbecue	1 ea	32	58	53	<1	12	<1	<1	.05	.13	2.4
1231	Sweet & sour	1 ea	32	57	55	<1	14	<1	<1	.1	.1	.3
	Low-fat (frozen yogurt) milk shakes:											
1232	Chocolate	1 ea	293	71	346	13	66	<1	5	3.5	.1	.7
1233	Strawberry	1 ea	293	72	342	12	63	<1	5	3.4	.1	.6
1234	Vanilla	1 ea	293	75	308	12	54	<1	5	3.3	.1	.6
	Low-fat (frozen yogurt) sundaes:											
1237	Hot caramel	1 ea	168	56	283	6	58	<1	3	2	.5	1.5
1235	Hot fudge	1 ea	168	60	275	8	50	2	5	4.5	.5	2
1267	Strawberry	1 ea	168	65	226	6	49	1	1	.7	.2	.5
1238	Vanilla	1 ea	80	65	100	4	21	<1	1	.3	.2	.5
1239	Pie, apple	1 ea	83	35	286	3	34	1	14	3.7	4.5	2.8
	Muffins (fat-free)											
1266	Blueberry	1 ea	75	41	170	3	40	–	0	0	0	0
1240	Apple bran	1 ea	85	39	206	4	46	2	.77	.2	.14	.4
1241	Cookies, McDonaldland	1 ea	56	3	258	.03	41	<1	9	4.5	.9	.9
1242	Cookies, Chocolaty chip	1 ea	56	3	282	3	36	1	14	.7	.9	3.6
	Breakfast items:											
1243	English muffin with spread	1 ea	59	41	146	5	27	2	2	2.3	.6	.6
1244	Egg McMuffin	1 ea	138	57	292	18	29	1	13	6.1	1	4.1
1245	Hotcakes with marg & syrup	1 ea	176	44	442	8	80	2	11	1.9	4	4.6
1246	Scrambled eggs	1 ea	100	73	166	12	1	0	12	2	5	2
1247	Pork sausage	1 ea	48	45	193	8	<1	0	18	6	7	2
1248	Hashbrown potatoes	1 ea	53	55	130	1	15	1	7	1.4	7.3	2
1392	Sausage McMuffin	1 ea	117	42	377	13	28	2	24	8.6	8.5	3
1393	Sausage McMuffin with egg	1 ea	167	53	452	22	28	2	29	10.0	13.9	4
1394	Biscuit with biscuit spread	1 ea	75	32	257	5	32	1	13	9	1	3

(Computer code number is for West Diet Analysis program)

Chol (mg)	Calc (mg)	Iron (mg)	Magn (mg)	Phos (mg)	Pota (mg)	Sodi (mg)	Zinc (mg)	VT-A (RE)	Thia (mg)	Ribo (mg)	Niac (mg)	V-B6 (mg)	Fola (µg)	VT-C (mg)
15	60	.72	–	–	190	260	.6	40	.06	.07	2	–	–	–
0	200	.72	–	–	370	500	.4	–	.09	–	1.6	–	–	6
–	78	1.4	–	–	127	49	.6	–	.12	.06	1.6	–	–	–
76	201	4.3	45	266	454	928	4.8	–	.49	.43	6	.25	49	3
52	127	2.5	32	220	316	789	1	–	.9	.24	7.6	.39	36	1
57	126	4	38	218	517	780	4.7	–	.38	.34	7	.28	42	8
70	134	4	42	280	537	1005	–	150	.38	.34	7	–	–	6
68	123	4	33	281	394	672	–	40	.38	.26	7	.32	–	4
94	139	4	–	–	–	1132	–	150	.38	.34	7	.32	–	4
36	121	1.81	31	179	260	735	–	20	.3	.14	9.06	.1	–	<1
27	119	2.7	23	106	245	490	–	40	.3	.17	4	–	–	2
40	127	2.7	26	169	267	725	–	80	.3	.26	4	–	–	2
0	9	.53	26	88	469	110	–	0	.15	0	2	.18	–	9
65	15	1.08	26	306	323	580	–	0	.12	.14	8	.36	–	0
3	7	.8	–	18	29	85	–	2	.01	.01	.15	–	–	<1
0	4	0	–	7	51	277	–	40	.01	.01	.17	–	–	2
0	2	.17	–	7	8	158	–	60	0	.01	.08	–	–	1
24	369	.84	–	352	539	240	–	60	.12	.51	.4	.1	–	0
24	365	.29	–	327	540	169	–	60	.12	.51	.4	.11	–	0
24	360	.1	–	326	533	171	–	60	.12	.51	.31	–	–	0
7	227	.14	–	199	318	180	–	60	.09	.34	.27	–	–	0
5	242	.55	–	223	414	170	–	40	.09	.34	.29	–	–	0
5	209	.16	–	162	307	109	–	40	.06	.34	.25	–	–	1
3	95	.23	–	–	–	76	–	19	.03	.16	.38	–	–	0
0	17	1.2	7	37	68	175	.16	10	.12	.09	1.02	.03	3	1
0	80	.72	–	114	–	220	.37	–	.12	.14	.8	–	–	1
0	39	1.22	15	70	–	227	–	1	.17	.19	2.27	–	–	1
0	10	1.63	11	83	–	271	–	0	.13	.15	1.81	.03	–	0
3	28	1.6	4	–	–	249	–	0	.13	.15	1.78	–	–	0
6	126	2	13	67	65	362	.39	31	.24	.29	2.45	.03	16	1
235	152	2.76	4	272	–	726	–	102	.48	.34	3.79	.08	–	0
9	86	1.57	22	399	–	693	–	40	.3	.34	3.03	.11	–	0
416	49	1.8	10	169	–	290	–	100	.07	.26	.05	–	–	0
36	8	.6	7	66	–	346	–	0	.26	.11	2.23	–	–	0
0	7	.27	11	51	–	330	–	0	.06	.02	.8	–	–	1
49	138	2.34	23	163	–	667	–	35	.46	.22	4.33	.13	–	0
264	160	3.78	27	282	–	966	–	105	.56	.45	5.25	.21	–	0
0	67	1.44	9	349	–	730	–	0	.23	.1	1.65	.03	–	0

(For purposes of calculations, use "0" for t, <1, <.1, <.01, etc.)

Table I–1
Food Composition

Computer Code Number	Food Description	Measure	Wt (g)	H₂O (%)	Ener (cal)	Prot (g)	Carb (g)	Dietary Fiber (g)	Fat (g)	Fat Breakdown (g)		
										Sat	Mono	Poly
	McDONALD'S—Cont.											
	Breakfast items—Cont.:											
1395	Biscuit with sausage	1 ea	123	37	448	12	33	1	30	9	10	3
1396	Biscuit with sausage & egg	1 ea	180	48	548	19	34	1	37	11	14	4
1397	Biscuit with bacon, egg, cheese	1 ea	156	46	462	15	34	1	28	9	9	3
	Salads:											
1398	Chef salad	1 ea	283	86	186	18	8	3	10	4	3	1
1400	Garden salad	1 ea	213	92	77	5	6	2	4	1	1	1
1401	Chunky chicken salad	1 ea	250	86	138	24	7	3	4	1	1	1

Source: McDonald's Corporation.

Computer Code Number	Food Description	Measure	Wt (g)	H₂O (%)	Ener (cal)	Prot (g)	Carb (g)	Dietary Fiber (g)	Fat (g)	Sat	Mono	Poly
	PIZZA HUT											
	Pan Pizza:											
1657	Cheese	2 pce	205	48	492	30	57	5	18	8.6	5.5	2.7
1658	Pepperoni	2 pce	211	45	540	29	62	5	22	9.2	9.3	3.4
1659	Supreme	2 pce	255	54	589	32	53	7	30	13.8	11.9	4.3
1660	Super Supreme	2 pce	257	55	563	33	53	6	26	12	–	–
	Thin 'N Crispy:											
1649	Cheese Pizza	2 pce	148	43	398	28	37	4	17	10	4.6	2.3
1623	Pepperoni Pizza	2 pce	146	42	413	26	36	4	20	11	–	–
1622	Supreme Pizza	2 pce	200	53	459	28	41	5	22	11	–	–
1620	Super Supreme Pizza	2 pce	203	52	463	29	44	5	21	10	–	–
	Hand Tossed:											
1619	Cheese Pizza	2 pce	220	50	518	34	55	7	20	13.6	–	–
1618	Pepperoni Pizza	2 pce	197	47	500	28	50	6	23	12.9	–	–
1648	Supreme Pizza	2 pce	239	54	540	32	50	7	26	13.8	–	–
1617	Super Supreme Pizza	2 pce	243	53	556	33	54	7	25	13	–	–
	Personal Pan Pizza:											
1610	Pepperoni	1 ea	256	43	675	37	76	8	29	12.5	12.1	4.5
1609	Supreme	1 ea	264	47	647	33	76	9	28	11.2	12.4	4.4

Source: Pizza Hut.

Computer Code Number	Food Description	Measure	Wt (g)	H₂O (%)	Ener (cal)	Prot (g)	Carb (g)	Dietary Fiber (g)	Fat (g)	Sat	Mono	Poly
	TACO BELL											
	Breakfast burrito:											
1601	Bacon breakfast burrito	1 ea	99	48	291	11	23	–	17	4	–	–
1627	Country breakfast burrito	1 ea	113	53	281	10	26	–	16	5	–	–
1626	Fiesta breakfast burrito	1 ea	92	47	275	9	23	–	16	6	–	–
1625	Grande breakfast burrito	1 ea	177	52	457	14	46	–	24	8	–	–
1604	Sausage breakfast burrito	1 ea	106	49	303	11	23	–	19	6	–	–
	Burritos:											
1544	Bean with red sauce	1 ea	191	54	414	14	58	11	13	6.4	4.4	1.1
1545	Beef with red sauce	1 ea	191	53	457	23	44	4	19	9.7	6.9	.8
1546	Beef & bean with red sauce	1 ea	191	59	393	17	44	5	15	4.8	5.8	1.9
1552	Chicken burrito	1 ea	171	58	345	17	41	–	13	5	–	–
1547	Supreme with red sauce	1 ea	241	61	475	19	52	5	21	7.3	7.5	1.9
1569	Big beef burrito supreme	1 ea	298	64	525	25	51	–	25	11	–	–
1571	7 layer burrito	1 ea	234	60	458	14	55	8	20	5.9	–	–
1538	Chilito	1 ea	156	49	391	17	41	–	18	9	–	–
1549	Chilito, steak	1 ea	257	62	496	26	47	–	23	10	–	–

(Computer code number is for West Diet Analysis program)

Chol (mg)	Calc (mg)	Iron (mg)	Magn (mg)	Phos (mg)	Pota (mg)	Sodi (mg)	Zinc (mg)	VT-A (RE)	Thia (mg)	Ribo (mg)	Niac (mg)	V-B6 (mg)	Fola (µg)	VT-C (mg)
34	78	1.88	16	424	–	1084	–	0	.47	.18	4.17	.21	–	0
259	106	3	22	528	–	1244	–	62	.46	.36	4.1	.21	–	0
244	105	2.75	21	569	–	1238	–	102	.39	.35	2.04	.13	–	0
161	142	1.54	36	302	–	427	–	1067	.32	.28	4.27	–	–	22
27	48	1.62	22	370	–	79	–	1014	.1	.11	.45	–	–	24
64	45	1.06	37	569	–	225	–	1666	.22	.17	8.82	–	–	26
34	630	5.4	60	470	320	940	4.1	90	.56	.6	5.2	.17	–	7
42	520	6.3	56	440	405	1127	4.2	100	.63	.49	5.4	.17	0	8
48	500	5	76	460	580	1363	5.6	120	.81	.8	6	.31	–	10
55	540	6.7	72	470	532	1447	5.4	120	.75	.66	6.4	–	–	11
33	660	3.2	48	470	261	867	3.6	70	.39	.39	4.8	.16	–	5
46	450	3.2	44	370	287	986	3.5	70	.42	.43	5.2	–	–	6
42	430	5.9	68	400	544	1328	4.7	100	.6	.49	5.4	–	–	10
56	460	4.9	60	420	463	1336	4.5	100	.59	.44	5.4	–	–	8
55	750	5.4	72	550	396	1276	4.7	100	.48	.49	5.4	–	–	10
50	440	5	60	390	415	1267	3.8	100	.54	.53	5.6	–	–	7
55	480	8.1	80	460	578	1470	5.7	110	.69	.53	7.2	–	–	12
54	440	6.8	76	420	516	1648	4.8	110	.71	.58	7.4	–	–	12
53	730	5.8	60	450	408	1335	3.8	120	.56	.66	8.2	.2	–	10
49	520	6.7	60	400	487	1313	3.8	120	.59	.66	8	.32	–	11
181	80	1.8	–	–	–	652	–	310	–	–	–	–	–	–
173	80	3.42	–	–	–	627	–	310	–	–	–	–	–	–
27	60	1.44	–	–	–	680	–	260	–	–	–	–	–	–
183	200	3.6	–	–	–	1053	–	630	–	–	–	–	–	1
183	80	1.8	–	–	–	661	–	320	–	–	–	–	–	–
9	136	3.22	–	–	459	1064	–	46	.03	1.87	1.84	.29	–	49
53	106	3.46	–	–	352	1215	–	67	.37	1.98	3.19	.3	–	2
32	107	2.07	48	212	426	1095	2.58	77	.47	.4	2.98	.57	37	2
57	140	2.52	–	–	–	854	–	440	–	–	–	–	–	1
31	145	3.4	47	215	473	1116	–	118	.39	2	2.73	.33	–	24
72	200	4.5	–	–	–	1418	–	840	–	–	–	–	–	8
17	85	2.29	–	–	–	983	–	297	–	–	–	–	–	5
47	300	3.06	–	–	–	980	–	950	–	–	–	–	–	–
78	200	2.70	–	–	–	1313	–	970	–	–	–	–	–	2

(For purposes of calculations, use "0" for t, < 1, < .1, < .01, etc.)

Table I–1
Food Composition

Computer Code Number	Food Description	Measure	Wt (g)	H₂O (%)	Ener (cal)	Prot (g)	Carb (g)	Dietary Fiber (g)	Fat (g)	Fat Breakdown (g)		
										Sat	Mono	Poly
	TACO BELL—Cont											
1549	Enchirito with red sauce	1 ea	213	62	382	20	31	5	20	9.3	4.9	1.5
	Tacos:											
1551	Taco	1 ea	78	59	183	10	11	1	11	4.6	4.5	.8
1552	Taco Bellgrande	1 ea	163	63	355	18	18	1	23	10.9	9	1.3
1554	Soft taco	1 ea	92	54	225	12	18	1	12	5.4	4.3	1.2
1536	Soft taco supreme	1 ea	124	60	262	13	20	2	15	7.3	–	–
1568	Soft taco, chicken	1 ea	128	65	223	14	20	–	10	4	–	–
1572	Soft taco, steak	1 ea	100	56	217	12	21	–	9	4	–	–
1555	Tostada with red sauce	1 ea	156	69	243	9	27	5	11	4.1	5.5	.8
1558	Mexican pizza	1 ea	223	55	575	21	40	2	37	11.4	14	9.7
1559	Taco salad with salsa	1 ea	595	73	939	36	60	8	62	19	26.6	12.3
1560	Nachos, regular	1 ea	107	39	349	8	38	3	19	6.1	7.6	2.1
1561	Nachos, Bellgrande	1 ea	287	58	649	22	61	–	35	12.3	–	2.6
1562	Pintos & cheese with red sauce	1 ea	128	69	190	9	19	7	9	3.6	4	.8
1563	Taco sauce, packet	1 ea	4	96	1	< 1	< 1	< 1	< 1	0	0	0
1564	Salsa	1 ea	10	42	18	1	4	–	< 1	0	0	0
1565	Cinnamon twists	1 ea	47	3	231	3	32	1	11	5.4	3.5	1.2
1628	Caramel roll	1 ea	85	19	353	6	46	–	16	4	–	–
	Border Light menu:											
1749	Bean burrito	1 ea	198	–	330	14	55	8	6	2	–	–
1750	Burrito supreme	1 ea	248	–	350	20	50	4	8	3	–	–
1744	7 layer burrito	1 ea	276	–	440	19	67	10	9	3.5	–	–
1745	Taco	1 ea	78	–	140	11	11	2	5	1.5	–	–
1746	Taco supreme	1 ea	106	–	160	13	14	2	5	1.5	–	–
1747	Soft taco	1 ea	99	–	180	13	19	2	5	2.5	–	–
1748	Soft taco supreme	1 ea	128	–	200	14	23	2	5	2.5	–	–
1742	Taco salad without chips	1 ea	464	–	330	30	35	10	9	4.5	–	–
1743	Taco salad with chips	1 ea	535	–	680	35	81	10	25	8	–	–

Source: Taco Bell Corporation.

	WENDY'S											
	Hamburgers:											
1566	Single on white bun, no toppings	1 ea	119	44	350	21	29	< 1	16	–	–	–
1568	Double on white bun, no toppings	1 ea	197	44	560	41	32	< 1	34	7.4	12.5	8
1569	Big Classic	1 ea	241	63	470	26	36	–	25	–	–	–
	Cheeseburgers:											
1570	Bacon cheeseburger	1 ea	147	46	460	29	23	< 1	28	13	13	2
1571	Double with lettuce & tomato	1 ea	215	50	548	30	32	2	33	12.9	11.8	5.4
1572	Double with all toppings	1 ea	291	50	735	48	27	2	47	18.4	18	5.9
1730	Chicken sandwich, grilled	1 ea	177	62	290	24	35	2	7	1.5	–	–
	Baked potatoes:											
1573	Plain	1 ea	250	75	250	6	52	4	< 1	t	t	.1
1574	With bacon & cheese	1 ea	350	71	570	19	57	4	30	11.8	11.4	5.6
1575	With broccoli & cheese	1 ea	365	74	500	13	54	5	25	9.2	8.3	4.5
1576	With cheese	1 ea	350	71	590	16	55	4	34	12.5	12.7	7.1
1577	With chili & cheese	1 ea	400	72	510	22	63	8	20	13	6.8	.9
1578	With sour cream & chives	1 ea	310	71	460	6	53	4	24	10	7.9	3.3
1579	Chili	1 ea	256	81	230	21	16	–	9	–	–	–

(Computer code number is for West Diet Analysis program)

Chol (mg)	Calc (mg)	Iron (mg)	Magn (mg)	Phos (mg)	Pota (mg)	Sodi (mg)	Zinc (mg)	VT-A (RE)	Thia (mg)	Ribo (mg)	Niac (mg)	V-B6 (mg)	Fola (µg)	VT-C (mg)
54	269	2.84	–	–	423	1243	–	100	.26	.42	2.3	1	–	28
32	84	1.07	–	–	159	276	–	24	.05	.14	1.2	.12	–	1
56	182	1.9	–	–	334	472	–	40	.11	.29	2.02	.21	–	5
32	116	2.27	–	–	196	554	–	30	.39	.22	2.74	.1	–	1
44	78	1.74	–	–	–	533	–	291	–	–	–	–	–	2
58	60	1.44	–	–	–	553	–	540	–	–	–	–	–	2
31	50	1.08	–	–	–	569	–	130	–	–	–	–	–	–
16	179	1.53	–	–	401	596	–	95	.06	.17	.63	.26	–	45
52	257	3.74	80	400	408	1031	5.4	215	.32	.33	2.96	1.11	60	31
82	405	7.22	–	–	1066	1307	–	407	.52	.77	4.88	.57	–	78
9	193	.91	52	262	161	403	1.7	88	.17	.16	.69	.19	10	2
36	297	3.48	–	–	674	997	–	40	.1	.34	2.17	–	–	58
16	156	1.42	110	156	384	642	2.17	87	.05	.15	.4	.21	68	52
0	1	.02	–	–	4	42	–	6	0	<.01	.02	<.01	–	<1
0	36	.6	–	–	376	376	–	7	.02	.14	0	–	–	2
1	37	.49	–	–	36	316	–	0	.14	.05	.96	.05	–	1
15	60	1.44	–	–	–	312	–	330	–	–	–	–	–	4
5	100	3.6	–	–	–	1340	–	400	–	–	–	–	–	2
25	80	2.7	–	–	–	1300	–	600	–	–	–	–	–	9
5	250	4.5	–	–	–	1430	–	350	–	–	–	–	–	5
20	0	0	–	–	–	280	–	40	–	–	–	–	–	0
20	0	0	–	–	–	340	–	100	–	–	–	–	–	2
25	40	1.08	–	–	–	550	–	40	–	–	–	–	–	0
25	40	1.08	–	–	–	610	–	100	–	–	–	–	–	2
50	100	2.7	–	–	–	1610	–	1200	–	–	–	–	–	27
50	250	3.6	–	–	–	1620	–	1800	–	–	–	–	–	27
65	100	4.5	–	–	265	420	–	0	.38	.34	6	–	–	–
125	48	6.3	42	339	431	575	8.35	0	.22	.43	9	.47	29	<1
80	40	4.5	–	–	470	900	–	60	.3	.25	5	–	–	12
65	136	3.6	33	296	332	860	5.14	82	.26	.28	5.7	.23	25	1
84	177	4	33	339	430	864	4.41	111	.34	.35	5.29	.25	28	5
165	180	5.4	50	470	620	883	8.8	112	.36	.53	10	.46	31	5
55	100	2.8	–	–	–	720	–	20	–	–	–	–	–	6
0	40	2.7	66	169	1360	60	.65	0	.27	.1	3.82	.7	67	36
22	200	3.7	80	406	1380	180	2.53	150	.22	.17	4.64	.87	33	36
22	250	3.6	83	373	1550	430	.86	350	.3	.25	4	.86	66	90
22	350	3.6	78	50	1380	450	.61	200	.22	.25	3.3	.8	33	36
22	250	6.13	111	498	1590	810	3.78	172	.3	.26	4.1	.9	50	36
15	40	2.7	70	185	1420	230	.9	100	.22	.14	3	.79	32	36
–	60	4.5	–	–	565	960	–	200	.12	.17	3	–	–	9

(For purposes of calculations, use "0" for t, <1, <.1, <.01, etc.)

Table I-1
Food Composition

Computer Code Number	Food Description	Measure	Wt (g)	H₂O (%)	Ener (cal)	Prot (g)	Carb (g)	Dietary Fiber (g)	Fat (g)	Fat Breakdown (g) Sat	Mono	Poly
	WENDY'S—Cont.											
1580	French fries	1 ea	106	43	306	4	38	1	15	7	5	2
1581	Frosty dairy dessert	1 c	216	35	354	7	53	0	13	5	3	2
1582	Chocolate chip cookies	1 ea	64	4	320	3	40	1	17	5.5	5.8	4.9
	Source: Wendy's International.											
	CONVENIENCE FOODS & MEALS											
	ALPINE LACE											
	Cheese spread, free'n lean:											
1926	Cheddar	1 oz	28	–	30	5	1	–	0	0	0	0
1928	Cream cheese	1 oz	28	–	30	5	1	–	0	0	0	0
1929	Garden vegetable	1 oz	28	–	30	5	1	–	0	0	0	0
1932	Garlic herb	1 oz	28	–	30	5	1	–	0	0	0	0
1933	Horseradish	1 oz	28	–	30	5	1	–	0	0	0	0
	BUDGET GOURMET											
1695	Chicken cacciatore	1 ea	312	80	300	20	27	–	13	–	–	–
1694	Sweet & sour chicken with rice	1 ea	284	72	350	18	53	–	7	–	–	–
1689	Teriyaki chicken	1 ea	340	77	360	20	44	–	12	–	–	–
1692	Linguini & shrimp	1 ea	284	77	330	15	33	–	15	–	–	–
1691	Scallops & shrimp	1 ea	326	79	320	16	43	–	9	–	–	–
1693	Sirloin tips with country gravy	1 ea	284	80	310	16	21	–	18	–	–	–
1690	Veal parmigiana	1 ea	340	75	440	26	39	–	20	–	–	–
1696	Yankee pot roast	1 ea	312	77	380	27	22	–	21	–	–	–
	Source: The All American Gourmet Company.											
	HAAGEN DAZS											
	Sorbet:											
1758	Lemon	½ c	113	–	140	0	35	–	0	0	0	0
1760	Orange	½ c	113	–	140	0	36	–	0	0	0	0
1759	Raspberry	½ c	113	–	110	0	27	–	0	0	0	0
	Yogurt, frozen:											
1753	Chocolate	½ c	98	–	170	8	26	–	4	2	2	0
1754	Strawberry	½ c	98	–	170	6	27	–	4	2	2	0
1755	Vanilla almond	1 ea	107	–	370	6	26	–	27	14	10	3
	Yogurt extra, frozen:											
1752	Brownie nut	½ c	101	–	220	8	29	–	9	4	4	1
1751	Raspberry rendezvous	½ c	101	–	132	4	26	–	2	1	1	0
	HEALTHY CHOICE											
	Entrees:											
1628	Chicken Chow Mein	1 ea	241	78	220	18	31	–	3	.8	–	.8
1630	Fillet of Fish Florentine	1 ea	273	80	220	26	13	–	7	3	–	2
2112	Fish, lemon pepper	1 ea	303	78	290	14	47	7	5	1	–	–
1624	Lasagna	1 ea	284	78	260	18	37	–	5	–	–	–
2111	Meatloaf, traditional	1 ea	340	79	320	16	46	7	8	4	–	–
1629	Seafood Newburg	1 ea	227	80	200	13	30	–	3	.8	–	.8
1625	Spaghetti	1 ea	284	77	280	14	42	–	6	–	–	–
2104	Zucchini lasagna	1 ea	397	80	330	20	58	11	2	1	–	–

(Computer code number is for West Diet Analysis program)

Chol (mg)	Calc (mg)	Iron (mg)	Magn (mg)	Phos (mg)	Pota (mg)	Sodi (mg)	Zinc (mg)	VT-A (RE)	Thia (mg)	Ribo (mg)	Niac (mg)	V-B6 (mg)	Fola (µg)	VT-C (mg)
15	13	1.02	45	197	689	105	.51	0	.15	.04	2.96	.26	33	12
44	257	.86	43	238	518	194	.92	143	.11	.45	.31	.12	17	<1
5	10	1.09	15	62	100	235	.46	0	.06	.07	.4	.03	6	0
5	100	–	–	–	30	165	–	–	–	–	–	–	–	–
5	100	–	–	–	30	165	–	–	–	–	–	–	–	–
5	100	–	–	–	30	165	–	–	–	–	–	–	–	–
5	100	–	–	–	30	165	–	–	–	–	–	–	–	–
5	100	–	–	–	30	165	–	–	–	–	–	–	–	–
60	150	1.8	–	–	–	810	–	40	.23	.51	5	–	–	21
40	60	.72	–	–	–	640	–	80	.12	.34	3	–	–	2
55	80	1.4	–	–	–	610	–	300	.15	.34	6	–	–	12
75	10	3.6	–	–	–	1250	–	1000	.3	.17	3	–	–	2
70	150	.72	–	–	–	690	–	150	–	.26	3	–	–	12
40	60	.36	–	–	–	570	–	150	.15	.17	4	–	–	2
165	30	4.5	–	–	–	1160	–	1000	.45	.6	6	–	–	6
70	150	1.8	–	–	–	690	–	600	.15	.43	7	–	–	6
0	–	–	–	–	30	20	–	–	–	–	–	–	–	7
0	–	–	–	–	80	20	–	–	–	––	–	–	–	20
0	–	–	–	–	60	15	–	–	–	–	–	–	–	7
40	146	.7	–	146	240	45	–	20	–	.17	–	–	–	–
50	146	–	–	146	140	45	–	20	.03	.17	–	–	–	–
90	160	.38	–	107	220	85	–	160	–	.18	–	–	–	–
55	152	.73	–	152	250	60	–	20	–	.14	–	–	–	–
20	81	–	–	61	97	25	–	0	–	.1	–	–	–	5
45	20	1.4	–	290	290	440	–	81	.15	.14	4	–	–	4
65	150	.72	58	–	780	590	1.2	500	.15	.34	2	.14	<1	1
25	20	1.08	–	–	–	360	–	100	–	–	–	–	–	30
20	100	2.7	–	210	500	420	–	150	.3	.26	2	–	–	2
35	40	1.8	–	–	–	460	–	150	–	–	–	–	–	54
55	60	1.1	–	160	270	440	–	3	.12	.14	1.2	–	–	4
20	6	3.6	–	160	540	480	–	250	.38	.26	2	–	–	5
10	200	2.7	–	–	–	310	–	250	–	–	–	–	–	0

(For purposes of calculations, use "0" for t, <1, <.1, <.01, etc.)

Table I–1
Food Composition

Computer Code Number	Food Description	Measure	Wt (g)	H₂O (%)	Ener (cal)	Prot (g)	Carb (g)	Dietary Fiber (g)	Fat (g)	Fat Breakdown (g)		
										Sat	Mono	Poly
	HEALTHY CHOICE—Cont.											
	Dinners:											
2110	Pasta shells marinara	1 ea	340	74	360	25	59	5	3	1.5	–	–
1627	Sirloin Tips	1 ea	334	81	280	23	30	–	8	–	–	–
1626	Sole Au Gratin	1 ea	312	80	270	16	40	–	5	–	–	–
	Low-fat ice milk:											
1601	Berry	½ c	113	–	120	3	23	–	2	1	–	0
1604	Chocolate	½ c	113	–	130	3	24	–	2	1	–	0
1608	Cookie & Cream	½ c	113	–	130	4	24	–	2	–	–	0
1621	Vanilla	½ c	113	–	120	4	21	–	2	1	–	0
	Low-fat ice cream:											
973	Brownie	½ c	71	61	120	3	22	2	2	1	–	.7
650	Chocolate chip	½ c	71	62	120	3	21	1	2	1	–	0
259	Butter pecan	½ c	71	61	120	3	22	1	2	1	–	.7
45	Rocky road	½ c	71	53	140	3	28	2	2	1	–	0
391	Vanilla fudge	½ c	71	62	120	3	21	1	2	1.5	–	.7
	Source: ConAgra Frozen Foods, Omaha, NE.											
	HEALTH VALLEY											
	Soups, fat-free:											
2001	Beef broth, no salt added	6.9 oz	196	98	15	4	0	0	0	0	0	0
2073	Beef broth, w/salt	6.9 oz	196	98	15	4	0	0	0	0	0	0
2016	Black bean & vegetable	7.5 oz	213	93	70	7	12	11	0	0	0	0
2017	Chicken broth	7.5 oz	213	97	22	4	1	0	0	0	0	0
2018	14 garden vegetable	7.5 oz	213	92	50	5	6	5	0	0	0	0
2015	Lentil & carrot	7.5 oz	213	86	90	8	14	7	0	0	0	0
2014	Split pea & carrot	7.5 oz	213	86	90	8	14	7	0	0	0	0
2013	Tomato vegetable	7.5 oz	213	90	50	5	8	6	0	0	0	0
	LA CHOY											
2100	Egg rolls, mini, chicken	1 ea	106	53	220	8	35	3	6	1.5	–	–
2099	Egg roles, mini, shrimp	1 ea	106	56	210	7	35	3	4	1	–	–
	LEAN CUISINE											
	Dinners:											
1639	Baked Cheese Ravioli	1 ea	241	77	240	13	30	3	8	3	3	.5
1640	Chicken Cacciatore	1 ea	308	80	280	22	31	4	7	2	–	1
1632	Chicken Chow Mein	1 ea	255	78	240	14	34	–	5	1	–	1
1633	Lasagna	1 ea	291	79	260	19	34	2	5	2	2	.5
1634	Macaroni & Cheese	1 ea	255	74	290	15	37	–	9	4	–	.5
1631	Spaghetti w/Meatballs	1 ea	269	75	280	19	35	11	7	2	2.6	1
	Pizza:											
1635	French Bread Cheese Pizza	1 ea	145	52	300	17	38	<1	9	3	5	.5
1638	French Bread Deluxe Pizza	1 ea	174	56	320	22	39	2	8	3	3	.5
1637	French Bread Pepperoni Pizza	1 ea	149	51	330	19	38	2	11	3	5.4	1
1636	French Bread Sausage Pizza	1 ea	170	55	330	22	40	2	9	3	4.3	.5
	Source: Stouffer's Foods Corp, Solon, OH.											
	TASTE ADVENTURE SOUPS											
1905	Black bean	8 oz	227	–	130	6	26	6	1	–	–	–
1903	Curry lentil	8 oz	227	–	130	6	28	5	1	–	–	–
1906	Lentil chili	8 oz	227	–	170	10	31	6	1	–	–	–
1903	Split pea	8 oz	227	–	130	5	25	5	1	–	–	–

(Computer code number is for West Diet Analysis program)

Chol (mg)	Calc (mg)	Iron (mg)	Magn (mg)	Phos (mg)	Pota (mg)	Sodi (mg)	Zinc (mg)	VT-A (RE)	Thia (mg)	Ribo (mg)	Niac (mg)	V-B6 (mg)	Fola (µg)	VT-C (mg)
25	400	1.8	–	–	–	390	–	100	–	–	–	–	–	4
65	20	2.7	–	190	540	370	–	700	.15	.17	5	.35	–	42
55	80	1.1	–	260	430	470	–	–	.23	.17	1.6	–	–	6
5	100	–	–	10	160	60	–	–	.03	.17	–	–	–	–
5	100	–	–	10	191	70	–	–	.03	.17	–	–	–	–
5	150	–	–	10	180	80	–	–	.03	.17	–	–	–	–
5	150	–	–	10	180	60	–	–	.06	.25	–	–	–	–
3	80	0	–	113	268	55	–	40	–	–	–	–	–	0
3	100	0	–	141	240	50	–	40	–	–	–	–	–	0
3	100	0	–	113	212	60	–	40	–	–	–	–	–	0
3	100	0	–	9	168	60	–	40	.03	.15	–	–	–	0
3	100	0	–	141	296	50	–	40	–	–	–	–	–	0
0	–	–	–	–	160	60	–	–	–	–	.8	–	–	–
0	–	–	–	–	160	290	–	–	–	–	.8	–	–	–
0	60	4.5	–	–	600	290	–	1000	.3	.1	1.2	.2	120	0
0	–	.39	–	43	130	315	–	–	–	.03	2.17	–	–	–
0	40	1.08	–	–	360	250	–	1000	.23	.07	2	.16	24	6
0	60	4.5	–	–	390	270	–	1000	.09	.14	5	.4	24	0
0	60	4.5	–	–	390	270	–	1000	.09	.14	5	.4	–	0
0	40	.72	–	–	540	230	–	1000	.09	.07	2	.12	32	9
5	20	1.44	–	–	–	460	–	20	–	–	–	–	–	0
5	20	1.44	–	–	–	510	–	20	–	–	–	–	–	0
55	200	1.44	42	168	380	590	1.5	60	.06	.25	1.2	.2	48	36
45	40	1.44	47	–	560	570	.97	100	.22	.17	6	–	–	9
30	40	1.08	30	–	350	530	1.1	60	.15	.17	5	–	–	6
25	150	1.8	44	–	700	590	2.9	100	.15	.25	3	.32	–	6
30	250	.72	–	–	160	550	–	20	.12	.25	1.2	–	–	0
35	100	1.8	47	–	500	490	2.5	60	.15	.25	3	.2	–	4
15	250	2.7	34	–	320	590	1.6	60	.37	.34	4	.1	–	6
40	200	1.44	38	–	440	860	2.08	150	.45	.51	5	.16	–	6
25	200	3.6	34	–	390	790	1.8	100	.45	.42	5	.07	–	6
40	250	2.7	39	–	440	860	2.2	80	.45	.51	5	.07	–	6
–	–	–	–	–	609	530	–	–	–	–	–	–	–	–
–	–	–	–	–	440	550	–	–	–	–	–	–	–	–
–	–	–	–	–	609	420	–	–	–	–	–	–	–	–
–	–	–	–	–	450	550	–	–	–	–	–	–	–	–

(For purposes of calculations, use "0" for t, < 1, < .1, < .01, etc.)

Table I–1
Food Composition

Computer Code Number	Food Description	Measure	Wt (g)	H₂O (%)	Ener (cal)	Prot (g)	Carb (g)	Dietary Fiber (g)	Fat (g)	Fat Breakdown (g)		
										Sat	Mono	Poly
	WEIGHT WATCHERS											
1981	Baked beans	5 oz	142	74	100	9	18	9	0	0	0	0
	Cheese, fat free:											
1978	Cheddar, sharp	2 pce	21	60	30	5	2	0	0	0	0	0
1980	Swiss	2 pce	21	59	30	5	2	0	0	0	0	0
1977	White	2 pce	21	59	30	5	2	0	0	0	0	0
1979	Yellow	2 pce	21	59	30	5	2	0	0	0	0	0
	Dinners:											
1641	Beef Stroganoff	1 ea	238	73	290	22	26	3	9	4	3	2
1646	Oven Fried Fish	1 ea	198	79	240	20	23	–	7	–	5	2
1647	Fried Chicken Patty	1 pce	184	73	270	16	14	–	16	8	6	2
1654	Chicken Burrito w/Vegetable	1 ea	216	68	330	15	36	–	14	4	6	3
2029	Chicken chow mein	1 ea	255	81	200	12	34	3	2	.5	–	–
1656	Pasta Primavera	1 ea	238	75	260	15	22	2	11	.8	8	3
1972	Margarine, reduced fat	1 tbs	14	50	60	0	0	0	7	1.5	–	–
	Pizza:											
1653	Cheese Pizza	1 ea	164	56	300	22	37	2	7	3	3	1
1650	Deluxe Combination Pizza	1 ea	200	64	330	26	35	3	10	3	5	2
1651	Sausage Pizza	1 ea	175	60	320	24	35	2	10	2	6	2
1652	Pepperoni Pizza	1 ea	171	56	320	26	31	–	10	3	5	2
	Desserts:											
1645	Apple pie	1 ea	98	49	200	2	39	–	5	1	2	2
1643	Boston cream pie	1 ea	85	48	170	4	35	1	4	1	1	2
1644	Chocolate brownie	1 ea	35	29	100	3	17	<1	4	1	2	1
2024	Chocolate eclair	1 ea	60	45	150	3	24	2	5	1.5	–	–
1642	Strawberry cheesecake	1 ea	109	62	180	7	28	–	5	1	1	2
2027	Triple chocolate cheesecake	1 ea	89	52	200	7	32	1	5	2.5	–	–
1655	Chocolate mousse	1 ea	70	46	170	6	24	<1	6	–	4	2
	Sweet Success:											
	Drinks, prepared:											
1776	Chocolate chip	1 c	265	81	180	15	30	6	3	1.6	–	–
1777	Chocolate fudge	1 c	265	81	180	15	30	6	2	–	–	–
1774	Chocolate mocha	1 c	265	81	180	15	30	6	1	1	–	–
1778	Milk chocolate	1 c	265	81	180	15	30	6	2	1	–	–
1775	Vanilla	1 c	265	81	180	15	33	6	1	.6	–	–
	Drinks, ready to drink:											
2147	Chocolate mint	10 oz	284	82	179	11	34	5	3	0	–	–
2148	Strawberry	10 oz	284	82	179	11	34	5	3	0	–	–
	Shakes:											
1771	Chocolate almond	1¼ c	313	82	200	12	38	6	3	1.1	1.6	.3
1773	Chocolate fudge	1¼ c	313	82	200	12	38	6	5	1.1	1.6	.3
1768	Chocolate mocha	1¼ c	313	82	200	12	38	6	3	.8	.8	1.3
1769	Chocolate raspberry truffle	1¼ c	313	82	200	12	38	6	3	1.1	1.6	.3
1770	Vanilla creme	1¼ c	313	82	200	12	38	6	3	.8	1.8	.4
	Snack bars:											
1767	Chocolate brownie	1 ea	33	8	120	2	23	3	4	2	.5	.6
1766	Chocolate chip	1 ea	33	8	120	2	23	3	4	2	.4	.5
1765	Peanut butter	1 ea	33	8	120	2	23	3	4	2	.6	.6
1921	Oatmeal raisin	1 ea	33	7	120	2	23	3	4	2	–	–

Source: Foodway National Inc., Boise, ID.

(Computer code number is for West Diet Analysis program)

Chol (mg)	Calc (mg)	Iron (mg)	Magn (mg)	Phos (mg)	Pota (mg)	Sodi (mg)	Zinc (mg)	VT-A (RE)	Thia (mg)	Ribo (mg)	Niac (mg)	V-ß6 (mg)	Fola (µg)	VT-C (mg)
0	60	2.7	–	–	329	190	–	–	.2	.1	1.2	–	–	12
0	100	0	–	–	65	310	–	57	–	–	–	–	–	0
0	100	0	–	–	75	280	–	57	–	–	–	–	–	0
0	100	0	–	–	65	310	–	57	–	–	–	–	–	0
0	100	0	–	–	65	310	–	57	–	–	–	–	–	0
25	80	2.7	–	–	350	600	–	60	.23	.26	4	.32	–	4
15	20	.72	–	–	340	380	–	100	.09	.14	1.6	–	–	5
70	39	1.7	–	–	350	610	–	75	.19	.18	4	–	–	6
65	56	2.3	–	–	390	800	–	38	.52	.39	5.9	–	–	3
25	40	.72	–	–	360	430	–	300	–	–	–	–	–	36
5	300	1.8	–	–	260	800	–	350	.23	.26	3	.18	–	18
0	0	0	–	–	5	130	–	50	–	–	–	–	–	0
35	450	1.4	–	–	420	630	–	200	.3	.51	3	.06	–	12
25	350	1.8	–	–	490	650	–	350	.3	.51	3	.2	–	21
35	300	1.8	–	–	470	630	–	250	.3	.51	3	.06	–	18
35	400	1.8	–	–	420	710	–	200	.23	.51	3	–	–	15
5	20	1.1	–	–	80	280	–	–	.06	.07	.4	–	–	1
5	65	.6	–	–	120	290	–	14	.03	.02	.3	.08	–	1
10	19	.9	–	–	120	150	–	14	.06	.03	.2	.03	–	1
0	40	0	–	–	65	150	–	0	–	–	–	–	–	0
20	80	.36	–	–	140	210	–	40	.06	.07	1.6	–	–	2
10	80	1.08	–	–	170	200	–	0	–	–	–	–	–	0
5	60	1.1	–	–	210	190	–	–	.03	.03	.4	.06	–	5
6	500	6.3	140	350	600	288	5.25	–	.53	.6	7	.7	140	21
6	500	6.3	140	350	750	336	5.25	–	.53	.6	7	.7	140	21
6	500	6.3	140	350	800	336	5.25	–	.53	.6	7	.7	140	21
6	500	6.3	140	350	750	336	5.25	–	.53	.6	7	.7	140	21
6	500	6.3	140	350	830	312	5.25	–	.53	.6	7	.7	140	21
6	449	5.67	125	315	502	215	4.82	314	.48	.54	6.24	.62	125	19
6	449	5.67	125	315	502	188	4.82	314	.48	.54	6.24	.62	125	19
5	500	6.3	140	350	540	240	5.25	–	.53	.6	7	.7	140	21
4	500	6.3	140	350	520	220	5.25	–	.53	.6	7	.7	140	21
5	500	6.3	140	350	1490	220	5.25	–	.53	.6	7	.7	140	21
5	500	6.3	140	350	520	220	5.25	–	.53	.6	7	.7	140	21
5	500	6.3	140	350	350	220	5.25	–	.53	.6	7	.7	140	21
5	150	2.71	8	50	140	35	.01	–	.22	.25	3	.3	60	9
5	150	2.71	8	150	110	40	.01	–	.22	.25	3	.3	60	9
5	150	2.71	8	150	125	35	.01	–	.22	.25	3	.3	60	9
5	2	2.71	–	–	–	30	–	–	–	–	–	–	–	9

(For purposes of calculations, use "0" for t, < 1, < .1, < .01, etc.)

Table I–1
Food Composition

Computer Code Number	Food Description	Measure	Wt (g)	H₂O (%)	Ener (cal)	Prot (g)	Carb (g)	Dietary Fiber (g)	Fat (g)	Fat Breakdown (g)		
										Sat	Mono	Poly
BABY FOODS												
1720	Apple juice	4 fl oz	125	88	59	0	15	–	< 1	–	–	–
1721	Applesauce, strained	1 tbs	14	89	6	< 1	2	–	< 1	–	–	–
1716	Carrots, strained	1 tbs	14	92	4	< 1	1	–	< 1	–	–	–
1718	Cereal, mixed, millk added	1 tbs	14	75	16	1	2	–	< 1	–	–	–
1719	Cereal, rice, milk added	1 tbs	14	75	16	1	2	–	< 1	–	–	–
1723	Chicken and noodles, strained	1 tbs	14	88	7	< 1	1	–	< 1	–	–	–
1722	Peas, strained	1 tbs	14	88	6	1	1	–	< 1	–	–	–
1717	Teething biscuits	1 ea	11	6	43	1	8	–	< 1	–	–	–

(Computer code number is for West Diet Analysis program)

Chol (mg)	Calc (mg)	Iron (mg)	Magn (mg)	Phos (mg)	Pota (mg)	Sodi (mg)	Zinc (mg)	VT-A (RE)	Thia (mg)	Ribo (mg)	Niac (mg)	V-B6 (mg)	Fola (μg)	VT-C (mg)
–	5	.71	4	6	114	4	.04	3	.01	.02	.1	.04	< 1	72
–	1	.03	< 1	1	10	< 1	< .01	< 1	< .01	< .01	.01	< .01	< 1	6
–	3	.05	1	3	28	5	.02	164	< .01	.01	.07	.01	2	1
–	31	1.49	4	20	28	7	.1	3	.06	.08	.82	.01	2	–
–	34	1.73	6	25	27	7	.09	4	.07	.07	.74	.02	1	–
–	3	.06	1	3	6	2	.04	16	< .01	.01	.07	.01	1	< 1
–	3	.14	2	6	16	< 1	.05	8	.01	.01	.14	.01	4	1
–	29	.39	4	18	36	40	.1	1	.03	.06	.48	.01	2	1

(For purposes of calculations, use "0" for t, < 1, < .1, < .01, etc.)

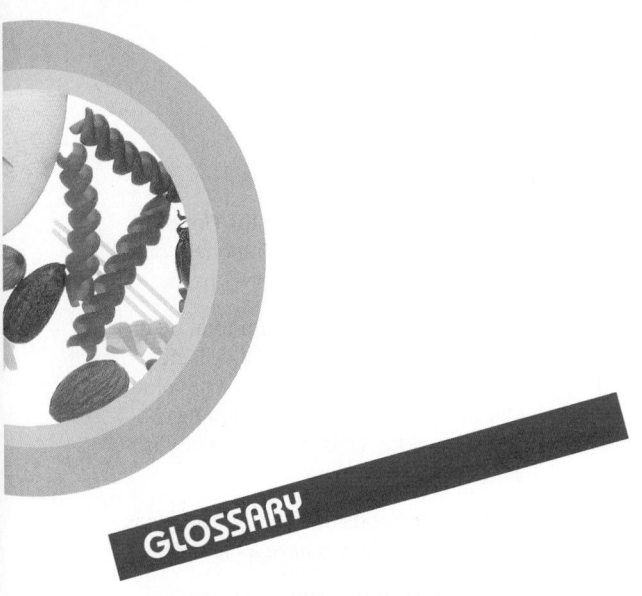

ACCREDITATION approval; in the case of hospitals or university departments, approval by a professional organization of the educational program offered. There are phony accrediting agencies; the genuine ones are listed in a directory called *Accredited Institutions of Postsecondary Education.*

ACESULFAME K (AY-see-sul-fame) a derivative of acetoacetic acid approved for use in the United States in 1988 (approval in Canada is still under consideration). Since it is not metabolized by the body, acesulfame K does not contribute calories and is excreted from the body unchanged. It is currently approved for use in more than 70 countries and found in more than 100 international products, including chewing gums, gelatins, nondairy creamers, powdered drink mixes, and puddings.

ACETALDEHYDE (ass-et-AL-duh-hide) a substance to which drinking alcohol (ethanol) is metabolized.

ACID-BASE BALANCE equilibrium between acid and base concentrations in the body fluids.

ACIDOSIS (a-sih-DOSE-iss) blood acidity above normal, indicating excess acid.

ACIDS compounds that release hydrogens in a watery solution; acids have a low pH.

ACQUIRED IMMUNE DEFICIENCY SYNDROME (AIDS) an immune system disorder caused by the human immunodeficiency virus (HIV). Its attack on the individual's immune cells (T-cells) results in a decreased ability to fight for-

eign organisms, thus increasing the individual's susceptibility to a variety of opportunistic infections. AIDS is transmitted to a person through direct contact of the person's body fluids with contaminated body fluids. It is most often transmitted through sexual intercourse, contaminated needles, contaminated blood products, or from mother to infant during pregnancy or lactation. Since the early 1980s, AIDS has become a major public health problem.

ACTIVITIES OF DAILY LIVING (ADL) include bathing, dressing, grooming, transferring from bed to chair, going to the bathroom, and feeding oneself.

ADEQUACY characterizes a diet that provides all of the essential nutrients, fiber, and energy (calories) in amounts sufficient to maintain health.

AEROBIC requiring oxygen.

AFLATOXIN a poisonous toxin produced by molds.

AGAVE a plant with spiny-margined leaves and flowers.

ALCOHOL DEHYDROGENASE a liver enzyme that converts ethanol to acetaldehyde. The MEOS also oxidizes alcohol.

ALCOHOLISM a dependency on alcohol marked by compulsive uncontrollable drinking with negative effects on physical health, family relationships, and social health.

ALKALOSIS (al-kah-LOH-sis) blood alkalinity above normal.

ALLYL SULFIDES compounds in garlic that may help lower blood cholesterol levels and protect against some types of cancer.

ALTERNATIVE SWEETENERS nutritive (calorie-containing) sweeteners such as fructose, sorbitol, mannitol, and xylitol.

AMARANTH a golden-colored grain.

AMINE (a-MEEN) **GROUP** the nitrogen-containing portion of an amino acid.

AMINO (a-MEEN-o) **ACIDS** building blocks of protein; each is a compound with an amine group at one end, an acid group at the other, and a distinctive side chain.

ANABOLIC STEROID synthetic male hormones with a chemical structure similar to that of cholesterol; such hormones have wide-ranging effects on body functioning.

ANAEROBIC not requiring oxygen.

ANEMIA any condition in which the blood is unable to deliver oxygen to the cells of the body. Examples include a shortage or abnormality of the red blood cells. Many nutrient deficiencies and diseases can cause anemia.

ANOREXIA NERVOSA literally "nervous lack of appetite"; a disorder (usually seen in teenage girls) involving self-starvation to the extreme.
   an = without
   orexis = appetite

ANTIBODIES large proteins of the blood and body fluids, produced by one type of immune cell in response to invasion of the body by unfamiliar molecules (mostly foreign proteins). Antibodies inactivate the foreign substances and so protect the body. The foreign substances are called antigens.

anti = against
gen = producer

ANTIOXIDANT (anti-OX-ih-dant) a compound that protects other compounds from oxygen by itself reacting with oxygen; a substance, such as a vitamin, that is "anti-oxygen"—that is, it helps to prevent damage done to the body as a result of chemical reactions that involve the use of oxygen.

APPENDICITIS inflammation and/or infection of the appendix, a sac protruding from the large intestine.

APPETITE the psychological desire to find and eat food, experienced as a pleasant sensation, often in the absence of hunger.

APPROPRIATE TECHNOLOGY a technology that utilizes locally abundant resources in preference to locally scarce resources. Developing countries usually have a large labor force and little capital; the appropriate technology would therefore be labor intensive.

AROUSAL heightened activity of certain brain centers associated with excitement and anxiety.

ARTESIAN WATER or **ARTESIAN WELL WATER** water drawn from a well that taps a confined water-bearing rock or rock formation.

ARTIFICIAL SWEETENERS nonnutritive sugar replacements such as acesulfame K, aspartame, and saccharin.

ASPARTAME a dipeptide containing the amino acids aspartic acid and phenylalanine and used in the United States and Canada since 1981. While it is digested as protein and supplies calories, it is so sweet that only small amounts, which contribute negligible calories, are needed to sweeten foods. Thus, it is classified as a nonnutritive

sweetener. Often sold under the trade name NutraSweet, aspartame is blended with lactose and an anticaking agent and sold commercially as Equal.

ATHEROSCLEROSIS (ATH-er-oh-scler-OH-sis) a type of cardiovascular disease; the most common kind of hardening of the arteries characterized by the formation of fatty deposits, or plaques, in their inner walls.

ATHLETIC AMENORRHEA cessation of menstruation associated with strenuous athletic training.

ATROPHIC GASTRITIS an age-related condition characterized by the stomach's inability to produce acid, which in turn leads to vitamin B_{12} deficiencies. In severe cases, the condition limits the ability to make intrinsic factor as well.

ATROPHY a decrease in size in response to disuse.

BAKE to cook in an oven surrounded by heat.

BALANCE a feature of a diet that provides a number of types of foods in balance with one another, such that foods rich in one nutrient do not crowd out of the diet foods that are rich in another nutrient.

BALANCED MEAL a meal containing sufficient but not excessive amounts of foods from each of the food groups and therefore sufficient but not excessive amounts of carbohydrates, fat, protein, vitamins, and minerals.

BALANCE STUDY a laboratory study in which a person is fed a controlled diet to measure the intake and excretion of a nutrient. If the nutrient is not changed in the body and a person excretes more of it than is consumed over time, the person slips into *negative balance.*

BALLISTIC STRETCHES stretches characterized by short, choppy, sometimes painful movements that often pull connective tissues beyond their elastic limits.

BASAL METABOLIC RATE (BMR) the rate at which the body spends energy to

support its basal metabolism. The BMR accounts for the largest component of a person's daily energy (calorie) needs.

BASAL METABOLISM the sum total of all the chemical activities of the cells necessary to sustain life, exclusive of voluntary activities—that is, the ongoing activities of the cells when the body is at rest.

BASES compounds that accept hydrogens from solutions; bases have a high pH.

BEHAVIOR MODIFICATION a process developed by psychologists for helping people make lasting behavior changes.

BENZOCAINE an anesthetic found in gum or candy form that numbs the taste buds and reduces the desire for food.

BERIBERI the thiamin deficiency disease, characterized by irregular heartbeat, paralysis, and extreme wasting of muscle tissue.

BETA-CAROTENE an orange pigment found in plants that is converted into vitamin A inside the body. Beta-carotene is also an antioxidant.

BIALY a flat breakfast roll that is softer than a bagel.

BIFIDUS FACTOR (BIFF-id-us) a factor in colostrum and breast milk that favors the growth in the infant's intestinal tract of the "friendly" bacteria *Lactobacillus bifidus* so that other, less desirable intestinal inhabitants will not flourish.

BILE a mixture of compounds, including cholesterol, made by the liver, stored in the gallbladder, and secreted into the small intestine. Bile emulsifies lipids to ready them for enzymatic digestion and helps transport them into the intestinal wall cells.

BINDERS in foods, chemical compounds that can combine with nutrients (especially minerals) to form complexes the body cannot absorb. Examples of such binders are phytic (FIGHT-ic) acid and oxalic (ox-AL-ic) acid.

BING thin pancakes.

BIOELECTRICAL IMPEDANCE estimation of body fat content made by measuring how quickly electrical current is conducted through the body.

BIOLOGICAL VALUE (BV) a measure of protein quality, assessed by determining how well a given food or food mixture supports nitrogen retention.

BLACK, CUBAN, or **TURTLE BEANS** medium-size black-skinned ovals that have a rich, sweet taste. They are best served in Mexican and Latin American dishes or thick soups and stews.

BLACK-EYED PEAS small and oval shaped, creamy white legumes with a black spot. They have a vegetable flavor with mealy texture. Use in salads with rice and greens.

BLOOD LIPID PROFILE a test that determines the amounts and kinds of lipids in the blood, normally as part of a diagnosis for cardiovascular disease risk.

BODY MASS INDEX (BMI) an index of degree of obesity derived from the height and weight.

BOK CHOY a vegetable with broad, white or greenish-white stalks and dark green leaves; also called Chinese chard.

BOLILLO a roll-like bread often used instead of tortillas or to make sandwiches.

BRAISE to cook by browning in fat and then simmering in a covered container with a little liquid.

BRAN the fibrous protective covering of a whole grain and the chief source of fiber in grain (removed during refining). The bran covering actually includes four outer layers of the whole grain—primarily the *aleurone* and *pericarp* layers.

BROIL to cook quickly over or under a direct source of intense heat, allowing fats to drip away.

BROWN RICE SYRUP similar to honey in taste and consistency; also available as a powder.

BROWN SUGAR white sugar with molasses added; about 95 % pure sucrose.

BUFFERS compounds that help keep a solution's acidity (amount of acid) or alkalinity (amount of base) constant.

BULIMIA NERVOSA, BULIMAREXIA (byoo-LEE-me-uh, byoo-lee-ma-REX-ee-uh) binge eating (literally, "eating like an ox"), known popularly as pigging out. Combined with an intense fear of becoming fat and sometimes followed by self-induced vomiting or the taking of laxatives, this form of eating behavior has also been called the binge-purge syndrome.
buli = ox

BURRITOS warm flour tortillas stuffed with a mixture of egg, meat, beans, and/or avocado.

CAFFEINE a type of compound, called a methylxanthine, found in coffee beans, cola nuts, cocoa beans, and tea leaves. A central nervous system stimulant, caffeine's effects include increasing the heart rate, boosting urine production, and raising the metabolic rate.

CAFFEINE DEPENDENCE SYNDROME dependence on caffeine characterized by at least three of the four following criteria: withdrawal symptoms such as headache and fatigue; caffeine consumption despite knowledge that it may be causing harm; repeated, unsuccessful attempts to cut back on caffeine; and tolerance to caffeine.

CALORIE the unit used to measure energy. Technically, when we see the term *calorie* on food labels or talk about the amount of calories our bodies need, we are referring to *kilocalories* (*kcal*)—the amount of heat required to raise the temperature of one kilogram of water one degree Celsius. Use of the term *kilocalorie*, however, tends to be reserved for laboratories and technical journals. Throughout this book, we will use the term *calorie* rather than kilocalorie.
calor = heat

CALORIE CONTROL control of consumption of energy (calories); a feature of a sound diet plan.

CARBOHYDRATES compounds made of single sugars or multiples of them and composed of carbon, hydrogen, and oxygen atoms.
carbo = carbon (C)
hydrate = water (H_2O)

CARDIOVASCULAR CONDITIONING or **TRAINING EFFECT** the effect of regular exercise on the cardiovascular system—including improvements in heart, lung, and muscle function and increased blood volume.

CARDIOVASCULAR DISEASE (CVD) disease of the heart and blood vessels. The two most common forms of CVD are atherosclerosis and hypertension.

CARRAGEENAN a seaweed derivative used by food manufacturers to add "body" to numerous products, including ice cream, frozen yogurt, and salad dressings.

CASSAVA a starchy root that is never eaten raw because it must be cooked to eliminate its bitter smell.

CELLOPHANE NOODLES thin, translucent noodles made from mung beans.

CENTRAL OBESITY excess fat on the abdomen and around the trunk. Peripheral obesity is excess fat on the arms, thighs, hips, and buttocks.

CHALLAH an egg-containing yeast bread, often braided, and served on the Sabbath and holidays.

CHERIMOYA a fruit with a rough green outer skin and sherbetlike flesh.

CHILAQUILES tortilla casserole often made with eggs or meat.

CHILES RELLENOS roasted mild green chili pepper stuffed with cheese, dipped in egg batter, and fried.

CHINESE BROCCOLI a green leafy vegetable often stir-fried; also called Chinese kale.

CHITTERLINGS (chitlins) pig intestine.

CHLOROFLUOROCARBONS (CFCs) chemicals once used in aerosol sprays and other products and that seem to contribute to the destruction of the earth's ozone layer.

CHLOROPHYLL the green pigment of plants that traps energy from sunlight and uses this energy in photosynthesis (the synthesis of carbohydrate by green plants).

CHOLESTEROL (koh-LESS-ter-all) one of the sterols, manufactured in the body for a variety of purposes and also found in animal-derived foods.

CHORIZO spicy beef or pork sausage.

CHOY SUM a bright-green vegetable commonly stir-fried; also called field mustard or Chinese flowering cabbage.

CHYLOMICRON (KIGH-loh-MY-cron) a type of lipoprotein (very low in density) made by the cells of the intestinal wall; serves as a means of transporting newly digested fat from the intestine through lymph and blood. Chylomicrons donate lipids to all body cells, and the remnants are ultimately cleared from the blood by liver cells.

CIRRHOSIS (seer-OH-sis) advanced liver disease, often associated with alcoholism, in which liver cells have died and hardened and have permanently lost their function.

CLUB SODA artificially carbonated water containing added salts and minerals.

COENZYMES enzyme helpers; small molecules that interact with enzymes and enable them to do their work. Many coenzymes are made from water-soluble vitamins.

COFACTOR a mineral element that, like a coenzyme, works with an enzyme to facilitate a chemical reaction.

COLLAGEN the characteristic protein of connective tissue.
 kolla = glue
 gennan = to produce

COLON CANCER cancer of the large intestine (colon), the terminal portion of the digestive tract (see Appendix B).

COLOSTRUM (co-LAHS-trum) a milklike secretion from the breast, rich in protective factors, present during the first day or so after delivery and before milk appears.

COMPLEMENTARY PROTEINS two or more food proteins whose amino acid assortments complement each other in such a way that the essential amino acids limited in or missing from each are supplied by the others.

COMPLETE PROTEINS proteins containing all the essential amino acids in the right proportion relative to need. The *quality* of a food protein is judged by the proportions of essential amino acids that it contains relative to our needs. Animal proteins are the highest in quality.

COMPLEX CARBOHYDRATES long chains of sugars (glucose) arranged as starch or fiber. Also called polysaccharides.
 poly = many
 saccharides = sugar unit

COMPULSIVE OVEREATING an eating disorder characterized by uncontrolled chronic episodes of overeating (binge eating) without other symptoms of eating disorders. If the episodes of binge eating occur at least twice a week on average for a period of six months or more, the behavior is referred to as binge-eating disorder.

CONCENTRATED FRUIT JUICE SWEETENER a concentrated sugar syrup made from dehydrated, deflavored fruit juice, commonly grape juice, used to sweeten products such as jams and cookies that can then claim to be "all fruit."

CONFECTIONERS SUGAR finely powdered sucrose; 99.9% pure sucrose.

CONSTIPATION hardness and dryness of bowel movements associated with discomfort in passing them.

CONTAMINANTS potentially dangerous substances, such as lead, that can accidentally get into foods.

CONTAMINATION IRON iron found in foods as the result of contamination by inorganic iron salts from iron cookware, iron-containing soils, and the like.

CORN SWEETENERS corn syrup and sugars derived from corn.

CORN SYRUP a syrup produced by the action of enzymes on cornstarch; contains mostly glucose.

CORRESPONDENCE SCHOOL a school from which courses can be taken and degrees granted by mail. Schools that are accredited offer respectable courses and degrees.

CORTICAL BONE the dense outer ivory-like layer of bone that provides an exterior shell over trabecular bone.

CRETINISM (CREE-tin-ism) severe mental and physical retardation of an infant caused by iodine deficiency during pregnancy.

CROSS-CONTAMINATION the inadvertent transfer of bacteria from one food to another that occurs, for instance, by chopping vegetables on the same cutting board used to skin poultry.

CULTURE knowledge, beliefs, customs, laws, morals, art, and literature acquired by members of a society and passed along to succeeding generations.

DAILY VALUES the amount of fat, sodium, fiber, and other nutrients health experts say should make up a healthful diet. The % Daily Values that appear on food labels tell you the percentage of a nutrient that a serving of the food contributes to a healthful diet.

DEGENERATIVE DISEASE chronic disease characterized by deterioration of body organs as a result of misuse and neglect; poor eating habits, smoking, lack of exercise, and other lifestyle habits often contribute to degenerative diseases, including heart disease, cancer, osteoporosis, and diabetes.

DELANEY CLAUSE a provision in the 1958 Food Additives Amendment that prohibits manufacturers from using any substance that is known to cause cancer in animals or humans at any dose level.

DENATURATION the change in shape of a protein brought about by heat, alcohol, acids, bases, or other agents. Many well-known poisons are salts of heavy metals such as mercury and silver; these salts alter the structure of proteins wherever they touch them.

DENTAL CARIES decay of the teeth, or cavities.
  caries = rottenness

DENTAL PLAQUE a colorless film, consisting of bacteria and their by-products, that is constantly forming on the teeth.

DESIGNER FOODS foods "fortified" with phytochemicals or plants bred to contain high levels of phytochemicals; also known as "future foods."

DEXTROSE another name for glucose.

DIABETES (dye-uh-BEET-eez) a disorder (technically termed *diabetes mellitus*) characterized by insufficiency or relative ineffectiveness of insulin, which renders a person unable to regulate the blood glucose level normally.

DIM SUM steamed or fried dumplings stuffed with pork, shrimp, beef, sweet paste, or preserves and steamed or fried.

DIPEPTIDES (dye-PEP-tides) protein fragments two amino acids long. A peptide is a strand of amino acids.

DIPLOMA MILL a correspondence school that grinds out degrees—sometimes worth no more than the cost of the paper they are printed on—the way a grain mill grinds out flour.

DISABILITY any restriction on or impairment in performing an activity in the manner or within the range considered normal for a human being.

DIURETICS (dye-you-RET-ics) medications causing increased water excretion.
  dia = through
  ouron = urine

DIVERTICULOSIS (dye-ver-tic-you-LOCE-iss) outpocketings of weakened areas of the intestinal wall, like blowouts in a tire, that can rupture, causing dangerous infections.

DRINK a dose of any alcoholic beverage that delivers one-half ounce of pure ethanol:
  5 ounces of wine
  12 ounces of beer
  1.5 ounces of hard liquor (whiskey, gin, rum, or vodka)

DRUGS substances that can modify one or more of the body's functions.

DYSENTERY (DISS-en-terry) an infection of the digestive tract that causes diarrhea.

EATING DISORDER general term for several conditions (anorexia nervosa, bulimia nervosa, bulimarexia, compulsive overeating, obesity, and excessive dieting) that exhibit an excessive preoccupation with body weight, a fear of body fatness, and a distorted body image.

ECLAMPSIA a severe extension of preeclampsia characterized by convulsions.

EDEMA (eh-DEEM-uh) swelling of body tissue caused by leakage of fluid from the blood vessels, seen in (among other conditions) protein deficiency.

ELECTROLYTES compounds that partially dissociate in water to form ions; examples are sodium, potassium, and chloride.

EMPTY-CALORIE FOODS a phrase used to indicate that a food supplies calories but negligible nutrients. When many empty-calorie foods are eaten regularly, they displace nutrient-dense foods from the diet and contribute to both poor nutritional health and obesity.

EMULSIFIER a substance that mixes with both fat and water and can break fat globules into small droplets, thereby suspending fat in water.

ENDOSPERM the bulk of the edible part of a grain; contains starch grains embedded in a protein matrix.

ENDURANCE the ability to sustain an effort for a long time. One type, muscle endurance, is the ability of a muscle to contract repeatedly within a given time without becoming exhausted. Another type, cardiovascular endurance, is the ability of the cardiovascular system to sustain effort over a period of time.

ENERGY the capacity to do work, such as moving or heating something.

ENRICHED refers to a process by which the B vitamins thiamin, riboflavin, and niacin and the mineral iron are added to refined grains and grain products at levels specified by law. After enrichment, a grain product has approximately the same amount of thiamin, niacin, and iron and about twice as much riboflavin as the original whole-grain product had.

ENRICHED FOODS wheat flour, cornmeal, grits, and polished rice.

ENTEROTOXIN a toxic compound, produced by microorganisms, that harms the gastrointestinal tract.
  entero = intestine

ENZYMES protein catalysts. A catalyst facilitates a chemical reaction without itself being altered in the process.

EOSINOPHILIA-MYALGIA (ee-o-sin-o-FIL-ia my-AL-jia) **SYNDROME (EMS)** a disease characterized primarily by a high level of eosinophils, a type of white blood cell, as well as myalgia—that is, muscle pain and weakness.

EPITHELIAL (ep-ih-THEE-lee-ul) **TISSUE** those cells that form the outer surface of the body and line the body cavities and the principal passageways leading to the exterior. Examples include the cornea, digestive tract lining, respiratory tract lining, and skin.

ERGOGENIC AIDS anything that helps to increase the capacity to work or exercise.
  ergo = work
  genic = give rise to

ESSENTIAL AMINO ACIDS amino acids that cannot be synthesized by the body or that cannot be synthesized in amounts sufficient to meet physiological need.

ESSENTIAL FATTY ACID a fatty acid that cannot be synthesized in the body in amounts sufficient to meet physiological need.

ESSENTIAL NUTRIENTS nutrients that must be obtained from food because the body cannot make them for itself.

ESTROGEN a major female hormone—important in connection with nutrition because it maintains calcium balance and because its secretion abruptly declines at menopause.

ETHNIC CUISINE the traditional foods eaten by the people of a particular culture.

EUPHORIA (you-FORE-ee-uh) a feeling of great well-being that people often seek through the use of drugs such as alcohol.

eu = good
phoria = bearing

EXCHANGE LISTS lists of foods with portion sizes specified; the foods on a single list are similar with respect to nutrient and calorie content and so can be mixed and matched in the diet.

EXERCISE STRESS TEST a test that monitors heart function during exercise to detect abnormalities that may not show up under ordinary conditions; exercise physiologists and trained physicians or health-care professionals can administer the test.

EXTERNAL CUE THEORY the theory that some people eat in response to such external factors as the presence of food or the time of day rather than to such internal factors as hunger.

FAMINE widespread lack of access to food caused by natural disasters, political factors, or war; characterized by a large number of deaths due to starvation and malnutrition.

FARTLEK speed play; alternating periods of fast and slow exercise.

FAT CELL THEORY states that during the growing years, fat cells respond to overfeeding by producing additional fat cells (hyperplastic obesity); the number of fat cells eventually becomes fixed, and overfeeding from this point on causes the body to enlarge existing fat cells (hypertrophic obesity).

Hypertropic obesity is the more common type, and is usually seen in adults.

FATS lipids that are solid at room temperature.

FATTY ACIDS basic units of fat composed of chains of carbon atoms with an acid group at one end and hydrogen atoms attached all along their length.

FATTY LIVER an early stage of liver disease seen in several conditions (kwashiorkor, alcoholic liver disease), characterized by accumulation of fat in the liver cells.

FETAL ALCOHOL SYNDROME (FAS) the cluster of symptoms seen in an infant or child whose mother consumed excess alcohol during pregnancy, including retarded growth, impaired development of the central nervous system, and facial malformations.

FIBERS the indigestible residues of food, composed mostly of polysaccharides. Thus fibers are the nonstarch polysaccharides in foods. The term *dietary fiber* refers to nutritionally significant fiber in food—that is, the fiber that resists human digestive enzymes.

FIRST AMENDMENT the amendment to the U.S. Constitution that guarantees freedom of the press.

FITNESS the body's ability to meet physical demands, composed of four components: flexibility, strength, muscle endurance, and cardiovascular endurance.

FLEXIBILITY the ability to bend or extend without injury; flexibility depends on the elasticity of the muscles, tendons, and ligaments and on the condition of the joints.

FLUID BALANCE distribution of fluid among body compartments.

FLUOROSIS (floor-OH-sis) discoloration of the teeth from ingestion of too much fluoride during tooth development.

FOAM CELLS macrophage cells from the immune system containing scavenged

oxidized LDL-cholesterol that are thought to initiate plaque formation and the development of atherosclerosis.

FOOD ADDITIVE any substance added to food, including substances used in the production, processing, treatment, packaging, transportation, or storage of food.

FOOD BANKS nonprofit community organizations that collect surplus commodities from the government and edible but often unmarketable foods from private industry for use by nonprofit charities, institutions, and feeding programs at nominal cost.

FOODBORNE ILLNESS or **FOOD POISONING** illness occurring as a result of eating food contaminated with disease-producing microorganisms, such as bacteria, viruses, or parasites, or toxic substances such as chemicals.

FOODBORNE INFECTION illness caused by eating a food containing bacteria or other microorganisms capable of growing and thriving in a person's tissues.

FOOD COMPOSITION TABLES tables that list the nutrient profile of commonly eaten foods.

FOOD GROUP PLAN a diet-planning tool, such as the Food Guide Pyramid, that groups foods according to similar origin and nutrient content and then specifies the number of foods from each group that a person should eat.

FOOD INSECURITY the inability to acquire or consume an adequate quality or sufficient quantity of food in socially acceptable ways, or the uncertainty that one will be able to do so.

FOOD INTOXICATION illness caused by eating food that contains a harmful toxin.

FOOD PANTRIES centers usually attached to existing nonprofit agencies that distribute bags or boxes of groceries to people experiencing food emergencies. Foods distributed by pantries are prepared and consumed elsewhere. Referrals or proof of need is often required. There are roughly two food pantries to every soup kitchen.

FOOD SECURITY access by all people at all times to enough food for an active and healthy life. Food security has two aspects: ensuring that adequate food supplies are available and ensuring that households whose members suffer from undernutrition have the ability to acquire food, either by producing it themselves or by being able to purchase it.

FORTIFIED FOOD a food to which manufacturers have added 10 percent or more of the Daily Value for a particular nutrient.

FORTIFIED FOODS foods to which nutrients have been added. Examples: margarine with added vitamin A, milk with added vitamin D, certain brands of orange juice, and bread with added calcium.

FRAME SIZE the size of a person's bones and musculature. A person with a large frame can weigh more than one the same height with a small frame without increased risks.

FREE RADICAL highly toxic compound created in the body as a result of chemical reactions that involve oxygen. Environmental pollutants such as cigarette smoke and ozone also prompt the formation of free radicals.

FROM A COMMUNITY WATER SYSTEM or **FROM A MUNICIPAL SOURCE** statement that must appear on bottles containing water derived from a municipal water supply. The phrase must conspicuously precede or follow the name of the brand.

FRUCTOSE (FROOK-toce) fruit sugar—the sweetest of the single sugars. Another single sugar, galactose (ga-LACK-toce), occurs bonded to glucose in the sugar of milk. A double sugar is known as a disaccharide.
  di = two

FUSION CUISINE a term used to describe food that combines the elements of two or more cuisines—say, European and Oriental—to create a new one.

GARBANZO BEANS or **CHICK-PEAS** large, round, and tan-colored legumes. They have a nutty flavor and crunchy texture. Use in soups and stews and puréed for dips.

GASTROPLASTY surgery on the stomach (also called stomach stapling) that reduces its volume to less than two ounces (the size of a shot glass) to prevent overeating.

GELFILTE FISH a chopped fish mixture often made with pike and whitefish as well as matzoh crumbs, eggs, and seasonings.

GENETIC ENGINEERING the process of altering the genes of a plant in an effort to create a new plant with different traits. This process of recombining genes is also known as recombinant DNA.

GERM the nutrient-rich and fat-dense inner part of a whole grain (removed during refining).

GESTATIONAL DIABETES the appearance of abnormal glucose tolerance during pregnancy, with a return to normal following pregnancy.

GLUCAGON (GLUE-cuh-gon) insulin's opposing hormone, released by the pancreas when blood glucose is too low; it draws forth glucose and other fuels from storage, making them available to supply energy to cells.

GLUCOSE (GLOO-koce) the building block of carbohydrate; a single sugar used in both plant and animal tissues as quick-energy currency. A single sugar is known as a monosaccharide.
  mono = one

GLUTINOUS RICE short-grained, opaque, white rice that turns sticky when cooked.

GLYCEROL (GLISS-er-all) an organic compound, three carbons long, of interest here because it serves as the backbone for triglycerides.

GLYCOGEN (GLY-co-gen) a polysaccharide composed of chains of glucose, manufactured in the body and stored in liver and

muscle. As a storage form of glucose, glycogen can be broken down by the liver to maintain a constant blood glucose level when carbohydrate intake is inadequate.

GOBI an acronym formed from the elements of UNICEF's Child Survival campaign—**G**rowth charts, **O**ral rehydration therapy, **B**reast milk, and **I**mmunization.

GOITER (GOY-ter) enlargement of the thyroid gland caused by iodine deficiency.

GRANULATED SUGAR common table sugar; crystalline sucrose—99.9% pure sucrose.

GRAS (GENERALLY RECOGNIZED AS SAFE) LIST a list of ingredients, established by the FDA, that had long been in use and were believed safe. The list is subject to revision as new facts become known.

GRAZING eating small amounts of food at intervals throughout the day rather than —or in addition to—eating regular meals.

GREAT NORTHERN BEANS medium white and kidney shaped beans. Enjoy the delicate flavor and firm texture in salads, soups, and main dishes.

GRITS coarsely ground cornmeal.

GROUND WATER water that comes from an underground body of water that does not come into contact with any surface water.

GUAVA a sweet juicy fruit with green or yellow skin and red or yellow flesh.

HAZARD state of danger; used to refer to any circumstance in which harm is possible.

HDL (high-density lipoprotein) carries cholesterol in the blood back to the liver for recycling or disposal.

HEALTH CLAIM a statement on the food label linking the nutritional profile of a food to a reduced risk of a particular disease, such as osteoporosis or cancer. Manufacturers must adhere to strict government guidelines when making such claims.

HEALTH FRAUD conscious deceit practiced for profit, such as the promotion of a false or an unproven product or therapy.

HEAT STROKE an acute and dangerous reaction to heat buildup in the body.

HEAVY METALS any of a number of mineral ions, such as mercury and lead, so named because of their relatively high atomic weight. Many heavy metals are poisonous.

HEME (HEEM) **IRON** the iron-holding part of the hemoglobin protein, found in meat, fish, and poultry. About 40% of the iron in meat, fish, and poultry is bound into heme. Meat, fish, and poultry also contain a factor (MFP factor) other than heme that promotes the absorption of iron, even of the iron from other foods eaten at the same time as the meat.

HEMOGLOBIN (HEEM-oh-globe-in) the oxygen-carrying protein of the blood; found in the red blood cells.
  hemo = blood
  globin = spherical protein

HEMORRHOIDS (HEM-or-oids) swollen, hardened (varicose) veins in the rectum, usually caused by the pressure resulting from constipation.

HIGH-FRUCTOSE CORN SYRUP (HFCS) the predominant sweetener used in processed foods and beverages; contains mostly fructose, with some glucose and maltose.

HOMINY hulled, dried corn kernels with certain parts removed.

HOMOCYSTEINE a chemical that appears to be toxic to the blood vessels of the heart. High blood levels of homocysteine have been associated with low blood levels of vitamin B_{12}, vitamin B_6, and folate.

HONEY primarily a mixture of glucose and fructose made by bees from the sucrose in nectar.

HORMONES chemical messengers. Hormones are secreted by a variety of glands in the body in response to altered conditions. Each affects one or more target tissues or organs and elicits specific responses to restore normal conditions.

HUNGER the physiological drive to find and eat food, experienced as an unpleasant sensation.

HUSK the outer, inedible covering of a grain.

HYDROGENATION (high-droh-gen-AY-shun) the process of adding hydrogen to unsaturated fat to make it more solid and more resistant to chemical change.

HYDROSTATIC WEIGHING or **UNDERWATER WEIGHING** a weighing method in which the less a person weighs underwater compared to the person's out-of-water weight, the greater the proportion of body fat (fat is less dense or more buoyant than lean tissue).

HYPERGLYCEMIA an abnormally high blood glucose concentration, often a symptom of both types of diabetes.

HYPERTENSION sustained high blood pressure.
  hyper = too much
  tension = pressure

HYPERTROPHY an increase in size in response to use.

HYPOGLYCEMIA (HIGH-po-gligh-SEEM-ee-uh) an abnormally low blood glucose concentration—below about 60 to 70 mg/100 ml.

HYPOTHALAMUS (high-poh-THALL-ah-mus) a part of the brain that senses a variety of conditions in the blood, such as temperature, salt content, and glucose content, and then signals other parts of the brain or body to change those conditions when necessary.

IMMUNITY specific disease resistance derived from the immune system's memory of prior exposure to specific disease agents and its ability to mount a swift response against them.

INCIDENTAL FOOD ADDITIVES (or indirect additives) substances that accidentally get into food as a result of contact with it during growing, processing, packaging, storing, or some other stage before the food is consumed.

INCOMPLETE PROTEIN a protein lacking or low in one or more of the essential amino acids.

INGREDIENTS LIST a listing of the ingredients in a food, with items listed in descending order of predominance by weight. All food labels are required to bear an ingredients list.

INORGANIC being or composed of matter other than plant or animal.

INSOLUBLE FIBER includes the fiber types called cellulose, hemicellulose, and lignin; insoluble fibers do not dissolve in water.

INSULIN a hormone secreted by the pancreas in response to high blood glucose levels; it assists cells in drawing glucose from the blood.

INTEGRATED PEST MANAGEMENT the use of biological controls, crop rotation, genetic engineering, and other tactics to reduce chemical use in the growing of crops.

INTENTIONAL FOOD ADDITIVES substances intentionally added to food. Examples include nutrients, colors, spices, and herbs.

INTESTINAL FLORA the normal bacterial inhabitants of the digestive tract.
  flora = plant inhabitants

INTRINSIC FACTOR a compound made in the stomach that is necessary for the body's absorption of vitamin B_{12}.

INVERT SUGAR a mixture of glucose and fructose formed by splitting sucrose in processing; sold in liquid form and used as an additive to prevent crystallization of sucrose in candies and other confections.

IONS (EYE-ons) electrically charged particles, such as sodium (positively charged) and chloride (negatively charged).

IRON-DEFICIENCY ANEMIA a reduction of the number and size of red blood cells and a loss of their color because of iron deficiency.

IRON OVERLOAD a condition in which the body contains more iron than it needs or can handle; excess iron is toxic and can damage the liver.

IRRADIATION the process of exposing a substance to low doses of radiation to kill insects, bacteria, and other potentially harmful microorganisms.

ISOFLAVONES compounds found in many fruits, vegetables, and soy-based foods that are thought to play a role in fighting breast cancer by blocking the action of the hormone estrogen.

JICAMA a crisp, bean root vegetable that is tan outside and white inside and is always eaten raw; jicama is as popular in Mexico as the potato is in the United States.

JUJUBE Chinese date.

KASHA cracked buckwheat, barley, millet, or wheat that is served as a cooked cereal or potato substitute.

KASHRUT biblical ordinances regarding which foods are fit to eat.

KETOSIS (kee-TOE-sis) an adaptation of the body to prolonged (several days') fasting or carbohydrate restriction: body fat is converted to ketones, which can be used as fuel for some brain cells.

KIDNEY BEANS large, red, and kidney-shaped beans (the white variety is called cannellini). They have a bland taste and soft texture but tough skins. Use in chili, bean stews, and Mexican dishes for red; Italian dishes for white.

KNISH a potato pastry filled with ground meat, potato, or kasha.

KOSHER fit, proper, or in accordance with religious law.

KWASHIORKOR (kwash-ee-OR-core) a deficiency disease caused by inadequate protein in the presence of adequate food energy.

LACTOFERRIN (lak-toe-FERR-in) a factor in breast milk that binds iron and keeps it from supporting the growth of the infant's intestinal bacteria.

LACTOSE a double sugar composed of glucose and galactose; commonly known as milk sugar.

LACTOSE INTOLERANCE inability to digest milk sugar as a result of a lack of the necessary enzyme lactase; a genetic flaw that can occur at any age. Symptoms include nausea, abdominal pain, diarrhea, or excessive gas that occurs anywhere from 30 minutes to a couple of hours after consuming milk or milk products.

LDL (low-density lipoprotein) carries cholesterol (much of it synthesized in the liver) to body cells. A high blood cholesterol level usually reflects high LDL.

LECITHIN (LESS-ih-thin) a phospholipid, a major constituent of cell membranes, manufactured by the liver and also found in many foods.

LEGUMES (leg-GYOOMS) plants of the bean and pea family having roots with nodules that contain bacteria that can trap nitrogen from the air in the soil and make it into compounds that become part of the seed. The seeds are rich in high-quality protein compared with those of most other plant foods.

LENTILS These legumes are small, flat, and round. Usually brown colored, lentils also can be green, pink, or red. They have a mild taste with firm texture. Best used when combined with grains or vegetables in salads, soups, or stews.

LEVULOSE another name for fructose.

LIFESTYLE DISEASES conditions that may be aggravated by modern lifestyles that include too little exercise, poor diets, and excessive drinking and smoking. Lifestyle diseases are also referred to as diseases of affluence.

LIMA or **BUTTER BEANS** limas are soft and mealy in texture. They are flat, oval shaped, and white tinged with green. The smaller variety has a milder taste. Use in soups and stews.

LIMITING AMINO ACID a term given to the essential amino acid in shortest supply (relative to the body's need) in a food protein; it therefore *limits* the

body's ability to make its own proteins.

LINOLEIC (lin-oh-LAY-ic) **ACID, LINOLENIC** (lin-oh-LEN-ic) **ACID** polyunsaturated fatty acids, essential for human beings.

LIPIDS a family of compounds that includes triglycerides (fats and oils), phospholipids (lecithin), and sterols (cholesterol).

LIPOPROTEINS (LIP-oh-PRO-teens) clusters of lipids associated with protein that serve as transport vehicles for lipids in blood and lymph. The four main types of lipoproteins are chylomicrons, VLDL, LDL and HDL.

LIPOSUCTION a type of surgery (also called lipectomy) that vacuums out fat cells that have accumulated, typically in the buttocks and thighs. If the person continues to eat more calories than are expended through physical activity, fat will return to the fat cells that remain in those regions.

LITCHI small, round fruits with orange-red skin and opaque, white flesh; also called litchee or lychee.

LONGAN a small, round fruit with smooth brown skin and clear pulp.

LOW BIRTHWEIGHT (LBW) a birthweight of 5½ lb (2,500 g) or less, used as a predictor of poor health in the newborn and as a probable indicator of poor nutrition status of the mother during and/or before pregnancy. Normal birthweight for a full-term baby is 6½ to 8¾ lb (about 3,000 to 4,000 g). LBW infants are of two different types. Some are premature (they are born early). Others have suffered growth failure in the uterus; they may or may not be born early, but they are small.

LOX smoked salmon.

L-TRYPTOPHAN an essential amino acid that has been sold in tablets, capsules, and powders as a dietary supplement.

LYMPH (LIMF) the body fluid that moves from the bloodstream into tissue spaces and then travels in its own lymphatic vessels, which transport the products of fat digestion toward the heart and eventually drain back into the bloodstream; lymph consists of the same components as blood except red blood cells.

MAJOR MINERAL an essential mineral nutrient found in the human body in amounts greater than 5 grams.

MALNUTRITION any condition caused by an excess, deficiency, or imbalance of calories or nutrients.

MALTITOL, MANNITOL, SORBITOL, XYLITOL sugar alcohols that can be derived from fruits or commercially produced from dextrose; absorbed more slowly and metabolized differently than other sugars in the human body. The sugar alcohols are not readily used by ordinary mouth bacteria and therefore are associated with less cavity formation. Although the sugar alcohols are used as sugar substitutes, they add the same amount of calories as sugar does to a food product. They are found in a wide variety of chewing gums, candies, and dietetic foods.

MALTOSE a double sugar composed of two glucose units.

MANTOU steamed bread.

MAPLE SYRUP a concentrated form of sucrose purified from the sap of the sugar maple tree; maple sugar is made from the syrup.

MARASMUS (ma-RAZ-mus) an energy-deficiency disease; starvation.

MARGIN OF SAFETY from a food safety standpoint, the margin is a zone between the maximum amount of a substance that appears to be safe and the amount allowed in the food supply.

MATZOH a crackerlike bread eaten most often at Passover.

MEAT REPLACEMENT a textured vegetable protein product formulated to look and taste like meat, fish, or poultry. Many of these are designed to match the known nutrient content of animal protein foods.

MEGADOSE a dose of ten or more times the amount normally recommended in the RDA. An overdose is an amount high enough to cause toxicity symptoms. Megadoses taken over a long period often result in an overdose.

MENOPAUSE the time of life at which a woman's menstrual cycle ceases, usually at about 45 to 50 years of age.

MEOS (MICROSOMAL ETHANOL-OXIDIZING SYSTEM) a system of enzymes in the liver that oxidize not only alcohol but also several classes of drugs. (The microsomes are tiny particles of membranes with associated enzymes that can be collected from broken-up cells.)
micro = tiny
soma = body

MFP FACTOR a factor in **M**eat, **F**ish, and **P**oultry that promotes the absorption of nonheme iron present in the same foods or in other foods eaten at the same time.

MILK ALLERGY the most common food allergy; caused by the protein in raw milk. Milk allergy is sometimes overcome by cooking the milk to denature the protein; it is sometimes alleviated by an abstinence from and a gradual reintroduction to milk.

MILK ANEMIA iron-deficiency anemia caused by drinking so much milk that iron-rich foods are displaced from the diet.

MINERALS small, naturally occurring, inorganic, chemical elements; the minerals serve as structural components and in many vital processes in the body.

MINERAL WATER water that is drawn from an underground source and that contains at least 250 parts per million of dissolved solids. If the water contains between 250 and 500 parts per million total dissolved solids, the statement "low mineral content" must appear. If it contains more than 1,500 parts per million, the statement "high mineral content" must appear. If a cup of the water contains at least 20 milligrams of calcium, .36 milligrams of iron, or 5 milligrams of sodium, the product must carry nutrition labeling.

MODERATION the attribute of a diet that provides no unwanted constituent in excess.

MOLASSES a thick brown syrup; a leftover from the process of refining sucrose from sugar cane; blackstrap molasses contains certain minerals—notably iron—picked up from the machinery used to process it.

MONOGLYCERIDE (mon-oh-GLISS-er-ide) one of the products of digestion of lipids; a glycerol molecule with one fatty acid attached to it.

MONOUNSATURATED FAT a triglyceride in which one or more of the fatty acids is monounsaturated.

MONOUNSATURATED FATTY ACID (sometimes abbreviated MUFA) a fatty acid containing one point of unsaturation.

MULTINATIONAL CORPORATIONS international companies with direct investments and/or operative facilities in more than one country. U.S. oil and food companies are examples.

MUTUAL SUPPLEMENTATION the strategy of combining two protein foods in a meal so that each food provides the essential amino acid or amino acids lacking in the other.

NARCOTIC (nar-KOT-ic) any drug that dulls the senses, induces sleep, and becomes addictive with prolonged use.

NATURAL FOOD one that has been altered as little as possible from the original farm-grown state. As used on labels, this term may misleadingly imply unusual power to promote health; it has no legal definition.

NATURAL SWEETENER a term without a legal definition; refers to any sugar or sweetener other than refined table sugar.

NEURAL TUBE DEFECTS birth defects including spina bifida—the incomplete closing of the bony casing around the spinal cord—and anencephaly—a condition in which major parts of the brain are missing.

NEUROTOXIN a poisonous compound that disrupts the nervous system.

neuro = nerve

NIACIN EQUIVALENTS (NEs) the amount of niacin present in food, including the niacin that can theoretically be made from tryptophan contained in the food.

NIGHT BLINDNESS slow recovery of vision following flashes of bright light at night; an early symptom of vitamin A deficiency.

NONHEME IRON the iron found in plant foods.

NURSING BOTTLE SYNDROME (also called baby bottle tooth decay) decay of all the upper and sometimes the back lower teeth that occurs in infants given carbohydrate-containing liquids when they sleep. The syndrome can also develop in babies given bottles of liquid to carry around and sip all day.

NUTRIENT CONTENT CLAIMS claims such as "low-fat" and "low-calorie" used on food labels to help consumers who don't want to scrutinize the Nutrition Facts panel get an idea of a food's nutritional profile. These claims must adhere to specific definitions set forth by the Food and Drug Administration.

NUTRIENT DENSE refers to a food that supplies large amounts of nutrients relative to the number of calories it contains. The higher the level of nutrients and the fewer the number of calories, the more nutrient dense the food is.

NUTRIENTS substances obtained from food and used in the body to promote growth, maintenance, and repair.

NUTRITION FACTS PANEL a detailed breakdown of the nutritional content of a serving of a food that must appear on virtually all packaged foods sold in the United States.

NUTRITIONAL (BREWER'S) YEAST a fortified food supplement containing B vitamins, iron, and protein that can be used to improve the quality of a vegetarian diet.

NUTRITIONIST a person who claims to be capable of advising people about their diets. Some nutritionists are registered dietitians, whereas others are self-described experts whose training is questionable.

OBESITY conventionally defined as weight 20% or more above the desirable weight for height. Morbid obesity is a weight of at least 100 pounds above "ideal" weight for height.

OILS lipids that are liquid at normal room temperature.

OLESTRA an artificial fat derived from vegetable oils and sugar combined in such a way that the body cannot break them down. Sold under the brand name Olean®, olestra does not contribute calories to food. It can, however, prevent absorption of some nutrients. Thus, the FDA requires all products made with it to bear this warning: "This Product Contains Olestra. Olestra may cause abdominal cramping and loose stools. Olestra inhibits the absorption of some vitamins and nutrients. Vitamins A, D, E, and K have been added."

OMEGA the last letter—the far end—of the Greek alphabet (ω), used by chemists to refer to the position of the end-most double bond in a fatty acid. The omega-6 fatty acids have their end-most double bonds after the sixth carbon in the chain; the omega-3 acids, after the third.

OPPORTUNISTIC INFECTIONS infections produced by organisms that do not affect people whose immune systems are working normally. An example is the unusual form of pneumonia caused by *Pneumocystis carinii*, often seen in individuals with AIDS.

ORAL REHYDRATION THERAPY (ORT) the treatment of dehydration (usually due to diarrhea caused by infectious disease) with an oral solution; ORT as developed by UNICEF is intended to enable a mother to mix a simple solution for her child from substances that she has at home.

ORGANIC of, related to, or containing carbon compounds.

ORGANIC HALOGENS compounds that contain one or more of a class of atoms called halogens, including fluorine, chlorine, iodine, or bromine.

ORIENTAL RADISH large, cylindrically shaped vegetables with smooth skin; also called daikon.

OSTEOMALACIA (os-tee-o-mal-AY-shuh) the disease resulting from vitamin D deficiency in adults. (Its counterpart in children is called rickets.) Osteomalacia can also be caused by calcium deficiency (see Chapter 7); it is characterized by bowed legs and a curved spine.

OSTEOPOROSIS (OSS-tee-oh-pore-OH-sis) also known as adult bone loss; a disease in which the bones become porous and fragile.

osteo = bones
poros = porous

OVERLOAD an extra physical demand placed on the body. A principle of training is that for a body system to improve, its workload must be increased by increments over time.

OVERNUTRITION calorie or nutrient overconsumption severe enough to cause disease or increased risk of disease; a form of malnutrition.

OVERWEIGHT conventionally defined as weight between 10% and 20% above the desirable weight for height.

OXIDIZED LDL-CHOLESTEROL (o-LDL) the cholesterol in LDLs that is attacked (oxidized) by reactive oxygen molecules inside the walls of the arteries; o-LDL is taken up by scavenger cells which are deposited in arterial plaque.

PASTEURIZATION the process of sterilizing food via heat treatment.

PELLAGRA (pell-AY-gra) niacin deficiency characterized by diarrhea, inflammation of the skin, and, in severe cases, mental disorders.

PEPTIDE BOND a bond that connects one

PEPTIDE BOND a bond that connects one amino acid with another.

PERIODONTAL DISEASE inflammation or degeneration of the tissues that surround and support the teeth.

PESTICIDES chemicals applied intentionally to plants, including foods, to prevent or eliminate pest damage. Pests include all living organisms that destroy or spoil foods: bacteria, molds and fungi, insects, and rats and other rodents, to name a few.

pH the concentration of hydrogen ions. The lower the pH, the stronger the acid; pH 2 is a strong acid; pH 7 is neutral; and a pH above 7 is alkaline.

PHENYLKETONURIA an inborn error of metabolism, detectable at birth, in which the body lacks the enzyme needed to convert the amino acid phenylalanine to the amino acid tyrosine. As a result, derivatives of phenylalanine accumulate in the blood and tissues, where they can cause severe damage, including mental retardation.

PHENYLPROPANOLAMINE HYDROCHLORIDE (PPA) a stimulant of the central nervous system available in over–the–counter weight-loss products used to suppress appetite.

PHOSPHOLIPIDS (FOSS-foh-LIP-ids) one of the three main classes of lipids; a lipid similar to a triglyceride but containing phosphorus.

PHOTOSYNTHESIS a process in which plants use the green pigment chlorophyll to trap the energy of the sun and produce glucose from carbon dioxide and water.

PHYTOCHEMICALS chemicals found in plants that are not nutrients but that appear to help fight diseases such as cancer.
  phyto = plant

PICA the craving of nonfood items such as clay, ice, and laundry starch. Pica does not appear to be limited to any particular geographic area, race, sex, culture, or social status.

PIGMENT a molecule capable of absorbing certain wavelengths of light. Pigments in the eye permit us to perceive different colors.

PINTO BEANS medium oval legumes that are mottled beige and brown with an earthy flavor. They are most often used in Mexican dishes, such as refried beans, stews, or dips.

PLACEBO (plah-SEE-bo) a sham treatment given to a control group; an inert, harmless "treatment" that the group's members cannot recognize as different from the real thing. This will minimize the chance that an effect of the treatment will appear to have occurred due to the placebo effect—the healing effect that the belief in the treatment, rather than the treatment itself, often has.

PLACEBO EFFECT an improvement in a person's sense of well-being or physical health in response to the use of a placebo (a substance having no medicinal properties or medicinal effects).

PLACENTA (pla-SEN-tuh) the organ inside the uterus in which the mother's and fetus's circulatory systems intertwine and in which exchange of materials between maternal and fetal blood takes place. The fetus receives nutrients and oxygen across the placenta; the mother's blood picks up carbon dioxide and other waste materials to be excreted via her lungs and kidneys.

PLANTAIN a greenish, starchy banana; because it is starchy even when ripe, it is never eaten raw and is usually pan-fried.

POACH to cook foods (fish, an egg without its shell, etc.) in water near the boiling point.

POINT OF UNSATURATION a site in a molecule where the bonding is such that additional hydrogen atoms can easily be added.

POLYPHARMACY the taking of three or more medications regularly; occurs in one-third of those over 65 years.

POLYUNSATURATED FAT a triglyceride in which one or more of the fatty acids is polyunsaturated.

POLYUNSATURATED FATTY ACID (sometimes abbreviated PUFA) a fatty acid in which two or more points of unsaturation occur.

POSTNATAL after birth.

POVERTY the state of having too little money to meet minimum needs for food, clothing, and shelter. The U.S. Department of Health and Human Services defines the poverty level in the United States as an annual income of $14,350 for a family of four.

PRECURSOR a compound that can be converted into another compound. For example, beta-carotene is a precursor of vitamin A.
  pre = before
  cursor = runner, forerunner

PREECLAMPSIA a condition characterized by hypertension, fluid retention, and protein in the urine.

PREGNANCY-INDUCED HYPERTENSION (PIH) high blood pressure that develops during the second half of pregnancy.

PREMENSTRUAL SYNDROME (PMS) a cluster of physical, emotional, and psychological symptoms that some women experience seven to ten days before menstruating. Symptoms can include acne, anxiety, food cravings (especially for sweets), back pain, breast tenderness, cramps, depression, fatigue, headaches, irritability, moodiness, water retention, and weight gain. Because a clear-cut treatment for the symptoms of PMS has not been identified, women who suffer from the problem rank as prime targets for unproved nutritional remedies for the condition.

PRENATAL prior to birth.

PREPARED AND PERISHABLE FOOD PROGRAMS (PPFPs) nonprofit programs that help to feed people in need by linking sources of unused, unserved cooked and fresh food—such as caterers, restaurants, hotel kitchens, and cafeterias—with social service agencies that serve meals to people who would otherwise go hungry. *Foodchain* is the national network of over 125 community-based PPFPs in 41 states and Canada.

PRO-OXIDANT a compound that stimulates free radical damage.

PROTEIN DIGESTIBILITY-CORRECTED AMINO ACID SCORE (PDCAAS) a measure of protein quality; the PDCAAS takes into account both the amino acid balance of a food and its digestibility.

PROTEIN-ENERGY MALNUTRITION (PEM), also called **PROTEIN-CALORIE MALNUTRITION (PCM)** the world's most widespread malnutrition problem, including both kwashiorkor and marasmus as well as the states in which they overlap.

PROTEIN QUALITY a measure of the essential amino acid content of a protein relative to the essential amino acid needs of the body.

PROTEINS compounds—composed of atoms of carbon, hydrogen, oxygen, and nitrogen—arranged as strands of amino acids. Some amino acids also contain atoms of sulfur.

PROTEIN-SPARING a description of the effect of carbohydrate and fat, which, by being available to yield energy, allow amino acids to be used to build body proteins.

PROTEIN SYNTHESIS the process by which cells assemble amino acids into proteins. Each individual is unique because of minute differences in the ways his or her body proteins are made. The instructions for making every protein in a person's body are transmitted in the genetic information the person receives at conception.

PURIFIED WATER (also know as **DEMINERALIZED WATER, DISTILLED WATER, DEIONIZED WATER,** or **REVERSE OSMOSIS WATER**) water from which all the minerals have been removed, thereby eliminating the possibility that the minerals might corrode, say, a steam iron.

PURSLANE leafy vegetable that can be used in salads or cooked like spinach.

QUACKERY fraud. A quack is a person who practices health fraud.
  quack = to boast loudly

QUESO BLANCO, FRESCO, or **MEXICANO** soft white cheese made of part-skim milk.

RAW SUGAR the first crystals produced during the sugar refining process; not sold in the United States because of the presence of "filth" (dirt, insect fragments).

RECOMMENDED DIETARY ALLOWANCES (RDA) a set of daily nutrient and calorie consumption levels intended to meet the nutritional needs of virtually all healthy people living in the United States.

RECOMMENDED NUTRIENT INTAKES (RNI) nutrition guidelines set forth by the Canadian government for the Canadian people; similar to the RDA used in the United States. (See Appendix C for a full listing of the RNI.)

RED BEANS versatile beans that are medium-size, dark red ovals. The taste and texture are similar to kidney beans. Use in soups and stews and serve with rice.

REFERENCE DAILY INTAKES (RDI) a table devised in 1968 listing one suggested daily intake for vitamins, minerals, and protein. The RDI are not intended as nutritional goals that everyone should meet. Rather, they are for use on food labels to help people get an idea of the amount of nutrients a serving of the product contributes to the diet. The RDI were known as the U.S. RDA (the U.S. Recommended Daily Allowances) until the food labels were revamped in 1993.

REFERENCE DOSE the estimated amount of a chemical that could be consumed daily without causing harmful effects.

REFERENCE PROTEIN egg white protein, the standard with which other proteins are compared to determine protein quality.

REFINED refers to the process by which the coarse parts of food products are

removed. For example, the refining of wheat into flour involves removing three of the four parts of the kernel—the chaff, the bran, and the germ—leaving only the endosperm (starch, with only a little protein).

REGISTERED DIETITIAN (R.D.) a professional who has graduated from a program of dietetics approved by the American Dietetic Association (ADA), has passed a registration examination, has served an internship program or the equivalent to gain practical skills, and maintains competencies through continuing education. Some states require licensing for dietitians; that is, they have legislation in place obligating anyone who wants to use the title "dietitian" to receive permission by passing a state examination. Other states do not require dietitians to be licensed. R.D. (the abbreviation for registered dietitian) is often used to refer to such a professional in the same way M.D. designates a medical doctor.

REGULATION a legal mandate that must be obeyed. Failure to follow a regulation brings about serious legal consequences.

REQUIREMENT the minimum amount of a nutrient in the diet that will prevent the development of deficiency symptoms. Requirements differ from the RDA, which include a substantial margin of safety to cover the requirements of different individuals.

RETINA (RET-in-uh) the paper-thin layer of light-sensitive cells lining the back of the inside of the eye.

RETINAL (RET-in-al) one of the active forms of vitamin A that functions in the pigments of the eye. Other active forms of vitamin A include retinol.

RETINOL one of the active forms of vitamin A.

RETINOL EQUIVALENTS (RE) a measure of the amount of retinol the body will derive from a food containing preformed vitamin A or beta-carotene. Note that some tables list vitamin A in terms of *International Units (IU)*. See

Appendix D for methods of converting from one measure to another.

RICE STICKS flat, opaque, wide noodles made from rice flour.

RICE VERMICELLI thin, white noodles made from rice flour.

RICKETS a disease that occurs in children as a result of vitamin D deficiency and that is characterized by abnormal growth of bone, which in turn leads to bowed legs and an outward-bowed chest.

RISK the harm a substance may confer. Scientists estimate risk by assessing the amount of a chemical that each person in a population might consume over time (also called *exposure*) and by considering how toxic the substance might be (*toxicity*).

  risk = exposure × toxicity
  exposure = amount of substance in
    food × amount of food eaten

ROUGHAGE (RUFF-edge) the rough parts of food; an imprecise term that has been largely replaced by the term *fiber*. The best known of the fibrous polysaccharides are cellulose, hemicellulose, pectin, and gums.

SACCHARIN a zero-calorie sweetener discovered in 1879 and used in the United States since the turn of the century. A possible link to bladder cancer has led to saccharin's being banned as a food additive in Canada, although it is available there as a tabletop sweetener; it is used with a warning label in the United States and is the sweetening agent in Sweet 'N Low.

SALT a pair of charged mineral particles, such as sodium (Na+) and chloride (Cl−), that associate together. In water, they dissociate and help to carry electric current—that is, they become electrolytes.

SALT SENSITIVE the tendency for blood pressure to rise in proportion to salt consumption that certain people seem to have from birth.

SATIETY the feeling of fullness or satisfaction that people feel after meals.

SATURATED FATTY ACID a fatty acid carrying the maximum possible number of hydrogen atoms (having no points of unsaturation). A saturated fat is one that is made up primarily of saturated fatty acids.

SAUTÉ (saw-TAY, the French word for stir-fry) to cook in a pan using little fat; foods are stirred frequently to prevent sticking.

SCHMALTZ chicken fat.

SCURVY the vitamin-deficiency disease characterized by bleeding gums, tooth loss, and even death in severe cases.

SECOND HARVEST a national food banking network to which the majority of food banks belong.

SELTZER tap water injected with carbon dioxide and containing no added salts.

SERVING the amount of food a person might eat, similar to a helping.

SET-POINT THEORY the theory that the body tends to maintain a certain weight by adjusting hunger, appetite, and food energy intake on the one hand and metabolism (energy output) on the other so that a person's conscious efforts to alter weight may be foiled.

SIMPLE CARBOHYDRATES (sugars) the single sugars (monosaccharides) and the pairs of sugars (disaccharides) linked together.

SIMPLESSE® the trade name for a protein-based, low-calorie artificial fat, approved by the FDA for use in foods such as frozen desserts; cannot be used for frying or baking.

SKINFOLD TEST a clinical test of body fatness in which the thickness of a fold of skin on the back of the arm (the triceps), below the shoulder blade (subscapular), or in other areas is measured with an instrument called a caliper. Obesity is defined by triceps skinfold thickness equal to or greater than 18–19 mm in adult men or 25–26 mm in women.

SOCIAL GROUP a group of people, such as a family, who depend on one another and share a set of norms, beliefs, values, and behaviors.

SOLUBLE FIBER includes the fiber types called pectin, gums, and mucilages; soluble fibers either dissolve or swell when placed in water. Psyllium seed husk is an ingredient in certain bulk-forming laxatives and contains soluble fiber.

SOPA rice or pasta that is fried and cooked in consomme.

SOUL FOOD a term coined in the mid-1960s to promote ethnic pride and solidarity among African-Americans.

SOUP KITCHEN small feeding operations attached to existing organizations such as churches, civic groups, or nonprofit agencies that serve prepared meals that are consumed on site. Soup kitchens generally do not require clients to prove need or show identification.

SOURCE REDUCTION (also called precycling) reducing waste by using fewer materials to begin with.

SOYBEANS You can find these creamy white ovals in numerous food products, such as tofu, flour, grits, and milk. They have a firm texture and bland flavor. The fat content of soybeans is the highest of all legumes.

SPARKLING BOTTLED WATER water whose carbon dioxide (the ingredient that makes soda pop bubbly) is naturally present. That is, carbonation is not added from an outside source.

SPLIT PEAS green or yellow, these small halved peas supply an earthy flavor with mealy texture. They are best used in soups and with rice or grains.

SPRING WATER water derived from an underground formation from which water flows naturally to the surface of the earth and to which minerals have not been added or taken away. It may be collected either at the spring itself or through a hole tapping the underground formation feeding the spring.

STAPLE FOOD a food used frequently or daily in the diet—for example, potatoes (in Ireland) or rice (in the Far East).

STAPLE GRAIN a grain used frequently or daily in the diet—for example, corn (in Mexico) or rice (in Asia).

STARCH a plant polysaccharide composed of glucose, digestible by human beings.

STATIC STRETCHES stretches that lengthen tissues without injury; characterized by long-lasting, painless, pleasurable stretches.

STEAM to cook foods suspended over boiling water.

STEROLS (STEER-alls) one of the three main classes of lipids; a lipid with a structure similar to that of cholesterol.

STRENGTH the ability of muscles to work against resistance.

STRESS any threat, be it physical or psychological, to a person's well-being.

STRESS FRACTURE bone damage or breakage caused by stress on bone surfaces during exercise.

STRESS RESPONSE the body's response to stress, initially mediated by both nerves and hormones. It begins with an alarm reaction, proceeds through a stage of resistance, and ends with recovery or, if prolonged, exhaustion.

SUCROSE (SOO-crose) a double sugar composed of glucose and fructose.

TARGET HEART RATE the heartbeat rate that will achieve a cardiovascular conditioning effect for a given person—fast enough to push the heart but not so fast as to strain it.

TARO a starchy vegetable with brown, hairy skin and a pink-purple interior.

TOFU (TOE-foo) a curd made from soybeans, rich in protein and calcium (when a calcium salt is used as the curdling agent), used in many Asian and vegetarian dishes in place of meat. *Firm* tofu is dense and solid and holds up well in stir-fry dishes, soups, or on the grill—anywhere that you want the tofu to maintain its shape; *Soft* tofu is a better choice for recipes that call for blended tofu. *Silken* tofu is made by a different process that results in a creamy, custardlike product that works well in pureed or blended recipes.

TOLERANCE the maximum amount of a particular substance allowed on food.

TOXICANTS poisons, that is, agents that cause physical harm or death when present in large amounts.

TOXICITY the ability of a substance to harm living organisms. All substances are toxic if present in high enough concentrations.

TRABECULAR (tra-BECK-you-lar) **BONE** the lacy inner network of calcium-containing crystals—spongelike in appearance—that supports the bone's structure.

TRACE MINERAL an essential mineral nutrient found in the human body in amounts less than 5 grams.

TRANS FATTY ACID a type of fatty acid created when an unsaturated fat is hydrogenated. Found primarily in margarines, shortenings, commercial frying fats, and baked goods, trans fatty acids have been implicated in preliminary research as culprits in heart disease.

TRIGLYCERIDES (try-GLISS-er-ides) the major class of dietary lipids, including fats and oils. A triglyceride is made up of three units known as fatty acids and one unit called glycerol.

TRIMESTER one-third of the normal duration of pregnancy; the first trimester is 0 to 13 weeks, the second is 13 to 26 weeks, and the third trimester is 26 to 40 weeks.

TRIPEPTIDES (try-PEP-tides) protein fragments three amino acids long.

TURBINADO SUGAR raw sugar that has been washed to remove the filth.

UNDER-FIVE MORTALITY RATE (U5MR) the number of children who die before the age of five for every 1,000 live births.

UNDERNUTRITION severe underconsumption of calories or nutrients leading to disease or increased susceptibility to disease; a form of malnutrition. Also, a term that describes the domestic and world food problem of a continuous lack of the food energy and nutrients necessary to achieve and maintain health and protection from disease.

UNDERWEIGHT weight 10% or more below the desirable weight for height.

UNICEF the United Nations International Children's Emergency Fund, now referred to as the United Nations Children's Fund.

UNIQUE RADIOLYTIC PRODUCTS substances unique to irradiated food and apparently created during the process of irradiation.

UNSATURATED FATTY ACID a fatty acid in which one or more points of unsaturation occur. An unsaturated fat is a triglyceride in which one or more of the fatty acids is unsaturated.

UNSPECIFIED EATING DISORDERS some people suffer from unspecified eating disorders; that is, they exhibit some but not all of the criteria for specific eating disorders.

UREA (yoo-REE-uh) the principal nitrogen-excretion product of metabolism, generated mostly by the removal of amine groups from unneeded amino acids or from those amino acids being sacrificed to a need for energy.

VARIETY a feature of a diet in which different foods are used for the same purposes on different occasions—the opposite of *monotony*.

VITAMIN a potent, indispensable compound that performs various bodily functions that promote growth and reproduction and maintain health. Vitamins are organic, meaning that they contain or are related to carbon compounds. Contrary to popular belief, vitamins do not supply calories.
   vita=life
   amine =containing nitrogen

VLDL (very-low-density lipoprotein) carries fats packaged or made by the liver to various tissues in the body.

WELL WATER water derived from a rock formation by way of a hole bored, drilled, or otherwise constructed in the ground.

WHITE NAVY BEANS These beans are small, white ovals and are best used in soups and stews and as baked beans.

WHITE SUGAR pure sugar; made by dissolving, concentrating, and recrystallizing raw sugar.

WHOLE FOOD a food that is altered as little as possible from the plant or animal tissue from which it was taken—such as beets, milk, or oats.

WHOLE GRAIN refers to a grain that is milled in its entirety (all but the husk), not refined. Whole grains include wheat, corn, rice, rye, oats, amaranth, barley, buckwheat, sorghum, and millet; two others—bulgur and couscous—are processed from wheat grains.

XEROPHTHALMIA (ZEER-ahf-THALL-me-uh) a severe form of eye disease in which the cornea hardens and may cause blindness. The problem results from vitamin A deficiency.

YARD-LONG BEANS thin, tender string beans that grow to as long as 18 inches.

ZAPOTE an apple-size fruit with green skin and black flesh.

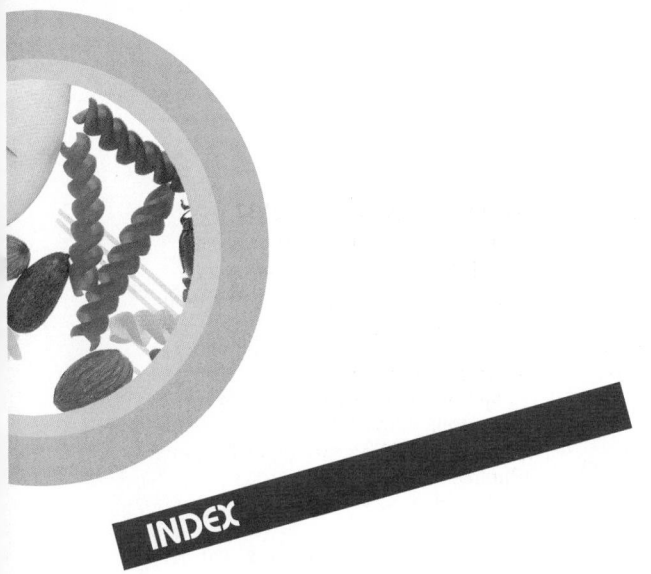

INDEX

Opportunistic infection, **173**
Oral rehydration therapy, 450, **454**
Organically grown produce, 440–41
Organic halogens, **434**
Osteomalacia, **219**
Osteoporosis, 54, **235**, 242–46
Overload, **319**
Overnutrition, **5**
Overweight, **271**
Oxalic acid, **236**
Oxidation, 119
Oxidized LDL-cholesterol, **130**

P

PABA (para-aminobenzoic acid), 223
Pantothenic acid, 199, 209
Pasteur, Louis, 444
Pasteurization, **416**, 444–45
Pauling, Linus, 210
PBBs (polybrominated biphenyl), 434
PCBs (polychlorinated biphenyl), 434, 435
Pellagra, **5**, 9, **198**
Peptide bond, **166**
Periodontal disease, **73**
Pesticides, **437**-41
pH, **174**
Phenylketonuria (PKU), **76**
Phenylpropanolamine (PPA) hydrochloride, **292**
Phospholipids, 114, **115**, 123
Phosphorus, 232, 247–48
Photosynthesis, **63**
Physical activity scorecard, 325
Physical conditioning, 318–20
Phytic acid, **236**
Phytochemicals, **225**, 226, 227
Pica, **369**
Picnics, foods at, 427–28
Pigment, **216**
Placebo, **76**
Placebo effect, **342**
Placenta, **363**
Point of unsaturation, **116**
Polypharmacy, 399
Polyunsaturated fats, **118**
Polyunsaturated fatty acid, **116**
Postnatal, **364**
Potassium, 232, 248–53
Poverty
    defined, **454**
    hunger and, 449
Precursor, **217**
Preeclampsia, **371**
Preformed vitamin A, **216**
Pregnancy
    adolescent, 372
    alcohol consumption during, 370
    caffeine consumption during, 369

diabetes, 371–72
drugs taken during, 370
folate/folic acid and, 205–6, 366
food guide for, 367
how nutrients reach the fetus, 363–64
-induced hypertension (PIH), **371**
malnutrition and, 364
nutrient supplementation in, 367–68
nutritional needs during, 365–68
nutritional readiness scorecard for, 365
nutrition-related problems during, 370–72
practices to avoid during, 369–70
weight gain in, 368–69
Premenstrual syndrome (PMS), **207**
Prenatal, **364**
Procter & Gamble, 141
Pro-oxidant, **225**
Protein(s)
    See also Amino acids
    antibodies, **172**-73
    biological value of, **177**
    as buffers, 174
    calcium and, 236
    calories in, 32
    complementary, **176**
    complete, **176**
    composition of, 165–70
    consumption scorecard for, 185
    content on food labels, 179
    cost of supplements, 170
    defined, **165**
    denaturation, **167**
    digestibility-corrected amino acid score (PDCAAS), **177-78**
    energy from, 175
    -energy malnutrition (PEM), **180**-82
    enzymes, 171
    fitness and, 332–33
    fluid balance and, **173**-74
    formed from amino acids, 166–67
    functions of, 171–75
    growth and, 171
    health and, 180–83, 187
    hormones and, **172**
    how the body handles, 175–76
    incomplete, **176**
    misinformation about supplements, 168–70
    as a nutrient, 30
    pregnancy and, 366
    quality of, in foods, 176–78, **177-78**
    recommendation intakes, 178, 180, 182, 183
    reference, **177**
    sources of, 183–84, 187
    -sparing, **175**
    synthesis, **166**
    transport, 174–75
Pulse, how to take your, 329

Q

Quakery, defined, **4**

R

Recommended Dietary Allowances (RDA)
    for calories, 36–37
    defined, **34**
    for nutrients, 35–36
    for protein, 178, 180, 182
    purpose of, 34–35
Recommended Nutrient Intakes (RNI), **34**, 37
Recycling, 431–33
Reference Daily Intakes (RDI), 54, **57**
Reference dose, **439**
Reference protein, **177**
Refined grain, **85**
Refrigeration times and temperatures for foods, 425
Registered dietitian (R.D.), **22**, 23
Regulations, **438**
Religious dietary practices, 17
Requirement, **35**
Retina, **216**
Retinal, **216**
Retinol, **217**
Retinol equivalents (REs), **217**
Riboflavin, 199, 203
Rickets, **198**, 219
Risk, **438**
Roughage, **87**

S

Saccharin
    cancer and, 75
    defined, **75**
Safety issues
    chemical agents, 434–36
    food additives, 442–44
    foodborne illnesses/poisoning, agents that cause, 415–23
    foods at picnics, 427–28
    food storage and preparation, 423–30
    genetic engineering, **446**-48
    irradiation, **445**-46
    microwaving, 427
    pesticides, 437–41
    scorecard, 430
    seafood, 428–29
Salmonellosis/*Salmonella*, 417, 418, 421
Salt, **250**
Salt, table. *See* Sodium
Salt sensitive, **255**
Satiety, 114
Saturated fatty acids
    defined, **116**
    versus unsaturated, 115–16

Photo Credits

Chapter opening photos Tom McCarthy
Chapter 1 5 Michael Newman/PhotoEdit; 13 Robert Brenner/PhotoEdit; 16 Merritt Vincent/PhotoEdit; 22 Marilyn Herbert; 23 Michael Newman/PhotoEdit.
Chapter 2 30 Mary Kate Denny/PhotoEdit; 32 Felicia Martinez/PhotoEdit; 39 Felicia Martinez/PhotoEdit.
Chapter 3 64 Felicia Martinez/PhotoEdit; 65 Tony Freeman/PhotoEdit; 70 Felicia Martinez/PhotoEdit; 75 Felicia Martinez/PhotoEdit; 82 Felicia Martinez/PhotoEdit; 83 Felicia Martinez/PhotoEdit; 85 Alan Oddie/PhotoEdit; 86 Juan Pablo Lira/The Image Bank, Courtesy of USDA; 87 Dan McCoy/The Stock Market.
Chapter 4 113 David R. Frazier; 118 Quest Photographics, Inc.; Michael Newman/PhotoEdit; 133 Felicia Martinez/PhotoEdit; 138 Thomas Harm & Tom Peterson/Quest Photographics, Inc.; 139 Quest Photographics, Inc.; Felicia Martinez/PhotoEdit; 153 Reproduced by permission of ICI Pharmaceuticals Division, Cheshire, England; 158 Ray Stanyard.
Chapter 5 170 Jean Marc Barey/Photo-Researchers, Inc.; 171 Felicia Martinez/PhotoEdit; 181 Courtesy of Dr. Robert S. Goodhard, M.D.; 185 Felicia Martinez/PhotoEdit; 191 Tony Freeman/PhotoEdit (top 3 photos); Leslye Borden/PhotoEdit (bottom left); Tony Freeman/PhotoEdit (bottom middle & bottom right).
Chapter 6 197 Anthony Vannelli; 198 Biophoto Associates/Science Source/Photo Researchers; 203 Thomas Harm & Tom Peterson/Quest Photographics, Inc.; 204 Quest Photographics, Inc.; 205 Quest Photographics, Inc.; 206 © 1990 National Medical Slide/Custom Medical Stock; 207 Quest Photographics, Inc.; 208 Quest Photographics, Inc.; 210 Quest Photographics, Inc.; 211 Quest Photographics, Inc.; 214 David R. Frazier; Quest Photographics, Inc.; 217 Quest Photographics, Inc.; 218 Quest Photographics, Inc.; 220 Quest Photographics, Inc.; 223 Quest Photographics, Inc.
Chapter 7 237 Quest Photographics, Inc. 238 Courtesy of Gjon Mill; With permission from Dempster et. al., J. Bone Min. Res 1: 15, 1986; 246 Cindy Charles/PhotoEdit; 248 Quest Photographics, Inc.; 252 Quest Photographics, Inc.; 254 Quest Photographics, Inc.; 255 Charles Feil/Stock Boston; 258 Quest Photographics, Inc.; 259 Quest Photographics, Inc.; 260 Nutrition Today Magazine, P.O. Box 1829 Annapolis, MD 21404, March 1968; 261 Quest Photographics, Inc.; 262 L. V. Bergman & Assoc.; 264 Camera M.D. Studios; 266 Michael A. Keller/The Stock Market.
Chapter 8 271 Tony Freeman/PhotoEdit; 274 David Young-Wolff/PhotoEdit; 274 Tony Freeman/PhotoEdit; Alan Oddie/PhotoEdit; 300 David Young Wolff/PhotoEdit; 308 George S. Zimbel/Monkmeyer; 310 Michael Newmann/PhotoEdit; Felicia Martinez/PhotoEdit.
Chapter 9 317 Richard Hutchings/PhotoEdit; 318 Tony Freeman/PhotoEdit; 324 David Young-Wolff/PhotoEdit; 326 PhotoResearchers; 330 1&2 - PhotoEdit; 3 - PhotoResearchers, Inc.; 331 Pascal/Explorer/Photo Researchers, Inc.; Tim Davis/Photo Researchers, Inc.; 332 Tony Freeman/PhotoEdit; 333 David Young-Wolff/PhotoEdit; 335 E. Webber/Visuals Unlimited; 336 David Young-Wolff/PhotoEdit; 337 Michael Newman/PhotoEdit; 345 John Bahlik; 347 Felicia Martinez/PhotoEdit; 351 Richard Hutchings/PhotoEdit.
Chapter 10 369 Robert Brenner/PhotoEdit; 371 Jones, K.L., Smith, D.W., Ulleland, C.N., & Steissguth, A.P. The Lancet, June 9 19732, pp. 1267-1271; 376 Reprinted with permission from J. Brown, Nutrition Now, (St. Paul, MN: West Publishing Company, 1994); 377 Myrleen Ferguson Cate/PhotoEdit; 378 J. Gerard Smith/Photo Researchers, Inc.; 380 Robert Brenner/PhotoEdit; 383 Anthony Vannelli; 385 Robert Brenner/PhotoEdit; 387 Jeff Greenberg/PhotoResearchers, Inc.; 390 Myrleen Ferguson Cate/PhotoEdit; 391 Tony Freeman/PhotoEdit; 396 Michael Newman/PhotoEdit; Bill Bachmann/PhotoEdit; 409 Karl Weidmann/Photo-Researchers; 411 David R. Frazier.
Chapter 11 415 Roy Morsch/The Stock Market; 420 Martin Chaffer/Tony Stone Images; 424 Felicia Martinez/PhotoEdit; 426 David Young-Wolff/PhotoEdit; 433 David Young-Wolff/PhotoEdit; 434 Phil Borden/PhotoEdit; 436 David Young-Wolff/PhotoEdit; 437 George Loun/VisualsUnlimited; 448 Antonio Montaner/Smithsonian; 449 Joe Sohn/Chromosohn 1990/The Stock Market; Bruce Brander/Photo Researchers, Inc.